D1750192

Dr. med. Michael Pruggmayer
Dipl. Biol.
Frauenarzt - Medizinische Genetik
Zytogenetisches Labor
Bahnhofstr. 5 - Tel. (0 51 71) 37 75
D-3150 Peine

Cancer
of the
Ovary

Cancer of the Ovary

Editors

Maurie Markman, M.D.
*Director
The Cleveland Clinic Cancer Center
Chairman
Department of Hematology and
Medical Oncology
The Cleveland Clinic Foundation
Cleveland, Ohio*

William J. Hoskins, M.D.
*Chief
Gynecology Service
Department of Surgery
Memorial Sloan-Kettering Cancer Center
New York, New York*

Raven Press ◆ New York

Raven Press, Ltd., 1185 Avenue of the Americas, New York, New York 10036

© 1993 by Raven Press, Ltd. All rights reserved. This book is protected by copyright. No part of it may be reproduced, stored in a retrieval system, or transmitted, in any form or by any means, electronic, mechanical, photocopying, recording, or otherwise, without prior written permission of the publisher.

Made in the United States of America

Library of Congress Cataloging-in-Publication Data

Cancer of the ovary / editors, Maurie Markman, William J. Hoskins.
   p. cm.
   Includes bibliographical references and index.
   ISBN 0-88167-970-4
   1. Ovaries—Cancer. I. Markman, Maurie. II. Hoskins, William J., 1940– .
   [DNLM: 1. Ovarian Neoplasms. WP 322 C215]
RC280.08C36 1993
616.99′465—dc20
DNLM/DLC
for Library of Congress   92-49712
                                                                                                                             CIP

   The material contained in this volume was submitted as previously unpublished material, except in the instances in which some of the illustrative material was derived.
   Great care has been taken to maintain the accuracy of the information contained in the volume. However, neither Raven Press nor the editors can be held responsible for errors or for any consequences arising from the use of the information contained herein.
   Materials appearing in this book prepared by individuals as part of their official duties as U.S. Government employees are not covered by the above-mentioned copyright.

9 8 7 6 5 4 3 2 1

To our wives, Tomes Markman and Iffath Abbasi Hoskins.

Contents

Contributors		ix
Preface		xiii
Acknowledgments		xv
1	Normal Ovarian Development and Function *Gail F. Whitman, Thomas E. Nolan, and Donald G. Gallup*	1
2	The Histopathology of Malignant Ovarian Tumors *Patricia E. Saigo*	21
3	Immunobiology of Ovarian Epithelial Cancer *Kenneth O. Lloyd*	47
4	Growth Factors, Oncogenes, and Tumor-Suppressor Genes *Andrew Berchuck and Robert C. Bast, Jr.*	61
5	The Epidemiology of Ovarian Cancer *Susan Harlap*	79
6	Hereditary/Familial Ovarian Cancer *Iffath Abbasi Hoskins and Harry Ostrer*	95
7	Prognostic Factors in Ovarian Cancer *Thomas B. Hakes*	115
8	Early Diagnosis of Epithelial Ovarian Cancer *J. R. van Nagell, Jr. and P. D. DePriest*	127
9	Radiologic Evaluation of Ovarian Cancer *D. David Dershaw and David M. Panicek*	133
10	Diagnosis and Staging of Epithelial Ovarian Cancer *John P. Curtin*	153
11	Primary Cytoreduction *William J. Hoskins*	163
12	Second-Look Laparotomy in Ovarian Cancer *Stephen C. Rubin*	175
13	Secondary Cytoreduction of Ovarian Malignancies *Laura L. Williams*	187
14	Central Venous and Intraperitoneal Access in Patients with Ovarian Cancer *Luis Vaccarello and William J. Hoskins*	205
15	Palliative Surgery in Ovarian Cancer *Carol L. Brown and John L. Lewis, Jr.*	217

16	The Role of Radiotherapy in the Management of Epithelial Ovarian Cancer *Borys R. Mychalczak and Zvi Fuks*	229
17	In Vitro Evaluation of Chemotherapeutic Agents *Charles E. Welander*	243
18	Dose Intensity in the Treatment of Ovarian Carcinoma *Leslie Levin*	251
19	Drug Resistance in Ovarian Cancer *Robert F. Ozols, Peter J. O'Dwyer, and Thomas C. Hamilton*	261
20	Chemotherapy in the Management of Celomic Epithelial Carcinoma of the Ovary *J. Tate Thigpen*	277
21	Experimental Agents (Nonbiological) in Ovarian Cancer *William P. McGuire*	287
22	Immunotherapy of Ovarian Cancer *Otoniel Martínez-Maza and Jonathan S. Berek*	301
23	Intraperitoneal Chemotherapy *Maurie Markman*	317
24	High-Dose Chemotherapy with Autologous Bone Marrow Support for the Treatment of Epithelial Ovarian Cancer *Elizabeth J. Shpall, Salomon M. Stemmer, Scott I. Bearman, Robert C. Bast, Jr., William P. Peters, Maureen Ross, and Roy B. Jones*	327
25	Hormone Therapy in Ovarian Cancer *Peter E. Schwartz and Joseph T. Chambers*	339
26	Complications of Chemotherapy *Maurie Markman*	349
27	Management of Early Stage Ovarian Cancer *Robert C. Young*	359
28	Management of Germ Cell Tumors of the Ovary *Stephen D. Williams and David M. Gershenson*	375
29	Sex Cord-Stromal Tumors of the Ovary *Walter B. Jones*	385
30	Metastatic Tumors to the Ovary *Richard R. Barakat*	407
31	Epithelial Ovarian Tumors of Low Malignant Potential *Edward L. Trimble and Cornelia Liu Trimble*	415
Subject Index		431

Contributors

Richard R. Barakat, M.D. Gynecology Service, Department of Surgery, Memorial Sloan-Kettering Cancer Center, 1275 York Avenue, New York, New York 10021

Robert C. Bast, Jr., M.D. Departments of Medicine and Microbiology/Immunology, Duke University Medical Center and The Duke Comprehensive Cancer Center, Durham, North Carolina 27710

Scott I. Bearman, M.D. Bone Marrow Transplant Program, University of Colorado Health Sciences Center, 4200 East Ninth Avenue, Denver, Colorado 80262

Andrew Berchuck, M.D. Department of Obstetrics and Gynecology, Division of Gynecologic Oncology, Duke University Medical Center and The Duke Comprehensive Cancer Center, Durham, North Carolina 27710

Jonathan S. Berek, M.D. Gynecologic Oncology Service, Department of Obstetrics and Gynecology, Division of Gynecology, UCLA School of Medicine and Jonsson Comprehensive Cancer Center, Los Angeles, California 90024

Carol L. Brown, M.D. Gynecology Service, Department of Surgery, Memorial Sloan-Kettering Cancer Center, 1275 York Avenue, New York, New York 10021

Joseph T. Chambers, M.D., Ph.D. Department of Obstetrics and Gynecology, Division of Gynecologic Oncology, Yale University School of Medicine, P.O. Box 3333, 333 Cedar Street, New Haven, Connecticut 06510

John P. Curtin, M.D. Gynecology Service, Department of Surgery, Memorial Sloan-Kettering Cancer Center, 1275 York Avenue, New York, New York 10021

P.D. DePriest, M.D., Ph.D. Department of Obstetrics and Gynecology, Division of Gynecologic Oncology, University of Kentucky Medical Center, 800 Rose Street, Room MN 308, Lexington, Kentucky 40536

D. David Dershaw, M.D. Department of Radiology, Memorial Sloan-Kettering Cancer Center, 1275 York Avenue, New York, New York 10021

Zvi Fuks, M.D. Department of Radiation Oncology, Memorial Sloan-Kettering Cancer Center, 1275 York Avenue, New York, New York 10021

Donald G. Gallup, M.D. Department of Obstetrics and Gynecology, Section of Gynecologic Oncology, The Medical College of Georgia, CK-166, 1120 Fifteenth Street, Augusta, Georgia 30912

David M. Gershenson, M.D. Department of Gynecology, The University of Texas M.D. Anderson Cancer Center, 1515 Holcom Boulevard, Houston, Texas 77030

Thomas B. Hakes, M.D. Department of Medicine, Solid Tumor Service, Memorial Sloan-Kettering Cancer Center, 1275 York Avenue, New York, New York 10021

Thomas C. Hamilton, Ph.D. Fox Chase Cancer Center, 7701 Burholme Avenue, Philadelphia, Pennsylvania 19111

Susan Harlap, M.D., B.S. Department of Epidemiology and Biostatistics, Memorial Sloan-Kettering Cancer Center, 1275 York Avenue, New York, New York 10021

Iffath Abbasi Hoskins, M.D. *Department of Obstetrics and Gynecology, Division of Maternal Fetal Medicine, New York University Medical Center, 550 First Avenue, Room 9N1, New York, New York 10016*

William J. Hoskins, M.D. *Gynecology Service, Department of Surgery, Memorial Sloan-Kettering Cancer Center, 1275 York Avenue, New York, New York 10021*

Roy B. Jones, M.D., Ph.D. *Bone Marrow Transplant Program, University of Colorado Health Sciences Center, 4200 East Ninth Avenue, Denver, Colorado 80262*

Walter B. Jones, M.D. *Gynecology Service, Department of Surgery Memorial Sloan Kettering Cancer Center, 1275 York Avenue, New York, New York 10021*

Leslie Levin, M.D., F.R.C.P.C. *Department of Oncology, University of Western Ontario and London Regional Cancer Centre, 790 Commisioners Road East, London, Ontario, Canada N6A 4L6*

John L. Lewis, Jr., M.D. *Gynecology Service, Department of Surgery, Memorial Sloan-Kettering Cancer Center, 1275 York Avenue, New York, New York 10021*

Kenneth O. Lloyd, Ph.D. *Department of Immunology, Memorial Sloan-Kettering Cancer Center, 1275 York Avenue, New York, New York 10021*

Maurie Markman, M.D. *The Cleveland Clinic Cancer Center, Department of Hematology and Medical Oncology, The Cleveland Clinic Foundation, 9500 Euclid Avenue, Cleveland, Ohio 44195*

Otoniel Martínez-Maza, Ph.D. *Departments of Obstetrics and Gynecology and Microbiology and Immunology, UCLA School of Medicine, Los Angeles, California 90024*

William P. McGuire, M.D. *Department of Oncology, The Johns Hopkins Oncology Center, 600 North Wolfe Street, Room 173, Baltimore, Maryland 21205*

Borys R. Mychalczak, M.D. *Department of Radiation Oncology, Memorial Sloan-Kettering Cancer Center, 1275 York Avenue, New York, New York 10021*

Thomas E. Nolan, M.D. *Departments of Obstetrics and Gynecology and Internal Medicine, Section of General Obstetrics and Gynecology, The Medical College of Georgia, CJ-120, 1120 Fifteenth Street, Augusta, Georgia 30912*

Peter J. O'Dwyer, M.D. *Fox Chase Cancer Center, 7701 Burholme Avenue, Philadelphia, Pennsylvania 19111*

Harry Ostrer, M.D. *Department of Pediatrics, Division of Human Genetics, New York University Medical Center, 550 First Avenue, New York, New York 10024*

Robert F. Ozols, M.D., Ph.D. *Fox Chase Cancer Center, 7701 Burholme Avenue, Philadelphia, Pennsylvania 19111*

David M. Panicek, M.D. *Department of Radiology, Memorial Sloan-Kettering Cancer Center, 1275 York Avenue, New York, New York 10021*

William P. Peters, M.D. *Bone Marrow Transplant Program, Duke University Medical Center, Durham, North Carolina 27710*

Maureen Ross, M.D. *Bone Marrow Transplant Program, Duke University Medical Center, Durham, North Carolina 27710*

Stephen C. Rubin, M.D. *Gynecology Service, Department of Surgery, Memorial Sloan-Kettering Cancer Center, 1275 York Avenue, New York, New York 10021*

Patricia E. Saigo, M.D. *Department of Gynecology, Memorial Sloan-Kettering Cancer Center, 1275 York Avenue, New York, New York 10021*

Peter E. Schwartz, M.D. *Department of Obstetrics and Gynecology, Division of Gynecologic Oncology, Yale University School of Medicine, P.O. Box 3333, 333 Cedar Street, New Haven, Connecticut 06510*

Elizabeth J. Shpall, M.D. *Department of Medicine, University Hospital, University of Colorado Health Sciences Center, Box B190, 4200 East Ninth Avenue, Denver, Colorado 80262*

Salomon M. Stemmer, M.D. *Bone Marrow Transplant Program, University of Colorado Health Sciences Center, Box B190, 4200 East Ninth Avenue, Denver, Colorado 80262*

J. Tate Thigpen, M.D. *Department of Medicine, Division of Oncology, University of Mississippi School of Medicine, 2500 North State Street, Jackson, Mississippi 39216*

Cornelia Liu Trimble, M.D. *Department of Gynecologic Pathology, The Johns Hopkins Hospital, 600 North Wolfe Street, Pathology 709, Baltimore, Maryland 21205*

Edward L. Trimble, M.D., M.P.H. *Clinical Investigation Branch, Cancer Therapy Evaluation Program, Division of Cancer Treatment, National Cancer Institute, Executive Plaza North Suite 741, Bethesda, Maryland 20892*

J.R. van Nagell, Jr., M.D. *Department of Obstetrics and Gynecology, Division of Gynecologic Oncology, University of Kentucky Medical Center, 800 Rose Street, Room MN308, Lexington, Kentucky 40536*

Luis Vaccarello, M.D. *Gynecology Service, Department of Surgery, Memorial Sloan-Kettering Cancer Center, 1275 York Avenue, New York, New York 10021*

Charles E. Welander, M.D. *Department of Gynecologic Oncology, Medical Center Hospital of Vermont, Shepardson South #419, Burlington, Vermont 05401*

Gail F. Whitman, M.D. *Department of Obstetrics and Gynecology, Section of Reproductive Endocrinology, Infertility, and Genetics, The Medical College of Georgia, CK-159, 1120 Fifteenth Street, Augusta, Georgia 30912*

Laura L. Williams, M.D. *Department of Obstetrics and Gynecology, Vanderbilt University Medical Center, B-1100 Vanderbilt Medical Center North, Nashville, Tennessee 37232*

Stephen D. Williams, M.D. *Department of Medicine, Indiana University School of Medicine, 926 West Michigan Street, Room N262, Indianapolis, Indiana 46202*

Robert C. Young, M.D. *Fox Chase Cancer Center, 7701 Burholme Avenue, Philadelphia, Pennsylvania 19111*

Preface

In women in the United States, ovarian cancer is the leading cause of death from gynecologic malignancies and the fifth leading cause of all cancer mortalities. Of the 21,000 new cases diagnosed each year in this country, there will be approximately 13,000 deaths. Even though ovarian cancer is less common in the population than cancers of the cervix or endometrium, it is responsible for more deaths than these two malignancies combined.

Despite these distressing figures, a number of important new developments hold considerable promise for the future. Clinical investigative efforts directed at the ability to diagnose ovarian cancer at an early stage, when the disease can be cured with surgery, have begun to bear fruit. New drugs, such as taxol, and new therapeutic modalities, such as bone marrow transplantation and intraperitoneal chemotherapy, have raised the very real possibility that a greater number of women with advanced ovarian cancer can experience long-term disease-free survival and even cure. Finally, recent basic laboratory and clinical research efforts involving the epidemiology, genetics, and biology of ovarian cancer have led to important advances in our understanding of this difficult malignancy. Thus, there is legitimate reason to be hopeful regarding progress in the prevention, diagnosis, and management of this disease.

To succeed at this remarkable task requires that those who care for women with ovarian cancer be knowledgeable in a broad range of topics. Since the training of the obstetrician/gynecologist, the gynecologic oncologist, the medical oncologist, or the radiation oncologist may not provide sufficient depth to allow complete understanding of this disease, the editors have attempted to create an ultimate reference text for ovarian cancer. The topics have been chosen to provide a depth of material not possible in a general text of gynecology or oncology. Each chapter has been written by individuals who are recognized as experts in their fields. No other major textbook focuses exclusively on the many facets of this fascinating and extremely serious malignancy.

Readers of this book should come away with a new understanding of the extraordinary biology of ovarian cancer and, we hope, will begin to share our enthusiasm and anticipation that major advances in the management of this disease will be forthcoming.

M. Markman
W. J. Hoskins

Acknowledgments

We wish to acknowledge the very able assistance of our editorial assistants in the Academic Office of the Gynecology Service, Department of Surgery, Memorial Sloan-Kettering Cancer Center. Guillermo Metz and Denise Haller managed the entire preparation of this book at Memorial Sloan-Kettering, including communications with authors and Raven Press. Above all, they meticulously edited the entire manuscript. We are very grateful for their assistance.

M. Markman
W. J. Hoskins

CHAPTER 1

Normal Ovarian Development and Function

Gail F. Whitman, Thomas E. Nolan, and Donald G. Gallup

Ovarian cancer is one of the greatest challenges faced by gynecologists in the 1990s. In contrast to the declining death rates for cervical and uterine cancer, the annual reported death rates for ovarian cancer have risen by 250% since 1930 (1). It is the fifth leading cause of cancer death in women, exceeded only by cancers of the breast, colon, lung, and pancreas.

An understanding of the pathogenesis of ovarian cancer is likely to be of benefit in the ongoing search for effective treatment. In this chapter, we will review the development and function of normal ovaries, followed by a discussion of ovarian tumor histogenesis. The histogenesis of some ovarian tumors is becoming better defined, particularly with regard to the role of the Y chromosome in certain germ cell tumors.

ORGANOGENESIS

Gonadal Differentiation

To understand the evolution of certain ovarian neoplasms, it is important to review gonadal development. Sex chromosomes within the zygote determine the direction in which the gonad will differentiate. Gonadal differentiation is the first of three major stages in human sexual development. Chronologically, the other two stages are the differentiation of the internal genitalia (accessory structures) and differentiation of the external genitalia.

The gonad begins as a stratification of coelomic epithelium on the medial aspect of the urogenital ridge (mesonephric kidney). It consists of both somatic and germ cells. Somatic cells are derived from the ridge mesoderm. Primordial germ cells originate outside the presumptive gonad region. These cells arise from the inner cell mass of the early human blastocyst and, if successful, ultimately give rise to gametes (2).

By the fourth week of gestation, primitive germ cells (gonocytes) begin to migrate by ameboid movement from the yolk sac entoderm, through the hindgut, and into the mesoderm of the dorsal mesentary. They come to rest in the coelomic epithelium of the genital ridges (3). Gonocytes undergo several cycles of mitosis during this mass migration period (4). Once they have reached the genital ridge, they lose motility, become associated with coelomic epithelial cells, and move into the underlying mesenchyme. Failure of active mitosis and/or migration at this stage has been postulated as a cause of gonadal agenesis, a condition in which the "streak" gonads contain embryonic stroma but no germ cells (5).

At five to six weeks of intrauterine life, the primitive gonad can be recognized, but it is histologically indistinguishable as either ovary or testis. At this point, the gonad consists of three distinct cell types: gonocytes in mitosis, coelomic epithelium, and stroma derived from the original mesenchyme of the gonadal ridge. Surviving gonocytes are progenitors of adult oocytes, spermatogonia, and germ cell tumors (6). The coelomic epithelium, which invaginates over the embryonic gonadal ridge, becomes surface epithelium in adult ovaries. Approximately 75% to 80% of all ovarian malignancies arise from the coelomic epithelium, or mesothelium (7). These tumors can be classified as differentiated or undifferentiated, with varying amounts of contributions from the gonadal mesenchyme (8).

Several salient differences exist between germ cell differentiation in the male and in the female. Male gonocytes undergo mitotic arrest after reaching the genital ridge and become prespermatogonia. These cells do not enter meiosis until puberty, when the per-

---

G. F. Whitman, T. E. Nolan, and D. G. Gallup: Sections of Reproductive Endocrinology Infertility, and Genetics; General Obstetrics and Gynecology; and Gynecologic Oncology, Department of Obstetrics and Gynecology, Medical College of Georgia, Augusta, Georgia 30912-3345

petual production of haploid gametes continues through senescence. In contrast, female gonocytes ultimately respond to the somatic cell environment of the genital ridge by entering meiosis (6). At about eight weeks of intrauterine life, female germ cells within a single ovary undergo any of the following: mitosis, meiosis, and oogonial atresia (9). This fundamental concept becomes important in adult life; the male continually reproduces germ cells from puberty on, and the female has a finite pool of oocytes from birth.

Sexual dimorphism is seen in the somatic cell contribution to the gonad. The indifferent gonad consists of a cortex and medulla, with coelomic epithelial cells and mesenchyme clustered around germ cells until sexual differentiation takes place. If the gonad differentiates toward masculinization, the medullary region becomes predominant. Testicular determination is currently believed to be triggered by a gene product transcribed from the Y chromosome region, the sex-determining region of Y (SRY) (10). The male gonad undergoes an earlier differentiation than the female gonad, which prevents subsequent ovarian differentiation. The formation of Sertoli cells and spermatogenic cords takes place in the six- to seven-week embryo. These cords later envelop the germ cells, and thus represent the progenitors of adult seminiferous tubules (11).

The gonad that fails to develop in the male direction maintains the somatic cell pattern that was established in the indifferent gonad until midgestation, when ovarian cortical dominance is established (discussed later in this chapter). The absence of testicular development beyond seven weeks gestation indicates that the gonad will differentiate toward feminization (11).

Development of Accessory Structures

After gonadal differentiation, the embryo must develop the appropriate internal accessory structures and external genitalia for successful sexual function. The internal accessory structures are determined by müllerian and wolffian duct development (12). Müllerian derivatives become the uterus, fallopian tubes, and upper one-third of the vagina. Wolffian duct derivatives give rise to the epididymis, vas deferens, and seminal vesicle (Fig. 1).

Müllerian and wolffian duct development begins in all embryos, but final development of these structures is modified by the presence of substances produced by the developing testis. By the seventh week of gestation, the developing testis has seminiferous tubules with Sertoli cells. The Sertoli cells produce high levels of müllerian-inhibiting substance (MIS) or antimüllerian hormone (13). This protein acts locally to cause regression of the müllerian ducts in male embryos. Regression is complete by the eighth week of gestation. Because this hormonal action is local, an individual gonad controls the regression of the ipsilateral müllerian duct. The human gene for MIS has been cloned, sequenced, and mapped to an autosome—chromo-

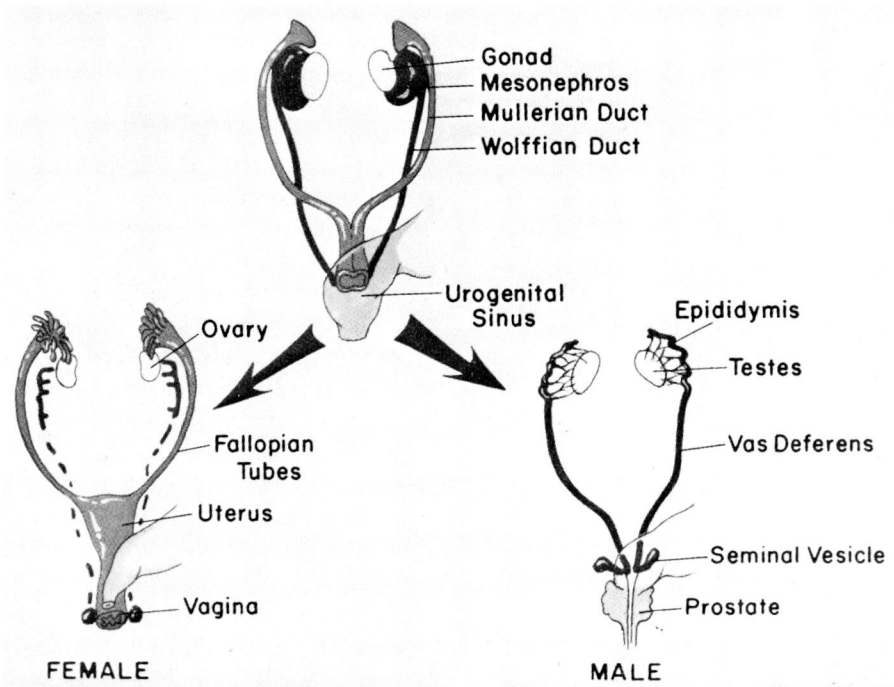

FIG. 1. The development of internal accessory structures from embryo (top) in the male and female (From Dr. J Wilson and WB. Saunders Company, with permission.)

some 19 subband p 13.2-13.3 (14,15). Investigators are currently evaluating recombinant human MIS protein for potential use as an antineoplastic agent against müllerian-derived malignancies (16).

By the eighth week of gestation, Leydig cells within the developing testis begin to produce high levels of testosterone. Maternal human chorionic gonadotropin (HCG) levels, which peak at this time, appear to be the primary stimulus for initiating steroidogenesis within the Leydig cells (17). Gonadal testosterone effects the development of the ipsilateral wolffian duct, which progresses only under the direct effect of testosterone (12,13). Another substance, androgen binding protein (ABP), is produced at this time by the Sertoli cells (18). ABP may aid in the maintenance of the high local testosterone levels necessary for continued wolffian duct development.

Each gonad is responsible for the development of its own internal accessory structures; the effects of MIS and testosterone are both local and unilateral. In the absence of local testosterone, wolffian derivatives fail to complete development. The presence or absence of local action has profound implications. An abnormal gonad may be unable to appropriately direct the development of accessory structures, and it is not surprising that a variable array of duct structures may be present in certain pathologic states.

Differentiation of the external genitalia is the third chronologic stage of human sexual differentiation. The external genitalia develop in the female direction unless local levels of testosterone are converted to intracellular dihydrotestosterone (DHT) (19). Masculinization of the external genitalia results in labioscrotal fusion, extension of the urethral grove into the genital tubercle, and elongation of the genital tubercle (Fig. 2). This process is completed by the fifteenth week of gestation (20). Testicular descent is controlled by a number of endocrine and morphologic factors, of which local testicular androgen production and gonadotropin stimulation appear to be highly significant (21). Testicular descent is usually not completed until after the thirty-second week of gestation.

Cortical Dominance

When gonadal differentiation fails to move toward the male direction, many of the gonadal ridge gonocytes (oogonia) continue to proliferate mitotically for several cycles (6). Between the fifth and fifteenth weeks of gestation, the number of oogonia increases to a maximal endowment of six to seven million. This profound proliferation has been attributed to elevated fetal gonadotropin levels, which peak between the sixteenth and eighteenth week of gestation (22). Gonadotropin stimulation ensures an appropriate local environment for the extensive folliculogenesis that actively occurs in the cortex at midgestation.

To allow the future reproductive competence, the female gonad must establish cortical dominance and salvage an adequate number of germ cells. These goals are usually achieved, but not without struggle! Many

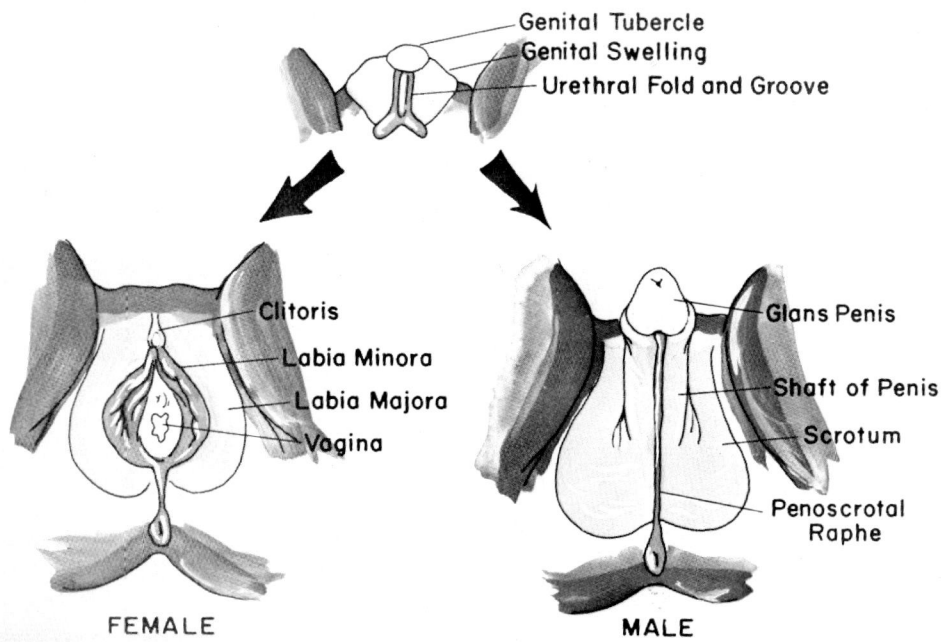

FIG. 2. The development of external genitalia from embryo (top) in the male and female (From Dr. J Wilson and WB. Saunders Company, with permission.)

oogonia are lost to the peritoneal cavity by migration through ovarian surface epithelium (23). Additionally, at about the fifteenth week of gestation, waves of follicular atresia begin to rapidly deplete the existing germ cell endowment (24). Successful preservation of the germ cell endowment requires ovarian determinant gene action. This gene action probably controls the development of a mantle of follicular cells and compact stroma that envelops and protects differentiating germ cells from atresia (9).

Oogonia become primary oocytes as they leave mitosis, begin meiosis, and arrest in prophase. This process can be seen in some germ cells as early as the eighth week of gestation (9). By the twentieth week of gestation, the female gonad is composed of a sheet of oogonia and primary oocytes residing in an enlarged cellular cortex. The cortex becomes vascularized from the medulla. Perivascular cells of epithelial and mesenchymal origin invade with blood vessels to surround the primary oocytes. These primary oocytes become individually isolated with the invading cells and form functional units called primordial follicles. The conversion of mitotically dividing oogonia to primary oocytes must be completed by the seventh month of gestation, or oogonial atresia will occur (9). Additionally, the primary oocytes must be enveloped by the mantle cells that organize the primordial follicles, or they too will undergo premature atresia (11). No primordial follicles are formed after six weeks of neonatal life (9).

The primordial follicles have two important components. First, they serve as a home for the resting oocyte by providing protection from the forces of premature atresia. Second, they ultimately serve as the single most important source of gonadal sex steroids in the female. Primordial follicles consist of a single arrested oocyte at meiotic prophase I (dictyate state) surrounded by a single layer of epithelial cells (pregranulosa cells). This unit resides in an outer matrix of mesenchymal cells (pretheca cells). Primordial follicles represent the first stage of follicular growth and differentiation. These follicles exist in a continuum that is independent of gonadotropin stimulation. They are present in the ovary until after menopause (9).

Some fetal primordial follicles are recruited to leave the resting state and undergo further differentiation. The first sign of this differentiation is a change in the morphologic appearance of the pregranulosa cell layer, which changes from squamous to columnar (25). The tiny follicles, now called primary follicles, may grow and differentiate, becoming preantral or antral follicles (Fig. 3). Ultimately, however, they will undergo follicular atresia because the extragonadal mechanism necessary for full follicular development and ovulation will not reach maturity until late puberty. At birth, the female neonate possesses bilateral, fully differentiated, dynamic ovaries that contain one to two million oocytes (26,27). These oocytes reside in follicle units at various stages of follicular growth, differentiation, and follicular atresia.

Normal ovarian development appears to require the following: the absence of genetically active Y chromosomal material and the presence of two intact and ge-

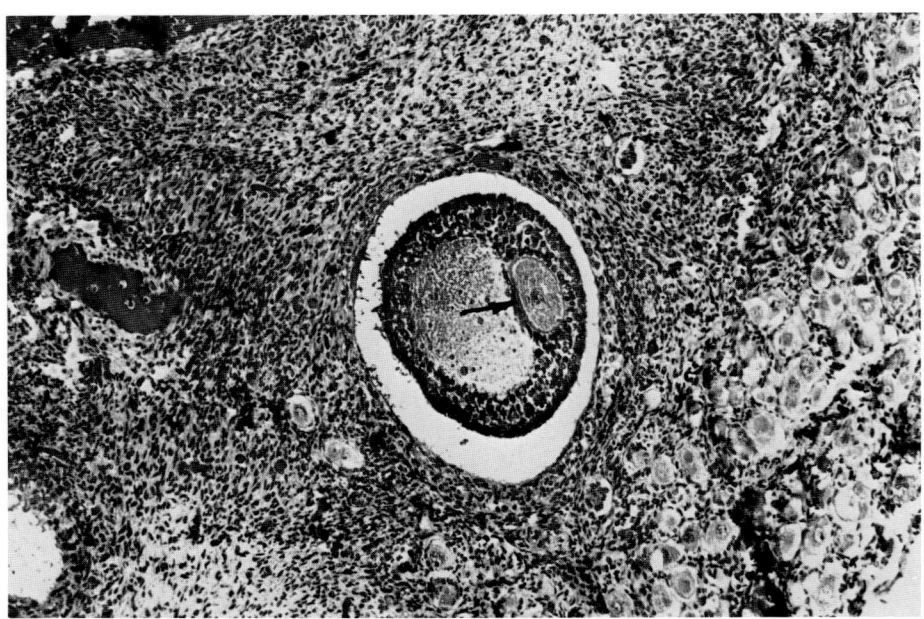

FIG. 3. Representative section from a human fetal ovary at term obtained at autospy. Note the large antral follicle (*arrow*) containing an oocyte. Several tiny primordial follicles are present at the lower periphery (Courtesy of Dr. C. Pantazis, Department of Pathology, Medical College of Georgia).

netically active X chromosomes in the germ cell line, germ cell migration to the genital ridges, mitotic activity of germ cells in the ridge, development of the granulosa cell mantle, normal transformation of the oogonium into a primary oocyte, with controlled arrest and development at the dictyotene state (arrested meiotic prophase), and physiologic response of the primary follicle to fetal follicle stimulating hormone (FSH).

ABNORMAL DEVELOPMENT

The following examples of abnormal gonadal development are not intended to comprise an all-inclusive list. These conditions are stressed here because they have the potential to give rise to ovarian malignancy.

46,XY Pure Gonadal Dysgenesis (Swyers Syndrome)

In pure gonadal dysgenesis, "male" gonocytes have failed to migrate to the genital ridge, have failed to replicate there, or were destroyed very early in embryonic development. Whether this condition is the result of teratogenesis, repressed gene action on testicular determinants, or abnormal gonadal receptors for determinant gene products is unknown. These phenotypic female patients have streak gonads, a eunuchoid habitus, primary amenorrhea, and persistent sexual infantilism at puberty. Gonadotropins are persistently in the castrate range at puberty.

Disruption of testicular development prior to the production of MIS and testosterone allows for the maintenance of müllerian structures. Patients with pure gonadal dysgenesis have a normal uterus, fallopian tube, and upper one-third of the vagina. Because these patients lack the obvious physical signs of Turner's or other syndromes, most present with delay in the onset of puberty. Unfortunately, intraabdominal "male streak" gonads are abnormal and at high risk for malignant degeneration. This tendency toward malignancy exists throughout life. Germ cell tumors often arise in these individuals during early childhood. Patients with pure gonadal dysgenesis are at the highest risk for genital ridge tumors. Gonadoblastoma and dysgerminoma are most common (Fig. 4) (28).

Gonadal Dysgenesis Caused by Sex Chromosome Aneuploidy

Numerical and structural abnormalities of the sex chromosomes can lead to abnormal gonadal development. These conditions are associated with normal germ cell migration and endowment. However, privation of ovarian determinants on the X chromosome can lead to incomplete formation of the granulosa cell man-

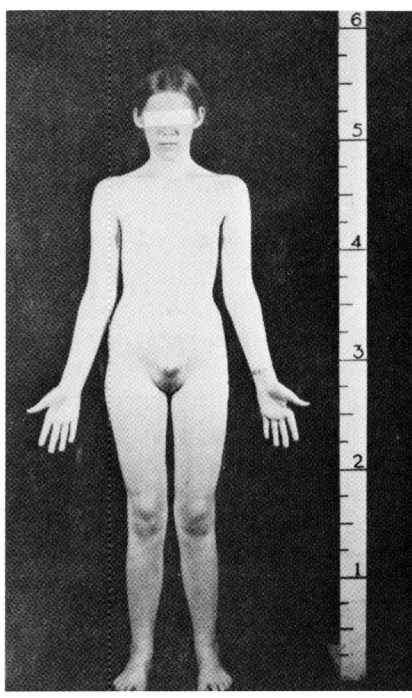
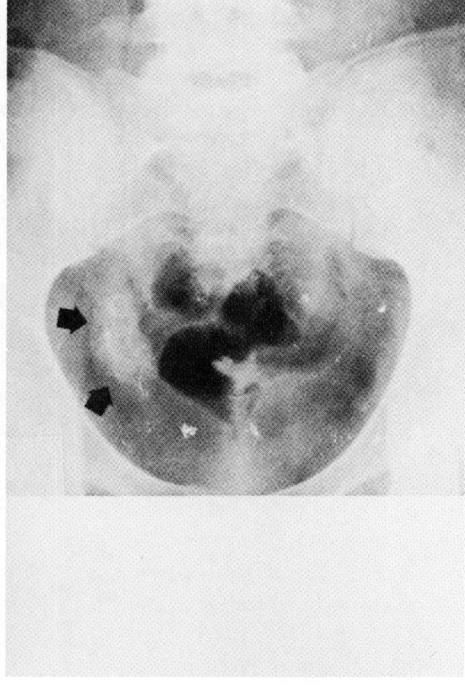

FIG. 4. A 19-year-old girl with 46,XY gonadal dysgenesis, normal stature, sexual infantilism, and bilateral gonadoblastoma. The right gonadoblastoma was larger than the left and was more extensively calcified. A floccular calcification is visualized in the region of the right gonadal tumor (*arrows*). (From McDonough PG, Simmons RG, and Obstet Gynecol), with permission.

tle that surrounds and protects oocytes while cortical dominance is established. Unarrested meiotic activity and accelerated atresia of primary oocytes occur during the second half of gestation. The absence of Y chromosomal material and the presence of two normal X chromosomes and an unidentified autosome are required for the ovarian determinant gene action that is needed to complete ovarian development (29).

45,X Gonadal Dysgenesis (Classic Turner's Syndrome)

This syndrome is diagnosed in approximately 1 in 2700 newborn girls. Intrauterine growth retardation, low birth weight, and high infant mortality rates are common. Because of phenotypic abnormalities, Turner's syndrome is usually diagnosed in the nursery. Thirty percent of the newborns have lymphedema of the upper and lower extremities. Webbed neck, high arched palate, low-set, prominent ears, low posterior hairline, epicanthal folds, a tendency toward micrognathia, cubitus vulgus, shield chest with wideset nipples, hypoplastic nailbeds, and shortening of the fourth and fifth digits may also be present. These individuals are at risk for a variety of renal and cardiovascular anomalies, particularly coarctation of the aorta, which is an unusual condition in females (30). They also have an increased risk of diabetes mellitus and Hashimoto's thyroiditis, particularly if an isochromosome of long arm of X–46,X,i(Xq) is present (31). At puberty, patients with classical Turner's syndrome are short (under 60 inches), experience primary amenorrhea, display persistent sexual infantilism, and have persistently elevated gonadotropins (32).

The most common human chromosomal anomaly is 45,X. Point eight percent of all zygotes have it, but less than 3% of these survive to delivery (33). Most 45,X fetuses die in utero. Many of the abortuses have lymphedematous collars, which are presumed to be forerunners of the webbed neck (29). The 45,X karyotype was originally thought to arise as a result of a paternal meiotic error (34). In this scenario, a null paternal gamete would inseminate a maternal haploid oocyte, resulting in a 45,X embryo with one cell line.

Recent evidence suggests that 45,X individuals arise as the result of postsegmentation mitotic cleavage errors in normal 46,XX or 46,XY embryos (35). All these individuals would therefore be mosaic for a second cell line in some organ or tissue. The high intrauterine wastage seen in this condition is thought to be secondary to the absence of a second cell line with two sex chromosomes. Because the second cell line may be present in very low numbers, it may go unidentified during routine cytogenetic procedures. Unfortunately, problems may arise if a covert Y cell line is present. At our institution, an adolescent with a 45,X karyotype diagnosed by a count of 50 cells was noted to have developed a unilateral dysgerminoma with a contralateral gonadoblastoma. After surgery, a repeat karyotype was done, and 150 cells were counted. On this occasion, two cells were found to be 46,XY. This minority cell population was overlooked on two previous karyotype screenings!

Turner's patients must be closely followed for the possibility of germ cell tumor formation. Annual serum β-HCG and alpha fetoprotein (AFP) may be helpful. Anteroposterior films of the pelvis may identify gonadoblastoma calcifications. The recent development of DNA probe systems capable of detecting a minority cell population with Y chromosomal material not easily detected by cytogenetics may also be of benefit (discussed later in this chapter) (36,37). To date, studies of 45,X putative mosaics to detect covert YDNA have identified only a few individuals not identified by standard cytogenetic technique. Prophylactic gonadectomy is not recommended when the cytogenetic diagnosis of X chromosome aneuploidy is clear and a covert Y cell line is not suspected.

Mosaic Sex Chromosome Deletion Syndromes

These conditions arise as the result of mitotic cleavage errors in the very early embryo (38) that lead to the development of additional cell lines. A wide range of cytogenetic findings are common.

X Chromosome Aneuploidy

Karyotypes with 45,X/46,XX; 45,X/47,XXX; 45,X/46,X,i(Xq); and 45,X/46,Xdel(X) are a few of the possibilities. These individuals have lost various amounts of X chromosomal material. The absence of overt Y is detected by cytogenetic techniques. These patients may or may not have the signs of classic Turner's syndrome. Because they have a full complement of germ cells until mid-gestation, incomplete follicular depletion by atresia may occur. Some individuals may actually have a few remaining follicles capable of responding to the high gonadotropin levels produced at puberty (39). Some evidence of estrogenic activity and some estrogen-dependent secondary sexual development can occur. The relative ratio of 46,XX stem line cells to postsegmentation–derived 45,X cells may impact on individual gonadal function. Though most individuals have bilateral streak gonads and short stature, limited estrogenic function can be present in up to 12% (39). Dysfunctional uterine bleeding and painful ovarian cysts may be related to the remaining follicles present. Rarely, pregnancy may occur in these individuals (28). Every conceptus has a 50% chance of aneuploidy, and genetic amniocentesis should be offered. Some of these individuals present in their late twenties or early thirties as premature ovarian failure cases (40). As with classic Turner's syndrome, consideration must be given to the possibility of covert Y material and the associated risk of germ cell malignancy (discussed later in this chapter).

Y Chromosome Aneuploidy

This group includes a variety of conditions from 45,X/46,XY to 45,X/46,X variant Y. These individuals carry one monosomic X cell line and a second cell line with a normal X chromosome and a normal or variant Y chromosome. 45,X/46,XY is the most common form of sex chromosome mosaicism (28). These individuals begin as normal 46,XY embryos. However, during an early mitosis, one of the Y chromatids fails to migrate to the daughter cell (anaphase lag). This creates a 45,X cell line in addition to the 46,XY line. Gonadal development varies. Individuals may have bilateral rudimentary streak gonads, a unilateral streak with contralateral intraabdominal or scrotal testis, or (rarely) bilateral scrotal testes (41). The phenotype and sex assignment from birth may be that of a nonmasculinized female, a female with clitoral enlargement, a newborn with sexual ambiguity, or (rarely) an azoospermic male with bilateral scrotal testes (41). Most of these individuals are raised as females. Although they may masculinize or develop clitoral enlargement at puberty, most present with female sexual infantilism. They may also present to puberty with a germ cell malignancy. Fifteen to twenty-five percent of patients with asymmetric gonadal dysgenesis (45,X/46,XY) develop gonadal tumors if the gonads are left in place (Fig. 5) (28). Therefore, the gonads should be removed as soon as the diagnosis of gonadal dysgenesis is made.

Clearly, the minority XY cell population in putative 45,X classic Turner's syndrome needs to be identified. The origin of suspect sex chromosome fragments that may be ambiguous should also be clarified by standard cytogenetic techniques. DNA technology has recently been used in clinical decision-making. Any fragment of Y that is mitotically stable, regardless of size, must contain DNA target sequences that correspond to the Y centromere because centromere activity is necessary for normal cell division. A DNA probe for repetitive copy sequences present in alphoid satellite sequences in the Y centromere region, probe Y 97, is highly sensitive and specific for YDNA (36). This probe may be used to determine the origin of suspect sex chromosomes and may identify minority covert Y cell lines with the aid of polymerase chain reaction (37).

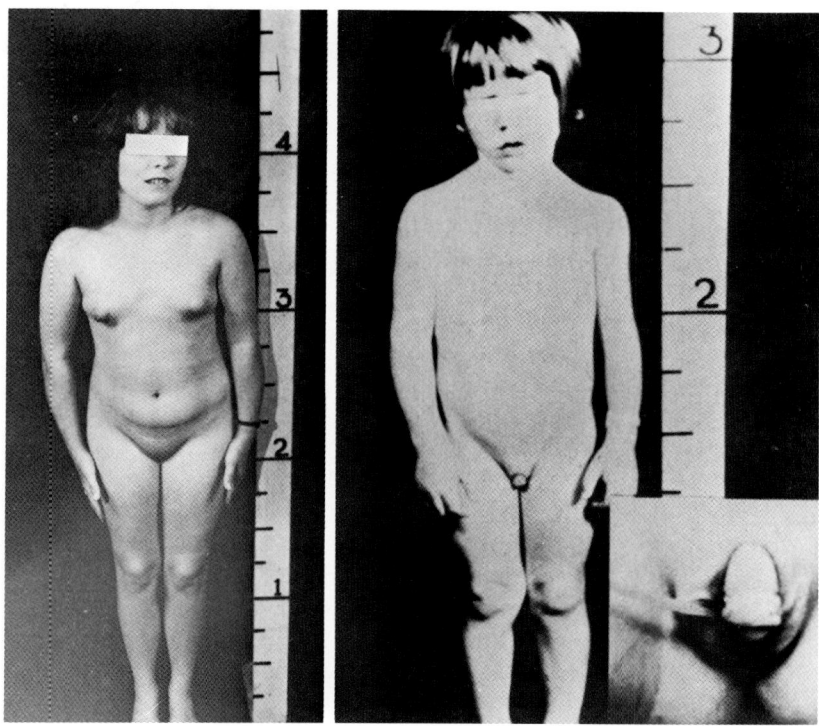

FIG. 5. Two individuals with 45,X/46,XY gonadal dysgenesis. On the left is a 14-year-old with bilateral rudimentary streak gonads. On the right is a 5-year-old with marked clitoromegaly and empty labioscrotal pouches. The child's left rudimentary streak and right testis were both intraabdominal (From McDonough PG, Simmons RG, and Obstet Gynecol), with permission.

True Hermaphroditism

This very rare condition is defined as the coexistence of ovarian and testicular tissue within one individual (42). Both tissues may be present in a single gonad (ovotestis) or in opposite gonads. The nature of internal or external genitalia does not affect the diagnosis. The presence of an ovotestis on one side and an ovary or testis on the opposite side (unilateral true hermaphroditism) is the most common presentation and occurs in 50% of the cases (42). In 30% of the cases, a single ovary is present on one side and a testis is present on the contralateral side (lateral true hermaphroditism) (42). Both gonads are usually associated with appropriate internal accessory structures. In 20% of the cases, bilateral ovotestes are present (bilateral true hermaphroditism) (42).

True hermaphrodites have a wide variety of possible clinical presentations. The external genitalia are often ambiguous. Most are raised as males because of the size of the phallus or the presence of scrotal gonad at birth. Many have hypospadias in various degrees ranging from perineal to penile, accompanied by incomplete labioscrotal fusion. Cryptorchidism is common. Inguinal hernias with a gonad or accessory structure may be present. Seventy percent of these individuals are 46,XX; less frequently, 46,XY and 46,XX/46,XY are found on cytogenic evaluation (43). Although most of these individuals are raised as males, most have a uterus, and two-thirds will eventually menstruate. Cyclic hematuria may occur. Many have significant breast development. Ovulation occurs frequently. Spermatogenesis is rare. At least six pregnancies have been reported (28).

Current controversy exists about the tendency toward germ cell tumor formation in this group and whether or not gonadal extirpation is necessary. Treatment to date has been based on presenting phenotype, social adjustment, and preservation of reproductive function (when feasible). Pregnancy is usually attainable by individuals with normal ovarian function. The presence of a uterus may also allow donor oocyte and future reproduction in individuals raised as females.

Intraabdominal Testis in 46,XY Phenotypic Females

Steroid-enzyme-deficient 46,XY patients have normal testicular development and an elaboration of MIS. In these patients, however, the fetal Leydig cells do not elaborate optimal levels of testosterone; testosterone is produced but is not recognized due to receptor defects, or testosterone is not converted to intracellular DHT (44,45). Deficiencies of testosterone or testosterone and DHT or their action affect wolffian ducts and masculinization of external genitalia. Deficiency of only DHT or its action affects only the external genitalia and leads to pseudovaginal, perineoscrotal hypospadias (46). These patients have intraabdominal testes and are at risk for tumors associated with cryptorchidism (mainly seminoma) (28).

The most common condition in this category is complete testicular feminization syndrome (complete androgen insensitivity syndrome). These 46,XY individuals have normal testicular determination and development (28,44,45). Endocrine development proceeds, including normal elaboration of MIS and regression of the müllerian duct. Although testosterone is elaborated, receptors are unable to recognize it or its converted product (DHT). Internal and external genitalia development goes in the female direction. Müllerian structures are absent, and the testes remain intraabdominal. These individuals have adequate height and breast development at puberty, but scant sexual hair and primary amenorrhea (Fig. 6).

Recently, the issue of timing in regard to the removal of dysgenetic gonads and intraabdominal testes has been considered. A recent review concerning dysgenetic gonads revealed that amenorrhea was present in

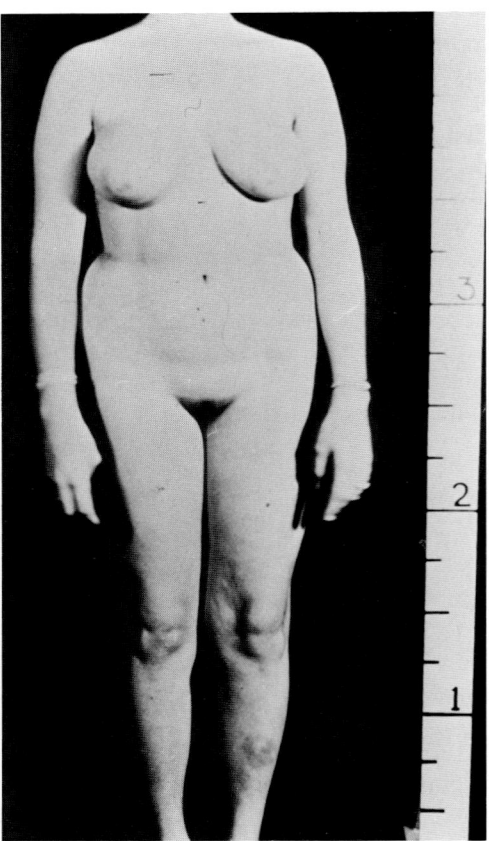

FIG. 6. Patient with androgen insensitivity. She presented with primary amenorrhea, and was found to have a 46,XY karyotype, a blind vaginal pouch, and bilateral intraabdominal testes. Note the absence of sexual hair.

94.5% of affected patients (47). The mean age of diagnosis was 18 years and 8 months. Approximately 10% of affected patients were diagnosed prior to ten years of age. Most of the tumors associated with dysgenetic gonads are gonadoblastomas or dysgerminomas, but multiple cell types have been described, including choriocarcinomas and immature teratomas. Dysgenetic gonads should be removed as soon as the diagnosis is made. However, the intraabdominal testes seen in association with the steroid enzyme deficiency syndromes are genetically normal. Although they are associated with malignant transformation, as documented in males with cryptorchidism, a delay in surgery until completion of secondary sexual development has been advocated in these patients (28). Endogenous gonadal steroids may ensure a more normal puberty than steroid replacement therapy. Malignant transformation rarely occurs before the adult years, and it does so at the same rate as cryptorchid testes. The tumors that result are usually seminomas (28).

NORMAL OVARIAN STRUCTURE

Normal Anatomy

The normal adult ovary is gray-white in color and measures approximately 4 cm in length, 3 cm in width, and 1.5 to 3 cm in thickness. It is divided into two major histologic areas, the outer cortex and the inner medulla. The surface epithelium consists of a single layer of flattened cuboidal or low columnar epithelium and is referred to as germinal epithelium. These cells become continuous with the peritoneum at the mesovarium. The outer cortex is made up of condensed, connective tissue stroma that is called the *tunica albuginea*. The stroma of the ovary has tightly packed cells (theca cells) that surround follicles in various stages of development. Atretic follicles and active and regressive corpus luteum are present. The medulla consists of a highly vascular area and specialized polyhedral hilar cells that are similar to testicular interstitial cells.

The blood supply to the ovary arises from several sources. The ovarian artery originates from the aorta below the renal artery and courses in the retroperitoneum. After crossing the psoas muscle anteriorly, the artery courses over the iliac vessels. It then courses through the infundibulopelvic ligament, enters the mesovarium from the posterior surface of the broad ligament, and enters the ovarian hilum. The ovarian veins originate in a pampiniform plexus that coalesces and drains through the hilum. The ovarian veins course with the arteries; the right ovarian vein empties into the inferior vena cava, and the left vein enters the left renal vein. The second major source of blood supply is the ovarian branch of the uterine artery, which enters the mesovarium superior to the ovarian ligament. Both of the arterial blood supplies anastomose in the ovary.

The lymphatic drainage to the ovary is primarily to the aortic chain and rarely to the closer iliac nodes. Nerves of the ovary enter through the infundibulopelvic ligament and connect to the hypogastric and aortic plexus. The ovary is attached in the pelvis by three major ligaments. The primary attachment is the infundibulopelvic ligament which attaches at the posterior lateral wall of the pelvis. The mesovarian ligament is the lateral attachment of the ovary, which contains the anastomoses of the utero-ovarian blood supply and the ovarian artery. The ovarian ligament is a prominent fibromuscular structure that courses from the lower pole of the ovary to the uterus. In the nulliparous patient, the ovary sits in the ovarian fossa, an indentation in the posterior peritoneum.

The size of the ovary changes during a normal menstrual cycle and may enlarge to 5 cm at ovulation. Follicular cysts may be as large as 6 to 7 cm without any associated pathology. The weight of the ovary varies between 3 and 6 grams, dependent on the timing of the menstrual cycle and the patient's age. With advancing age, the number of follicles decrease, and the amount of scarring from healed ovulation sites increases. The size and weight of the ovary slowly decreases. A postmenopausal ovary that can be palpated is a significant clinical finding. The average postmenopausal ovary is 1.5 cm x 1 cm x 0.5 cm. In a postmenopausal patient with a palpable ovary, the possibility of malignancy must be considered.

The concept of the postmenopausal palpable ovary syndrome (PMPO) was first suggested as a means of diagnosing ovarian cancer in the early stages and improving survival (48). The overall prognosis of ovarian cancer is poor because it is usually in an advanced stage at diagnosis. The incidence of malignancy in patients with PMPO is estimated to be approximately 10%, with Brenner tumors and fibromas most commonly found (49). However, few series give actual numbers, and interpretation is difficult because of the limited number of patients. In one series of patients who met the original criteria outlined by Barber and Graber, ovarian cancer was found in less than 10% (n = 1/11) (50). A more recent study reported an incidence of 15% (n = 3/20) (51). The total reported cases have been inadequate for further recommendations.

The role of ultrasound, especially transvaginal ultrasonography, is currently being evaluated in the early recognition of malignancy (52). In a pilot study of twenty-nine patients, benign cysts were found in all cases in which the following criteria were met: unilateral simple cysts without septations, no solid components, a diameter less than 5 cm, and no free peritoneal fluid (53). Tumor markers such as CA-125 may also contribute to earlier diagnosis. A large study combining CA-125, transabdominal ultrasound, and pelvic exam reached 100% sensitivity in the recognition of ovarian carcinoma (54). As screening procedures evolve, the concept of the PMPO syndrome may become less important. Presently, when a palpable ovary is found in a postmenopausal woman, it should be evaluated by imaging, tumor markers, and laparoscopy or laparotomy with oophorectomy (55,56).

Accessory Ovaries

Congenital abnormalities of the ovary are rare and limited to case reports. Most reported cases involve ectopic ovarian tissue. The most common abnormality is the accessory ovary, but less than two dozen cases have been reported in the world literature.

Accessory ovaries are usually small (less than 1 cm in diameter). They are commonly identified as lymph nodes at the time of surgery, and the actual diagnosis is not apparent until histological examination. The definitive diagnosis of an accessory ovary requires that normal ovarian tissue be present and the accessory ovary be close to the normal ovary. It may also be connected to the broad, utero-ovarian or infundibulopelvic ligaments (57). The accessory ovary is formed from the same primordium as the primary ovary.

Supernumerary Ovaries

A supernumerary ovary is defined as normal ovarian tissue with no connection to ovaries in their normal position (58). It is distinguished from the accessory ovary by its location and probably arises at a different time during fetal development. The supernumerary ovary is thought to arise from an independent embryologic source. A plausible explanation for this phenomena is that a separate primordium arises from arrested gonocytes during mass migration to the genital ridge. The location of most supernumerary ovaries is in the retroperitoneum, omentum, or the mesentary, which supports the migration theory (57).

Accessory ovaries and supernumerary ovaries may be important etiologic factors in cases of epithelial cancer that arise after prophylactic oophorectomy in familial ovarian cancer situations (59). An increase in associated defects of the urogenital ridge has been described with both anomalies. These defects include accessory fallopian tubes, bicornate uterus, and renal agenesis (57).

NORMAL OVARIAN FUNCTION

The Extragonadal Constraining Mechanism

From birth, the human ovary is intrinsically capable of completing all the steroidogenic and gametogenic functions necessary for female reproduction (60). Nature wisely provides a constraint on this process via an extragonadal mechanism. This mechanism must be induced to maturation before ovulation and conception can take place. Puberty is the usual time for the commencement of this induction.

Ovarian function is always under the control of the pituitary follicle stimulating hormone (FSH) and luteinizing hormone (LH). These gonadotropins are released in a pulsatile manner from cells in the pituitary gland called *gonadotropes*. Gonadotropes manufacture, store, and secrete gonadotropins. The signals that generate these activities are elicited by the activation of specific receptors that reside on the cell surface of gonadotropes. These receptors are activated when they become occupied by gonadotropin-releasing hormone (GnRH), a neuropeptide that is released from nerve terminals in the hypothalamus.

Cell bodies synthesize GnRH in the arcuate nucleus of the medial basal hypothalamus (MBH) and release it from the median eminence (61). The median eminence is outside the blood brain barrier and is exposed to circulating hormones of high molecular weight. This environment is constantly under varying influences. Released GnRH is delivered to pituitary gonadotrope GnRH receptors via the hypothalamic-hypophyseal portal vessels.

The release of GnRH is pulsatile. The episodic release and subsequent delivery of GnRH to the pituitary is secondary to an as yet undefined pulse generator that triggers periodic discharges of the protein from its synthesizing neurons (62). This pulse generator is located in the MBH and receives input from higher centers in the CNS. Knobil demonstrated synchronism between the release of GnRH into portal blood and LH levels in peripheral blood (63). The neuromodulation of the GnRH pulse generator was identified and detailed by an elaborate series of experiments. Central catecholaminergic systems exert modulatory inputs on the system. A blockade of alpha adrenergic input by phentolamine or dopaminergic activity by metaclopramide inhibits the frequency of pulse generation (64). The activity of this unit is also influenced by opioidergic input. Morphine and endogenous opioids have an inhibitory effect on pulse frequency that can be abruptly reversed by the administration of naloxone, an opiate antagonist (64). Additionally, peripherally administered corticotrophin-releasing hormone suppresses GnRH pulse generator activity (61,63). This inhibition is mediated through the activation of endogenous opiates (61,63). Thus, the hypothalamus and pituitary gland function together as a unit for the appropriate release of FSH and LH. The activity of this unit is principally mediated by a central catecholaminergic mechanism, and it is modified by both circulating ovarian sex steroids and hypothalamic opioidergic neuron activity.

By midgestation, the human fetus has an active hypothalamic GnRH pulse generator and functioning pituitary gonadotropes (65,66). This unit maintains the appropriate FSH and LH levels necessary for normal gonadal development and function. Serum concentrations and pituitary levels of immunoreactive LH at midgestation are significantly greater in the female fetus than in the male fetus (67). This dimorphism is believed to be secondary to negative feedback action by testicular factors that weaken pituitary sensitivity to GnRH stimulation (sex steroid and inhibin). The elevated levels of gonadotropin in the female fetus at midgestation aid in the completion of ovarian development, with retention of the germ cell endowment and folliculogenesis.

Because the ovary is under gonadotropin control throughout life, a review of the ontogeny of gonadotropin secretion helps to explain normal physiologic events that occur in the ovary at specific developmental stages. Often, these events go unappreciated until clinical decisions must be made about an ovarian mass. Too often, patients undergo surgery by physicians who are unfamiliar with temporal events that influence normal ovarian function.

The Neonatal Period

The ontogeny of gonadotropin secretion from fetal life through adolescence is illustrated in Fig. 7. Note the acute rise of gonadotropin levels shortly after birth. In female infants, serum FSH and LH levels continue to rise until about three months of age. FSH levels may reach the castrate levels seen in postmenopause. Gonadotropin levels later undergo a slow decline and reach a nadir between ages two and three.

The postnatal gonadotropin surge elicits a response in the young ovary. An increased number of large steroid-producing follicles is associated with a rise in serum estradiol levels (68). Estradiol, produced by the granulosa cells of the large follicles, may cause breast enlargement. The ovaries may develop functional cysts in response to elevated FSH levels in the newborn period (68).

The postnatal gonadotropin surge appears to be initiated by the sudden removal of the placental steroids that inhibit fetal gonadotropin levels through negative feedback mechanisms (65,66). These negative feedback mechanisms involve a principal direct action on the pituitary gland and secondary influence on GnRH neuronal activity mediated through neighboring systems

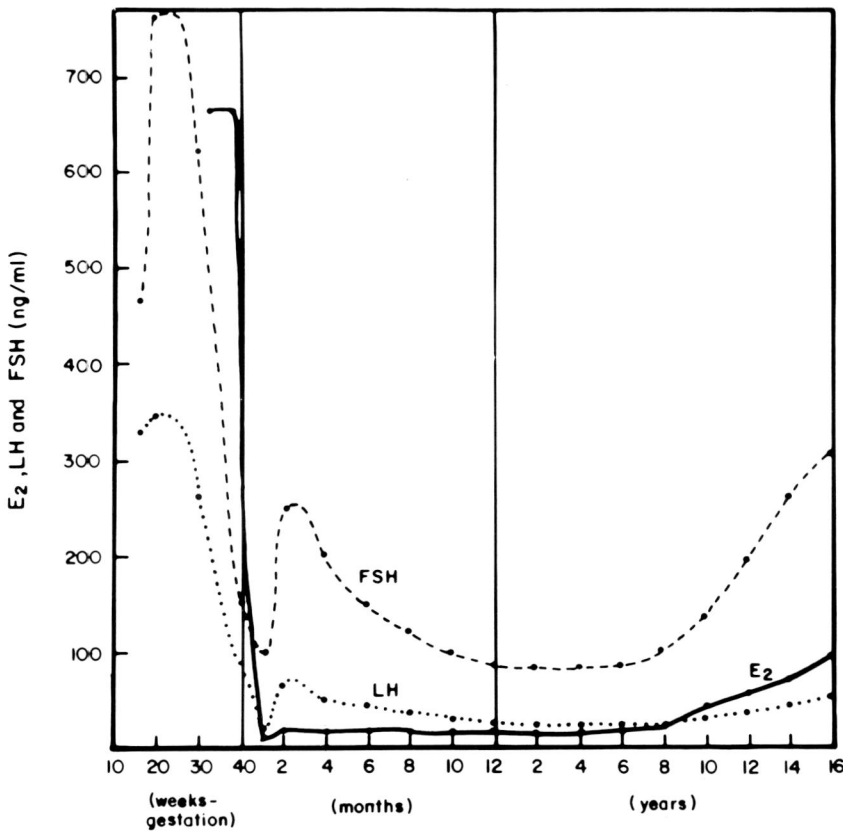

FIG. 7. The ontogeny of gonadotropin secretion from fetal life through adolescence. LH, luteinizing hormone; FSH, follicle stimulating hormone. From Lee, with permission (114).

within the MBH (69). Neighboring systems are probably dopaminergic and β-endorphinergic in nature, because they both maintain axo-axonal synapses with GnRH neurons (69). These systems have the ability to influence the GnRH pulse generator, GnRH secretion, and response to sex steroid feedback action.

The Resting Stage

From about age two to age seven, a subsequent decline occurs in pituitary gonadotropin levels. This decline is the result of active inhibition of GnRH secretion and not the result of gonadal steroid inhibition or other ovarian input; it is also seen in agonadal children (70). The baseline levels of serum FSH and LH overlap between eugonadal and agonadal children at ages four to seven. The neuroendocrine mechanism responsible for this active inhibition of GnRH secretion is viewed conceptually as two interacting components: an intrinsic CNS inhibitory mechanism that suppresses pulsatile GnRH release, and a highly sensitive, tonically negative sex steroid feedback mechanism (71,72).

An ovary in the resting stage maintains an intrinsic ability to carry out reproductive function but fails to do so because of extragonadal constraint. Exceptions include the ovarian stimulation with ovulation seen in some children with central precocious puberty (73). Normal children in this age group have quiescent ovaries with follicles in varying stages of differentiation and atresia. Ovarian masses in this age group are generally associated with pathology. Adnexal masses 2 cm or greater in prepubertal patients must be investigated (74). During investigation special caution must be taken to rule out primary hypothyroidism, because high elevations of thyroid stimulating hormone can stimulate multifollicular cyst formation (75). Because patients in this age group are at risk for germ cell tumors, a chest X-ray (to rule out lung metastasis), serum HCG, serum alpha fetoprotein (AFP), and liver function tests should be ordered. A karyotype should also be done because of the propensity of these tumors to arise in dysgenetic gonads (74).

Puberty

Between eight and eleven years of age, most girls experience an enhanced secretion of LH associated with an increased pulse frequency during sleep (71). This pattern is an expression of CNS maturation and hypothalamic control of pituitary gonadotropin release. Amplification of GnRH pulsing is critical to the activation of pituitary stimulated gonadal function (64). The onset of puberty is associated with an increase in opioidergic tone and enhanced proopiomelanocortin (POMC) gene expression in the arcuate nucleus (76,77). An increase in the pulsatile release of hypothalamic GnRH results in increases in pulsatile gonadotropin levels. This feature is independent of sex steroid action; a disinhibition of gonadotropin pulses occurs in both eugonadal and agonadal states during this period (70). Eventually, agonadal children demonstrate higher gonadotropin levels than eugonadal children (70). Agonadal children cannot produce the sex steroids that limit the level of gonadotropins via negative feedback mechanisms. Eugonadal children exhibit an enhanced ovarian production of sex steroids that initiate and sustain the development of estrogen-dependent adult secondary sexual characteristics. The final stage of puberty involves full maturation of the hypothalamic-pituitary unit. Maturity is manifested by the ability to mount an LH surge in response to high circulating levels of estradiol (71). This positive feedback response permits ovulation and reproduction.

The Mature Axis

One result of the operating GnRH pulse generator and its influence on pituitary stimulation of gonadal function is the establishment and maintenance of repetitive menstrual cycles in sexually mature female individuals. This cyclicity is associated with structural and functional changes of target tissues in the reproductive tract. The changing pattern of circulating gonadotropin concentrations before, during, and after the female reproductive period is illustrated in Fig. 8. In the absence of appropriate sex steroid levels, the amount of circulating FSH is greater than that of LH. During the reproductive years, the FSH/LH ratio is markedly reduced. Prepubertal gonadotropin levels are low because of insufficient GnRH stimulation (71). Postmenopausal gonadotropin levels are high principally because of a decline in the negative feedback effect of ovarian sex steroids and inhibin (72,78).

Pulsatile GnRH release is tonically inhibited by neighboring opioidergic neurons (76). The degree to which this inhibition occurs depends on ovarian steroid levels. When these levels are low, dissociation of the inhibition results in an increase in the pulse amplitude of gonadotropin release (72). Modulation of the GnRH pulse generator by inhibition and disinhibition of opioid tone is important for the maintenance of ovulation and menstrual cyclicity.

As stated, maturation of the hypothalamic-pituitary-gonadal axis is manifested by the ability to mount an LH surge in response to high circulating estradiol levels (71). This ability is acquired in the female during late puberty and remains intact until death. The mechanism includes an increase in the GnRH receptor concentration on pituitary gonadotropes, which allows more syn-

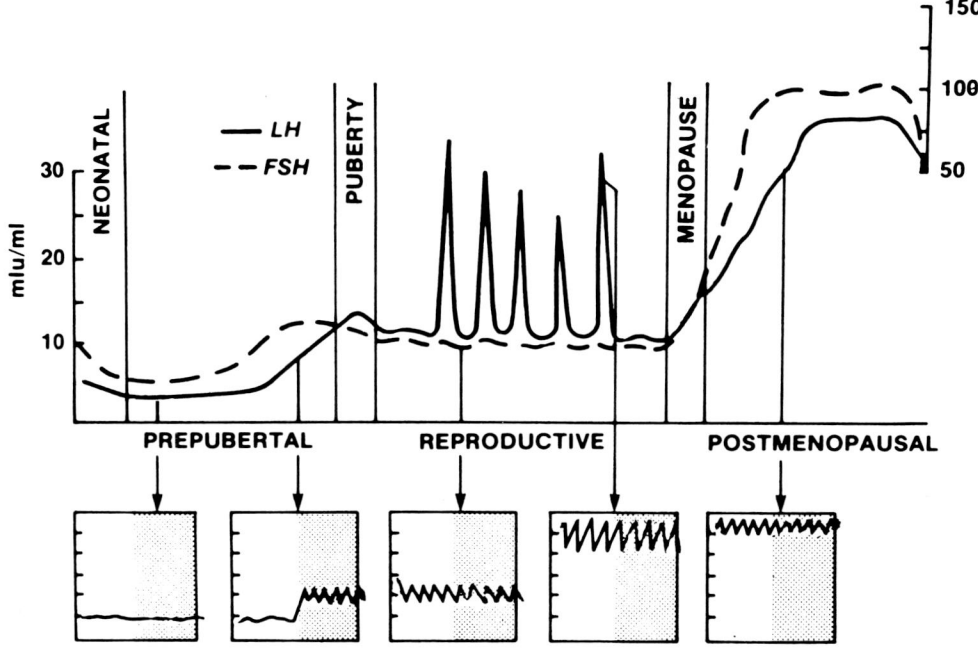

FIG. 8. Changing pattern of circulating gonadotropin levels during the human female life cycle. From Yen, with permission (115).

thesis and secretion of gonadotropin at that particular time (63).

The Reproductive Ovary

Ovarian function is dependent on gonadotropin stimulation. Events that occur during the menstrual cycle are related to cyclic alterations in gonadotropin, estradiol, and progesterone levels. These levels are a function of follicular development, ovulation, and postovulatory events. In the reproductive ovary, gonadotropins act synergistically to stimulate follicular growth and development, oocyte growth and maturation, and steroidogenesis in the stromal elements.

Although many steroid products are secreted by the reproductive ovary, estradiol, progesterone, and androstenedione are the most significant (9). Ovarian stromal cells and thecal interstitial cells primarily produce androgens. Androstenedione is the principal androgen secreted by these cells. Granulosa cells are the source of estradiol. Because the number of granulosa cells increases with follicular growth and maturity, estradiol levels are correlated to follicular maturity. Progesterone is a product of luteinized cells and is made abundantly by the corpus luteum. Ovarian sex steroid production is a function of the number and developmental stages of all follicles present in the ovary at any given point.

The two-cell–two-gonadotropin concept of ovarian follicle maturation and estradiol synthesis has received wide acceptance (9). In thecal cells, LH stimulates conversion of cholesterol to androstenedione and testosterone. Thecal cells always have LH receptors, so this process continues whenever LH is present. Granulosa cells must acquire FSH receptors and aromatase enzyme activity early in follicular development. They are stimulated by FSH to convert thecal androstenedione and testosterone to estradiol and some estrone. Estradiol acts locally to induce granulosa cell proliferation, additional FSH receptors, and enhanced follicular growth and differentiation (Fig. 9). Estradiol production increases, resulting in higher serum estradiol levels and the presence of this steroid in antral follicular fluid. Initially, higher serum estradiol levels cause circulating gonadotropin levels to fall (71,72). Granulosa cells also secrete inhibin, a protein that exerts direct effect on the pituitary gland to lower the secreted level of FSH (78). Thus, less gonadotropin becomes available for the growing follicles, and many are pushed toward atresia instead of continued growth (79,80).

The follicular microenvironment determines whether a given follicle grows or becomes atretic (79). Successful growth requires that a given follicle convert the androgenic environment generated by thecal androgens to an estrogenic environment. Follicles grow from preantral to antral follicles. A cohort is selected to undergo rapid development (80). Out of this cohort, a single follicle becomes dominant as it grows ahead of the pack. This dominant follicle will provide the signals necessary for meiotic reactivation of the oocyte, a pro-

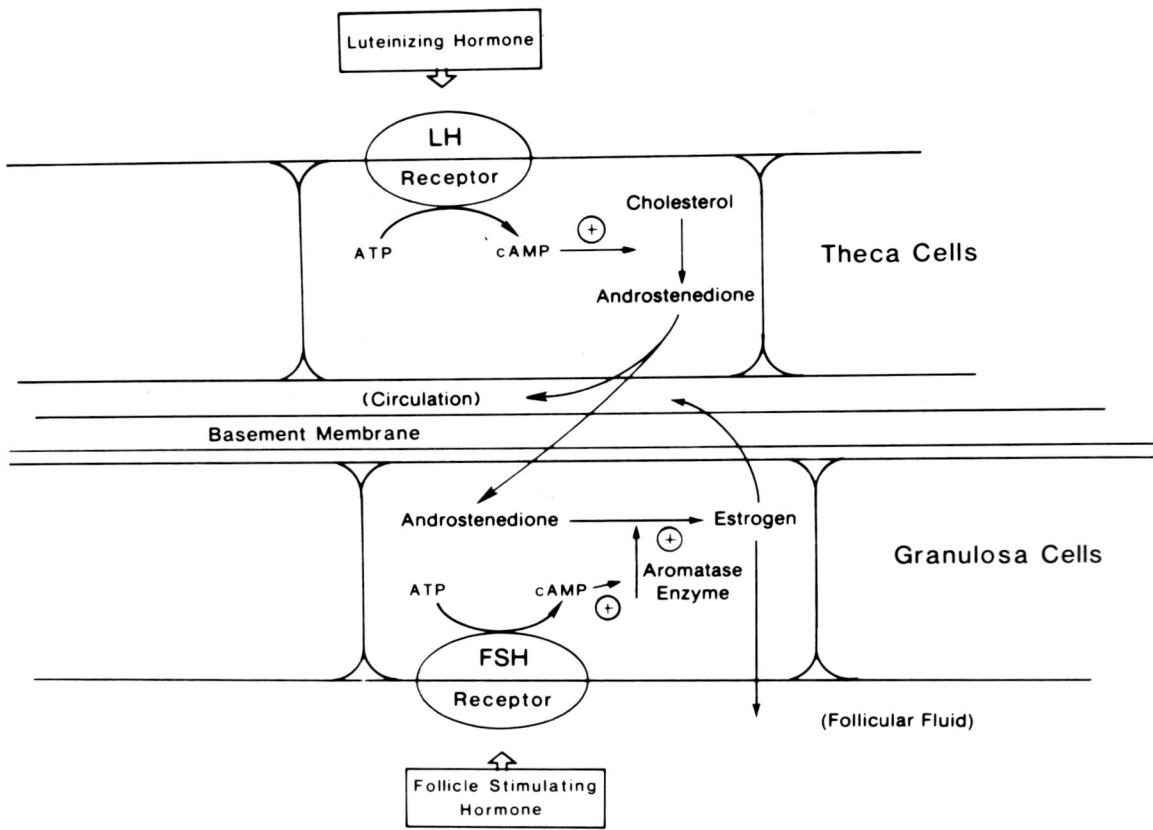

FIG. 9. Two-cell theory of follicular estrogen production. LH binds (*arrows, top*) to specific membrane receptors on theca cells and stimulates cAMP production and the conversion of cholesterol to androstenedione. Androstenedione diffuses (*arrows, center*) into the circulation and across the basement membrane into follicle granulosa cells. FSH binds (*arrows, bottom left*) to specific granulosa cell receptors, and stimulates cAMP production, which leads to increased aromatase enzyme and the conversion (*arrows, right*) of theca androgen to estrogen. From Yen, with permission (115).

cess that has been arrested since fetal development, and for the initiation of ovulatory events (9). Follicular dominance is established by the fifth day of the menstrual cycle (81). FSH eventually induces LH receptor formation on the granulosa cells of the dominant follicle, which by now is producing a large amount of estradiol (82). Estradiol levels peak about 24–36 hours before ovulation (83). By this time, many LH receptors are present on the granulosa cells of the dominant follicle, and the associated theca is richly vascularized. Circulating estradiol levels rise to approximately 200–300 pg/ml. Eighty percent of the total estradiol that is produced is from the dominant follicle, and the remaining twenty percent comes from other follicles and the peripheral conversion of testosterone and estrone.

In response to persistently elevated estradiol levels, LH secretion increases in women who have completed the required hypothalamic-pituitary maturation at puberty (63,71,83). The estradiol level necessary to achieve this gonadotropin surge is over 200 pg/ml for about 50 hours (84). In the dominant follicle, a small amount of progesterone is produced by luteinizing cells, stimulated by rising LH levels (85). This progesterone production occurs about 12–24 hours before ovulation and signals both the rapid and marked surge in LH secretion and the associated midcycle FSH peak (85,86). Thus, the dominant follicle emits its own trigger for ovulation.

The midcycle LH surge initiates completion of the first meiotic division of the oocyte (9,84). Granulosa cells become luteinized and make progesterone in high quantities. Prostaglandin synthesis is also initiated and will contribute to follicular rupture. The FSH peak stimulates plasminogen activator, which converts plasminogen to the proteolytic enzyme plasmin. This enzyme helps to free the cumulus cells from parietal granulosa cells so the oocyte can be extruded with cumulus intact. Once the oocyte has ovulated, the remaining follicle wall, which consists of parietal granulosa cells on a basement membrane and theca interstitial cells, involutes (9,84). These cells are luteinized, and they incorporate lutein, a yellow pigment. The granulosa cell layer becomes fully vascularized, and serum progesterone levels increase dramatically.

Progesterone and estradiol production continues from the early postovulatory phase and peaks approximately seven days later (9,84). The uterine endometrium, made lush by this hormonal milieu, is ready to support a conceptus if successful fertilization of the ovulated oocyte occurs.

When implantation occurs, HCG from trophoblasts at the implantation site rescues the corpus luteum until placental function is established later in the first trimester of pregnancy (84). Chronically elevated levels of HCG have a powerful luteinizing effect on the theca cells that surround atretic follicles and on the interstitial stroma. When the stromal compartment is particularly sensitive to normal amounts of HCG, or when high amounts of HCG are produced by molar pregnancies or multiple gestations, thecal hyperplasia with luteinization can occur (87). This hyperplasia can result in the formation of a discrete mass called a *pregnancy luteoma* (87). These "tumors" are associated with increased androgen production, occasional maternal virilization, and possible virilization of a female fetus. Pregnancy luteomas regress after delivery.

Circulating levels of estradiol and progesterone modulate the GnRH pulse generator and associated pituitary secretion of gonadotropin. In the absence of conception, the corpus luteum undergoes luteolysis. The resulting decline in sex steroid levels is associated with a rise in FSH levels and the beginning of the selection process for a new dominant follicle (84).

Many other modulators of the ovulatory process exist but are not described here. Numerous intraovarian autocrine and paracrine mechanisms and additional central influences participate in this finely tuned process. The reader is referred to a number of excellent texts on this subject (9,84,87).

The Senescent Ovary

At a genetically predetermined time period, accelerated atresia of remaining follicles ensues. Fewer primary follicles are available for gonadotropin-induced growth and differentiation. The individual may begin to experience symptoms consistent with estrogen deprivation as follicular steroidogenesis declines and levels of estradiol (the most bioactive estrogen) begin to wane. Eventually, follicular and gametogenic functions cease. However, the senescent ovary is not inactive. It maintains extensive gonadotropin-dependent androgen production (9,87). Androstenedione and testosterone are the principal sex steroids produced at this time. The senescent ovary contributes no more than 20% of the androstenedione produced daily, but circulating testosterone levels are only minimally lower than before menopause (9). The adrenal production and contribution of androstenedione increases dramatically at this time. Estrogen production is exclusively caused by extraglandular aromatization of androstenedione to estrone. Because peripheral aromatization is a function of body weight, some obese women experience problems associated with relative estrogen excess, despite low circulating estradiol levels (87).

Histologically, the ovary appears small and has a yellow, lusterless cast. The medulla assumes dominance as the cortex becomes thin and devoid of follicles. Old corpora albicantia are present and act as stromal cells. Hilar cells, analogues of testicular Leydig cells, become prominent and are responsive to high circulating gonadotropin levels (87). It is not uncommon for stromal hyperthecosis to develop and produce symptoms of virilization in some postmenopausal women (87). Peripheral conversion of androgen may lead to endometrial hyperplasia and carcinoma. Hilus cell hyperplasia may occur, less commonly as a result of high circulating postmenopausal LH levels (87). Hilar cells preferentially produce testosterone that can present as both virilization and endometrial hyperplasia.

OVARIAN TUMOR HISTOGENESIS

Epithelial Tumors

Most ovarian neoplasms are of coelomic epithelial origin. One-half to two-thirds of the benign neoplasms that occur before menopause and 80% of those that occur after menopause are also of this origin (88). Malignant epithelial tumors of the ovary account for 85% of all ovarian cancers (88). If the mechanism(s) of coelomic epithelial tissue transformation were to be identified, more effective treatment strategies for this tumor category might be developed.

Various theories have been postulated for the histogenesis of epithelial ovarian tumors. Epidemiologic data suggests that risk is related to reproductive status (89). Single, nulliparous, or relatively infertile women are at higher risk. The infrequency of the disease before puberty and its high rate of occurrence after menopause suggest a hormonal relationship. Oral contraceptive use and high parity appear to have a protective effect.

Fathalla proposed a model for tumorigenesis that suggested that the repetitive ovarian trauma associated with ovulation is causative (90). Cramer and Welch also supported the notion of trauma-related tumorigenesis (91). "Incessant ovulation" predisposes individuals to the formation of germinal inclusion cysts. With each ovulation, coelomic epithelium extends into the ruptured follicle. This epithelium proliferates under local estrogenic influence. During the healing process, a bud of epithelium is burrowed into the ovarian substance. The resulting germinal inclusion undergoes extensive squamous metaplasia and may become the focus of a benign or malignant process. Factors that cause the differentiation and proliferation of inclusion cysts by direct estrogen stimulation may be implicated because some ovarian cystadenomas and adenocarcinomas have estrogen receptors (92). The estrogen responsiveness of coelomic epithelial cells during ovarian organogenesis tends to support this mechanism. Between 16 and 20 weeks of gestation, these cells undergo extensive proliferation (93). Proliferative activity ceases by week 24, when the epithelium exists as the single cell layer in adult women. Peak proliferative activity during the intrauterine period occurs when intraovarian sex steroids are at high levels (22). The specific growth regulatory factors that initiate or terminate epithelial cell proliferation are unknown, and few clues can be obtained from the clinical literature. Only a few studies have evaluated the incidence of ovarian cancer in patients who take estrogen replacement therapy. La Vecchia and associates reported that endometrioid cancer and clear cell carcinoma of the ovary were more common in patients who used hormones (94). Weiss and colleagues also reported an increase in endometrioid tumors but noted no correlation with the duration of hormone use (95).

Some population-based studies suggest a role for environmental carcinogens. Because coelomic epithelium is analogous to mesothelium, many have postulated that asbestos-like substances may be involved in epithelial tumorigenesis. Talc, silicon, magnesium, and environmental exposure to cigarette smoke and ionizing radiation have been implicated (96). Theories that relate galactose metabolism, dietary fat, and food preparation (i.e., frying) have also been proposed (97,98,99).

Ovarian cancer has been associated with Peutz-Jeghers syndrome, basal cell nevus syndrome, consanguinity, and family pedigrees with primary carcinomas of the colon, lung, ovary, and prostate glands (100,101,102).

The inactivation of one or more tumor suppressor genes may contribute to ovarian cancer development. Cytogenetic studies of invasive ovarian cancer have demonstrated a variety of aneuploid karyotypes in these tumors (103,104). However, to date, no consistent cytogenetic abnormalities have been pathognomonic in ovarian epithelial cancers.

Germ Cell Tumors

Germ cell tumors represent 15% to 20% of all primary ovarian neoplasms, which makes them second only to epithelial tumors in incidence (74,88). The mean age at diagnosis is nineteen years. Benign cystic teratoma (dermoid) is the most common tumor, followed by dysgerminoma, endodermal sinus tumor, immature teratoma, embryonal carcinoma, choriocarcinoma, and polyembryoma. Ten to fifteen percent of these tumors will be of the mixed cell type (74,88).

Despite the fact that no consistent cytogenetic abnormalities have been pathognomonic for ovarian epithelial cancers, quite the opposite can be said for some of the germ cell tumors. Substantial evidence supports the notion that dermoid tumors arise from the parthenogenetic reactivation of arrested primary oocytes (105). A single reactivated oocyte extrudes the first polar body and becomes a secondary oocyte in early meiosis II as shown in Fig. 3. This oocyte does not ovulate. It remains in the ovary and cannot be inseminated. Instead, it undergoes centromere separation, retaining both sister chromatids. This diploid 46,XX ovum becomes the progenitor cell of the dermoid. Dermoid tumors represent a complete duplication of the maternal haploid genome that arise from a meiotic II gametogenic error. Cytogenetically, these tumors are 46,XX.

The disorganized development of the dermoid tumor may be related to its homozygosity for certain lethal mutations (105). It is estimated that every individual carries six to eight lethal single gene mutations. These mutations are usually carried in the genome in a heterozygous state and go unnoticed. However, because dermoid tumors carry two identical copies of one or more lethal mutations in a single genome, homozygous gene expression may allow the uncontrolled embryonic development seen in these tumors. Propensity to malignant degeneration may be related to the number of copies of homozygous lethal mutations that exist in the tumor genome. Three to four mutations may be less ominous than six to eight, etc. Immature teratomas are usually trisomic. Trisomy 20 is the most common aneuploidy found, although trisomy 3, 12, 14, 21, and X have been reported (106).

Malignant germ cell tumors represent less than 5% of all ovarian cancers (74,88). The epidemiology of these tumors demonstrates a higher prevalence in oriental and black societies, in which they may represent up to 15% of all ovarian malignancies (74,88). These tumors tend to be aggressive and tragically, they affect the young. In the first two decades of life, 70% of ovarian malignancies fall into this category. These cancers rarely occur after the third decade.

Gonadoblastomas are unusual, premalignant lesions. They arise almost exclusively in cases of intersex pure gonadal dysgenesis, mixed gonadal dysgenesis, and testicular feminization (107). Ninety percent of the patients with these tumors are sex chromatin negative, and the most common karyotypes are 46,XY and 45,X/46,XY (107). Twenty-five percent of the patients are phenotypic males, but ambiguous genitalia are commonly present. Often, patients with female phenotypes show some evidence of masculinization. Calcification may be present on pelvic X-ray. Gonadoblastomas represent germ cells that are intimately mixed with indifferent sex cord elements and resemble immature granulosa and Sertoli cells. Leydig cells may be present in the stroma. The tumors are usually small and may be bilateral in up to one-third of the cases. Most importantly, half of the reported cases were associated with malignant degeneration. Dysgerminoma is the most commonly associated tumor, followed by an occasional choriocarcinoma, endodermal sinus tumor, and mixed germ cell tumor (107). Because these tumors can occur in the first decade of life, they should be removed as soon as they are discovered because of the high frequency of malignant degeneration. Prepubertal ovaries are very difficult to evaluate grossly, and it is extremely important to obtain a karyotype of these patients before surgery (107).

Dysgerminomas are the most common malignant germ cell tumors. They represent 30% to 40% of all germ cell malignancies (74). Seventy-five percent of the cases occur between the ages of ten and thirty years (74). Dysgerminomas represent 20% to 30% of the ovarian cancer that arise during pregnancy (74). These tumors are rare in patients over age fifty (74).

Five percent of all dysgerminomas occur in phenotypic females with abnormal gonads (pure gonadal dysgenesis 45,XY with bilateral streak gonads, mixed gonadal dysgenesis 45,X/46,XY unilateral streak gonad with contralateral testis, and androgen insensitivity syndrome 46,XY with bilateral testis) (74,88). Synctiotrophoblastic cells are present in some dysgerminomas and can induce isosexual pseudoprecocious puberty in children or menstrual irregularities in older females (108). In most patients with gonadal dysgenesis, dysgerminomas arise in gonadoblastoma (88). If the gonadoblastoma is left in situ, 50% will undergo malignant degeneration (108).

Sex Cord-Stromal Tumors

Five to eight percent of all ovarian malignancies are sex cord-stromal tumor. These tumors are derived from sex cords and mesenchyme (88). They may occur at any age, although the peak incidence is during the postmenopausal years (mean age of 50 at diagnosis) (107). Less than 5% will occur before puberty. Because of their rarity, these tumors are frequently misdiagnosed, which makes epidemiologic study difficult. They also have a tendency toward delayed recurrence.

Factors that indirectly affect the differentiation and proliferation of inclusion cysts through gonadotropin-induced stromal proliferation may be implicated in the histogenesis of granulosa cell tumors. Davy demonstrated the presence of FSH receptors in a granulosa cell tumor (109). Goldston proposed suppression of FSH receptors with exogenous estrogen therapy as treatment (110). Schwartz reported ten months of stable disease in a patient with a recurrent granulosa cell tumor who was treated with progesterone (111). More recently, Martikainen reported a partial response in a patient with metastatic granulosa cell carcinoma treated with the GnRH agonist leuprolide (112). After stimulating an initial gonadotropin release, this agonist induces castrate estrogen levels and prevents subsequent secretion of gonadotropins by pituitary gonadotropes (113).

CONCLUSION

The ovary is a complex organ with an ever-changing, heterogeneous population of cells programmed for different functions. Malignant transformation can arise in any of the various cell types. Cancer therapy and diagnosis must address this heterogeneity. For example, although many highly undifferentiated tumors behave in an unpredictable, bizarre fashion, tumors differentiated enough to acquire and maintain gonadotropin receptors might respond to therapy based on endocrine logic. An understanding of the development and function of the normal ovary is essential if we are to understand how ovarian cancers develop. Our challenge in the 1990s is to inquire at both the cellular and molecular level into the behavior and control mechanisms of normal ovarian cells. Only in this way can we begin to decipher the behavior of deviant ovarian cells.

REFERENCES

1. Morrow CP, Townsend DE. Tumors of the ovary: general considerations; classification; the adnexal mass. In: Morrow CP, Townsend DE, eds. *Synopsis of Gynecologic Oncology*, 3rd ed. New York: John Wiley & Sons, 1987;231–255.
2. Hertig AR, Adams EC, McKay DG, Rock J, Mulligan WJ, Merkin M. A description of 34 human ova within the first 17 days of development. *Am J Anat* 1956;98:435–493.
3. Fujimoto T, Miyayama Y, Fuyuta M. The origin, migration and fine morphology of human primordial germ cells. *Anat Rec* 1977;188:315–330.
4. Donovan PJ, Stott D, Cairns LA, Heasman J, Wylie CC. Migratory and postmigratory mouse primordial germ cells behave differently in culture. *Cell* 1986;44:831–836.

5. Novak ER, Woodruff JD, Embryology and histology of ovaries. In: Novak ER, Woodruff JD, eds. *Novak's Gynecologic and Obstetric Pathology*, 7th ed. Philadelphia: WB Saunders Co, 1974;328–347.
6. Hogan B, Costantini F, Lacy E. *Manipulating the Mouse Embryo*. New York: Cold Spring Harbor Laboratory, 1986;1–77.
7. Parmley TH, Woodruff JD. The ovarian mesothelioma. *Am J Obstet Gynecol* 1974;120:234–241.
8. Novak ER, Woodruff JD. Ovarian Neoplasia: stromo-epithelial lesions—primarily epithelial. In: Novak ER, Woodruff JD, eds. *Novak's Gynecologic and Obstetric Pathology*, 7th ed. Philadelphia: WB Saunders Co, 1974;367–393.
9. Adashi EY. The ovarian life cycle. In: Yen SCC, Jaffe RB, eds. *Reproductive Endocrinology*, 3rd ed. Philadelphia: WB Saunders, 1991;181–237.
10. Sinclair AH, Berta P, Palmer MS, et al. A gene from the human sex-determining region encodes a protein with homology to a conserved DNA-binding motif. *Nature* 1990;346:240–244.
11. Jirasek JE. Principles of reproductive embryology. In: Simpson JL, ed. *Disorders of Sexual Differentiation*, New York: Academic Press, 1976;51–110.
12. Jost A. Problems in fetal endocrinology: the gonadal and hypophyseal hormones. *Recent Prog Horm Res* 1953;8:379–418.
13. Jost A, Vigier B, Prépin J, Perchellet JP. Studies on sex differentiation in mammals. *Recent Prog Horm Res* 1973;29:1–41.
14. Cate RL, Mattaliano RJ, Hession C, et al. Isolation of the bovine and human genes for müllerian inhibiting substance and expression of the human gene in animal cells. *Cell* 1986;45:685–698.
15. Cohen-Haguenauer O, Picard JY, Mattei MG, et al. Mapping of the gene for anti-Müllerian hormone to the short arm of human chromosome 19. *Cytogenet Cell Genet* 1987;44:2–6.
16. Wallen JW, Cate RL, Kiefer DM, et al. Minimal antiproliferative effect of recombinant müllerian inhibiting substance on gynecological tumor cell lines and tumor explants. *Cancer Research* 1989;49:2005–2011.
17. Huktaniemi IT, Korenbrot CC, Jaffe RB. HCG binding and stimulation of testosterone biosynthesis in the human fetal testis. *J Clin Endocrinol Metab* 1977;44:963–967.
18. Ritzen EMS, Neyfeh SN, French FS, Dobbins MV. Demonstration of androgen-binding components in rat epididymis cytosol and comparison with binding components in prostate and other tissues. *Endocrinology* 1971;89:143–151.
19. Wilson JD, Lasnitzki I. Dihydrotestosterone formation in fetal tissues of the rabbit and rat. *Endocrinology* 1971;89:659–668.
20. Wilson JD. Embryology of the genital tract. In: Harrison JH, Gittes RF, Perlmutter AD, Stamey TA, Walsh PC, eds. *Urology*, Vol 2. 4th ed. Philadelphia: WB Saunders, 1979;1469–1483.
21. Gier HT, Marion GB. Development of the mammalian testis and genital ducts. *Biol Reprod* 1969;1:1–23.
22. Gulyos BJ, Hodgen GD, Tullner WW, Ross GT. Effects of fetal or maternal hyposphyectomy on endocrine organs and body weight in infant rhesus monkeys with particular emphasis on oogenesis. *Biol Reprod* 1977;16:216–227.
23. Boonilla-Musoles F, Renau J, Hernandez-Yago J, Torres YJ. How do oocytes disappear? *Arch Gynaekol* 1975;218:233–241.
24. Peters H. Intrauterine gonadal development. *Fertil Steril* 1976;27:493–500.
25. Weakly BS. Electron microscopy of the oocyte and granulosa cells in the developing ovarian follicles of the golden hamster. *J Anat* 1966;100:503–534.
26. Himelstein-Braw R, Byskov AG, Peters H, Farber M. Follicular atresia in the infant human ovary. *J Reprod Fertil* 1976;46:55–59.
27. Lintern-Moore S, Peters H, Moore GPM, Farber M. Follicular development in the infant human ovary. *J Reprod Fertil* 1974;39:53–64.
28. Rhinedollar RH, Tho SPT, McDonough PG. Abnormalities of sexual differentiation: evaluation and management. *Clin Obst Gynecol* 1987;30:697–713.
29. Singh RP, Carr DH. The anatomy and histology of XO human embryos and fetuses. *Anat Rec* 1966;155:369–383.
30. Friedman WF. Congenital heart disease. In: Braunwald E, Isselbacher KJ, Petersdorf RG, Wilson JD, Martin JB, Fauci AS, eds. *Harrison's Principles of Internal Medicine*, Vol 1. New York: McGraw-Hill Book Company, 1987;948.
31. Fialkow PJ, Uchida IA. Antibodies in Down's syndrome and gonadal dysgenesis. *Ann NY Acad Sci* 1968;155:759–769.
32. Turner HH. A syndrome of infantilism, congenital webbed neck, and cubitus valgus. *Endocrinology* 1938;23:566–574.
33. Carr DH. Chromosome studies in selected spontaneous abortions and early pregnancy loss. *Obstet Gynecol* 1971;31:570–574.
34. Sanger R, Tippett P, Gavin J, Teesdale P, Daniels GL. Xg groups and sex chromosome abnormalities in people of northern European ancestry. [An addendum] *J Med Genet* 1977;14:210–211.
35. Hook EB, Warburton D. The distribution of chromosomal genotypes associated with Turner's syndrome: livebirth prevalence rates and evidence for diminished fetal mortality and severity in genotypes associated with structural X abnormalities or mosaicism. *Hum Genet* 1983;64:24–27.
36. Tho SP, Behzadian A, Byrd JR, McDonough PG. Use of human alpha-satellite deoxyribonucleic acid to detect Y-specific centromeric sequences. *Am J Obstet Gynecol* 1988;159:1553–1557.
37. Witt M, Erickson RP. A rapid method for detection of Y chromosomal DNA from dried blood specimens by the polymerase chain reaction. *Hum Genet* 1989;82:271–274.
38. Reindollar RH, Byrd JR, McDonough PG. Delayed sexual development: a study of 252 patients. *Am J Obstet Gynecol* 1981;140:371–380.
39. McDonough PG, Byrd JR, Tho PT, Mahesh VB. Phenotypic and cytogenetic findings in eighty-two patients with ovarian failure-changing trends. *Fertil Steril* 1977;28:638–641.
40. Layman LC. The genetics of ovarian failure. *Obstetrics and Gynecology Report* 1990;2:363–375.
41. Gantt PA, Byrd JR, Greenblatt RB, McDonough PG. A clinical and cytogenetic study of 15 patients with 45,X/46,XY gonadal dysgenesis. *Fertil Steril* 1980;34:216–221.
42. van Nielerk WA, Retief AE. The gonads of human true hermaphrodites. *Hum Genet* 1981;58:117–122.
43. Simpson JL. True hermaphroditism: etiology and phenotype considerations. *Birth Defects* 1978;14:9–35.
44. New MI. Male pseudohermaphroditism due to 17 alpha hydroxylase deficiency. *J Clin Invest* 1970;49:1930–1941.
45. Saez JM, Morera AM, de Peretti E, Bertrand J. Further in vitro studies in male pseudohermaphroditism with gynecomastia due to a testicular 17-ketosteroid reductase defect (compared to a case of testicular feminization). *J Clin Endocrinol Metab* 1972;34:598–600.
46. Peterson RE, Imperato-McGinley J, Gautier T, Sturnba E. Male pseudohermaphroditism due to steroid 5 alpha-reductase deficiency. *Am J Med* 1977;62:170–191.
47. Troche V, Hernandez E. Neoplasia arising in dysgenetic gonads. *Obstet Gynecol Surv* 1986;41:74–79.
48. Barber HRK, Graber EA. The PMPO syndrome (postmenopausal palpable ovary syndrome) (Editorial). *Obstet Gynecol* 1971;38:921–923.
49. The adnexal mass and early ovarian cancer. In: Disaia PJ, Creasman WT, eds. *Clinical Gynecologic Oncology* 3rd ed. St Louis: C.V. Mosby Co; 1989,310–311.
50. Flynt JR, Gallup DG. The postmenopausal palpable ovary syndrome: a fourteen-year review. *Milit Med* 1981;146:686–688.
51. Miller RC, Nash JD, Weiser EB, Hoskins WJ. The postmenopausal palpable ovary syndrome: a retrospective review with histopathologic correlates. *J Repro Med* 1991;36:568–571.
52. Rulin MC, Preston AL. Adnexal masses in postmenopausal women. *Obstet Gynecol* 1987;70:578–581.
53. Schoenfeld A, Levavi H, Hirsch M, Pardo J, Ovadia J. Transvaginal sonography in postmenopausal women. *J Clin Ultrasound* 1990;18:350–358.
54. Jacobs I, Stabile I, Bridges J, et al. Multimodal approach to screening for ovarian cancer. *Lancet* 1988;1:268–271.
55. Hall D, McCarthy K. The significance of the postmenopausal simple adnexal cyst. *J Ultrasound Med* 1986;5:503–505.
56. Parker WH, Berek JS. Management of selected cystic adnexal

56. masses in postmenopausal women by operative laparoscopy: a pilot study. *Am J Obstet Gynecol* 1990;163:1574–1577.
57. Pearl M, Plotz EJ. Supernumerary ovary: report of a case. *Obstet Gynecol* 1963;21:253–256.
58. Wharton LR. Two cases of supernumerary ovary and one of accessory ovary, with an analysis of previously reported cases. *Am J Obstet Gynecol* 1959;78:1101–1119.
59. Lynch HT, Bewtra C, Lynch JF. Familial peritoneal ovarian carcinomatosis: a new clinical entity? *Med Hypotheses* 1986;21:171–177.
60. Peters HR, Himelstein-Braw R, Faber M. The normal development of the ovary in childhood. *Acta Endocrinol (kbh)* 1976;82:617–630.
61. Knobil E. Electrophysiological approaches to the hypothalamic GnRH pulse generator. In: Yen SSC, Vale W, eds. *Symposium on Neuroendocrine Regulation of Reproduction*, Norwell, Mass: Serono Symposia, USA, 1990;3–9.
62. Knobil E. The electrophysiology of the GnRH pulse generator. *J Steroid Biochem* 1989;33:669–671.
63. Knobil E. Neuroendocrine control of the menstrual cycle. *Rec Prog Horm Res* 1980;36:53–88.
64. Yen SSC. The hypothalamic control of pituitary hormone secretion. In: Yen SCC, Jaffe RB, eds. *Reproductive Endocrinology*, 3rd ed. Philadelphia: WB Saunders, 1991;65–104.
65. Takagi S, Yoshida T, Tsubata K, et al. Sex differences in fetal gonadotropins and androgens. *J Steroid Biochem* 1977;8:609–620.
66. Ronnekleiv OK, Resko JA. Ontogeny of gonadotropin-releasing hormone-containing neurons in early fetal development of rhesus macaques. *Endocrinology* 1990;126:498–511.
67. Reyes RI, Boroditsky RS, Winter JSD, Faiman C. Studies on human sexual development: II. fetal and maternal serum gonadotropin and sex steroid concentrations. *J Clin Endocrinol Metab* 1974;38:612–617.
68. Kulin HE, Reiter EO. Gonadotropins during childhood and adolescence: a review. *Pediatrics* 1973;51:260–271.
69. Yen SSC. The human menstrual cycle: neuroendocrine regulation. In: Yen SCC, Jaffe RB, eds. *Reproductive Endocrinology*, 3rd ed. Philadelphia: WB Saunders, 1991;273–292.
70. Boyar RM, Finkelstein J, Roffwarg H, Kapen S, Weitzman ED, Hellman L. Twenty-four-hour luteinizing hormone and follicle-stimulating hormone secretory patterns in gonadal dysgenesis. *J Clin Endocrinol Metab* 1973;37:521–525.
71. Lemarchand-Beraud T, Zufferey M-M, Reymond M, Rey I. Maturation of the hypothalmo-pituitary-ovarian axis in adolescent girls. *J Clin Endocrinol Metab* 1982;54:241–246.
72. Yen SSC, Tsai CC, Naftolin F, Vandenberg G, Ajabor L. Pulsatile patterns of gonadotropin release in subjects with and without ovarian function. *J Clin Endocrinol Metab* 1972;34:671–675.
73. Reiter EO, Kaplan SL, Conte FA, Grumbach MM. Responsivity of pituitary gonadotropes to luteinizing hormone-releasing factor in idiopathic precocious puberty, precocious thelarche, precocious adrenarche. *Pediatr Res* 1975;9:111–116.
74. Berek JS. Nonepithelial ovarian and tubal cancers. In: Berek JS, Hacker NF, eds. *Practical Gynecologic Oncology*. Baltimore: Williams and Wilkins, 1989;365–390.
75. Pringle PJ, Stanhope R, Hindmarsh P. Abnormal pubertal development in primary hypothyroidism. *Clinical Endocrinology* 1988;28:479–486.
76. Petraglia F, Bernasconi S, Iughetti L, et al. Naloxone-induced luteinizing hormone secretion in normal, precocious, and delayed puberty. *J Clin Endocrinol Metab* 1986;63:1112–1116.
77. Wiemann JN, Clifton DK, Steiner RA. Pubertal changes in gonadotropin-releasing hormone and proopiomelanocortin gene expression in the brain of the male rat. *Endocrinology* 1989;124:1760–1767.
78. Rivier C, Rivier J, Vale W. Inhibin-mediated feedback control of follicle stimulating hormone secretion in the female rat. *Science* 1986;234:205–208.
79. Ross GT. Gonadotropins and preantral follicular maturation in women. *Fertil Steril* 1974;25:522–543.
80. Gougeon A. Dynamics of follicular growth in the human: a model from preliminary results. *Human Reprod* 1986;1:81–87.
81. Di Zerega GS, Marut EL, Turner CK, Hodgen GD. Asymmetrical ovarian function during recruitment and selection of the dominant follicle in the menstrual cycle of the rhesus monkey. *J Clin Endocrinol Metab* 1980;51:689–701.
82. Erickson GF, Wang C, Hsueh AJW. FSH induction of functional LH receptors in granulosa cells cultured in a chemically defined medium. *Nature* 1979;279:336–338.
83. Pauerstein CJ, Eddy CA, Croxatto HD, Hess R, Siler-Khodr TM, Croxatto HB. Temporal relationships of estrogen, progesterone, and luteinizing hormone levels to ovulation in women and infrahuman primates. *Am J Obstet Gynecol* 1978;130:876–886.
84. Speroff L, Glass RH, Kase NG. Regulation of the menstrual cycle. In: Speroff L, Glass RH, Kase NG, eds. *Clinical Gynecologic Endocrinology and Infertility*, 4th ed. Baltimore: Williams & Wilkins, 1989;91–119.
85. March CM, Marrs RP, Goebelsmann U, Mishell DR. Feedback effects of estradiol and progesterone upon gonadotropin and prolactin release. *Obstet Gynecol* 1981;58:10–16.
86. Liu JH, Yen SSC. Induction of midcycle gonadotropin surge by ovarian steroids in women: a critical evaluation. *J Clin Endocrinol Metab* 1983;57:797–802.
87. Jansen RPS. Endocrine consequences of female genital tract neoplasia. In: Shearman RP, ed. *Clinical Reproductive Endocrinology*, Edinburgh: Churchill Livingstone, 1985;697–726.
88. Scully RE. *Tumors of the ovary and maldeveloped gonads*, Fasicle 16. Washington, DC: Armed Forces Institute of Pathology, 1979.
89. Silverberg E. *Statistical and epidemiological information on gynecological cancer*. New York: American Cancer Society, 1986.
90. Fathalla MF. Factors in the causation and incidence of ovarian cancer. *Obstet Gynecol Surv* 1972;27:751–768.
91. Cramer D, Welch W. Determinants of ovarian cancer risk. II. Inferences regarding pathogenesis. *Journ Natl Cancer Inst* 1983;71:717–721.
92. Slotman B, Rao B. Ovarian carcinoma (review). *Anticancer Res* 1988;8:417–434.
93. Gondos B. Surface epithelium of the developing ovary. *Am J Pathol* 1975;81:303–320.
94. LaVecchia C, Liberati, Franceschi S. Noncontraceptive estrogen use and the occurrence of ovarian cancer. *JNCI* 1982;69:1207.
95. Weiss NS, Lyon JL, Krishnamurthy S, Dietert SE, Liff JM, Daling JR. Noncontraceptive estrogen use and the occurrence of ovarian cancer. *JCNI* 1982;68:95–98.
96. Cramer DW, Welch WR, Scully RE, Wojciechowski CA. *Cancer* 1982;52:372–376.
97. Cramer DW. Epidemiologic aspects of early menopause and ovarian cancer. *Ann NY Acad Sci* 1990;592:363–375.
98. Armstrong B, Doll R. Environmental factors and cancer incidence and mortality in different countries with special reference to dietary factors. *Int J Cancer* 1975;15:617–631.
99. Showdon DA. Diet and ovarian cancer. *JAMA* 1985;254:356–357.
100. Humphries AL Jr, Shephard MH, Peters HJ. Peutz-Jeghers syndrome with colonic adenocarcinoma and ovarian tumor. *JAMA* 1966;197:296–298.
101. Berlin NI, YanScott EJ, Clendenning WE, et al. Basal cell nevus syndrome. Combined clinical staff conference at the National Institute of Health. *Ann Intern Med* 1966;64:403–411.
102. Cramer DW, Hutchison GB, Welsch WR, Scully RE, Ryan KJ. Determinants of ovarian cancer risk. 1. Reproductive experiences and family history. *JNCI* 1983;71:711–716.
103. Lee JH, Kavanagh JJ, Wildrick DM, Wharton JT, Blick M. Frequent loss of heterozygosity on chromosomes 6q, 11, and 17 in human ovarian carcinomas. *Cancer Res* 1990;50:2724–2728.
104. Tanaka K, Boice CR, Testa JR. Chromosome aberrations in nine patients with ovarian cancer. *Cancer Genet Cytogenet* 1989;43:1–14.
105. McDonough PG. Cytogenetics in reproductive endocrinology. In: Yen SCC, Jaffe RB, eds. *Reproductive Endocrinology*, 3rd ed. Philadelphia: WB Saunders, 1991;462–479.
106. Butler MG, Dev VG, Phillips JA III. Genetics and cytogenetics.

In: Jones HW III, Wentz AC, Burnett LS, eds. *Novak's Textbook of Gynecology*, 11th ed. Baltimore: Williams & Wilkins, 1988;101–139.
107. Morrow CP, Townsend DE. Tumors of the ovary: sex cord stromal tumors and germ cell tumors. In: Morrow CP, Townsend DE, eds. *Synopsis of Gynecologic Oncology*, 3rd ed. New York: John Wiley & Sons, 1987;305–333.
108. Kurman RJ, Norris HJ. Malignant mixed germ cell tumors of the ovary. A clinical and pathologic analysis of 30 cases. *Obstet Gynecol* 1976;48:579–589.
109. Davy M, Torjesen PA, Aakvaag A. Demonstration of an FSH receptor in a functioning granulosa cell tumor. *Acta Endocrinologica* 1977;85:615–623.
110. Goldston WR, Johnston WW, Fetter BF, Parker RT, Wilbanks GD. Clinicopathologic studies in feminizing tumors of the ovary. I. Some aspects of the pathology and therapy of granulosa cell tumors. *Am J Obstet Gynecol* 1972;112:422–429.
111. Schwartz PE, MacLusky N, Sakamoto H, et al. Steroid-receptor proteins in nonepithelial malignancies of the ovary. *Obstet Gynecol* 1983;15:305–315.
112. Martikainen H, Penttinen J, Huhtaniemi I, et al. Gonadotropin-releasing hormone agonist analog therapy effective in ovarian malignancy. *Gynecol Oncol* 1989;35:406–408.
113. Karten MJ, Rivier JE. Gonadotropin-releasing hormone analog design. Structure-function studies toward the development of agonists and antagonists: Rationale and perspective. *Endocr Rev* 1986;7:44–66.
114. Lee PA. Neuroendocrine maturation. In: Lavery JP, Sanfilippo JS, eds. *Pediatric and adolescent obstetrics and gynecology*. New York: Springer-Verlag, 1985:13.
115. Yen SCC. The human menstrual cycle. In: Yen SSC, Jaffe RB, eds, 2nd edition. *Reproductive endocrinology*. Philadelphia: WB Saunders, 1986:202.

CHAPTER 2

The Histopathology of Malignant Ovarian Tumors

Patricia E. Saigo

The vast array of ovarian neoplasms makes a discussion of each type overwhelming. This chapter will focus on the malignant tumors, with inclusion of benign conditions and tumors when pertinent. The most common type of malignant tumors are epithelial, accounting for 90% of the malignant tumors of the ovary (1). Others, including sex cord-stromal tumors, germ cell tumors, and tumors of uncertain histogenesis, comprise a smaller but important group of malignant tumors.

PRIMARY CARCINOMAS OF THE OVARY

The carcinomas of the ovary are thought to originate from the cells of the surface epithelium, which is embryologically related to the coelomic epithelium from which the lining of the fallopian tubes, the endometrial cavity, and the endocervical canal is derived. In these locations, the epithelium gives rise to tumors with a particular histologic pattern predominant in that site but not exclusive to it. In the ovary, if the carcinomas are derived from the surface epithelium, there must be a mechanism for that epithelium to enter the cortical stroma because most of the carcinomas arise within the substance of the ovary rather than from its surface. The theoretical model suggests that the surface epithelium invaginates into the cortical stroma, eventually detaching itself from the surface and forming cortical cysts. The carcinomas that arise in the ovary are similar histologically to those originating in the endometrium, uterine cervix, and proximal vagina. Distinguishing the tissue of origin may be difficult, if not impossible, in cases of extensive disease involving several organs from which such a tumor may have derived. Occasionally, there are histologically similar tumors which arise simultaneously in two organs, such as in the uterus and the ovary. Criteria for the determination of simultaneous primary tumors is subjective, based on the degree of invasion as an indicator of the metastatic potential of the tumor in each location.

The four most common histologic subtypes are serous, mucinous, endometrioid, and clear cell carcinoma. Of these, the most common type of carcinoma of the ovary is serous as compared to the 10% of endometrial carcinomas with a similar histologic pattern (2). Simultaneous serous carcinomas of the ovary and endometrium are rare. Mucinous carcinomas account for 6% to 16% of ovarian carcinomas, while this histologic type is found in nearly half of endocervical carcinomas (3). Endometrioid carcinomas of the ovary constitute about a fourth of primary carcinomas; this is the predominant pattern in the endometrium. Clear cell carcinoma constitutes as much as 11% of primary ovarian carcinomas and is the predominant type in the vagina. All of the ovarian tumors can have more than one histologic pattern. Most of the tumors are classified according to the predominant type and are graded according to the degree of differentiation in the primary tumor in the ovary. The most differentiated tumors, deviating little from their benign counterpart, are the carcinomas of low malignant potential (LMP) or borderline tumors. All other carcinomas are graded on the degree of differentiation: well-differentiated or grade 1, moderately differentiated or grade 2, and poorly differentiated or grade 3 carcinomas.

Serous Carcinomas

The most common epithelial carcinoma is serous, accounting for about 40% of the malignant epithelial

---

P. E. Saigo: Department of Gynecology, Memorial Sloan-Kettering Cancer Center, New York, New York 10021

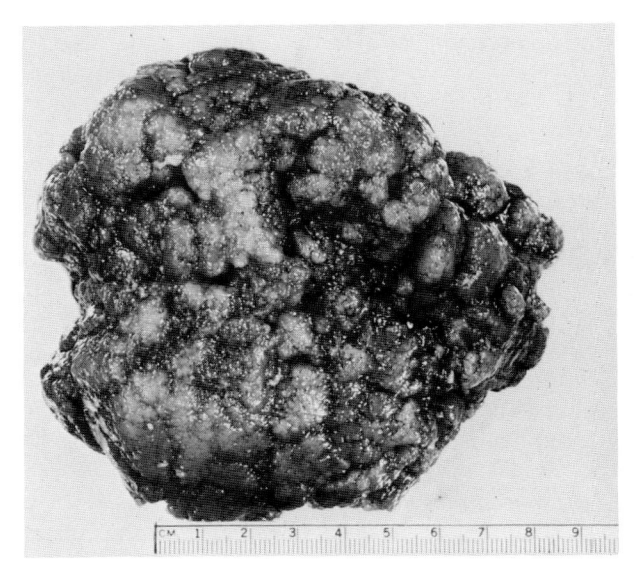

FIG. 1. The lining of the cysts of this papillary serous carcinoma of low malignant potential is covered with papillary excrescences.

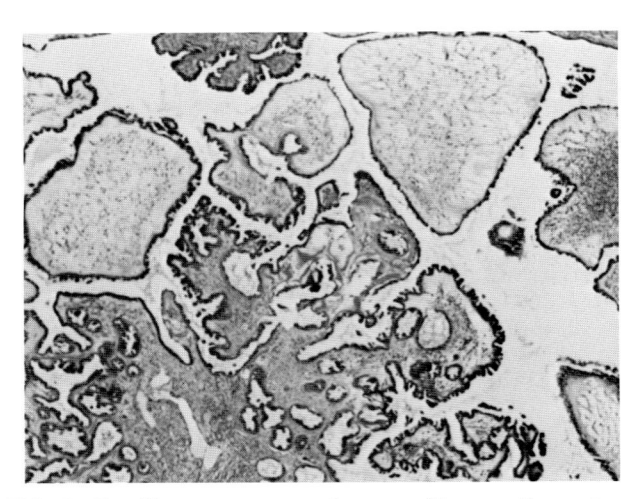

FIG. 2. Papillary serous carcinoma of low malignant potential is characterized by proliferation of the epithelium covering fibrovascular cores (H&E, ×100).

tumors, occurring most frequently in the 40- to 60-year age group (4). About half of them involve the ovaries bilaterally.

Gross examination. These tumors are frequently multicystic with papillary projections partially or entirely lining the cystic spaces (Fig. 1). The fluid may be straw-colored, clear, and thin, blood-stained, or viscid. The latter may be misconstrued as mucin. In large tumors, areas of necrosis are present as yellow or dark red-brown, soft, semisolid areas in otherwise tan or white firm tumor tissue. The external surface of the ovary is smooth unless the tumor has grown through the capsule or the tumor is adherent to adjacent organs. Over half of the tumors have been reported to be larger than 15 cm (5).

Histologic examination. The cytology of these tumors is characterized by small cuboidal cells with eosinophilic cytoplasm. These cells form multiple layers as they cover the fibrovascular cores of the papillae. As the tumors become less differentiated, the cells become larger and more anaplastic, often forming giant tumor cells; the papillary growth pattern is obliterated by areas of tumor present in solid sheets.

Serous Carcinomas of LMP

The most common type of carcinoma of LMP is serous carcinoma of LMP. This type accounts for as much as 82% of all carcinomas of LMP and 15% of serous tumors (6,7). A third to nearly two-thirds of serous carcinomas of LMP are limited to one ovary (7).

Microscopic examination. The tumors are characterized by proliferating small cuboidal cells with little pleomorphism, scant eosinophilic cytoplasm, and oval nuclei containing small, inconspicuous nucleoli covering fibrotic, often edematous papillations (Fig. 2). Mitotic figures are rare. The cell layers may create a thickened covering and small groups of tumor cells may become detached from the surface and lie free in the cystic space (Fig. 3). Some cells may be larger with more abundant eosinophilic cytoplasm. When these cells detach, they resemble those of the mesothelium, a feature that may confound the evaluation of ascitic fluid or pelvic washings.

Differentiating these tumors from a grade I serous carcinoma requires the identification of areas of invasion. When invasion is noted either by the presence of eosinophilic glands (Fig. 4) or papillations invading the stroma, the tumor is no longer classified as LMP.

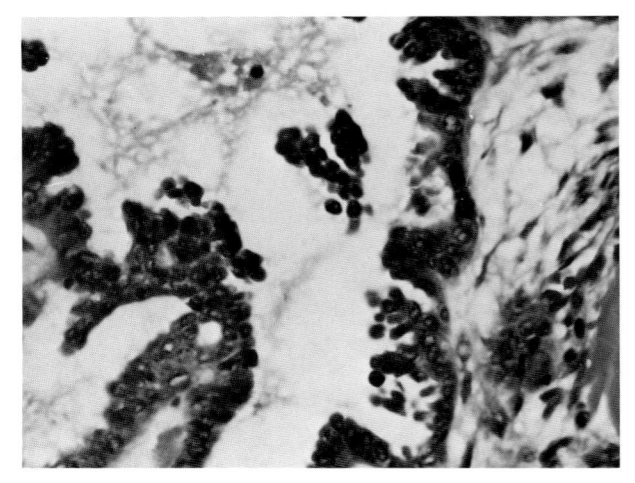

FIG. 3. The epithelial cells are small, cuboidal and uniform. Some of the proliferating epithelial clusters become detached from the surface (H&E, ×400).

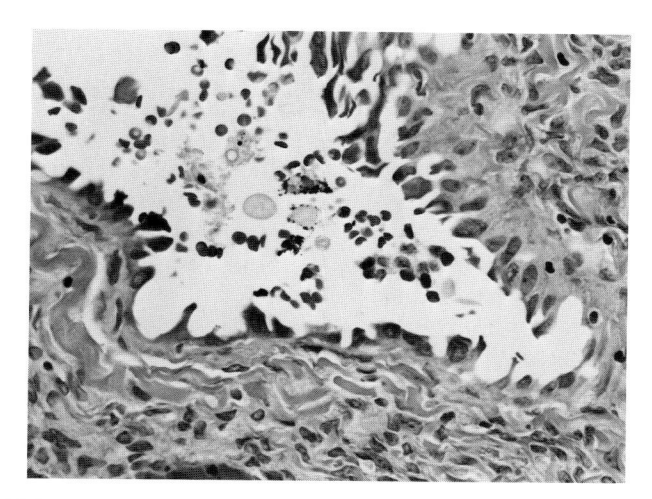

FIG. 4. This area of invasion shows eosinophilic cells infiltrating into the desmoplastic stroma (H&E, ×400).

There are occasions when discrimination between invasion and invagination of the papillary fronds is difficult, if not impossible. In general, the presence of papillary tumor within a space lined by the same type of uniform cuboidal cells suggests invagination as compared to the presence of papillary tumor in a stromal space without such a lining (Fig. 5).

As nearly half of these patients will have extraovarian intraperitoneal spread, attempts have been made to identify histologic predictors of prognosis. Among these have been the separation of invasive from noninvasive implants. The descriptions of the differences between the two are often vague. Noninvasive implants are those without any destruction of the surrounding tissue, although there may be an associated desmoplasia (8). Invasive implants are those that destroy the tissues with irregularly spaced glands invading the desmoplastic stroma (8). Some investigators have found no prognostic differences between the two types (9), while others have found that those with invasive implants are more likely to succumb to their disease (8).

Although the disease tends to remain within the peritoneum, it can metastasize to more distant sites (6). Because the number of patients dying of this disease is small and because there were a number of other variables involved (cytologic atypia, mitoses, residual disease), the authors advise caution. Currently, consistency in separating the two types has not yet been established and the problem is made more difficult as both types may be found in a given patient. Data from more studies must be collected before a conclusion as to the import of these findings can be established.

Differential diagnosis. Benign serous tumors rarely have the extent of epithelial proliferation that characterize the LMP carcinomas. Occasionally a benign serous cystadenoma may have many papillations, but the epithelial covering is a single layer of cuboidal cells. Serous cystadenofibromas may have many more infoldings of the epithelium, but the single layer of uniform cells indicates a benign tumor. Serous carcinomas of LMP have, however, been found in association with cystadenofibromas in which they have the same histologic appearance as those without this association, e.g., proliferation of the epithelium on edematous fibrovascular cores.

DNA analysis. Because these tumors are so well differentiated and because they have a generally indolent course, it would be beneficial to have objective means of discriminating these tumors and to have an indicator of favorable and unfavorable prognoses. The presumption is that those with unfavorable characteristics would be treated with chemotherapy. To this end, there has been investigation into DNA analysis by flow cytometry. To date the number of cases examined by this technique has been limited. Most of the tumors have been diploid or tetraploid (10,11). Although there are few tumors which are aneuploid, this finding does not appear to adversely affect prognosis (13). It has also been noted that differentiating the carcinomas from normal ovaries or from cystadenomas by this technique is possible by evaluating the proliferating fraction or the S-phase fraction, but that the separation of carcinomas of LMP from frank carcinomas is not feasible (13). The potential of this technique to aid in prognosis is currently tentative and is yet to be extensively explored.

Other techniques. Attempts to discriminate the serous carcinomas of LMP by methods other than subjective evaluation have employed nuclear analysis. In one study, analysis of the nuclear area, nuclear perimeter, and the nucleolar organizer region discriminated between these tumors (12). Other investigators have used counts of the nucleolar organizer regions to discrimi-

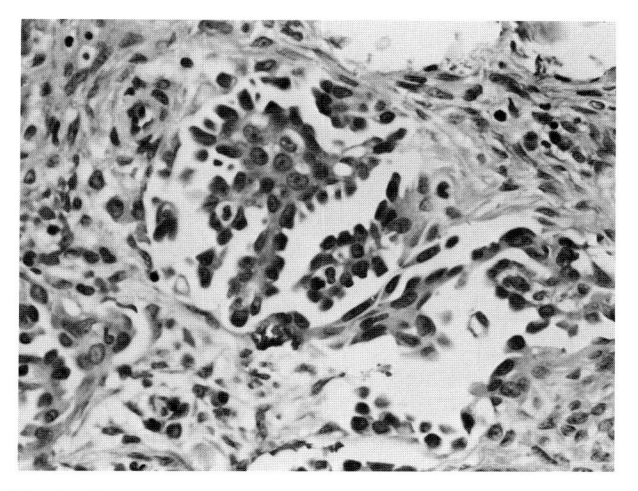

FIG. 5. These papillary clusters have invaded into the stroma (H&E, ×400).

nate between cystadenomas, carcinomas of LMP, and carcinomas. One study found this method effective in identifying carcinomas of LMP (92%), but one was classified as a cystadenoma and another as a well-differentiated carcinoma (13). They found that this method could distinguish among these three entities as a group, but could not always differentiate a carcinoma of low malignant potential from a well-differentiated adenocarcinoma and could not predict prognosis (13).

Other investigative techniques have combined these modalities with others. In studying diploid serous tumors by flow cytometry and the gene product of the *ras* oncogene p21, one group found that normal ovary and cystadenoma could be distinguished from carcinoma of LMP and frank carcinoma, but that separation within the latter group was not possible (14).

Serous Carcinomas

These histologically malignant tumors are graded according to the degree of differentiation. In these papillary tumors, the well-differentiated carcinomas contain many papillae covered by uniform, eosinophilic tumor cells with oval nuclei containing small, prominent nucleoli (Fig. 6). The nuclear abnormalities are much more pronounced than in the carcinomas of LMP, and the tumor invades the stroma. Mitoses are more numerous. The fibrovascular cores are thinner and rarely edematous. As the tumor becomes less differentiated, the spaces between papillations decreases; in the poorly differentiated carcinomas the papillations are very close together, nearly devoid of any space, or the tumor grows as a solid sheet. With the loss of architectural differentiation, the cytology becomes more anaplastic with the appearance of tumor giant cells, marked cytologic and nuclear pleomorphism, and an increase in mitoses.

DNA analysis. Attempts to identify prognostic features by DNA analysis have been employed with serous carcinomas (10,11,12,15). Such analyses have not been successful in predicting outcome, particularly in advanced disease, but may be useful in those with limited disease (stages I and II) (15). Another study of analysis of tumor cells in ascites found longer survival in those with diploid tumors (15 months) as compared to those with aneuploid tumors (6 months) (16).

Other techniques. Flow cytometry combined with the protein product of *ras* oncogene p21, was not predictive of stage (14). In a study of *neu* protein over expression, those with histologic grade III tumors which were strongly positive had a shorter disease-free interval than those with weakly staining tumors or negative ones, although the findings did not reach statistical significance (17). This study also found that carcinomas of LMP were more likely to be negative for *neu*, as were mesodermal mixed tumors. One case of a benign tumor reacted strongly.

Mucinous Carcinomas

Mucinous carcinomas constitute about 6% to 16% of the primary carcinomas of the ovary (4). The age groups most commonly affected are in the 30- to 50-year category. These tumors are characterized by tall columnar cells (similar to endocervical type cells) which secrete mucus. Another type of cell is the intestinal type of mucinous cell which includes goblet cells.

Gross examination. These tumors are often multiloculate cystic tumors. From the gross appearance, it is difficult, if not impossible, to predict the degree of histologic abnormality. There may be visible excrescences lining the cyst wall. Tumor involving the surface is uncommon. The fluid contained within the loculi is very thick and viscid.

Mucinous Carcinomas of LMP

The most common type of gross appearance of the mucinous carcinomas of LMP is a multiloculated cystic tumor (Fig. 7). About 8% are bilateral (18). In the series reported by Hart and Norris, 14% of the stage I mucinous ovarian tumors were carcinomas of LMP and 6% were carcinomas; the remaining 80% were benign cystadenomas (18).

Histologic evaluation. The evaluation and classification of mucinous tumors is more difficult than for serous carcinomas of LMP, for the abnormalities are more subtle. The histologic criteria described by Hart and Norris have been most frequently applied (18). These require presence of stratified layers of cells with

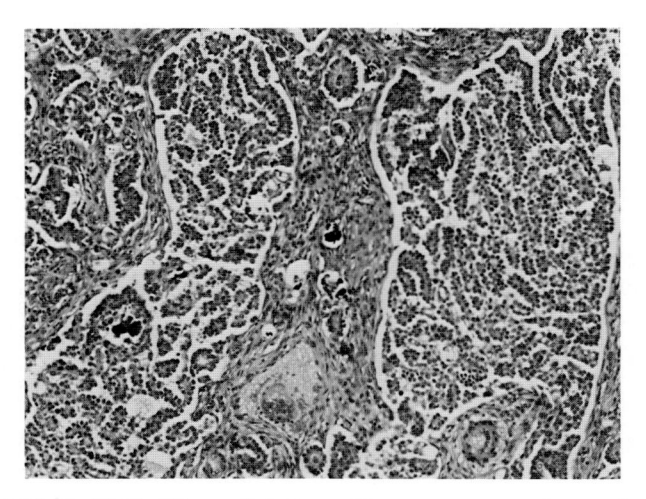

FIG. 6. Well-differentiated papillary serous carcinoma is composed of numerous papillations and psammoma bodies (H&E, ×40).

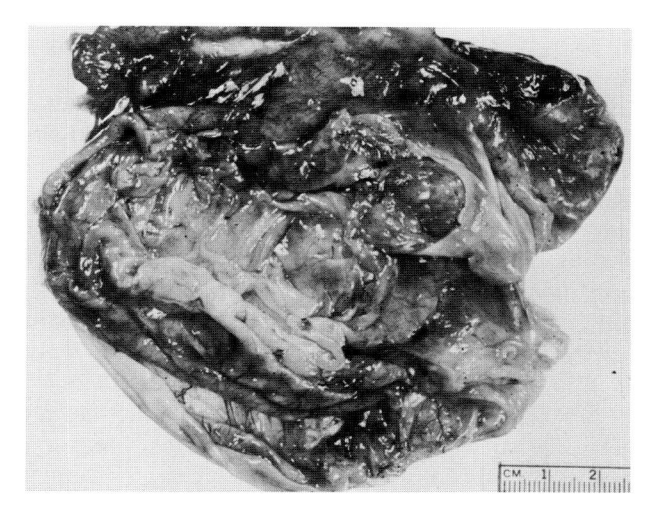

FIG. 7. The lining of this multiloculated mucinous carcinoma of low malignant potential is smooth with occasional areas of thickening.

enlarged, slightly hyperchromatic nuclei and prominent nucleoli not exceeding three layers and no stromal invasion (Fig. 8). A subset of these carcinomas are called *müllerian* are mucinous papillary cystadenomas of borderline malignancy (20). These tumors are found in younger women, average age 34 years, as compared to the intestinal type, average age 52 years. Other differences were that 40% were bilateral synchronously and 30% were associated with endometriosis. Twenty-three percent had extra-ovarian spread, including two with lymph node metastases, but no patient had pseudomyxoma peritonei.

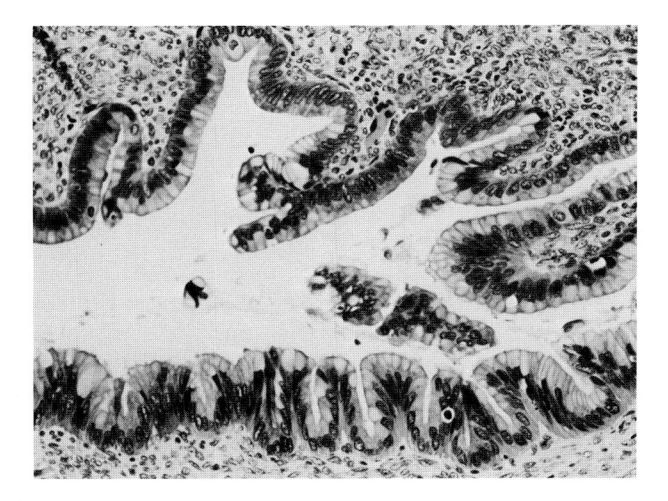

FIG. 8. Mucinous carcinoma of low malignant potential is composed of tall columnar cells showing areas three cell layers thick adjacent to other areas with a single cell layer. The cells have nuclei which are larger than those in a mucinous cystadenoma. Several of the cells are goblet cells indicating that this is the intestinal type of mucinous carcinoma (H&E, ×200).

One group of investigators analyzed 53 tumors graded according to the number of cell layers, nuclear features as compared to the stromal cells, and the mitotic count per ten high power fields (19). They found that the three deaths due to disease were among those whose tumors were grade 4, i.e., they showed evidence of proliferative activity and cytologic atypia. The criteria employed in this study is relatively less subjective and is not based on identifying stromal invasion as the hallmark of a carcinoma, which is often difficult to determine in these well-differentiated tumors.

Mucinous Carcinomas

Microscopic examination. These often well-differentiated tumors are composed of tall columnar, mucin-secreting cells forming stratified layers and complex glands (Fig. 9). Invasion is present when the tumor is present in desmoplastic stroma or the papillations are devoid of intervening stroma. The presence of stromal invasion separates the well-differentiated carcinomas from those of LMP. Well-differentiated carcinomas may not have any identifiable invasion. As the tumor becomes less well-differentiated, the glands invade as smaller, often irregular acini crowded together with little intervening stroma or as single cells. The cells often retain their columnar shape.

The presence of invasion may be clinically relevant. In one study, only two of twelve patients with invasive cancers survived, one with stage Ia and the other with stage IIc disease as compared to those with non-invasive carcinomas, of whom one of fifteen with stage I carcinomas died, as did four of five with stage III tumors (21). In this as well as in another study, tumors with invasion were of a higher stage (21,22).

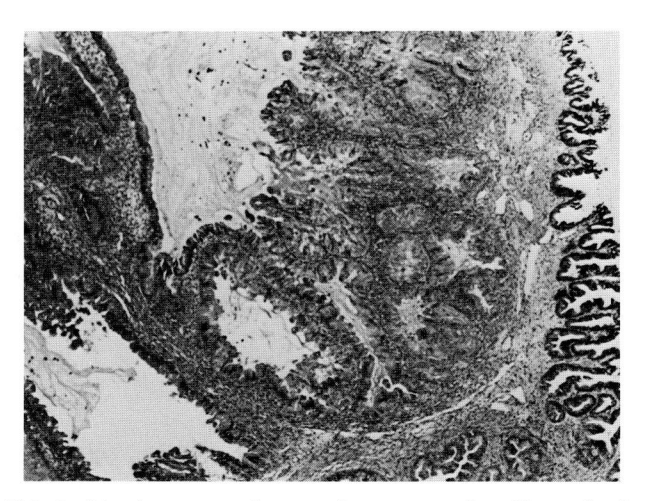

FIG. 9. Mucinous carcinomas have areas lined by a single layer of cells adjacent to others which are frankly malignant (H&E, ×100).

Occasionally, mucinous carcinomas of LMP or which are well-differentiated have areas of anaplastic carcinoma (23,24,25,28) which may resemble sarcomas or sarcoma-like nodules (24,25,26,27,29). The sarcomas have been fibrosarcoma, undifferentiated sarcoma, and rhabdomyosarcoma (26,29). Immunohistochemical studies by two groups have shown that in some cases there is a transition between the carcinomatous and sarcomatous elements; they have also demonstrated that some spindle-cell areas have immunologic patterns of reactivity that are consistent with carcinoma rather than sarcoma (24,25). The presence of anaplastic carcinoma has conferred a poor prognosis to these tumors while this has not been shown for those with sarcomatous areas (23).

A report of Zollinger-Ellison syndrome associated with well-differentiated mucinous adenocarcinoma has been reported (30).

Differential diagnosis. Consideration of a metastasis from a mucinous carcinoma of the gastrointestinal tract or from the pancreas should be entertained. In primary mucinous tumors, there is often a spectrum of histologic patterns, ranging from areas resembling a mucinous adenoma to carcinoma. Metastatic carcinomas, even the well-differentiated ones, are homogeneous. Metastatic carcinomas are more likely to be bilateral.

Pseudomyxoma Peritonei

A complication of mucinous tumors of the ovary as well as from other identified sites (such as the appendix) or unidentified sites is pseudomyxoma peritonei. The abdomen is filled with thick, viscid mucus containing few columnar cells. This complication from ovarian mucinous tumors is small, but may be as high as 17%, and may result from benign as well as malignant mucinous tumors (20,21,31).

The presence of mucinous tumors of the appendix and ovary simultaneously in patients with pseudomyxoma peritonei has been reported (31,32). There has been some debate as to whether these tumors represent independent primaries or metastases from one organ to the other. A cogent argument for origin in the appendix with metastasis to the ovary(ies) has been made by Young et al. (32). Their most salient point is that it would be extraordinarily rare to have simultaneous, histologically similar primary tumors in organs embryologically unrelated. But the issue remains speculative.

Endometrioid Carcinomas

Endometrioid Carcinomas of LMP

These are uncommon tumors which are usually associated with endometrioid adenofibromas. The criteria separating these from those classified as proliferating endometrioid adenofibromas are insufficiently distinct. No consistent criteria and terminology has yet been developed to permit comparison of cases from the several studies in the literature (33,34,35). In the report by Bell and Scully (34), those classified as representing carcinomas of low malignant potential had the histologic features of complex endometrial hyperplasia, while the criteria applied by Snyder et al. requires an area of at least 5 mm of noninvasive, cytologically malignant epithelium to be considered a tumor of LMP (Fig. 10) (35). In the latter series, there was one patient with an extrauterine metastasis who survived 8.9 years free of disease. There have been cases associated with endometriosis which may have been misinterpreted as

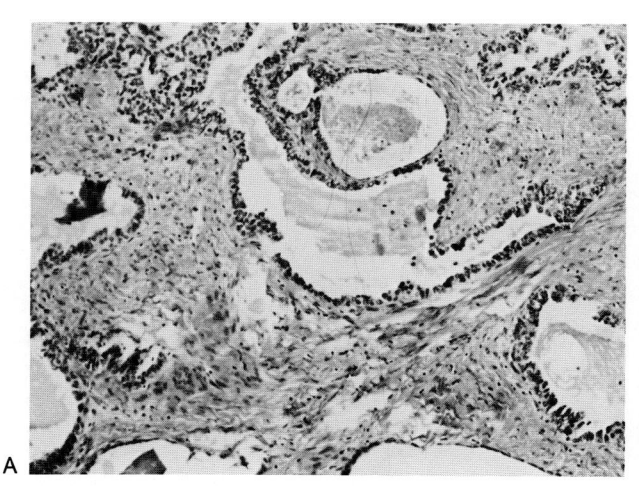

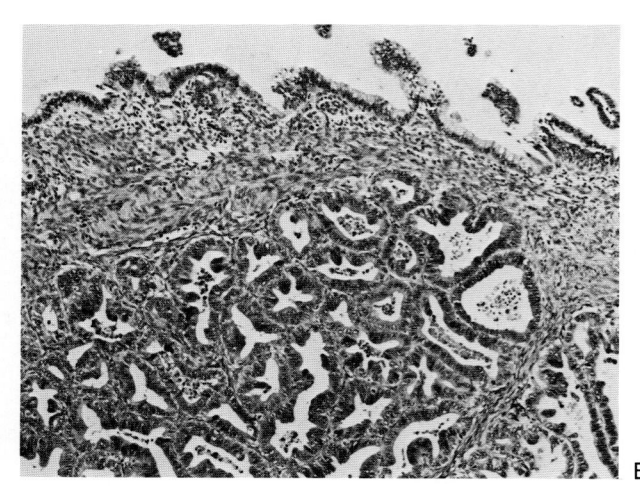

FIG. 10. This endometrioid adenofibroma (a) has areas of endometrioid carcinoma of low malignant potential (b) (H&E, ×100, ×200).

recurrent disease and others with endometrioid carcinoma developing in the contralateral ovary leading to the demise of the patient. Most of the reports of this entity are associated with adenofibromas, except for that of Colgan and Norris (36).

Endometrioid Carcinomas

These tumors comprise about 15% to 25% of the primary carcinomas of the ovary (4). Most patients are in their fifth and sixth decades (4). They may be associated with endometriosis, although the rate of malignant transformation in endometriosis is very low, estimated at less than 2% (37,38).

Gross examination. The gross examination of these tumors reveals a cystic mass, often with areas of hemorrhage (Fig. 11). The solid areas are brown or tan. In some, papillary excrescences are noted in the cystic cavities. About 30% to 50% are bilateral (1,39).

Histologic examination. These tumors resemble the endometrioid type of adenocarcinoma of the endometrium. The cells are columnar with oval, relatively uniform nuclei forming acini (Fig. 12). In the ovary, these tumors are often papillary with thin fibrovascular cores (Fig. 13). There may be secretory changes (Fig. 14). Psammoma bodies may be present. In the less well-differentiated types, the cytologic features may become more anaplastic with scattered tumor giant cells and the histologic pattern assumes a sheet-like arrangement. The acinar, papillary, and sheet-like arrangements may be present in the same tumor.

Squamous differentiation may occur in these tumors. In the well-differentiated tumors, the squamous differentiation often has a bland appearance. When the squamous component resembles that of squamous car-

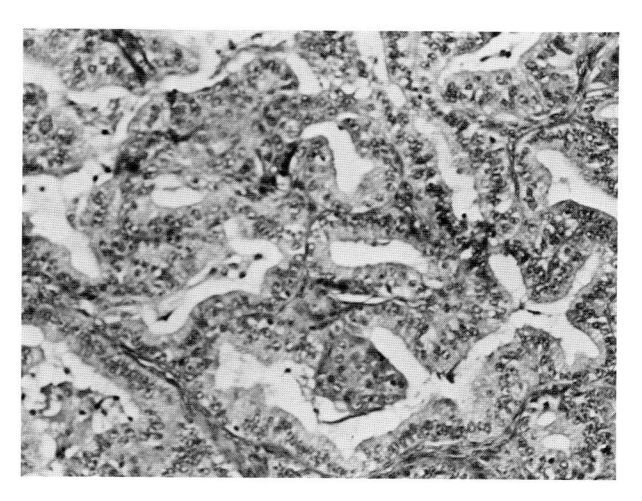

FIG. 12. Well-differentiated endometrioid carcinoma may have areas of squamous metaplasia as noted in the acinus at the bottom of the field (H&E, ×400).

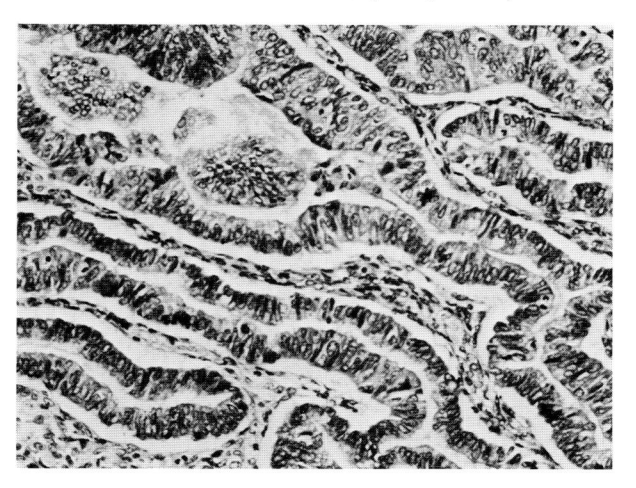

FIG. 13. Another pattern of endometrioid carcinoma is papillary with thin fibrous cores (H&E, ×200).

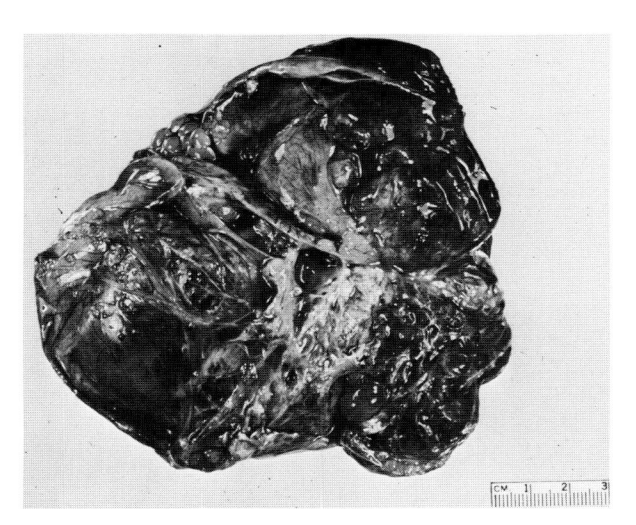

FIG. 11. Endometrioid carcinoma is often cystic with solid areas which may be necrotic.

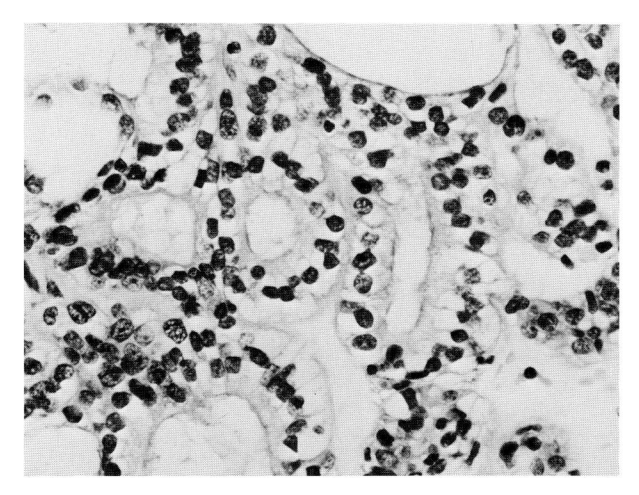

FIG. 14. Endometrioid carcinoma may show secretory changes with subnuclear vacuoles (H&E, ×400).

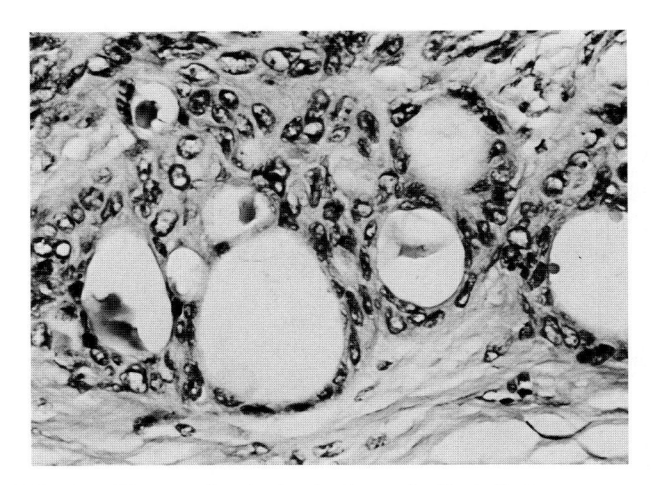

FIG. 15. The small tubules in the spindle cell stroma suggest sex cord-stromal tumors. Mucin stain showed apical and intracytoplasmic mucin (H&E, ×400).

cinoma, the tumor is classified as an adenosquamous carcinoma.

A peculiar histologic presentation is one that resembles sex cord-stromal tumors of the ovary (Fig. 15) (40,41). This is an uncommon histologic finding which requires the use of special studies such as a mucin stain to demonstrate mucin in these cells. Sampling the tumor generously may reveal areas of conventional endometrioid carcinoma or areas of squamous metaplasia and thus confirm the diagnosis of an endometrioid carcinoma.

Differential diagnosis. The most common mimicker of endometrioid carcinoma is metastatic colorectal carcinoma. The presence of squamous differentiation or spindly cell areas supports the diagnosis of an endometrioid carcinoma. The presence of extremely elongated nuclei and nuclei with very coarse chromatin suggests metastatic colorectal carcinoma. While both tumors, especially when they achieve large size, may have necrosis, colorectal carcinomas are more likely to have necrosis in the lumina of acini, even when the tumor is small.

In about 14% to 50% of endometrioid carcinomas, a concomitant endometrial adenocarcinoma will be present (39,42). It is sometimes difficult to determine whether these represent independent primary carcinomas or whether the ovarian tumors are metastases. If the endometrial carcinoma is limited to the endometrium or if the myometrial infiltration is superficial and limited in extent, it is likely that the ovarian carcinomas are independent, simultaneous primary carcinomas. The ovarian and endometrial carcinomas are often similar in grade and histologic pattern. When there is extensive involvement of many structures, it may not be possible to determine the origin of the disease.

Mesodermal Mixed Tumors of the Ovary

An unusual form of ovarian carcinoma is mesodermal mixed tumor (MMT). These tumors are composed of a mixture of malignant epithelial and sarcomatous elements. When the sarcomatous components are those of stroma or smooth muscle, these tumors have been classified as homologous or carcinosarcoma. When the sarcomatous elements are other types, such as rhabdomyosarcoma or osteosarcoma, these tumors have been classified as heterologous. A recent report noted the presence of immature neural elements similar to those found in immature teratoma (43).

Most of the women are postmenopausal (44,45,46). A few have been associated with endometriosis and with synchronous endometrioid carcinoma of the contralateral ovary (47).

Gross examination. The tumors may be solid or cystic, especially if there is much necrosis. If there is a significant sarcomatous component, the tissue is grayish and fleshy.

Microscopic examination. The epithelial component is commonly endometrioid, often papillary, although there may be other histologic types like clear cell carcinoma as well. The carcinoma is well-demarcated from the underlying sarcoma (Fig. 16), which differentiates this from a poorly differentiated carcinoma in which the clearly identifiable carcinoma merges imperceptibly with the solidly growing carcinoma. The heterologous sarcomatous elements are commonly rhabdomyosarcoma (Fig. 17) or chondrosarcoma (Fig. 18).

Adenosarcoma

A more unusual form of mesodermal mixed tumor is adenosarcoma. In this tumor, the epithelial component

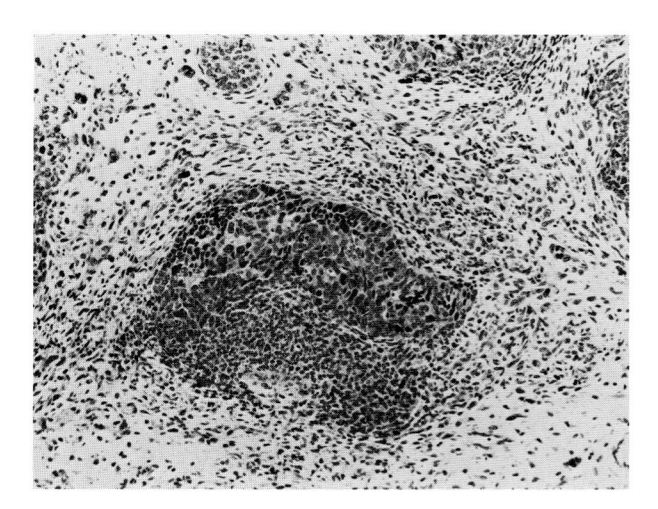

FIG. 16. The epithelial component of mesodermal mixed tumor is well-demarcated from the surrounding sarcomatous component (H&E, ×100).

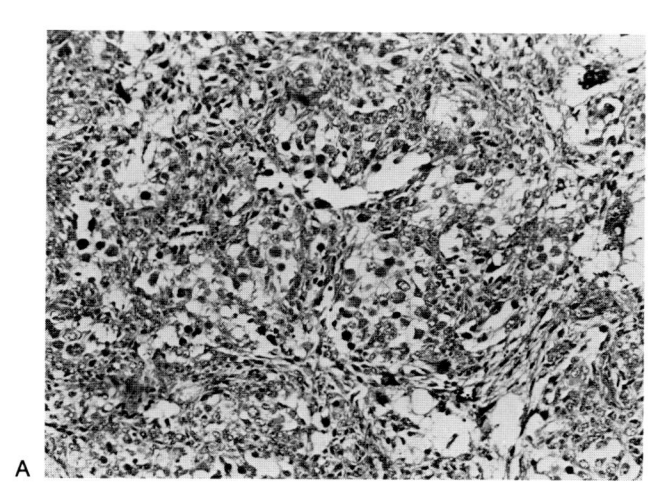

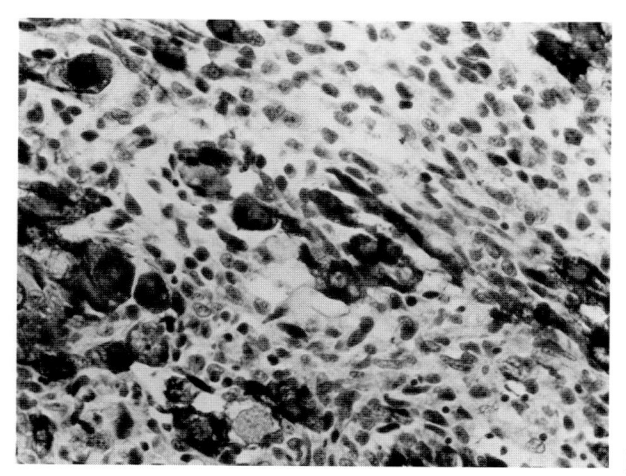

FIG. 17. Rhabdomyosarcoma, a frequent component of mesodermal mixed tumors, is represented here. A: as rhabdomyoblasts and as elongated cells (H&E, ×100). The tumor cells display a strong reaction for muscle common actin. B: Diaminobenzedine, ×250.

is benign while the sarcomatous component resembles a low-grade stromal sarcoma (48,49).

Clear Cell Carcinomas

Clear Cell Carcinomas of LMP

These are very rare tumors which are adenofibromatous (50,51). In general, the few published series have reported excellent prognoses, except for one case in which pulmonary metastases were evident four years after diagnosis (51). Extensive sampling of the tumor is in order before the diagnosis of clear cell carcinoma of LMP is made to exclude the possibility of an obvious area of clear cell carcinoma.

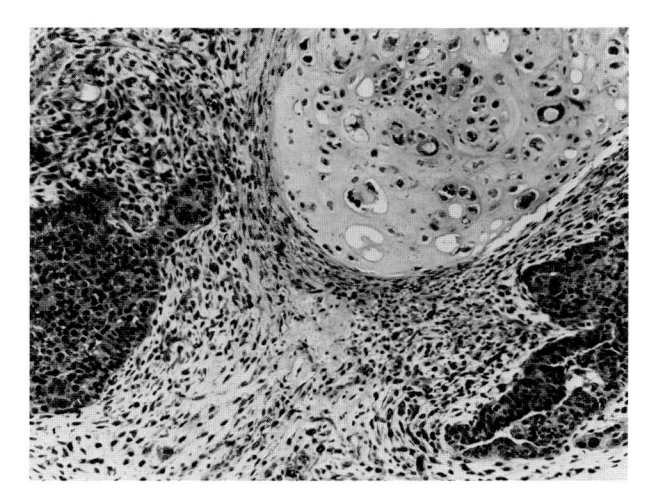

FIG. 18. Chondrosarcoma, undifferentiated sarcoma, and poorly differentiated carcinoma are noted in this field (H&E, ×100).

Clear Cell Carcinomas

Clear cell carcinoma is a malignant tumor that is derived from the müllerian epithelium. This premise is strengthened by the association of this carcinoma with endometriosis in 8% to 53% of cases, a finding more likely with this histologic type than with the other carcinomas (52,53).

Clear cell carcinoma is found in 5% to 11% of primary ovarian carcinomas. The age range is from 40 to 78 years with a mean age of 54 years (52,53).

Gross examination. The tumors are often cystic with areas of necrosis. The solid portions are yellow, cream, or hemorrhagic. As many as half the cases are bilateral (53).

Microscopic examination. There are three microscopic patterns: papillary, acinar, and solid. A tumor may have one or more patterns. The cells are cuboidal with either clear (Fig. 19) or eosinophilic granular cytoplasm (54). The distinctive nuclei are hyperchromatic, round or oval with prominent nucleoli. In some acinar tumors, the central space may be filled with eosinophilic material that resembles colloid (Fig. 20). The cells at the periphery become attenuated and flattened, sometimes barely perceptible. Many of these tumors will have hyalinized, eosinophilic stroma. This stromal change is rarely observed in any of the other carcinomas. Another interesting finding is the presence of PAS-positive globules of eosinophilic material associated with the tumor cells. These mimic similar structures noted in endodermal sinus tumors. In the former, immunohistochemical stain for alpha fetoprotein (AFP) is negative, while it is positive in the latter.

Differential diagnosis. The one tumor that resembles this best is endodermal sinus tumor. As this germ cell tumor is found in patients much younger than those

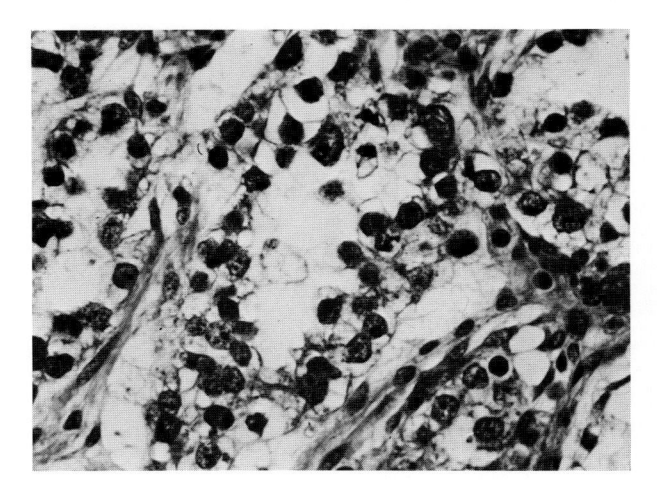

FIG. 19. The acini are formed by cells with clear cytoplasm and nuclei with prominent nucleoli (H&E, ×400).

with clear cell carcinoma, the problem is rarely encountered. Resolution is possible using stains for AFP.

Brenner Tumors

Brenner tumors are common, accounting for 2% to 3% of ovarian neoplasms (55,56,57,58,59,60,61). They are present as incidental findings in ovaries removed for other reasons. The tumor is often unilateral, although as many as 10% have been bilateral (62,63). Most of the tumors are benign, although it has been reported that 5% of those which are palpable are more likely to be proliferative or malignant (56).

Gross examination. The tumor is nodular, firm, and gray-white. The sizes range from microscopic to 8 cm in diameter. About 10% to 25% are present as nodules in the wall of the mucinous cystadenomas (62).

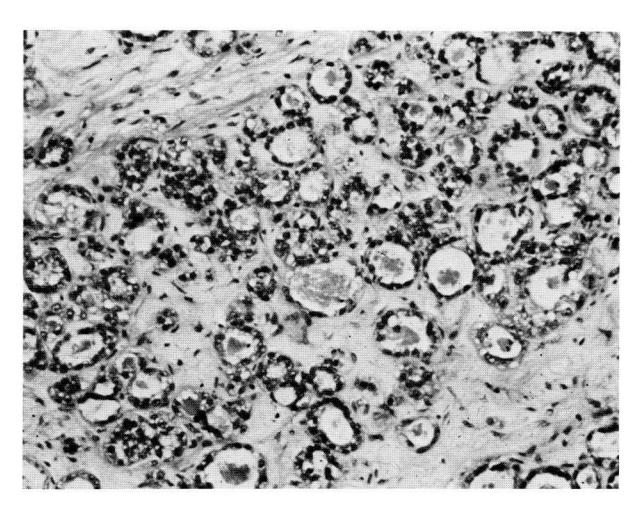

FIG. 20. The round acini lying in hyalinized stroma contain eosinophilic material and mimic thyroid follicles (H&E, ×100).

Microscopic examination. These tumors are composed of two types of cells. The epithelial cells, which resemble urothelial cells, are polygonal with abundant, clear or pale pink cytoplasm and oval nuclei with a longitudinal groove, the "coffee bean" nuclei. The central areas may be cystic, and the cells surrounding the space may be flat to tall columnar, mucinous cells. Mucin may be present in the central cystic space or in the lumen. The stroma in which these nests are embedded is collagenous with spindly cells.

Proliferating or Borderline Brenner Tumors

Grossly, these are more likely to be palpable and to be cystic than other Brenner tumors. Histologically, the cells covering the projecting fronds resemble those of a transitional cell carcinoma, grade I. No stromal invasion is identified. Areas of typical Brenner tumor will be found adjacent to these proliferating or borderline areas (55,56,57,58,59).

Malignant Brenner Tumors

To qualify as a malignant Brenner tumor, the tumor should resemble a high-grade transitional cell carcinoma and have identifiable Brenner tumor in adjacent areas (60,61,64,65). If the latter is missing, the tumor is better classified as a transitional cell carcinoma of the ovary (61,66).

Transitional Cell Carcinomas

These are tumors that resemble transitional cell carcinoma of the urinary bladder; they are unaccompanied by Brenner tumor. This type of carcinoma may comprise the entire tumor or a part of it. Classification is of importance, for patients whose tumors and their metastases were composed of this histologic type had a more favorable prognosis than the cohort that had this as a minor component (66).

Undifferentiated Carcinomas

These are primary carcinomas of the ovaries which have no evidence of differentiation. They are often bilateral, solid masses composed of pleomorphic cells, including tumor giant cells.

SEX CORD-STROMAL TUMORS

The group of sex cord-stromal tumors accounts for 6% of the ovarian neoplasms and are the most common of those which are clinically functional (67). However, the most common among these, the fibroma, is endocrinologically inactive.

Granulosa Cell Tumors

Granulosa cell tumors comprise 15% of all ovarian neoplasms (68) and 6% of all ovarian malignant tumors (69). Of those which are hormonally active, three-fourths are estrogenic and the remainder androgenic (70,71,74). The latter are often cystic.

These tumors are most common among postmenopausal women and less than 5% are found in prepubertal girls, most of whom present with isosexual pseudoprecocity.

The patients present with endocrinologic symptoms or with an abdominal mass or swelling. Rupture with hemoperitoneum has been reported in about ten percent (72,74). About 10% of the tumors have been found during surgery for abnormal uterine bleeding (73).

Gross examination. These tumors are most commonly unilateral solid or cystic masses averaging 12.5 cm in diameter (73,74).

Microscopic examination. Areas composed of granulosa cells and those of theca cells are often combined in varying proportions. There may also be areas of stromal luteinization. The granulosa cells are small and uniform with significant pleomorphism found in no more than 2% (75). The round or oval nuclei are commonly grooved (Fig. 21). These cells are arranged in four major patterns: follicular with microcysts and/or macrocysts (Fig. 22), insular with groups of cells, trabecular with cells arranged in linear cords (Fig. 23), and diffuse with no particular arrangement.

A distinctive type of granulosa cell tumor occurring in the first two decades of life is the juvenile granulosa cell tumor. Over 80% present with isosexual pseudoprecocity (76). Most of the tumors are unilateral; less than three percent are bilateral (76). Another unusual feature is an association with Ollier's disease and Maffucci's syndrome (76). In one series of 125 patients, eight patients had these or other soft tissue tumors.

These tumors are histologically very unique. They are composed of large cells in sheets or nodular aggregates with theca cells interspersed. There may be areas of recognizable adult type granulosa cell tumor, but the cytology of these is one of marked cellular pleomorphism in which the tumor cells have round nuclei, abundant cytoplasm, and many mitoses (Fig. 24). Because of the pleomorphism, the high mitotic rate, and the solid growth pattern, recognition of this histologic pattern as a granulosa cell tumor may not be readily evident. In some areas, however, there will be the mi-

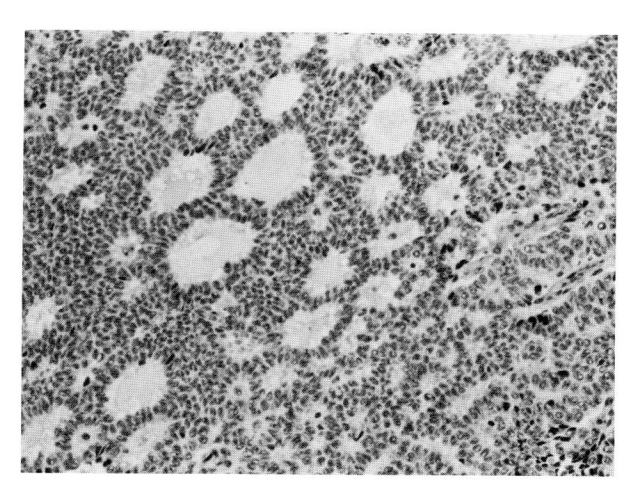

FIG. 22. The microfollicular pattern recapitulates the appearance of developing follicles (H&E, ×100).

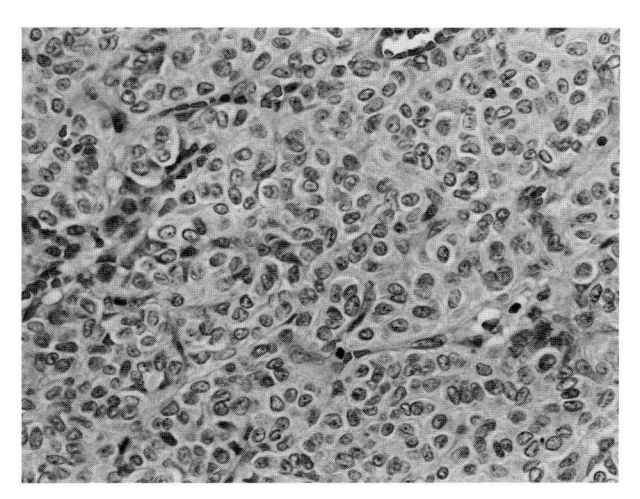

FIG. 21. Nuclear grooves are present in many of the cells in this granulosa cell tumor, which has a diffuse pattern (H&E, ×600).

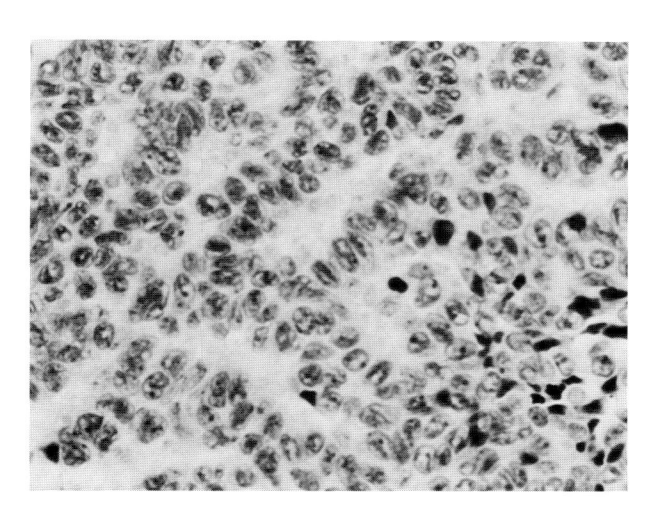

FIG. 23. Some of the granulosa cells forming the linear arrangement have nuclear grooves (H&E, ×600).

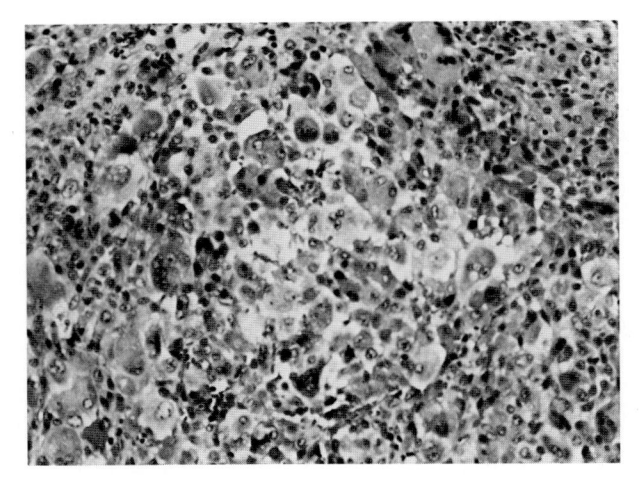

FIG. 24. Very anaplastic, pleomorphic cells are noted in juvenile granulosa cell tumor (H&E, ×400).

crocystic or microfollicular pattern of the more typical granulosa cell tumor (Fig. 25). Because of their unusual histology and the young age of the patient, they may be misinterpreted as embryonal carcinoma, thecoma, Sertoli-Leydig cell tumor, small cell carcinoma or clear cell carcinoma. The youthful age of the patient and the identification of adult granulosa cells are helpful in the classification of these tumors.

Thecomas/Fibromas

Thecomas

These tumors comprise 0.5% of ovarian neoplasms. The patients may present with symptoms referable to estrogen production and of these 84% are postmenopausal (81,82,83). Three percent are bilateral (84).

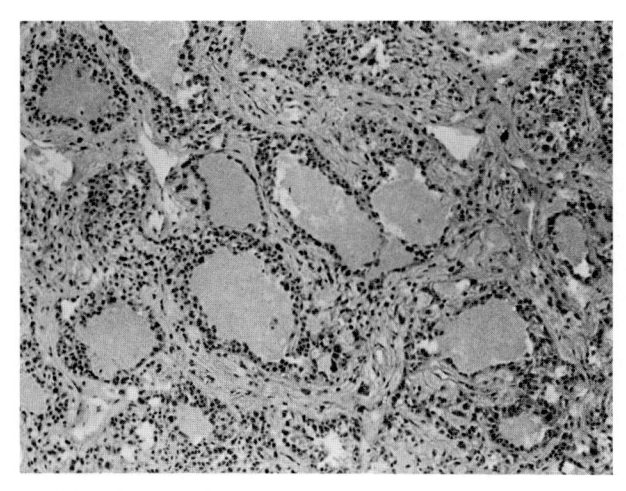

FIG. 25. Macrofollicles in juvenile granulosa cell tumor assist in classification (H&E, ×100).

Gross examination. The tumor forms bright yellow solid tissue. Some tumors with fibrous areas may have gray-white areas. Tumors with prominent luteinization will be more yellow.

Microscopic examination. The tumor is composed of large round cells containing lipid. Demonstration of lipid requires stain for fat performed on fresh tissue. Fibrous tissue, comprising a small component, may be found interspersed among these cells, and hyalinized fibrous plaques may also be present. Rarely, the tumors are calcified. When the tumor is composed of a mixture of thecomatous and fibrous tissue, the tumor is classified as a fibrothecoma.

Luteinized thecomas are found among younger women, about half of whom show symptoms of hyperestrogenism and about 10% androgenic stimulation (85).

Fibromas

These tumors are found in women over the age of 40 years with an average age of 48 years (77). They are unilateral but may be bilateral, particularly in those with basal cell nevus syndrome (78). In tumors larger than 10 cm, 40% are associated with ascites and 1% with Meigs' syndrome (79,80).

Gross examination. These tumors, which average 6 cm, are composed of solid firm white tissue that forms a distinct nodule.

Microscopic examination. Bland spindle cells are storiform patterned with areas of hyalinized collagen between bundles. In some tumors, the hyalinized collagen may form large plaques. Edematous areas may also be present.

Clinically, these tumors are endocrinologically inactive and are benign.

Sertoli Cell and Sertoli-Leydig Cell Tumors

Sertoli Cell Tumors

The average age of patients with Sertoli cell tumors (SCT) is 27 years (86). About two-thirds have symptoms related to estrogen secretion and occasionally to isosexual pseudoprecocity (86,87,88,89). The tumors are unilateral and very rarely malignant.

Gross examination. The tumors average 9 cm and are solid yellow masses.

Microscopic examination. SCT tumors are composed of tubules which may be hollow or solid. The former are lined by columnar or cuboidal cells with slightly eosinophilic cytoplasm. The cells in the latter have cytoplasm rich in lipid.

Sertoli-Leydig Cell Tumors

Sertoli-Leydig cell tumors (SLT) are rare ovarian neoplasms accounting for less than 0.2% of the primary ovarian tumors (90,91,92,93,94). The peak incidence is during the reproductive years and about half of the patients are either hirsute or virilized, or both (93).

Gross examination. These generally unilateral tumors are composed of solid yellow-tan tissue and average 10 cm in diameter. Those which are cystic are associated with heterologous elements or with a retiform component. About two percent are bilateral (93).

Microscopic examination. The Sertoli cell component may show differing degrees of differentiation. When this component is well differentiated, the tumor cells are similar to the Sertoli cell tumors with the formation of hollow or solid tubules. As the tumor becomes less differentiated, these cells become more spindly, resembling the cells of fibrosarcoma. The Sertoli cells are associated with the more polygonal eosinophilic Leydig cells (Fig. 26).

A unique subtype of SLT is that with the retiform pattern, comprising 10% of SLT (95). These tumors have small uniform cells lining slit-like spaces and covering papillae. In other areas, the tubules are lined by the more conventional type of Sertoli cell. While this pattern may be misinterpreted as representing an endodermal sinus tumor or a papillary epithelial tumor, the clinical data, particularly the age of the patient and evidence of virilization, would preclude consideration of these other entities.

About 20% (96,97,98,99) of SLT contain heterologous elements, most commonly intestinal epithelium (Fig. 27) (96,97). Other types of heterologous elements include cartilage and skeletal muscle. A low-grade adenocarcinoma or carcinoid tumor may be present (96,97) (Fig. 28).

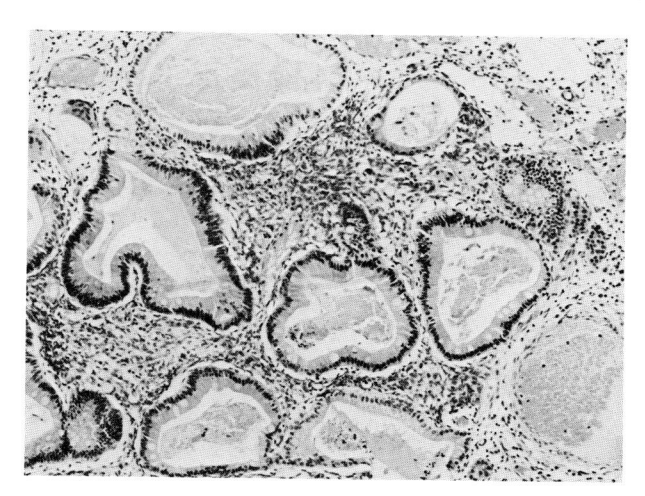

FIG. 27. Heterologous elements in Sertoli-Leydig cell tumors are commonly of gastrointestinal type; note the Sertoli-Leydig cell component in between the intestinal-type glands (H&E, ×100).

Gynandroblastoma

Gynandroblastomas are rare tumors with a mixture of granulosa cell tumor and SLT. To be classified as a gynandroblastoma, the minor component (e.g., granulosa cell tumor) in a predominantly SLT should represent at least 10% of the tumor.

Unclassified Sex Cord-Stromal Tumors

This designation is assigned to those tumors with differentiation intermediate between granulosa cell

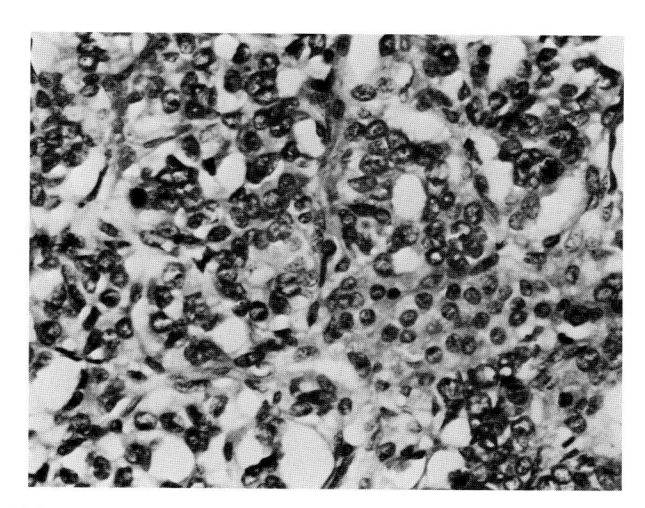

FIG. 26. Moderately differentiated Sertoli-Leydig cell tumor has small tubules whose cells are nuclei located antipodally and a small collection of Leydig cells forming a sheet (H&E, ×400).

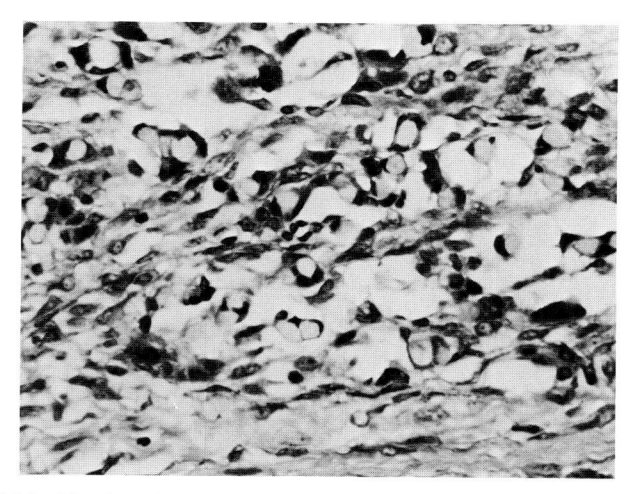

FIG. 28. Carcinoid tumor is also one of the common findings in heterologous tissue (H&E, ×400).

tumor and SLT. The difficulty in identifying a clear separation between these two tumors is particularly evident in tumors of pregnant women (100).

Sex Cord Tumor with Annular Tubules

The two forms of sex-cord tumor with annular tubules (SCTAT) are those in patients without Peutz-Jeghers Syndrome (PJS) and those found in patients with PJS (101,102,103). About 40% are associated with estrogen production (101).

Gross examination. In patients without PJS, the tumors are unilateral and large. In those with PJS, the tumors are usually multiple and are incidental findings (101). Calcification is rare in the former and common in the latter.

Microscopic examination. The tumor is formed of tubules surrounding thick, prominent collections of basement-membrane-like material. The cells forming the tubules have clear, lipid-rich cytoplasm and small, uniform nuclei distributed antipodally. These tumors may be associated with granulosa cell tumors or SCT (88,104). Because of the report of Böttcher's crystals in SCTAT, some have suggested that they represent a form of SLT (104).

GERM CELL TUMORS

Germ cell tumors account for 30% of all ovarian neoplasms, of which most are mature cystic teratomas. Malignant germ cell tumors account for 3% of the malignant ovarian tumors.

Dysgerminomas

About half of the malignant germ cell tumors are dysgerminomas. Eighty percent are found in women under the age of thirty; they are rarely present in girls younger than five years old or in women older than fifty (4). They represent 20% to 30% of the malignant ovarian tumors during pregnancy (4). Most of the tumors are unilateral and confined to the ovary (105,106,108). The patients typically present with signs and symptoms of an abdominal mass. In those tumors associated with gonadoblastoma, there may be signs of gonadal maldevelopment (4).

Gross examination. This solid tumor, ranging in size from 7–25 cm, average 15 cm, (108) is composed of gray-white to pink-tan fleshy tissue. There may be small areas of necrosis or hemorrhage. Eighty percent of the tumors are unilateral; about half of the remainder are bilateral, with gross disease apparent in the contralateral ovary in ten percent of those. In the other half, the tumor is present upon microscopic examination (4).

Microscopic examination. The tumor is composed of uniform cells with clear or eosinophilic cytoplasm and centrally-placed round or oval nuclei containing a prominent or several prominent nucleoli (Fig. 29). The cell borders are distinct. Sheets of tumor cells may be separated by fibrous bands of varying thickness. Infiltrates of lymphocytes may be present, occasionally in large numbers.

Large syncytiotrophoblastic-type cells may be found in 3% of dysgerminomas (107). These cells are immunoreactive for human chorionic gonadotropin (HCG), but the tumor should not be considered a mixed germ cell tumor with choriocarcinoma unless, after extensive sampling, areas of choriocarcinoma with syncytiotrophoblasts and cytotrophoblasts are found.

Differential diagnosis. The tumors that may be considered in the differential diagnosis are large cell lymphoma, clear cell carcinoma, and undifferentiated carcinoma. Large cell lymphomas have nuclei that are lobulated rather than round, and infiltrate rather than forming sheets of cells with distinct cell boundaries. Clear cell carcinoma will have areas of acinar or papillary growth; the surrounding stroma often show hyalinization. Undifferentiated carcinomas may be confused with dysgerminoma, but their cells are often more pleomorphic with nuclei that are eccentric.

DNA analysis. Studies to identify prognostic factors have included DNA analysis. In one study of twenty-three patients, three of whom had bilateral tumors, twenty-one percent were diploid and seventy-nine percent were nondiploid (108). There were no significant differences between these two groups with regard to stage of disease. Of the nondiploid tumors, sixteen

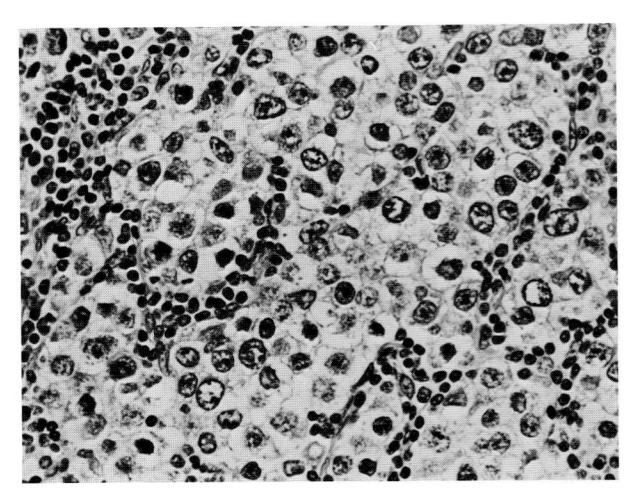

FIG. 29. The cells of dysgerminoma have distinct cell borders and centrally placed nuclei; lymphocytes often accompany the tumor cells (H&E, ×400).

were tetraploid and three aneuploid. Correlation with prognosis showed that one of the five patients, or twenty percent, with diploid tumors progressed as compared to the eight of sixteen tetraploid tumors, or fifty percent, and none of the aneuploid tumors. The one death due to disease in this study was a patient with a tetraploid tumor who had widespread disease at the time of presentation. Of the eight patients with peritoneal cytology, two had tumor cells present. Of these, one had a tetraploid tumor and the other had bilateral tumors (one diploid and one tetraploid); neither of these patients had a relapse. In another study using flow cytometry and computerized image analysis of twenty-five patients with dysgerminoma, the investigators found close correlation between these two techniques (109). In that population, there were no diploid tumors, eleven were tetraploid and fourteen aneuploid. There was no correlation with stage of disease or prognosis. Seven of nineteen patients, or thirty-seven percent with stage Ia1 tumors relapsed and one of these died of disease; the DNA index (DI) for this group was 1.29–3.23, median 1.94. There were no differences between those who did not relapse (DI range 1.29–2.69, median 1.93) and those who did (1.66–3.23, median 2.05). The one patient who died had a DI of 1.83. DNA analysis does not seem to have a role in predicting prognosis.

Endodermal Sinus Tumor (Yolk Sac Tumor)

Twenty percent of the malignant germ cell tumors are endodermal sinus tumors (EST) (4). It is common in girls and young adults, with an average age of 19 years. Rarely does it occur after age 40. Patients present with an abdominal mass and occasionally with the sudden onset of pain (110,111,112,113). Serum levels of AFP are elevated.

Gross examination. These tumors are usually unilateral. About a fourth of them are ruptured (111). The cut surface is composed of cystic and solid areas and in some there may be an associated cystic teratoma.

Microscopic examination. ESTs display a variety of histologic patterns. Among the more common are: the reticular pattern (Fig. 30), the pseudopapillary pattern (Fig. 31) with Schiller-Duval bodies, which is a central fibrous core containing a blood vessel covered by primitive cells lying in a space lined by similar primitive cells (Fig. 32), the polyvesicular vitelline pattern, and the solid pattern (Fig. 33). These histologic patterns may coexist in varying degrees and have no prognostic implication (111). The tumor cells may have abundant clear cytoplasm containing glycogen and in some fields will have the hobnail pattern similar to clear cell carcinomas. Some cells will have intracytoplasmic hyaline droplets containing AFP, and in other areas these hyaline globules will be extracellular (Fig. 34).

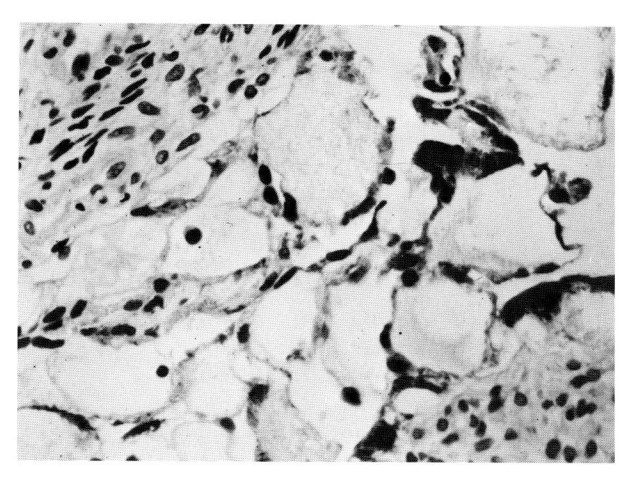

FIG. 30. The reticular pattern is formed by a lacy network; some of the cells have reacted with antibody for alpha fetoprotein characterized by dark cytoplasmic stain (Diaminobenzedine, ×400).

Other unusual patterns include the hepatoid (114,115) and the endometrioid-like patterns (Fig. 35) (116). Enteric-type glands are present in half of these tumors (111,113).

In one large series of seventy-one patients, ten patients had a mature cystic teratoma in the ovary with the endodermal sinus tumor; in two of these and in two other patients, mature teratoma was present in the contralateral ovary (111). Two patients had had benign tumors removed from the contralateral ovaries prior to the endodermal sinus tumor; one was a mature teratoma excised eleven years previously and the other was a mucinous cystadenoma removed six years prior

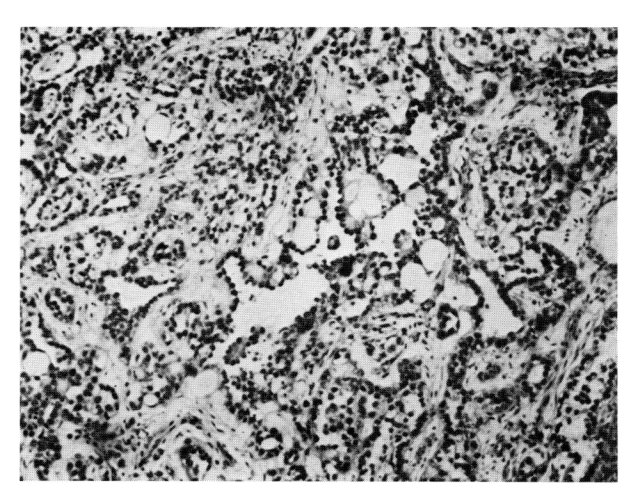

FIG. 31. The pseudopapillary pattern of endodermal sinus tumor can mimic a papillary carcinoma (H&E, ×100).

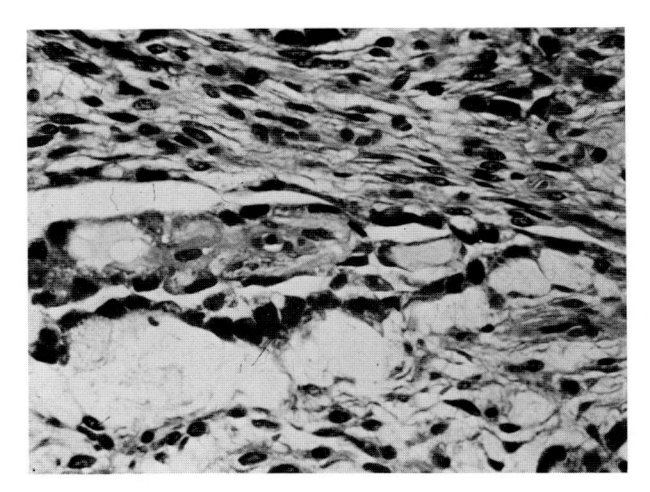

FIG. 32. A Schiller-Duval body lies within a tumor-lined space (H&E, ×400).

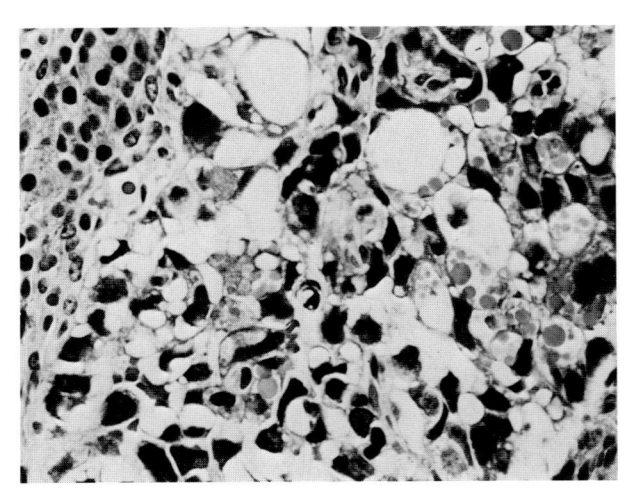

FIG. 34. Bright eosinophilic globules are present intracytoplasmically as well as in the stroma; these will stain for alpha fetoprotein (H&E, ×400).

to this series. Gonadoblastoma was noted microscopically adjacent to the endodermal sinus tumor in one case.

Embryonal Carcinoma

Embryonal carcinoma of the ovary is rare, accounting for 3% of the malignant germ cell tumors (117,118). They occur in children and young adults; the median age is 14 years (117). Half the patients have disorders related to sexual pseudoprecocity, abnormal uterine bleeding, or amenorrhea (117).

Gross examination. The tumors are unilateral, average 17 cm, and are composed of gray-white to yellow-tan tissue. Hemorrhage and necrosis are prominent.

Microscopic examination. The tumor cells have abundant clear or eosinophilic cytoplasm and hyperchromatic, slightly pleomorphic nuclei containing coarse chromatin and prominent nucleoli. They resemble the cells of dysgerminoma, but their nuclear features are more anaplastic (Fig. 36). While they form large sheets, they also form spaces and papillations. Necrosis and hemorrhage are prominent. Syncytiotrophoblastic-type giant cells may be found as well as mature teratoma and enteric glands (117). These tumors may stain for AFP.

Teratomas

Teratomas are the most common germ cell tumor of the ovary. They can be subclassified into mature teratoma, monodermal teratoma, and immature tera-

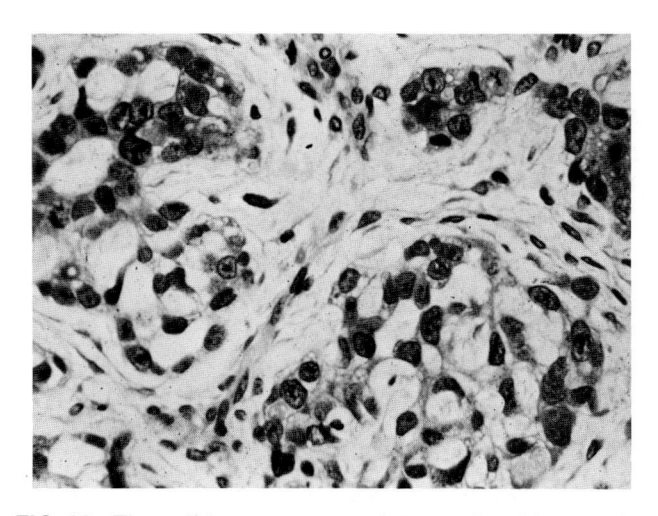

FIG. 33. The solid arrangement shows cells with granular cytoplasm, some with eccentric nuclei, and others with clear cytoplasm (H&E, ×400).

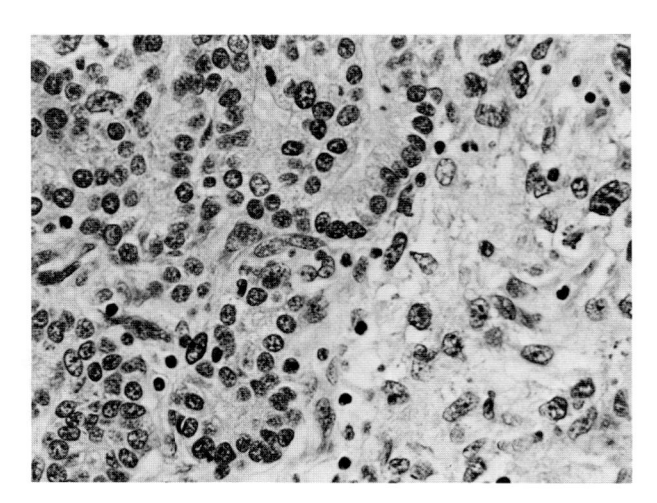

FIG. 35. This mixed germ cell tumor is composed of endodermal sinus tumor with the endometrioid pattern on the right half and embryonal carcinoma on the left (H&E, ×400).

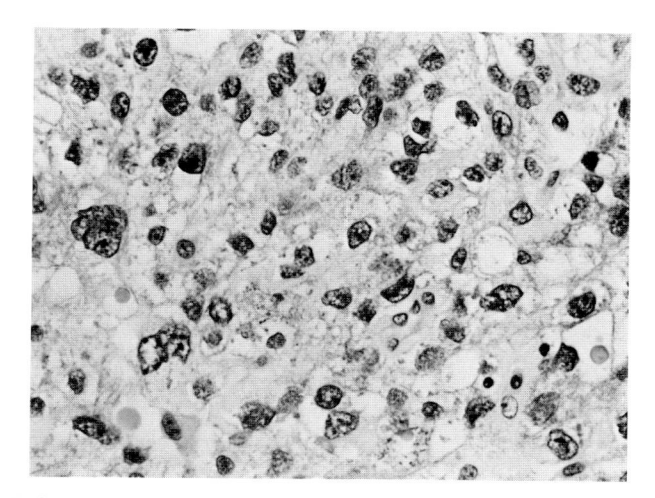

FIG. 36. The cells of embryonal carcinoma are pleomorphic and do not have sharply defined cell borders (H&E, ×400).

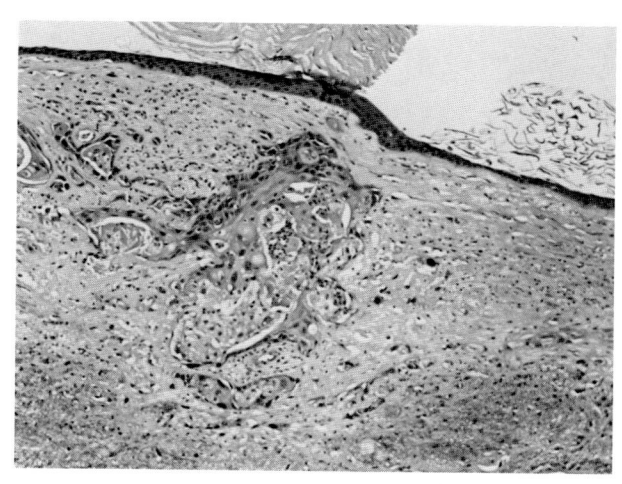

FIG. 37. Squamous carcinoma infiltrates into the stroma surrounding the squamous component of a mature teratoma (H&E, ×100).

toma. By definition, teratomas are composed of tissues derived from two or more embryologic tissues.

Mature Teratomas

Mature teratomas are composed of histologically mature tissue only. They comprise about 30% of all ovarian tumors, about 30% of all benign ovarian tumors, and about two-thirds of all tumors in girls under the age of 15 years (4).

Gross examination. The tumors are often cystic with grumous material and hair in the cysts. Teeth and bone are often present. Areas representing brain, thyroid, or mucinous tissues may be identified grossly. Rarely, a homunculus or well-developed organs such as the eye may be present (119,120). About 12% are bilateral (121). In the 1% to 2% of tumors with a malignant component, there may be nodules or plagues of solid tissue in the cyst wall (122). These areas may be hemorrhagic or necrotic.

Microscopic examination. The most common type of epithelium is squamous, often accompanied by the adnexal structure of the skin. Other ectodermally derived constituents include mature neural tissue, glia, and choroid plexus. Endodermal tissues include respiratory mucosa, gastrointestinal epithelium, and thyroid tissue. Tissue representing mesoderm are bone, cartilage, fat, and smooth muscle.

The most common type of malignant tumor arising in a mature teratoma is squamous carcinoma (Fig. 37). Adenocarcinomas, sarcomas, and melanomas have also been reported (123,124,125,126,127,128).

Immature Teratomas

Immature teratomas are those teratomas with any immature tissue, usually immature glial tissue. These tumors account for 20% of the germ cell tumors, and 10% to 20% of the malignant ovarian tumors in the first two decades of life (4).

Gross examination. These tumors are likely to be large, predominantly solid masses with areas of soft, fleshy, pale pink or tan tissue. The contralateral ovary may be involved if there is extraovarian spread, but these tumors are rarely bilateral. In 10%, the contralateral ovary contains another benign ovarian tumor (121).

Microscopic examination. These tumors contain histologically mature tissues, similar to those seen in mature teratoma. The hallmark is the presence of immature tissues, most commonly immature neuroectodermal tissue (Fig. 38). They may form tubules as well as rosettes resembling neuroblastoma or glioblastoma.

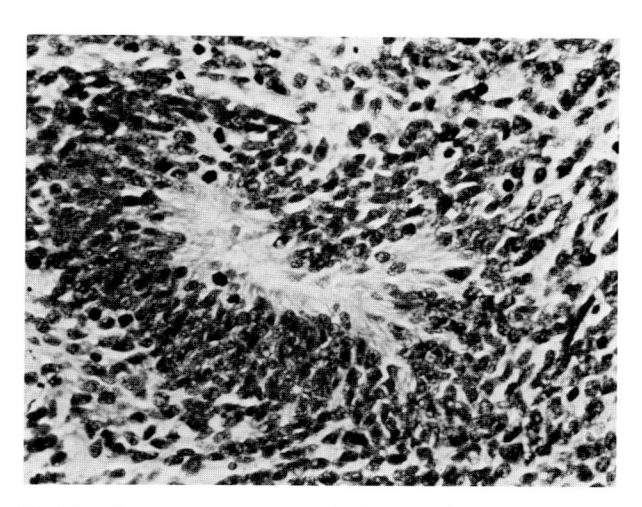

FIG. 38. The immature neural element has many mitotic figures and a rosette arrangement (H&E, ×400).

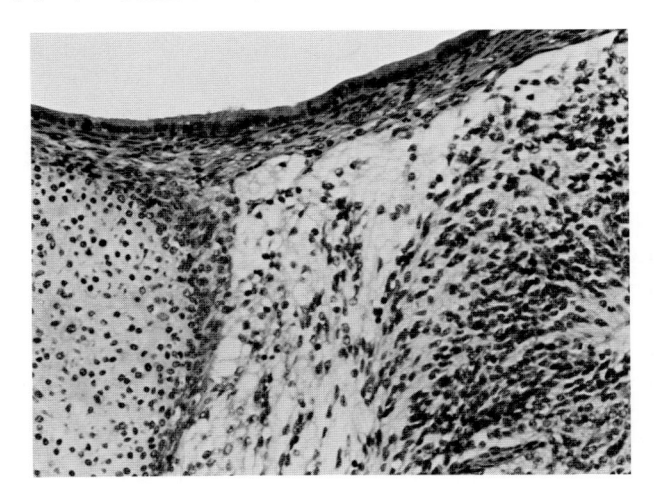

FIG. 39. Mature glandular tissue is present next to immature cartilage and neural tissue (H&E, ×200).

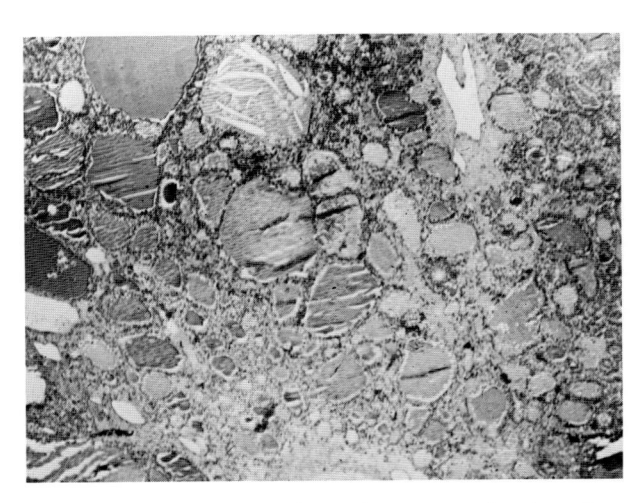

FIG. 40. Mature thyroid tissue is present in abundance (H&E, ×40).

Other forms of immature mesenchymal tissues may be present, particularly immature cartilage (Fig. 39).

The tumors are graded according to the amount of immature tissue present. Grade 1 tumors have immature glial tissue occupying less than one low power field, grade 2 tumors have immature glial tissue in two to three low power fields in one slide, and grade 3 tumors have four or more fields in one slide (129,130,131).

Peritoneal seeding from these tumors may be represented by mature glial seeding, or gliomatosis. Peritoneal gliomatosis from a gastric teratoma in a two-day-old boy has been reported (132).

Monodermal Teratomas

Monodermal teratomas are tumors composed almost exclusively of one type of tissue. The most common of these is thyroid tissue and carcinoid tumor.

Struma ovarii. Tumors composed predominantly of thyroid tissue are the most common type of monodermal teratoma. Only rarely is there an associated hyperthyroidism (4). About 5% to 10% are considered malignant, but only 40% of these have been associated with extraovarian spread (133,134,135,136).

Gross examination. These tumors are cystic with areas of brown or green-brown glistening tissue.

Microscopic examination. The tumor is composed of mature thyroid tissue constituting at least 20% of the total neoplastic tissue (Fig. 40), which may also contain oxyphil cells and areas that resemble thyroid adenomas. The criteria for making the diagnosis of carcinoma have not been established, but follow those for the thyroid gland, i.e., vascular invasion, cytologic atypia in papillary tumors.

Strumal carcinoids. Carcinoids are the second most common monodermal teratoma. They are subclassified into insular and trabecular pure carcinoids, strumal carcinoids, and mucinous carcinoids. About a third of the patients with insular carcinoid have the carcinoid syndrome (137) and a case of strumal carcinoid has also been reported (138). Less than 5% of these tumors metastasize, but those that do are most commonly of the insular or mucinous type (137,139,140,141,142).

Gross examination. These tumors are usually solid, yellow, unilateral masses. In 15%, a benign tumor (cystic teratoma, Brenner tumor, or mucinous tumor) is present in the contralateral ovary (139,142).

Microscopic examination. Insular carcinoids resemble midgut carcinoids with the formation of nests of acini in a fibrous stroma. The cells are uniform with oval, basally placed nuclei which may contain small punctate nucleoli. In some, there may be red granules in the cytoplasm.

The trabecular pattern, reminiscent of the foregut and hindgut carcinoids, is characterized by ribbons of similar cells forming rows one or two cells thick. The ribbons are closely packed and separated by a thin band of fibrous tissue.

Strumal carcinoids are composed of an admixture of both thyroid and carcinoid tissue, the latter most commonly represented by the trabecular pattern (139,143,144). These tumors contain argentaffin granules.

Mucinous carcinoids are similar to adenocarcinoids of the appendix (Fig. 41). The goblet cells have large mucin vacuoles and may form pools of mucin. The nuclei are oval and eccentrically placed. The cytoplasm may have fine red granules which when stained appropriately are argyrophilic (Fig. 42).

Immunohistochemical studies have shown the pres-

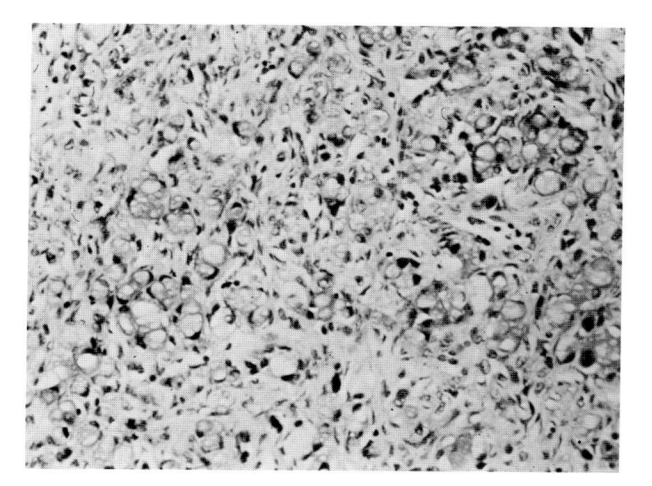

FIG. 41. Metastatic adenocarcinoid from the appendix is characterized by signet ring cells and granular pink cytoplasm (H&E, ×200).

ence of a variety of polypeptides in these tumors. Serotonin has been demonstrated in insular (137), mucinous (141), and strumal carcinoids (143,144). Other polypeptides include pancreatic polypeptide, glucagon, enkephalin, and somatostatin (145). Neuron-specific enolase has been noted in insular and strumal carcinoids (146). In strumal carcinoids, thyroglobulin has been reported in the follicular cells and on occasion in trabecular cells (143,144).

Other Monodermal Teratomas. Other rare monodermal teratomas include the malignant neuroectodermal tumors (147,148,149,150), sebaceous gland tumors (151), tumors resembling the retinal anlage tumor (152), cysts lined by ependyma (153,154) or respiratory epithelium (155).

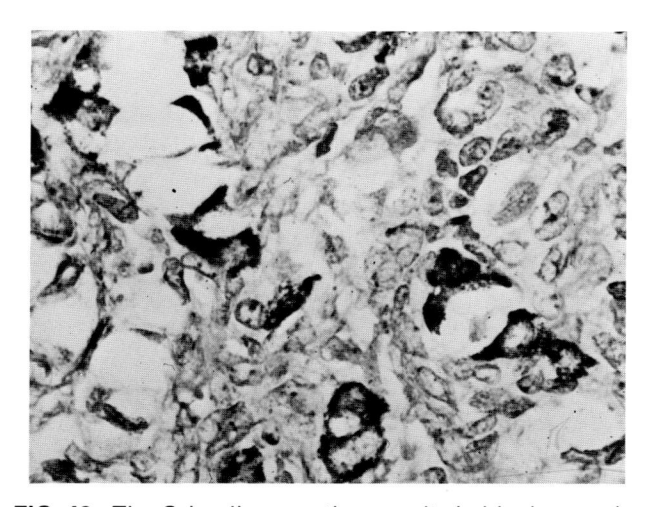

FIG. 42. The Grimelius reaction results in black granules in the cytoplasm, indicating argyrophil granules (×400).

Mixed Germ Cell–Sex Cord-Stromal Tumors

Gonadoblastomas

Gonadoblastoma, a rare tumor, is found in children and young adults, most commonly with female phenotype, with an underlying gonadal disorder. It accounts for two-thirds of the tumors in the group of mixed germ cell-sex cord-stromal tumors (156). Pure or mixed gonadal dysgenesis is present in those with a sexual disorder, and a Y chromosome has been detected in 90% of cases (4). If no germ cell tumor is present, the tumor is benign; however, malignant germ cell tumors are frequently associated with gonadoblastoma (4).

Gross examination. Pure gonadoblastomas are 8 cm or less and a third are bilateral (4). They vary from soft and fleshy to cartilaginous or calcified (4). The germinoma may overgrow the gonadoblastoma so that it may be present in rare foci or not be evident at all. The gonad in which these tumors arise is of unknown type in 60%, in an abdominal or inguinal testis in 20%, and in a gonadal streak in 20% (4). Rarely, these tumors have been found in apparently normal ovaries (4).

Microscopic examination. These tumors are composed of the germ cell component, cells resembling germinoma mixed with small cells of the sex cord type, resembling granulosa or Sertoli cells. The sex cord cells may surround eosinophilic basement-membranelike material or may surround germ cells. The eosinophilic material is calcified in a large percentage of gonadoblastomas (4). The stromal cells may be luteinized or may be Leydig cells (4). A malignant germ cell tumor is present in 60%, of which 80% are germinomas. Other less common tumors are endodermal sinus tumor, embryonal carcinoma, choriocarcinoma, or immature teratoma (157,158).

Differential diagnosis. Gonadoblastomas may be confused with SCTAT because of the eosinophilic material and calcification; however no germ cells are present in SCTAT. These tumors may superficially resemble granulosa cell tumors, but the grooved nuclei of the typical granulosa cell tumors are absent.

SARCOMAS

Pure sarcomas of the ovary are rare. There are reported cases of fibrosarcoma (159,160,161,162, 163,164), leiomyosarcoma (165,166), malignant peripheral nerve sheath tumor (167), lymphangiosarcoma (160), and angiosarcoma (168). Adequate sampling of the tumor should be performed to exclude origin from mesodermal mixed tumor, cystic teratoma, Sertoli-Leydig cell tumor with heterologous elements, or ovarian myxoma (169).

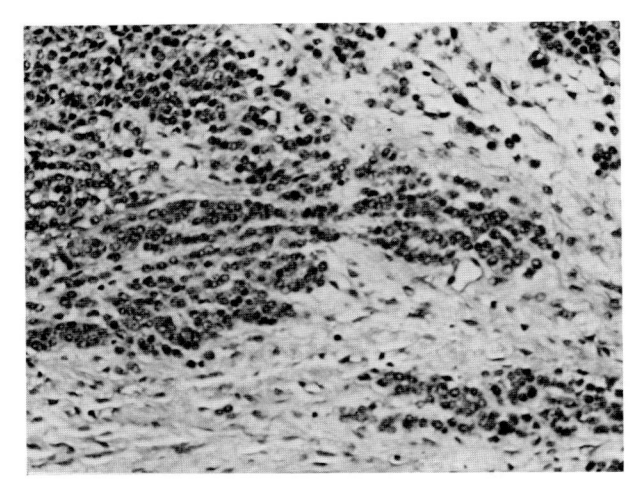

FIG. 43. Small cell carcinoma shows no differentiation (H&E, ×200).

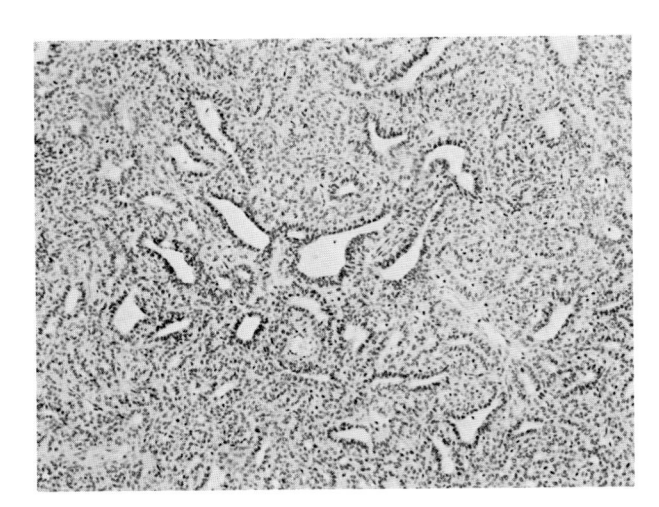

FIG. 45. Adnexal tumor of probable wolffian origin has many spaces producing the sieve-like effect (H&E, ×40).

SMALL CELL CARCINOMA OF THE OVARY

Small cell carcinoma of the ovary is a distinctive tumor found in young women between 10 and 42 years of age, of whom two-thirds will have an associated hypercalcemia (170).

Gross examination. These unilateral tumors are large, solid, tan masses with areas of necrosis and hemorrhage.

Microscopic examination. The tumor is composed of small cells with scant cytoplasm (Fig. 43). These cells form linear arrays, sheets, and follicles. The chromatin is coarsely granular and nucleoli are present. No nuclear grooves are evident. Mitoses are numerous. A fourth of the tumors have cells with large eosinophilic cytoplasm (Fig. 44).

Differential diagnosis. These tumors may be misinterpreted as adult granulosa cell tumors, but their nuclei are too anaplastic to be compatible with granulosa cell nuclei. Mitotic activity is also too prominent. They may also be confused with lymphoma, but the nuclear features, the follicle formation, and the presence of large eosinophilic cells and occasionally mucinous cells precludes the diagnosis of lymphoma.

OTHER RARE TUMORS OF UNCERTAIN CELL TYPE

There are other rare tumors that have been reported. Among these is hepatoid carcinoma which is a tumor that resembles hepatocellular carcinoma and the gastric hepatoid tumors (171). Another is the ovarian tumor of probable wolffian origin (Fig. 45), which has been reported in the ovary as well as in the broad ligament (172,173).

METASTATIC TUMORS

That a tumor is metastatic to the ovaries is a consideration in patients with a known malignant tumor and in those with synchronous tumors, particularly when the ovarian involvement is bilateral. An estimated 15% to 20% of the bilateral ovarian tumors are metastatic.

Krukenberg Tumors

Krukenberg tumors have distinctive signet ring cell infiltrates. The primary carcinoma may be in the stomach, breast, gallbladder, or elsewhere. The ovarian tumors (Fig. 46) may present several years before the primary carcinoma is identified. These tumors tend to be found in young women, mean 45 years of age (174,175,176,177,178). There may be endocrine mani-

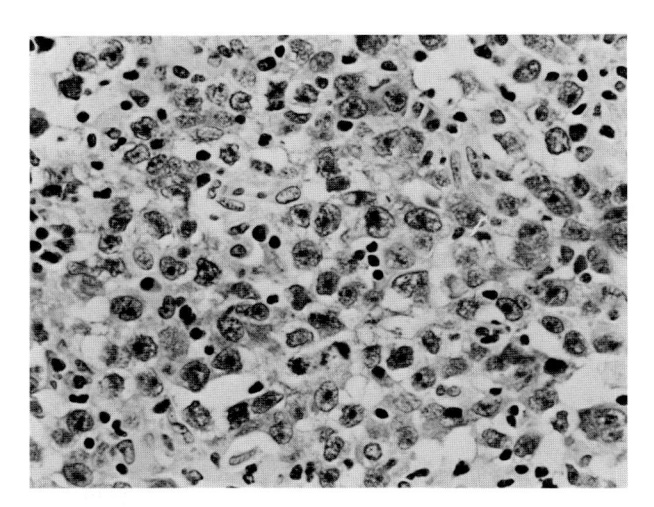

FIG. 44. Small cell carcinoma may have eosinophilic cytoplasm and the cells may be larger (H&E, ×400).

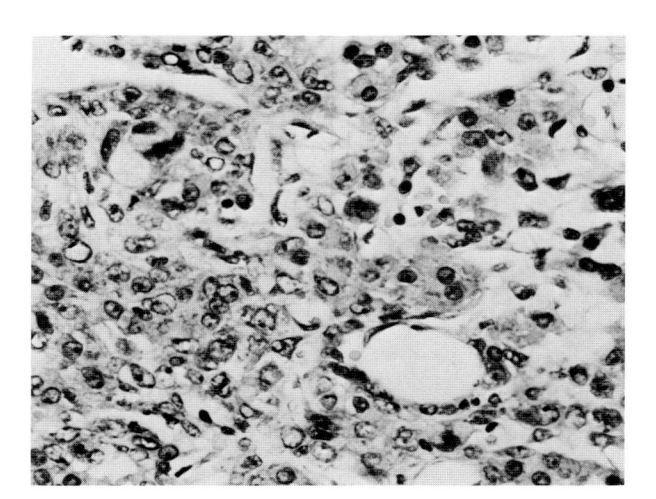

FIG. 46. The stroma surrounding the metastatic gastric carcinoma is luteinized (H&E, ×400).

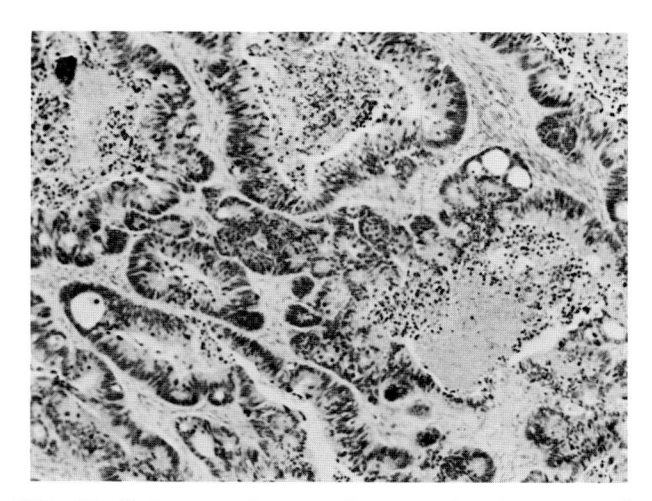

FIG. 47. Colon carcinoma shows extensive necrosis; note that the arrangement of some of the smaller acini could mimic endometrioid carcinoma (H&E, ×40).

festations, particularly during pregnancy, because of stromal luteinization (179). Rarely, no other carcinoma is identified after many years; these cases may represent true primary Krukenberg tumors of the ovary (179).

Colorectal Carcinomas

Most colorectal carcinoma patients will have had a resection of their colorectal carcinoma and then present with ovarian metastases (50% to 75%) (180,181, 182,183,184,185). A smaller proportion, 3% to 20%, have the ovarian metastases synchronously with their intestinal carcinoma or present with ovarian tumors prior to the identification of their primary tumor.

Gross examination. These tumors are soft with abundant yellow necrotic tissue. The solid areas are white or yellow with mucinous secretions.

Microscopic examination. Colorectal carcinomas are composed of tall columnar cells with eosinophilic (Fig. 47) or mucinous cytoplasm with goblet cells interspersed. The nuclei are oval and occasionally very elongated and narrow. Necrosis within the tumor nests is common and prominent. The stroma may be very fibrous or may be luteinized.

Differential diagnosis. When the tumor is very mucinous, it may be misinterpreted as a mucinous tumor of the ovary. However, bilateral mucinous carcinomas of the ovary are uncommon and have areas that range from benign-appearing epithelium to malignant cells. Metastatic tumors generally have one type of tumor tissue, that which is frankly malignant. The other consideration is that the tumor is an endometrioid carcinoma. In general, the latter is not accompanied by necrosis, the cells are not as columnar, goblet cells are not a feature of endometrioid carcinoma, and the distribution of the tumor in the stroma is usually one of sheets of tumor infiltrating the ovarian stroma rather than islands of tumor in a fibrous stroma.

Breast Carcinomas

About a third of breast cancer patients have ovarian metastases (186). In about two-thirds the ovaries are of normal size and appearance (187). Lobular carcinomas (Fig. 48) are more likely to metastasize than are ductal cancers, but the latter are more common (188).

Endometrial Carcinomas

With endometrial carcinoma, there is always the question of whether the ovarian and endometrial carci-

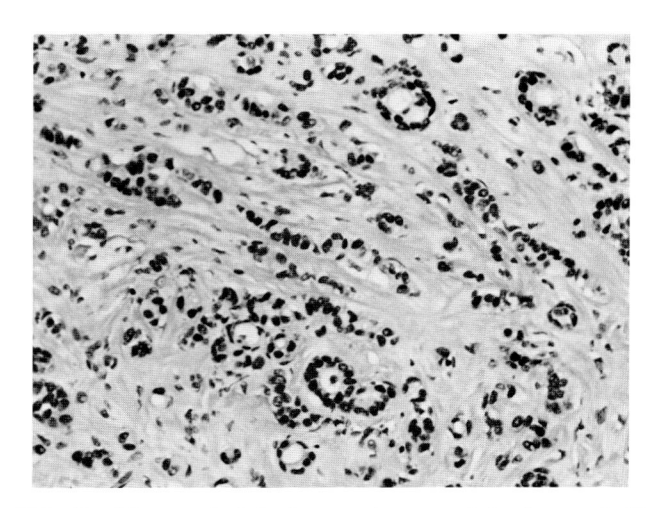

FIG. 48. Metastatic lobular carcinoma of the breast infiltrates in a linear arrangement and in small glands (H&E, ×200).

nomas are synchronous primary cancers or do the ovarian tumors represent metastatic spread from the endometrium The tumors are likely to be independent primary carcinomas if the endometrial carcinoma is confined to the endometrium or if the myometrial invasion is superficial. The ovarian carcinomas are likely to be metastases if the endometrial carcinoma is deeply invasive, lymphovascular permeation is present, luminal tumor emboli are noted in the fallopian tubes, tumor emboli are noted in the ovarian vessels, or the tumor involves only the surface of the ovaries.

Adenocarcinomas of the Cervix

Independent primary mucinous adenocarcinomas of the cervix and the ovary have been reported in ten percent of patients (189,190). However, it may not be possible to determine whether the tumors are independent or whether the ovarian ones represent metastases in some cases. Criteria similar to those applied to endometrial tumors may be useful.

Squamous Carcinomas of the Cervix

Less than 1% of the squamous carcinomas of the cervix metastasize to the ovary (191). Consideration of an independent ovarian squamous carcinoma is usual (192,193,194,195).

Lymphomas and Leukemia

Lymphomas

In a study of 1467 patients with nondisseminated extranodal lymphomas, 1% were primary in the female

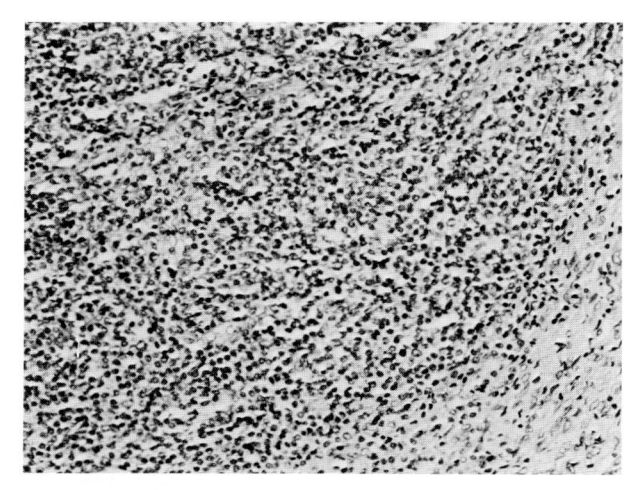

FIG. 49. Malignant lymphoma is composed of small uniform cells infiltrating in a diffuse pattern (H&E, ×100).

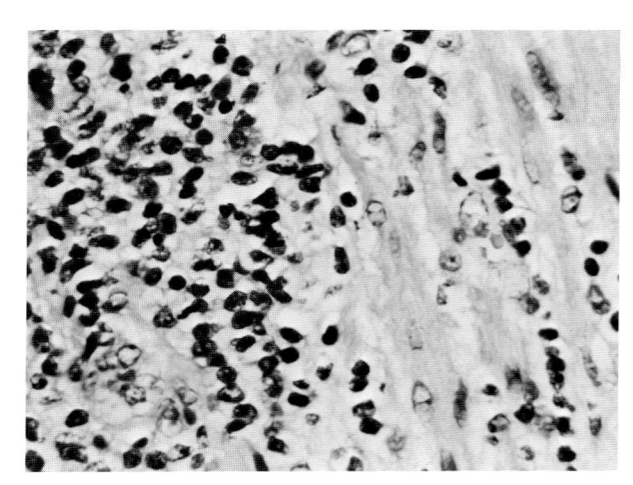

FIG. 50. The malignant lymphocytes infiltrate as single cells without intercellular associations (H&E, ×600).

genital tract (196). Of these, most were in the ovary. Involvement of the female genital organs is usually a manifestation of secondary involvement (197). In a series of forty cases with lymphoma and two with leukemia, fifty-five percent involved the ovaries bilaterally (198). Microscopically, six tumors were follicular and thirty-four diffuse; the latter were large cell immunoblastic (thirteen patients), small noncleaved lymphocytic (eleven patients), large cell noncleaved (five patients), intermediate grade large cell (three patients), and large cell cleaved lymphoma (two patients) (198).

The most common type of leukemia presenting as an ovarian tumor is granulocytic sarcoma (198,199). The ovaries were involved in six of eight patients with granulocytic sarcoma (200). Microscopically, the malignant cells are small and may be infiltrating in sheets (Fig. 49) or cords (Fig. 50), simulating the appearance of granulosa cell tumor or of an undifferentiated carcinoma. The nuclei of the malignant cells are often lobulated or reniform with large nucleoli. Immunohistochemical studies for the lymphoid markers will identify the nature of these cells. If granulocytic sarcoma is suspected, the chloracetate esterase stain will assist in defining the tumor cells.

In patients with disseminated disease, eighteen to forty percent will have involvement of the female genital organs (201).

REFERENCES

1. Scully RE. Recent progress in ovarian cancer. *Hum Pathol* 1970;1:73.
2. Hendrickson M, Ross J, Eifel P, Martinez A, Kempson R. Uterine papillary serous carcinoma. A highly malignant form of endometrial adenocarcinoma. *Am J Surg Pathol* 1982;6:93–108.
3. Saigo PE, Cain JM, Kim WS, Thompson R, Gainor J, Lewis JL Jr. Prognostic factors in cervical adenocarcinoma. *Cancer* 1986;57:1584–1593.

4. Scully RE. Tumors of the ovary and maldeveloped gonads. Washington, DC, Armed Forces Institute of Pathology. *Atlas of tumor pathology.* second series; 1979.
5. Allen MS, Hertig AT. Carcinoma of the ovary. *Am J Obstet Gynecol* 1949;58:640.
6. Barnhill D, Heller P, Brzozowski P, Advani H, Gallup D, Park R. Epithelial ovarian carcinoma of low malignant potential. *Obstet Gynecol* 1985;65:53–59.
7. Russell P. The pathological assessment of ovarian neoplasms. I. Introduction to the common "epithelial" tumors and analysis of benign "epithelial" tumors. *Pathol* 1979;11:5.
8. Bell DA, Weinstock MA, Scully RE. Peritoneal implants of serous borderline tumors: histologic features and prognosis. *Cancer* 1988;62:2212–2222.
9. Michael H, Roth LM. Invasive and noninvasive implants in ovarian serous tumors of low malignant potential. *Cancer* 1986;57:1240–1247.
10. Friedlander ML, Russell P, Taylor IW, Hedley DW, Tattersall MHN. Flow cytometric analysis of cellular DNA content as an adjunct to the diagnosis of ovarian tumours of borderline malignancy. *Pathol* 1984;16:301–306.
11. Dietel M, Arps H, Rohlff A, Bodecker R, Niendorf A. Nuclear DNA content of borderline tumors of the ovary: correlation with histology and significance for prognosis. *Virchows Arch* 1986;409:829–836.
12. Hytiroglou P, Harpaz N, Heller DS, Liu ZY, Deligdisch L, Gil J. Differential diagnosis of borderline and invasive serous cystadenocarcinomas of the ovary by computerized interactive morphometric analysis of nuclear features. *Cancer* 1992;69:988–992.
13. Khattech A, Spatz A, Prade M, Duvillard P, Charpentier P, Bognel Michel G, Lhomme C. Nucleolar organizer regions in ovarian tumors: Discrimination between carcinoma and borderline tumors. *Int J Gynecol Pathol* 1992;11:11–14.
14. Kotylo PK, Michael H, Fineberg N, Sutton G, Roth LM. Flow cytometric analysis of DNA content and ras p21 oncoprotein expression in ovarian neoplasms. *Inter J Gynecol Pathol* 1992;11:30–37.
15. Berchuck A, Boente MP, Kerns BJ, Kinney RB, Soper JT, Clarke-Pearson DL, Bast RC Jr, Bacus SS. Ploidy analysis of epithelial ovarian cancers using image cytometry. *Gynecol Oncol* 1992;44:61–65.
16. Rotmensch J, Atcher RW, Schwartz JL, Grdina DJ. Analysis of ascites from patients with ovarian carcinoma by flow cytometry. *Gynecol Oncol* 1992;44:10–12.
17. Kacinski BM, Mayer AG, King BL, Carter D, Chambers SK. Neu protein overexpression in benign, borderline, and malignant ovarian neoplasms. *Gynecol Oncol* 1992;44:245–253.
18. Hart WR, Norris HJ. Borderline and malignant mucinous tumors of the ovary. Histologic criteria and clinical behavior. *Cancer* 1973;31:1031.
19. Sumithran E, Susil BJ, Looi L-M. The prognostic significance of grading in borderline mucinous tumors of the ovary. *Hum Pathol* 1988;19:15–18.
20. Rutgers JL, Scully RE. Ovarian mucinous papillary cystadenomas of borderline malignancy. *Cancer* 1988;61:340–348.
21. Watkin W, Silva EG, Gershenson DM. Mucinous carcinoma of the ovary. Pathologic prognostic factors. *Cancer* 1992;69:208–212.
22. Chaitin BA, Gershenson DM, Evans HL. Mucinous tumors of the ovary. A clinicopathologic study of 70 cases. *Cancer* 1985;55:1958–1962.
23. Prat J, Young RH, Scully RE. Ovarian mucinous tumors with foci of anaplastic carcinoma. *Cancer* 1982;50:300–304.
24. Sondergaard G, Kaspersen P. Ovarian and extraovarian mucinous tumors with solid mural nodules. *Int J Gynecol Pathol* 1991;10:145–155.
25. Nichols GE, Mills SE, Ulbright TM, Czernobilsky B, Roth LM. Spindle cell mural nodules in cystic ovarian mucinous tumors. A clinicopathologic and immunohistochemical study of five cases. *Am J Surg Pathol* 1991;15:1055–1062.
26. Prat J, Scully RE. Sarcomas in ovarian mucinous tumors. A report of two cases. *Cancer* 1979;44:1327–1331.
27. Prat J, Scully RE. Ovarian mucinous tumors with sarcoma-like mural nodules. A report of seven cancers. *Cancer* 1979;44:1333–1344.
28. Czernobilsky B, Dgani R, Roth LM. Ovarian mucinous cystadenocarcinoma with mural nodule of carcinomatous derivation. A light and electron microscopic study. *Cancer* 1983;51:141–148.
29. Tsujimura T, Kawano K. Rhabdomyosarcoma coexistent with ovarian mucinous cystadenocarcinoma: A case report. *Int J Gynecol Pathol* 1992;11:58–62.
30. Cocco AE, Conway SJ. Zollinger-Ellison syndrome associated with ovarian mucinous cystadenocarcinoma. *N Engl J Med* 1975;293:485–486.
31. Kahn MA, Demopoulos RI. Mucinous ovarian tumors with pseudomyxoma peritonei: A clinicopathologic study. *Int J Gynecol Pathol* 1992;11:15–23.
32. Young RH, Gilks CB, Scully RE. Mucinous tumors of the appendix associated with mucinous tumors of the ovary and pseudomyxoma peritonei. A clinicopathological analysis of 22 cases supporting an origin in the appendix. *Am J Surg Pathol* 1991;15:415–429.
33. Roth LM, Czernobilsky B, Langley FA. Ovarian endometrioid adenofibromatous and cystadenomatous tumors: Benign, proliferating, and malignant. *Cancer* 1981;48:1838–1845.
34. Bell DA, Scully RE. Atypical and borderline endometrioid adenofibromas of the ovary. A report of 27 cases. *Am J Surg Pathol* 1985;9:205–214.
35. Snyder RR, Norris HJ, Tavassoli F. Endometrioid proliferative and low malignant potential tumors of the ovary. A clinicopathologic study of 46 cases. *Am J Surg Pathol* 1988;12:661–671.
36. Colgan JY, Norris HJ. Ovarian epithelial tumors of low malignant potential: A review. *Int J Gynecol Pathol* 1983;1:367–382.
37. Sampson JA. Endometrial carcinoma of ovary, arising in endometrial tissue in that organ. *Arch Surg* 1925;10:1–72.
38. Corner GW Jr, Hu C, Hertig AT. Ovarian carcinoma arising in endometriosis. *Am J Obstet Gynecol* 1950;59:760–774.
39. Czernobilsky B, Silverman BB, Mikuta JJ. Endometrioid carcinoma of the ovary. A clinicopathologic study of 75 cases. *Cancer* 1970;26:1141–1152.
40. Young RH, Prat J, Scully RE. Ovarian endometrioid carcinomas resembling sex cord-stromal tumors. A clinicopathologic analysis of 13 cases. *Am J Surg Pathol* 1982;6:513–522.
41. Roth LM, Liban E, Czernobilsky B. Ovarian endometrioid tumors mimicking Sertoli and Sertoli-Leydig cell tumors. Sertoliform variant of endometrioid carcinoma. *Cancer* 1982;50:1322–1331.
42. Dockerty MB. Primary and secondary ovarian adenoacanthoma. *Surg Gynecol Obstet* 1954;99:392.
43. Ehrmann RL, Weidener N, Welch WR, et al. Malignant mixed müllerian tumor of the ovary with prominent neuroecto-dermal differentiation (Teratoid carcinosarcoma). *Int J Gynecol Pathol* 1990;9:272–282.
44. Barwick KW, LiVolsi VA. Malignant mixed mesodermal tumors of the ovary. *Am J Surg Pathol* 1080;4:37–42.
45. Dinh TB, Slavin RE, Bhagavan BS, et al. Mixed mesodermal tumors of the ovary: A clinicopathologic study of 14 cases. *Obstet Gynecol* 1988;74:409–412.
46. Morrow CP, d'Ablaing D, Brady LW, et al. A clinical and pathologic study of 30 cases of malignant mixed müllerian epithelial and mesenchymal ovarian tumors: A Gynecologic Oncology Group study. *Gynecol Oncol* 1984;18:278–292.
47. Marchevsky AM, Kaneko M. Bilateral ovarian endometriosis associated with carcinosarcoma of the right ovary and endometrioid carcinoma of the left ovary. *Am J Clin Pathol* 1978;70:709–712.
48. Clement PB, Scully RE. Extrauterine mesodermal (müllerian) adenosarcoma. *Am J Clin Pathol* 1978;69:276–283.
49. Kao GF, Norris HJ. Benign and low grade variants of mixed mesodermal tumor (adenosarcoma) of the ovary and adnexal region. *Cancer* 1978;42:1314–1324.
50. Roth LM, Langley FA, Fox H, Wheeler JE, Czernobilsky B. Ovarian clear cell adenofibromatous tumors; benign, of low malignant potential, and associated with invasive clear cell carcinoma. *Cancer* 1984;53:1156–1163.

51. Bell DA, Scully RE. Benign and borderline clear cell adenofibromas of the ovary. *Cancer* 1985;56:2922–2931.
52. Brescia RJ, Dubin N, Demopoulos RI. Endometrioid and clear cell carcinoma of the ovary. Factors affecting survival. *Int J Gynecol Pathol* 1989;8:132–138.
53. Montag AG, Jenison EL, Griffiths CT, Welch WR, Lavin PT, Knapp RC. Ovarian clear cell carcinoma. A clinicopathologic analysis of 44 cases. *Inter J Gynecol Pathol* 1989;8:85–96.
54. Young RH, Scully RE. Oxyphilic clear cell carcinoma of the ovary. *Am J Surg Pathol* 1987;11:661–667.
55. Trebeck CE, Friedlander ML, Russell P, Baird PJ. Brenner tumors of the ovary: a study of the histology, immunohistochemistry and cellular DNA content in benign, borderline and malignant ovarian tumours. *Pathol* 1987;19:241–246.
56. Hallgrimson J, Scully RE. Borderline and malignant Brenner tumours of the ovary. A report of 15 cases. *Acta Pathol Microbiol Scand [A]* 1972;80 (Suppl);233:56–66.
57. Miles PA, Norris HJ. Proliferative and malignant Brenner tumors of the ovary. *Cancer* 1972;30:174–186.
58. Roth LM, Sternberg WH. Proliferating Brenner tumors. *Cancer* 1971;27:687–693.
59. Roth LM, Dallenbach-Hellweg G, Czernobilsky B. Ovarian Brenner tumors. I. Metaplastic, proliferating, and of low malignant potential. *Cancer* 1985;56:582–591.
60. Roth LM, Czernobilsky B. Ovarian Brenner tumors. II. Malignant. *Cancer* 1985;56:592–601.
61. Austin RM, Norris HJ. Malignant Brenner tumor and transitional cell carcinoma of the ovary. A comparison. *Int J Gynecol Pathol* 1987;6:29–39.
62. Waxman M. Pure and mixed Brenner tumors of the ovary. Clinicopathologic and histogenetic observations. *Cancer* 1979;43:1830–1839.
63. Shevchuk MM, Fenoglio CM, Richart RM. Histogenesis of Brenner tumors, I: Histology and ultrastructure. *Cancer* 1980;46:2607–2616.
64. Haid M, Victor TA, Weldon-Linne CM, Danforth DN. Malignant Brenner tumor of the ovary. Electron micro-scopic study of a case responsive to radiation and chemotherapy. *Cancer* 1983;51:498–508.
65. Seldenrijk CA, Willig AP, Baak JP, et al. Malignant Brenner tumor. A histologic, morphometrical immunohistochemical and ultrastructural study. *Cancer* 1986;58:754–760.
66. Silva EG, Robey-Cafferty SS, Smith TL, Gershenson DM. Ovarian carcinomas with transitional cell carcinoma pattern. *Am J Clin Pathol* 1990;93:457–465.
67. Young RH, Scully RE. Ovarian sex cord-stromal tumors. Recent advances and current status. *Clin Obstet Gynecol* 1984;11:93–134.
68. Hodgson JE, Dockerty MB, Mussey RD. Granulosa cell tumor of the ovary. A clinical and pathologic review of sixty-two cases. *Surg Gynecol Obstet* 1945;81:631–642.
69. Brennington JL, Ferguson BR, Haber SL. Incidence and relative frequency of benign and malignant ovarian neoplasms. *Obstet Gynecol* 1968;32:627–632.
70. Norris HJ, Taylor HB. Virilization associated with cystic granulosa cell tumors. *Obstet Gynecol* 1969;34:629–635.
71. Nakashima N, Young RH, Scully RE. Androgenic granulosa cell tumors of the ovary. A clinicopathologic analysis of 17 cases and review of the literature. *Arch Pathol Lab Med* 1984;108:786–791.
72. Stenwig JT, Hazekamp JT, Beecham JB. Granulosa cell tumors of the ovary. A clinicopathological study of 118 cases with long term follow-up. *Gynecol Oncol* 1979;7:136–152.
73. Fathalla MF. The occurrence of granulosa and theca tumors in clinically normal ovaries. *J Obstet Gynaecol Br Commonwealth* 1967;74:279–282.
74. Fox H, Agrawal K, Langley FA. A clinicopathologic study of 92 cases of granulosa cell tumor of the ovary with special reference to the factors influencing prognosis. *Cancer* 1975;35:231–241.
75. Young RH, Scully RE. Ovarian sex cord-stromal tumors with bizarre nuclei. A clinicopathologic analysis of seventeen cases. *Int J Gynecol Pathol* 1983;1:325–335.
76. Young RH, Dickersin GR, Scully RE. Juvenile granulosa cell tumor of the ovary. A clinicopathological analysis of 125 cases. *Am J Surg Pathol* 1984;8:575–596.
77. Dockerty MB, Masson JC. Ovarian fibromas: A clinical and pathologic study of two hundred and eighty-three cases. *Am J Obstet Gynecol* 1944;47:741–752.
78. Gorlin RJ. Nevoid basal cell carcinoma syndrome. *Medicine (Baltimore)* 1987;66:98–113.
79. Meigs JV. Fibroma of the ovary with ascites and hydrothorax-Meigs' syndrome. *Am J Obstet Gynecol* 1954;67:962–987.
80. Samanth KK, Black WC. Benign ovarian stromal tumors associated with free peritoneal fluid. *Am J Obstet Gynecol* 1970;107:538–545.
81. Geist SH, Gaines JA. Theca cell tumors. *Am J Obstet Gynecol* 1928;35:39–51.
82. Banner EA, Dockerty MB. Theca cell tumors of the ovary. A clinical and pathologic study of twenty-three cases (including thirteen new cases) with a review. *Surg Gynecol Obstet* 1945;81:234–242.
83. Sternberg WH, Gaskill CJ. Theca-cell tumors. With a report of twelve new cases and observations on the possible etiologic role of ovarian stromal hyperplasia. *Am J Obstet Gynecol* 1950;59:575–587.
84. Björkholm E, Silfverswärd C. Theca-cell tumors. Clinical features and prognosis. *Acta Radiol Oncol Radiat Phys Biol* 1980;19:241–244.
85. Zhang J, Young RH, Arseneau J, et al. Ovarian stromal tumors containing lutein or Leydig cells (luteinized thecomas and stromal Leydig cell tumors) — a clinico-pathological analysis of fifty cases. *Int J Gynecol Pathol* 1982;1:270–285.
86. Young RH, Scully RE. Ovarian Sertoli cell tumors. A report of ten cases. *Int J Gynecol Pathol* 1984;2:349–363.
87. Teilum G. Homologous ovarian and testicular tumors. III. Estrogen producing Sertoli cell tumors (androblastoma tubulare lipoides) of the human testis and ovary. *J Clin Endocrinol* 1949;9:301–318.
88. Tavassoli FA, Norris H. Sertoli tumors of the ovary. A clinicopathologic study of 28 cases with ultrastructural observations. *Cancer* 1980;46:2281–2217.
89. Solh HM, Azoury RS, Najjar SS. Peutz-Jeghers syndrome associated with precocious puberty. *J Pediatr* 1983;103:593–595.
90. O'Hern TM, Neubecker RD. Arrhenoblastoma. *Obstet Gynecol* 1962;19:758–770.
91. Roth LM, Anderson MC, Govan ADT, Langley FA, Gowing NFC, Woodcock AS. Sertoli-Leydig cell tumors. A clinicopathologic study of 34 cases. *Cancer* 1981;48:187–197.
92. Zaloudek C, Norris HJ. Sertoli-Leydig tumors of the ovary. A clinicopathologic study of 64 intermediate and poorly differentiated neoplasms. *Am J Surg Pathol* 1984;8:405–418.
93. Young RH, Scully RE. Ovarian Sertoli-Leydig cell tumors: a clinicopathological analysis of 207 cases. *Am J Surg Pathol* 1985;9:543–569.
94. Young RH, Scully RE. Well-differentiated ovarian Sertoli-Leydig cell tumors: clinicopathological analysis of 23 cases. *Int J Gynecol Pathol* 1984;3:277–290.
95. Young RH, Scully RE. Ovarian Sertoli-Leydig cell tumors with a retiform pattern: A problem in histopathologic diagnosis. A report of 25 cases. *Am J Surg Pathol* 1983;7:755–771.
96. Young RH, Prat J, Scully RE. Ovarian Sertoli-Leydig cell tumors with heterologous elements (i). Gastrointestinal epithelium and carcinoid; a clinicopathologic analysis of thirty-six cases. *Cancer* 1982;50:2448–2456.
97. Waxman M, Damjanov I, Alpert L, Sardinsky T. Composite mucinous ovarian neoplasms associated with Sertoli-Leydig and carcinoid tumors. *Cancer* 1981;47:2044–2052.
98. Prat J, Young RH, Scully RE. Ovarian Sertoli-Leydig cell tumors with heterologous elements (ii). Cartilage and skeletal muscle: a clinicopathological analysis of twelve cases. *Cancer* 1982;50:2465–2475.
99. Young RH, Perez-Atayde AR, Scully RE. Ovarian Sertoli-Leydig cell tumor with retiform and heterologous components. Report of a case with hepatocytic differentiation and elevated serum alpha-fetoprotein. *Am J Surg Pathol* 1984;8:709–718.
100. Young RH, Dudley AG, Scully RE. Granulosa cell, Sertoli-Leydig cell and unclassified sex cord-stromal tumors associ-

ated with pregnancy. A clinicopathological analysis of thirty-six cases. *Gynecol Oncol* 1984;18:181–205.
101. Young RH, Welch WR, Dickersin GR, Scully RE. Ovarian sex cord tumor with annular tubules: review of 74 cases including 27 with Peutz-Jeghers syndrome and four with adenoma malignum of the cervix. *Cancer* 1982;50:1384–1402.
102. Scully RE. Sex cord tumor with annular tubules. A distinctive ovarian tumor of the Peutz-Jeghers syndrome. *Cancer* 1970;25:1107–1121.
103. McGowan L, Young RH, Scully RE. Peutz-Jeghers syndrome with adenoma malignum of cervix. A report of two cases. *Gynecol Oncol* 1980;10:125–133.
104. Hart WR, Kumar N, Crissman JD. Ovarian neoplasms resembling sex cord tumors with annular tubules. *Cancer* 1980;45:2352–2363.
105. De Palo G, Lattuada A, Kenda R, et al. Germ cell tumors of the ovary: the experience of the national cancer institute of Milan. I. Dysgerminoma. *Int J Radiat Oncol Phys* 1987;13:853–860.
106. Thomas GM, Dembo AJ, Hacker NF, et al. Current therapy for dysgerminoma of the ovary. *Obstet Gynecol* 1987;70:268–275.
107. Zaloudek CJ, Tavassoli FA, Norris JH. Dysgerminoma with syncytiotrophoblastic giant cells. A histologically and clinically distinctive subtype of dysgerminoma. *Am J Surg Pathol* 1981;5:361–367.
108. Palmquist MB, Webb MJ, Lieber MM, Gaffey TA, Nativ O. DNA ploidy of ovarian dysgerminomas: correlation with clinical outcome. *Gynecol Oncol* 1992;44:13–16.
109. Oud PS, Soeters RP, Pahlplatz MM, et al. DNA Cytometry of pure dysgerminomas of the ovary. *Int J Gynecol Pathol* 1988;7:258–267.
110. Huntington RW, Bullock WK. Yolk sac tumors of the ovary. *Cancer* 1970;25:1357–1367.
111. Kurman RJ, Norris HJ. Endodermal sinus tumor of the ovary. A clinical and pathologic analysis of 71 cases. *Cancer* 1976;38:2404–2419.
112. Langley FA, Govan ADT, Anderson MC, et al. Yolk sac and allied tumours of the ovary. *Histopathol* 1981;5:389–401.
113. Ulbright TM, Roth LM, Brodhecker CA. Yolk sac differentiation in germ cell tumors. A morphologic study of 50 cases with emphasis of hepatic, enteric, and parietal yolk sac features. *Am J Surg Pathol* 1986;10:151–164.
114. Prat J, Bhan AK, Dickensin GR, Robboy SJ, Scully RE. Hepatoid yolk sac tumor of the ovary (endodermal sinus tumor with hepatoid differentiation). A light microscopic, ultrastructural and immunohistochemical study of seven cases. *Cancer* 1982;50:2355–2368.
115. Nakashima N, Fukatsu T, Nagasaki T, et al. The frequency and histology of hepatic tissue of germ cell tumors. *Am J Surg Pathol* 1987;11:682–692.
116. Clement PB, Young RH, Scully RE. Endometrioid-like yolk sac tumor of the ovary. A clinicopathological analysis of eight cases. *Am J Surg Pathol* 1987;11:767–778.
117. Kurman RJ, Norris HJ. Embryonal carcinoma of the ovary. A clinicopathologic entity distinct from endodermal sinus tumor resembling embryonal carcinoma of the adult testis. *Cancer* 1976;38:2420–2433.
118. Nakakuma K, Tashiro S, Uemura K, et al. Alpha-fetoprotein and human chorionic gonadotropin in embryonal carcinoma of the ovary. An 8-year survival case. *Cancer* 1983;52:1470–1472.
119. Woodfield B, Katz DA, Cantrell CJ, et al. A benign cystic teratoma with gastrointestinal tract development. *Am J Clin Pathol* 1985;83:236–240.
120. Abbott TM, Hermann WJ, Scully RE. Ovarian fetiform teratoma (homunculus) in a 9-year-old girl. *Int J Gynecol Pathol* 1984;2:392–402.
121. Yanai-Inbar I, Scully RE. Relation of ovarian dermoid cysts and immature teratomas: an analysis of 350 cases of immature teratoma and 10 cases of dermoid cyst with microscopic foci of immature tissue. *Int J Gynecol Pathol* 1987;6:203–212.
122. Krumerman MS, Chung A. Squamous carcinoma arising in benign cystic teratoma of the ovary. A report of four cases and review of the literature. *Cancer* 1977;39:1237–1242.
123. Genadry R, Parmley T, Woodruff JD. Secondary malignancies in benign cystic teratomas. *Gynecol Oncol* 1979;8:246–251.
124. Tsukamoto N, Matsukuma K, Matsumura M, et al. Primary malignant melanoma arising in cystic teratoma of the ovary. *Gynecol Oncol* 1986;23:395–400.
125. Peterson WF. Malignant degeneration of benign cystic teratomas of the ovary. A collective review of the literature. *Gynecol Oncol* 1957;12:793–830.
126. Ueda G, Sato Y, Yamasaki M, et al. Malignant fibrous histiocytoma arising in a benign cystic teratoma of the ovary. *Gynecol Oncol* 1975;5:313–322.
127. Climie ARW, Heath LP. Malignant degeneration of benign cystic teratomas of the ovary. Review of the literature and report of a chondrosarcoma and carcinoid tumor. *Cancer* 1968;22:824–832.
128. Seifer DB, Weiss LM, Kempson KL. Malignant lymphoma arising within thyroid tissue in a mature cystic teratoma. *Cancer* 1986;58:2459–2461.
129. Norris HJ, Zirkin HJ, Benson WL. Immature (malignant) teratoma of the ovary. A clinical and pathologic study of 58 cases. *Cancer* 1976;37:2359–2372.
130. Thurlbeck WM, Scully RE. Solid teratoma of the ovary. A clinicopathological analysis of 9 cases. *Cancer* 1960;13:804–811.
131. Steeper TA, Mukai K. Solid ovarian teratomas: an immunocytochemical study of thirteen cases with clinico-pathologic correlation. *Pathol Annu* 19;1984:81–92.
132. Coulson WF. Peritoneal gliomatosis from a gastric teratoma. *Am J Clin Pathol* 1990;94:87–89.
133. Gonzalez-Angulo A, Kaufman RH, Braungart CD, et al. Adenocarcinoma of thyroid arising in struma ovarii (malignant struma ovarii). Report of two cases and review of the literature. *Obstet Gynecol* 1963;21:567–576.
134. Hasleton PS, Kelehan P, Whittaker JS, et al. Benign and malignant struma ovarii. *Arch Pathol Lab Med* 1978;102:180–184.
135. Pardo-Mindan FJ, Vazquez JJ. Malignant struma ovarii. Light and electron microscopic study. *Cancer* 1983;51:337–343.
136. Yannopoulos D, Yannopoulos K, Ossowski R. Malignant struma ovarii. *Pathol Annu* 1976;11:403–413.
137. Robboy SJ, Norris HJ, Scully RE. Insular carcinoid primary in the ovary. A clinicopathologic analysis of 48 cases. *Cancer* 1975;36:404–418.
138. Ulbright TM, Roth LM, Ehrlich CE. Ovarian strumal carcinoid. An immunocytochemical and ultrastructural study of two cases. *Am J Clin Pathol* 1982;77:622–631.
139. Robboy SJ, Scully RE. Strumal carcinoid of the ovary: an analysis of 50 cases of a distinctive tumor composed of thyroid tissue and carcinoid. *Cancer* 1980;46:2019–2034.
140. Alenghat E, Okagaki T, Talerman A. Primary mucinous carcinoid tumor of the ovary. *Cancer* 1986;58:777–783.
141. Talerman A. Carcinoid tumors of the ovary. *J Cancer Res Clin Oncol* 1984;107:125–135.
142. Robboy SJ, Scully RE, Norris HJ. Primary trabecular carcinoid of the ovary. *Obstet Gynecol* 1977;49:202–207.
143. Stagno PA, Petras RE, Hart WR. Strumal carcinoids of the ovary. An immunohistologic and ultrastructural study. *Arch Pathol Lab Med* 1987;1:440–446.
144. Snyder RR, Tavassoli RA. Ovarian strumal carcinoid: immunohistochemical, ultrastructural, and clinicopathologic observation. *Int J Gynecol Pathol* 1986;5:187–201.
145. Sorrong B, Falkmer S, Robboy SJ, et al. Neurohormonal peptides in ovarian carcinoids: an immunohistochemical study of 81 primary carcinoids and of intraovarian metastases from six midgut carcinoids. *Cancer* 1982;49:68–74.
146. Inoue M, Ueda G, Nakajima T. Immunohistochemical demonstration of neuron-specific enolase in gynecologic malignant tumors. *Cancer* 1985;55:1683–1690.
147. Aguirre P, Scully RE. Malignant neuroectodermal tumor of the ovary, a distinctive form of monodermal teratoma. Report of five cases. *Am J Surg Pathol* 1982;6:283–292.
148. Dekmezian R, Sneige N, Ordonez NG. Ovarian and omental ependymomas in peritoneal washings: cytologic and immunocytochemical features. *Diagn Cytopathol* 1986;2:62–68.
149. Kleinman GM, Young RH, Scully RE. Neuroepithelial tumors

arising in the female genital tract [Abstract]. *J. Neuropathol Exp Neurol* 1980;39:367.
150. Kleinman GM, Young RH, Scully RE. Ependymoma of the ovary: report of three cases. *Hum Pathol* 1984;15:632–638.
151. Kaku T, Toyoshima S, Hackisuga T, et al. Sebaceous gland tumor of the ovary. *Gynecol Oncol* 1987;26:398–402.
152. King ME, Mouradian JA, Micha JP, et al. Immature teratoma of the ovary with predominant malignant retinal anlage component. A parthenogenically derived tumor. *Am J Surg Pathol* 1985;9:221–231.
153. Karten G, Sher JH, Marsh MR, et al. Neurogenic cyst of the ovary. A rare form of benign cystic teratoma. *Arch Pathol* 1968;86:563–567.
154. Tiltman AJ. Ependymal cyst of the ovary. *S Afr Med J* 1985;68:424–425.
155. Clement PB, Dimmick JE. Endodermal variant of mature cystic teratoma of the ovary. Report of a case. *Cancer* 1979;43:383–385.
156. Scully RE. Gonadoblastoma. A review of 74 cases. *Cancer* 1970;25:1340–1356.
157. Talerman A. Gonadoblastoma associated with embryonal carcinoma. *Obstet Gynecol* 1974;43:138–142.
158. Hart WR, Burkons DM. Germ cell neoplasms arising in gonadoblastomas. *Cancer* 1979;43:699–789.
159. Prat J, Scully RE. Cellular fibromas and fibrosarcomas of the ovary: a comparative clinicopathologic analysis of seventeen cases. *Cancer* 1981;47:2663–2670.
160. Talerman A. Nonspecific tumors of the ovary, including mesenchymal tumors and malignant lymphoma. In: Kurman RJ, ed. *Blaustein's Pathology of the Female Genital Tract*, 3rd edition. New York: Springer-Verlag; 1987:772–741.
161. Azoury RS, Woodruff JD. Primary ovarian sarcomas. Report of 43 cases from the Emil Novak Ovarian Tumor Registry. *Obstet Gynecol* 1971;37:920–941.
162. Nieminen V, von Numers C, Purola E. Primary sarcoma of the ovary. *Acta Obstet Gynecol Scand* 1969;48:423–432.
163. Kraemer BB, Silva EG, Sniege N. Fibrosarcoma of ovary. A new component in the nevoid basal-cell carcinoma syndrome. *Am J Surg Pathol* 1984;8:231–236.
164. Miles PA, Kiley KC, Mena H. Giant fibrosarcoma of the ovary. *Int J Gynecol Pathol* 1985;4:83–87.
165. Reddy SA, Poon TP, Ramaswamy G, Tchertkeff V. Leiomyosarcoma of the ovary. *NY State J Med* 1985;85:218–220.
166. Nogales FF, Ayala A, Ruiz-Avila I, Sirvent JJ. Myxoid leiomyosarcoma of the ovary: Analysis of three cases. *Hum Pathol* 1991;22:1268–1273.
167. Stone GC, Bell DA, Fuller A, et al. Malignant schwannoma of the ovary. Report of a case. *Cancer* 1986;58:1575–1582.
168. Ongkasuwan C, Taylor JE, Tang C-K, et al. Angiosarcomas of the uterus and ovary: clinicopathologic report. *Cancer* 1982;49:1469–1475.
169. Eichhorn JH, Scully RE. Ovarian myxoma: Clinicopathologic and immunocytologic analysis of five cases and a review of the literature. *Int J Gynecol Pathol* 1991;10:156–169.
170. Dickersin GR, Kline IW, Scully RE. Small cell carcinoma of the ovary with hypercalcemia. A report of eleven cases. *Cancer* 1982;49:188–197.
171. Ishikura H, Scully RE. Hepatoid carcinoma of the ovary; a report of five cases of newly described tumor. *Cancer* 1987;90:2775–2784.
172. Hughesdon PE. Ovarian tumours of wolffian or allied nature; their place in ovarian oncology. *J Clin Pathol* 1982;35:526–535.
173. Kariminejad MH, Scully RE. Female adnexal tumor of probable wolffian origin. A distinctive pathologic entity. *Cancer* 1973;31:671–677.
174. Diddle AW. Krukenberg tumors: Diagnostic problem. *Cancer* 1955;8:1026–1034.
175. Hale RW. Krukenberg tumor of the ovaries. A review of 81 records. *Obstet Gynecol* 1968;32:221–225.
176. Karsh J. Secondary malignant disease of the ovaries. A study of 72 autopsies. *Am J Obstet Gynecol* 1951;61:154–160.
177. Leffel Jr JM, Masson JC, Dockerty MB. Krukenberg tumors. A survey of forty-four cases. *Ann Surg* 1942;115:102–113.
178. Yakusshiji M, Tazaki T, Nishimura H, Kato T. Krukenberg tumors of the ovary; a clinicopathological analysis of 112 cases. *Acta Obstet Gynaecol Jpn* 1987;39:479–485.
179. Scully RE, Richardson GS. Luteinization of the stroma of metastatic cancer involving the ovary and its endocrine significance. *Cancer* 1961;14:827–840.
180. Ulbright TM, Roth LM, Stehman RB. Secondary ovarian neoplasia. A clinicopathologic study of 35 cases. *Cancer* 1984;53:1164–1174.
181. Burt CAV. Prophylactic oophorectomy with resection of the large bowel for cancer. *Am J Surg* 1951;82:571–577.
182. Cutait R, Lesser ML, Enker WE. Prophylactic oophorectomy in surgery for large-bowel cancer. *Dis Colon Rectum* 1983;26:6–11.
183. Graffner HOL, Alm POA, Oscarson JEA. Prophylactic oophorectomy in colorectal carcinoma. *Am J Surg* 1983;146:233–235.
184. Harcourt KF, Dennis DL. Laparotomy for "ovarian tumors" in unsuspected carcinoma of the colon. *Cancer* 1968;21:1244–1246.
185. Johansson H. Clinical aspects of metastatic ovarian cancer of extragenital origin. *Acta Obstet Gynecol Scand* 1960;39:681–697.
186. Lee YN, Hori JM. Significance of ovarian metastases in therapeutic oophorectomy for advanced breast cancer. *Cancer* 1971;27:1374–1378.
187. Lumb G, Mackenzie DH. The incidence of metastases in adrenal glands and ovaries removed for carcinoma of the breast. *Cancer* 1959;12:521–526.
188. Harris M, Howell A, Chrissohou M, Swindell RIC, Hudson M, Sellwood RA. A comparison of the metastatic pattern of infiltrating lobular carcinoma and infiltrating duct carcinoma of the breast. *Br J Cancer* 1984;50:32–40.
189. LiVolsi VA, Merino MJ, Schwartz PE. Coexistent endocervical adenocarcinoma and mucinous adenocarcinoma of ovary: a clinicopathologic study of four cases. *Int J Gynecol Pathol* 1983;1:391–402.
190. Kaminski PF, Norris HJ. Coexistence of ovarian neoplasms and endocervical adenocarcinoma. *Obstet Gynecol* 1984;64:553–556.
191. Ulbright TM, Roth LM. Metastatic and independent cancers of the endometrium and ovary: a clinicopathologic study of 34 cases. *Hum Pathol* 1985;16:28–34.
192. Black WC, Benitez RE. Nonteratomatous squamous cell carcinoma in situ of the ovary. *Obstet Gynecol* 1964;24:865–868.
193. Lele SM, Piver S, Barlow JJ, Tsukada Y. Squamous cell carcinoma arising in ovarian endometriosis. *Gynecol Oncol* 1978;6:290–293.
194. Shingleton HM, Middleton FF, Gore H. Squamous cell carcinoma in the ovary. *Am J Obstet Gynecol* 1974;120:556–560.
195. Tetu B, Silva EG, Gershenson DM. Squamous cell carcinoma of the ovary. *Arch Pathol Lab Med* 1987;111:864–866.
196. Freeman C, Berg JW, Cutler SJ. Occurrence and prognosis of extranodal lymphomas. *Cancer* 1972;29:252–260.
197. Lathrop JC. Malignant pelvic lymphomas. *Obstet Gynecol* 1967;30:137–145.
198. Osborne BM, Robboy SJ. Lymphomas or leukemia presenting as ovarian tumors. *Cancer* 1983;52:1933–1943.
199. Morgan ER, Labotka RJ, Gonzalez-Crussi F, et al. Ovarian granulocytic sarcomas as the primary manifestation of acute infantile myelomonocytic leukemia. *Cancer* 1981;48:1819–1824.
200. Liu PI, Ishimaru T, McGregor DH, et al. Autopsy study of granulocytic sarcoma (chloroma) in patients with myelogenous leukemia, Hiroshima-Nagasaki 1949–1969. *Cancer* 1973;31:948–955.
201. Castaldo TW, Ballon SC, Lagasse LD, Petrilli ES. Reticuloendothelial neoplasia in the female genital tract. *Obstet Gynecol* 1979;54:167–170.

CHAPTER 3

Immunobiology of Ovarian Epithelial Cancer

Kenneth O. Lloyd

Immunological studies of epithelial ovarian cancer have led to many insights into the biological nature of this cancer and to the development of practical approaches for diagnosis and therapy. This subject encompasses a wide range of topics, including humoral and cellular anti-tumor responses (specific and nonspecific), the identification of tumor antigens by antibodies and T-lymphocytes, the role of cytokines in cancer, and the use of immunological approaches to diagnosis and therapy. This chapter begins with a discussion of anti-tumor responses in patients with ovarian cancer but will concentrate mainly on the identification and analysis of tumor antigens in ovarian carcinoma by antibodies and the possible clinical uses of these antibodies.

EVIDENCE FOR AN IMMUNE RESPONSE TO OVARIAN CANCER

Two lines of evidence have been presented for the generation of specific, tumor-related immune responses in ovarian cancer patients: the detection of antibodies in serum and secretions that react with ovarian cancer cells, and the accumulation of lymphocytes and other immune cells within tumor tissue. Although this evidence is provocative, it is balanced by the difficulty involved in demonstrating the anti-tumor specificity of the responses. For example, some of the responses may be autoimmune in nature and not tumor-specific. Also, although ample evidence exists for antigenic changes in tumor cells, including ovarian cancer, the antigens have not yet been proven to be tumor-specific in the strictest sense of the term (1,2). Anti-tumor effects may also be nonspecific and carried out by natural killer (NK) lymphocytes (3) or macrophages (4). These cells may represent the first line of defense against tumors.

A number of studies have demonstrated that antibodies can be eluted from ovarian carcinoma cells or dissociated from immune complexes in ascitic fluid or serum. For example, Kutteh et al. (5,6) eluted antibodies from cystic or ascitic fluid cells by mild acid treatment and found that these antibodies reacted selectively with ovarian cancer cell lines and tissues. Earlier studies by Dorsett et al. (7) showed similar results. Another line of evidence for immunity to ovarian cancer comes from an analysis of antibodies in the sera of patients with paraneoplastic cerebellar degeneration syndrome. This disease is characterized by the loss of Purkinje neurons in some patients with small, often asymptomatic cancers, especially of the breast and ovary (8). High-titer autoimmune antibodies, which occur in about half of these patients, react with antigens found in Purkinje neurons and tumor tissue (9). A possible explanation for these findings is that Purkinje cells and some tumor cells have an antigen (or antigens) in common, and an immune response to the tumor results in concomitant damage to the brain.

Although tumor-infiltrating lymphocytes (TILs) are commonly found in human tumors, the significance of their presence is poorly understood. They may represent a true anti-tumor response, or alternatively their presence may be caused by a nonspecific inflammatory response. Their presence in malignant tumors and surrounding connective tissue and their absence in benign tumors favor a specific response. T-lymphocytes, macrophages, and, rarely, B cells are found in these infiltrates, although there is considerable variability from tumor to tumor. Lymphocytes that are freshly isolated from tumors have little or no cytolytic activity against tumor cells. Culture in the presence of tumor cells and/or IL-2 results in the proliferation of T cells, with cytotoxicity toward tumor cells. Also generated

---

K.O. Lloyd: Department of Immunology, Memorial Sloan-Kettering Cancer Center, New York, NY, 10021

are CD4-positive T cells, which have no cytotoxic effects on tumor cells. In a study of the surface phenotype of lymphocytes from freshly collected ascites of five ovarian cancer patients, Ionnides et al. (10) showed that cells with the $CD3^+$ $CD8^+$ phenotype (preferential cytotoxicity toward autologous tumor cells) and some clones with a wider specificity (non-MHC restricted) were generated. Other studies have shown that most T cells obtained from long-term cultures with IL-2 are of the nonspecific NK type (11). Recent work has shown that a combination of IL-2 and TNF-α may favor the proliferation of autotumor-reactive $CD3^+CD8^+$ cytotoxic cells in vitro (12,13). These studies are paving the way toward the use of adoptive immunotherapy of ovarian cancer with TILs, though more work is necessary before the generation of anti-tumor populations of T cells becomes routine.

ANTIGENIC MARKERS FOR OVARIAN SURFACE EPITHELIUM, PERITONEAL MESOTHELIUM, AND BENIGN TUMORS

The ovarian surface epithelium (OSE) and the mesothelial lining of the peritoneum have many characteristics in common presumably reflecting their common origin from the fetal coeloemic epithelium. Morphologically, the two tissues are very similar, but the peritoneal mesothelium shows some characteristic features which differentiate it from OSE (e.g., fewer cuboidal or columnar cells) (14). In addition, the OSE appears to be more proliferative than the peritoneal lining. Both tissues express many of the antigenic markers characteristic of epithelial cells. These markers include cytoskeletal filaments (e.g., low-molecular-weight keratins) and some surface antigens. Specific keratins (e.g., 4 and 13) may be useful in distinguishing mesothelial cells from benign and malignant ovarian tumors. Interestingly, OSE does not express many of the cell surface and secreted antigens that have been associated with ovarian tumors.

Several studies have attempted to identify antigenic markers that distinguish OSE and peritoneal mesothelium from their malignant counterparts. Van Niekerk, et al. (15) identified a number of ovarian carcinoma–associated antigens that were absent or showed only weak expression on OSE and mesothelium; these were OC-125, OV-TL-3, and OV-TL-10, and MOv18. Mattes et al. (16) identified monoclonal antibodies (mAbs) MH99, MX35, MW207 and MW162 using the same criteria. Other markers such as CEA, B72.3, and 19.9 (sialyl-Le^a blood group antigen) also exhibit this property, but they are not as often expressed on ovarian carcinomas. Another blood group antigen (Le^y) has been shown to be valuable in distinguishing malignant lung mesothelioma from pulmonary carcinomas (17), and this antigen should be examined in ovarian carcinomas.

The ovarian surface epithelium, which is normally composed of cuboidal epithelial cells, has a tendency to form columnar and ciliated cells, crypts, and inclusion cysts. These abnormal structures may be susceptible to further proliferative stimuli that lead eventually to adenomas and adenocarcinomas. Benign ovarian tumors such as adenomas and serous and mucinous cyst adenomas are a distinct clinical and pathological subset of ovarian neoplasms. Antigenically, however, this distinction is less clear. Benign tumors exhibit a complex spectrum of markers that overlap with both normal and malignant ovarian markers, although inclusion cysts and benign tumors express many of the antigens that are more closely associated with malignant tumors. Moreover, the development of morphologically abnormal mesothelial and OSE cells is accompanied by the expression of certain antigens [initially, epithelial surface antigen (ESA) followed by mucins] (C. Finstad and K. O. Lloyd—unpublished data). These observations appear to support the concept that malignant ovarian carcinomas develop from abnormal structures rather than from OSE directly.

ANTIGENIC MARKERS FOR OVARIAN CARCINOMAS

The heteroimmune antisera produced by the immunization of rabbits and other species with human ovarian tumor cells or their extracts produced the first evidence for the existence of ovarian tumor-associated antigens. However, only after the introduction of the hybridoma technique for the production of mAbs was substantial progress made in the identification of significant antigens. These mAbs provide potent reagents that have many applications in the study and treatment of cancer (Table 1). To date, over 50 mAbs have been produced by immunization with ovarian cancer cells, and a number of mAbs that were originally produced by immunization with other types of carcinomas react with ovarian carcinoma. Table 2 lists mouse mAbs raised against ovarian cancer cells and other mAbs that are of interest in the study of ovarian cancer.

CA125

Described by Bast et al. (18), in 1981, the antigen CA-125, which is recognizable by the mouse monoclonal antibody OC-125, the most significant and widely studied marker in epithelial ovarian cancer. The mAbOC-125 was developed after the immunization of mice with ovarian carcinoma cell line OVCA-433 (established from the ascites of a patient with papillary serous cystadenocarcinoma). OC-125 is expressed in

TABLE 1. *Uses of monoclonal antibodies in the study of ovarian cancer*

Basic studies on the biology of normal coelomic epithelium development and carcinogenesis.
Identification of tumor-associated antigens. Biochemical and molecular analysis of antigens.
Immunohistology
- differentiation of tumor from normal or benign tissues
- differentiation of carcinomas from nonepithelial tumors
- classificatin of ovarian tumors.

Serum assays
- sensitive assays for the diagnosis and monitoring of cancer.

Tumor localization
- radiolabeled antibody in the immunoscintographic detection of tumors.

Therapy
- unconjugated antibodies with suitable effector functions
- drug-antibody conjugates
- toxin-antibody conjugates
- bifunction antibodies to activate and target cytotoxic antibodies to tumors.

approximately 80% of ovarian tumors of the serous, endometrioid, clear cell, and undifferentiated types (19) and in a small proportion of mucinous tumors (20). CA-125 is expressed in the majority of endometrial adenocarcinomas (21). Although CA-125 is not strongly expressed on the OSE, it is found in other normal tissues such as the endocervix, endometrium, fallopian tube, goblet cells in respiratory tissues, and lung tissues (22). It is also detected in milk and saliva. Very high levels of CA-125 are found in cervical mucus (23). Although CA-125 has been described as a fetal differentiation antigen that becomes selectively expressed in certain Müllerian duct-derived adult tissues and tumors arising from these tissues, it clearly has a wider distribution. Despite the prominence of CA-125 as an ovarian tumor antigen, only one mAb in addition to OC-125 has been reported to recognize it. Produced by immunization with lung cancer cells, mAb 130-22 also reacts with the OC-125 antigen, but not with the same epitope (24).

The availability of commercial kits for the assay of CA-125 levels in serum has been a factor in its widespread study as a possible marker for diagnosis, monitoring, and prediction of prognosis in patients with ovarian carcinoma. Although CA-125 is not, for various reasons, effective in initial screening, it is widely used to monitor disease status in patients with known ovarian cancer.

Biochemically, CA-125 is a high molecular weight glycoprotein, but its exact molecular size is uncertain. By gel filtration in SDS-urea, CA-125 from OVCA 433 cell line was shown to have a molecular weight of 200,000 D, although SDS-polyacrylamide gel electrophoresis indicated a much larger mass of approximately one million daltons (25). An antigen sample prepared by immunoaffinity chromatography had a carbohydrate content of 24% and contained sialic acid, fucose, mannose, galactose, N-acetylglucosamine and N-acetylgalactosamine, with a buoyant density of 1.3 g/ml. These values are characteristic of a typical glycoprotein rather than a mucin. The nature of the determinant that is recognized by mAb OC-125 is unknown, although studies indicate that this determinant is probably conformationally dependent in the protein moiety rather than in the carbohydrate portion. Recent tests against a large panel of mucins, peptides, and carbohydrate structures failed to identify the precise epitope (26). Because CA-125 can be detected in a double-determinant immunoassay using a single antibody, the antigen must possess multiple identical epitopes. These epitopes may be either carbohydrate or peptide in nature. Considering the clinical significance of CA-125 as an ovarian tumor antigen, more detailed information on the biochemistry and gene structure of this molecule would be useful.

Mucins

Mucins can be defined as high molecular weight glycoproteins with a high characteristic carbohydrate content in which the carbohydrate chains are attached mainly to the serine and threonine residues of the peptide backbone by O-glycosidic bonds (27,28). Mucins differ from proteoglycans in the absence of uronic acid residues and a lower sulphate ester content. Mucins, which are characteristically found in secretions of the body, are produced by specialized secretory cells. They are also produced by carcinomas and, because of their altered levels, structure, and cellular location, they may serve as important tumor antigens.

The association of mucin expression and malignancy first became apparent through the use of mAbs (1,29,30). Numerous mouse mAbs produced against various carcinomas were found to react with mucins. Although a few anti-mucin mAbs have been generated by immunization with ovarian carcinoma cells, a larger number of antibodies that react with ovarian tumors have been produced by immunization with other antigens. These antibodies can be divided into three groups: those reacting with carbohydrate determinants; those reacting with the peptide core; and those that recognize combined protein-carbohydrate epitopes.

Numerous antibodies (more than 20) have been produced to human milk fat globule membranes (Table 3). While the antigen detected by these mAbs is found in many normal epithelia, it is also highly expressed in a wide range of carcinomas, including ovarian cancer. Another mAb (SM3), produced to deglycosylated

TABLE 2. Monoclonal antibodies reacting with ovarian carcinoma

A. Antibodies Developed by Immunization with Ovarian Cancer Cells

Antibody designation	Antigen designation	Antigen characteristics	Reference
OC125	CA125	High-molecular-weight glycoprotein (200,000 D)	18, 25
MH94		Glycolipid (?)	108
MH99[a]	ESA	Glycoprotein (38/32/6 kD)	59, 64
MF116		Glycoprotein (105 kD)	108
MT334		Mucin	37
OM1	SGA	Mucin	109
MW162		Mucin	16
MOv 1		Mucin	110
MOv 2		Mucin and glycolipid	110
MOv 18/19[b]	FBP	Glycoprotein (PI linked; 38 kD)	69, 70
B1		Le^y/H Type 2	46
B3		diLe^x, etc.	46
MA54, MA61		Mucin	112
MX35		NC	16
OV-TL-3	OA3	NC	111
OVB-3		NC	113
OM-A,B,C		NC	73
OV632		NC	114
CF511		NC	87
4C7, 3C2		NC	74
Ki-OC-I-6-2		NC	75
OVX1 and 2		NC	115

B. Antibodies Developed by Immunization with Other Tumor Types

Antibody designation	Antigen designation	Antigen characteristics	Reference
B72.3	TAG-72	Sialyl-Tn (mucin)	50, 52
CC49	TAG-72	Sialyl-Tn (mucin)	51
19.9	CA19.9	Sialyl-Le^a (mucin or glycolipid)	116
HMFG-1, -2[c]	HMFG[d]	Peptide determinant (MUC-1) in mucin	31
Anti-CEA[e]	CEA	Glycoprotein (180 kD)	38
Anti-PLAP	PLAP	Glycoprotein (67 kD)	76

Data compiled from refs. listed in table, with permission.
[a] A number of other monoclonal antibodies identifying this antigen have been developed [e.g., 17.1A, AUA1, KS ¼, and HEA125 (see refs. 60–62)].
[b] Monoclonal antibody MW 207 also identifies this antigen (see refs. 16, 53).
[c] A large number of monoclonal antibodies identifying overlapping peptide determinants on mucin (MUC-1) have been developed.
[d] Also known as episialin, MUC-1, polymorphic epithelial mucin (PEM) and epithelian membrane antigen (EMA).
[e] Numerous anticlonal antibodies to CEA have been developed (reviewed in ref. 40).

SGA, sebaceous gland antigen; ESA, epithelial surface antigen; FBP, folate-binding protein; PI, phosphatidyl inositol; CEA, carcinoembryonic antigen; PLAP, placental-type alkaline phosphatase; NC, not yet characterized.

HMFG, was reported to have an even greater specificity toward carcinomas. After molecular cloning of the gene coding for the mucin recognized by these mAbs (designated MUC-1), it was found that the antibodies are directed primarily against the peptide backbone of the mucins and that they recognize the repetitive amino acid sequence in this type of mucin (29,31). The MUC-1 antibodies differ in the precise amino acid sequences that they recognize and in the degree of involvement of carbohydrate residues to the epitope (Table 3). These mAbs therefore differ in their degree of selectivity for tumors over normal tissues. Studies have led to the concept that the peptide cores in mucins from tumors are more exposed than the peptide cores in normal mucins, which may result from underglycosylation of mucins in tumors. It should be noted that the high-molecular-weight glycoprotein with the MUC-1 peptide sequence is not a typical mucin in that it has a transmembrane sequence. Its relationship to more typical, secreted mucins is still being studied.

Detailed immunohistological studies have investigated the expression of the MUC-1 epitope in ovarian cancer (32). All studies reported that a high proportion of tumors were positive for these mAbs. Ward et al.,

TABLE 3. *Epitopes in MUC-1 mucin tandem repeat sequences recognized by monoclonal antibodies[a,b]*

Antibody	Epitope[c]
BC 1, 2, 3	APDTR
BrE-2	TRP
BrE-3	TRP
F36/22	RPAP
HMFG-1	PDTR
HMFG-2	DTR
OM-1	APDTRP
RINA 9/22	DTR
RINA 5/3	DTR
SM-3	PDTRP

[a] Repetitive sequence of MUC-1: -VTSAPDTRPAPGSTAPPAHG-. Single letter amino acid code: V, valine; T, threonine; S, serine; A, alanine; P, proline; D, aspartic acid, R, arginine; G, glycine; H, histidine; *, potential glycosylation sites.

[b] Other monoclonal antibodies, these include (e.g., DF3, E29, Mc5, 139H2, CU18, C595, and M15) are known to recognize this repeat structure, but the precise epitope has not been defined.

[c] Antibodies differ in the degree that glycosylation of the peptide influences their reactivity with the epitope.

(33) reported a relationship between antigen expression and tumor grade. Well-differentiated tumors were almost all positive (90%), whereas 78% of moderately differentiated tumors and only 40% of poorly differentiated tumors were positive. In breast cancer, patients with DF3-positive tumors had a superior disease-free survival that was related to the higher differentiation grade of their tumors (34). Normal ovarian epithelium was reported to be poorly reactive or nonreactive with these antibodies, but many other epithelial tissues were positive, including most glandular epithelial cells. Simple follicular and germinal inclusion cysts were nonreactive with mAb F36/22. Monoclonal antibody SM3 is better at distinguishing malignant tumors from benign lesions and normal OSE than the other mAbs (35,36), but it also appears to be a relatively weak antibody.

In contrast to the anti-peptide mAbs, the antibodies that react with carbohydrate structures on mucins have a wide spectrum of specificities. The majority of these are blood-group-related and will be discussed in a later section. Several other mAbs recognize well-defined determinants on mucins that seem to encompass both peptide and carbohydrate portions of the antigen or to require the three-dimensional conformation of the mucin to be intact. The latter group includes mAbs (e.g., MT334) that lose their reactivity with antigen when the disulfide bonds in the mucin are disrupted by reduction (37, and K.O. Lloyd, unpublished results). The MT334 antigen is expressed preferentially in benign mucinous cystadenomas and tumors of low malignant potential (LMP).

Carcinoembryonic Antigen

The carcinoembryonic antigen (CEA) is expressed in the majority of mucinous ovarian tumors (both benign and malignant) and in a proportion of endometrial carcinomas, but not generally in serous tumors (38). This antigen, first described as a colonic carcinoma marker, is a glycoprotein of 180,000 daltons. Gene cloning has demonstrated that CEA has a highly conserved repeating structure (39) and many antibodies to this antigen recognize the repeated epitopes (40). One of the first studies of radiolabelled antibodies in the localization of ovarian tumors used antibodies to CEA (41).

Blood Group Antigens

Blood group antigens, which are normally expressed on epithelia and in their secretions, often exhibit altered expression in carcinomas (42,43). Four types of alterations can occur: expression of blood group specificity in a tumor of which the tissue of origin does not normally express that antigen; overexpression of the antigenic specificity in a tumor; synthesis of a novel structure that is normally not or only minimally found in epithelia; and loss of a particular blood group specificity. In addition to these structural aspects, another factor that contributes to the role of blood group antigens (and mucins in general) as tumor markers results from a change in cellular distribution. Blood-group-bearing molecules are normally secreted in the lumen of ducts or are localized on the luminal surface of tissues. In tumors, this localization of mucins becomes altered, and the molecules appear in an intracellular localization as well as luminally. They are also secreted into the bloodstream. In the latter instance, they often serve as serum markers for malignancy.

Two families of blood antigens show significant alterations in carcinomas, including ovarian cancer: the A,B,O, Lewis family and the T/Tn family. Antigens of the first group are carried both by glycolipids and glycoproteins (particularly mucins), whereas antigens of the second group are found only on mucins. The structure of the antigenic determinants in these two blood group systems are summarized in Fig. 1. Changes in a number of these specificities have been associated with epithelial cancers. As shown in the figure above, in the T/Tn family the structures associated with cancer are intermediate or abnormal products in the biosynthesis of the normal, mature form.

As in some other carcinomas, ovarian carcinomas tend to show deletions in their A,B, and O(H) antigens (44,45). Whether these deletions in ovarian carcinomas are associated with aggressive tumors and poor prognoses, as they are in bladder cancer, is not known.

A, B, O, Lewis Family

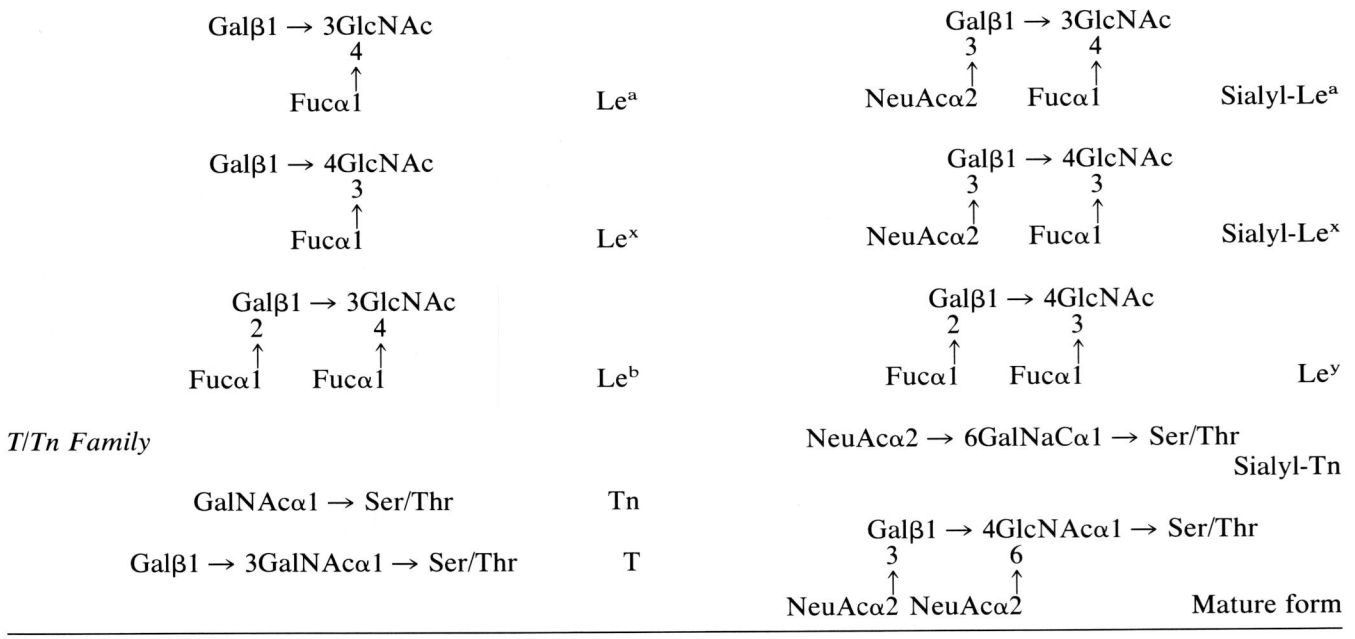

$$\begin{array}{c} Gal\beta1 \rightarrow 3GlcNAc \\ {}_{}4 \\ {}_{}\uparrow \\ Fuc\alpha1 \end{array} \quad Le^a$$

$$\begin{array}{c} Gal\beta1 \rightarrow 3GlcNAc \\ 34 \\ \uparrow\uparrow \\ NeuAc\alpha2Fuc\alpha1 \end{array} \quad Sialyl\text{-}Le^a$$

$$\begin{array}{c} Gal\beta1 \rightarrow 4GlcNAc \\ {}_{}3 \\ {}_{}\uparrow \\ Fuc\alpha1 \end{array} \quad Le^x$$

$$\begin{array}{c} Gal\beta1 \rightarrow 4GlcNAc \\ 33 \\ \uparrow\uparrow \\ NeuAc\alpha2Fuc\alpha1 \end{array} \quad Sialyl\text{-}Le^x$$

$$\begin{array}{c} Gal\beta1 \rightarrow 3GlcNAc \\ 24 \\ \uparrow\uparrow \\ Fuc\alpha1Fuc\alpha1 \end{array} \quad Le^b$$

$$\begin{array}{c} Gal\beta1 \rightarrow 4GlcNAc \\ 23 \\ \uparrow\uparrow \\ Fuc\alpha1Fuc\alpha1 \end{array} \quad Le^y$$

T/Tn Family

$$GalNAc\alpha1 \rightarrow Ser/Thr \quad Tn$$

$$Gal\beta1 \rightarrow 3GalNAc\alpha1 \rightarrow Ser/Thr \quad T$$

$$NeuAc\alpha2 \rightarrow 6GalNAc\alpha1 \rightarrow Ser/Thr \quad Sialyl\text{-}Tn$$

$$\begin{array}{c} Gal\beta1 \rightarrow 4GlcNAc\alpha1 \rightarrow Ser/Thr \\ 36 \\ \uparrow\uparrow \\ NeuAc\alpha2NeuAc\alpha2 \end{array} \quad Mature\ form$$

Gal, galactose; GlcNAc, N-acetylglucosamine; GalNAc, N-acetylgalactosamine; Fuc, fucose; NeuAc, N-acetylneuraminic acid

FIG. 1. Structures of Carbohydrate Epitopes of the A,B,O, Lewis and T/Tn Families.

Metoki et al. (44) showed that some O and B blood group patients express A blood group antigen in their tumors in an "incompatible" or "anomalous" situation. Lewis blood group antigens are also of interest in ovarian cancer. Rubin et al. (45) noted that only a subset of ovarian carcinomas show strong Le^a and Le^b expression, whereas most of the tumors expressed Le^y antigen. Two antibodies (B1 and B3) that react relatively with mucinous adenocarcinomas were shown to identify Le^y and Le^x-related antigens, respectively (46). Another mAb (BR96), raised against breast cancer, has been shown to identify a Le^y-related structure (47).

Sialylated forms of Lewis antigens also serve as markers for ovarian cancer. Monoclonal antibody 19-9, which detects the sialylated Le^a determinant, has received particular attention. CA19.9 is more highly expressed in mucinous adenocarcinomas and endometrioid carcinomas than in serous adenocarcinomas (38,48). Its expression closely follows that of CEA. Serum levels of CA19.9 are usually elevated in patients who show strong expression of the antigen in their tumors. The sialylated form of the Type 2 chain (i.e., sialyl-Le^x) has been studied as a serum marker for ovarian cancer, but lack of tumor specificity limits its diagnostic use (49).

In the T/Tn blood group system, mAbs B72.3 (50) and CC49 (51) have received the most study. These antibodies detect the sialylated form of the Tn structure (i.e., NeuAcα2→3GalNAcα1-Ser/Thr) (52) that is carried on high-molecular-weight mucins (TAG72). Monoclonal antibody B72.3 is reactive with a wide variety of carcinomas, including ovarian cancer. It is reactive with a few normal tissues, including small intestine, stomach, esophagus, and salivary gland (53). In a detailed study of the reactivity of mAb B72.3 with ovarian tumors of different histologic types, Thor et al. (54) showed that mAb B72.3 reacts with the majority of the samples tested, including serous and mucinous cyst adenocarcinomas and undifferentiated tumors. When tumors were defined as positive if more than 5% of their cells were reactive, 67% to 100% were classified as reactive, but when the limit was set as more than 25% reactive cells, this percentage fell to 33% to 86%. Mucinous tumors were more consistently positive than other tumor types. The expression of mAb B72.3 may be hormonally regulated (55). Benign ovarian tumors were generally not reactive with mAb B72.3, but all three mucinous cystadenocarcinomas of borderline malignancy were positive. Recombinant and chimeric forms of mAb B72.3 have been produced (56). Monoclonal antibody CC49 is a "second-generation" mAb to TAG72. It appears to recognize an epitope very similar to that recognized by mAb B72.3, but it has a higher avidity and stains a higher proportion of tumors with greater intensity (57). T antigen was reported to be present in 67% of ovarian carcinomas and to be poorly expressed or not expressed at all in benign tumors (58).

Epithelial Surface Antigen

Immunization of mice with a variety of human carcinomas, including ovarian carcinomas, has consistently resulted in the generation of mAbs that react with the glycoprotein ESA (also known as KSA, EPG, and GA733) of about 38,000 daltons. ESA is preferentially expressed on epithelial tissues and carcinomas. The mAbs that react with ESA include MH99 (developed by immunization with ovarian cancer cells (59)), 17-1A (developed by immunization with colon cancer (60)), KS1/4 (developed by immunization with lung cancer (61)), AUA1 (developed by immunization with colon cancer cells (62)), and HEA125 (developed by immunization with colon cancer cells (63)). ESA is expressed in the epithelial cells in all organs of the body. In some multilayered epithelia such as the skin and esophagus, only the basal layer is positive. Nonepithelial tissues and the tumors that are derived from them (e.g., sarcomas, melanomas, astrocytomas, neuroblastomas, leukemias and lymphomas) are ESA-negative. Although ESA has received considerable attention as a carcinoma-associated antigen, its enhanced expression in tumor cells is uncertain. The mAbs that react with ESA, unlike most anti-carcinoma mAbs, recognize a membrane antigen with a very uniform distribution in tumors. ESA is not shed or secreted from cells and is designated as a "surface" antigen (64). It serves as an important marker for distinguishing carcinomas from nonepithelial tumors.

A considerable amount of information is available on the biochemical and molecular structure of ESA. In cell lines, ESA occurs in two forms: a 38,000-dalton glycoprotein or a disulfide bond-linked dimer with 32,00 and 6,000 dalton subunits. Most cell lines contain both forms of ESA, and the 32 kD and 6 kD forms may result from proteolytic cleavage of the 38 kD form (64). Molecular cloning of ESA identified a gene coding for 314 amino acids, including a 23-amino-acid signal sequence with a transmembrane region and a short cytoplasmic tail (65,66). The protein has an arg-arg sequence at positions 80 and 81, which may represent a proteolytic cleavage site that results in the 32 kD and 6 kD forms of ESA. It has been suggested that ESA is a member of a family of adhesion molecules (67). A second gene related to ESA was cloned by Linnebach et al. (68), but this gene product is not recognized by any of the well-characterized mAbs to ESA.

Folate-Binding Protein

Three other mAbs raised to ovarian cancer (MOv-18, MOv-19, and MW207) also recognize a glycoprotein with a molecular weight of about 38,000 daltons (16,69). Although this antigen is expressed on a variety of normal epithelial tissues, it has a more restricted distribution on normal epithelia than ESA. MOv-18 and MOv-19 have been used in a variety of preclinical and clinical studies on ovarian cancer. The glycoprotein recognized by mAb MOv-18 has recently been shown to be anchored to the cell membrane through a glycosyl-phosphatidyl-inositol linkage (70). Isolation of a cDNA coding for this antigen (71) demonstrated its identity to folate-binding protein (FBP). Both membrane and soluble forms of FBP have previously been recognized. They are thought to act in the transport of folate across plasma membranes or to concentrate folate in fluid, respectively. The role of FBP in ovarian cancer is as yet unclear. Nevertheless, its possible role in conferring selective advantage to the proliferation of cancer cells and its regulation by hormonal levels encourages further study.

Other Ovarian Tumor Antigens

Many other mAbs to ovarian cancer have been developed, but most of them have not reached clinical studies. In some cases, the antigens recognized have not yet been characterized. A few of these will be discussed briefly here (see Table 2).

A number of mAbs that react selectively with mucinous ovarian tumors have been developed, including ID_3, which is derived by the immunization of mice with an ovarian cystadenocarcinoma extract (72). In one study, ID_3 reacted with all mucinous cystadenocarcinomas tested, but it did not react with the three benign mucinous cystadenomas. The mAb OM-A was reactive with the majority of mucinous tumors that were analyzed, including malignant, LMP, and benign tumors (73). Serous and clear cell tumors were negative, and two-thirds of endometrioid tumors were weakly positive. Normal tissues were not reactive. The biochemical nature of the antigen detected by mAb OM-A is unknown, but the epitope recognized is thought to be a carbohydrate structure. Monoclonal antibody 4C7 also reacts preferentially with mucinous tumors (74).

Monoclonal antibody Ki-OCI-6-2 is unusual because of its almost complete selectiveness for ovarian adenocarcinomas (75). Among normal cells, only epididymal epithelia were positive and, among tumors only one-fourth of hypernephromas were reactive.

Monoclonal antibody MX35 reacts with a very high proportion of ovarian carcinomas, and its distribution within tumors is relatively uniform (16,45). Both solid tumors and ascites cells show this type of reactivity. This antibody was among a panel selected for possible intraperitoneal (IP) use because of their lack of reactivity with the normal peritoneal lining. MX35 does, however, react with a number of other normal epithelia, including bronchus, kidney collecting ducts, fallopian tube, uterus and cervix. The biochemical nature of the antigen recognized is unknown.

Placental-type alkaline phosphatase (PLAP) has also received attention as a marker for ovarian epithelial cancer. This enzyme is present in a proportion of ovarian carcinomas and small amounts can be found in a number of normal tissues (76). Anti-PLAP antibodies have been used in radiolocalization studies (77).

Although a number of oncogene products show enhanced or abnormal expression in ovarian tumors, they are not, in general, suitable targets for immunological attack because of their intracellular location. One exception is the HER2 oncogene product p185. This glycoprotein, which is a truncated form of the epidermal growth factor receptor, is a cell-surface component that is expressed in a substantial proportion of ovarian cancers and in other tumors. Overexpression of HER2 is thought to be associated with poor survival in advanced ovarian cancer (78), and it could therefore serve as a target for antibodies in overexpressing tumors. In addition, the possible antiproliferative effects of anti-HER2 antibody on cultured tumor cells, and indications that its expression leads to enhanced cytokine and cisplatin killing will open new avenues of exploration (79).

HUMAN MONOCLONAL ANTIBODIES TO OVARIAN CANCER

Two incentives have encouraged the development of human mAbs that react with human tumors: the opportunity to examine the autologous antibody response to tumor antigens at the clonal level, and the generation of antibodies that could be used clinically without the drawbacks of mouse antibodies (e.g., a reduced anti-Ig response). Unfortunately, the technology for the production of human mAbs lags behind that for mouse mAbs. The two currently available approaches are the immortalization of B-lymphocytes by Epstein-Barr virus infection and the generation of human-human or human-mouse hybridomas, but neither is easy to apply (80). However, methods that use molecular cloning techniques hold some hope for the future (81). Thus far, only one human mAb has been developed from the lymphocytes of ovarian cancer patients (82). An IgG lambda antibody (14C1) developed from the lymph node cells of an ovarian cancer patient was shown to be reactive with 88% of the ovarian carcinoma tissues examined. A wide range of other normal and malignant tissues were unreactive. Monoclonal antibody 14C1 recognizes antigens of 26 kD and 32 kD in ovarian cancer cells. It carries out ADCC killing in vitro and may therefore be useful in the treatment of ovarian cancer.

SERUM MARKERS IN THE DIAGNOSIS AND MONITORING OF EPITHELIAL OVARIAN CANCER

One of the main goals in the search for ovarian tumor antigens is to develop serum markers that could be used in the diagnosis and monitoring of ovarian cancer. Unfortunately, of the numerous mAbs that have been developed, only OC-125 has provided a useful assay, and even this relatively specific antigen is unsuitable for the initial diagnosis of ovarian cancer. However, OC 125 has considerable utility in monitoring the clinical course of the disease and predicting recurrence. Other markers [e.g., CEA, B72.3, 19.9, CA-15-3, NB/70K, and MUC-1 (DF3)] have also been assessed for use in ovarian cancer. The use of two different markers may enhance specificity and sensitivity for the detection of ovarian cancer, although no combination has yet been found that is superior to OC-125 alone. Because tumors differ in the expression of a certain antigen, and individual tumors are usually heterogenous in their antigen expression, a combination of tumor markers seems to be a rational approach. The recently described marker CF511 seems promising; it was not elevated in 220 normal individuals, and it was detected in 42% to 96% of ovarian cancer patients (83). For detailed analysis of the clinical utility of serum markers in ovarian cancer, the reader is referred to other sources (84,85).

ANTIBODIES IN THE RADIOLOCALIZATION OF TUMORS

The use of radiolabeled antibodies for the detection of occult cancer is currently an active area of investigation. The detection during surgery of occult tumor lesions and the early detection of recurrence would have important clinical implications. Although the use of radiolabeled mAbs for these purposes is an extremely attractive idea, many obstacles must be overcome before the method can be used in routine practice. The selective specificity of the mAb for tumor is the most obvious parameter to be considered. Other parameters are the ability to radiolabel the antibody, the use of intact Ig versus $F(ab')_2$ or Fab fragments, the choice of radionuclide, and the isotype and affinity of the antibody. Other factors that become considerations in vivo include the size of the tumor, the antigen heterogeneity and density, the internalization of the antigen-antibody complex, the degree of elicitation of an antimouse Ig response, the route of inoculation, and the degree of penetration of antibody into the tumor. Although not all these problems have been solved or even examined completely, further progress can be expected in the near future in this rapidly evolving field. Advances in genetic engineering have already led to the production of "chimeric" or "humanized" antibodies that are less immunogenic in patients. Radiolabeling techniques continue to improve. A number of studies have emphasized the heterogeneity of antigen expression in ovarian carcinomas (86,87), thus supporting the use of a panel of antibodies in such studies. Conversely, the finding that multiple and recurrent tumors in the same patients retain a constant pattern of antibody reactivity has simplified the choice of antibody that is suitable for an individual patient (4,88).

A limited number of preclinical and clinical trials have been carried out on radiolabeled mAbs in the localization of ovarian cancer. Ward and Wallace (89) studied the localization of ^{131}I-labeled mAb HMFG-2 and compared IP versus intravenous routes of administration in nude mice. They concluded that, for ascites cells, the IP route was most efficient, but the IP route had relatively little advantage for solid tumors. In a similar study, Thédrez, et al. (90) analyzed the IP biodistribution of ^{111}In-labeled mAb OC-125 in nu/nu mice that carried the ovarian cancer cell line OVCAR-3 intraperitoneally. High, specific uptake after IP injection of the antibody was found. Wahl and coworkers (91) reached similar conclusions. Although the IP route of administration of antibody gives initial high concentrations of antibody in the peritoneal cavity, antibody levels eventually equilibrate with the blood pool. Various methods have been examined to reduce the levels of antibody that escape into the blood, thus optimizing the IP effect and avoiding exposure of extraperitoneal sites to radiation. Mattes (92) showed that conjugation of galactose residues to antibody resulted in the rapid clearance of circulating antibody via the galactose-receptor of the liver, and IP injection of galactose-conjugated antibodies into mice bearing IP tumors resulted in very high tumor to nontumor ratios (93). The administration of an antimouse Ig second antibody achieves a similar effect, but it has the disadvantage of introducing another foreign protein into the system. A number of methods for improving tumor to nontumor ratios has also been examined, including two- and three-step procedures using biotin-coupled antibody with or without avidin to amplify the radioactive signal.

Radiolocalization studies have been carried out in ovarian cancer patients using a number of antibodies: anti-CEA, HMFG-1, HMFG-2, OC-125 and AUA1. The radioisotopes used in these studies were ^{125}I, ^{131}I, ^{123}I, ^{111}In or ^{90}Y. Each study reported positive scans and often obtained high sensitivity and specificity for the detection of ovarian tumors. For example, Hunter et al. (94), using ^{111}In-labeled OC-125, found a good correlation between antibody scans and the presence of tumor at second-look surgery (14 true-positive scans, 2 false-positive scans, 2 true-negative scans, and 2 false-negative scans). These studies and others have led to the conclusion that, although significant advances have been made, several problems must be overcome before this approach can be routinely used for the diagnosis of ovarian tumors or to replace second-look laparatomy for detecting recurrence.

IMMUNOTHERAPY OF OVARIAN CANCER USING ANTIBODIES

Three general approaches may be considered in the use of mAbs for the immunotherapy of cancer: (a) the use of unconjugated antibodies with the ability to kill cancer cells directly by activating complement or using antibody-dependent cytotoxicity, by inducing a nonspecific antiinflammatory response, or by interfering with growth in some way (e.g., by reacting with growth factor receptors); (b) the use of mAbs conjugated to agents that can kill cells (e.g., radioisotopes, drugs, or toxins); and (c) the use of bifunctional antibodies to redirect cytotoxic T-lymphocytes to the tumor in order to kill tumor cells.

The first approach has not been used extensively in ovarian cancer, possibly because the available mAbs lack suitable effector properties. An exception is the recent study by Goodman, et al. (95) of mAb L6 in nine ovarian cancer patients and a number of other carcinoma patients. The antibody (Ig2a subclass) was well-tolerated at quite high doses. No clinical responses were observed in the ovarian cancer patients, but a breast cancer patient achieved complete remission.

To circumvent the noncytotoxic nature of most mAbs, extensive efforts have been directed toward the production and testing of antibodies coupled with toxic agents. The use of plant and bacterial toxins for this purpose has received considerable attention because of the extreme toxicity of some of the agents (e.g., ricin, diphtheria toxin, pseudomonas toxin). Because these agents act internally in the cell, the antibody conjugate must be bound to the tumor relatively specifically and must be endocytosed and carried to its intracellular target. Considerable success has been achieved in constructing immunoconjugates that kill tumor cells in vitro, and a number of animal trials have also been successful. An antitransferrin receptor–ricin A chain conjugate inhibited the growth of OVCAR-3 cells in vivo (96). Likewise, Pastan and coworkers (97) showed the effectiveness of OVB3 antibody–Pseudomonas toxin conjugate in a mouse model system. However, the results of trials in patients with a variety of immunoconjugates have to date been disappointing. The problems involved have been pinpointed, and they may be overcome in the future. Recent advances in the field include the modification of toxins by recombinant DNA methods to reduce side effects and the use of similar methods to produce chimeric antibody-toxin molecules.

The use of drug-antibody conjugates capitalizes on the large number of drugs already in use for the treatment of cancer. The specificity of antibodies can guide drugs selectively to cancer cells. The design of these conjugates requires considerable effort and ingenuity. A particularly difficult problem is the need to regenerate free drug once the conjugate has attached to the tumor cell or become internalized. The design of cleavable linkers has attracted much attention. As with toxin conjugates, impressive killing has been achieved in vitro and in some mouse model systems (47,98). Clinical studies using drug-antibody conjugates have just begun; no studies appear to have been published on the use of these conjugates in ovarian cancer.

Radioimmunotherapy of ovarian cancer, on the other hand, has received considerable attention, particularly by Epenetos's group at the Hammersmith Hospital in London. This group recently reported the results of two trials on ovarian cancer, the first using ^{131}I-labeled antibodies (99) and the second using ^{90}Y-labeled antibodies (100). Antibodies were HMFG-1, HMFG-2, AUA1, and anti-PLAP were administered intraperitoneally. The ^{131}I study reported partial or complete responses in five of twenty-one patients with small lesions or microscopic disease. The ^{90}Y study was complicated by myelosuppression and bone marrow toxicity observed at relatively low doses of isotope (200 mCi). These complications were apparently caused by the instability of the yttrium conjugate in vivo. A number of problems with radioimmunotherapy are apparent. They include the need to improve the proportion of radiolabelled antibody that localizes to the tumor (i.e., higher percentage injected dose/g), the need for better and more stable isotope-antibody conjugates, and the need for methods of overcoming a human antimouse Ig response.

Bifunctional antibodies, with one arm directed to a tumor-associated antigen and the other to a T-lymphocyte antigen such as CD3, are designed to direct cytotoxic T cells to tumor cells irrespective of tumor specificity (101). Preclinical studies have examined the parameters involved in this novel approach to therapy. Several of these have been carried out on ovarian cancer cells either in vitro or using the OVCAR-3-bearing nu/nu mouse model (102,103). Garrido et al. (103) tested three different antibodies that were linked to an anti-CD3 antibody in combination with peripheral blood lymphocytes from normal donors. A significant increase in tumor-free mice in the treated animal group was reported. The mechanism of the effect was confirmed by the demonstration that, alone, anti-tumor antibody, anti-CD3 antibody, or lymphocytes were ineffective.

CELLULAR IMMUNOTHERAPY

The in vitro experiments discussed earlier on the generation of anti-tumor cell lymphocytes and macrophages opened the way to the application of adoptive cellular immunotherapy in the clinical treatment of cancer. A number of such trials have been carried out for ovarian cancer. The cytotoxic effects of IL-2-activated peripheral blood and tumor-infiltrating lymphocytes were compared (104). The lytic activity was present in an NK cell population. The IP administration of IL-2 as a method of generating cytotoxic cells in situ with the use of additional lymphokine-activated killer cells has also been examined (105,106). Minor or no anti-tumor responses were observed. These trials are associated with the dose-limiting toxicities of IL-2. Methods of overcoming this problem must be developed before cellular immunotherapy can be used successfully in the clinical treatment of ovarian cancer. Ferrini et al. (107) targeted T-lymphocytes bearing the gamma/delta T cell receptor on the basis of their uniform cytotoxic properties. Bifunctional antibodies with anti-$\gamma\delta/\beta$ t-cell receptor and anti-FBP (MOv-19) showed specific cytolytic activity against ovarian cancer cells in vitro. Future developments in this area will include the use of humanized antibodies or antibody fragments, cytokine therapy, and methods for improving the trafficking of lymphocytes to solid tumors.

REFERENCES

1. Lloyd KO. Molecular characteristics of tumor antigens. *Immunol Allergy Clinics of N America* 1990;10:765–779.
2. Oettgen HF, Rettig WJ, Lloyd KO, Old LJ. Serologic analysis of human cancer. *Immunol Allergy Clinics of N America* 1990;10:607–637.
3. Whiteside TL, Herberman RB. Characteristics of natural killer cells and lymphokine-activated killer cells: Their role in the biology and treatment of human cancer. *Immunol Allergy Clinics of N America* 1990;10:663–704.
4. Esgro JJ, Whitworth P, Fidler IJ. Macrophages as effectors of tumor immunity. *Immunol Allergy Clinics of N America* 1990;10:705–729.
5. Kutteh WH, Welander CE, Homesley HD, Doellgast GJ. Autologous antibodies eluted from membrane fragments isolated from the effusions of human ovarian epithelial neoplasm. I. Quantitation of antibodies. *Am J Obstet Gynecol* 1985;153:124–129.
6. Kutteh WH, Doellgast GJ. Autologous antibodies eluted from membrane fragments in human ovarian epithelial neoplastic effusions. II. Tissue specificity and reactivity. *JNCI* 1986;76:797–803.
7. Dorsett BH, Ioachim HL, Stolbach L, Walker J, Barber HRK. Isolation of tumor-specific antibodies from effusions of ovarian carcinomas. *Int J Cancer* 1975;16:779–780.
8. Anderson NE, Rosenblum MK, Posner JB. Paraneoplastic cerebellar degeneration: Clinical-immunological correlations. *Ann Neurol* 1988;24:559–567.
9. Furneaux HM, Dropcho EJ, Barbut D, et al. Characterization of a cDNA encoding a 34-kDa Purkinje neuron protein recognized by sera from patients with paraneoplastic cerebellar degeneration. *Proc Natl Acad Sci (USA)* 1989;86:2873–2877.
10. Ioannides CG, Platsoucas CD, Rashed S, Wharton JT, Ed-

wards CL, Freedman RS. Tumor cytolysis by lymphocytes infiltrating ovarian malignant ascites. *Cancer Res* 1991;51:4257–4265.
11. Heo DS, Whiteside TL, Kanbour A, Herberman RB. Lymphocytes infiltrating human ovarian tumors: I. Role of Leu-19 (NKH1)-positive recombinant IL-2-activated cultures of lymphocytes infiltrating human ovarian tumors. *J Immunol* 1988;140:4042–4049.
12. Wang YL, Lusheng S, Kanbour A, Herberman RB, Whiteside TL. Lymphocytes infiltrating human ovarian tumors: Synergy between tumor necrosis factor alpha and interleukin 2 in the generation of CD8+ effectors from tumor-infiltrating lymphocytes. *Cancer Res* 1989;49:5979–5985.
13. Vaccarello L, Wang YL, Whiteside TL. Sustained outgrowth of autotumor-reactive T-lymphocytes from human ovarian carcinomas in the presence of tumor necrosis factor alpha and interleukin 2. *Human Immunol* 1990;28:216–227.
14. Nicosia SV, Nicosia RF. Azar HA, eds. Neoplasms of the ovarian mesothelium. In: *Pathology of Human Neoplasms*. New York: Raven Press; 1989:435–486.
15. Van Niekerk CC, Boerman OC, Ramaekers FCS, Poels LG. Marker profile of different phases in the transition of normal human ovarian epithelium to ovarian carcinomas. *Amer J Pathol* 1991;138:455–463.
16. Mattes MJ, Look K, Furukawa K, et al. Mouse monoclonal antibodies to human epithelial differentiation antigens expressed on the surface of ovarian carcinoma ascites cells. *Cancer Res* 1987;47:6741–6750.
17. Jordon D, Jagirdar J, Kaneko M. Blood group antigens, Lewis^x and Lewis^y in the diagnostic discrimination of malignant mesothelioma versus adenocarcinoma. *Amer J Pathol* 1989;135:931–937.
18. Bast RC, Feeney M, Lazarus H, Nadler LM, Colvin RC, Knapp RC. Reactivity of a monoclonal antibody with human ovarian carcinoma. *J Clin Invest* 1981;68:1331–1337.
19. Kabawat SE, Bast RC, Welch WR, Knapp RC, Colvin RB. Immunopathologic characterization of a monoclonal antibody that recognizes common surface antigens of human ovarian tumors of serous, endometrioid, and clear cell types. *Amer J Clin Pathol* 1983;79:98–104.
20. Cordon Cardo C, Mattes MJ, Melamed MR, Lewis JL Jr, Old LJ, Lloyd KO. Immunopathologic analysis of a panel of mouse monoclonal antibodies reacting with human ovarian carcinomas and other human tumors. *Int J Gynecol Pathol* 1985;4:121–130.
21. Berchuck A, Soisson AP, Clarke-Pearson DL, et al. Immunohistochemical expression of CA125 in endometrial adenocarcinoma: Correlation of antigen expression with metastatic potential. *Cancer Res* 1989;49:2091–2095.
22. Kabawat SE, Bast RC Jr, Bhan AK, Welch WR, Knapp RC, Colvin RB. Tissue distribution of a coelomic-epithelium-related antigen recognized by the monoclonal antibody OC125. *Int J Gynecol Pathol* 1983;2:275–285.
23. de Bruijn HWA, Calkoen-Carpay TB, Jager S, Duk JM, Aalders JG, Fleuren GJ. The tumor marker CA125 is a common constituent of normal cervical mucus. *Am J Obstet Gynecol* 1986;154:1088–1091.
24. Matsuoka Y, Nakashima T, Endo K, et al. Recognition of ovarian cancer antigen CA125 by murine monoclonal antibody produced by immunization of lung cancer cells. *Cancer Res* 1987;47:6335–6340.
25. Davis HM, Zurawski VR, Bast RC, Sr., Klug TL. Characterization of the CA125 antigen associated with human epithelial ovarian cancer. *Cancer Res* 1986;46:6143–6148.
26. Taylor-Papadimitriou J. Report on the first international workshop on carcinoma-associated mucins. *Int J Cancer* 1991;49:1–5.
27. Carlstedt I, Sheenan J, Cornfeld AP, Gallagher JT. Mucus glycoproteins: A gel of a problem. *Essays Biochem* 1985;20:40–76.
28. Taylor-Papadimitriou J, Gendler SJ. Molecular aspects of mucins. *Cancer Rev* 1988;11–12:11–24.
29. Hilkens, J. Biochemistry and functions of mucins in malignant disease. *Cancer Rev* 1988;11–12:25–54.
30. Feizi T. Demonstration by monoclonal antibodies that carbohydrate structures of glycoproteins and glycolipids are oncodevelopmental antigens. *Nature* 1985;314:53–57.
31. Gendler S, Taylor-Papadimitriou J, Duhig T, Rothbard J, Burchell J. A highly immunogenic region of a human polymorphic epithelial mucin expressed by carcinomas is made up of tandem repeats. *J Biol Chem* 1988;263:12820–12823.
32. Zotter S, Hageman PC, Lossnitzer A, Mooi WJ, Hilgers J. Tissue and tumor distribution of human polymorphic epithelial mucin. *Cancer Rev* 1988;11–12:55–101.
33. Ward BG, Lowe DG, Shepherd JH. Patterns of expression of a tumor associated antigen, defined by the monoclonal antibody HMFG2, in human epithelial ovarian carcinoma: Comparison with expression of the HMFG1, AUA1, and F36/22 antigens. *Cancer* 1987;60:787–793.
34. Hayes DF, Mesa-Tejada R, Papsidero LD, et al. Prediction of prognosis in primary breast cancer by detection of a high molecular weight mucin-like antigen using monoclonal antibodies DF3, F36/22, and CU18: A cancer and leukemia group B study. *J Clin Oncol* 1991;9:1113–1123.
35. Girling A, Bartkova J, Burchell J, Gendler S, Gillett C, Taylor-Papadimitriou J. A core protein epitope of the polymorphic epithelial mucin detected by the monoclonal antibody SM-3 is selectively exposed in a range of primary carcinomas. *Int J Cancer* 1989;43:1072–1076.
36. Van Dam PA, Lowe DG, Watson JV, Jobling TW, Chard T, Shepherd JH. Multi-parameter flow cytometric quantitation of the expression of the tumor-associated antigen SM3 in normal and neoplasic ovarian tissues. *Cancer* 1991;68:169–177.
37. Mattes MJ, Look K, Lewis JL Jr, Old LJ, Lloyd KO. Three mouse monoclonal antibodies to human differentiation antigens: reactivity with two mucin-like antigens and with connective tissue fibers. *J Histochem Cytochem* 1985;33:1095–1102.
38. Charpin C, Bhan AK, Zurawski VR Jr, Scully RE. Carcinoembryonic antigen (CEA) and carbohydrate determinant 19-9 (A19-9) localization in 121 primary and metastatic ovarian tumors: An immunohistochemical study with the use of monclonal antibodies. *Int J Gynecol Pathol* 1982;1:231–245.
39. Thompson JA, Pande H, Paxton RJ, et al. Molecular cloning of a gene belonging to the carcinoembryonic antigen gene family and discussion of a domain model. *Proc Natl Acad Sci (USA)* 1987;84:2965–2969.
40. Hammarstrom S, Shively JE, Paxton RJ, et al. Antigenic sites in carcinoembryonic antigen. *Cancer Res* 1989;49:4852–4858.
41. van Nagell JR, Kim E, Casper S, et al. Radioimmunodetection of primary and metastatic ovarian cancer using radiolabeled antibodies to carcinoembryonic antigen. *Cancer Res* 1980;40:502–506.
42. Lloyd KO. Philip Levine award lecture. Blood group antigens as markers for normal differentiation and malignant change in human tissues. *Am J Clin Pathol* 1987;87:129–139.
43. Hakomori S. Tumor-associated carbohydrate antigens. *Annu Rev Immunol* 1984;2:103–126.
44. Metoki R, Kakudo K, Tsuji Y, Teng N, Clausen H, Hakomori S. Deletion of histo-blood group A and B antigens and expression of incompatible A antigen in ovarian cancer. *JNCI* 1989;81:1151–1157.
45. Rubin SC, Finstad CL, Hoskins WJ, et al. Analysis of antigen expression at multiple tumor sites in epithelial ovarian cancer. *Am J Obstet Gynecol* 1991;164:558–563.
46. Pastan I, Lovelace ET, Gallo MG, Rutherford AV, Magnani JL, Willingham MC. Characterization of monoclonal antibodies B1 and B3 that react with mucinous adenocarcinomas. *Cancer Res* 1991;51:3781–3787.
47. Hellstrom I, Garrigues HJ, Garrigues U, Hellstrom KE. Highly tumor-reactive, internalizing, mouse monoclonal antibodies to Lewis^y-related case surface antigens. *Cancer Res* 1990;50:2183–2190.
48. Scharl A, Crombach G, Vierbuchen M, Göhring U-J, Göttert T, Holt JA. Antigen CA 19-9: Presence in mucosa of non-diseased müllerian duct derivatives and marker for differentiation in their carcinomas. *Obstet Gynecol* 1991;77:580–585.
49. Inoue M, Shimizu C, Sasagawa T, Shimizu H, Saito J, Tanizawa O. Sialyl Lewis-Xi antigen in patients with gynecologic tumors. *Obstet Gynecol* 1989;73:79–83.

50. Colcher D, Hand PH, Nuti M, Schlom J. A spectrum of monoclonal antibodies reactive with human mammary tumor cells. *Proc Natl Acad Sci (USA)* 1981;78:3199–3203.
51. Muraro R, Kuroki M, Wunderlich D, et al. Generation and characterization of B72.3 second generation monoclonal antibodies reactive with the tumor-associated glycoprotein 72 antigen. *Cancer Res* 1988;48:4588–4596.
52. Gold DM, Mattes MJ. Monoclonal antibody B72.3 reacts with a core region structure of O-linked carbohydrates. *Tumour Biol* 1988;9:137–144.
53. Stein R, Goldenberg DM, Mattes MJ. Normal tissue reactivity of four anti-tumor monoclonal antibodies of clinical interest. *Int J Cancer* 1991;47:163–169.
54. Thor A, Gorstein F, Ohuchi N, Szpak CA, Johnston WW, Schlom J. Tumor-associated glycoprotein (TAG-72) in ovarian carcinomas defined by monoclonal antibody B72.3. *JNCI* 1986; 76:995–1006.
55. Cajigas HE, Fariza E, Scully RE, Thor AD. Enhancement of tumor-associated glycoprotein-72 antigen expression in hormone-related ovarian serous borderline tumors. *Cancer* 1991; 68:348–354.
56. Colcher D, Milenic D, Roselli M, et al. Characterization and biodistribution of recombinant and recombinant/chimeric constructs of monclonal antibody B72.3. *Cancer Res* 1989;49: 1738–1745.
57. Molinolo A, Simpson JF, Thor A, Schlom J. Enhanced tumor binding using immunohistochemical analyses by second generation anti-tumor-associated glycoprotein 72 monoclonal antibodies versus monclonal antibody B72.3 in human tissue. *Cancer Res* 1990;50:1291–1298.
58. Ghazizadeh M, Oguro T, Sasaki Y, Aihara K, Araki T, Springer GF. Immunohistochemical and ultrastructural localization of T antigen in ovarian tumors. *Amer J Clin Pathol* 1990;93:315–321.
59. Mattes MJ, Cairncross JG, Old LJ, Lloyd KO. Monoclonal antibodies to three widely distributed human cell surface antigens. *Hybridoma* 1983;2:253–264.
60. Herlyn M, Streplewski Z, Herlyn D, Koprowski H. Colorectal carcinoma-specific antigen: Detection by means of monoclonal antibodies. *Proc Natl Acad Sci (USA)* 1979;76:1435–1442.
61. Varki NM, Reisfeld RA, Walker LE. Antigens associated with tumor lung carcinoma defined by monoclonal antibodies. *Cancer Res* 1984;44:681–687.
62. Durbin H, Rodrigues N, Bodmer WF. Further characterization, isolation and identification of the epithelial cell-surface antigen defined by monoclonal antibody AUA1. *Int J Cancer* 1990;45:562–565.
63. Moldenhauer G, Momburg F, Möller P, Schwartz R, Hämmerling GJ. Epithelium-specific surface glycoprotein of Mr 34,000 is a widely distributed human carcinoma marker. *Br J Cancer* 1987;56:714–721.
64. Thampoe IJ, Ng JSC, Lloyd KO. Biochemical analysis of a human epithelial surface antigen: Differential cell expression and processing. *Arch Biochem Biophys* 1988;267:342–352.
65. Perez MS, Walker LE. Isolation and characterization of a cDNA encoding the KS1/4 epithelial carcinoma marker. *J Immunol* 1989;142:3662–3667.
66. Strand J, Hamilton AE, Beavers LS, et al. Molecular cloning and characterization of a human adenocarcinoma/epithelial cell surface antigen complementary DNA. *Cancer Res* 1989;49: 314–317.
67. Simon B, Podolsky DK, Moldenhauer G, Isselbacher KJ, Gattoni-Celli S, Brand SJ. Epithelial glycoprotein is a member of a family of epithelial cell surrface antigens homologous to nidogen, a matrix adhesion protein. *Proc Natl Acad Sci (USA)* 1990; 87:2755–2759.
68. Linnebach AJ, Wojcierowski J, Wu S, et al. Sequence investigation of the major gastrointestinal tumor-associated antigen gene family, GA733. *Proc Natl Acad Sci (USA)* 1989;88:27–31.
69. Miotti S, Canevari S, Ménard S, et al. Characterization of human ovarian carcinoma-associated antigens defined by novel monoclonal antibodies with tumor-restricted specificity. *Int J Cancer* 1987;39:297–303.
70. Alberti S, Miotti S, Fornaro M, et al. The Ca-MOv18 molecule, a cell-surface marker of human ovarian carcinomas, is anchored to the cell membrane by phosphatidylinositol. *Biochem Biophys Res Commun* 1990;171:1051–1055.
71. Campbell IG, Jones TA, Foulkes WD, Trowsdale J. Folate-binding protein is a marker for ovarian cancer. *Cancer Res* 1991;51:5329–5338.
72. Gangopadhyay A, Bhattacharya M, Chatterjee SK, Barlow JJ, Tsukada Y. Immunoperoxidase localization of a high-molecular-weight mucin recognized by monoclonal antibody 1D$_3$. *Cancer Res* 1985;45:1744–1752.
73. Sakakibara K, Ueda R, Ohta M, Nakashima N, Tomoda Y, Takahashi T. Three novel mouse monoclonal antibodies, OM-A, OM-B, and OM-C, reactive with mucinous type ovarian tumors. *Cancer Res* 1988;48:4639–4645.
74. Tsuji Y, Suzuki T, Nishiura H, Takemura T, Isojima S. Identification of two different surface epitopes of human ovarian epithelial carcinomas by monoclonal antibodies. *Cancer Res* 1985; 45:2358–2362.
75. Mettler L, Radzun J, Salmassi A, et al. Six new monoclonal antibodies to serous, mucinous, and poorly differentiated ovarian adenocarcinomas. *Cancer* 1990;65:1525–1532.
76. McDicken IW, McLaughlin PJ, Tromaus PM, Luesley DM, Johnson PM. Detection of placental-type alkaline phosphatase to ovarian cancer. *Br J Cancer* 1985;52:59–64.
77. Epenetos AA, Houker G, Durbin H. Indium-111 labelled monoclonal antibody to placental alkaline phosphatase in the detection of neoplasms of testis, ovary and cervix. *Lancet* 1985;2: 350–353.
78. Berchuck A, Kamel A, Whitaker R, et al. Overexpression of HER-2/neu is associated with poor survival in advanced epithelial ovarian cancer. *Cancer Res* 1990;50:4087–4091.
79. Hancock MC, Langton BC, Chan T, et al. A monoclonal antibody against the c-erbB-2 protein enhances the cytotoxicity of cis-diaminedichloroplatinum against human breast and ovarian tumor cell lines. *Cancer Res* 1991;51:4575–4580.
80. Lloyd KO, Old LJ. Human monoclonal antibodies to glycolipids and other carbohydrate antigens: Dissection of the humoral immune response in cancer patients. *Cancer Res* 1989;49: 3445–3451.
81. Waldmann TA. Monoclonal antibodies in diagnosis and therapy. *Science* 1991;252:1657–1662.
82. Gallagher G, Al-Azzawi F, Walsh LP, Wilson G, Handley J. Multiple epitopes of the human ovarian cancer antigen 14C1 recognized by human IgG antibodies: Their potential in immunotherapy. *Br J Cancer* 1991;64:35–40.
83. Ohkawa K, Takada K, Hatano T, et al. An evaluation of ovarian carcinoma-associated antigen defined by murine monoclonal antibody CF511 in sera from patients with ovarian carcinoma. *Br J Cancer* 1991;64:259–262.
84. Onsrud M. Tumour markers in gynaecologic oncology. *Scand J Clin Lab Invest* 1991;51[Suppl 206]:60–70.
85. Berchuck A, Rodriguez G, and Bast RC. Recent advances in immunodiagnosis and immunotherapy. In: Greer BE, ed. *Current topics in obstetrics and gynecology*. Elsevier; 1991:33–55.
86. Mattes MJ, Major PP, Goldenberg DM, Dion AS, Hulter RV, Klein KM. Patterns of antigen distribution in human carcinomas. *Cancer Res* 1990;50:880–884.
87. Berchuck A, Olt GJ, Soisson AP, et al. Heterogeneity of antigen expression in advanced epithelial ovarian cancer. *Am J Obstet Gynecol* 1990;162:883–888.
88. Rubin SC, Finstad CL, Hoskins WJ, Federici MG, Lloyd KO, Lewis JL. A longitudinal study of antigen expression in epithelial ovarian cancer. *Gynecol Oncol* 1989;34:389–394.
89. Ward BG, Wallace K. Localization of the monoclonal antibody HMFG2 after intravenous and intraperitoneal injection into nude mice bearing subcutaneous and intraperitoneal human ovarian cancer xenografts. *Cancer Res* 1987;47:4714–4718.
90. Thédrez P, Saccavini J-C, Nolibé D, et al. Biodistribution of indium-111-labelled OC 125 monoclonal antibody after intraperitoneal injection in nude mice intraperitoneally grafted with ovarian carcinoma. *Cancer Res* 1989;49:3081–3086.
91. Wahl R, Piko C. Intraperitoneal (IP) delivery of radiolabelled monoclonal antibody to IP-included xenografts of ovarian cancer. *Proc Amer Assoc Cancer Res* 1985;26:298.
92. Mattes MJ. Biodistribution of antibodies after intraperitoneal

or intravenous injection and effect of carbohydrate modifications. *JNCI* 1987;79:855–863.
93. Ong GL, Ettenson D, Sharkey RM, et al. Galactose-conjugated antibodies in cancer therapy: properties and principles of action. *Cancer Res* 1991;51:1819–1826.
94. Hunter RE, Doherty P, Griffin TW, et al. Use of indium-111-labelled OC125 monoclonal antibody in the detection of ovarian cancer. *Gynecol Oncol* 1987;27:325–337.
95. Goodman GE, Hellström I, Brodzinsky L, et al. Phase I trial of murine monoclonal antibody L6 in breast, colon, ovarian, and lung cancer. *J Clin Oncol* 1991;8:1083–1092.
96. FitzGerald DJ, Bjorn MJ, Ferris RJ, et al. Anti-tumor activity of an immunotoxin in a nude mouse model of human ovarian cancer. *Cancer Res* 1987;47:1407–1410.
97. Willingham MC, Fitzgerald DJ, Pastan I. Pseudomonas extoxin coupled to monoclonal antibody against ovarian cancer inhibits the growth of human ovarian cancer cells in a mouse model. *Proc Natl Acad Sci (USA)* 1987;84:2474–2479.
98. Apelgren LD, Zimmerman DL, Briggs SL, Bumol TF. Antitumor activity of the monoclonal antibody-Vinca alkaloid immunoconjugate LY 203725 (KS1/4-4-diacetylvinblastine-3-carboxyhydrazide) in a nude mouse model of human ovarian cancer. *Cancer Res* 1990;50:3540–3544.
99. Stewart JSW, Hird V, Snook D, et al. Intraperitoneal radioimmunotherapy for ovarian cancer: Pharmacokinetics, toxicity, and efficacy of I-131 labelled monoclonal antibodies. *Int J Radiat Oncol Biol Phys* 1989;16:405–413.
100. Hird V, Stewart JSW, Snook D, et al. Intraperitoneally administered 90Y-labelled monoclonal antibodies as a third line of treatment in ovarian cancer. A phase 1-2 trial: Problems encountered and possible solutions. *Br J Cancer* 1990;62:48–51.
101. Nelson H. Targeted cellular immunotherapy with bifunctional antibodies. *Cancer Cells* 1991;3:163–172.
102. Mezzanzanica D, Garrido MA, Neblock DS, et al. Human T-lymphocytes targeted against an established human ovarian carcinoma with a bispecific F(ab')$_2$ antibody prolong host survival in a murine xenograft model. *Cancer Res* 1991;51:5716–5721.
103. Garrido MA, Valdayo MJ, Winkler DF, et al. Targeting human T-lymphocytes with bispecific antibodies to react against human ovarian carcinoma cells growing in nu/nu mice. *Cancer Res* 1990;50:4227–4232.
104. Stewart JA, Belison LJ, Moore AL, et al. Phase I trial of intraperitoneal recombinant interleukin-2/lymphokine-activated killer cells in patients with ovarian cancer. *Cancer Res* 1990;50:6302–6310.
105. Lotzova E, Savary CA, Freedman RS, Edwards CL, Morris M. Comparison of recombinant interleukin-2-activated peripheral blood and tumor-infiltrating lymphocytes of patients with epithelial ovarian carcinoma: cytotoxicity, growth kinetics, and phenotype. *Cancer Immunol Immunother* 1990;31:169–175.
106. Sleis RG, Urba WJ, Vandermolen LA, et al. Intraperitoneal lymphokine-activated killer cell and interleukin-2 therapy for malignancies limited to the peritoneal cavity. *J Clin Oncol* 1990;8:1618–1629.
107. Ferrini S, Prigione I, Mammoliti S, et al. Re-targeting of human lymphocytes expressing the T-cell receptor gamma/delta to ovarian carcinoma cells by the use of bispecific monoclonal antibodies. *Int J Cancer* 1989;44:245–250.
108. Mattes MJ, Cordon Cardo C, Lewis JL Jr, Old LJ, Lloyd KO. Cell surface antigens of human ovarian and endometrial carcinoma defined by mouse monoclonal antibodies. *Proc Natl Acad Sci (USA)* 1984;81:568–572.
109. de Kretser TA, Thorne HJ, Picone D, Jose DG. Biochemical characterization of the monoclonal antibody-defined ovarian carcinoma-associated antigen SGA. *Int J Cancer* 1986;37:705–712.
110. Miotti S, Aguanno S, Canevari S, et al. Biochemical analysis of human ovarian cancer-associated antigens defined by murine monoclonal antibodies. *Cancer Res* 1985;45:826–832.
111. Poels LG, Peters D, van Megen Y, et al. Monoclonal antibody against human ovarian tumor-associated antigens. *JNCI* 1986;76:781–791.
112. Nozawa S, Yajima M, Kojima K, et al. Tumor-associated mucin-type glycoprotein (CA54/61) defined by two monoclonal antibodies (MA54 and MA61) in ovarian cancers. *Cancer Res* 1989;49:493–498.
113. Willingham MC, FitzGerald DJ, Pastan I. Pseudomonas exotoxin coupled to a monoclonal antibody against ovarian cancer inhibits the growth of human ovarian cancer cells in a nude mouse model. *Proc Natl Acad Sci (USA)* 1987;84:2474–2478.
114. Fleuren GJ, Coerkamp EG, Nap M, Broek LJCM, Warnaar SO. Immunohistological characterization of a monoclonal antibody (OV632) against epithelial ovarian carcinomas. *Virchows Arch* 1987;410:481–486 (abst).
115. Xu F-J, Yu Y-H, Li B-Y, et al. Development of two new monoclonal antibodies reactive to a surface antigen present on human ovarian epithelial cancer cells. *Cancer Res* 1991;51:4012–4019.
116. Magnani JL, Nilsson B, Brockhaus M, et al. A monoclonal antibody-defined antigen associated with gastrointestinal cancer is a ganglioside containing sialylated lacto-N-fuco-pentaose II. *J Biol Chem* 1982;257:14305–14309.

CHAPTER 4

Growth Factors, Oncogenes, and Tumor-Suppressor Genes

Andrew Berchuck and Robert C. Bast, Jr.

Although recent advances in molecular and cellular biology have dramatically increased our understanding of the biomolecular events involved in growth regulation and transformation, it has been known for some time that proliferation of human cells is the result of replication of chromosomal DNA (cDNA) followed by cytokinesis. This sequence of events known as the cell cycle can be divided into several distinct phases, including gap 1 (variable number of hours), the DNA synthesis phase (8–30 hours), gap 2 (1 hour), and mitosis (0.5–1.5 hours). Cell cycle times for human tumors have been reported to range from 12 hours to 5 days. In most normal tissues and neoplasms, however, the majority of cells are in a nonproliferative, resting state. The portion of cells that are in the cell cycle is referred to as the growth fraction. The growth rate of a tumor depends not only on the cell cycle time and the growth fraction, but also on the fraction of cells that are destined to die because of hypoxia or genetic abnormalities.

In normal cells, proliferation is closely regulated, and the growth fraction varies between different types of cells. Some cells, such as neurons, are terminally differentiated and rarely divide; others, such as hepatocytes, proliferate only in response to injury; still others, such as bone marrow cells, divide constantly. Regardless of the intrinsic rate of proliferation, normal cells exhibit contact inhibition so that proliferation ceases when cells grow to high density. In contrast, cancer cells are not contact-inhibited and can inappropriately proliferate to form a neoplasm. Other features of malignant growth include development of the ability to proliferate in culture without attachment to a solid surface (anchorage-independent growth) and tumor formation in immunocompromised nude mice. In most cases, tumor growth occurs as a result of an increased growth fraction and loss of contact inhibition rather than decreased cell cycle time.

Although cell cycle kinetics have been well described, the factors that regulate entry into the cell cycle remain poorly understood. During the past two decades, however, studies in the areas of growth factors, proto-oncogenes, and tumor-suppressor genes have begun to elucidate the complex molecular events involved in normal growth regulation and malignant transformation. Although the close relationship between the fields of cancer-causing genes and peptide growth factors is now apparent, these areas of investigation originally evolved independently. In this chapter, the role of specific peptide growth factors in the regulation of normal and malignant ovarian epithelial cells will be discussed first. The latter portion of the chapter will examine the role of proto-oncogenes and tumor-suppressor genes in ovarian cancer.

PEPTIDE GROWTH FACTORS

Peptide growth factors are glycoprotein hormones that stimulate proliferation or differentiation by binding to specific cell-membrane receptors. Although they are considered hormones, unlike steroids and gonadotropins, they are not often secreted by endocrine organs into the circulation to travel to specific target organs. Rather, they usually act in the local environment via autocrine, paracrine, or juxtacrine mechanisms (Fig. 1). In an autocrine pathway, a cell secretes growth factor into the extracellular space. The growth

---

A. Berchuck and R.C. Bast, Jr.: Departments of Obstetrics and Gynecology, Division of Gynecologic Oncology; and Medicine and Microbiology/Immunology, Duke Comprehensive Cancer Center, Duke University, Durham, North Carolina, 27710

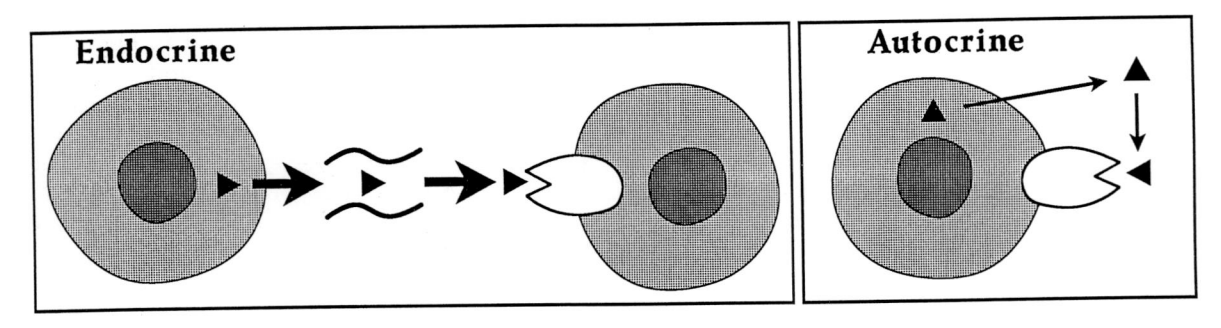

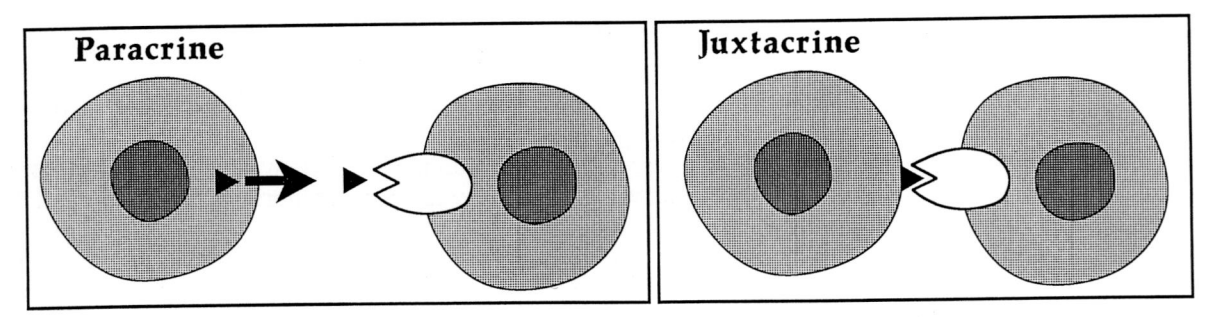

FIG. 1. Endocrine, autocrine, paracrine, and juxtacrine growth regulatory mechanisms.

factor then interacts with receptors on the same cell. Autocrine growth stimulation may be an important mechanism by which cancer cells gain a proliferative advantage relative to normal cells. In the paracrine model, growth factors secreted by one type of cell bind to receptors on other nearby cells of a different type. Paracrine mechanisms may contribute to communication between epithelial and stromal cells, thereby facilitating coordinated action within normal tissues. In the juxtacrine model, growth factor inserted into the cell membrane binds to receptors on immediately adjacent cells. Although peptide growth factors are thought to play a role in development, tissue regeneration, and wound healing, their precise role in individual organ systems remains largely unknown.

Most peptide growth factors that have been implicated in cancer interact with receptors that contain an extracellular ligand-binding domain, a hydrophobic, membrane-spanning region, and an inner tyrosine kinase domain (Table 1)(1,2). Binding of growth factor to its receptor results in activation of the tyrosine kinase, which then phosphorylates its intracellular domain (autophosphorylation) and other proteins on tyrosine residues. Although tyrosine phosphorylation represents considerably less than 1% of total cellular phosphorylation, it is thought to be of signal importance in propa-

TABLE 1. *Peptide growth factors that interact with tyrosine kinase receptors*

Growth factor	MW	Chromosome (growth factor gene)	Receptor/Receptor MW	Chromosome (receptor gene)
EGF	6 kD	4q25-27	EGF receptor/170 kD	7p12-14
TGF-α	6 kD	2p12-13	EGF receptor/170 kD	7p12-14
PDGF	28 kD–35 kD	A-7p21-22 B-22q11	PDGF receptor/165 kD	α-4q11-12 β-5q31-32
Acidic FGF	15.5 kD	5q31-33	FGF receptor/125 kD	unknown
Basic FGF	18 kD–29 kD	4q25	FGF receptor/125 kD	unknown
IGF-1	7.5 kD	12q23	Type 1 IGF receptor α-130 kD β-95 kD	15q25
IGF-2	7.5 kD	11p15	Type 1 IGF receptor α-130 kD β-95 kD	15q25
M-CSF	70 kD	5q33.1	*fms*/165 kD	5q33.2-34

MW, molecular weight; EGF, epidermal growth factor; TGF-α, transforming growth factor-α; PDGF, platelet-derived growth factor; FGF, fibroblast growth factor; IGF, insulin-like growth factor; M-CSF, macrophage colony-stimulating growth factor.

gating mitogenic stimuli. Ligand binding usually is also associated with internalization of the receptor-ligand complex via clatherin-coated pits with resultant downregulation of cell-surface receptor levels. Subsequent signal transduction is clearly complex, and the relative importance of events such as calcium flux, phospholipid metabolism, and activation of other kinases remains poorly understood.

Epidermal Growth Factor Family

Epidermal growth factor (EGF) was among the first peptide growth factors discovered. Its name derives from its ability to stimulate development of epidermal structures, including the eyelids, teeth, and hair in newborn mice (3,4). EGF is a 53-amino-acid molecule that is maintained in a folded form due to the presence of three disulfide bonds between cysteine residues; reduction of the disulfide bonds leads to loss of biologic activity. Mature EGF is produced from a larger precursor form that is inserted into the cell membrane. Cleavage from this precursor is required to release EGF into the extracellular environment, but the membrane-associated growth factor is active and may participate in juxtacrine stimulation of adjacent cells. In addition, soluble EGF acts as a mitogen for a wide range of cells in culture.

More recently, transforming growth factor-α (TGF-α) has been shown to be a 50-amino-acid protein that is highly homologous to EGF, is produced as a membrane-inserted protein, binds to the EGF receptor, and has biological effects barely distinguishable from those of EGF (5,6). Although TGF-α initially was named for its ability to act in concert with transforming growth factor-β (TGF-β) to transform some types of cells in culture, it is produced by normal cells as well.

The EGF receptor is a 170 kD glycosylated membrane-spanning protein that has served as the prototype for studies of tyrosine kinase receptors (1,2). Most normal cells, with the notable exception of hematopoietic cells, have 10^4–10^5 EGF receptors/cell, and proliferation is stimulated by EGF or TGF-α. Paradoxically, when cells express greater than 10^6 EGF receptors/cell, treatment with EGF inhibits rather than stimulates cellular proliferation. Both EGF and TGF-α bind to the extracellular domain of the EGF receptor with equivalent affinity. Ligand binding is believed to lead to dimerization of EGF receptors, which may be involved in optimal activation of the intracellular tyrosine kinase domain.

Several lines of evidence implicate the EGF family in malignant transformation (7). First, the viral *erb*B oncogene represents a truncated EGF receptor that is constitutively activated. Second, some cancer cells secrete EGF or TGF-α into the local environment, which might act in an autocrine fashion to stimulate tumor growth. Elevated levels of EGF and TGF-α also frequently are detected in malignant effusions and urine of patients whose tumors secrete these growth factors (8). In addition, EGF receptor levels are abnormal in some human cancers (7). In squamous cancers, overexpression of the EGF receptor frequently occurs (9). In some cases, overexpression is due to gene amplification, while in other instances, there is increased transcription of the EGF receptor gene. Conversely, a portion of adenocarcinomas appear to have decreased EGF receptor expression. In breast cancer, EGF receptor expression has been shown to relate inversely to estrogen receptor expression and to correlate with poor clinical outcome (10).

We examined the expression of EGF receptor in frozen tissue samples of normal and malignant human ovaries (11). In the normal ovary, EGF receptor was observed in both the epithelium and the underlying stroma. Among advanced stage epithelial ovarian cancers, EGF receptor was detectable immunohistochemically in 77% of cases. As with breast cancer, survival of patients with EGF receptor-negative ovarian cancers was significantly better than that of patients with EGF receptor-positive cancers. Likewise, Kohler (12) and coworkers found that 40% of ovarian cancers with the highest EGF receptor levels had the worst prognosis. On the other hand, Bauknecht et al. (13) found that EGF receptor expression in ovarian cancers was associated with favorable survival. In this study, however, all histologic types and stages of ovarian cancer were combined. Further studies are needed to clarify the relationship between EGF receptor expression and the biologic behavior of ovarian cancers.

Insulin-like Growth Factors

The insulin-like growth factors (IGFs) are so named because of their close structural similarity to insulin (14). IGF-1 originally was named *Somatomedin-C* and was thought to be produced in the liver and other tissues in response to growth hormone as a mediator of skeletal growth. Mature IGF-1 (70 amino acids) and IGF-2 (67 amino acids) each contain 3 disulfide bonds and are produced by processing of precursor molecules. IGFs can act both as local autocrine/paracrine factors and as circulating hormones. In the circulation and other body fluids such as amniotic fluid, IGFs are carried by binding proteins that prevent interaction with the IGF receptor. Several different binding proteins, some of which are growth hormone inducible, have been characterized and are thought to be involved in regulating IGF action. Two different IGF receptors have been identified. The Type I IGF receptor is a heterodimeric receptor that, similar to the insulin receptor, is composed of two α-subunits and two β-subunits. It binds insulin weakly and binds IGF-1 with higher affinity than IGF-2. Ligand binding leads to activation of the intracellular tyrosine kinase. The mitogenic effect of both IGFs is thought to be mediated by the Type I receptor. The Type II IGF receptor has a completely different structure, does not contain tyrosine kinase activity, and has a much higher affinity for IGF-2.

Although IGFs are expressed in many tissues and are thought to be involved in the physiologic growth of the fetus, child, and adult, their precise role remains poorly defined. In addition, IGFs may have important nonmitogenic effects. For example, in the ovary, IGFs act synergistically with gonadotropins to stimulate steroidogenesis of granulosa cells (15). Production of IGF-1 by cancers is rare for the most part. However, it has been reported that some ovarian cancers produce mRNA for IGF-1, IGF-1 binding protein, and Type 1 IGF receptor (16). Thus, it is possible that IGF-1 may act as an autocrine growth factor for some ovarian cancer cells. In addition, many types of tumors secrete IGF-2, and the paraneoplastic syndrome of hypoglycemia that is seen in association with some sarcomas has been shown to be related to production of IGF-2 (14).

Fibroblast Growth Factor Family

The fibroblast growth factors (FGFs) were originally described as mitogenic peptides extracted from brain and pituitary (17,18). Further study of these proteins led to the characterization of acidic and basic FGF, both of which are potent mitogens for fibroblasts, endothelial cells, smooth muscle cells, astrocytes, and granulosa cells. FGFs are not the only peptide growth factors that act as mitogens for these cells, however. More recently, the FGF family has grown to include the less well-characterized FGF-like molecules encoded by the *int, hst,* and FGF-5 proto-oncogenes and keratinocyte growth factor.

FGFs are produced by many of the same types of mesenchymal cells that are responsive to FGFs. Mature acidic and basic FGFs are made up of 154-amino-acid peptides. Although FGFs do not appear to be glycosylated, variable truncation of these molecules during processing of their precursors yields heterogeneous molecular weight species. Serum levels of FGFs are insignificant, and it is thought that FGFs normally act in the local environment. Many tissues have relatively large amounts of FGFs bound to the extracellular matrix due to their affinity for heparin and other glycosaminoglycans. FGFs bind to a specific membrane-spanning receptor which contains intrinsic tyrosine kinase activity. Receptor numbers vary from 2,000 to 80,000 per cell. Both high- and low-affinity species of receptor are present, but the mitogenic effect of FGFs can only be transmitted via the high-affinity binding sites. Basic FGF has a higher affinity for the FGF receptor, consistent with its 10–100-fold higher activity relative to acidic FGF in biologic systems.

FGFs are thought to play a role in normal development, tissue regeneration, and wound healing. In addition, FGF bound to the extracellular matrix may serve as a growth factor reservoir that is released when destruction of tissue occurs due to trauma or infection. Free FGF can then stimulate proliferation of fibroblasts and vascular endothelial cells that are required for healing. Because basic FGF is present in ovarian follicular fluid, it may be involved in stimulating vascularization of the corpus luteum after ovulation. In addition, although epithelial cells are not thought to respond to FGFs, FGFs are found in human carcinomas where they may act to promote neovascularization, which is requisite for tumor growth.

Platelet-Derived Growth Factor

Though originally discovered in serum as a platelet product, platelet-derived growth factor (PDGF) is also produced by a wide range of normal and malignant cells (19,20). It is a potent mitogen for connective tissue cells such as fibroblasts, glial cells, and smooth muscle cells. The PDGF molecule is a dimer composed of A and B chains that are held together by disulfide bonds. Both homodimers (AA, BB) and heterodimers (AB) are produced, and they frequently differ in their biologic activities in various systems. Both the A and B chains are produced following processing of larger precursor molecules. Similar to the FGFs, differential processing leads to size heterogeneity, and mature PDGF ranges in size from 28 kD to 35 kD. PDGF contains 4–7% carbohydrate and glycosylation also contributes to molecular weight heterogeneity. The PDGF receptor structure is not completely understood, but is thought to involve coalescence of α and β subunits in the presence of PDGF. As with other growth factor receptors, ligand binding leads to activation of the intracellular tyrosine kinase domain. In general, PDGF receptors are present on connective tissue cells and are not expressed on epithelial cells.

Expression of PDGF by normal cells is usually tightly regulated. Similar to FGFs, PDGF is thought to play a role in wound healing. In this model, platelet release of chemotactic factors and PDGF into the wound would lead to both recruitment and mitogenic stimulation of cells involved in tissue repair. It has also been postulated that PDGF may be involved in pathologic tissue repair processes such as atherosclerosis, in which abnormal proliferation of intimal smooth muscle cells leads to vessel occlusion (21).

The Simian sarcoma virus (*sis*) oncogene is derived from the gene that encodes the B chain of PDGF. In this context, PDGF B chain is secreted, binds to PDGF receptors on monkey fibroblasts, and stimulates autocrine proliferation and tumor formation. Since human connective tissue cells express PDGF and its receptor, PDGF may play a role in the growth of some human sarcomas (22). PDGF is also expressed by many transformed epithelial cells, including human ovarian cancer cell lines, but these cells usually are not responsive to PDGF (23). Although PDGF is not thought to participate in autocrine growth stimulation in this setting, it may evoke the surrounding desmoplastic reaction.

Macrophage Colony-Stimulating Factor

Macrophage colony-stimulating factor (M-CSF) is a peptide growth factor that stimulates proliferation and functional responses of macrophages (24). It is a homodimer whose two 112-amino-acid subunits are held together by disulfide bonds. As with many other peptide growth factors, glycosylation of M-CSF (70 kD) results in a greater molecular weight than would be predicted on the basis of the amino acid sequence. The M-CSF receptor is a tyrosine kinase that was first discovered as the transforming gene in feline sarcoma viruses (*v-fms*). The transforming ability of the viral *fms* gene product is due to constitutive activation of the tyrosine kinase domain as a result of different point mutations. The normal "M-CSF receptor" is encoded by the cellular homolog of the viral oncogene, referred to as c-*fms*.

Although M-CSF initially was thought to be a lineage-specific growth factor restricted to macrophages, it has been shown that other tissues including trophoblast may produce M-CSF. In addition, normal ovarian epithelium (25) and ovarian cancer cell lines produce M-CSF (26), and serum levels of M-CSF are elevated in some patients with ovarian cancer (27). Because it has been reported that *fms* is expressed by many ovarian cancers (28) but not by normal ovarian epithelium (unpublished observation), M-CSF and *fms* may comprise an autocrine growth stimulatory pathway in some ovarian cancers. In addition, M-CSF may act in a paracrine fashion to stimulate recruitment and activation of macrophages. Because macrophage products such as interleukin-1 (IL-1), IL-6, and tumor necrosis factor-α stimulate proliferation of some ovarian cancer cell lines (29), the potential for paracrine stimulation of the cancer by macrophages also exists. Finally, *fms* expression in endometrial cancer is associated with increased myometrial invasion (30). Perhaps *fms* expression by ovarian cancers also augments invasiveness.

Because M-CSF is produced by ovarian cancers and detectable levels are present in serum, we and others have investigated its utility as a tumor marker in patients with ovarian cancer (26). The group at Yale first reported that M-CSF levels are elevated in most women with active ovarian cancer relative to normal, healthy women (27). Since CA-125 has been the most useful serum marker in this disease, we examined whether M-CSF would prove complementary to CA-125 (31). Overall, sixty-nine percent of patients with active ovarian cancer had elevated M-CSF levels. Among twenty-four of these patients in whom CA-125 levels were normal, fifty-four percent had elevated M-CSF levels. In addition, thirty-two percent of patients who had a positive second-look laparotomy despite a normal CA-125 level had elevated M-CSF levels. Thus, M-CSF deserves further consideration as a complementary marker to CA-125.

Transforming Growth Factor-β Family

Although transforming growth factor-β (TGF-β) was named for its ability to act in concert with TGF-α to transform some types of cells in culture, TGF-β inhibits proliferation of normal epithelial cells (32–34). Proliferation of mesenchymal cells may be either stimulated or inhibited by TGF-β depending upon the culture conditions and specific cell type. Three closely related forms of TGF-β encoded by separate genes have subsequently been discovered: TGF-β1 on chromosome 19q13, TGF-β2 on chromosome 1q41, and TGF-β3 on chromosome 14q24. All three forms of TGF-β are 25 kD homodimers in which the subunits are bound together by disulfide bonds. TGF-β is ubiquitous and is produced in particularly large quantities by platelets, kidney, and placenta. TGF-β is secreted from cells in an inactive form bound to a portion of its precursor molecule, from which it must be cleaved to release biologically active TGF-β. The factors that regulate activation of TGF-β are not well understood, however. Although TGF-β interacts with at least three different high-affinity cell-surface receptors, these receptors and their biochemical mechanisms of signal transduction remain obscure. Unlike stimulatory growth factor receptors, TGF-β receptors do not have tyrosine kinase activity.

A number of other peptides that are homologous with TGF-β, including activin, inhibin, and müllerian-inhibitory substance, comprise the TGF-β family (32). It is thought that members of the TGF-β family are involved in growth inhibition of many types of normal cells, including epithelial cells and hepatocytes, when proliferation is inappropriate. In contrast, however, TGF-β has stimulatory effects on various mesenchymal cells involved in remodeling of bone and wound repair. More recently, a number of nonmitogenic effects of TGF-β have also been discovered. These include increased production of extracellular matrix and modulation of immune function (35). In the ovary, TGF-β is produced by theca cells (36) and acts in a paracrine fashion to augment granulosa-cell lutenizing hormone receptor levels (37) and steroidogenesis (38).

Growth Regulation of Normal and Malignant Ovarian Epithelium

To test the autocrine hypothesis in ovarian cancer, we asked whether ovarian cancer cell lines respond to exogenous peptide growth factors and whether they secrete growth factors (39). For these experiments, we utilized several human epithelial ovarian cancer cell lines that had been established previously in our laboratory. Although proliferation of the ovarian cancer cell lines was unaffected by FGF and PDGF, a varied response was noted to EGF. Proliferation of one cell line was stimulated two- to three-fold, two cell lines were stimulated 50–100%, and two cell lines were not affected by EGF. When the ovarian cancer cell lines were treated with TGF-β, one was markedly inhibited (more than 95%), two were modestly inhibited (15–20%), and one was unaffected. In addition, some of the ovarian cancer cell lines were modestly responsive to tumor necrosis factor-α, IL-1, and IL-6, but none were responsive to granulocyte colony-stimulating factor (G-CSF), granulocyte macrophage-CSF (GM-CSF), or M-CSF (29). In summary, each of the ovarian cancer cell lines had a different pattern of responsiveness to the growth factors tested. In the ovarian cancer cell lines that were responsive to growth factors, however, the magnitude of the response was usually less than that of the normal control cells.

In addition, the ovarian cancer cell lines were tested for production of several peptide growth factors (39). The cancer cells were cultured in serum-free medium, which was then tested for its effect on proliferation of cell lines that are known to respond to various growth factors. Using these bioassays, EGF, PDGF, and FGF were not detected in any of the conditioned media. In contrast to our studies in which an autocrine loop involving EGF was not demonstrated, however, other investigators have found that EGF (40) and TGF-α (41) are produced by some ovarian cancers that also express EGF receptors (42). These findings have been interpreted as suggestive of the presence of an autocrine growth stimulatory pathway. In these experiments, however, growth factor was proven to be associated with the cells but secretion was not examined. In addition, in one paper, treatment of ovarian cancer cells with monoclonal antibodies that inhibit binding of TGF-α to the EGF receptor inhibited proliferation (42). Again, this was interpreted as proof of an autocrine loop. The apparent difference between our studies and the others could be reconciled, however, by the juxtacrine hypothesis. If ovarian cancers were producing the membrane-bound form of EGF or TGF-α that was stimulating proliferation of adjacent cells by binding to EGF receptors, but release of growth factor from the cell surface was not occurring, this would lead to the findings reported in the seemingly contradictory studies.

Most, but not all, of the ovarian cancer cell lines that we studied secreted latent TGF-β into their culture medium, which could be activated by heating. One cell line also produced biologically active TGF-β. The production of TGF-β was confirmed with the ribonuclease (RNase) protection assay using cDNA probes for the three different forms of TGF-β (43). Four of the five ovarian cancer cell lines were found to produce TGF-β1 and TGF-β2 mRNA, while none of the ovarian cancer cell lines produced TGF-β3. Since ovarian cancer cell lines both produced and responded to TGF-β, we tested its role as an autocrine growth factor. Ovarian cancer cell lines were grown in the presence of an antisera that neutralizes the biologic effect of TGF-β. Growth of ovarian cancer cell lines that either do not produce TGF-β or produce only latent TGF-β was unaffected by anti-TGF-β antibody. On the other hand, the one cell line that both secreted active TGF-β and was inhibited by exogenous TGF-β was stimulated by the anti-TGF-β antibody. Therefore, it appears that TGF-β acts as an autocrine growth-inhibitory factor in this one cell line. This was the only example of an autocrine loop that we were able to demonstrate, however.

Most ovarian cancers in adults arise from the surface epithelium or underlying inclusion cysts. To define alterations that occur during oncogenesis, we examined the role of peptide growth factors in growth regulation of normal human ovarian epithelium. The method of Auersperg (44) was adapted to grow normal human ovarian epithelial cells from ovaries removed during surgery for benign gynecological diseases. Proliferation of monolayers of ovarian epithelial cells was strikingly stimulated by EGF twofold to fivefold (45), whereas the ovarian cancer cell lines had previously been found to be relatively resistant to EGF (39). In addition, although IGF-1 and IGF-2 alone had no effect on proliferation of ovarian epithelial cells, treatment with EGF in combination with either IGF resulted in greater stimulation of proliferation than when EGF was used alone. Since it has been shown that both EGF and IGFs are present in follicular fluid (46,47), these growth factors may act in a paracrine fashion to stimulate regrowth of the ovarian epithelium following disruption of the ovarian surface at ovulation. Alternatively, the epithelial cells themselves or the underlying stromal cells could produce autocrine- or paracrine-acting growth factors that stimulate regeneration of the epithelial surface.

Since a fraction of adenocarcinomas appear to have lost EGF receptor expression (7), we determined whether the relative decrease in responsiveness of ovarian cancer cell lines to EGF was due to a decrease in numbers of cell surface EGF receptors or to changes in receptor affinity (45). Normal human ovarian epithelial cells were found to have approximately 1×10^5 EGF receptors/cell with a linear Scatchard curve, which is indicative of a single class of high-affinity receptor. The ovarian cancer cell lines had similar numbers of high-affinity cell-surface EGF receptors, as do normal ovarian epithelial cells. There was no relationship between EGF receptor number or affinity and responsiveness to EGF. Thus, decreased receptor expression does not appear to be the mechanism by which ovarian cancer cell lines lose responsiveness to EGF.

In addition, we examined the role of TGF-β in the growth regulation of normal ovarian epithelium. TGF-β inhibited proliferation of normal ovarian epithelial cells from 40% to 70% (43). Like most of the ovarian cancer cell lines, normal ovarian epithelial cells were found to produce TGF-β1 and TGF-β2 mRNA. In addition, normal ovarian epithelial cells are able to process TGF-β into its biologically active form. These data suggest that TGF-β might normally act as an autocrine growth-inhibitory factor in normal ovarian epithelium which, under most circumstances, is thought to be relatively quiescent. Conversely, since we found that most ovarian cancers either fail to produce, activate, or respond to TGF-β, loss of this growth-inhibitory pathway might play a role in the development of some ovarian cancers.

In addition to the studies of our group, other researchers have taken somewhat different approaches to investigating the role of peptide growth factors in ovarian center. Mills and coworkers (48) have shown that ascites of patients with ovarian cancer contains factor(s) that stimulate proliferation of both fresh ovarian cancer cells and ovarian cancer cell lines. In addition, growth of an ovarian cancer cell line in nude mice was shown to occur in the presence of ovarian cancer ascites but not in the presence of benign ascites (49). Efforts are underway to identify this growth factor, which appears unrelated to any known factor. In addition, it has been shown that benign and malignant ovarian cysts contain activity that stimulates proliferation of an ovarian cancer cell line (50). This is particularly intriguing because it is thought that some ovarian cancers develop in small epithelial inclusion cysts that arise as the result of entrapment of epithelial cells following ovulation. The presence of growth factors in these cysts might play a role in stimulating further proliferation and transformation.

ONCOGENES

It is now known that cancer occurs due to abnormalities in expression of genes that encode the proteins normally involved in growth-regulatory pathways, including: growth factors and their receptors, cytoplasmic molecules involved in signal transduction, and nuclear transcriptional regulatory factors. Two classes of genes, proto-oncogenes and tumor-suppressor genes, have been described (51–53). Proto-oncogenes encode proteins that normally are part of growth stimulatory pathways. Since alterations in only a single allele of a proto-oncogene can transform cells when such genes are activated by mutation, deletion, overexpression, or translocation, oncogenes are considered dominant transforming genes. The second class of cancer-causing genes, the tumor-suppressor genes (antioncogenes) encode proteins that inhibit proliferation. Because these genes inhibit rather than stimulate proliferation, inactivation of both copies of a tumor-suppressor gene is required to produce malignant transformation. Thus, tumor-suppressor genes act as recessive transforming genes.

Although much remains to be learned about the role of oncogenes and tumor-suppressor genes in the development of human cancers, several general concepts have emerged. First, studies of cells in culture have shown that transformation usually requires the cooperative effort of two or more cancer-causing genes acting in concert (52). For example, mutant p53 genes markedly augment the ability of mutant *ras* genes to transform cells in culture. Activation of as many as four or five different genes may be required for the development of a clinically-recognizable human cancer. Second, specific oncogenes appear to be activated in some, rather than all, types of cancers. For example, translocation of the *myc* and *abl* oncogenes is seen in some hematologic malignancies, but not in solid tumors. Finally, in a given type of cancer, tumors from different patients differ with respect to which cancer-causing genes are activated. Epithelial ovarian cancer probably occurs due to activation of several different combinations of genes, which may produce cancers that vary in their biologic and clinical characteristics.

Oncogenes were first discovered in retroviruses, which are viruses containing ribonucleic acid (RNA) that induce tumors in a wide range of animals (52). Initially, the viral *src* (v-*src*) oncogene, which encodes a tyrosine kinase, was shown to be responsible for the transforming activity of the Rous sarcoma virus. Several dozen oncogenes subsequently have been found in various other retroviruses. These viral oncogenes have been shown to be homologous to vertebrate genes that are normally involved in growth regulation. It is thought that the viral oncogenes have been acquired from animal hosts and activated to forms that possess transforming activity. For example, the v-*sis* oncogene of the Simian sarcoma virus encodes one chain of PDGF. The v-*erb*B oncogene of the avian erythroblastosis virus encodes a truncated version of the EGF receptor that is constitutively activated. Although few human cancers are caused by retroviruses, the same genes (proto-oncogenes) are often activated in human malignancies. To date, over 60 proto-oncogenes have been described, and an equal number of tumor-suppressor genes are suspected to exist. Detailed studies of these molecules have led to the classification of oncogenes into families, the members of which share structural and functional properties (Table 2).

TABLE 2. *Classification of oncogene families*

Peptide growth factors		
sis		
int		
hst		
FGF-5		
Tyrosine Kinases		
Receptor	Non-receptor	
EGF receptor (*erb*B)	*src* family	*abl* family
HER-2/*neu* (*erb*B-2)	src	abl
CSF-1 receptor (*fms*)	yes	arg
met	fgr	
trk	lck	miscellaneous
kit	fyn	fes
sea	lyn	
ret	hck	
ros		
Serine/threonine kinases		
raf family	miscellaneous	
c-*raf*-1	mos	
A-*raf*	pim-1	
B-*raf*		
protein kinase C family		
PKC beta-1		
PKC gamma		
G proteins		
ras family		
N-*ras*		
H-*ras*		
Ki-*ras*		
miscellaneous		
gip		
gsp		
Nuclear oncogenes		
AP-1 transcription factor components	miscellaneous	
jun	myb	
jun-B	ets-1	
jun-D	ets-2	
fos	ski	
fos-B	rel	
fra-1		
myc family	hormone receptors	
c-*myc*	erbA	
L-*myc*		

Tyrosine Kinases

The largest family of oncogenes are the tyrosine kinases, which act to transfer a phosphate from adenosine triphosphate (ATP) to tyrosine residues on specific cellular proteins (51–54). Following binding of peptide growth factors to their receptors, tyrosine phosphorylation of various cellular proteins is an integral part of the complex cascade of events that eventually culminates in proliferation. Ordinarily, the level of tyrosine phosphorylation is tightly controlled by the opposing effect of phosphatases, which remove phosphate from tyrosine residues (55). Inappropriate tyrosine kinase activity, due to oncogenically activated species, is thought to contribute to transformation by tipping this balance toward increased cellular tyrosine phosphorylation.

Two types of tyrosine kinases have been described. The first are those that act as receptors for growth factors (1,2). These membrane-spanning tyrosine kinases were discussed in the section on peptide growth factors. In addition to autophosphorylation of their intracellular domains, many of these receptors phosphorylate other intracellular substrates involved in signal transduction. For example, phosphorylation of phospholipase C-γ activates this enzyme to cleave diacylglycerol from membrane phospholipids (56). Diacylglycerol is then involved in activation of protein kinase C, another important molecule in signal transduction pathways. The second class of tyrosine kinases, exemplified by the *src* family, are found anchored to the inner surface of the cell membrane. These tyrosine kinases also phosphorylate cellular proteins involved in signal transduction. In contrast to the receptor kinases, which are regulated by peptide growth factors, relatively less is known regarding regulation of the nonreceptor tyrosine kinases.

In addition to the large family of tyrosine kinases that are involved in growth regulation, several of the cytoplasmic serine/threonine kinases also play a role in transduction of mitogenic stimuli from the periphery of the cell to the nucleus (52–54). Several of these kinases, which phosphorylate cellular proteins on serine and threonine residues, including the *raf* family, the protein kinase C family, *mos*, and *pim*-1 can be oncogenically activated in retroviruses or under experimental conditions in vitro. Although cytoplasmic serine/threonine kinases are thought to be critical in transmission of signals initiated by cell-membrane-associated tyrosine kinases and G proteins, their role in human cancers remains largely unknown, and we are unaware of any studies that have examined their expression in ovarian cancer.

Although the role of the vast majority of tyrosine kinases in ovarian cancer remains unexplored, a number of studies have examined expression of the EGF receptor and HER-2/*neu* in ovarian cancer. HER-2/*neu* is postulated to be a growth factor receptor due to its close structural similarity to the EGF receptor: including a cysteine-rich extracellular ligand binding domain, a hydrophobic membrane-spanning region and an intracellular tyrosine kinase domain (57–60). The name *HER-2* is an abbreviation for human epidermal growth factor receptor-2. The name *neu* refers to the fact that this gene was originally identified as the transforming gene in neuroblastomas that arise in rats exposed to a chemical carcinogen. The EGF receptor gene is called *erb*B and is located on chromosome 7p; the HER-2/*neu* gene is called *erb*B-2 and is located on chromosome 17q. Binding of both EGF and TGF-α to the EGF receptor results in activation of the inner tyrosine kinase domain. Likewise, ligands of 30 kD and 70 kD that bind to HER-2/*neu* have been described; however, these proteins have not yet been completely characterized (61).

Although the transforming HER-2/*neu* gene in carcinogen-stimulated rat neuroblastomas is activated by virtue of a mutation that causes an amino acid substitution in the membrane-spanning region (62), mutations have not been found in the HER-2/*neu* gene in human cancers (63). Slamon and coworkers (64,65) have demonstrated, however, that approximately one-third of human breast cancers have from twofold to 40-fold increased levels of structurally normal HER-2/*neu* protein. Overexpression of HER-2/*neu* is usually due to amplification of the number of copies of the HER-2/*neu* gene, but in 10% of cancers, overexpression of HER-2/*neu* protein occurs despite the presence of only a single gene copy. In Slamon's studies, overexpression of HER-2/*neu* in breast cancer was associated with aggressive biologic behavior and poor survival. Subsequently, several but not all (66) large studies have confirmed the relationship between overexpression of HER-2/*neu* and poor survival in breast cancer (66–70).

The reason for the relationship between HER-2/*neu* overexpression and poor prognosis is not known. Since this relationship is so striking, however, studies have been undertaken to determine what role HER-2/*neu* overexpression plays in the development of cancer. In this regard, it has been shown that normal cells in culture acquire a malignant phenotype when they are transfected with and overexpress HER-2/*neu* (71,72). In addition, transgenic mice in which HER-2/*neu* is overexpressed develop breast cancer (73,74). Finally, the finding that HER-2/*neu* is amplified in some cases of carcinoma-in-situ of the breast (66,75) is consistent with this being an early event in tumorigenesis. Although all of these studies suggest that overexpression of HER-2/*neu* is a critical event, much remains unclear, including the role, if any, of the availability of ligand.

Slamon (65) performed a comparative analysis of the various methods used to assess HER-2/*neu* expression in human tumor samples. In breast cancers, there was a close correlation between the levels of HER-2/*neu* DNA on Southern blots, RNA on Northern blots, protein on Western blots, and immunohistochemical staining in frozen sections. Slamon concluded that immunohistochemical analysis of fresh frozen tissue was the preferred method for evaluating HER-2/*neu* expression in clinical samples because the admixture of tumor cells and benign elements differs between samples. Such differences cannot be taken into account with methods such as the Southern, Northern, and Western blot techniques, in which tissue homogenates are assayed, whereas expression of HER-2/*neu* by individual cancer cells can be evaluated directly with immunohistochemistry. The main disadvantage of immunohistochemical techniques is that they have been only semi-quantitative in the past. Recently, however, image analysis technology has been successfully used to quantitate immunohistochemical staining (76). Immunohistochemistry with image analysis may be the most practical method for assessing HER-2/*neu* expression in cancer specimens from patients.

The HER-2/*neu* oncogene is also amplified in some ovarian cancers. Slamon (65) reported the first large study of HER-2/*neu* expression in ovarian cancer. He found that, as with breast cancer, HER-2/*neu* was overexpressed in approximately one-third of ovarian cancers, and overexpression was associated with poor survival. Two smaller studies by other investigators also found amplification of HER-2/*neu* in 3 of 15 (20%) and in 10 of 30 (33%) epithelial ovarian cancers (77,78). To investigate further the relationship between HER-2/*neu* expression and the clinical biology of ovarian cancer, we used an immunohistochemical technique to localize HER-2/*neu* in frozen sections of a larger number of advanced stage ovarian cancers (79). Monoclonal antibody TA1, which is specifically reactive with the extracellular domain of HER-2/*neu* (80), was used as the primary antibody. The intensity of staining in the cancers was compared to that seen in normal ovaries. In the normal ovary, light to moderate staining was seen in the epithelium, while staining in the underlying stroma was absent. Similarly, 50 of 73 stage III/IV epithelial ovarian cancers that we examined also exhibited light to moderate staining for HER-2/*neu*. In contrast, 23 of the cancers (32%) exhibited strong staining consistent with overexpression.

In several ovarian cancers, we examined HER-2/*neu* expression in the primary tumor and multiple metastases (79). Regardless of the level of expression, the intensity of staining was similar between various sites in a given patient. In addition, in a given patient, the intensity of staining for HER-2/*neu* did not change between initial surgery and second-look operation. Similarly, HER-2/*neu* expression has been noted to be consistent between primary, metastatic, and recurrent breast cancers (75,81). Thus, it appears that immunohistochemical assessment of a single viable frozen tissue specimen is sufficient to predict the level of HER-2/*neu* expression in ovarian cancer nodules throughout the peritoneal cavity.

We also examined the relationship between HER-2/*neu* overexpression and other known prognostic factors in ovarian cancer (79). There was no relationship between overexpression and either histologic grade or the ability to perform optimal cytoreductive surgery. Patients whose cancers had normal HER-2/*neu* expression were fivefold more likely to achieve a negative second-look laparotomy, however, than those patients whose cancers overexpressed HER-2/*neu*. In addition, the median survival of patients whose cancers overexpressed HER-2/*neu* was strikingly worse (16 months) than that of patients whose cancers had normal HER-2/*neu* expression (32 months) (Fig. 2). The molecular mechanisms underlying the relationship between HER-2/*neu* overexpression and poor survival remain unknown. It has been shown, however, that down-regulation of cell surface levels of HER-2/*neu* in breast and ovarian cancer cells that overexpress this proto-oncogene can increase sensitivity to cis-platinum (82). Currently, responsiveness to cis-platinum is probably the most important determinant of survival in patients with advanced epithelial ovarian cancer. Thus, if overexpression of HER-2/*neu* is associated with cis-platinum resistance, this might contribute to the poor survival of this subset of patients.

Since it has been shown that HER-2/*neu* can be detected in serum (83), we have investigated its utility as a serum tumor marker in patients with ovarian cancer. Using an enzyme-linked immunoassay that employs monoclonal antibody TA1, which reacts with an epitope on the extracellular domain, we were able to detect HER-2/*neu* in serum from both apparently healthy individuals and patients with ovarian cancer (84). Elevated levels were detected in fourteen percent of patients with ovarian cancer, and there was a significant correlation between elevated serum levels of HER-2/*neu* and overexpression of HER-2/*neu* in tissue. Although overexpression in tissue correlated better with prognosis than did serum levels, further studies are needed to determine whether serum HER-2/*neu* levels complement CA-125 in predicting disease status.

In addition, our group and others are exploring the therapeutic potential of HER-2/*neu* overexpression in ovarian and breast cancer. Specifically, it has been shown that unconjugated antibodies and immunotoxins that bind to this receptor can down-regulate and kill breast and ovarian cancer cells that overexpress it (85,86). Treatment of cancer cells that overexpress HER-2/*neu* with unconjugated antibodies has resulted in up to 90% inhibition of both anchorage-dependent and independent proliferation (87). Similar inhibition of tumor growth has been reported in nude mouse models (85). Although some normal cells also express HER-2/*neu*, an acceptable therapeutic index may be achieved in cancers that overexpress it.

G Proteins

Like tyrosine kinases, the membrane-associated G proteins represent an important mechanism by which cell-surface receptors are coupled to intracellular effectors (51–54). The best described system in which G proteins are known to participate is that of hormones such as gonadotropins that activate adenylate cyclase.

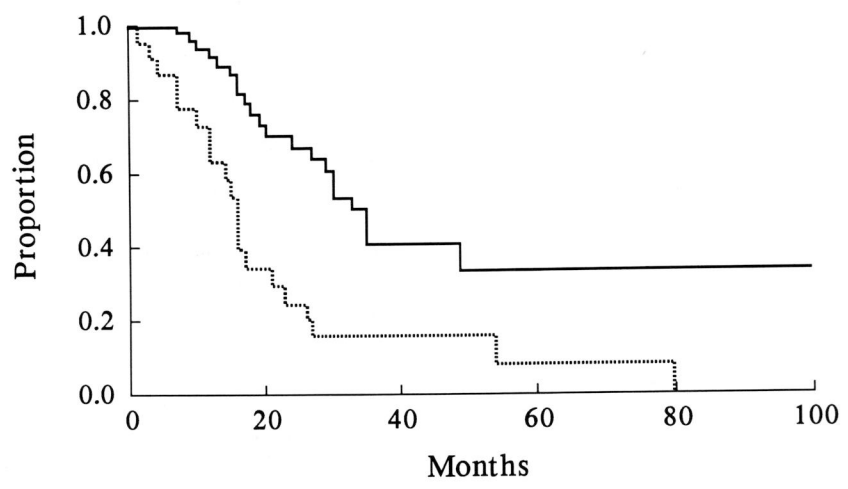

FIG. 2. Survival in advanced stage ovarian cancer patients with normal HER-2/*neu* expression (———) and HER-2/*neu* overexpression (·····).

In the resting state, the three subunits of the G$_s$ protein (α, β, γ) are bound to the gonadotropin receptor in a complex with GDP. Binding of hormone to its receptor results in exchange of guanosine triphosphate (GTP) for GDP, which leads to dissociation of the α subunit. The free α subunit is then capable of interacting with and activating adenylate cyclase, resulting in transduction of the hormonal signal. Activation of the α subunit is terminated by hydrolysis of GTP and reassociation with the β and γ subunits.

Several different G proteins have been found to be activated in human cancers due to point mutations (51,52,54). The most ubiquitous of these are the *ras* family of oncogenes (N-*ras*, Ki-*ras*, H-*ras*) (53). These closely related proteins of 188 or 189 amino acids bind GTP and have intrinsic GTPase activity similar to other G proteins. In addition, it has been shown that mutations in codons 12, 13, or 61 result in constitutive activation of *ras* by inhibiting hydrolysis of bound GTP, which traps *ras* in its active GTP-bound state. Mutations in *ras* genes have been noted in a significant fraction of a wide range of human malignancies including colon (88) and pancreatic carcinomas (Ki-*ras*) and leukemias (N-*ras*). Mutant *ras* genes infrequently are found in epithelial ovarian cancers, however (89). Although mutant *ras* genes have been noted in some mucinous ovarian cancers, these tumors comprise a small fraction of epithelial ovarian cancers (89). In two studies in which the ability of ovarian-cancer-derived DNA to transform NIH 3T3 cells was used to detect activated *ras* genes, one of five cystadenocarcinomas was found to have a mutant Ki-*ras* gene (90) and one of 18 was found to have a mutant N-*ras* gene (91).

It has also been shown that Ki-*ras* may be amplified in approximately 5–10% of epithelial ovarian cancers (92). In two small studies, amplification of the Ki-*ras* gene was found in three of seven (93) and two of eight (94) ovarian cancers using Southern hybridization. By contrast, in two larger studies, only 1 of 23 ovarian cancers had amplification of the H-*ras* gene (95), and only 3 of 37 ovarian cancers had amplification of Ki-*ras* (96). Using an immunohistochemical technique that recognized all of the *ras* gene products, Rodenburg and coworkers (97) showed that some epithelial ovarian cancers had higher expression of *ras* than normal cells. The level of *ras* expression was not found to correlate with histologic grade or survival. Amplification of *ras* genes also has been described in other types of cancers, including bladder (H-*ras*, Ki-*ras*), lung (Ki-*ras*), and breast (N-*ras*) carcinomas (51,52). Similar to receptor tyrosine kinases, increased levels of nonmutated proto-oncogene products such as *ras*, which transduce growth stimulatory signals, may lead to transformation. Transformation associated with *ras* amplification likely requires cooperation with other classes of activated oncogenes.

In addition to *ras* mutations, the α-subunits of G$_s$ and G$_i$, which also are G proteins, have been shown to be mutated in some endocrine tumors (98,99). The G$_s$ gene was found to be mutated in growth-hormone-secreting pituitary tumors and thyroid tumors, while G$_i$ mutations were present in three of ten granulosa/theca tumors as well as in some adrenocortical tumors (98). The G$_i$ mutations in ovarian and adrenal tumors were all at codon 179 and resulted in substitution of either cysteine or histidine for arginine. Similar to *ras* mutations, it is thought that G$_s$ and G$_i$ mutations result in constitutive activation of the products of these genes by inhibiting the intrinsic GTPase activity of the α-subunits, which normally act to hydrolyze GTP and turn off these G proteins. Thus, although abnormalities of these genes have not been found in epithelial cancers, they do appear to be a common genetic change in granulosa\theca tumors and in some other types of tumors arising in endocrine cells that secrete hormones that activate adenylate cyclase.

Nuclear Transcription Factors

The oncogenes that encode cell-membrane and cytoplasmic proteins such as growth factor receptors and G proteins transmit extracellular mitogenic stimuli to the nucleus. Ultimately, however, if proliferation is to occur, these peripheral signals must impact on gene expression and lead to the initiation of DNA synthesis. In this regard, a family of nuclear genes whose products bind to DNA and regulate transcription has been described (51–54). Transcription of several of these genes, including *myc* and *fos,* increases dramatically within minutes of treatment of normal cells in culture with peptide growth factors. Once induced, the products of these genes presumably bind to specific DNA-regulatory elements and result in transcription of genes involved in DNA synthesis and division of normal cells. Conversely, when inappropriately overexpressed, these transcription factors can act as oncogenes.

Among the nuclear transcription factors, oncogenic activation has been observed most often in the *myc* oncogene family (c-*myc*, N-*myc*, L-*myc*). The c-*myc* oncogene may be activated in Burkitt's lymphoma due to translocation from chromosome 8 to 14, but translocation of *myc* genes has not been noted in epithelial cancers. In contrast, amplification of *myc* genes is a common finding in a number of solid tumors, including small cell lung cancer, breast cancer, neuroblastoma, and cervical cancer. In early stage cervical cancer, c-*myc* is amplified in 33% of cases and has been shown to be associated with an increased risk of relapse following primary therapy (100). A relationship between *myc* amplification and poor survival also has been reported in neuroblastoma and breast cancer.

Amplification of the c-*myc* oncogene has also been reported to occur in epithelial ovarian cancer. In four small studies, c-*myc* was reported to be amplified in a total of 17 of 52 cases (33%) (93,101–103). In one other study, amplification of c-*myc* was not seen in any of 13 cancers examined (104). None of these reports included enough patients to determine whether a relationship exists between c-*myc* amplification and biologic behavior of ovarian cancers. Larger studies that include early stage and borderline lesions are needed to clarify this issue. In addition, studies are needed to address the role, if any, of L-*myc* and N-*myc* in ovarian cancer. Similarly, there are a significant number of other nuclear oncogenes that have not yet been studied in ovarian cancer (see Table 2) (51–53).

TUMOR-SUPPRESSOR GENES

Tumor-suppressor genes encode proteins that normally act to restrain proliferation at times when it is inappropriate. Expression of these genes likely plays a role in density-dependent inhibition of growth of normal cells (contact inhibition). Conversely, loss of tumor-suppressor function appears to play a role in immortalization of cells in culture and malignant transformation. Loss of suppressor function may occur at several levels, including deletion of both copies of a gene, mutations or partial deletions that cripple the gene product, lack of transcription, and inactivation of the protein. Among the best characterized instances in which inactivation of tumor-suppressor gene products is known to occur is that of the single-strand DNA tumor viruses. It has been shown that the transforming activity of these viruses is due to binding of specific viral proteins (SV40 T antigen, adenovirus Ela and Elb, human papilloma virus E7 and E6) to the retinoblastoma (Rb) and p53 tumor-suppressor gene products (105). The interaction between viral oncoproteins and Rb and p53 is thought to neutralize normal suppressor function. Studies are needed to clarify the implications of these observations in cervical cancer, which is associated with human papilloma virus in greater than 80% of cases.

Although Rb and p53 encode nuclear DNA-binding proteins, it is thought that other tumor-suppressor genes may encode cytoplasmic and cell-membrane associated molecules. Theoretically, any protein that normally is involved in inhibition of proliferation could conceivably be a tumor-suppressor. In this regard, the family of phosphatases that normally oppose the action of the tyrosine kinases by dephosphorylating tyrosine residues are appealing candidates (55). Recently, it has been shown that there is loss of expression of protein tyrosine phosphatase-γ (PTP-γ), a membrane-spanning phosphatase, in some renal and breast cancers (106). Studies of PTP-γ have not been reported in ovarian cancer. The DCC gene (deleted in colon carcinoma) is another example of a non-nuclear protein that is thought to act as a tumor-suppressor (107). The DCC gene was identified as a genetic locus on chromosome 18q that frequently is lost in patients with hereditary polyposis and colon cancer. Molecular cloning has revealed homology between DCC and cell-surface adhesion molecules. Although loss of DCC function also has been reported in endometrial cancer cell lines (108), loss of DCC has not been found in ovarian cancers. Because the field of tumor-suppressor genes is a relatively new one, it is likely that many additional suppressor genes will be discovered in the next several years.

Retinoblastoma

The retinoblastoma gene (Rb gene) was the first tumor-suppressor gene discovered. In hereditary retinoblastoma, affected individuals inherit one defective copy of the Rb gene as a germ-line defect. Since one intact copy of the Rb gene is still present in each cell, however, a cancer does not develop until the second copy of the gene is inactivated in a single cell. Retinoblastoma is a rare cancer, but it has been shown that loss of both copies of the Rb gene also may occur in some sarcomas and other solid tumors (51–53,109). In one study of gynecologic cancers, loss of Rb expression was not observed in 19 ovarian or endometrial cancers (110).

p53 Gene

The most extensively studied tumor-suppressor gene in solid tumors is p53, a 53-kD nuclear phosphoprotein with a short half-life that is present in small amounts in most normal cells (111,112). Like the oncogenes that encode nuclear transcription factors, p53 also binds to DNA and is thought to act as a transcriptional regulator (113). Several lines of evidence are suggestive that p53 normally acts as a tumor-suppressor gene. First, transfection of normal wild-type p53 into some transformed cells suppresses the malignant phenotype (114,115). Conversely, deletion of both copies of the wild-type p53 gene is associated with transformation of cells in culture. In addition, however, there is evidence that p53 can act as a dominant transforming oncogene. First, transfection of cells with mutant p53 genes that encode proteins with increased stability can produce transformation (116). The increased stability of these mutant forms of p53 is due to decreased degradation of the mutant protein. In addition, it has been shown that mutant p53 protein complexes with wild-type p53, which may lead to inactivation of the suppressor function of wild-type p53 protein (117).

Mutation of the p53 gene is the most frequent genetic change to be described in human cancers thus far (118,119). Mutant p53 genes have been noted in 60% of colon (120) and lung cancers (121) and in 20–25% of breast (122) and endometrial cancers (123). In addition, p53 mutations often are associated with loss of the other wild-type p53 allele (124). Mutations of the p53 have been shown to be diverse, but most occur in highly conserved regions of the gene that are of presumably functional importance (125). Since mutant p53 genes encode proteins with a prolonged half-life, mutation of the p53 gene usually leads to relative overexpression of p53 protein.

Recently, we have examined expression of the p53 gene in epithelial ovarian cancer (126). For these studies, snap-frozen tissue samples were obtained from 9 ovaries that were normal or had benign epithelial tumors and from 107 epithelial ovarian cancers. An avidin-biotin peroxidase immunohistochemical technique was used to localize p53 in frozen sections. The primary antibody (PAb) 1801, is a murine monoclonal antibody specifically reactive with p53 (127). Consistent with prior studies of normal and benign tissues, we did not find immunohistochemically detectable p53 in any of the nine normal ovaries or benign ovarian tumors because the small amounts of p53 present in most cells are below the threshold of detection. Similar to normal tissues, immunohistochemically detectable p53 was not seen in 53 (50%) of the ovarian cancers. In contrast, 54 of 107 cancers (50%), had strong nuclear staining in the majority of malignant cells, consistent with overexpression.

We also examined the relationship between p53 expression and prognostic factors in patients with ovarian cancer (126). Overexpression of p53 was seen with equal frequency in early stage (I/II) cancers (53%) and advanced stage (III/IV) cancers (50%). In this study, however, many of the tissue samples from early stage cancers were obtained at the time of recurrence. Therefore, this group of early stage cancers was biased toward more virulent lesions. Further studies of larger numbers of early stage cancers are needed. Among patients with stage III/IV disease, there was no relationship between histologic grade, optimal debulking or survival, and p53 overexpression. We did, however, observe a significant relationship between ploidy and p53 overexpression. Overall, 23% of the ovarian cancers were diploid, while 77% were aneuploid. We found that p53 overexpression was significantly more common in aneuploid cancers (58%) than in diploid cancers (30%).

To determine if overexpression of p53 in ovarian cancer is associated with mutation of the p53 gene, sequence analysis of the p53 gene was performed in several ovarian cancers following amplification using the polymerase chain reaction (126). Of three cancers in which immunohistochemically detectable p53 was not seen, all were found to have a normal wild-type p53 sequence. In contrast, three cancers that demonstrated high levels of p53 protein all contained point mutations that altered the coding sequence. In the cancer shown in Fig. 3, there was a mutation at codon 278 that changed the sequence from the wild-type CCT to CGT, with a resulting substitution of arginine for proline. No wild-type allele was seen. In two other cancers, we observed point mutations that resulted in amino acid substitutions at codons 282 and 216. Wild-type allele was clearly absent in one tumor while in the other a faint band corresponding to the wild-type sequence also was seen. The relatively faint intensity of this band suggested contamination with a small amount of DNA from normal cells rather than the presence of a copy of the wild-type allele in the cancer. All three mutations that we found were in evolutionary conserved areas of the gene (125) where mutations have been reported in other cancers (128).

Although we and others have found a close relationship between overexpression of p53 protein and point mutations in the p53 gene, it has been shown that nonsense mutations, which result in a truncated p53 mole-

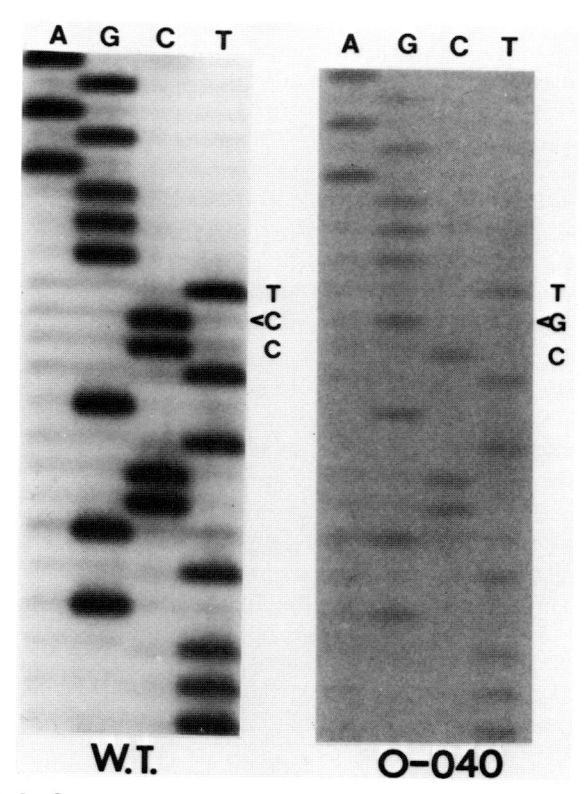

FIG. 3. Sequence analysis of the p53 gene from an ovarian cancer that overexpresses p53 protein. Point mutation (C to G) at codon 278 (arrows) changes proline to arginine.

cule that does not have an increased half-life, may also be present in some cancers (128). If one allele was lost and the other allele contained a nonsense mutation, complete loss of p53 tumor-suppressor function would result, which may contribute to the transformed phenotype. Thus, immunohistochemical staining may underestimate the frequency of p53 involvement in ovarian cancers.

The DNA-sequencing data that we have presented suggests that p53 mutations are often associated with loss of the other wild-type allele in ovarian cancer. Also consistent with this hypothesis are studies by other investigators that have shown allelic loss on chromosome 17p, where the p53 gene resides, in from one-third to three-fourths of epithelial ovarian cancers (129–133). Although it is thought that wild-type p53 normally acts as a transcriptional regulator (134,135), further studies are needed to determine the molecular mechanisms by which loss of wild-type p53 facilitates transformation.

More recently, three other reports have appeared in the literature that confirm the high frequency of allele loss and mutation and overexpression of p53 in ovarian cancer. In one study from the United Kingdom, overexpression of p53 was seen in 50% of 22 ovarian cancers (132). In another paper from Japan, p53 mutations were observed in 29% of 31 ovarian cancers (131). A French study found p53 mutations in 11 of 30 (36%) cases (136). None of these studies was large enough to further clarify the relationship between p53 expression and clinicopathologic features of ovarian cancers, however.

Similar to other common cancers associated with aging (colon, lung, breast, endometrium), p53 mutations in ovarian cancers do not appear to occur at a single codon, but rather throughout large conserved regions of the gene. By contrast, in esophageal and liver cancers, caused by known dietary carcinogens in certain areas of the world, a single codon has consistently been found to be mutated (137). These and other findings have led to speculation that mutations that occur in p53, ras, and other genes in cancers of aging are not due to environmental carcinogens. Rather, it is thought that these mutations are due to errors in DNA synthesis that occur at a low frequency during DNA replication associated with normal cellular proliferation (138–140). Thus, the longer one is alive, the higher the probability of accumulating cells that have acquired the multiple activated cancer-causing genes required for the development of a clinically recognizable tumor. This hypothesis is certainly appealing in the case of epithelial ovarian cancer, since no environmental carcinogens have been convincingly associated with this disease, despite numerous studies.

Another important issue is whether p53 mutations are early causative events in ovarian carcinogenesis or late events that occur due to genetic instability associated with the malignant phenotype. Data from other tumors appear to indicate that activation of p53 may occur at different stages of tumorigenesis in different tumor types. For example, although it appears that p53 mutation is a late event in colon carcinogenesis that is seen infrequently in premalignant colonic adenomas (141), p53 mutations have been found in carcinoma-in-situ of the breast (142). In addition, the finding that patients with Li-Fraumeni Familial Cancer Syndrome who develop multiple cancers at a young age have inherited mutant p53 genes is suggestive that p53 mutation may be an early event in the development of some human cancers (143). Alternatively, the accumulation of multiple activated genes in a cell may be more important than the order in which they occur.

CONCLUSION

The discovery of cancer-causing genes has provided us with the exciting opportunity to begin to understand the molecular pathology of ovarian cancer. Activation of several of these genes, including HER-2/neu, c-myc, ras, and p53, has been described in some ovarian cancers (Table 3). In addition, since some proto-oncogenes such as the EGF receptor (erbB) and the M-CSF receptor (fms) are expressed along with their respective ligands in some ovarian cancers, autocrine, paracrine, or juxtacrine growth-stimulatory pathways may exist in some cases. For every proto-oncogene and tumor-suppressor gene that has been studied in ovarian cancer, however, there are at least a half-dozen that remain unexplored.

In the future, a better understanding of the molecular pathology involved in the development of ovarian cancer will improve our ability to predict the clinical behavior of a patient's cancer. It is likely that epithelial

TABLE 3. Oncogenes and tumor-suppressor genes activated in ovarian cancer

Gene	Class	Activation	Frequency
HER-2/neu	tyrosine kinase	amplification/overexpression	32%
Ki-ras	G protein	mutation	rare
		amplification	5–10%
c-myc	nuclear transcription	amplification	33%
p53	tumor-suppressor	mutation/overexpression	50%

ovarian cancer actually comprises several subsets of cancers of varying virulence that can be defined on the basis of abnormalities in various cancer-causing genes. The pathology report of the future will likely provide information on the status of these genes, in addition to the histologic description of the appearance of the cancer, which is of limited value beyond identifying the cell type of origin. In addition, insights into the molecular mechanisms of ovarian carcinogenesis should lead to improvements in diagnosis, treatment, and eventually to prevention of ovarian cancer.

REFERENCES

1. Czech M, Clairmont K, Yagaloff K, Corvera S. Properties and regulation of receptors for growth factors. In: Sporn MB, Roberts AB, eds. *Peptide growth factors and their receptors I.* Berlin: Springer-Verlag; 1990:37–65.
2. Ullrich A, Schlessinger J. Signal transduction by receptors with tyrosine kinase activity. *Cell* 1990;61:203–212.
3. Carpenter G, Wahl MI. The epidermal growth factor family. In: Sporn MB, Roberts AB, eds. *Peptide growth factors and their receptors I.* Berlin: Springer-Verlag; 1990:69–171.
4. Carpenter G, Cohen S. Epidermal growth factor. *J Biol Chem* 1990;265:7709–7712.
5. Massague J. Transforming growth factor-α: A model for membrane-anchored growth factors. *J Biol Chem* 1990;265:21393–21396.
6. Derynck R. Transforming growth factor-α. *Cell* 1988;54:593–596.
7. Gullick WJ. Prevalence of aberrant expression of the epidermal growth factor receptor in human cancers. *Br Med Bull* 1991;47:87–98.
8. Hanauske AR, Arteaga CL, Clark GM, et al. Determination of transforming growth factor activity in effusions from cancer patients. *Cancer* 1988;61:1832–1837.
9. Hendler FJ, Ozanne BW. Human squamous cell lung cancers express increased epidermal growth factor receptors. *J Clin Invest* 1984;74:647–651.
10. Sainsbury JR, Farndon JR, Needham GK, Malcolm AJ, Harris AL. Epidermal-growth-factor receptor status as predictor of early recurrence of and death from breast cancer. *Lancet* 1987;1:1398–1402.
11. Berchuck A, Rodriguez GC, Kamel A, et al. Epidermal growth factor receptor expression in normal ovarian epithelium and ovarian cancer: I. Correlation of receptor expression with prognostic factors in patients with ovarian cancer. *Am J Obstet Gynecol* 1991;164:669–674.
12. Kohler M, Janz I, Wintzer HO, Wagner E, Bauknecht T. The expression of EGF receptors, EGF-like factors and c-*myc* in ovarian and cervical carcinomas and their potential clinical significance. *Anticancer Res* 1989;9:1537–1547.
13. Bauknecht T, Runge M, Schwall M, Pfleiderer A. Occurrence of epidermal growth factor receptors in human adnexal tumors and their prognostic value in advanced ovarian carcinomas. *Gynecol Oncol* 1988;29:147–157.
14. Rechler MM, Nissley SP. Insulin-like growth factors. In: Sporn MB, Roberts AB, eds. *Peptide growth factors and their receptors I,* Berlin: Springer-Verlag; 1990:263–367.
15. Adashi EY, Resnick CE, D'Ercole AJ, Svoboda ME, Van Wyk JJ. Insulin-like growth factors as intraovarian regulators of granulosa cell growth and function. *Endocr Rev* 1985;6:400–420.
16. Yee D, Morales FR, Hamilton TC, Von Hoff DD. Expression of insulin-like growth factor I, its binding proteins, and its receptor in ovarian cancer. *Cancer Res* 1991;51:5107–5112.
17. Baird A, Bohlen P. Fibroblast growth factors. In: Sporn MB, Roberts AB, eds. *Peptide growth factors and their receptors I,* Berlin: Springer-Verlag; 1990:369–418.
18. Burgess W, Maciag T. The heparin-binding (fibroblast) growth factor family of proteins. *Annu Rev Biochem* 1989;58:575–606.
19. Raines EW, Bowen-Pope DF, Ross R. Platelet-derived growth factor. In: Sporn MB, Roberts AB, eds. *Peptide growth factors and their receptors I,* Berlin: Springer-Verlag; 1990:173–262.
20. Westermark B. The molecular and cellular biology of platelet-derived growth factor. *Acta Endocrinol* 1990;123:131–142.
21. Libby P, Warner S, Salomon RN, Birinyi LK. Production of platelet-derived growth factor-like mitogen by smooth-muscle cells from human atheroma. *N Engl J Med* 1988;318:1493–1498.
22. Westermark B, Heldin CH. Platelet-derived growth factor in autocrine transformation. *Cancer Res* 1991;51:5087–5092.
23. Sariban E, Sitaras NM, Antoniades HN, Kufe D, Pantazis P. Expression of platelet-derived growth factor (PDGF)-related transcripts and synthesis of biologically active PDGF-like proteins by human malignant epithelial cell lines. *J Clin Invest* 1988;82:1157–1164.
24. Sherr CJ, Stanley ER. Colony-stimulating factor 1 (macrophage colony-stimulating-factor). In: Sporn MB, Roberts AB, eds. *Peptide growth factors and their receptors I,* Berlin: Springer-Verlag; 1990:667–698.
25. Lidor YJ, Xu FJ, Martinez-Maza O, et al. Constitutive production of macrophage colony stimulating factor and interleukin-6 by human ovarian surface epithelial cells, (submitted).
26. Ramakrishnan S, Xu FJ, Brandt SJ, Niedel JE, Bast RC Jr, Brown EL. Constitutive Production of Macrophage Colony-Stimulating Factor by Human Ovarian and Breast Cancer Cell Lines. *J Clin Invest* 1989;83:921–926.
27. Kacinski BM, Stanley ER, Carter D, et al. Circulating levels of CSF-1 (M-CSF) a lymphohematopoietic cytokine may be a useful marker of disease status in patients with malignant ovarian neoplasms. *Int J Radiat Oncol Biol Phys* 1989;17:159–164.
28. Kacinski BM, Carter D, Mittal K, et al. Ovarian adenocarcinomas express *fms*-complementary transcripts and *fms* antigen, often with coexpression of CSF-1. *Am J Pathol* 1990;137:1:135–147.
29. Wu S, Rodabaugh K, Martinez-Maza O, Berek JS, Boyer CM and Bast RC. Stimulation of ovarian tumor cell proliferation with monocyte products including interleukin-1-alpha, interleukin-6 and tumor necrosis factor-alpha, 1991 (submitted).
30. Kacinski BM, Carter D, Kohorn EI, et al. High level expression of *fms* proto-oncogene mRNA is observed in clinically aggressive endometrial adenocarcinomas. *Int J Radiat Oncol Bio Phys* 1988;15:823–829.
31. Xu FJ, Ramakrishnan S, Daly L, et al. Increased serum levels of macrophage colony-stimulating factor in ovarian cancer. *Am J Obstet Gynecol* 1992;165:1356–1362.
32. Roberts AB, Sporn MB. The transforming growth factor-β. In: Sporn MB, Roberts AB, eds. *Peptide growth factors and their receptors I,* Berlin: Springer-Verlag; 1990:419–472.
33. Wakefield L, Sporn MB. Suppression of carcinogenesis: a role for TGF-β and related molecules in prevention of cancer. In: Klein G, ed. *Tumor Suppressor Genes,* New York: Marcel Dekker, Inc.; 1990:217–243.
34. Moses HL, Yang HY, Pietenpol JA. TGF-β stimulation and inhibition of cell proliferation: New mechanistic insights. *Cell* 1990;63:245–247.
35. Sporn MB, Roberts AB. Peptide growth factors are multifunctional. *Nature* 1988;332:217–218.
36. Mulheron GW, Danielpour D, Schomberg DW. Rat thecal/interstitial cells express transforming growth factor-β Type 1 and 2, but only Type 2 is regulated by gonadotropin in vitro. *Endocrinol* 1991;129:368–374.
37. Blair EI, Kim IC, Estes JE, Keski-Oja J, Schomberg DW. Human platelet-derived growth factor preparations contain a separate activity which potentiates follicle-stimulating hormone-mediated induction of luteinizing hormone receptor in cultured rat granulosa cells: Evidence for transforming growth factor-β. *Endocrinol* 1988;123:2003–2008.
38. Adashi EY, Resnick CE, Hernandez ER, May JV, Purchio AF, Twardzik DR. Ovarian transforming growth factor-beta (TGF-β): cellular site(s), and mechanism(s) of action. *Mol Cell Endocrinol* 1989;61:247–256.
39. Berchuck A, Olt GJ, Everitt L, Soisson AP, Bast RC Jr, Boyer

CM. The role of peptide growth factors in epithelial ovarian cancer. *Obstet Gynecol* 1990;75:255–262.
40. Bauknecht T, Kiechle M, Bauer G, Siebers JW. Characterization of growth factors in human ovarian carcinomas. *Cancer Res* 1986;46:2614–2618.
41. Kommoss F, Wintzer HO, Von Kleist S, et al. In situ distribution of transforming growth factor-α in normal human tissues and in malignant tumours of the ovary. *J Pathol* 1990;162:223–230.
42. Morishige K, Kurachi H, Amemiya K, et al. Evidence for the involvement of transforming growth factor-α and epidermal growth factor receptor autocrine growth mechanism in primary human ovarian cancers in vitro. *Cancer Res* 1991;51:5322–5328.
43. Berchuck A, Rodriguez GC, Olt GJ, et al. Regulation of growth of normal ovarian epithelial cells and ovarian cancer cell lines by transforming growth factor-β. *Am J Obstet Gynecol* 1992;166:676–684.
44. Kruk PA, Maines-Bandiera SL, Auersperg N. A simplified method to culture human ovarian surface epithelium. *Lab Invest* 1990;63:132–136.
45. Rodriguez GC, Berchuck A, Whitaker RS, Schlossman D, Clarke-Pearson DL, Bast RC Jr. Epidermal growth factor receptor expression in normal ovarian epithelium and ovarian cancer. II. Relationship between receptor expression and response to epidermal growth factor. *Am J Obstet Gynecol* 1991;164:745–750.
46. Hofmann GE, Scott RT, Brzyki RG, Jones HW. Immunoreactive epidermal growth factor concentrations in follicular fluid obtained from in vitro fertilization. *Fertil Steril* 1990;54:303–307.
47. Eden JA, Jones J, Carter GD, Alaghband-Zadeh J. Follicular fluid concentrations of insulin-like growth factor 1, epidermal growth factor, transforming growth factor-α and sex-steroids in volume matched normal and polycystic human follicles. *Clin Endo* 1990;32:395–405.
48. Mills GB, May C, McGill M, Roifman CM, Mellors A. A putative new growth factor in ascitic fluid from ovarian cancer patients: identification, characterization, and mechanism of action. *Cancer Res* 1988;48:1066–1071.
49. Mills GB, May C, Hill M, Campbell S, Shaw P, Marks A. Ascitic fluid from human ovarian cancer patients contains growth factors necessary for intraperitoneal growth of human ovarian adenocarcinoma cells. *J Clin Invest* 1990;86:851–855.
50. Wilson AP, Fox H, Scott IV, Lee H, Dent M, Golding PR. A comparison of the growth promoting properties of ascitic fluids, cyst fluids and peritoneal fluids from patients with ovarian tumours. *Br J Cancer* 1991;63:102–108.
51. Bishop JM. Molecular themes in oncogenesis. *Cell* 1991;64:235–248.
52. Hunter T. Cooperation between oncogenes. *Cell* 1991;64:249–270.
53. Cooper JM. *Oncogenes*, Boston: Jones and Bartlett; 1990.
54. Cantley LC, Auger KR, Carpenter C, et al. Oncogenes and signal transduction. *Cell* 1991;64:281–302.
55. Hunter T. Protein-tyrosine phosphatases: The other side of the coin. *Cell* 1989;58:1013–1016.
56. Meisenhelder J, Suh PG, Rhee SG, Hunter T. Phospholipase C-gamma is a substrate for the PDGF and EGF receptor protein-tyrosine kinases in vivo and in vitro. *Cell* 1989;57:1109–1122.
57. Schechter AL, Hung MC, Vaidyanathan L, et al. The *neu* gene: an *erb*B-homologous gene distinct from and unlinked to the gene encoding the EGF receptor. *Science* 1985;229:976–978.
58. Coussens L, Yang-Feng TL, Liao YC, et al. Tyrosine kinase receptor with extensive homology to EGF receptor shares chromosomal location with *neu* oncogene. *Science* 1985;230:1132–1139.
59. Schechter AL, Stern DF, Vaidyanathan L, et al. The *neu* oncogene: an *erb*-B-related gene encoding a 185,000-Mr tumour antigen. *Nature* 1984;312:513–516.
60. Bargmann CI, Hung MC, Weinberg RA. The *neu* oncogene encodes an Epidermal Growth Factor Receptor-related protein. *Nature* 1986;319:226–230.
61. Lupu R, Colomer R, Zugmaier G, et al. Direct interaction of a ligand for the *erb*B2 oncogene product with the EGF receptor and p^{185} *erb*B2. *Science* 1990;249:1552–1555.
62. Bargmann CI, Hung MC, Weinberg RA. Multiple independent activations of the *neu* oncogene by a point mutation altering the transmembrane domain of p185. *Cell* 1986;45:649–657.
63. Lemoine NR, Staddon S, Dickson C, Barnes DM, Gullick WJ. Absence of activating transmembrane mutations in the c-*erb*B-2 proto-oncogene in human breast cancer. *Oncogene* 1990;5:237–239.
64. Slamon DJ, Clark GM, Wong SG, Levin WJ, Ullrich A, McGuire WL. Human breast cancer: Correlation of relapse and survival with amplification of the HER-2/*neu* oncogene. *Science* 1987;235:177–182.
65. Slamon DJ, Godolphin W, Jones LA, et al. Studies of HER-2/*neu* proto-oncogene in human breast and ovarian cancer. *Science* 1989;244:707–712.
66. van de Vijver MJ, Peterse JL, Mooi WJ, et al. *Neu*-protein overexpression in breast cancer. Association with comedotype ductal carcinoma in situ and limited prognostic value in stage II breast cancer. *N Engl J Med* 1988;319:1239–1245.
67. Borg A, Tandon AK, Sigurdsson H, et al. HER-2/*neu* amplification predicts poor survival in node-positive breast cancer. *Cancer Res* 1990;50:4332–4337.
68. Paterson MC, Dietrich KD, Danyluk J, et al. Correlation between c-*erb*B-2 amplification and risk of recurrent disease in node-negative breast cancer. *Cancer Res* 1991;51:556–567.
69. Tandon AK, Clark GM, Chamness GC, Ullrich A, McGuire WL. HER-2/*neu* oncogene protein and prognosis in breast cancer. *J Clin Oncol* 1989;7:1120–1128.
70. Paik S, Hazan R, Fisher ER, et al. Pathologic findings from the National Surgical Adjuvant Breast and Bowel Project: prognostic significance of *erb*B-2 protein overexpression in primary breast cancer. *J Clin Oncol* 1990;8:103–112.
71. Di Fiore PP, Pierce JH, Kraus MH, Segatto O, King CR, Aaronson SA. *erb*B-2 is a potent oncogene when overexpressed in NIH/3T3 Cells. *Science* 1987;237:178–182.
72. Hudziak RM, Schlessinger J, Ullrich A. Increased expression of the putative growth factor receptor p185HER2 causes transformation and tumorigenesis of NIH 3T3 cells. *Proc Natl Acad Sci USA* 1987;84:7159–7163.
73. Bouchard L, Lamarre L, Tremblay PJ, Jolicoeur P. Stochastic appearance of mammary tumors in transgenic mice carrying the MMTV/c-*neu* oncogene. *Cell* 1989;57:931–936.
74. Muller WJ, Sinn E, Pattengale PK, Wallace R, Leder P. Single-step induction of mammary adenocarcinoma in transgenic mice bearing the activated c-*neu* oncogene. *Cell* 1988;54:105–115.
75. Iglehart JD, Kraus MH, Langton BC, Huper G, Kerns BJ, Marks JR. Increased *erb*B-2 gene copies and expression in multiple stages of breast cancer. *Cancer Res* 1990;50:6701–6707.
76. Bacus SS, Ruby SG, Weinberg DS, Chin D, Ortiz R, Bacus JW. HER-2/*neu* oncogene expression and proliferation in breast cancers. *Am J Pathol* 1990;137:103–111.
77. Zhang X, Silva E, Gershenson D, Hung MC. Amplification and rearrangement of c-*erb* B proto-oncogenes in cancer of human female genital tract. *Oncogene* 1989;4:985–989.
78. Zheng J, Robinson WR, Ehlen T, Yu MC, Dubeau L. Distinction of low grade from high grade human ovarian carcinomas on the basis of losses of heterozygosity on chromosomes 3, 6, and 11 and HER-2/*neu* gene amplification. *Cancer Res* 1991;51:4045–4051.
79. Berchuck A, Kamel A, Whitaker R, et al. Overexpression of HER-2/*neu* is associated with poor survival in advanced epithelial ovarian cancer. *Cancer Res* 1990;50:4087–4091.
80. McKenzie SJ, Marks PJ, Lam T, et al. Generation and characterization of monoclonal antibodies specific for the human *neu* oncogene product, p185. *Oncogene* 1989;4:543–548.
81. Lacroix H, Iglehart JD, Skinner MA, Kraus MH. Overexpression of *erb*B-2 or EGF receptor proteins present in early stage mammary carcinoma is detected simultaneously in matched primary tumors and regional metastases. *Oncogene* 1989;4:145–151.
82. Hancock MC, Langton BC, Chan T, et al. A monoclonal antibody against the c-*erb*B-2 protein enhances the cytotoxicity of

cis-Diamminedichloroplatinum against human breast and ovarian tumor cell lines. *Cancer Res* 1991;51:4575–4580.
83. Langton BC, Crenshaw MC, Chao LA, Stuart SG, Akita RW, Jackson JE. An antigen immunologically related to the external domain of gp185 is shed from nude mouse tumors overexpressing the c-*erb*B-2 (HER-2/*neu*) oncogene. *Cancer Res* 1991;51: 2593–2598.
84. McKenzie S, Hollis D, DeSombre K, et al. Serum levels of HER-2/*neu* (c-*erb*B-2) correlate with overexpression of the proto-oncogene in human ovarian cancer (submitted).
85. Stancovski I, Hurwitz E, Leitner O, Ullrich A, Yarden Y, Sela M. Mechanistic aspects of the opposing effects of monoclonal antibodies to the ERBB2 receptor on tumor growth. *Proc Natl Acad Sci USA* 1991;88:8691–8695.
86. Myers JN, Drebin JA, Wada T, Greene MI. Biological effects of monoclonal antireceptor antibodies reactive with *neu* oncogene product p185/*neu*. *Methods Enzymol* 1991;198:277–290.
87. Xu FJ, Rodriguez GC, Whitaker R, et al. Antibodies against immunochemically distinct domains on the extracellular domain of HER-2/*neu* (c-*erb*B-2) inhibit growth of breast and ovarian cancer cell lines. *Proc Am Assoc Cancer Res* 1991;32: 260.
88. Vogelstein B, Fearon ER, Hamilton SR, et al. Genetic alterations during colorectal-tumor development. *N Engl J Med* 1988; 319:525–532.
89. Enomoto T, Inoue M, Perantoni AO, Terakawa N, Tanizawa O, Rice JM. K-*ras* activation in neoplasms of the human female reproductive tract. *Cancer Res* 1990;50:6139–6145.
90. Feig LA, Bast RC Jr, Knapp RC, Cooper GM. Somatic activation of *ras*K gene in a human ovarian carcinoma. *Science* 1984; 223:698–701.
91. Haas M, Isakov J, Howell SB. Evidence against *ras* activation in human ovarian carcinomas. *Mol Biol Med* 1987;4:265–275.
92. Filmus J, Trent JM, Pullano R, Buick RN. A cell line from a human ovarian carcinoma with amplification of the K-*ras* gene. *Cancer Res* 1986;46:5179–5182.
93. Zhou DJ, Gonzalez-Cadavid N, Ahuja H, Battifora H, Moore GE, Cline MJ. A unique pattern of proto-oncogene abnormalities in ovarian adenocarcinomas. *Cancer* 1988;62:1573–1576.
94. Fukumoto M, Estensen RD, Sha L, et al. Association of Ki-*ras* with amplified DNA sequences, detected in human ovarian carcinomas by a modified in-gel renaturation assay. *Cancer Res* 1989;49:1693–1697.
95. Boltz EM, Kefford RF, Leary JA, Houghton CR, Friedlander ML. Amplification of c-*ras*-Ki oncogene in human ovarian tumours. *Int J Cancer* 1989;43:428–430.
96. van't Veer LJ, Hermens R, van den Berg-Bakker LAM, et al. *ras* oncogene activation in human ovarian carcinoma. *Oncogene* 1988;2:157–165.
97. Rodenburg CJ, Koelma IA, Nap M, Fleuren GJ. Immunohistochemical detection of the *ras* oncogene product p21 in advanced ovarian cancer. Lack of correlation with clinical outcome. *Arch Pathol Lab Med* 1988;112:151–154.
98. Lyons J, Landis CA, Harsh G, et al. Two G protein oncogenes in human endocrine tumors. *Science* 1990;249:655–659.
99. Bourne HR, Sanders DA, McCormick F. The GTPase superfamily: a conserved switch for diverse cell functions. *Nature* 1990;348:125–132.
100. Bourhis J, Barros L, Jeannel GD, et al. Prognostic value of c-*myc* proto-oncogene overexpression in early invasive carcinoma of the cervix. *J Clin Oncol* 1990;8:1789–1796.
101. Baker VV, Borst MP, Dixon D, Hatch KD, Shingleton HM, Miller D. c-*myc* amplification in ovarian cancer. *Gynecol Oncol* 1990;38:340–342.
102. Serova DM. Amplification of c-*myc* proto-oncogene in primary tumors, metastases and blood leukocytes of patients with ovarian cancer. *Eksp Onkol* 1987;9:25–27.
103. Sasano H, Garrett CT, Wilkinson DS, Silverberg S, Comerford J, Hyde J. Proto-oncogene amplification and tumor ploidy in human ovarian neoplasms. *Hum Pathol* 1990;21:382–391.
104. Tyson FL, Boyer CM, Kaufman R, et al. Overexpression and amplification of the HER-2/*neu* (c-*erb*B-2) proto-oncogene in epithelial ovarian tumors and cell lines. *Am J Obstet Gynecol* 1991;165:640–646.
105. Levine AJ. The p53 protein and its interactions with the oncogene products of the small DNA tumor viruses. *Virology* 1990; 177:419–426.
106. LaForgia S, Morse B, Levy D, et al. Receptor protein-tyrosine phosphatase gamma is a candidate tumor suppressor gene at human chromosome region 3p21. *Proc Natl Acad Sci USA* 1991;88:5036–5040.
107. Fearon E, Cho K, Nigro J, et al. Identification of a chromosome 18q gene that is altered in colorectal cancers. *Science* 1990;247: 49–56.
108. Boyd J, Risinger JI, Walmer DK, Cho KR, Vogelstein B, Barrett JC. Altered structure and expression of the DCC gene in human endometrial carcinoma. *Proc Am Assoc Cancer Res* 1991;32:309.
109. Levine AJ, Momand J. Tumor suppressor genes: the p53 and retinoblastoma sensitivity genes and gene products. *Biochim Biophys Acta* 1990;1032:119–136.
110. Sasano H, Comerford J, Silverberg SG, Garrett CT. An analysis of abnormalities of the retinoblastoma gene in human ovarian and endometrial carcinoma. *Cancer* 1990;66:2150–2154.
111. Lane DP, Benchimol S. p53: oncogene or anti-oncogene? *Genes Dev* 1990;4:1–8.
112. Levine AJ, Momand J, Finlay CA. The p53 tumour suppressor gene. *Nature* 1991;351:453–456.
113. Kern SE, Kinzler KW, Bruskin A, et al. Identification of p53 as a sequence-specific DNA-binding protein. *Science* 1991;252: 1708–1711.
114. Baker SJ, Markowitz S, Fearon ER, Willson JK, Vogelstein B. Suppression of human colorectal carcinoma cell growth by wild-type p53. *Science* 1990;249:912–915.
115. Finlay CA, Hinds PW, Levine AJ. The p53 proto-oncogene can act as a suppressor of transformation. *Cell* 1989;57:1083–1093.
116. Hinds P, Finlay C, Levine AJ. Mutation is required to activate the p53 gene for cooperation with the *ras* oncogene and transformation. *J Virol* 1989;63:739–746.
117. Kraiss S, Quaiser A, Oren M, Montenarh M. Oligomerization of oncoprotein p53. *J Virol* 1988;62:4737–4744.
118. Harris AL. Mutant p53—the commonest genetic abnormality in human cancer? *J Pathol* 1990;162:5–6.
119. Nigro JM, Baker SJ, Preisinger AC, et al. Mutations in the p53 gene occur in diverse human tumour types. *Nature* 1989;342: 705–708.
120. Rodrigues NR, Rowan A, Smith ME, et al. p53 mutations in colorectal cancer. *Proc Natl Acad Sci U S A* 1990;87: 7555–7559.
121. Iggo R, Gatter K, Bartek J, Lane D, Harris AL. Increased expression of mutant forms of p53 oncogene in primary lung cancer. *Lancet* 1990;335:675–679.
122. Davidoff AM, Humphrey PA, Iglehart JD, Marks JR. Genetic basis for p53 overexpression in human breast cancer. *Proc Natl Acad Sci U S A* 1991;88:5006–5010.
123. Kohler MF, Berchuck A, Davidoff AM, et al. Overexpression and mutation of p53 in endometrial carcinoma. *Cancer Res* 1992;52:1622–1627.
124. Baker SJ, Fearon ER, Nigro JM, et al. Chromosome 17 deletions and p53 gene mutations in colorectal carcinomas. *Science* 1989;244:217–221.
125. Soussi T, Caron de Fromentel C, Mechali M, May P, Kress M. Cloning and characterization of a cDNA from Xenopus laevis coding for a protein homologous to human and murine p53. *Oncogene* 1987;1:71–78.
126. Marks JR, Davidoff AM, Kerns BJ, et al. Overexpression and mutation of p53 in epithelial ovarian cancer. *Cancer Res* 1991; 51:2979–2984.
127. Banks L, Matlashewski G, Crawford L. Isolation of human-p53-specific monoclonal antibodies and their use in the studies of human p53 expression. *Eur J Biochem* 1986;159:529–534.
128. Hollstein M, Sidransky D, Vogelstein B, Harris CC. p53 mutations in human cancers. *Science* 1991;253:49–53.
129. Eccles DM, Cranston MG, Steel CM, et al. Allele losses on chromosome 17 in human epithelial ovarian carcinoma. *Oncogene* 1990;5:1599–1601.
130. Russell SEH, Hickey GI, Lowry WS, et al. Allele loss from

chromosome 17 in ovarian cancer. *Oncogene* 1990;5: 1581–1583.
131. Okamoto A, Sameshima Y, Yokoyama S, et al. Frequent allelic losses and mutations of the p53 gene in human ovarian cancer. *Cancer Res* 1991;51:5171–5176.
132. Eccles D, Cranston G, Gruber L, et al. Allele losses in human epithelial ovarian carcinoma (EOC) and immunohistochemical detection of mutant p53 protein. *Proc Am Soc Clin Oncol* 1991; 10:81.
133. Sato T, Saito H, Morita R, Koi S, Lee JH, Nakamura Y. Allelotype of human ovarian cancer. *Cancer Res* 1991;51:5118–5122.
134. Fields S, Jang SK. Presence of a potent transcription activating sequence in the p53 protein. *Science* 1990;249:1046–1049.
135. Raycroft L, Wu HY, Lozano G. Transcriptional activation by wild-type but not transforming mutants of the p53 anti-oncogene. *Science* 1990;249:1049–1051.
136. Mazars R, Pujol P, Maudelone T, Jeanteur P, Theillet C. p53 mutations in ovarian cancer: a late event? *Oncogene* 1991;6: 1685–1690.
137. Hsu IC, Metcalf RA, Sun T, Welsh JA, Wang NJ, Harris CC. Mutational hotspots in the p53 gene in human hepatocellular carcinoma. *Nature* 1991;350:427–428.
138. Cohen SM, Ellwein LB. Cell proliferation in carcinogenesis. *Science* 1990;249:1007–1011.
139. Preston-Martin S, Pike MC, Ross RK, Jones PA, Henderson BE. Increased cell division as a cause of human cancer. *Cancer Res* 1990;50:7415–7421.
140. Ames BN, Gold LS. Too many rodent carcinogens: Mitogenesis increases mutagenesis. *Science* 1990;249:970–971.
141. Baker SJ, Preisinger AC, Jessup JM, et al. p53 gene mutations occur in combination with 17p allelic deletions as late events in colorectal tumorigenesis. *Cancer Res* 1990;50:7717–7722.
142. Davidoff AM, Kerns BJ, Iglehart JD, Marks JR. Maintenance of p53 alterations throughout stages of breast cancer progression. *Cancer Res* 1991;51:2605–2610.
143. Malkin D, Li FP, Strong LC, et al. Germ line p53 mutations in a familial syndrome of breast cancer, sarcomas, and other neoplasms. *Science* 1990;250:1233–1238.

CHAPTER 5

The Epidemiology of Ovarian Cancer

Susan Harlap

The ovary is the sixth most common site of cancer in women after the breast, lung, colon, rectum, and endometrium. Cancer of the ovary affects about 4% of the more than half a million women diagnosed each year with cancer in the US (1), and 3–7% of women with cancer in other countries (2). Approximately 20,000 deaths occur annually in the US as a result of this disease. Some 1–2% of women can expect to be diagnosed with ovarian cancer during their lifetime (3).

PATTERNS OF INCIDENCE

Geographic

There are up to sevenfold differences in the annual incidence of ovarian cancer among different countries; estimates vary from 2–4 per 100,000 population in certain developing countries (4) and rural areas of Japan (4,5) to 14–15 in some European countries (4). In Europe there is a north-south gradient, age-adjusted incidence rates being highest in Scandinavian countries (13.9–15.3 per 100,000 annually), intermediate in the United Kingdom, France, Switzerland, and Germany (7.8–13.2 per 100,000) and lowest in countries and areas bordering the Mediterranean (5.4–11.7 per 100,000). A reversed south-north gradient is seen in South America (2). In the US, the annual incidence, age-adjusted to the world population, is 12–13 per 100,000, with only minor variations between states. Incidence rates are similar in Canada (4,6). While the very low incidence of ovarian cancer in developing countries and in urban versus rural areas (7) may be partly explained by incomplete reporting, most of the differences between geographic areas are explained by socioeconomic development, particularly the effect of that development on patterns of fertility.

Race and Religion

In the US, the age-adjusted incidence of ovarian cancer has been consistently higher in whites compared with blacks (1,4,5). The difference between blacks and whites diverges progressively with increasing age (1) and is due to variations in the incidence of epithelial cancers (8). Below age 45, blacks show higher rates of ovarian cancer than whites due to an excess of nonepithelial tumors (8).

Racial and religious variations in ovarian cancers in adults are generally consistent with group differences in fertility and/or socioeconomic status. Thus, lower incidence rates in American Indians and in Hispanic versus non-Hispanic women in New Mexico (9), and lower rates in Catholics and Mormons (10,11) compared with other white Americans, are consistent with the higher fertility of these groups. In Israel, the incidence of ovarian cancer in Jewish emigrants from Europe or the Americas is among the highest in the world (12,13), compatible with the extremely low fertility of Jews in those countries (14). By contrast, Israeli Arabs and Jewish groups emigrating from countries of North Africa and the Asian Near East (groups with high fertility) have shown very low incidence of the disease (13).

Time Trends

Judging from autopsy series, ovarian cancer seems to have been extremely rare in the nineteenth century (15,16). Mortality rates from this disease increased in many industrial countries during the early 1900s (17), stabilizing in the second half of the century. Since 1950, mortality rates have been arising in Japan, France,

---

S. Harlap: Department of Epidemiology and Biostatistics, Memorial Sloan-Kettering Cancer Center, New York, New York, 10021

Italy, and Ireland, which were formerly "low risk" countries (9). The rise in mortality from ovarian cancer has been substantial in these countries—about 1 per 100,000 per decade, representing roughly 50–100% increase in mortality over a 20-year period (9).

On the other hand, both mortality and incidence rates were rather stable between 1950 and 1985 in Sweden, Denmark, the Netherlands, the US (whites) and Canada (9). But these cross-sectional rates have masked more complex changes associated with cohort year of birth and age that have been occurring in developed countries. The lifetime incidence of ovarian cancer rose for women born in successive birth cohorts between 1861 and 1901, both in the US and in England and Wales; it reached a maximum among women born around the turn of the century, but fell somewhat in women born since then (18). Similarly, in Sweden, the lifetime incidence of ovarian cancer increased for women born in the last few decades of the 1800s; but for women born since 1920 the risk has been decreasing in successive birth cohorts (19). Similar trends can be inferred from vital statistics in Denmark and in the Netherlands, in which there were falling mortality rates from ovarian cancer in the late 1970s and early 1980s in women under age 45 (9). In England and Wales, younger women also showed decreases in the incidence and mortality from ovarian cancer during the 1970s and 1980s, at a time when these were still rising in older women. The same trends have been seen in the US (20).

The increasing risk of ovarian cancer in older women born in successively later cohorts of the late 1800s has been attributed to decreasing fertility (18) or to other effects of industrialization. It is consistent with the rising incidence of ovarian cancer in: Japanese immigrants to the US (21), immigrants to Israel from North Africa and Asia (13) and formerly low-risk areas such as Quebec, Brazil, and Singapore (9). On the other hand, the decreasing risk of ovarian cancer in recent birth cohorts in developed countries has been attributed to oral contraceptives (7,19,22) and to other factors, such as tubal sterilizations and oophorectomies that may also have contributed to these changes.

Age

Knowledge of the cohort effects described above is needed to interpret cross-sectional patterns of incidence and mortality by age. The probability of ovarian cancer being diagnosed in an individual woman rises with age (19,23). In the middle of this century, cross-sectional data from the US suggested that incidence rates rose with age to a maximum around age 50, thereafter falling with increasing age. This is an artifact due to a cohort effect; risks are lower in cohorts born progressively earlier, but within each birth cohort there is little evidence to support the notion that incidence rates for ovarian cancer actually decrease with age. Adami et al. (19) have calculated incidence rates in Sweden adjusted for cohort effects and for trends according to year of diagnosis. According to that report, ovarian cancer increases in an almost linear fashion between ages 30–50; thereafter there is a continued rise with age, though with a lower gradient. Thus, the pattern of incidence by age is similar to that observed for breast cancer (23,24).

Histologic Type

The three main types of ovarian cancers—epithelial, germ cell, and sex cord-stromal tumors—have differing patterns of incidence by age (Fig. 1). Epithelial tumors increase in incidence with increasing age but are less common in older than in middle-aged women due to the cohort effects described above. Germ cell tumors peak in incidence in early postpubertal life and occur roughly constantly at older ages. Sex cord and stromal tumors increase in incidence with increasing age (25). The prevalence of the three different types of ovarian tumors seen at different ages is shown in Fig. 2. In children, ovarian cancers are germ cell tumors, or (more rarely) sex cord-stromal neoplasms. Epithelial tumors occur after puberty and account for an increasing proportion of ovarian cancers with increasing age; above age 35, some 90–95% of ovarian tumors are epithelial (8). Among epithelial tumors, there are some variations in the prevalence of different subtypes at different ages, but these variations are small (Fig. 3) (2,25). The statistics shown in Figs. 1–3 are derived from population-based data from the US that were collected in the 1970s; more recent data are not available. Statistics based on cases seen in specific hospitals can be misleading and should not normally be used to draw inferences about patterns of incidence because patterns of referral to hospitals can distort the prevalence of different histologic types seen at different ages.

As mentioned earlier, the incidence of ovarian cancers remained rather stable in the US over the years 1950–1985. However, there was an increase in the late 1960s and early 1970s in the incidence of epithelial tumors classified as endometrioid or clear cell. Other types of epithelial ovarian tumors, i.e., those classified as serous, mucinous, or other types, showed no change in incidence during this time (25). The increase in endometrioid cancers (a doubling) does not seem to be accounted for by a reduction in categories of "unknown" or "other" epithelial types. Some of the change may be explained by increased surveillance associated with the increased interest in endometrial cancer at that time, and associated with use of "unopposed" estro-

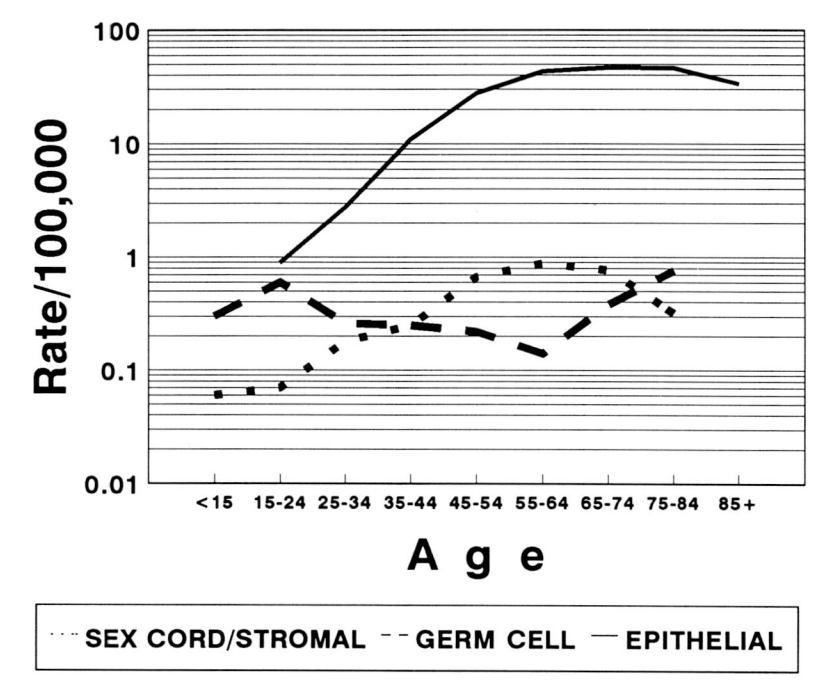

FIG. 1. Incidence of ovarian cancers by age and histologic type. Source: SEER 1975–77. Drawn from data tabulated in (25).

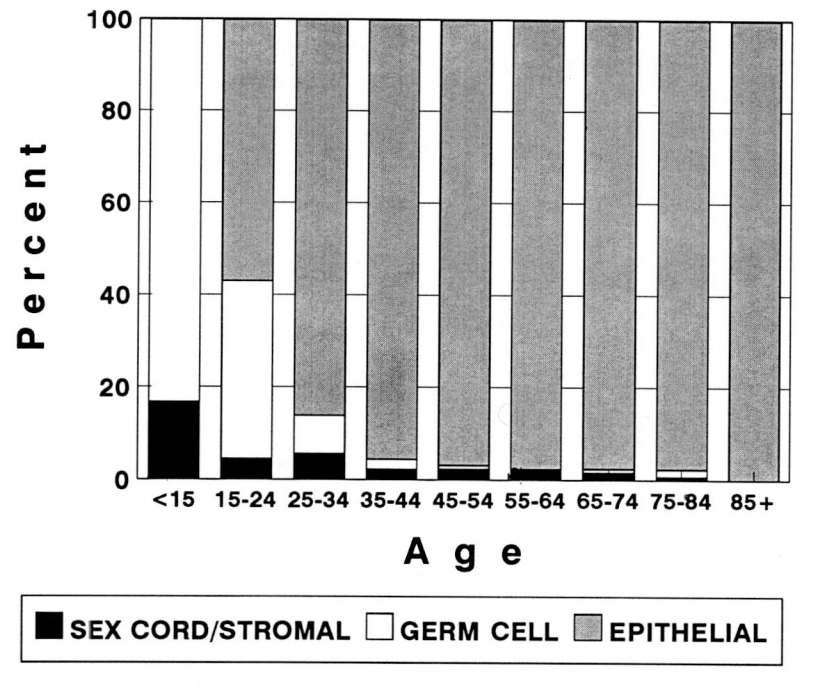

FIG. 2. Prevalence (percent) of different types of ovarian cancer, by age. Source: SEER 1975–77. Drawn from data tabulated in (25).

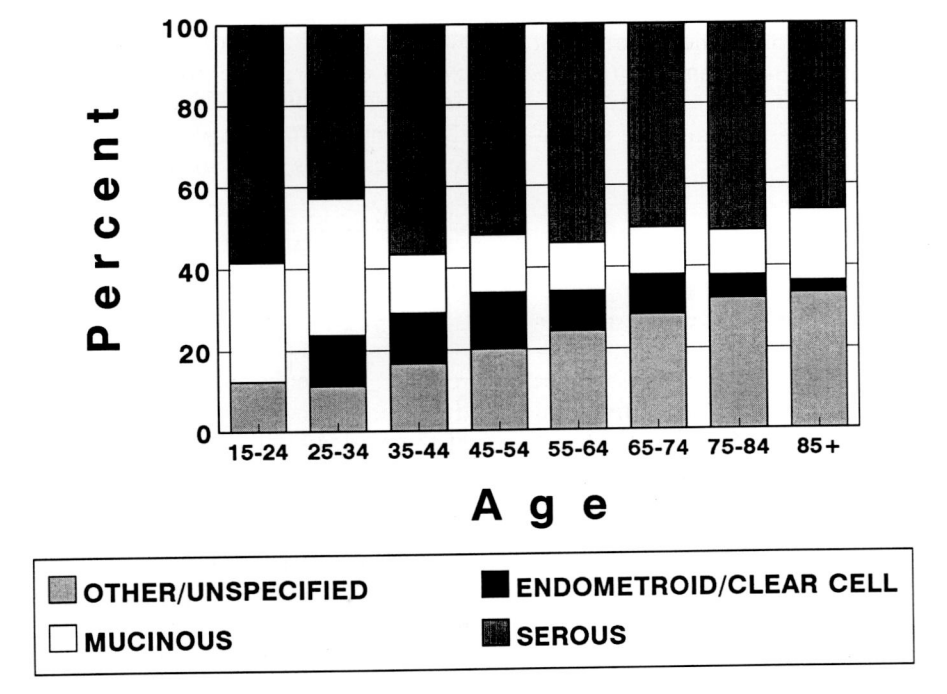

FIG. 3. Prevalence (percent) of different subtypes of epithelial ovarian cancers, by age. Source: SEER 1975–77. Drawn from data tabulated in (25).

gens in sequential oral contraceptives and postmenopausal hormone therapy (25,26).

RISK FACTORS FOR NONEPITHELIAL OVARIAN TUMORS

Relatively little is known of the epidemiology of nonepithelial tumors of the ovary. Germ cell malignancies have been the subject of two recent case-control studies (27,28), and others based on surveillance data (8,27, 29–32), and those studies demonstrate the anticipated similarity between the epidemiology of these tumors and testicular neoplasms. The two main types of germ cell tumors, ovarian teratomas and dysgerminomas, differ in respect to the pattern of incidence by age. Although both peak at ages 15–19, the incidence of dysgerminomas decreases with age thereafter and remains low, while teratomas show a second, broad peak in women aged 60–75 (31).

During the 1970s and early 1980s in England and Wales, ovarian teratomas increased slightly in incidence in women aged under 45, which was associated with an apparent cohort effect of year of birth (31). In older women, they decreased slightly over time. Similar trends have been seen in ovarian teratoma in the US (30), as well as for testicular cancer in the US, Denmark, and Israel (31,33).

In a recent case-control study, ovarian teratomas and dysgerminomas were grouped together and compared with community controls (27). Increased relative risks were observed for a maternal history of breast cancer, in utero exposure to exogenous sex hormones, and in association with a raised body mass index in the subject's mother prior to conception. These risk factors are similar to those observed for testicular cancer (27). In another study that also included other nonepithelial ovarian tumors, occupational exposure to paint was associated with a raised relative risk (28).

One epidemiologic study is available for benign ovarian teratomas (34), also showing some similarities between this condition and testicular cancer. Cases were of a higher social class, had more often married late or not at all, exercised more, and drank more alcohol (34).

RISK FACTORS FOR EPITHELIAL OVARIAN TUMORS

Until recently, studies of risk factors for ovarian cancer did not distinguish between the different histologic types. Because virtually all studies have concentrated on tumors in adults, most of which are epithelial, studies of risk factors, unless otherwise specified, reflect the epidemiology of epithelial cancers. Most studies done in the 1980s and later have excluded germ cell and stromal tumors, however, to focus specifically on epithelial cancers. Most authors have stated that they have included borderline tumors, though some have specifically excluded them (28,35). A few studies have focused *only* on borderline tumors (36), though a few have compared risk factors for borderline tumors with those that are fully malignant or have compared different types of epithelial tumors (37–42). In general, the different types of epithelial tumors seem to be similar epidemiologically.

Reproductive and Menstrual Factors

Numerous studies have focused on the contribution of a woman's menstrual and reproductive characteristics to the risk of ovarian cancer, including age at menarche and menopause (37,40–52), age at first and last pregnancies (43,44,46,47,49,50,52–63); measures of fertility (18,22,35,36,38,41,44–47,49,52,54,58,60,61, 64–71), infertility and fetal loss (35,40,41,44,46,50–53, 55,58,62–64,69,71–74); and lactation (36,41,43,47, 50–52,58,75). For earlier reviews see Weiss, 1988 (70) and Parazzini et al., 1991 (7). Earlier studies were often unable to separate the confounding effects of one variable on another, but more recent ones, including meta-analyses provided by Whittemore (76), have achieved increasing methodologic sophistication, allowing investigation of independent effects of these variables. The risk of ovarian cancer is weakly related to age at menarche (the risk decreases as the age of menarche increases), but hardly, if at all, to age at menopause (76). Nulliparous women are at increased risk, and increasing parity beyond the first birth is associated with a progressive reduction in subsequent incidence of ovarian cancer. In addition, lactation is protective.

Recent research has focused on two related questions for investigation: first, to what extent are epidemiologic findings due to the cumulative number of ovulations in a woman's lifetime; and second, is there evidence for an independent effect of infertility and/or treatment for anovulation? The risk of ovarian cancer increases in relation to the total number of ovulatory cycles in a woman's lifetime (35,50,74) and the time spent in a nonpregnant state using no method of birth control (35,50,55). Conversely, segments of a woman's life when she has not ovulated because she has been pregnant (35,50,74), whether to full term or with incomplete pregnancies (50,74); lactating (50,51,74); or using oral contraceptives (see below) each protect against the disease. One study (51) has suggested that, month for month, periods of anovulatory life spent in pregnancy may be more protective than those spent using the pill or lactating. Furthermore, pregnancy may have more impact on the risk of ovarian cancer in younger women compared with older ones (51,71).

Research on the relationship of infertility to ovarian cancer has been unsatisfactory because investigators have not been able to separate male from female infertility or effects of tubal, endocrine, and other forms (70). A recent analysis (51) found "medically diagnosed" infertility unrelated to the risk of epithelial ovarian cancer, once effects of parity, lactation, and oral contraceptive use were taken into account. Others (28,77) have linked ovarian cancer to hormone therapy for infertility, specifically treatment with ovulation-inducing agents.

Oral Contraceptives

Women who have used oral contraceptives have a reduced incidence of ovarian cancer, and this reduction is one of the strongest and most consistent features of the epidemiology of the disease (18,28,36,39,40,44, 46,47,49–51,58,64,67,69,78–82) (Fig. 4). For recent reviews, see Parazzini et al., 1991 (7) and Stanford, 1991 (5). Eighteen of twenty studies have demonstrated the protective effect of the pill, and in eleven of the individual studies the effects of oral contraceptives were statistically significant. One study found no protective effects of the pill (58). Another study in China suggested that women who had used the pill had a raised risk of the disease (28); however, reanalysis of the data without adjusting for ovarian cysts (whose incidence is reduced by oral contraceptive use) showed a less increased relative risk, suggesting that the original finding was an artifact (Shu XO, personal communication).

Women who have used the pill at any time have a relative relative risk of ovarian cancer of about 0.6 compared to nonusers (26), as shown in (Fig. 4). In the US, "ever users" have used oral contraceptives for 4–5 years on average. The protective effect of the pill has been observed in some studies after durations of use as short as 1–3 years (40,46,67,69,80), though some

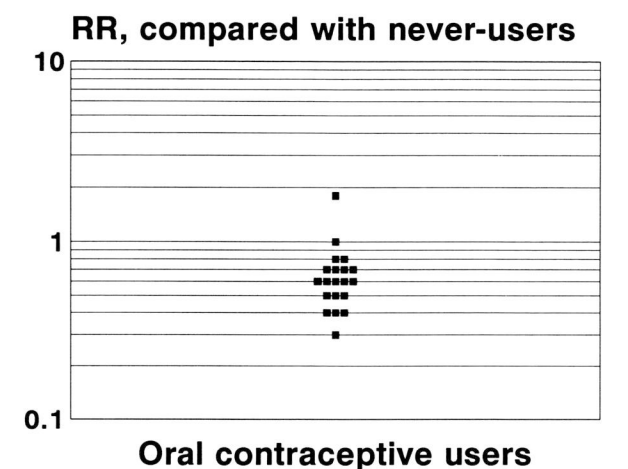

FIG. 4. Relative risk of ovarian cancer in women who have ever used oral contraceptives in 20 studies. From refs. 18,28,36,39,40,44,46,47,49,51,58,64,67,69,78,80,81, 89,103.

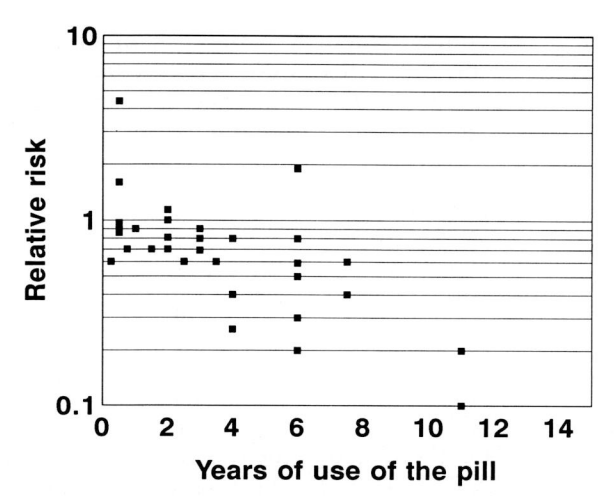

FIG. 5. Relative risk of ovarian cancers by duration of use of the pill. Data from 10 studies. From refs. 28,36,40,46, 50,58,67,69,80,103.

research groups have detected no change in risk for such short durations (49,79). Others (28,58) have detected a temporarily raised risk of ovarian cancer after very short durations of use. Figure 5 depicts a clear "dose-response" effect after longer durations of use, the risk of ovarian cancer decreasing progressively with increasing duration of use (28,49,50,62,80,83).

Although the effects of duration of pill use are not ambiguous, effects of latency and recency are controversial. It is not clear how soon after starting to use the pill its effect becomes obvious. Two large and reliable studies, the Cancer and Steroid Hormones (CASH) study done by the Centers for Disease Control (69) and another done by the World Health Organization (WHO) (80) suggested that the pill's protective effect on ovarian cancer was barely discernible until ten or more years after starting. Other, smaller, studies (56,58), however, have pointed to a much shorter latent effect. There is no clear effect of recency of pill use on ovarian cancer incidence (Fig. 6). The pill offers long-term protection from ovarian cancer that continues for many years after a woman has discontinued use. For the periods that it has been possible to study, this protection seems not to have decreased with time (28,39, 50,67,69,80).

Research on latency and recency is confounded, at least theoretically, by effects of dose and composition of oral contraceptives. Pills used more recently have contained lower doses of both estrogen and progestin (84), and different types of progestin (85). However, the dose of estrogen and the type of progestin in combined oral contraceptives has no detectable effect on ovarian cancer risk (66,78). Regarding other types of hormonal contraceptives, sequential pills were also found to protect against ovarian cancer, though less than combined ones (67,69,80). Progestin-only injectable contraceptives, however, are believed not to change the risk of ovarian cancer (86).

Other topics investigated in relation to the effects of the pill have been the age at which women started

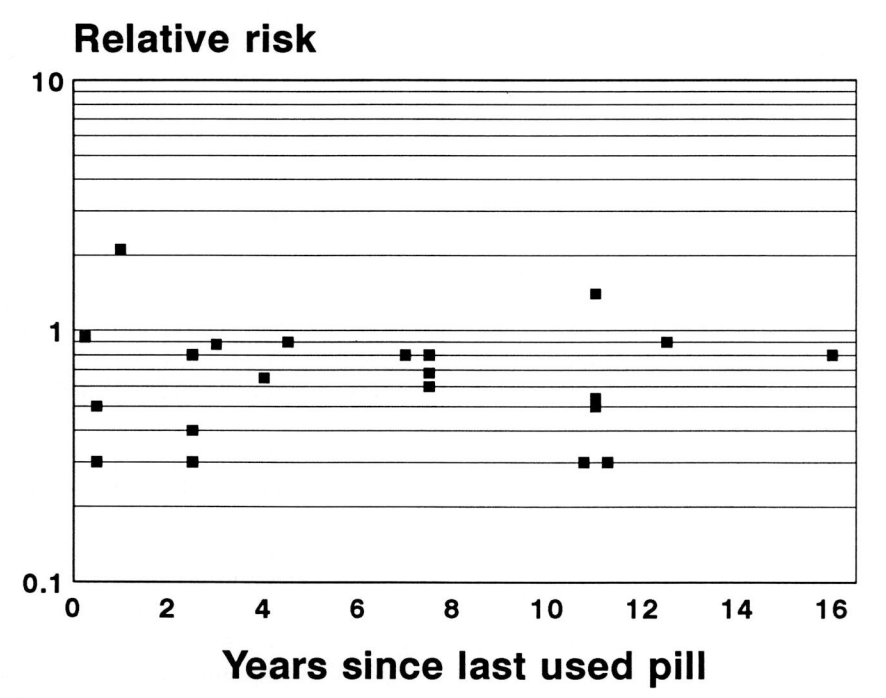

FIG. 6. Relative risk of ovarian cancers by recency of use of oral contraceptives. Data from 6 studies. From refs. 40,50,58,67,80,87.

to use oral contraceptives (39,50,87), age at diagnosis (18,39,46,50,56,58,67,69,80,87), and parity (39,46,50,56,67,70,80,87). While each has generated controversy as to whether the pill protects equally in these subgroups, it seems likely that some measure of protection is present in women using oral contraceptive therapy, whatever their age, parity, and at whatever age such therapy was begun.

Regarding different histologic types, some (36,44,69,80), but not all, studies (38) show that the pill protects against borderline tumors; the protection may be somewhat less than that afforded against fully malignant ovarian tumors. The pill protects against serous, endometrioid, and clear cell subtypes (39,69,78,80), but there is some debate as to whether the risk is equally reduced in mucinous tumors. Some studies find the pill protective (69,78), others do not (39,80). The pill gives no protection against nonepithelial tumors, at least in younger women (28,34,78).

Regarding benign tumors, there has been little research into effects of the pill. Benign tumors classified as cystadenomas and teratomas were recorded in the Walnut Creek (88) and Oxford Family Planning studies (89) and another study in Oxford (34); no relationship was detected between benign tumors and oral contraceptives. Regarding ovarian cysts, functional ovarian cysts are believed to be less common in women using the pill (82,88,90,91); however, this belief is based on studies done in the 1970s, when pills contained high doses of steroids. One study has suggested a role for the dose of estrogen and/or progestin in preventing ovarian cysts (92). Since low-dose pills were introduced, however, there has been no change detected in the incidence of functional ovarian cysts, judging from hospital admissions (93).

Prevention of epithelial ovarian cancer is a noncontraceptive side effect of the pill that has, apparently, a strong public health benefit. The incidence of ovarian cancer has been falling in cohorts of women exposed to the pill in many industrialized countries (9,22,23,25); in spite of its progressive rise in earlier cohorts (9,21), not exposed to the pill. Using the data on relative risks to estimate incidence rates, Harlap et al. (94) have calculated that a hypothetical cohort of 100,000 US women would experience 28 fewer cases of ovarian cancer annually at ages 50–54 if they had used the pill for 10 years in the past, compared with women who had never used it. The cumulative benefit from any use of the pill would be about 200 cases of ovarian cancer averted per 100,000 women by age 55. If, as seems possible, there is little reduction in the protective effect of the pill with increasing time since ceasing use, the number of ovarian cancers averted by the pill may be larger.

Oral contraceptives are recommended for women with a family history of epithelial ovarian cancer (95), but the basis of this recommendation is empirical. An analysis from the CASH study suggests that the pill may not protect such women, but the data are too sparse to conclude this with certainty (96).

Other Contraceptives

A few reports have mentioned investigating methods of birth control other than oral contraceptives (38,39,41,47,50,55,61,73,97), but the data are often not shown, making the results difficult to interpret. Diaphragms and condoms have been studied by researchers interested in a role for talc (see below) but have not been consistently related to the risk of ovarian cancer. Similarly, IUDs (39,50,61) and vasectomies (50) have not shown any significant relationship to ovarian cancer. On the other hand, tubal sterilization has been strongly and consistently associated with a reduced risk (41,50,72,73,98), as has hysterectomy with oophorectomy (73,99). One explanation suggested for this is that these operations give an opportunity for screening the ovaries, and/or that an elective oophorectomy can be done at the time of hysterectomy in women at high risk by virtue of a family history. Women with intact ovaries after hysterectomy may therefore be a select group with a lower-than-average risk of ovarian cancer. Against this hypothesis is the finding that the protection associated with hysterectomy and tubal sterilization is long-lived, continuing for at least 20 years; however, it may wane thereafter (73). Another possibility is that because tubal ligation and hysterectomy cause a physical barrier between the lower genital tract and the ovary, they prevent the passage of carcinogens such as talc (see below).

Postmenopausal Estrogen Therapy

Knowledge of the protection offered by oral contraceptives, together with an understanding that ovarian cancer cells contain estrogen and progesterone receptors (100–102), led some to question whether hormone therapy given to post-menopausal women would influence the risk of ovarian cancer. Estrogen replacement therapy appears to have no affect (Fig. 7). Eleven case-control studies have shown relative risks varying from 0.5 to 1.6 (36,40,45,47,49,50,52,58,103,105). While one study has suggested an increased risk for estrogen used for more than five years (52), six others have shown no such trend (45,47,49,58,103,104). Four studies have focused specifically on endometrioid tumors, the rationale being that because the epidemiology of these tumors shows some features similar to those of endometrial cancer and because postmenopausal estrogens are strongly related to the risk of endometrial cancer (26), estrogens might also influence endometrioid can-

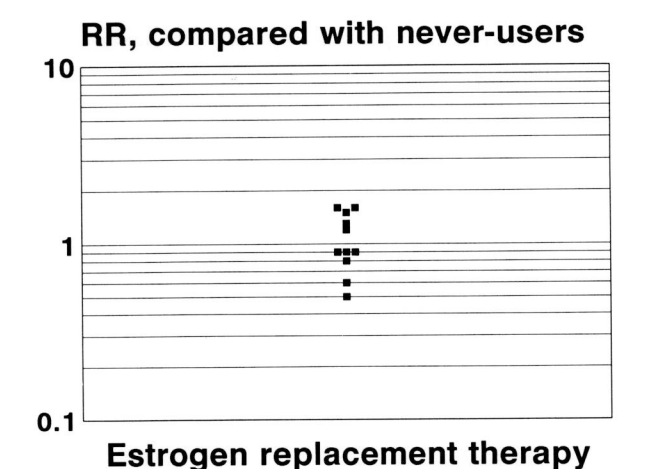

FIG. 7. Relative risks of ovarian cancer in women who have ever used estrogen replacement therapy. Data from 11 studies. From refs. 36,41,45,47,49,50,52.

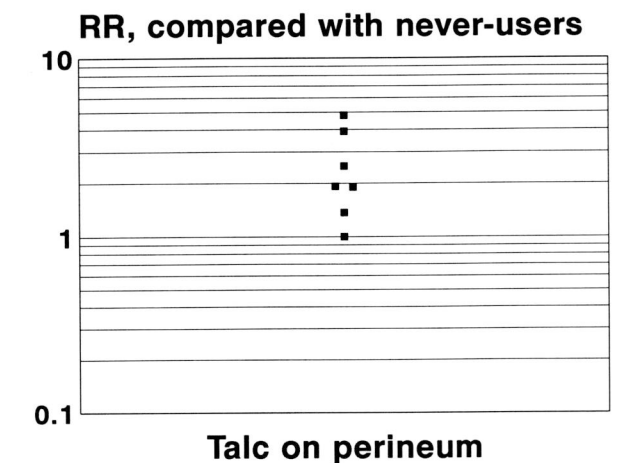

FIG. 8. Relative risks of ovarian cancer in women with exposure to talc on the perineum. Data from seven studies in refs. 38,50,61,98,117,119.

cers. Although two studies did find a significantly increased risk of endometrioid tumors in estrogen users, the relative risks were low—2.3 (103) and 3.1 (105). Two more recent studies had findings suggesting a reduced risk of endometrioid tumors associated with estrogen therapy, with relative risks of 0.5 (58) and 0.9 (104). Taken together, these four studies suggest no effect of estrogens on epithelial tumors of the endometrioid subtype.

Eight of the eleven case-control studies investigating ovarian cancer and postmenopausal estrogens have been done in the US and pertain to the use of conjugated equine estrogens (Premarin) used continuously. There is less certainty about the long-term safety of other estrogens, of estrogen-progestin combinations, or of preparations used cyclically. These other forms of hormone replacement therapy have been used more commonly in Europe than in the US; there is no obvious difference between the results of studies from the US (36,45,47,49,52,58,103,104) and those from Europe (40,50,105). An association of ovarian cancer with stilbestrol has been suggested (28,106).

Talc

Interest in talc as an etiologic factor in ovarian carcinoma occurred as a result of a histologic resemblance, or confusion, of epithelial ovarian tumors with abdominal mesotheliomas (107) [For a review, see Lingeman 1974 (108)]. Talc and asbestos are closely related chemically and often occur together in nature, and asbestos was a contaminant of talcum powder prior to the mid-1970s (109,111). Asbestos is an accepted cause of mesothelioma (112). Asbestos injected experimentally into the peritoneal cavity has caused atypical papillary hyperplasia of ovarian epithelium in guinea pigs and rabbits (109). In humans, ovarian cancer is more common in women with asbestosis (113,114).

Occupational exposure to talc has been associated with lung disease indistinguishable from that caused by asbestos, but with a longer latent period (115). There is some controversy as to whether this is an independent condition actually caused by talc or asbestosis caused by contamination of the talc with asbestos (116). Thus, it is not clear whether talc per se induces disease in humans (111).

Figure 8 shows the results from six case-control studies that have detected raised relative risks of ovarian cancer associated with exposure to talc on the perineum (38,50,61,98,117–119) and one other that found no increase in risk (50). Three of four studies (38,50,98,118) showed trends suggesting a dose-response effect, either with duration of use or with frequency of use. Talc (and/or asbestos as a contaminant) is presumed to enter the peritoneal cavity by retrograde migration up the genital tract (120). The protective effects of hysterectomy and of tubal ligation against ovarian cancer are consistent with this hypothesis; the effects of pregnancy may also be protective.

Diet

In contrast to the large number of investigations of diet in relation to other neoplasias, few reports deal with ovarian cancer and diet. Five case-control studies have explored the subject, using food frequency questionnaires (61,68,121–123); others have taken a more qualitative approach (41,122) or reported on very specific features of diet (124,125). Taken together, these studies suggest a raised risk of ovarian cancer associated with increased intakes of total fat (68,122,123), including animal fat (121,123), butter (121,122), or fried foods (122), before adjustment for calories. Similarly, they suggest protective roles for dietary fish (122-123), vegetables (61,122,123), grains or carbohydrates (122,123), and skim milk (41,125), with an increased risk associated with whole milk (121,125), meat (122,123), or total protein (68,123). These associations are weak, for the most part, and have not been adjusted for total calorie intake; there are too few studies to draw any firm conclusions. The findings, as they stand, suggest that epithelial ovarian cancers may share many of the associations with diet that have been found in other cancers.

Coffee, Alcohol, and Smoking

Coffee drinking is associated with reduced fertility and fecundity (126,127). Aggregate results from eight case-control studies suggest that coffee drinking increases the risk of ovarian cancer, although the relationship is weak and most studies individually have found no significant effect (40,68,118,121,128-131). Although some research groups have reported that the relative risk rises with the number of cups of coffee drunk per day (131), or with years of drinking it (118,128), there is no clear trend when all studies are considered together (Fig. 9). Smoking and alcohol do not explain the effects of coffee (40,121).

Alcohol is only weakly related to ovarian cancer, if at all. Two studies have suggested that it may be protective (68,132), especially in young women (68), while others found slightly raised relative risks associated with drinking for many years (40), drinking greater amounts of alcohol (58), or in drinkers who were also smokers (121). Most of these findings are likely to be due to chance. The large population-based CASH study (133) found no effects of alcohol.

In contrast, findings for smoking are more consistent and suggest a protective effect against ovarian cancer, though this is also weak and, in most studies, is likely to be due to chance (40,58,68,72,123,131,132,134,135). The few research groups that have sought a dose-response effect with the number of cigarettes and/or the duration of smoking have found none (40,68,134).

Lactose Intolerance

In 1983, Cramer et al. (124,136) proposed that dietary galactose consumption could be an etiologic factor in ovarian cancer. They argued that dietary galactose (and a key metabolizing enzyme, galactose-1-phosphate uridyl transferase) has been causally linked to hypogonadotropic gonadism; the latter has been proposed as an antecedent to epithelial ovarian cancer (137). Galactose is one of the two sugars that constitute lactose, the principal carbohydrate of milk. Women will be "exposed" to more galactose if they possess gut bacteria that digest lactose (138); if they have a hereditary inability to produce the transferase enzyme (139); if, as adults, they continue to produce the jejunal enzyme lactase [most adults of non-European descent lose this ability with age (140)]; or if they eat fermented milk products such as yogurt or certain cheeses. A small body of epidemiologic, ecologic, and experimental evidence supports this argument (124,136,141).

Cramer et al. (124) found a significantly doubled relative risk of ovarian cancer in women with low transferase activity, combined with a high consumption of lactose. However, in another study, Mettlin and Piver (125) found evidence that consumption of skim milk products was unrelated to the risk of ovarian cancer, whereas whole milk, animal fat, and total fat increased the risk. They argued that Cramer's original observation was likely explained by an effect of fat intake. At present, this controversy is unresolved.

Mumps and Other Infectious Diseases

Several research groups have explored the relationship of ovarian cancer to past history of infectious diseases. Most have focused on mumps (28,40,43,44,58, 61,64,66,74,75,142,146), but rubella (43,57,60,74), measles (39,43,57,60,74), influenza/pneumonia (51), chicken pox (57,60), and shingles (57) have also been investigated. A rationale for these studies has been that mumps and other viruses may infect the ovary (149), leading to permanent damage that results in premature ovarian failure. No information is available to indicate whether mumps or any other viruses can remain latent

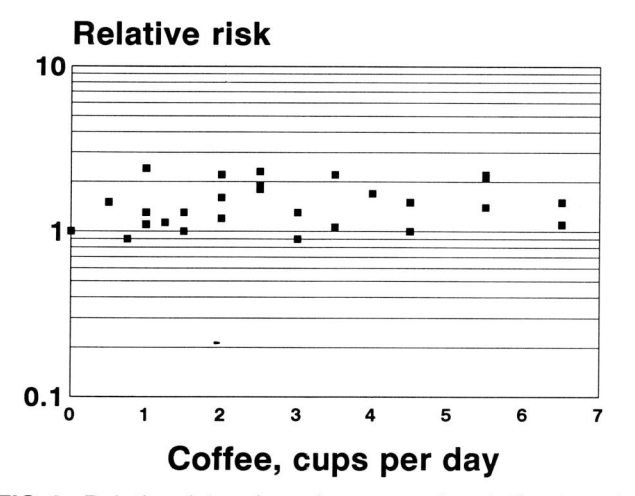

FIG. 9. Relative risks of ovarian cancer in relation to coffee consumption. Data from N studies. Sources: (37,40, 68,118,128-131).

in ovarian tissue or give rise to any active chronic infection at this site beyond the acute phase of the initial infection. Several groups have recorded a lower recall of mumps in cases compared to controls (42,60,63,74, 143,150), especially in postmenopausal subjects (147,151). Others have not (28,39,43,57,71,99). One group in Israel demonstrated lower mumps antibody titers in women with ovarian cancer, but their findings cannot be evaluated because they included some patients after chemotherapy (142). Another group in China found higher antibody titers to mumps viruses in women with ovarian cancer compared with controls (61).

Association with Other Primary Neoplasias

There are many anecdotal reports of an excess of other primaries, particularly breast cancer, in women with ovarian cancer (43). Most such publications originate in tertiary-care cancer centers where Berksonian bias (149) may cause a referral pattern that brings in patients with double primaries who would normally have been seen in community hospitals. Perhaps because of this, anecdotal reports have suggested a strong association between ovarian and other cancers in the same woman, while population-based studies show only weak associations.

Case-control (41,58,68) and follow-up (150,155) studies have confirmed that breast and ovarian cancer occur in the same woman more often than would be expected by chance. Retrospective studies of ovarian cancer patients have suggested that the risk is increased up to fourfold for women with a prior history of breast cancer (41,45,58) and up to threefold for those with a prior history of benign breast disease (68). Population-based follow-up studies of women with breast cancer give relative risks of developing ovarian cancer to be 1.3–1.7 (154), with somewhat higher risk in women whose breast cancer was diagnosed prior to age 54, compared with women who were older at diagnosis (151). These are likely to be substantial underestimates, however, since such population-based studies have been unable to separate women with and without oophorectomy following a diagnosis of breast cancer.

For women with ovarian cancer, the relative risk of developing breast cancer is also raised by 10–40% [relative risk is 1.1–1.4 overall and 1.5–1.9 within 1–4 years after diagnosis (154–156)]. Part of this increase may be due to more careful screening for breast cancer following a diagnosis of ovarian cancer and to the shared association with major risk factors such as reduced parity. Again, these data do not take into account the expected reduction in breast cancer that follows oophorectomy, so that the true association between breast and ovarian cancers must be underestimated.

Other second primaries occurring with greater frequency than expected in women with ovarian cancer include those of colon, kidney, bladder, and acute non-lymphocytic leukemias (156), a pattern that is obviously likely to reflect radiation-induced cancers. Endometrial and cervical cancer have also been associated with ovarian cancer in anecdotal reports (43).

Population-based studies find an increased relative risk of ovarian cancer after a diagnosis of endometrial cancer that is strongest in the first year of follow-up, suggesting a role for surveillance bias (154). Risk for cervical cancer is temporarily increased following radiotherapy for ovarian cancer (RR = 1.6, $p < .05$); this change is not seen in patients who are not irradiated (157).

Association Within Families

In contrast to the weak associations with other primary neoplasms in the same patient, ovarian cancer is strongly associated with other cancers within families, especially with ovarian (40,47,52), prostate (52,72), breast (41,44,47,52,72,158–161), colorectal (40,159), lung (52), and any reproductive cancer in a first-degree female relative (41,44,159), as well as with any type of cancer in first-degree relatives of either sex (41,52). Consanguinity also increases the risk (52). Relative risk estimates for women who have a first-degree relative with ovarian cancer have ranged from 0.9 to infinity in retrospective studies, with a mean around 4–6 (Fig. 10). For women who have a first-degree relative with

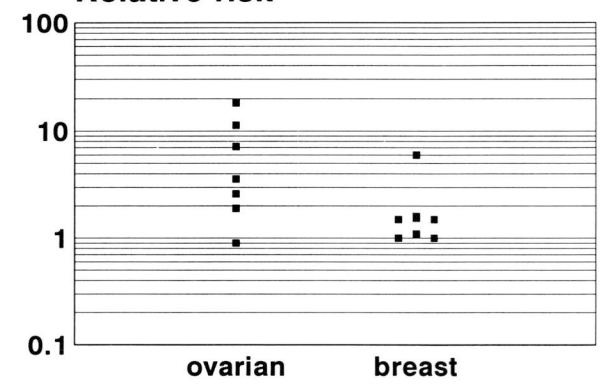

FIG. 10. Relative risks of ovarian cancer in women with a family history of ovarian or breast cancer. Data from studies of a family history of the specific cancer ■ in first-degree relatives; ● in first or second degree relatives, ▽ in any relatives; △ family history of any remote reproductive cancers; and + family history of cancer.

breast cancer, relative risk estimates have varied from 0.6 to 6.1 (47,52,72,158,161); most are above one. One population-based study explored differences in histologic type and found that a family history of ovarian cancer raised the risk of all epithelial malignancies of the ovary, whether serous, mucinous, or endometrioid, but was not associated with a change in the risk of borderline tumors (159). However, numbers available for the study were small, and these findings require confirmation from further studies. Further, a family history of endometrial cancer probably does not raise the risk of ovarian cancer (96), though some studies have suggested that it may (40,47).

Aggregations of ovarian cancer in families in which relatives have ovarian or other cancers are consistent with an increase in literature addressing hereditary cancer syndromes, including site-specific ovarian cancer, breast/ovarian cancer syndrome, and other syndromes (167–165). More than one and perhaps several loci may be involved in the breast/ovarian syndrome (165). Analysis of pedigrees of affected families has suggested early onset of ovarian cancer and a lifetime risk close to 50% in syndromes involving a locus on chromosome 17q21 (165–166). However, since the families in these studies were ascertained, i.e., "selected" for early-onset disease, it is not clear whether such early onset is a true feature of the syndrome. Epidemiologic studies thus far (74,96) tend to challenge the hypothesis that age of onset modifies the relative risks of ovarian cancers within families having ovarian or breast cancers, although earlier analysis of the crude relative risks had suggested that it did (96).

Familial occurrence of ovarian cancer is rare, and some of it is bound to occur by chance. In the population-based CASH study, 7% of patients aged 20–54 reported having any relative with ovarian cancer, but only 3.2% had an affected first-degree relative, and only 0.6% had more than one relative affected (42,159). In a large Italian case-control study, only 2% of patients knew of a first-degree relative with ovarian cancer (161). Case series based on tertiary-care referral centers are likely to report higher proportions.

Whether classical risks factors alter the lifetime incidence or timing of hereditary ovarian cancers is unknown. Data from the CASH study suggest that oral contraceptives may not protect against ovarian cancer in women with a family history of the disease (69), but the data are too sparse to conclude this with certainty.

Pharmaceutical Agents and Exposure to Industrial Chemicals

There are several reports of an increased risk of epithelial and other ovarian cancers in women using psychotropic drugs, including: triamcinolone (167); prochlorperazine (167); antidepressants (40), including tricyclic compounds (121); and anticonvulsants (168), including barbiturates (121,167). Information bias may account for some of these associations. On the other hand, some of these drugs have affinities for steroid receptors (169,170), interfere with hepatic metabolism of steroids or other compounds, or change the pattern of gonatropin-releasing hormone (GnRH) and gonadotropins.

Industrial and environmental chemicals have been studied little in relation to ovarian cancer (28,171). One study in China has shown women occupationally exposed to paint to have a relative risk of 2.2, but this was likely to be due to chance (28); similarly, raised relative risks associated with metal working (1.5) and exposure to benzene (1.4) were not statistically significant. Asbestos exposure was not a risk factor for ovarian cancer in this study.

ETIOLOGIC HYPOTHESES FOR EPITHELIAL OVARIAN CANCERS

Epidemiologic research in ovarian cancer has been dominated over the past two decades by two opposing hypotheses that attempt to explain the etiology of this cancer. The first, the "incessant ovulation" hypothesis (158,172), postulates that the risk of epithelial ovarian cancer is a function of the epithelial tearing and regenerating that occurs with each ovulation. This hypothesis accords with the view that the rate of cell turnover is a determinant of neoplasia (173), dividing cells being vulnerable to mutations caused by carcinogens, chance, or from failure to repair DNA. The epidemiologic findings in relation to pregnancy, lactation, and oral contraceptive use have been invoked to support this hypothesis. However, direct estimates of the number of ovulations and the length of the menstrual cycle (28) suggest this is not so. Furthermore, the finding by Gwinn et al. (57) that the early months of lactation and oral contraception protect more than later months, and the suggestion of a time-dependent effect of pregnancy (51,71) mean that this hypothesis is an oversimplification. The results of Gwinn et al. suggest instead that the risk of mutation is "turned off" at some stage by events in a woman's reproductive life.

The effects of pregnancy, lactation, and oral contraception are also consistent with the second hypothesis, which postulates a role for gonadotropins (124,136,137). Premature ovarian failure brought on by damage to oocytes through infection (such as mumps), radiation, cytotoxic drugs, or environmental toxins may result in a breakdown of the normal ovarian-hypothalamic feedback, leading to an excess of gonadotropins. Evidence in support of this hypothesis is tenuous, and it has received less attention from epidemiologists than the "incessant ovulation" hypothesis. Evidence for the gonadotropin hypothesis has been explored by Cramer et al. in relation to a role for dietary consumption of fermented milk products and a role for red-cell galactose-1-phosphate uridyl transferase, both of which would be expected to raise gonadotropin levels (124). Also supporting this hypothesis is the observation that rodents treated with oocyte toxins (174) or with congenital absence of oocytes (175) develop ovarian tumors; however, these are mainly stromal types.

A third hypothesis postulates a role for carcinogens that gain access to the ovarian epithelium via the genital tract. Talc is the only agent that has been investigated in detail in this context (38,50,61,98,117–119). The protective effect of tubal ligation (41,50,72,73,98) and hysterectomy (73,98,99) is consistent with this hypothesis. The protective effect of oral contraceptives against ovarian cancers is not inconsistent with this hypothesis, if one can postulate that spermatozoa can act as a vector for carcinogens (such as talc) or pathogens, or act directly as irritants to the ovarian epithelium. The pill's action would be through its role in altering cervical mucous (176), making it impenetrable to spermatozoa, or by altering tubal motility (177).

REFERENCES

1. National Cancer Institute, Division of Cancer Prevention and Control Surveillance Program. *Cancer Statistics Review, 1973–86.* Washington, DC: Department of Health and Human Services, 1989.
2. Parkin DM, Laara E, Muir CS. Estimates of the world wide frequency of sixteen major cancers in 1980. *Int J Cancer* 1988; 41:184–197.
3. Piver MS, Baker TR, Piedmonte M, Sandecki AM. Epidemiology and etiology of ovarian cancer. *Sem Oncol* 1991;18: 177–185.
4. Muir CS, Waterhouse J, Mack T, Powell J, Whelan S. Cancer incidence in five continents, V. *IARC Sci pub no. 88.* Lyon: IARC, 1987.
5. Waterhouse J, Muir C, Shanmugaratnam K, Powell J, Peacham D, Whelan S. Cancer incidence in five continents, IV. *IARC Sci pub no. 42.* Lyon: IARC, 1982.
6. Ayiomamitis A. The epidemiology of malignant neoplasms of the ovary, fallopian tube, and broad ligament in Canada: 1950–1984. *Obstet Gynecol* 1989;73:1017–1021.
7. Parazzini F, Franceschi S, La Vecchia C, Fasoli M. The epidemiology of ovarian cancer. *Gynecol Oncol* 1991;43:9–23.
8. Weiss NS, Homonchuk T, Young JL. Incidence of the histologic types of ovarian cancer: the U.S. third national cancer survey, 1969–1971. *Gynecol Oncol* 1977;5:161–167.
9. Hanai A. Trends and differential in ovarian cancer: incidence, mortality and survival experience. *APMIS* 1990;12:1–20.
10. Lyon JL, Gardner JW, West DW. Cancer incidence in Mormons and non-Mormons in Utah during 1967–1975. *JNCI* 1980; 654:1055–1061.
11. Lyon JL, Klauber MR, Gardner JW, et al. Cancer incidence in Mormons and non-Mormons in Utah, 1966–1970. *N Engl J Med* 1976;294:129–133.
12. Parkin DM. Cancers of the breast, endometrium and ovary: geographic correlations. *Eur J Cancer Clin Oncol* 1989;25: 1917–125.
13. Steinitz R, Parkin DM, Young JL. Cancer Incidence in Jewish Migrants to Israel, 1961–1981. *IARC Sci Pub No.98.* Lyon: IARC, 1989.
14. Ben Porath Y. *Economic analysis of fertility in Israel: point and counterpoint.* [Research Paper No. 34.] Jerusalem: Falk Institute, 1973.
15. Andreizen WL, Leitch A. Cancers of the uterus, vagina and vulva. A statistical study of the records of the Middlesex Hospital. *Arch Middlesex Hosp* 1906;7:165–188.
16. Ogilvie R. Autopsy data, the Royal infirmary, Endinburgh, Scotland. 1849–1860 and 1949–1960. *Personal communication* cited by Graham and Graham, 1967.
17. Kurihara M, Aoki K, Tominaga S. *Cancer mortality statistics in the world.* University of Nagoya Press: Nagoya, 1984.
18. Beral V, Fraser P, Chilvers C. Does pregnancy protect against ovarian cancer? *Lancet* 1978;1:1083–1087.
19. Adami H-O, Bergström R, Persson I, Sparén. The incidence of ovarian cancer in Sweden, 1960–1984. *Am J Epidemiol* 1990; 132:446–452.
20. Devesa SS, Silverman DT, Young YL, et al. Cancer incidence and mortality trend among whites in the United States 1947–1984. *JNCI* 1987;79:701–770.
21. Haenszel W, Kurihara M. Studies of Japanese migrants. I. Mortality from cancer and other diseases among Japanese in the United States. *JNCI* 1968;40:43–68.
22. Villard-Mackintosh L, Vessey MP, Jones L. The effects of oral contraceptives and parity on ovarian cancer trends in women under 55 years of age. *Br J Obstet Gynaecol* 1989;96:783–788.
23. Decarli A, LaVecchia C, Mezzanote G, Cislagi C. Birth cohort, time and age effects in Italian cancer mortality. *Cancer* 1987; 59:1221–1232.
24. Moolgavkar SH. Carcinogenesis modeling: from molecular biology to epidemiology. *Ann Rev Publ Health* 1986;7:151–169.
25. Cramer DW, Devesa SS, Welch WR. Trends in the incidence of endometrioid and clear cell cancers of the ovary in the United States. *Am J Epidemiol* 1981;114:201–208.
26. Prentice FL, Thomas DB. On the epidemiology of oral contraceptives and disease. *Adv Cancer Res* 1987;49:285.
27. Walker AH, Ross RK, Haile RWC, Henderson BE. Hormonal factors and risk of ovarian germ cell cancer in young women. *Br J Cancer* 1988;57:418–422.
28. Shu XO, Brinton LA, Gao YT, Yuan JM. Population-based case-control study of ovarian cancer in Shanghai. *Cancer Res* 1989;49:3670–3674.
29. Li FP, Fraumeni JF, Jr, Dalager N. Ovarian cancers in the young. *Cancer* 1973;32:969–972.
30. Walker AH, Ross RK, Pike MC, Henderson BE. A possible rising incidence of malignant germ cell tumors in young women. *Br J Cancer* 1984;49:669.
31. dos Santos Silva I, Swerdlow AJ. Ovarian germ cell malignancies in England: epidemiological parallels with testicular cancer. *Br J Cancer* 1991;63:814–818.
32. Stalsberg H, Bjarnason O, Carvalho ARL, et al. International comparisons of histologic types of ovarian cancer registry material. In: Stalsberg H, ed. *An international survey of distributions of histologic types of tumors of the testis and ovary.* Geneva: International Union Against Cancer, 1983; UICC Technical Report No 75: 247.
33. Osterlind A. Diverging trends in incidence and mortality of testicular cancer in Denmark, 1943–82. *Br J Cancer* 1986;53:501.
34. Westoff C, Pike M, Vessey M. Benign ovarian teratomas: A population-based case-control study. *Br J Cancer* 1988;58: 93–98.
35. Whittemore AS, Wu ML, Paffenbarger RS Jr, et al. Epithelial ovarian cancer and the ability to conceive. *Cancer Res* 1989; 49:4047–4052.
36. Harlow BL, Weiss NS, Roth GJ, Chu J, Daling JR. Case-control study of borderline ovarian tumors: reproductive history and exposure to exogenous female hormones. *Cancer Res* 1988;48:5849–5852.
37. Szamborski J, Czerwinski W, Gadomska H, Kowalski M, Wacker-Pujdak B. Case control study of high-risk factors in ovarian carcinomas. *Gynecol Oncol* 1981;11:8–16.
38. Cramer DW, Welch WR, Scully RE, Wojciechowski CA. Ovarian cancer and talc: A case-control study. *Cancer* 1982;50: 372–376.
39. Cramer DW, Hutchinson GB, Welch WR, Scully RE, Knapp

RC. Factors affecting the association of oral contraceptives and ovarian cancer. *N Engl J Med* 1982;307:1047–1051.
40. Tzonou A, Day NE, Trichopoulos D, et al. The epidemiology of ovarian cancer in Greece: a case-control study. *Eur J Cancer Clin Oncol* 1984;20:1045–1052.
41. Mori M, Kiyosawa H, Miyake H. Case-control study of ovarian cancer in Japan. *Cancer* 1984;53:2746–2752.
42. Schildkraut JM, Thompson WD. Familial ovarian cancer: a population-based case-control study. *Am J Epidemiol* 1988;128:456–466.
43. Wynder EL, Dodo H, Barber HRK. Epidemiology of cancer of the ovary. *Cancer* 1969;23:352–370.
44. McGowan L, Parent L, Lednar W, Norris HJ. The woman at risk for developing ovarian cancer. *Gynecol Oncol* 1979;7:325–344.
45. Annegers JF, Strom H, Decker DG, Dockerty MB, O'Fallon WM. Ovarian cancer. *Cancer* 1979;43:723–729.
46. Willett WC, Bain C, Hennekens CH, Rosner B, Speizer FE. Oral contraceptives and risk of ovarian cancer. *Cancer* 1981;48:1684–1687.
47. Hildreth NG, Kelsey JL, LiVolsi VA, et al. An epidemiologic study of epithelial carcinoma of the ovary. *Am J Epidemiol* 1981;114:398–405.
48. Franceschi S, La Vecchia C, Booth M, et al. Pooled analysis of 3 European case-control studies of ovarian cancer: II. Age at menarche and at menopause. *Int J Cancer* 1991;49:57–60.
49. Wu ML, Whittemore AS, Paffenbarger RS Jr, et al. Personal and environmental characteristics related to epithelial ovarian cancer. *Am J Epidemiol* 1988;128:1216–1227.
50. Booth M, Beral V, Smith P. Risk factors for ovarian cancer: a case-control study. *Br J Cancer* 1989;60:592–598.
51. Gwinn ML, Lee NC, Rhodes PH, Layde PM, Rubin GL. Pregnancy, breast feeding, and oral contraceptives and the risk of epithelial ovarian cancer. *J Clin Epidemiol* 1990;43:559–568.
52. Cramer DW, Hutchinson GB, Welch WR, Scully RE, Ryan KJ. Determinants of ovarian cancer risk. I. Reproductive experiences and family history. *JNCI* 1983;71:711–716.
53. Joly DJ, Lilienfeld AM, Diamond EL, Bross IDJ. An epidemiologic study of the relationship of reproductive experience to cancer of the ovary. *Am J Epidemiol* 1974;99:190–209.
54. Franceschi S, La Vecchia C, Helmrich SP, Mangioni C, Tognoni G. Risk factors for epithelial ovarian cancer in Italy. *Am J Epidemiol* 1982;115:714–719.
55. Nasca PC, Greenwald P, Chorost S, Richard R, Caputo T. An epidemiologic case-control study of ovarian cancer and reproductive factors. *Am J Epidemiol* 1984;119:605–613.
56. La Vecchia C, Franceschi S, Decarli A. Oral contraceptive use and the risk of epithelial ovarian cancer. *Br J Cancer* 1984;50:31–34.
57. Lesher L, McGowan L, Hartge P, Hoover R. Age at first birth and risk of eipthelial ovarian cancer [Letter]. *JNCI* 1985;74:1361–1363.
58. Hartge P, Schiffman MH, Hoover R, McGowan L, Lesher L, Norris HJ. A case-control study of epithelial ovarian cancer. *Am J Obstet Gynecol* 1989;161:10–16.
59. Chen Y, Wu BZ. Risk factors for epithelial ovarian cancer in China—a case-control study [Abstract]. *Am J Epidemiol* 1990;132:777–778.
60. Miller AB, Barclay THC, Choi NW, et al. A study of cancer, parity and age at first pregnancy. *J Chron Dis* 1980;33:595–605.
61. Chen Y, Wu P-C, Lang J-H, Hartge P, Brinton LA. Risk factors for epithelial ovarian cancer in Peking, China. *Int J Epidemiol* 1992;21:23–29.
62. Kvale G, Heuch I, Nilssen S, Beral V. Reproductive factors and risk of ovarian cancer: A prospective study. *Int J Cancer* 1988;42:246–251.
63. Voigt LF, Harlow BL, Weiss NS. The influence of age at first birth and parity on ovarian cancer risk. *Am J Epidemiol* 1986;124:490–491.
64. Newhouse ML, Pearson RM, Fullerton JM, Boesen EAM, Shannon HS. A case control study of carcinoma of the ovary. *Br J Prev Soc Med* 1977;31:148–153.
65. Demopoulos RI, Seltzer V, Dubin N, Gutman E. The association of parity and marital status with the development of ovarian carcinoma: clinical implications. *Obstet Gynecol* 1979;54:150–155.
66. Cramer DW, Welch WR, Cassells S, Scully RE. Mumps, menarche, menopause, and ovarian cancer. *Am J Obstet Gynecol* 1983;147:1–6.
67. Rosenberg L, Shapiro S, Slone D, et al. Epithelial ovarian cancer and combination oral contraceptives. *JAMA* 1982;247:3210–3212.
68. Byers T, Marshall J, Graham S, Mettlin C, Swanson M. A case-control study of dietary and nondietary factors in ovarian cancer. *JNCI* 1983;71:681–686.
69. The Cancer and Steroid Hormone Study of the Centers for Disease Control and the National Institute of Child Health and Human Development. The reduction in risk of ovarian cancer associated with oral-contraceptive use. *N Engl J Med* 1987;316:650–655.
70. Weiss NS. Measuring the separate effects of low parity and its antecedents on the incidence of ovarian cancer. *Am J Epidemiol* 1988;128:451–455.
71. Negri E, Franceschi S, Tzonou A, et al. Pooled analysis of 3 European case control studies: I. Reproductive factors and risk of epithelial ovarian cancer. *Int J Cancer* 1991;49:50–56.
72. Koch M, Jenkins H, Gaedke H. Risk factors of ovarian cancer of epithelial origin: A case control study. *Cancer Det Prev* 1988;13:131–136.
73. Irwin K, Weiss N, Lee N, Peterson H. Tubal sterilization, hysterectomy, and the subsequent occurrence of epithelial ovarian cancer. *Am J Epidemiol* 1991;134:362–369.
74. Risch HA, Weiss NS, Lyon JL, Daling JR, Liff JM. Events of reproductive life and the incidence of epithelial ovarian cancer. *Am J Epidemiol* 1983;117:128–139.
75. West RO. Epidemiologic study of malignancies of the ovaries. *Cancer* 1966;19:1001–1007.
76. Whittemore - metanalysis.
77. Dietl J. Ovulation and ovarian cancer. *Lancet* 1991;338:445.
78. Casagrande JT, Pike MC, Henderson BE. Oral contraceptives and ovarian cancer. *N Engl J Med* 1983;308:843–844.
79. Weiss NS, Sayvetz TA. Incidence of endometrial cancer in relation to the use of oral contraceptives. *N Engl J Med* 1980;302:551–554.
80. WHO Collaborative Study of Neoplasia and Steroid Contraceptives. Epithelial ovarian cancer and combined oral contraceptives. *Int J Epidemiol* 1989;18:538–545.
81. Parazzini F, La Vecchia C, Negri E, Bocciolone L, Fedele L, Franceschi S. Oral contraceptive use and the risk of ovarian cancer: an Italian case-control study. *Eur J Cancer* 1991;27:594–598.
82. Vessey M, Metcalfe A, Wells C, McPherson K, Westhoff C, Yates D. Ovarian neoplasms, functional ovarian cysts, and oral contraceptives. *Br Med J* 1987;294:1518–1520.
83. Schlesselman JJ. Cancer of the breast and reproductive tract in relation to oral contraceptives. *Contraception* 1989;40:1–38.
84. Piper JM, Kennedy DL. Oral contraceptives in the United States. Trends in content and potency. *Int J Epidemiol* 1987;16:215–221.
85. Diczfalusy E. The history of steroidal contraception: What is past and what is present. In: Michael F, ed. Safety Requirements for Contraceptive Steroids. Cambridge: Cambridge University Press, 1989:1–18.
86. [Anonymous.] Depot-medroxyprogesterone acetate (DMPA) and cancer: [Memorandum] *Bull WHO* 1986;64:375–382.
87. Franceschi S, Parazzini F, Negri E, et al. Pooled analysis of 3 European case-control studies of epithelial ovarian cancer: III. Oral contraceptive use. *Int J Cancer* 1991;49:61–65.
88. Ramcharan S, Pellegrin FA, Ray R, Hsu J-P. The Walnut Creek Contraceptive Drug Study. *A prospective study of the side effects of oral contraceptives,* Vol III. Bethesda: National Institutes of Health, 1981.
89. Vessey M, Doll R, Peto R, Johnson B, Wiggins PA. Long-term follow-up study of women using different methods of contraception—an interim report. *J Biosoc Sci* 1976;8:373–427.
90. Ory HW, Boston Collaborative Drug Surveillance Programme. Functional ovarian cysts and oral contraceptives: negative association confirmed surgically. *JAMA* 1974;228:68.

91. Royal College of General Practitioners. Oral Contraceptives and Health. In: *An interim report from the oral contraception study of the Royal College of General Practitioners.* London: Pitman, 1974.
92. Holt VL, Daling JR. Low vs. high estrogen oral contraceptives and ovarian cyst risk [Abstract]. *Am J Epidemiol* 1990;132:768.
93. Grimes DA, Hughes JM. Use of multiphasic oral contraceptives and hospitalizations of women with functional ovarian cysts in the United States. *Obstet Gynecol* 1989;73:1037.
94. Harlap S, Kost K, Forrest JD. *Preventing pregnancy, protecting health.* New York: The Alan Guttmacher Institute, 1991.
95. Hatcher RA, Stewart FH, Trussell J, Kowal D, Guest FJ, Stewart GK, Cates W Jr. *Contraceptive technology, 1990–1992.* New York: Irvington Publishers, Inc., 1990:246.
96. Schildkraut JM, Risch N, Thompson WD. Evaluating genetic association among ovarian, breast, and endometrial cancer: evidence for a breast/ovarian cancer relationship. *Am J Hum Genet* 1989;45:521–529.
97. Stewart HL, Dunham LJ, Casper J, et al. Epidemiology of cancers of uterine cervix and corpus, breast and ovary in Israel and New York City. *JNCI* 1966;37:1–95.
98. Rosenblatt KA, Szklo M, Rosenshein NB. Mineral fiber exposure and the development of ovarian cancer [*in press*].
99. Siddle N, Sarrell P, Whitehead M. The effect of hysterectomy on the age of ovarian failure: Identification of a subgroup of women with premature loss of ovarian function and literature review. *Fertil Steril* 1987;47:94–100.
100. Friberg LG, Kullander S, Persijn JP, Korsten CP. On receptors for estrogens (E2) and androgens (DHT) in human endometrial and ovarian tumors. *Acta Obstet Gynecol Scand* 1978;57:261–264.
101. Holt JA, Caputo TA, Kelly KM, et al. Estrogen and progestin binding in cytosol of ovarian carcinoma. *Obstet Gynecol* 1979;53:50–58.
102. Galli MC, DeGiovanni BS, Nicolletti G, et al. The occurrence of multiple steroid hormone receptors in disease-free and neoplastic human ovary. *Cancer* 1981;47:1297–1302.
103. Weiss NS, Lyon JL, Krishnamurthy S, Dietert SE, Liff JM, Daling JR. Noncontraceptive estrogen use and the occurrence of ovarian cancer. *JNCI* 1982;68:95–98.
104. Kaufman DW, Kelly JP, Welch WR, Rosenberg L, Stolley PD, Warshauer ME, Lewis J, Woodruff J. Noncontraceptive estrogen use and epithelial ovarian cancer. *JNCI* 1982;69:1207.
105. La Vecchia C, Liberati A, Franceschi S. Noncontraceptive estrogen use and the occurrence of ovarian cancer. *JNCI* 1982;69:1207.
106. Hoover R, Gray LA, Fraumeni JF Jr. Stilboestrol (Diethylstilbestrol) and the risk of ovarian cancer. *Lancet* 1977;2:533–534.
107. Graham J, Graham R. Ovarian cancer and asbestos. *Environ Res* 1967;1:115–128.
108. Lingeman CH. Etiology of cancer of the human ovary: A review. *JNCI* 1974;53:1603–1618.
109. Cralley LJ, Key MM, Groth DH, Lainhart W, Ligo RM. Fibrous and mineral content of cosmetic talcum products. *Am Ind Hyg Assoc J* 1968;29:350–354.
110. Rohl AN, Langer AM, Selikoff IJ, et al. Consumer talcums and powders: mineral and chemical characterization. *J Toxicol Environ Hlth* 1976;2:255–285.
111. Hildick-Smith GY. The biology of talc. *Br J Ind Med* 1976;33:217–229.
112. Selikoff IJ, Churg J, Hammond EC. Relation between exposure to asbestos and mesothelioma. *N Engl J Med* 1965;272:560–565.
113. Keal EE. Asbestosis and abdominal neoplasms. *Lancet* 1960;2:1211.
114. Newhouse ML, Berry G, Wagner JC, Turok ME. A study of the mortality of female asbestos workers. *Br J Ind Med* 1972;29:134–141.
115. Kleinfeld M, Messite J, Kooyman O, Zaki MH. Mortality among talc miners and millers in New York State. *Arch Environ Hlth* 1967;14:663–667.
116. Longo DL, Young RC. Cosmetic talc and ovarian cancer. *Lancet* 1979;2:349–351.
117. Hartge P, Hoover R, Lesher LP, McGowan L. Talc and ovarian cancer [Letter]. *JAMA* 1983;250:1844.
118. Whittemore AS, Wu ML, Paffenbarger RS Jr, et al. Personal and environmental characteristics related to epithelial ovarian cancer. II. Exposures to talcum powder, tobacco, alcohol and coffee. *Am J Epidemiol* 1988;128:1228–1240.
119. Harlow BL, Weiss NS. A case-control study of borderline ovarian tumors: the influence of perineal exposure to talc. *Am J Epidemiol* 1989;130:390–394.
120. Egli GE, Newton M. The transport of carbon particles in the human female reproductive tract. *Fertil Steril* 1961;12:151–155.
121. Cramer DW, Welch WR, Hutchinson GB, Willett W, Scully RE. Dietary animal fat in relation to ovarian cancer risk. *Obstet Gynecol* 1984;63:833–838.
122. La Vecchia C, Decarli A, Negri E, et al. Dietary factors and the risk of epithelial ovarian cancer. *JNCI* 1987;79:663–669.
123. Shu XO, Gao YT, Yuan JM, Ziegler RG, Brinton LA. Dietary factors and epithelial ovarian cancer. *Br J Cancer* 1989;59:92–96.
124. Cramer DW, Willett WC, Bell DA, et al. Galactose consumption and metabolism in relation to the risk of ovarian cancer. *Lancet* 1989;2:66–271.
125. Mettlin CJ, Piver S. A case-control study of milk-drinking and ovarian cancer risk. *Am J Epidemiol* 1990;132:871–876.
126. Christianson RE, Oechsli FW, Van Den Berg BJ. Caffeinated beverages and decreased fertility. *Lancet* 1989;1:378.
127. Wilcox AJ, et al. . . . *Lancet* 1988;ii:1453.
128. Trichopoulous D, Papapostolou M, Polychronopoulou A. Coffee and ovarian cancer. *Int J Cancer* 1981;28:691–693.
129. Hartge P, Lesher LP, McGowan L, Hoover R. Coffee and ovarian cancer. *Int J Cancer* 1982;30:531–532.
130. Miller DR, Rosenberg L, Kaufman DW, et al. Epithelial ovarian cancer and coffee drinking. *Int J Epidemiol* 1987;16:13–17.
131. La Vecchia C, Franceschi S, Decarli A, et al. Coffee drinking and the risk of epithelial ovarian cancer. *Int J Cancer* 1984;332:559–562.
132. Kato I, Tominaga S, Terao C. Alcohol consumption and cancers of hormone-related organs in females. *Jpn J Clin Oncol* 1989;19:202–207.
133. Gwinn ML, Webster LA, Lee NC, et al. Alcohol consumption and ovarian cancer risk. *Am J Epidemiol* 1986;123:759–766.
134. Franks AL, Lee NC, Kendricks JS, Rubin GL, Layde PM, and the Cancer and Steroid Hormone Study Group. Cigarette smoking and the risk of epithelial ovarian cancer. *Am J Epidemiol* 1987;126:112–117.
135. Parazzini F, La Vecchia C, Franceschi S, Negri E, Cecchetti G. Risk factors for endometrioid, mucinous and serous benign ovarian cysts. *Int J Epidemiol* 1989;18:108–112.
136. Cramer DW, Welch WR. Determinants of ovarian cancer risk. II. Inferences regarding pathogenesis. *JNCI* 1983;71:717–721.
137. Gardner WU. Hormonal imbalances in tumorigenesis. *Cancer Res* 1948;8:397–411.
138. Savaiano DA, Abou E, Anouar A, et al. Lactose malabsorption from yogurt, pasteurized yogurt, sweet acidophilus milk and cultured milk in lactose-deficient individuals. *Am J Clin Nutri* 1984;40:1219–1223.
139. Gitzelman R, Hansen RG. Galactose metabolism, hereditary defects and their clinical significance. In: Burman, Holteon JB, Pennoch CA, eds. *Inherited disorders of carbohydrate metabolism.* Baltimore: University Park Press, 1980.
140. Sahi T, Isokoshi M, Jussela J, et al. Recessive inheritance of adult-type lactose malabsorption. *Lancet* 1973;iii:623–630.
141. Cramer DW. Lactase persistance and milk consumption as determinant of ovarian cancer risk. *Am J Epidemiol* 1989;130:904–910.
142. Menczer J, Modan M, Ranon L, Golan A. Possible role of mumps virus in the etiology of ovarian cancer. *Cancer* 1979;43:1375–1379.
143. Rosenblatt KA, Rosenshein NB. Mumps parotitis and ovarian cancer [Letter]. *Am J Obstet Gynecol* 1984;149:472–473.
144. Cramer DW. Reply to Rosenblatt and Rosenshein (Correspondence). *Am J Obstet Gynecol* 1984;149:473–474.
145. Schiffman MH, Hartge P, Lesher LP, McGowan LM. Mumps

and postmenopausal ovarian cancer [Letter]. *Am J Obstet Gynecol* 1985;152:116–117.
146. Cramer DW. Mumps and postmenopausal ovarian cancer [Letter]. *Am J Obstet Gynecol* 1985;152:117–118.
147. Reed D, Brown G, Merrick R, Sever J, Feltz E. A mumps epidemic on St. George Island, Alaska. *JAMA* 1967;199:113–117.
148. Golan A, Joosting ACC, Orchard ME. Mumps virus and ovarian cancer. *S Afr Med J* 1979;56:18.
149. Schlesselman JJ. *Case-control studies*. New York: Oxford University Press, 1982:136.
150. Schottenfeld D, Berg J. Incidence of multiple primary cancers. IV. Cancers of the female breast and genital organs. *JNCI* 1971;46:161–170.
151. Harvey EB, Brinton LA. Second cancer following cancer of the breast in Connecticut, 1935–1982. *Natl Cancer Inst Monogr* 1985;68:99–112.
152. Storm HH, Ewertz M. Second cancer following cancer of the female genital system in Denmark, 1943–1980. *Natl Cancer Inst Monogr* 1985;68:331–340.
153. Curtis RE, Hoover RN, Kleinerman RA, Harvey ED. Second cancer following cancer of the female genital system in Connecticut, 1935–1982. *Natl Cancer Inst Monogr* 1985;68:113–137.
154. Ewertz M, Storm HH. Multiple primary cancers of the breast, endometrium and ovary. *Eur J Cancer Clin Oncol* 1989;25:1927–1932.
155. Schoenberg BS. *Multiple primary malignant neoplasms: the Connecticut experience, 1935–1964*. Berlin: Springer-Verlag, 1977.
156. Prior P, Pope DJ. Subsequent primary cancers in relation to treatment of ovarian cancer. *Br J Cancer* 1989;59:453–459.
157. Kleinerman RA, Curtis RE, Boice JD Jr, Flannery JT, Fraumeni JF Jr. Second cancers following radiotherapy for cervical cancer. *JNCI* 1982;69:1027–1033.
158. Casagrande JT, Pike MC, Ross RK, Louie EW, Roy S, Henderson BE. "Incessant ovulation" and ovarian cancer. *Lancet* 1979;2:170–173.
159. Schildkraut JM, Thompson WD. Relationship of epithelial ovarian cancer to other malignancies within families. *Genetic Epidemiol* 1988;5:355–367.
160. Thompson WD, Schildkraut JM. Family history of gynecological cancers: relationships to the incidence of breast cancer prior to age 55. *Int J Epidemiol* 1991;20:595–602.
161. Parazzini F, Negri E, La Vecchia C, Restelli C, Franceschi S. Family history of reproductive cancers and ovarian cancer risk: an Italian case-control study. *Am J Epidemiol* 1992;135:35–40.
162. Lynch JF, Lynch PM, Campbell A. Surveillance and management of patients of high genetic risk for ovarian carcinoma. *Obstet Gynecol* 1982;59:589–596.
163. Lynch HT, Albano W, Black L, Lynch JF, Recabaren J, Pierson R. Familial excess of cancer of the ovary and other anatomic sites. *JAMA* 1981;245:261–264.
164. Piver MS, Mettlin CJ, Tsukada Y, Nasca P, Greenwald P, McPhee ME. Familial ovarian cancer registry. *Obstet Gynecol* 1984;64:195–199.
165. Narod SA, Lynch HT, Conway T, et al. Familial breast-ovarian cancer locus on chromosome 17q12-q23. *Lancet* 1991;338:82–83.
166. Hall JM, Lee MK, Newman B, et al. Linkage of early-onset familial breast cancer to chromosome 17q21. *Science* 1990;250:1684–1689.
167. Friedman GD, Ury HK. Initial screening for carcinogenicity of commonly used drugs. *JNCI* 1980;65:723–733.
168. Schweisguth O, Gerard-Marchant R, Plainfosse B, Lemerle J, Watchi JM, Seringe P. Bilateral nonfunctioning thecoma of the ovary in epileptic children under anticonvulsant therapy. *Acta Pædiat Scand* 1971;60:6–10.
169. Sutherland RL, Watts CK, Hall RE, et al. Mechanisms of growth inhibition by nonsteroidal antiestrogens in human breast cancer cells. *J Steroid Biochem* 1987;27:891.
170. Watts CK, Sutherland RL. Studies on the ligand specificity and potential identity of microsomal antiestrogen binding sites. *Mol Pharmacol* 1987;31:541.
171. Spinelli JJ, Gallagher RP, Band PR, et al. Multiple myeloma, leukemia, and cancer of the ovary in cosmetologists and hairdressers. *Am J Ind Med* 1984;6:97–102.
172. Fathalla MF. Incessant ovulation—A factor in ovarian neoplasia? *Lancet* 1971;2:163.
173. Preston-Martin S, Pike MC, Ross RK, Henderson BE. Epidemiologic evidence for the increased cell proliferation model of carcinogenesis. *Prog Clin Biol Res* 1991;369:21–34.
174. Howell JS, Marchant J, Orr JW. The induction of ovarian tumors in mice with 9–10 dimethyl 1:2-benzanthracene. *Br J Cancer* 1954;8:635–646.
175. Murphey ED, Russell ES. Ovarian tumorigenesis following genic deletions of germ cells in hybrid mice. *Acta Un Int Cancer* 1963;19:779–782.
176. Fotherby K. Low doses of gestagens as fertility regulating agents. In: Diczfalusy E, ed. *Regulation of Human Fertility*. Copenhagen: Scriptor, 1977:283–321.
177. Jacobovits A, Gesce A, Piukovich I, Szontagh F, Karady I. Effects of 19-nor steroids on the motility of human fallopian tubes. *Int J Fertil* 1970;15:36.

CHAPTER 6

Hereditary/Familial Ovarian Cancer

Iffath Abbasi Hoskins and Harry Ostrer

Ovarian cancer, the sixth most common malignancy, is a prevalent and silent killer. It is the fourth leading cause of death from cancer, representing 5% of all cancer deaths. The increase in frequency over the last few decades, especially in industrialized Western countries, has made it the leading cause of death from gynecologic malignancies. Ovarian cancer is now responsible for more than 50% of these deaths. This rate is greater than that from cervical and endometrial cancers combined (1). Approximately 20,000 new cases are diagnosed each year, of which 65% are advanced (stages III and IV) at initial presentation. Because ovarian cancer is a leading killer of women and because it is so difficult to diagnose, concentrated efforts are being made to identify the individuals at highest risk for developing the disease.

SCREENING FOR OVARIAN CANCER

A major reduction in the mortality from ovarian cancer can occur only if it can be prevented or identified in its earliest stages when the chances for survival are greatest. For instance, the relative five-year survival rate for advanced disease (stages III and IV) is 20% to 30%, whereas the rate is 80% to 90% for stage I disease (2,3).

Early detection of any disease is best accomplished by the application of screening techniques designed to identify the disease at its earliest occurrence. In order for screening techniques to be useful in any population, certain criteria apply (Table 1). The incidence of the disease, the mortality rate, and the identity of high risk subgroups should be known. The screening test should be cost-effective, with a high sensitivity (percent of test results that are positive in women with disease) and specificity (percent of test results that are negative in women without disease). It should be acceptable to the patient and to the care provider.

Factors associated with increased risks for ovarian cancer include: age greater than 60 years, European descent, positive family history of ovarian cancer, previous history of breast cancer, and nulliparity (2,3). The age-specific incidence of ovarian cancer in the general population is greater than 15 per 100,000 women over 40 years of age. It rises to 25 per 100,000 women by 45 years of age, and to 50 per 100,000 in women aged 70 years (4). At present, similar information is not available for patients with familial ovarian cancer who are at increased risk of developing the disease. Therefore, until new strategies to determine these figures are completed, such information must be surmised from existing data.

To estimate the effect, if any, of screening on survival, one must assume that women whose cancers are detected in this way would have improved survival rates over those who were not screened. Of the approximately 20,000 new cases per year in the general population, there will be approximately 7,600 five-year survivors. Westhoff, et al. (5) stated that if a screening test having a sensitivity of 80% (similar to that of a Papanicolaou smear or mammogram) is applied to the general population, the number of five-year survivors would increase to 14,400. There would be one additional survivor for every 440 women screened. Nearly all of these would be in women over 45 years of age. This approach gives a simplistic assessment of the number of lives that might be saved by screening. It does not address any possible adverse effects of screening, such as the emotional and economic consequences. Obtaining such information requires randomized controlled trials.

As discussed below, current screening methods may

I. A. Hoskins: Department of Obstetrics and Gynecology, New York University Medical Center, New York, NY 10016.
H. Ostrer: Department of Pediatrics, New York University Medical Center, New York, NY 10016

TABLE 1. *Criteria for screening test*

The prevalence of the disease should be known.
Reliable screening tests should be available.
Early indicators of disease (precursors) should be known.
Duration of early disease should be known.
There should be increased morbidity with occurrence of the disease.

---

not identify early stage ovarian cancer in a large number of individuals. Such guidelines are currently unresolved, with no one technique having been shown to be beneficial either in the general population or in those considered to be at increased risk. In order to have a significant impact on reducing the mortality of this disease, a new screening paradigm is required. One approach may be to screen those with a family history of disease. However, many at-risk individuals would still be missed. A second approach may be the development of genetic tests to identify those at higher risk. The methods currently available are sonography, Doppler velocimetry, and serum CA-125 levels.

Sonography

Though pelvic examination is a commonly used procedure to assess the ovaries, it is imprecise; enlargements or abnormalities can be missed if they are too small to be felt (6). The use of ultrasonography to visualize the pelvis allows more accurate and specific evaluation of the ovaries.

Transabdominal sonography (TAS) has been widely used for this purpose. Unfortunately, low-frequency transducers are needed to clearly image structures inside the pelvis, resulting in loss of image quality due to attenuation of the ultrasound beam. Since the introduction of transvaginal sonography (TVS), the transducer can be placed closer to the pelvic structures, and image quality is improved because higher frequencies are used.

The efficacy of sonography to assess pelvic viscera has been described previously. Andolf et al. (7) prospectively compared clinical and sonographic examinations with operative findings in patients undergoing surgery for pelvic pathology. When correlated with operative findings, TAS had a sensitivity of 83% versus 67% for pelvic exams. The specificities were 96% and 94%, respectively. Similar results have been obtained with the use of TVS (8,9).

Sonography has also been proposed to screen for occult ovarian cancer. Campbell et al. (10) evaluated 5,479 self-referred, asymptomatic women annually for 3 years to detect abnormal ovaries or persistent masses. They found 326 abnormal scans in these women, including morphologic (hyperechogenic or hypoechogenic), outline (regular or irregular), and volume (greater than 20 cc) abnormalities of the ovaries. All underwent laparotomy. Nine had ovarian cancer (five primary, four metastatic), for an incidence of one cancer per 67 abnormal scans and a positive predictive value of 1.5%. Bourne et al. (11) used TVS to screen 776 asymptomatic women who had either a first- or second-degree relative with ovarian cancer. The sensitivity of TVS for detecting ovarian cancer was 100%, the specificity was 94.8%, and the positive predictive value was 7.7%. Others have reported similar results with this technique (12–13,106–107) (Table 2).

Color-flow Doppler velocimetry allows detection of the intratumoral neovasculature that accompanies malignant tumors. The underlying hypothesis is that flow characteristics of malignant tumors are different from those of benign tissues. Determination of the pulsatility index (PI) (end diastolic Doppler shift subtracted from the peak systolic Doppler shift divided by mean maximum Doppler shift over the cardiac cycle) can help to determine the benign or malignant nature of a tumor. This is especially useful when neovascularization precedes tumor growth. Several authors have reported on its use for predicting ovarian malignancy (11,14–15,16) (Table 3).

Although TVS can reliably evaluate pelvic viscera, the low predictive values suggest that further studies are needed before it can be used as a screening technique for ovarian cancer. The chance that an ovarian tumor is malignant increases 12-fold between the ages of 30 years and 70 years, being 13% if a woman is premenopausal and 45% after menopause. Therefore, the applicability of this test to different age groups with

TABLE 2. *Sensitivity, specificity, and predictive values of sonography to assess pelvic viscera*

Author, year	No. of patients	Menopausal status	Sens %	Spec %	PPV %
Campbell S., 1989	5479	pre & post	100	97.7	1.5
Andolf E, 1990	801	pre & post	100	79.1	5.5
Van Nagell J., 1991	1300	post	100	98	11.1
Bourne T., 1991	1000	pre & post	100	94.8	7.7
Sassone A., 1991	143	pre & post	83	100	37.0
Granberg S., 1988	132	pre & post	0	99	0

Sens, sensitivity; Spec, specificity; PPV, positive predictive value; NA, data not available.

TABLE 3. *Sensitivity, specificity, and predictive value of color flow velocimetry for predicting ovarian malignancies*

Author, year	No. of patients	Menopausal status	Sens %	Spec %	PPV %
Bourne T., 1989	50	pre & post	80	71	40
Bourne T., 1989	1000	pre & post	100	94.8	7.7
Kawai M., 1992	24	pre & post	88	60	57
Weiner Z., 1992	62	pre & post	94	97	94

Sens, sensitivity; Spec, specificity; PPV, positive predictive value.

vastly different incidences of ovarian cancer should be evaluated further with large scale screening programs before it can be offered to the general population. Additionally, issues such as the emotional cost of positive findings, the management and follow-up of false-positive results and the degree of reassurance allowed with negative findings should be addressed.

Serum CA-125 Levels

In past years, the use of tumor markers has been suggested to detect ovarian cancer. To date, none has significantly improved clinical detection or identification of relapse of disease. The ideal tumor marker would be one that is expressed in large amounts by all tumor cells in an easily accessible body compartment (e.g., blood) with levels that accurately reflect the presence and amount of tumor so as to distinguish benign from malignant disease. Most currently available markers do not have the degree of sensitivity or specificity required of a screening test for detection of early stage cancer. Additionally, they are elevated not only with many different kinds of malignancies but also with many benign conditions.

Several antigens associated with ovarian cancer have been reported. One such marker is cancer antigen-125 (CA-125), an antigenic determinant defined by the monoclonal antibody OC-125 (17). It is not produced by normal ovarian tissue but can be detected in fallopian tube, endometrium, endocervix and mesothelial surfaces (peritoneum, pleura, pericardium) (18). Ninety-nine percent of healthy women have serum levels less than 35 U/ml and 99.7% have levels less than 65 U/ml (20). Eighty-two percent of patients with epithelial ovarian cancer (EOC) exhibit levels above 35 U/ml (18). For most CA125-positive ovarian tumors, the serum concentration reflects tumor burden even when there is no clinical evidence of disease. However, a normal level does not reliably predict absence of disease (19–22).

CA-125 is not specific for ovarian carcinoma. Other gynecologic malignancies, including adenocarcinomas of the fallopian tube, endometrium, and cervix can also exhibit levels greater than 35 U/ml, as can breast, lung, pancreas, and colon cancers (18). Several benign conditions can also be associated with elevated CA-125 levels (23–27) (Table 4).

Despite this, several authors have described the use of CA-125 in evaluating patients at increased risk for developing ovarian cancer (17,26,28–31) (Table 5). Most of them agree that though the high sensitivity of the serum CA-125 assay lends credence to its value in detecting ovarian malignancy, the low specificity warrants further evaluation before the test can be offered for screening the general population.

Creasman and DiSaia (32) evaluated the usefulness of combining serum CA-125 levels and ultrasonography to screen the general population for ovarian cancer. They calculated the increased financial burden incurred (approximately $14 million) if every woman over the age of 45 was screened. The authors stated that to offer such interventions as standard screening

TABLE 4. *Conditions associated with elevated CA-125 levels*

Malignant

Gynecologic cancers:

  ovary
  fallopian tube
  endometrium
  cervix

Nongynecologic cancers:

  breast
  lung
  pancreas
  colon

Benign

Gynecologic:

  menstruation
  pelvic inflammatory disease
  endometriosis, adenomyosis
  ectopic pregnancy
  pregnancy, first trimester
  leiomyoma uteri
  cystadenoma, ovary

Nongynecologic:

  liver disease
  pancreatitis
  peritonitis
  renal failure

TABLE 5. *Sensitivity, specificity, and predictive values of serum CA-125 levels*

Author, year	No. of patients	Menopausal status	Sens %	Spec %	PPV %
Einhorn N.,* 1986	100	NA	77	89	61
Vasilev S., 1988	182	pre & post	73	81	77
Finkler N.,* 1988	131	pre & post	68	74	65
Malkasian G.,* 1988	158	pre & post	78	78	73
Zurawski V., 1990	1082	post	100	97	2.8

* Includes CA125 assay cutoff values >35 U/ml
Sens, sensitivity; Spec, specificity; PPV, positive predictive value; NA, data not available.

procedures with no evidence to date that the ovarian cancer death rate would be lowered, is premature. However, even though there are no currently available data to justify this action, such screening may be offered to the small subset of patients (less than 5%) who are at extremely high risk for developing ovarian cancer so as to provide these patients some reassurance.

Currently, the development and evaluation of effective screening tests for ovarian cancer detection in the general population require additional study with special emphasis on testing those subgroups that have increased risks for developing this disease. Highly specific, inexpensive tests should be sought. At present, there are no suitable techniques available for such screening (33).

GENETIC BASIS FOR OVARIAN CANCER

Relatives of ovarian cancer patients have long been known to be at increased risk for developing ovarian cancer, but the genes that predispose to this have not been identified. Familial ovarian cancer is considered to be transmitted in an autosomal dominant fashion with transmission occurring from both males and females. First-degree female relatives of cancer patients may have up to a 50% chance of developing ovarian cancer as compared to the background risk of 1.4%. In one study (11), 776 women with positive family histories of ovarian cancer were followed. This study found a tenfold increased risk of a woman developing cancer if she has a close relative with the disease. Such women may also have increased risks for other cancers (breast, colon, endometrium) resulting from an inherited genetic susceptibility of the target tissues. Conversely, female relatives of persons with these other tumors may be at increased risk for developing ovarian cancer.

During the past decade, significant advances in the understanding of the genetic basis of cancer have been made. Most if not all cancers have been shown to result from stable genetic changes that occur at the cellular level. Some of these changes may be inherited through the germ line, whereas others originate from somatic mutations. It has been estimated that four to six such changes are required for the transformation to malignant progression (34–35).

Some of the genes that play a role in cellular transformation were identified on the basis of their having homologues in tumor viruses that could transform cells (35). Others were "rescued" from tumor cells on the basis of their ability to transform NIH 3T3 mouse cells. This is a cell type that has become immortalized, but does not manifest the lack of contact inhibition that is characteristic of the transformed phenotype (36) (Fig. 1). Still other genes have been identified by virtue of their link to the development of the phenotype in certain cancer family syndromes (Fig. 2).

The first of these to be cloned was the retinoblastoma (Rb) gene. This has served as the model for identifying genes in the family cancer syndromes. The location of such a gene was postulated from the observation that many sporadic retinoblastomas were associated with deletion of band q13 on the long arm of chromosome 13. Inherited deletions of this region were observed in nonfamilial cases. A linked genetic marker, esterase D_1, was identified (37). Within a family with multiple cases of retinoblastoma, specific alleles of the esterase D_1 gene correlated with the development of the tumor. The linkage to esterase D_1 proved that inheritance of a specific gene caused retinoblastoma. This marker could also be used in a predictive way to identify those at risk.

A molecular basis for the action of such a gene was developed by Knudson in the early 1970s (38). Based on the distribution of inherited versus sporadic tumors, he postulated that two genetic hits were required for these tumors to develop. In inherited cases, one of the hits was transmitted through the germ line and the other was acquired through somatic mutation. In sporadic cases, both hits were the result of somatic mutation. By comparing the pattern of polymorphic DNA markers on chromosome 13 from blood and from tumor tissue, Cavanee and coworkers (39) demonstrated how these two hits occur. They developed the term *loss of heterozygosity* to explain their observation that one of the two naturally occurring markers is lost in these tumors (Fig. 3). There can be a mutation (deletion or substitution) of chromosome 13 in the region of the retinoblastoma gene as one of the hits. The second hit may involve a mutation of the other normal gene by deletion, insertion, or alteration of a single nucleotide

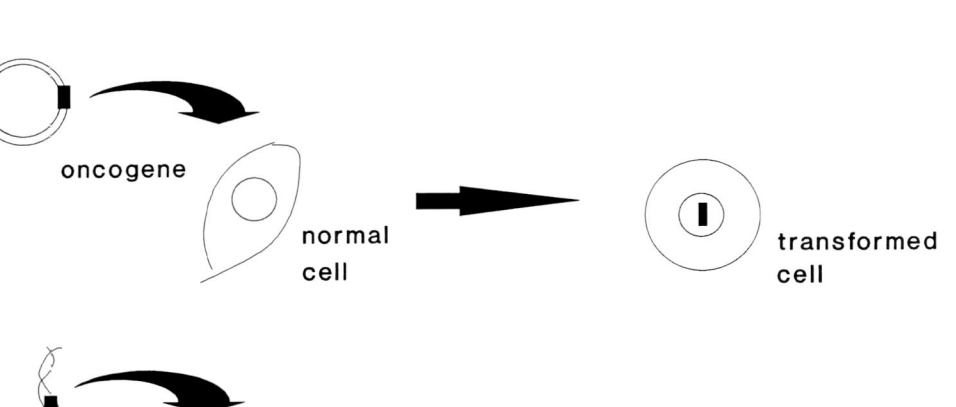

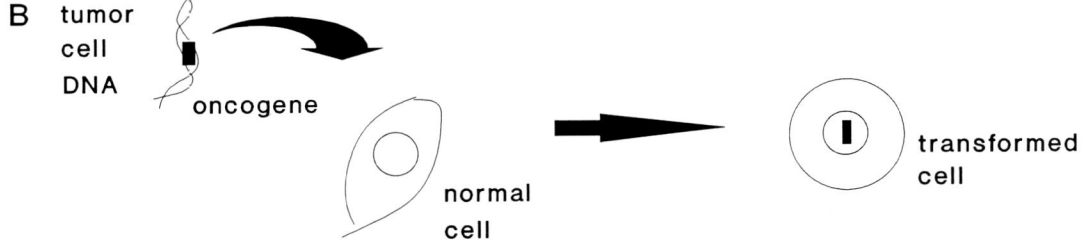

FIG. 1. Methods for identifying dominantly acting oncogenes. A: Transformation by tumor virus DNA. B: Transformation by tumor cell DNA.

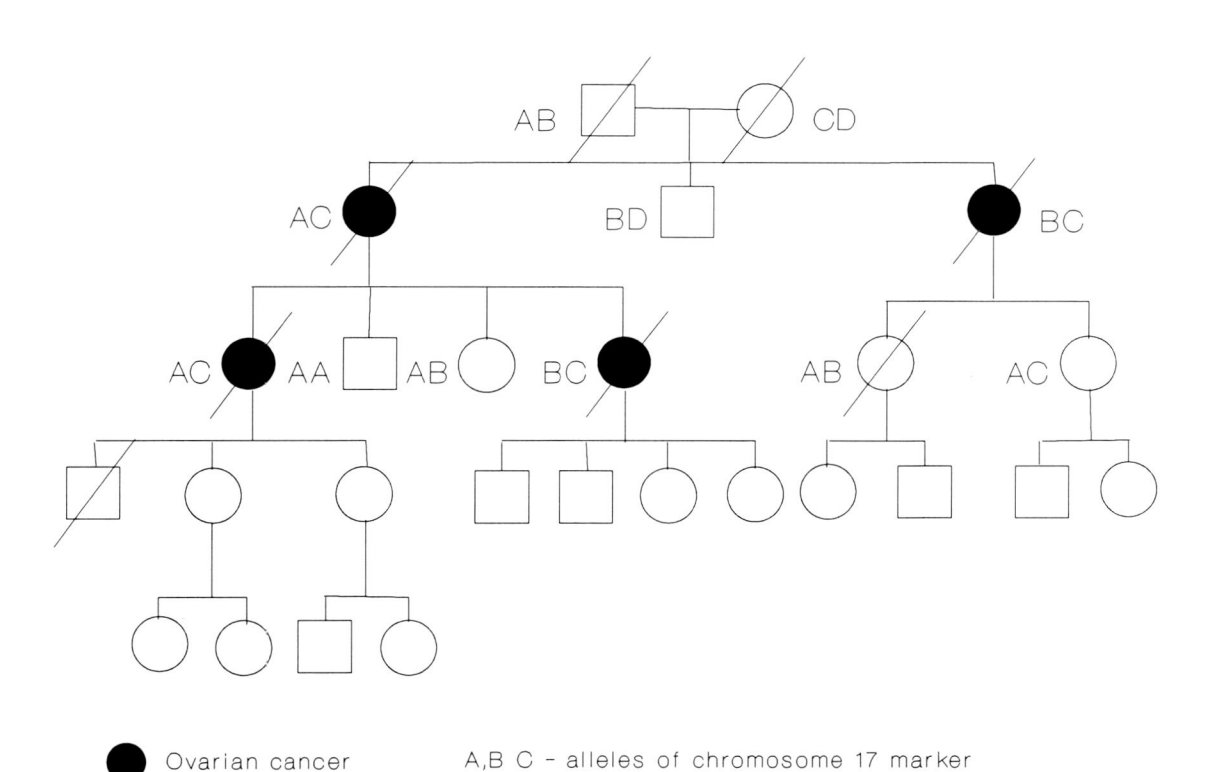

FIG. 2. Pedigree with site-specific ovarian cancer depicting identification of cancer-predisposing genes by linkage analysis. In this hypothetical pedigree with multiple members affected with ovarian cancer, the predisposition to inheriting cancer is transmitted with allele C of the chromosome 17 marker.

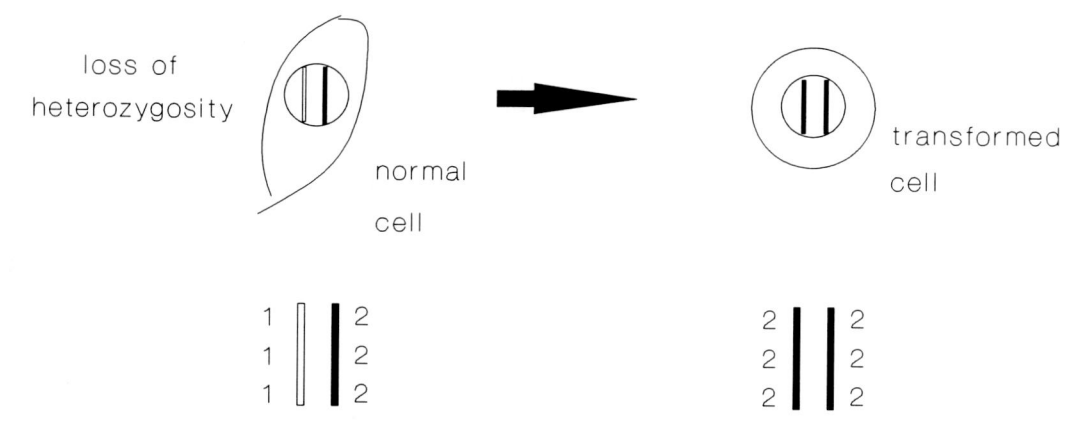

FIG. 3. Identification of oncogenes from loss of heterozygosity. Through this mechanism, one of the two alleles of a chromosome in a given pair is lost.

of DNA in the somatic cells. Alternatively, the second hit may involve loss of the normal chromosome 13, somatic recombination, or gene conversion between the chromatids of the normal and the deletion-bearing chromosomes (Fig. 4).

The identification of loss of heterozygosity suggested that the development of retinoblastoma was a recessive phenotype because two hits were required for the tumor to develop. It explained why some individuals who inherit an allele for retinoblastoma do not develop the disease. Such nonpenetrance results from the absence of a second hit. It also suggested the mechanism of action for the Rb gene. In its natural form, i.e., the wild-type, it acted as a tumor-suppressor gene. With complete inactivation of this gene, the suppressive effect on unregulated growth was removed and tumors could develop. With identification of the Rb protein, this mechanism of action has proven to be correct (40).

Retinoblastomas were observed to be associated with osteogenic sarcomas in individuals who survived the disease. Whereas this was initially thought to be the effect of treatment with radiation and/or chemotherapy, detailed analysis has demonstrated that the same genetic mechanism operates in the bone as in the retina. Loss of heterozygosity has been demonstrated in osteogenic sarcomas, although there is preferential loss of the paternal alleles in these tumors, suggesting that the paternal and maternal copies of this gene are not functionally equivalent (41). The molecular basis for this difference is not clearly understood. The Rb gene has been found to play a role in other tumors,

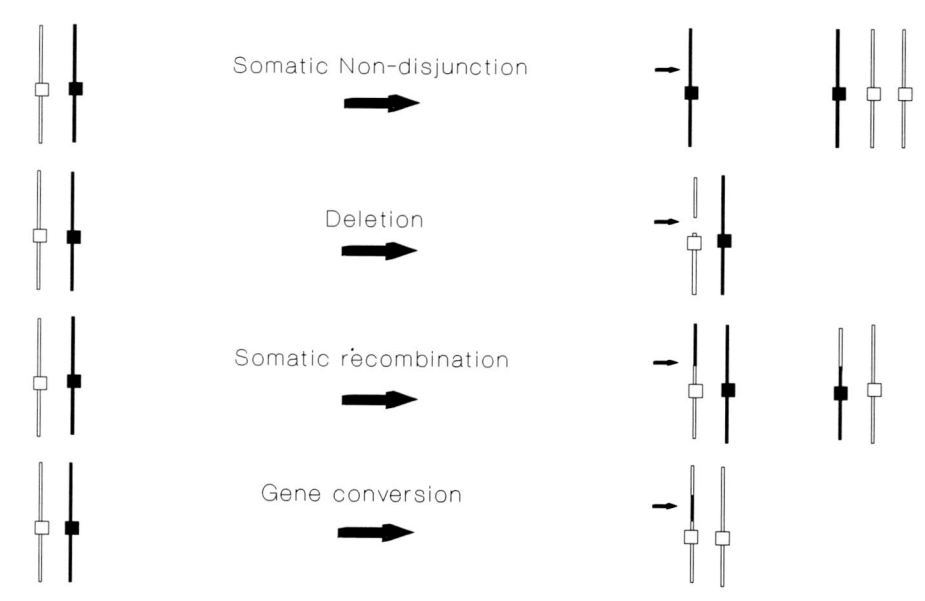

FIG. 4. Mechanisms of somatic mutation resulting in loss of heterozygosity. These include somatic non-disjunction, deletion, somatic recombination, and gene conversion.

including small cell carcinoma of the lung. This demonstrates that mutation in a single gene may be associated with several different tumors.

Loss of heterozygosity has been implicated in the development and progression of a host of other tumors, including such common solid tumors as colon, lung, and breast (42–44). Several genes have been identified whose transmission is associated with tumor development. These include familial colon cancer, Li-Fraumeni Syndrome, Wilms tumor, and neurofibromatosis (45–48).

A body of evidence has been mounting to demonstrate a genetic basis for ovarian cancer. Though specific genetic changes have not been identified, certain consistent chromosomal changes have been observed, along with loss of heterozygosity on certain chromosomes. Several different genetic conditions have been associated with increased frequency of ovarian tumors, including familial ovarian cancer. It is likely that the genes that are transmitted through these families may represent some of the first hits in the development of ovarian cancer.

Cytogenetic Studies

Cytogenetic studies of ovarian cancer have demonstrated marked variability in the chromosomal constitution of the tumors. These include modal numbers that are hypodiploid (less than 46 chromosomes) or hyperdiploid (60–100 chromosomes), and the presence of multiple chromosomal markers and cells with spontaneous chromosome breaks (49). Much of the data on ovarian cancer have been obtained from metastatic tumors and malignant ascites or pleural fluid. These tumors may be indicative of the karyotypes of the primary tumors. A more favorable prognosis is associated with tumors that have a near-diploid chromosome number (50). Cultured ovarian tumor cell lines have been observed to undergo progressive karyotypic changes (51).

Two consistent sets of changes have been observed in ovarian cancer, i.e., those involving chromosomes 1 and 6. In the study by Whang-Peng et al. (52), the short arm of chromosome 1 (1p) was found to be the most frequent site of translocations. The long arm of this chromosome (1q), especially the region between bands q21→44, was commonly involved in deletions and translocations. Chromosome 1 is also commonly involved in other carcinomas (53). It has been suggested that this region plays a role in tumor progression rather than tumor initiation (49). This mechanism of progression may be common to a wide variety of different tumors.

Deletions and translocations of the long arm (q) of chromosome 6 have been reported in several cytogenetic studies of ovarian cancer (54–55). The commonly affected region involves bands q15→21. Wake (55) suggested that a specific translocation between the long arms of chromosomes 6 and 14 [t(6;14)(q15;q24)] was involved in papillary serous cystadenocarcinomas. He found that five tumors had this translocation and four had either a deletion of the long arm of chromosome 6 (6q⁻) or an addition onto the long arm of chromosome 14 (14q⁺) (Fig. 5). In the study on malignant pleural or ascitic fluids from patients with ovarian carcinoma (48), about 40% of the tumors had alterations of 6q

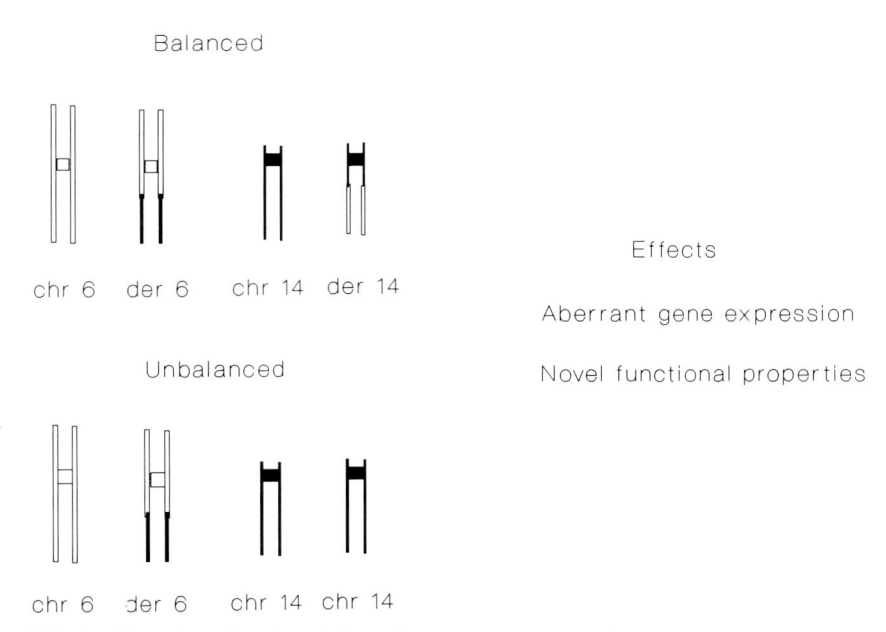

FIG. 5. Translocation involving chromosomes 6 and 14 in ovarian cancer.

that were demonstrable cytogenetically. Of these, 70% were missing the long arm of chromosome 6 (6q−).

Loss of Heterozygosity

Each DNA marker or gene in a given pair of chromosomes is referred to as an *allele*. Using molecular techniques, the two alleles can be identified. Loss of one of these alleles, or loss of heterozygosity, is shown in Fig. 4. Several studies have demonstrated loss of heterozygosity for alleles on different chromosomes. In one study of 17 matched pairs of ovarian tumors and white blood cell samples from the same patients, 10 had DNA markers that could distinguish the two alleles of the oncogene c-Ha-*ras* 1 on chromosome II (56). Five of these ten informative cases demonstrated loss of one of the c-Ha-*ras* 1 alleles. When this study was extended to other chromosomes (57), 9 of 14 cases had loss of heterozygosity for the estrogen receptor locus on 6q. This was the first demonstration of loss of heterozygosity at this chromosomal region for any tumor, and confirmed the cytogenetic studies implicating this region in the development of ovarian carcinoma. Loss of heterozygosity was also demonstrated on the short arm of chromosome 17 at the locus, D17S28, in 6 of 8 cases; and at the locus, D17S30, in 9 of 14 cases. Loss of heterozygosity has not been observed for loci on chromosomes 1, 2, 5, 6, 7, 11, 12, 19, and 22, suggesting that this is not a generalized phenomenon. It has been found on both the short and long arms of chromosome 17 in epithelial ovarian cancer (EOC) (58). In a study that used minisatellite DNA sequences for "DNA fingerprinting" to compare ovarian tumor and white blood cell DNA from the same subjects, the most common findings were loss or decrease in relative intensity of a band. These findings are most compatible with loss of heterozygosity, but the technique is not sensitive enough to identify the sites at which this occurs (59).

The sites at which loss of heterozygosity has been observed may themselves be involved in the pathogenesis of these tumors. Alternatively, they may be carried along as markers. In that case, these markers would show a less frequent loss of heterozygosity than the linked genes that play a role in cancer development. Mechanisms such as gene conversion and deletion may encompass oncogenes, but not linked markers. As noted earlier, regions demonstrating loss of heterozygosity can be further evaluated for an etiologic role by testing for linkage in families that transmit the phenotype and by demonstrating that specific mutations in these genes can be correlated with the tumor phenotype. It is possible that certain genes, such as the one on chromosome 6, are specific to ovarian cancer, whereas others are shared by ovarian cancer and other tumors.

Gene Amplification

One mechanism of modulating gene expression is gene amplification, i.e., increasing the copy number. As with breast cancer, amplification of the HER-2/*neu* oncogene has been found in ovarian cancer (60). This is located on chromosome 17, q12–q22. Of 120 primary ovarian malignancies studied by Solomon et al. (60), 26% showed evidence of HER-2/*neu* amplification. Of these, twenty-three were amplified twofold to fivefold, and eight were amplified greater than fivefold. The cumulative survival was inversely proportional to the degree of amplification of this gene. The median survivals for the unamplified, twofold to fivefold and greater than fivefold amplified groups were 1,879, 959, and 243 days respectively. Hence, the degree of amplification serves as a prognostic factor for ovarian cancer. In contrast, amplification of another oncogene, c-*ras*-Ki, which is located on chromosome 12, p11-p12, has been rarely observed in epithelial ovarian carcinoma and does not seem to correlate with outcome (61).

The HER-2/*neu* oncogene has structural and sequence similarity with the epidermal growth factor receptor. This suggests that it is the receptor for an as yet undetermined growth factor. Cultured ovarian carcinoma cell lines that overexpress the HER-2/*neu* oncogene are relatively resistant to the cytotoxic effects of tumor necrosis factor and lymphokine-activated killer cells (62), but can have their proliferation inhibited by gamma interferon (63). The gamma interferon directly inhibits the expression of the HER-2/*neu* gene product, suggesting that proliferation is mediated by the overexpression of the HER-2/*neu* gene.

CANCER FAMILY SYNDROMES

Several cases of familial cancer have been reported. Some investigators have suggested that, because cancers are a common occurrence (one in four persons), clustering in families may be due to chance alone. Because these families have a common environment, they may share a carcinogenic agent that may predispose to the development of these tumors. Alternatively, there may be a genetic basis for the occurrence and transmission of cancers in these families.

Multiple investigators have described the familial transmission of ovarian cancer and suggested the existence of genetic cancer family syndromes (2–3,64). Individuals with these syndromes have an earlier age of onset of disease, a greater incidence of bilaterality, multifocal affected sites, and multiple primary cancers occurring in the same individual. Additionally, numerous members over several generations in a family may have the same features, suggesting autosomal dominant transmission. Five-year survival periods in these

TABLE 6. *Cardinal features of familial cancer*

Earlier age of onset.
Clusters of ovary, breast, proximal colon, and endometrium cancers, either in the same individual or in several members of the same pedigree.
Increased incidence of bilaterality.
Advanced stages of cancer at time of diagnosis.
Greater likelihood of papillary serous cystadenocarcinomas in those who have ovarian cancer.
Lower five-year survival rates.

patients are generally shorter than in those with sporadic cancers (Table 6).

Familial cancer syndromes that involve epithelial ovarian carcinoma include: (a) familial site-specific epithelial ovarian cancer alone; (b) familial epithelial ovarian and breast cancer; (c) familial proximal colon cancer along with other cancers, (breast, ovary, endometrium, stomach, urinary tract), also called the Lynch Cancer Family Syndrome II (65–66) (Figs. 6–8).

When familial ovarian cancer is associated with familial breast cancer, the pedigree may show mixtures of first- and second-degree relatives demonstrating either one or both these cancers. As in site-specific familial ovarian cancer, these patients also have a tendency toward earlier (premenopausal) age of onset of the disease, increased incidence of bilaterality, and frequent occurrence of both cancers in the same individual. Patients belonging to such pedigrees and developing either ovarian or breast cancer will have significantly higher chances of developing cancers in the other associated sites (breast or ovary).

Schoenberg et al. (67) determined that women with primary breast or gynecologic cancers had a 50% or greater risk of developing a second primary cancer in the colon, endometrium, or ovary. They suggested that, because a common etiology seems to exist for these cancers, women with breast or genital tract cancers should receive careful follow-up screening for early detection of second primary cancers. Waterhouse et al. (68) stated that patients with premenopausal breast cancer had a threefold increased incidence of subsequently developing ovarian cancer.

Linkage Studies

Linkage studies have reinforced the idea of a genetic basis for cancer family syndromes. Such studies were performed in 17 families with both breast and ovarian cancer occurring in the same family (69). Linkage was demonstrated to the Rhesus (Rh) gene on chromosome 1. Generally, likelihood of development (LOD) scores of three or more are taken as proof of linkage. The maximal LOD scores (i.e., likelihood of linkage) were 1.228 and 1.876, respectively, at zero recombination. The higher value was associated with susceptibility to fibrocystic disease. If higher penetrance (LOD, given inheritance of the susceptibility gene) and gene frequency values were assumed, the LOD scores were 1.35 and 2.28, respectively. There was no suggestion of heterogeneity among the different pedigrees studied. Though these findings require further validation, they may reflect the common occurrence of chromosome 1

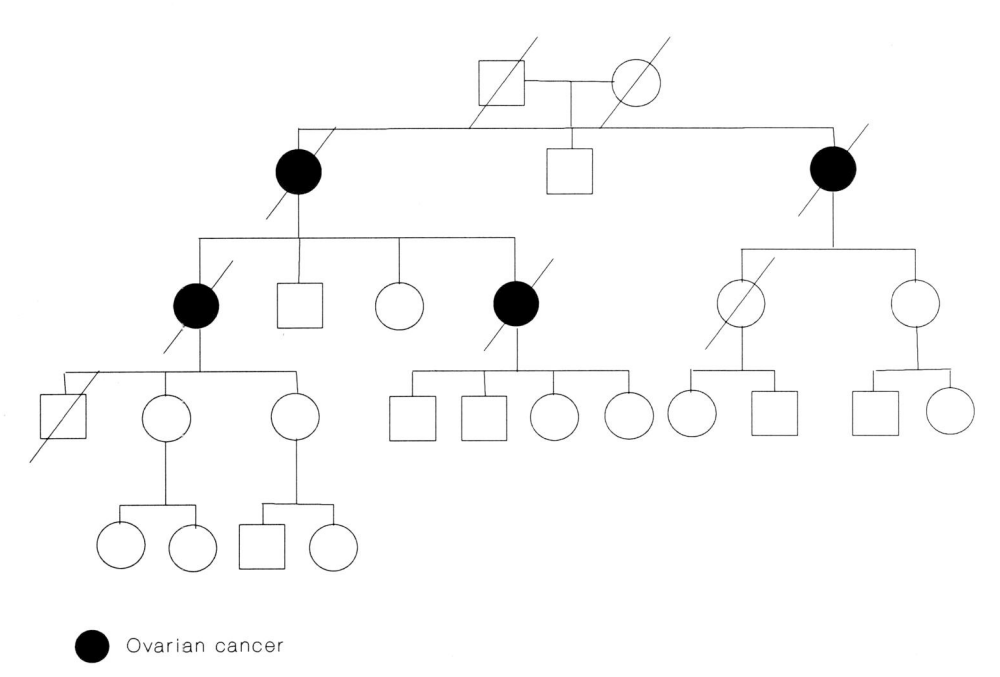

FIG. 6. Pedigree with site-specific ovarian cancer.

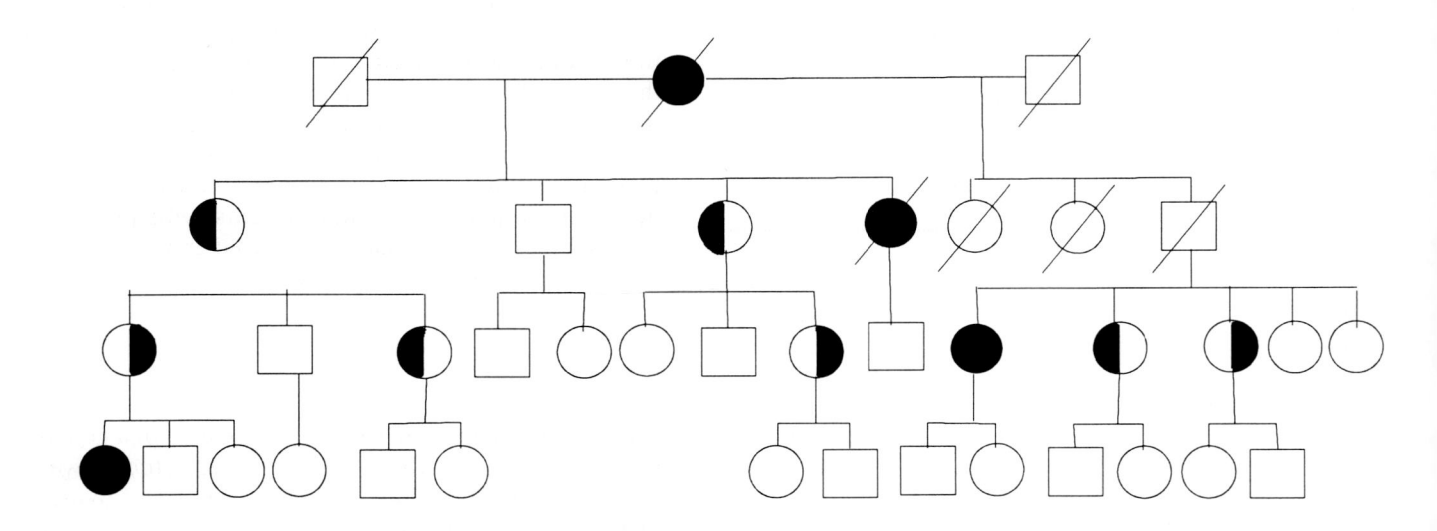

104 / CHAPTER 6

◐ breast cancer

◐ ovarian cancer

● breast/ovarian cancer

FIG. 7. Pedigree with breast/ovarian cancer syndrome.

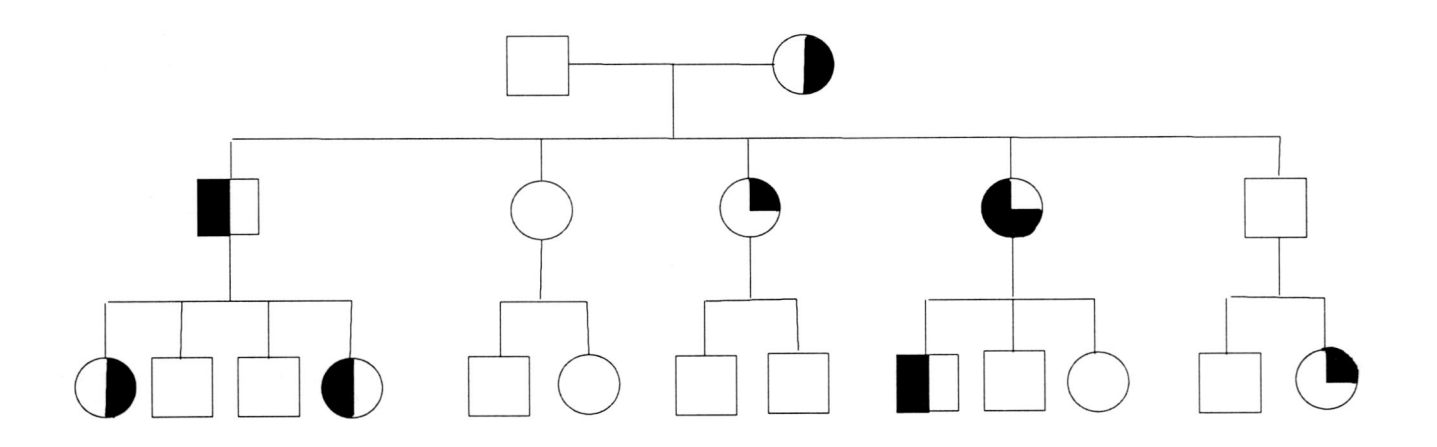

◔ ovarian cancer

◴ breast cancer

◐ non-adenomatous colon cancer

FIG. 8. Pedigree with Lynch Cancer Family Syndrome II. This includes breast, ovarian, and non-adenomatous colon cancer.

involvement in ovarian carcinoma, as judged by cytogenetic analysis of the tumors.

Linkage has also been described between the Lynch cancer family syndrome II (ovary, breast, colon, endometrium) and the Kidd blood group at an LOD score of 3.19. (70). The Kidd blood group has been mapped to chromosome 18, q11–q12. Through additional linkage studies, other genetic markers may be found for these cancer family syndromes.

GENETIC CONDITIONS THAT PREDISPOSE TO CANCER

Several other genetically determined conditions can be associated with ovarian tumors. Typically, these tumors do not involve the epithelial cells of the more common adenocarcinomas discussed in this chapter. They include Peutz-Jeghers syndrome (PJS), basal cell nevus syndrome, and gonadal dysgenesis. These conditions should be considered when a familial clustering of nonepithelial ovarian tumors is found in a pedigree.

PJS is a hamartosis transmitted in an autosomal dominant fashion. The syndrome is characterized by (a) the occurrence of hamartomatous polyps in the intestinal tract, especially in the jejunum; (b) melanin spots of the lips and buccal mucosa; and (c) in women, granulosa cell tumors of the ovary (71). These are benign, estrogen-producing tumors. If they occur early in life, isosexual precocious puberty may develop. The intestinal polyps may cause rectal bleeding and intussusception.

Follow-up was obtained for 72 patients with PJS in the St. Mark's polyposis registry (72). Among these individuals, nine developed gastrointestinal tumors; seven developed nongastrointestinal tumors. Granulosa cell tumors were found in 1.4% of females with PJS. Males with PJS may develop sex cord-stromal tumors. These may produce estrogen and cause gynecomastia.

The basal cell nevus syndrome is transmitted in an autosomal dominant fashion, with 40% of cases representing new mutations (73). Large numbers of basal cell nevoid epitheliomas appear, starting at puberty. These are locally destructive and may metastasize to the brain and lungs. Bone abnormalities may occur, especially keratocysts of the jaw. These patients are at increased risk for developing medulloblastomas. Ovarian cysts and fibromas commonly occur and may become quite large and calcify.

Individuals with intact or fragmented Y chromosomes and maldeveloped gonads (mixed gonadal dysgenesis) are at a significantly increased risk for developing cancer of those gonads, specifically gonadoblastomas (74). These tumors are composed of germ cells and sex cord derivatives which resemble immature granulosa and Sertoli cells (75). The cumulative incidence of gonadal tumors in mixed gonadal dysgenesis rises with age, being 10% at 15 years and 25% at 26 years (76). The epidemiological evidence suggests that the risk factor gene is located on the Y chromosome. These tumors may undergo malignant degeneration. Prophylactic removal of dysgenetic gonads is generally recommended if a Y chromosome is present in the intact, fragmented, or mosaic state. Familial cases of gonadal dysgenesis have been reported.

Genetic Testing

Genetic testing for ovarian cancer will provide a new approach to identifying those at high risk prior to the development of disease. Currently, high risk individuals can be identified only on the basis of family history. In the future, screening for ovarian cancer can take two forms: detecting germ line mutations in blood or other tissues to identify those who are at increased risk for developing cancer; and screening of blood or other tissues for the presence of specific mutations or chromosomal rearrangements that are indicative of circulating cancer cells. These tests can use the polymerase chain reaction to amplify specific genes and identify mutations or rearrangements. Other tests can use "chromosome painting" to demonstrate abnormal numbers of chromosomes or chromosome regions in cancer cells.

Screening for ovarian cancer may become a two-stage procedure. First, individuals who are at increased risk for developing cancer will be identified by the presence of germ line mutations. Such screening may be aimed at the general population or at those who have a family history of cancer. Once individuals with germ line mutations have been identified, they may be monitored for development of tumors by interventions such as TVS, serum CA-125 levels, or by screening for the presence of circulating cells with specific mutations or chromosomal rearrangements.

These tests must be subjected to the same scrutiny that has been applied to other screening tests, such as Papanicolaou smears and mammography, to determine their sensitivity and specificity. In addition, screening tests such as TVS and serum CA-125 levels should be reexamined in high-risk populations to determine whether their sensitivities and specificities are similar to those of the general population. If that is the case, the predictive value of a positive result may become higher because of the individual's greater likelihood of developing the cancer. Such a screening system may reduce or eliminate the need for prophylactic surgery in those defined to be at low risk by these interventions. Alternatively, these screening tests may prove to be ineffective for identifying ovarian cancer in its earliest stages; oral contraceptive use and/or prophylatic oophrectomy may become the only forms of prevention that can be offered to these high-risk patients.

PREVENTION OF OVARIAN CANCER: ORAL CONTRACEPTIVES

One of the potential causes of ovarian cancer is put forth by the "incessant ovulation" hypothesis. Investigators have reported increased mortality rates from ovarian cancer in nuns. Others (77–78) have hypothesized that ovarian cancer may result from trauma or mitotic stimulation of ovarian epithelium that has been subjected to prolonged ovulation. Still others (79–80) have suggested that exposure of the ovarian epithelium to persistent, high gonadotropin levels increases their likelihood of becoming cancerous. It is widely recognized that pregnancy, breast feeding, and use of oral contraceptives (OCP) all protect against the development of EOC. These effects are probably mediated by causing prolonged periods of anovulation or by suppressing pituitary gonadotropin secretion.

Gwinn et al. (81) described the risk of EOC in women over 55 years of age in relation to pregnancy, breast feeding, and OCP use. They evaluated 436 women between the ages of 20 and 54 years who had histologically confirmed ovarian cancer, and compared them to 3,833 age-matched controls. All three factors were more prevalent and were associated with reduced risk for EOC in the study group. Estimated relative risk for ovarian cancer was 0.5 in the group with a history of OCP use. There was a 0.8% reduction in this risk with each month of OCP use. They also found that a considerable degree of protection was conferred with just a few months of OCP use.

The investigators in the Cancer and Steroid Hormone (CASH) Study group (82) studied 546 women between 20 and 54 years of age with ovarian cancer. There were 4,228 control women for comparison. The relative risk of EOC with OCP use was 0.6. This protection was seen with as little as three to six months of use. Even though the protective effect took five to ten years to become apparent, it lasted up to fifteen years after the pills had been discontinued. There was no correlation between the type of OCP used and the histologic subtype of EOC.

Others have described a 50% reduction in EOC risk with five years of OCP use. This increases to 60–80% with use lasting seven years or more. On the other hand, Whittemore et al. (83) have not found any additional protection conferred by OCP use beyond six years.

The "artificial" suppression of ovulation produced by OCPs may be offered to women who have significantly increased risks of ovarian cancer but who have not yet completed their childbearing. This intervention would appear to be more effective in decreasing EOC death rates than any of the screening techniques which can only test patients after the cancer has already occurred.

PREVENTION OF OVARIAN CANCER: PROPHYLACTIC SURGERY

Because of the poor prognosis of this disease, prophylactic oophorectomy has become an important cancer control strategy for selected women at high genetic risk for ovarian carcinoma. If childbearing is not an issue, prophylactic removal of the uterus, tubes, and ovaries may be offered as a way of preventing the occurrence of cancer in these women.

Tobacman et al. (84) have challenged the efficacy of prophylactic oophorectomy in protecting these women. They state that in spite of such extensive surgery, a patient's risk of developing "ovarian" carcinoma may not be reduced to zero. They described the outcomes of twenty-eight women who underwent prophylactic surgery [total abdominal hysterectomy, bilateral salingo-oophorectomy (TAH.BSO)] because of their positions in sixteen familial cancer pedigrees. Three of these women subsequently (one, five, and eleven years later) developed disseminated intraabdominal carcinomatosis which was histologically indistinguishable from ovarian cancer. All three died of disease. These authors hypothesized that, in cancer-prone families, the tissues susceptible to cancer may involve not only the ovaries but also other coelomic epithelium derivatives, giving rise to primary peritoneal neoplasms. It is for this reason that they suggest that a detailed, meticulous ovarian cancer staging procedure should be an integral part of every prophylactic TAH.BSO performed for familial cancer prevention.

In a similar report, Chen et al. (85) reported the death of a patient due to disseminated intraabdominal carcinomatosis three years after prophylactic oophorectomy for familial ovarian cancer. However, retrospective serial sections on the resected ovaries revealed a small focus of ovarian carcinoma. They also concur with Tobacman's recommendations for meticulous staging surgery whenever a prophylactic TAH.BSO is performed.

Other authors (86–89) have described the outcome of an additional eighteen women who underwent prophylactic surgery for familial ovarian cancer histories. None developed extraovarian carcinomatosis. They concluded that although this can occur after prophylactic oophorectomy in cancer-prone patients, it appears to be a rare occurrence.

The benefit provided by prophylactic removal of the

When to Offer Prophylactic Oophorectomy?

X = level of risk at which to offer prophylactic oophorectomy

Z = risk of death from any cause in 5 years

.62 = risk of death in 5 years once cancer is detected

r = risk of death from prophylactic surgery

$$X = \frac{Z + r}{.62}$$

FIG. 9. Calculations for offering prophylactic oophrectomy.

ovaries may be due to removal of premalignant (e.g., hyperplastic) epithelial ovarian cells. Graham et al. (90) described the presence of foci of hyperplastic epithelium in ovaries removed prophylactically from a woman with a history of familial ovarian cancer. They believed that these foci were premalignant. Fraumeni et al. (91) described similar findings in three women following prophylactic oophorectomies for familial cancer. The ovaries showed excessive proliferative activity and hyperplastic foci of the epithelium. Demopoulos et al. (92) stated that, in a retrospective review of prophylactic oophorectomy cases performed in patients with breast cancer (before the availability of tamoxifen), approximately one-third had ovarian abnormalities (hyperplastic foci, metastases, etc.) in the absence of clinical involvement. Lynch and coworkers (93) stated that the insult that causes ovarian mesothelium to become cancerous can also make peritoneal mesothelium cancerous. This can occur not only in the patients at increased genetic risk for familial ovarian cancer, but also in women without such histories (94). However, both of these occurrences are extremely rare.

Unlike the situations with early stages of cervical and endometrial carcinomas, premalignant lesions for ovarian cancer have not been studied due to lack of availability of precursor tissues. Studying apparently grossly normal ovarian tissue removed at prophylactic surgery may provide some answers in these patients. Despite the reports of intraabdominal carcinomatoses occurring in some women following prophylactic oophorectomy, this intervention may be offered to selected women after they have completed childbearing (Fig. 9). When the ovaries are removed, serial sections should be meticulously examined to identify any microscopic malignant or premalignant foci. Also, the surgery should be performed in the same manner as an ovarian cancer staging operation and include biopsies of all peritoneal surfaces, gutters, diaphragm, etc.

SCREENING FOR OTHER CANCERS

As stated previously, patients with familial cancer pedigrees are at increased risk for developing other cancers such as breast, colon, and endometrium. Therefore, screening for these related cancers should be incorporated into the surveillance plan for these women. Male members in such pedigrees may also have an increased risk (up to 50%) for developing these cancers and should be counseled and screened accordingly.

Breast

At present, one in nine women will develop breast cancer (1). Approximately eighteen percent of women with breast cancer will die in 1992 (1). Some women who are at risk for developing ovarian cancer are also at risk for developing breast cancer. It is evident that early detection significantly improves survival, because patients with small, localized tumors have better survival rates.

Frequent breast self-examinations (BSE) and mammography whenever indicated have been shown to be effective for early detection of this disease; up to 73% of breast cancers are self-discovered (95). Several authors report statistically significant survival advantages in patients whose cancers are detected by BSE when compared to women who do not perform BSE. This has been attributed to the small size and lack of spread of tumors associated with early diagnosis. Though recent surveys (96) have shown that only a small number (35% in one survey) of women perform

TABLE 7. *Proposed screening guidelines for patients at risk for familial cancer*

Test or Procedure	Age (yrs)	Frequency
Sigmoidoscopy	At age 50 and thereafter	Every one to three years based on history
Colonoscopy	At age 40 and thereafter	Every six months
Stool guaiac test	After age 50	Every year
Rectal examination	After age 40	Every year
Papanicolaou smear and pelvic examination	After age 18 and/or sexually active	Every year
Endometrial biopsy	Age 35	Based on advice of physician
Breast self-examination	At age 20 and thereafter	Monthly
Mammography	At age 35 and thereafter	Every six months
Cancer checkup: (examination for cancer of thyroid, ovaries, lymph nodes, oral region, skin)	Age 30	Every year

Modified from American Cancer Society recommendations for early detection of cancer in asymptomatic people.

monthly BSE, this intervention should be offered as an effective, inexpensive, simple technique which has significant benefits.

Mammography was introduced by Soloman et al. (97) in 1913, and has since provided a means to facilitate early detection of breast cancer, thereby improving patient survival (98). Not only have the techniques improved over time, but the radiation dose per exam has markedly decreased to the current level of less than 1rad (99). Thus, a patient would have to undergo 13 annual mammograms to produce a 1% increased risk of developing breast cancer in her lifetime (99).

The recommendations made by the American Cancer Society for universal breast cancer screening can be modified to survey these women. Six-monthly mammograms coupled with monthly BSE can be offered to intensify their surveillance (Table 7).

Colon

Colorectal cancer is the second most common cancer in the US, accounting for 14% of all cancers by site (1). Approximately 13% of women with colorectal cancer will die in 1992 (1). The incidence has been increasing over the last decade due to a combination of environmental, dietary, and genetic causes. Women who are at increased risk for developing ovarian cancer may also be at risk for developing colon cancer.

As with ovarian cancer, a major problem associated with this disease is early detection. At present there are no immunologic or biochemical precursors that provide evidence of a patient's high risk status. Surveillance programs should focus on high-risk groups to improve the cost-effectiveness of screening. Lynch et al. (100) state that, due to the early age of onset and increased predilection for right-sided colonic lesions, routine colon cancer screening after age 50 years with colonoscopy alone is inadequate. They suggest that, from age 20 years onward, all these patients should undergo six-monthly stool guaiac examinations and biennial colonoscopy or proctosigmoidoscopy with barium enema after age 25 years. All polyps should be removed to prevent the occurrence of invasive cancer in these sites.

Endometrium

Women at risk for ovarian cancer may also be at increased risk for developing endometrial cancer. Because of the increased incidence of endometrial cancer in these high risk groups, they should be offered six-monthly bimanual pelvic examinations, coupled with sonography to assess pelvic pathology. Additionally, they should be offered yearly endometrial biopsies to rule out endometrial hyperplasia or other precancerous pathology. Fractional dilatation and curettage (D&C) is indicated when menstrual abnormalities occur, in order to rule out cancer.

Recently, TVS has been utilized for screening these patients. Granberg et al. (101) used endometrial thickness as measured by TVS as an indicator of endometrial abnormality. In 205 postmenopausal women with vaginal bleeding, no endometrial cancer was found on D&C if the endometrium was less than 9 mm in thickness. The mean endometrial thickness was 18.2 mm in women with endometrial cancer, versus 3.4 mm in those with atrophic endometrium. Goldstein et al. (102) studied thirty women with postmenopausal bleeding using TVS prior to obtaining an endometrial tissue biopsy. All eleven patients with endometrial echoes of 5 mm or less had scant or insufficient tissue on biopsy. The seventeen patients with endometrial echoes of 6 mm or more had a variety of pathologic diagnoses, including one case of endometrial cancer. They suggested that further interventions to rule out cancer may be obviated when "pencil-thin" endometrial echoes are found on TVS.

PREVENTION OF RELATED CANCERS WITH PROPHYLACTIC SURGERY

Prophylactic surgical mastectomy with bilateral removal of superficial breast tissue can be offered to familial cancer patients as an alternative approach to the surveillance plan which involves frequent BSEs and physician breast exams; yearly mammograms with aspiration of any suspicious cysts or masses; and cytologic analysis of any nipple discharge. The remaining subcutaneous tissue should undergo six-monthly surveillance, even if prophylactic surgery is chosen.

Women who have unilateral breast cancer are known to have an increased risk of developing the disease in the contralateral breast. This risk may be further compounded if they are members in familial cancer pedigrees. In this circumstance, prophylactic contralateral mastectomy may be considered.

If a woman belongs to a pedigree which puts her at high risk for both breast and ovarian cancer, removal of both sets of organs may be offered. The issue of prophylactic oophorectomy at the time of prophylactic mastectomy is a difficult one to resolve. The obvious advantage is removal of the estrogen hormone which is known to be associated with the occurrence (and spread) of breast cancer. The disadvantages are the known adverse sequelae of estrogen deprivation, including cardiovascular and skeletal compromise. Sometimes, despite a patient's wishes, intensive surveillance for breast cancer may not be an option. Prophylactic bilateral mastectomy may be the only choice for women with severe fibrocystic disease where breast exams and mammography would be useless.

DNA BANKING

DNA analysis for clinical purposes is becoming an important source of genetic information. The long-term stability of DNA permits its banking for performance of tests long after its procurement. This facilitates storage of genetic information on diseased individuals. DNA can be banked from both normal and cancerous tissues, including blood. With the anticipated development of genetic tests over the next few years, banked DNA can be used to identify specific mutations in tumors and to test at-risk family members for the presence of these mutations. When counseling patients with familial cancer, this option may be offered (102). There are several such facilities in the country where blood or tumor tissue can be stored for nominal fees. Banked DNA is the property of the depositor unless otherwise stated. The results of DNA tests are subject to the traditional principles of patient confidentiality that apply to all medical tests.

REGISTRIES

Cancer registries have been established for the purpose of obtaining information about familial cancers. One such registry for familial ovarian cancer is at Roswell Park (103-104). Another is the Hereditary Cancer Institute Registry for all cancers. The purpose is to obtain and record all disease and cancer information on individuals in familial cancer pedigrees. This allows patients to access information to determine their risks for specific cancers. Such registries also create research databases for calculation of genetic and epidemiologic risks. Ideally, all information in such registries should be verified by pathology and autopsy reports (93). This will minimize the chances of disseminating inaccurate and incomplete information for use in making decisions. As with DNA banking, information recorded in these registries is subject to the traditional rules of medical confidentiality.

COUNSELING

Delineation of hereditary cancers requires detailed and extensive pedigree documentation. Ideally, the information obtained should cover at least three to four generations, including maternal and paternal grandparents, aunts, and uncles, with special emphasis on older relatives. It must be kept in mind that in all such pedigrees, male members may either be affected themselves or may transmit the gene to their offspring. Some pedigrees may be quite informative and contain several of the cardinal features that constitute hereditary cancer. In such cases it becomes quite easy to calculate risk status for the proband and/or her relatives. Often, however, such information is sketchy.

All counseling regarding patients' increased risks for ovarian, breast, endometrial, and colorectal cancers in familial cancer syndromes should be based on the knowledge of the lifetime general population risks for developing these diseases. These are 1.2%, 11%, 8%, and 5%, respectively. Examples of such calculations are provided in Figure 10.

Delayed age of onset of certain cancers may obscure the fact that multiple family members are at increased risk for the development of these particular cancers. Empiric figures have been derived for individuals with a family history of ovarian cancer (86,103). A woman whose mother and sister have had ovarian cancer has a 50% chance of developing the disease. If her mother and daughter have the disease, she is considered an obligate gene carrier, and her risk now increases to 100%. If the affected members are one first-degree relative and one second-degree relative, her chance of developing ovarian cancer is approximately 25%. A woman with one affected first-degree relative has only

	Has disease	Does not have disease
General population		
Positive test		
Prior probability	.01	.99
Conditional probability	.90	.20
Joint probability	.009	.198
Posterior probability	.009 / (.009 + .198) = 1/23 = 0.04	.198 / (.009 + .198) = .96
Negative test		
Prior probability	.01	.99
Conditional probability	.10	.80
Joint probability	.001	.792
Posterior probability	.001 / (.001 + .792) = 1/793 = .0013	.792 / (.001 + .792 + .999)
AD, positive test		
Prior probability	.50	.50
Conditional probability	.90	.20
Joint probability	.45	.10
Posterior probability	.45 / (.10 + .45) = 0.82	.10 / (.10 + .45) = 0.18

FIG. 10. Risk calculations using Bayes Theorem. AD, autosomal dominant.

a 10% chance of developing the disease. If she has one affected second-degree relative, her risk of developing ovarian cancer may approach that of the general population (105).

Houlston et al. (108) studied 462 pedigrees of unaffected women who had one or more close relatives with ovarian cancer. The overall risk of developing ovarian cancer in these individuals was increased four and a half times over that of the general population. The relative risk was highest (7.4) for relatives of women whose cancers had developed before the age of 55. It was 3.7 in those women whose relatives had developed ovarian cancer later in life. If two or more first-degree relatives were affected, the relative risk was 39.1.

Patients with such histories and risks would benefit most from a surveillance or management protocol. The protocol should include a detailed and accurate history, verification of all cancer diagnoses, preferably by pathology or autopsy reports, and extension of the pedigree to include information on at least three to four generations. The patient and her family members should be educated regarding their risks for developing cancer. Figure 10 shows such risk calculations based on the results of a hypothetical (and as yet unavailable) screening test in combination with a patient's own history. If she is from the general population and has a positive screening test result, her chance of developing ovarian cancer is low (0.04%). On the other hand, if she is a member of a familial cancer pedigree, her risk of having ovarian cancer with a positive screening test result would be very high (82%).

Once such risk figures have been calculated, if the patient desires children, she may be offered OCPs. Alternatively, she may elect to complete her childbearing earlier than originally planned. If childbearing is not an issue, she can be offered prophylactic surgery, e.g., TAH.BSO with the caveat that removal of these organs does not guarantee freedom from future cancers. When prophylactic surgery is being offered to a woman based on her status in a familial cancer pedigree, all risk calculations should be based only on histologically verified cancers in that pedigree. Figure 9 shows a suggested equation to calculate the level of risk at which prophylactic oophorectomy can be offered to a woman with familial ovarian cancer.

A woman at risk must be counseled that each decision has its associated burdens. If she chooses surveillance, she will have to undergo frequent exams, tests, and occasional biopsies, while living with the associated fear and worry. If surgery is chosen, she will still require serial surveillance. She may also need to address the financial and emotional costs of reconstructive surgery. If surgery is declined, she can be offered serial screening for ovarian cancer (sonography, serum CA-125 levels, pelvic exams), though these interventions are controversial and have not been shown to be beneficial in the screening of asymptomatic women for the detection of ovarian cancer.

If there is evidence for a genetic predisposition to breast cancer in her family, prophylactic bilateral mastectomies can be offered. If surgery is declined, breast cancer screening (serial BSE and mammography) can be offered. Following prophylactic surgery, similar screening may be offered to evaluate the residual subcutaneous tissues.

If she is at risk for colon cancer, she can be screened with serial rectal and guaiac exams, and colonoscopy. The guidelines provided by the American Cancer Society for screening asymptomatic individuals could be incorporated for such screening (see Table 7). When possible, tissue and DNA banking should be offered for future analysis. The option of entering her pedigree into a cancer registry for future data collection should also be provided.

When a patient or her relative are being evaluated and counseled, attention must be paid to issues of confidentiality. She should be guaranteed that screening results will not be released to others, such as insurance and mortgage companies, or to employers without her consent. All information about risks for cancer should be made available only to the patient herself. Provision of this information to others such as relatives, doctors, and friends can only be done with her permission and knowledge. If conflicts arise where knowledge of increased cancer risks are identified in individuals otherwise unknown to the counselor, the patient's rights of confidentiality must override all other concerns.

REFERENCES

1. Boring CC, Squires TS, Tong T. Cancer Statistics, 1992. *Ca-A Journal for Clinicians,* 1992;42,19–38.
2. Piver S, Child M. Familial cancer in the general population. *Cancer* 1977;40:1674–9.
3. Lynch HT, Harris RE, Guirgis HA, et al. Familial association of breast/ovarian carcinoma. *Cancer* 1978;41:1543–9.
4. Office of Population Census Survey [OPCS] Monitor; 1981. *Deaths by Cause;* DH281/1.
5. Westhoff C, Randall MC. Ovarian cancer screening: potential effect on mortality. *Am J Obstet Gynecol* 1991;165–502.
6. Andolf E, Svalenius E, Astedt B. Ultrasonography for early detection of ovarian carcinoma. *Br J Obstet Gynecol.* 1986;93:1286–9.
7. Andolf E, Jorgensen C. A prospective comparison of clinical ultrasound and operative examination of the female pelvis. *J Ultrasound Med* 1988;7:617.
8. Tessler FN, Schiller VL, Perella RR, et al. Transabdominal versus endovaginal pelvic sonography: prospective study. *Radiology* 1989;170:553.
9. Frederick JL, Paulson RJ, Sauer MV. Routine use of vaginal ultra sonography in the preoperative evaluation of gynecologic patient. *J Reprod Med* 1991;36(11):779–782.
10. Campbell S, Bhan V, Royston P, et al. Transabdominal ultrasound screening for early ovarian cancer. *Br Med J* 1989;299:1363–7.
11. Bourne TH, Whitehead MI, Campbells, Royston P, Bhan V, Collins WP. Ultrasound screening for familial ovarian cancer. *Gynecol Oncol* 1991;43:92–7.
12. Granberg S, Wikland M. A comparison between ultrasound and gynecologic examination for detection of enlarged ovaries in a group of women at risk for ovarian carcinoma. *J Ultrasound Med* 1988;7:59.
13. Van Nagell JR, Higgins RV, Donaldson ES, et al. Transvaginal sonography as a screening method for ovarian cancer. *Cancer* 1990;65:573–577.
14. Kawai M, Kano T, Kikkawa F, Macda O, Oguchi H, Tomoda Y. Transvaginal Doppler ultrasound with color flow imaging in the diagnosis of ovarian cancer. *Obstet Gynecol* 1992;79:163–7.
15. Weiner Z, Thaler I, Beck D, Rottem S, Duetsch M, Brandes JM. Differentiating malignant from benign ovarian tumors with transvaginal color flow imaging. *Obstet Gynecol* 1992;79:159–62.
16. Bourne T, Campbell S, Steer C, Whitehead MI, Collins WP. Transvaginal color flow imaging: a possible new screening technique for ovarian cancer. *BMJ* 1989;299:1367–70.
17. Bast RC, Klug TL, St. John E, et al. A radioimmunoassay using a monoclonal antibody to monitor the course of epithelial ovarian cancer. *N Engl J Med* 1983;309:883–7.
18. Kabawat SE, Bast RC, Bhan AK, et al. Tissue distribution of a coelomic epithelium related antigen recognized by the monoclonal antibody OC125. *Int J Gynecol Pathol* 1983;2:275.
19. Bast RC, Feeney M, Lazarus H, et al. Reactivity of a monoclonal antibody with ovarian carcinoma. *J Clin Invest* 1981;68:1331.
20. Meier W, Stieber P, Eiermann W, Schneider A, Fathen-Maghadam A, Hepp H. Serum levels of CA125 and histological findings at second look laparotomy in ovarian carcinoma.
21. Zurawski VR, Sjovall K, Schoenfield DA, Broderick SF, Hall P, Bast RC, Eklund G, Mattson B, Connor RJ, Prorok PC, Knapp RC, Einhorn N. Prospective evaluation of serum CA125 levels in a normal population; Phase I: The specificities of single and serial determinations in testing for ovarian cancer. *Gynecol Oncol* 1990;36:292–305.
22. Khoo SK, Hurst R, Webb MJ, Dickie GJ, Kearsley JH, Mackay EV. Predictive value of serial CA125 antigen levels in ovarian cancer evaluated by second look laparotomy. 1986;765–771.
23. Pittaway DE, Fayez JA, The use of CA125 in the diagnosis and management of endometriosis. *Fertil Steril* 1986;46:790.
24. Pittaway DE, Fayez JA. Serum CA125 antigen levels increase during menses. *Am J Obstet Gynecol* 1987;156:75.
25. Niloff JM, Knapp RC, Schaetzl E, et al. CA125 antigen levels in obstetric and gynecologic patients. *Obstet Gynecol* 1984;64:703.
26. Vasilev SA, Schlaerth JB, Campeau J, et al. Serum CA125 levels in preoperative evaluation of pelvic mass. *Obstet Gynecol* 1988;71:751.
27. Renbal A, Encabo G, Capdevila JA, et al. CA125 serum levels in patients with liver disease. *Med Clin* (Barcelona) 1984;82:560.
28. Einborn N, Bast RC, Knapp RC, et al. Preoperative evaluation of serum CA125 levels in patients with primary epithelial ovarian cancer. *Obstet Gynecol* 1986;67:414.
29. Schwartz PE. The role of CA125 in the evaluation of palpable or enlarged postmenopausal ovaries. *Am J Obstet Gynecol* 1988;158:1072.
30. Malkasian GD, Knapp RC, Lavin PT, et al. Preoperative evaluation of serum CA125 levels in premenopausal and postmenopausal patients with pelvic masses: discrimination of benign from malignant disease. *Am J Obstet Gynecol* 1988;159:341.
31. Finkler NJ, Benacerraf B, Lavin PT, et al. Comparison of serum CA125, clinical impression and ultrasound in the preoperative evaluation of ovarian masses. *Obstet Gynecol* 1988;72:659.
32. Creasman WT, DiSaia PJ. Screening in ovarian cancer. *Am J Obstet Gynecol* 1991;165:7–10.
33. American College of Obstetrics/Gynecology Report of a task force on routine cancer screening. Washington, DC: *Am Coll Obstet Gynecol;* April 1989; ACOG Committee Opinion #68.
34. Fearon ER, Hamilton SR, Vogelstein B. Clonal analysis of human colorectal tumors. *Science* 1987;238:193–197.
35. Bishop JM. Cellular oncogenes and retroviruses. *Annu Rev Biochem* 1983;47:35–88.
36. Krontiris TG, Cooper GM. Transforming activity of human tumor DNAs. *Proc Natl Acad Sci USA* 1981;78:1181–1184.
37. Sparkes RS, Murphree AL, Lingua RW, et al. Gene for hereditary retinoblastoma assigned to human chromosome 13 by linkage to esterease D. *Science* 1983;219:971–975.
38. Knudson AG Jr. Mutation and cancer: Statistical study of retinoblastoma. *Proc Natl Acad Sci USA* 1971;68:820–823.
39. Cavenee W, Dryja T, Philips R, et al. Chromosome mecha-

nisms revealing recessive alleles in retinoblastoma. *Nature* 1983;305:779.
40. Goodrich DW, Lee WH. The molecular genetics of retinoblastoma. *Cancer Surv* 1990;9:529–554.
41. Leach RJ, Magewu AN, Buckley JD, et al. Preferential retention of paternal alleles in human retinoblastoma: evidence for genomic imprinting. *Cell Growth & Differentiation* 1990;1: 401–406.
42. Lundberg C, Skoog L, Cavenee WK, Nordenskjold M. Loss of heterozygosity in human ductal breast tumors indicates a recessive mutation on chromosome 13. *Proc Natl Acad Sci USA* 1987;84:2372–2376.
43. Naylor SL, Johnson BE, Minna JD, Sakaguchi AY. Loss of heterozygosity of chromosome 3p markers in small-cell lung cancer. *Nature* 1987;329:451–454.
44. Okamoto M, Sasaki M, Sugio K, et al. Loss of constitutional heterozygosity in colon carcinoma from patients with familial polyposis coli. *Nature* 1988;331:273.
45. Kinzler KW, Nilbert MC, Su L-K, et al. Identification of the *FAP* locus genes from chromosome 5q21. *Science* 1991;253: 661–665.
46. Malkin D, Li FP, Strong LC, et al. Germ line p53 mutations in a familial syndrome of breast cancer, sarcomas, and other neoplasms. *Science* 1990;250:1233–1238.
47. Call KM, Glaser T, Ito CY, et al. Isolation and characterization of a zinc finger polypeptide gene at the human chromosome 11 Wilms' tumor locus. *Cell* 1990;60:509–520.
48. Wallace M, Marchuk DA, Andersen LB, et al. Type 1 neurofibromatosis: identification of a large transcript disrupted in three NF1 patients. *Science* 1990;249:181–186.
49. Sandberg AA. *The chromosomes in human cancer and leukemia*. 2nd ed. New York: Elsevier, 1990.
50. Atkin NB. Prognostic value of cytogenetic studies of tumors of the female genital tract. *Adv Clin Cytol* 1984;2:103–121.
51. Smith A, van Haaften-Day C, Russell P. Sequential cytogenetic studies in an ovarian cancer cell line. *Cancer Genet Cytogenet* 1989;38:13–24.
52. Whang-Peng J, Knutsen T, Douglass EC, et al. Cytogenetic studies in ovarian cancer. *Cancer Genet Cytogenet* 1984;11: 91–106.
53. Atkin NB. Chromosome 1 aberrations in cancer. *Cancer Genet Cytogenet* 1986;21:279–285.
54. Trent JM, Salmon SE. Karyotypic analysis of human ovarian carcinoma cells cloned in short-term agar culture. *Cancer Genet Cytogenet* 1981;41:867–874.
55. Wake N, Hreshchyshyn MM, Piver SM, Matsui S, Sandberg AA. Specific cytogenetic changes in ovarian cancer involving chromosomes 6 and 14. *Cancer Res* 1980;40:4512–4518.
56. Lee JH, Kavanagh JJ, Wharton JT, Wildrick DM, Blick M. Allele loss at the c-Ha-ras 1 locus in human ovarian cancer. *Cancer Res* 1989;49:1220–1222.
57. Lee JH, Kavanagh JJ, Wildrick DM, Wharton JT, Blick M. Frequent loss of heterozygosity on chromosomes 6q, 11, and 17 in human ovarian carcinomas. *Cancer Res* 1990;50:2724–2728.
58. Eccles DM, Cranston G, Steel CM, Nakamura Y, Leonard RC. Allele losses on chromosome 17 in human epithelial ovarian carcinoma. *Oncogene* 1990;5:1599–1601.
59. Boltz EM, Harnett P, Leary J, Houghton R, Kefford RF, Friedlander ML. Demonstration of somatic rearrangements and genomic heterogeneity in human ovarian cancer by DNA fingerprinting. *Br J Cancer* 1990;62:23–27.
60. Solomon DJ, Godolphin W, Jones LA, et al. Studies of the HER-2/*neu* proto-oncogene in human breast and ovarian cancer. *Science* 1989;244:707–712.
61. Boltz EM, Kefford RF, Leary JA, Houghton CR, Friedlander ML. Amplification of c-ras-Ki oncogene in human ovarian tumours. *Int J Cancer* 1989;43:428–430.
62. Lichtenstein A, Berenson J, Gera JF, Waldburger K, Martinez-Maza O, Berek JS. Resistance of human ovarian cancer cells to tumor necrosis factor and lymphokine-activated killer cells: correlation with expression of HER-2/*neu* oncogenes. *Cancer Res* 1990;50:7364–7370.
63. Marth C, Müller-Holzner E, Greiter E, et al. Gamma-interferon reduces expression of the proto-oncogene c-*erb*B-2 in human ovarian carcinoma cells. *Cancer Res* 1990;50:7037–7041.
64. Fraumeni JF. *J Natl Cancer Inst* 1936;42:455.
65. Lynch HT. *Hereditary factors in carcinoma, recent results in cancer research*. New York: Springer-Verlag; 1967:186.
66. Lynch HT, Krush AJ. Hereditary and breast cancer: Implications for cancer detection. *Med Times* 1966;94:599.
67. Schoenberg BS, Greenberg RA, Eisenberg H. Occurrence of certain multiple primary cancers in females. *J Natl Cancer Inst* 1969;43:15–32.
68. Waterhouse JA, Prior MP. Letter: Breast cancer in young women. *Br Med J* 1975;3:434.
69. Ferrell RE, Anderson DE, Chidambaram A, Marino TR, Badzioch M. A genetic linkage study of familial breast-ovarian cancer. *Cancer Genet Cytogenet* 1989;38:241–248.
70. Lynch HT, Schuelke GS, Lynch JF. Biomarker studies in hereditary ovarian cancer. *Cancer Detec Prev* 1985;8:129–134.
71. Christian CD, McLoughlin TG, Cathcart ES, Eisenberg MM. Peutz-Jeghers syndrome associated with functioning ovarian tumor. *JAMA* 1964;190:935–938.
72. Gardiello FM, Welsh SB, Hamilton SR, et al. Increased risk of cancer in Peutz-Jeghers syndrome. *N Engl J Med* 1987;316: 1511–1514.
73. Gorlin RJ. Nevoid basal-cell carcinoma syndrome. *Medicine Baltimore* 1987;66:98–113.
74. Teter J, Boczkowski K. Occurrence of tumors in dysgenetic gonads. *Cancer* 1967;20:1301–1310.
75. Scully RE. Gonadoblastoma. *Cancer* 1970;25:1340–1356.
76. Manuel M, Katayama KP, Jones HW Jr. The age of occurrence of gonadal tumors in intersex patients with a Y chromosome. *Am J Obstet Gynecol* 1976;124:293–300.
77. Fathalla MF. Incessant ovulation—a factor in ovarian neoplasia? (Letter). *Lancet* 1971;2:163.
78. Fathalla MF. Factors in the causation and incidence of ovarian cancer. *Obstet Gynecol Surv* 1972;27:751–768.
79. Gardner WU. Tumorgenesis in transplanted irradiated and non-irradiated ovaries. *J Natl Cancer Inst* 1961;26:829–54.
80. Stadel BV. The etiology and prevention of ovarian cancer. *Am J Obstet Gynecol* 1975;123:772–774.
81. Gwinn ML, Lee NC, Rhodes PH, Layde PM, Rubing L. Pregnancy, breast feeding and oral contraceptives and the risk of epithelial ovarian cancer. *J Clin Endocrinol Metab* 1990;43:559.
82. The reduction in risk of ovarian cancer associated with oral contraceptive use. The Cancer and Steroid Hormone Study of the Centers for Disease Control and the National Institutes of Child Health and Human Development. *N Engl J Med* 1987; 316:650–655.
83. Whittemore AS, Harris R, Itmyre J and the Collaborative Ovarian Cancer Group. Characteristics relating to ovarian cancer risk. Collaborative analysis of twelve US Case-Control Studies IV. *The pathogenesis of epithelial ovarian cancer*, 1992.
84. Tobacman JK, Greene MH, Tucker MA, Costa J, Kase R, Fraumeni JR. Intra-abdominal carcinomatosis after prophylactic oophorectomy in ovarian cancer prone families. *Lancet* 1982;2:795–7.
85. Chen KTK, Schooley JL, Flam MS. Peritoneal carcinomatosis after prophylactic oophorectomy in familial ovarian cancer syndrome. *Obstet Gynecol* 1985;66:93S–94S.
86. Lewis ACL, Clare Davison BC. Familial ovarian cancer. *Lancet* 1969;2:235–7.
87. Lynch MT, Guinis MA, Albert S. Familial association of carcinoma of the breast and ovary. *Surg Gynecol Obstet* 1974;138: 717.
88. Skinner JL, Oats JJN, Segmonds EM. Familial ovarian carcinoma. *J R Coll Gen Pract* 1977;27:167.
89. Piver MS, Barton JJ, Sawyer D. Familial ovarian carcinoma—increasing in frequency? *Obstet Gynecol* 1982;60:397.
90. Graham J, Graham R. Ovarian cancer and asbestos. *Environ Res* 1967;1:115.
91. Fraumeni JF, Grunday GW, Creagan ET, et al. Six families prone to ovarian cancer. *Cancer* 1975;36:364.
92. Demopoulos R: *Personal communication*, 1992.
93. Lynch HT, Kullander S. In: *Cancer genetics in women*. Vol. I. Boca Raton: CRC Press; 1987:9–28.

94. Foyle A, Al-Jabi M, McCaughey WT. Papillary peritoneal tumors in women. *Am J Surg Pathol* 1981;5:241.
95. Nemoto T, Natarajan N, Smart CR, et al. Patterns of breast cancer detection in the United States. *J Surg Oncol* 1982;21:183.
96. Gallup Organization Inc, Princeton: [Survey] 1977.
97. Soloman A. Biethage Zur Pathologie und Klinik der Mammakarzinome. *Arch Klin Chir* 1913;101:573.
98. De Luca JT. A statistical comparison study of patients undergoing breast biopsy at a community hospital over a 16 year period. *J Radiol* 1974;112:315.
99. Dodd JD. Mammography—State of the art. *Cancer* 1984;53:652.
100. Lynch HT, Lynch JF. Lynch syndrome II. In: Lynch HT, Kullander S, eds. *Cancer genetics in women*. Boca Raton: CRC Press; 1987.
101. Granberg S, Wikland M, Karlsson B, Norstrom A, Friberg LG. Endometrial thickness as measured by endovaginal ultrasonography for identifying endometrial abnormality. *Am J Obstet Gynecol* 1991;164:47–52.
102. Ad Hoc Committee on DNA Technology. *DNA Banking and DNA analysis: points to consider*. American Society of Human Genetics: 1988.
103. Piver MS, Metlin CJ, Tsukada Y, et al. Familial ovarian cancer registry. *Obstet Gynecol* 1984;64:195.
104. Piver MS, Mettlin C, Tsukada Y, Nasca P, McPhee ME. Familial ovarian cancer registry, 1985 report. In: Lynch HT, Kullander S., eds. *Cancer Genetics in Women*, vol ii. Boca Raton: CRC Press; 1987.
105. Lynch HT: *Personal communication*, 1991.
106. Sassone AM, Timor-Tritsch IE, Artner A, Westhoff C, Warren WB. Transvaginal sonographic characterization of ovarian disease: evaluation of a new scoring system to predict ovarian malignancy. *Obstet Gynecol* 1991;78:70–76.
107. Andolf E, Jorgensen C, Astedt B. Ultrasound examination for detection of ovarian carcinoma in risk groups. *Obstet Gynecol* 1990;75:106–109.
108. Houlston RS, Collins A, Slack J, Campbell S, Collins WP, Whitehead MI, Morton NE. Genetic epidemiology of ovarian cancer: segregation analysis. *Ann Hum Genet* 1991;55:291–299.

CHAPTER 7

Prognostic Factors in Ovarian Cancer

Thomas B. Hakes

The topic of this chapter is prognostic factors that predict survival in epithelial ovarian cancer. Survival was chosen over other endpoints because it is the most frequent and unambiguous in the literature. Endpoints such as relapse-free survival (1), response to individual therapies (2), odds of achieving a negative second-look laparotomy (3), and likelihood of maintaining a complete remission (4), have been examined but lack either precision or a voluminous literature.

Our discussion is also limited to epithelial carcinomas, which comprise the vast majority of ovarian cancers. Histologies such as borderline malignancies, granulosa cell tumors, and germ cell tumors are discussed elsewhere in this book.

The literature addressing prognostic factors in epithelial ovarian cancer has a number of recurring problems, including poor definition or measurement, missing data, restricted groups, differing endpoints, mixed pretreatment and post-treatment information, and univariate analyses.

Prognostic factors are often loosely defined, difficult to measure, and reproduce poorly. Residual disease is an example of this. The very measurement of residual disease (e.g., diameter of largest residual mass) speaks to the problem. Though total volume of residual cancer may be a more important variable, it is too difficult to measure. We therefore make an approximation, classifying someone with a single 1.0 cm residual mass in the same group as someone with 50 such masses. Further, once this approximation is made, there is no agreement on standard measures. Among the papers reviewed in this chapter are comparisons using 0.5 cm, 1 cm, 2 cm, 3 cm, 5 cm, and 9 cm as significant break points for residual disease as well as categories of miliary, studding, some, none, measurable, nonmeasurable, large, and small.

Missing factors are common, especially in retrospective analyses. Often missing are major clinical variables such as amount of residual disease or performance status, both of which are difficult to define in retrospect. Pathologic factors such as histology and grade are not usually missing because they are easier to identify from retrospective chart or slide review.

Restricted study groups give a slanted view about the relative importance of prognostic factors. Studies restricted, for example, to stage I/II disease (5) or stage III/IV with residual disease of 3.0 cm or more (1) find residual disease to be a nonsignificant factor. In these examples, however, residual disease is uniform (i.e., absent in stage I/II and uniformly large in the second example).

Different endpoints may emphasize different prognostic factors. Grade is usually of low significance in predicting survival in stage III/IV (1,6) disease, but may be of major importance in predicting relapse after a negative second-look laparotomy (4).

Pretreatment and post-treatment factors are sometimes mixed. Ideal prognostic factors are pretreatment variables that permit prospective selection of appropriate treatment or stratification of patients based on risk. Examples of post-treatment variables are rate of fall of CA-125 (7) and degree of chemotherapy-induced myelosuppression (6).

Univariate analyses may generate hypotheses but cannot identify independent prognostic factors. For example, grade, S-phase fraction, hormone positivity, and age are interrelated factors and, according to some analyses, are predictors of survival. Which of these factors are more important? Multivariate analysis is the only way to answer this question. Once promising factors are identified in univariate analyses, they must be placed in perspective with other known factors by multivariate analysis.

Prediction of survival in epithelial ovarian cancer re-

T. B. Hakes: Department of Medicine, Memorial Sloan-Kettering Cancer Center, New York, NY 10021

mains a controversial subject, and some reasons for this controversy have been discussed. However, review of a large number of multivariate analyses suggests that the most important traditional factors in predicting survival are stage, residual disease, grade, and performance status, overshadowing other variables such as histology, mitoses, morphometrics, initial volume of disease, age, ascites, abdominal cytology, type of surgery, and others. Ploidy and DNA index stand out as important predictors among the newer variables, which also include S-phase fraction, estrogen receptor, progesterone receptor, androgen receptor, CA-125, HER-2/*neu* proto-oncogene, P-glycoprotein, clonogenic growth, and others which are appearing at an accelerating pace. With such a variety of traditional factors, their haphazard measurement and inclusion, along with the rapid appearance of new factors, it is not surprising that the relative importance of these factors is controversial.

STAGE AND ASSOCIATED FACTORS

Staging is the formal system of prognostic factors agreed upon for ovarian cancer. While it is a powerful tool, it is far from perfect, as evidenced by the wide range of additional factors discussed in this chapter. Staging is covered in detail in Chapter 10 in this book. However, several points deserve emphasis here.

The International Federation of Gynecology and Obstetrics (FIGO) recently modified the staging system (8,9) to include stage I patients with tumor capsule rupture or surface excrescences (penetration) under stage Ic and to recognize the importance of tumor bulk by categorizing stage III according to metastatic tumor size (i.e., IIIa, microscopic; IIIb tumor, 2.0 cm or smaller diameter; and stage IIIc tumor, greater than 2.0 cm diameter and/or presence of regional nodes). The changes regarding tumor size have some justification because residual cancer is perhaps the most powerful prognostic factor in ovarian cancer, as discussed later in this chapter. One small study found a close relationship between original cancer volume and both survival and residual disease after laparotomy (10), though others have found no relationship between original cancer volume and survival (11,12).

The changes regarding stage I disease seem less justified. Though some have suggested that capsule rupture and penetration are important predictors of survival (13,14), there are many more, including the FIGO annual report of treatment that suggests the far greater importance of grade (5,9,15,16,17).

Understaging of ovarian cancer is common, especially in stages I and II (18,19,20). In a systematic restaging of one hundred putative stage Ia–IIb patients, the Ovarian Study Group (19) found 31% to have been understaged, with three-quarters of these being reclassified as stage III. Reviewing 291 ovarian cancer operations in a variety of settings and by a variety of surgical specialists, McGowan, et al. (20) found that only 28% had received proper intraoperative evaluations and correct recording of stage. In retrospective study, the investigators were able to assign a stage to only 54%. Many older reviews, especially radiation series, have large numbers of stage I and II patients (16). It is not clear whether this represents referral bias (these stages are more suitable for radiation) or understaging.

Despite technical problems, stage is a powerful prognostic factor. Especially important is the division between stages I/II and III/IV (1,10,11,21–24). Also, prognostic factors vary by stage. Residual disease is an important prognostic factor in stages III/IV, where it is usually present, but it is not significant in stage I where, in its absence, grade assumes primary importance (17).

HISTOLOGY

Ovarian epithelium remains a pluripotent tissue, and the multiple histologic subtypes of epithelial ovarian cancers mirror the epithelium of many other portions of the genital tract. Serous histology is most common, followed by mucinous and endometrioid, with lesser numbers of clear cell, mixed, and undifferentiated cancers. It has been accepted for many years that histology impacts survival and survival decreases in the following histologic order: mucinous, endometrioid, serous, clear cell, and undifferentiated cancers (25,26). More recently, grade appears to be the more important variable (26,27). Favorable survival among mucinous cancer patients is due to their usually low-grade tumors and the poor survival among patients with serous cancers is due to their usually high-grade cancers. For example, Decker et al. (28) found 75% of mucinous ovarian cancers, but only 28% of serous cancers, to have low grade. However, this traditional view of prognosis has been challenged recently by several large studies of stage III/IV cancers which suggest that mucinous histology is a significant adverse risk factor (1,29).

Histologic classification of ovarian cancers is often difficult and variable (28,30,31). Multiple cell types are frequently present in a single specimen, as are large numbers of undifferentiated cells (28), leading to both interobserver and intraobserver variability in classifying ovarian cancers (30).

Most large series contain about 50–60% serous cancers, 10–20% endometrioid, and 5–15% mucinous, with variable numbers of other histologies. If a series contains stage I patients, there will be relatively more mucinous tumors, but if the series is limited to stages III/IV, there will be more clear cell and undifferentiated cancers. If histologic criteria are strictly applied and large numbers of a primary cell type are required to make a specific diagnosis, then the series will have an increased number of undifferentiated cancers (10,32,33). "Undifferentiated" in this context indicates indeterminate histology that is not poorly differentiated or of high grade.

Grade and Other Histologic Factors

Grade often appears to be a significant prognostic variable, especially in early stage ovarian cancer. In 1926, Broders (34), suggested a system for cytologic grading of squamous carcinomas based on percentage of undifferentiated cells, 0–25% being grade 1; 26–50%, grade 2; 51–75%, grade 3; and 76–100%, grade 4 (34). Numerous other grading systems have since been proposed. Among papers cited in this review are systems by Broders (34), Czernobilsky (35), Day et al. (27), Petterson et al. for the International Federation of Gynecology and Obstetrics (FIGO) (9), Ozols et al. (33), Russel (36), Sorbe et al. (37), Seroy et al. for the World Health Organization (WHO) (38), and others unspecified. There seem to be two major variations of grade: (a) a cytologic grade based on Broders's original four-grade system using percentages of undifferentiated cells, and (b) a pattern grade somewhat similar to the FIGO system for endometrial cancers (9), which stresses relative percentages of papillary/glandular areas versus solid areas. These systems are nicely summarized, photographed, and compared by Ozols et al. (33). The authors describe cytologic grade 1 as 0–25% undifferentiated cells with minimal malignant cytologic characteristics and few mitoses; they list grade 4 as 75–100% undifferentiated cells with a high degree of cytologic anaplasia and numerous mitoses. Conversely, they describe pattern grade 1 as a tumor composed wholly of papillary structures, while grade 3 is a tumor composed of solid sheets of malignant cells (Jacobs et al. (39) also provide useful descriptions and photographs of the pattern system.). Ozols et al. (33), while preferring cytologic grade, note a close correlation between the two systems. In their analysis, pattern grade 1 included mainly cytologic grade 1 and 2 cancers; pattern grade 2 contained cytologic grade 2, 3, and 4; and pattern grade 3 contained only cytologic grade 3 and 4 cancers. Swenerton et al. (16) describe a system which is a hybrid between the cytologic and pattern systems. Several authors (17,21,40) find a much stronger correlation between survival and grade among serous cancer patients than among those with mucinous, endometrioid, or clear cell cancers. To compound the problems of multiple grading systems and variable importance by histologic type is substantial interobserver and intraobserver variability in assigning grade (30,31).

Despite these problems, grade often appears to be a significant prognostic factor in multivariate analyses; low-grade cancers are associated with longer survival than high-grade cancers. Grade is the primary prognostic factor in most series of stage I/II ovarian cancers (5,16,17) but is of less or no significance in stage III/IV cancers (1,6,10,11,16,29,41,42,43). However, in stage III/IV patients who achieve a complete pathologic response, grade may be a significant factor in predicting relapse (4).

Numerous other histologic factors are claimed to have prognostic significance, including the ratio of lymphocytes to plasma cells (44,45), frequency of mitoses or mitotic activity index (23,46,47,48), mean nuclear area (23), volume percentage epithelium (23,49), and morphometric grade (23,48). In a number of small studies, a strong case is made for these factors. However, these determinations are time-consuming and complicated. Because we cannot agree on methodology to consistently reproduce something as simple as grade, it is doubtful that more complicated systems will play a meaningful role. These methods will likely be displaced by flow cytometry or other automated measurements.

RESIDUAL DISEASE

Diameter of the largest residual mass after initial laparotomy, more commonly referred to as "residual disease," is consistently one of the most important prognostic factors for survival in advanced ovarian cancer and virtually the only one the physician can modify. The power of this factor is manifest, despite the gross imprecision of its measurement. Patients are classified into groups by estimating the diameter of the largest remaining tumor mass on closing. Thus, as previously mentioned, a patient with a single 1.0 cm diameter mass is classed along with a patient with 50 such masses. Volume of tumor present on opening at the initial laparotomy has been examined and does not seem as important as residual disease, though the two are generally related (10,11,23,50). A small study by Redman et al. (10) examined the prognostic significance of the largest and total mass (volume in cc^3 of all the original tumor masses) on opening, as well as the largest and total residual mass on closing. They found total residual mass to have the most pronounced effect on survival and a strong correlation between total residual mass and the other three variables: largest original mass, total original mass, and largest residual mass.

Griffiths (51) was among the first to suggest that diameter of the largest residual mass was an important determinant of survival in ovarian cancer. In a univariate analysis, he demonstrated median survivals of 39 months for 0 cm residual, 29 months for 0–1.5 cm residual, 18 months for 0.6–1.5 cm residual, and 11 months for residual mass greater than 1.5 cm diameter. He also appropriately continued with a multivariate analysis, including an assortment of other clinical variables, and demonstrated (in order of importance) that high grade, clear cell histology, and large residual were adverse prognostic factors for survival. Most analyses since that time have shown residual disease to be an important determinant of survival in advanced ovarian cancer, usually the single most important variable.

It has also been argued that the important factor is not the residual disease itself but rather the biologic nature of the tumor that results in small residual disease or permits debulking to take place. Perhaps some cancers are less invasive of surrounding tissues, thus permitting debulking, while other cancers invade tissues and thwart debulking. It is this "invasive" factor which is of importance in determining outcome. It does not seem likely that this question will be answered soon, because most physicians consider elimination of all cancer cells necessary for cure of ovarian cancer.

AGE

Median age at diagnosis of ovarian carcinoma is 52 to 53 years. Age greater than 50 years has variously been reported to be: an adverse risk factor in multivariate analysis (1,12,21,22,29,41,43,52); an adverse factor in univariate analysis but of no significance in multivariate analysis (16); a factor of no significance (5,6,10,11,42,53), or (rarely) a favorable prognostic factor (54). Stage increases with age, there typically being five to twelve years between the mean ages for stage I and stage IV disease in the various histologic subtypes of ovarian cancer (9). Patients under 40 years of age have an increased incidence of good prognosis borderline (9) and poor prognosis small cell (55) ovarian cancers.

PERFORMANCE STATUS

Performance status, as measured by the Karnofsky scale (56) or the Eastern Cooperative Oncology Group (ECOG) scale (57), is a strong prognostic factor in many analyses (1,11,16,41,42,53,54), but is commonly missing in many others (5,6,7,12,13,17,21,22,23,24,43, 48,51,58). Performance status and age are the only host factors included in most studies. The remaining factors are tumor- or treatment-related. In several studies, performance status is a primary predictor of survival (1,11,42,53), with values below 60 or 70 (Karnofsky scale) being strongly adverse to survival.

ASCITES

The presence of ascites or positive peritoneal cytology is included in many analyses of prognostic factors (1,7,11,16,17,41,42,48,50,53). Some studies find it an adverse risk factor in stage I disease (9,15,17,48) but usually of limited (1,11,50) or no importance (7,16,48,51) in stage III/IV ovarian cancer. This variable is often poorly quantitated by its characterization as present or absent (1,7,11,16,48), though some authors are more precise (17,50).

PLOIDY, DNA INDEX, AND S-PHASE FRACTION

Ploidy refers to the number of copies of DNA carried by a cell. Normal cells are diploid (i.e., have two complete copies of DNA). Cancers often have cells of abnormal ploidy, such as triploid cells (with three copies of cellular DNA) or tetraploid cells (with four copies). Cells with some DNA content other than the normal diploid are called aneuploid and are generally held to carry a poorer prognosis for host survival (12,43,50,59). Aneuploid cancers typically have a mixture of cells, some being diploid and others aneuploid. If a cancer contains more than one aneuploid population it is called multiploid. Both fresh and paraffin-embedded tissue can be evaluated for the presence of cells with aberrant DNA content. Though technology for determining ploidy in fresh and fixed tissue has been available for many years (60), it is only with the more recent automated technology of flow cytometry that routine determination is practical (61). Ploidy determination involves preparation of a single cell suspension from fresh or paraffin-embedded tissue, staining of the DNA with a fluorescent dye (e.g., ethidium bromide or propidium iodide), and funneling of the cells single file through a flow cytometer which sorts cells into groups based on the intensity of their fluorescence and produces a *DNA histogram*. If the fluorescence of a diploid cell is taken as 1.0, then the fluorescence of a triploid cell would be 50% greater and have a *DNA index* of 1.5. Similarly, the fluorescence of a tetraploid cell would be 100% greater and have a DNA index of 2.0. However, the aberrant DNA need not be an integer multiple of the normal DNA, and incomplete copies of the genome or the presence of multiploid cells yield DNA indexes such as 1.79 or 2.60. Ploidy seems a stable characteristic of ovarian cancer. In general, comparison of tissues from the primary cancer, from metastases, and from second-look laparotomies shows no change in ploidy (12,50,62). There are, of course, the usual number of technical problems with measuring ploidy, which generally relate to distinguishing near-diploid aneuploid populations from normal diploid or G2 populations. These problems are decreasing as the resolution of flow cytometry improves (43). In general, aneuploid cancers are thought to have a poorer prognosis than diploid cancers (12,43,50,59); the higher the DNA index, the poorer the prognosis (except 2.0, the tetraploid DNA index) (59,63). It is not clear why patients with a tetraploid genome have nearly as favorable a prognosis as those with diploid genomes (59).

S-phase fraction refers to the number of cells in the DNA synthetic phase or S-phase of the cell cycle. It can be derived from the DNA histogram, though technical problems may occur in aneuploid or multiploid cancers. Flow cytometric S-phase measurements in ovarian cancer range from 2% to 20%, with aneuploid cancers having higher S-phase fractions than diploid cancers (e.g., 17.5% versus 10%) (59). Friedlander et al. (62) in an analysis of multiple areas of a single tumor or primary versus metastatic sites, found variations in S-phase fraction of greater than forty percent in eight of sixteen patients. The S-phase fraction seems a less stable tumor characteristic than ploidy, showing significant intratumoral and regional variation (62). However, Christov et al. (64) and Volm et al. (65), in a combined group of twelve patients, found a close correlation of S-phase fraction between primary and metastatic sites. S-phase fraction may also be measured by thymidine labeling index, an older, more time-consuming method which some claim is a more accurate reflection of proliferation and which gives values considerably lower than those determined by flow cytometry (66).

S-phase fraction is a measure of the rapidity of growth of a cancer. It does not present a complete picture because it does not consider rate of cell death, nor does it differentiate between stem cells, which can reproduce more or less ad infinitum, and differentiated cells, which will stop after several divisions. Therefore, S-phase fraction indicates the proliferative state but not the potential of a tumor. Quantification of stem cells, and hence the proliferative potential of a tumor, may be investigated through soft agar *stem cell assays* (67,68,69).

A number of papers have considered ploidy/DNA index (12,43,59,62,63,64,65,70,71) and S-phase fraction (59,64,65,66,70,72) as prognostic factors in ovarian cancer. Most find them powerful prognostic factors in univariate analyses, with aneuploidy, high DNA index, and high S-phase fraction associated with short survival. Small multivariate studies, which we will discuss later in this chapter, suggest ploidy may be a prognostic factor on par with residual disease and grade (12,43,50,59).

CA-125

CA-125, a circulating ovarian cancer antigen, is elevated in more than 75% of patients with epithelial ovarian cancer (73). Serum half-life is three to seven days. No correlation has been found between preoperative CA-125 levels and survival (7,73,74). However, postchemotherapy levels are predictive for survival in advanced ovarian cancer. Rustin et al. (2) found a two-year disease-free survival of 71% among those whose CA-125 levels had fallen sevenfold or more one month after starting chemotherapy as opposed to 11% among those whose CA-125 had dropped less quickly. A sevenfold drop of CA-125 per month would be equivalent to a drop at the half-life rate if we assume the average CA-125 half-life to be four days. Sevelda et al. (7) calculated that those whose CA-125 level had not normalized by the third month of chemotherapy had a risk of dying of 3.1 times greater than those whose levels had normalized; at this point the CA-125 level was a much more powerful predictor of survival than any initial factor such as stage or residual disease. Van der Berg et al. (74) found among patients whose CA-125 half-life on treatment was less than 20 days a median survival of 43 months, as opposed to 11 months for those with a half-life greater than 20 days. CA-125 seems to be a powerful posttreatment prognostic factor but is not useful in estimating survival at time of diagnosis.

HORMONE RECEPTORS

Approximately 50% of epithelial ovarian cancers are estrogen-receptor positive, 50% progesterone-receptor positive, and 35% positive for both receptors (24,75,76). Mean estrogen receptor values range from 19–54 fm/mg protein, and progesterone values range from 32–48 fm/mg protein. Receptor values for normal ovarian tissue fall in the same range (77). Unlike endometrial cancer, epithelial ovarian cancer (78,79) showed no correlation between histologic grade and receptor positivity. Nor was there any correlation between histologic grade any other variable such as histology, age, or stage (24,75,76,77). In univariate analysis, positive receptors are associated with longer survival; in two multivariate analyses, positive progesterone receptor ranked after stage and grade in one case (24), and positive estrogen receptor ranked after a residual disease and histology in another (76) as predictors of survival.

HER-2/*NEU* PROTO-ONCOGENE, P-GLYCOPROTEIN, AND CLONOGENIC ASSAY

Proto-oncogenes are normal cellular genes which bear a similarity to genes of known carcinogenic potential. HER-2/*neu* proto-oncogene is a normal cellular gene which appears to be closely related to the epidermal growth factor gene. It is a putative prognostic factor in breast cancer; tumors with an increased number of gene copies bearing a poorer prognosis (80). Slamon, et al. (80) analyzed 120 primary epithelial ovarian cancers for HER-2/neu and found the gene amplified in 31 (two to five gene copies in twenty-three patients and more than five copies in eight cases). Median survival diminished from approximately five years for those with a single HER-2/neu gene copy to eight months for those with five or more gene copies. No multivariate analyses have been done for this factor.

The multidrug resistance gene (MDR1) encodes P-glycoprotein, which is a plasma membrane glycoprotein associated with resistance to multiple chemotherapy drugs, possibly by accelerating their elimination from the cell. It has been suggested that MDR1 gene expression is increased in ovarian cancer, particularly after treatment (81,82). This might provide an explanation for the drug resistance which eventually develops in most ovarian cancers. No correlations between MDR1 and survival have been made. In fact, Rubin et al. (83) assayed 57 ovarian cancers (24 from chemotherapy-treated patients) for P-glycoprotein, the protein product of the MDR1 gene, and found it present in only 7% of cases. This factor appears less promising than the HER-2/neu proto-oncogene, but it is included as another example of a molecular marker under evaluation.

Dittrich et al. (69) examined 84 ovarian cancers in a soft agar clonogenic assay system. Single cell suspensions were prepared, and the cells were plated on soft agar and observed for colony formation. Survival was shorter among the thirty-five patients whose tumors manifested clonogenic growth as defined by the appearance of five or more colonies per plate. There was not, however, a linear relationship between number of soft agar colonies and survival. Multivariate analysis of standard prognostic factors identified the following factors, listed in descending order of significance, as independent variables associated with shorter survival: age, size of residual tumor, and clonogenic tumor growth.

Work on such molecular/biologic factors is in its infancy, and those mentioned above represent the first of many such markers we will see in the future. These markers are obviously much closer to the biology of ovarian cancer than our traditional clinical factors, and they offer hope for more specific and accurate prognostic indicators.

POST-TREATMENT VARIABLES AND SPECIALIZED ENDPOINTS

A number of variables which become apparent only after treatment is begun or finished exert a powerful influence on survival. Rate of fall of CA-125 serum levels, discussed earlier in this chapter, is an example.

Treatment-related myelosuppression and size of residual disease were the only two independent predictors of survival in a multivariate analysis of an Australian study of 369 stage III/IV ovarian cancer patients treated with chlorambucil or chlorambucil/cisplatin (6). Myelosuppression is likely related to dose intensity, though this was not analyzed in the aforementioned study. Levin and Hryniuk (84) have found dose intensity to be an important predictor of survival. They defined dose intensity as drug dose in mg/m^2 per unit time. In a review of multiple trials, survival increased with dose intensity, particularly with regard to cisplatin doses.

Negative second-look laparotomy is a powerful predictor of eventual survival, though not so powerful as in past years. In the era of alkylating agent therapy, second-look laparotomies were typically done at 18–24 months, and recurrence after negative laparotomy was rare (85). When duration of cisplatin therapy shortened, with second-look laparotomies taking place at six months, the recurrence rates rose to 40–60% (4,85,86,87). Examples of specialized predictive indexes surrounding second-look laparotomy include prediction of a negative laparotomy (3) and prediction of relapse after a negative laparotomy (4). In both instances, stage, residual disease, and grade were important predictors.

The post-treatment variables discussed above clearly predict survival, albeit in retrospect. They are useful but fall short in helping to select initial treatment, discuss survival, or stratify studies at the time of diagnosis.

MULTIVARIATE ANALYSES

We have discussed a large number of prognostic factors. All these factors have significance in predicting survival in univariate analyses, i.e., considered one at a time. However, univariate analysis does not identify related as opposed to independent factors, nor does it rank them in order of importance. As previously mentioned, the classic example is grade and histology. Both are important when considered individually, but grade is the significant and independent factor when considered together in multivariate analysis. Therefore, we will now consider what multivariate analysis can tell us about the relative importance of all the aforementioned factors. Significant factors for stage I ovarian cancer vary considerably from those for more advanced stages, and we will consider them separately.

Table 1 presents a number of multivariate analyses of stage I ovarian cancer. The table does not include all studies but is rather a cross-section chosen for their consideration of a wide range of variables and/or historic importance. The most striking observation is the universal agreement upon grade as the primary prog-

TABLE 1. Ranking of prognostic factors in multivariate analyses of stage I ovarian cancer

	Study				
	Webb	Swenerton	Sevelda	Dembo	Figo
Number of patients	271	123	204	489	1175
Rankings					
Ia, Ib	—	ns	ns	ns	ns
Ascites/Ic	—	ns	ns	3	2
Rupture	1	—	ns	ns	2
Penetration	1	—	—	ns	2
Adherence	1	—	—	2	—
Histology	ns	ns	ns	ns	ns
Grade	—	1	1	1	1
Age	—	ns	ns	ns	ns
Performance status	—	2	—	—	—
RT/Chemotherapy	—	ns	ns	ns	ns
USO vs. BSO	—	ns	2	—	—
Other factors	—	Weight loss	—	Size	

From Webb et al., ref. 13; Swenerton et al., ref. 16; Sevelda et al., ref. 5; Dembo et al., ref. 17; Pettersson et al. for International Federation of Gynecology and Obstetrics, ref. 9.

ns, not statistically significant; RT, radiation therapy; USO, unilateral salpingophorectomy; BSO, bilateral salpingophorectomy.

nostic factor. Grade is not only of first importance in virtually all studies, but within each study it is of far greater importance than second and third place factors. Swenerton et al. (16) noted that if the relative risk of death from stage I, grade 1 ovarian cancer is taken as 1.0, then the risk for grade 2 was 2.9; for grade 3, the relative risk is 6.4 times as great. Dembo et al. (17) noted risks of 1.0, 2.8, and 7.6 for the same groups. This corresponded to five-year disease-free survival rates of 91%, 71%, and 46% for grades 1, 2, and 3, respectively, in the first series (16); and 96%, 81%, and 58% in the other (17). There is no agreement on other factors of importance, especially those defining FIGO stage Ib and Ic (i.e., cyst rupture, capsular penetration by cancer, and cytologically positive ascites or pelvic washings). Webb et al. (13) found cyst rupture and capsular penetration to be significant risk factors; others have recently confirmed this (14). However, they did not consider grade in their analyses. The most recent FIGO annual report on treatment (9) notes grade to be of primary importance in prognosis and stage (Ia/b versus Ic) to be second in importance, but the report includes only sketchy information as to what portion of patients were Ic by virtue of capsular rupture, capsular penetration, ascites, or positive peritoneal cytology. However, three other large series specifically considered rupture, penetration, bilaterality, and cyst size and found no prognostic significance for any of these factors in either univariate or multivariate analyses (5,16,17). Which other prognostic factors ought to be considered in stage I remains unclear. While most series agree on grade as the prime factor predicting survival, they vary widely on secondary factors. Sevelda et al. (5) also found grade as the prime prognostic factor and USO (as opposed to BSO) of second importance, diminishing the five-year survival rate from 84% to 62%. Swenerton et al. (16) found ECOG performance status greater than zero to increase relative risk of death 3.4 times, while Dembo et al. (17) found large volume ascites (greater than 250 cc) to increase relative risk of death to 1.95 and dense adherence of the ovarian cancer to adjacent structures to increase relative risk to 2.5. As an interesting side note, Dembo et al. (17) attempt to resolve the issue of staging patients with otherwise stage I cancers which are adherent to adjacent structures. They suggest these patients be upstaged if the adherence is dense as defined by the need for sharp dissection, if a raw or oozing area is left in the location of the adherence, or if cyst rupture results from dissecting free the adherence. Relapse rate among those with dense adherence was 39% as opposed to 16% among those with minor or no adherence. Data as to the presence of malignant cells in the area of dense adherence was available in a portion of the population; the relapse rate among those with malignant cells was 38% as opposed to 35% for those with none. This seems to be a strong argument for upstaging to stage II those patients with dense adherence. Limited information is available on ploidy in stage I ovarian cancer. Approximately 50% to 60% stage I cancers are diploid (59,71), as opposed to 20% to 30% of stage III/IV cancers. Kallioniemi et al. (59), in an analysis of 77 stage I patients, found 52% to be diploid with a mean S-phase fraction of 11.4% for the group. Multivariate analysis showed ploidy and histology to be the independent predictors of survival, with risk of death increasing in the following order: (ploidy) diploid, aneuploid, multiploid; and (histology) mucinous, other, undifferentiated. Ploidy and S-phase fraction were related to grade, but in multivariate analysis, ploidy was the more important factor. The authors suggest that an additional advantage of ploidy over grade is the objective nature of the determination. Grade, as previously mentioned, is subject to wide variability in interpretation.

In summary, grade is the primary prognostic factor in stage I disease, with survival decreasing as grade increases. The role of other prognostic factors is unclear, including the traditional factors of bilaterality, rupture, penetration, ascites, and positive peritoneal cytology. The FIGO 1988 report (9) is the largest study to find stage Ic a significant prognostic factor, but it provides only minimal information on the relative importance of rupture versus penetration versus ascites or positive pelvic cytology. It does suggest that spontaneous rupture or ascites carry a more dire prognoses than capsular rupture by the surgeon (9). The reported number of patients with positive pelvic cytology or capsular penetration was too small to comment on risk. Newer factors such as ploidy, DNA index, and S-phase fraction have not been fully evaluated, though preliminary reports suggest ploidy may be a significant predictor of survival.

Few studies contain enough stage II patients for a multivariate analysis. However, Swenerton et al. (16) analyzed 177 stage II patients, including all the major clinical factors, and found substage (IIa, IIb, IIc), residual disease, histology, grade, age, ascites, performance status, and place of residence significant factors for survival in univariate analysis. In multivariate analysis, grade was of first importance and residual disease second, with all other factors dropping out.

Many studies have addressed prognostic factors in stage III/IV ovarian cancer. A number of reports considering the traditional clinical factors are summarized in Table 2. These studies were chosen because they included all major prognostic factors in their analyses. There are larger studies, but they do not include all factors. For instance, the FIGO multivariate analysis of 4,498 stage III/IV patients (9) lacks data on residual tumor and performance status, which are both important factors. In Table 2, residual disease seems consistently the major prognostic factor, with performance status of second importance and stage (III vs. IV) of third importance. Histology, grade, age, and ascites seem less important. In all of these studies, the therapy was either so variable or so similar that it did not appear as a prognostic factor. Major trials in which therapy is adequately evaluated either leave out major variables (6) or use restricted patient groups (1). A recent metanalysis of prognostic factors by Voest et al. (88) does permit evaluation of therapy. Sixty-six patient groups were analyzed, considering the following: stage (IIb/III vs. IV), histology, grade, residual disease (greater than vs. less than 2.0 cm), performance status, and chemotherapy (therapy containing cisplatin vs. other). Age is the only major variable missing. Significant factors predicting survival in univariate analysis were cisplatin therapy, residual disease, stage, and performance status. Multivariate analysis showed only cisplatin therapy and small residual disease to contribute, in roughly equal extent, to longer survival.

Several authors have constructed algorithms (6,10,11) or sought to define specific risk groups (16,21,41) based on multivariate analyses. They use traditional prognostic factors, including residual disease, stage, histology, grade, performance status, asci-

TABLE 2. *Ranking of older prognostic factors in multivariate analyses of stage III/IV ovarian cancer*

	Study				
	Marsoni	Swenerton	* Creaseman	Mangioni	v. Houwelingen
Number of Patients	852	256	406	167	268
Stage III	83%	76%	68%	78%	74%
Stage IV	17%	24%	32%	22%	26%
Rankings					
Stage	ns	2	ns	3	2
Residual	1	1	1	2	3
Ascites/cytology	—	ns	—	ns	6
Histology	2	ns	ns	ns	ns
Grade	ns	ns	ns	ns	5
Age	ns	ns	2	ns	ns
Performance Status	3	ns	ns	1	1
Chemotherapy	—	—	—	—	—
Other factors	hospital	hospital, weight loss	BSA	—	4-hospital, weight

From Marsoni et al., ref. 41; Swenerton et al., ref. 16; Creasman et al., ref. 52; Mangioni et al., ref. 53; v. Houwelingen et al., ref. 11.
  * residual disease ≥1.0 cm diameter.
  ns, not statistically significant.

TABLE 3. *Ranking of prognostic factors (including newer factors) in multivariate analyses of stage II/III/IV ovarian cancer*

	Study			
	Friedlander	Rodenberg	Blumenfeld	Kallioniemi
Number of patients	128	74	84	80
Stage II		14%	8%	15%
Stage III	76%	68%	68%	60%
Stage IV	24%	18%	24%	25%
Rankings				
Stage	2	ns	1	2
Residual	ns	ns	ns	—
Initial tumor bulk	—	ns	ns	—
Carcinomatosis	—	ns	—	—
Ascites/cytology	—	2	—	—
Histology	ns	ns	ns	3
Grade	ns	ns	ns	ns
Ploidy/DNA index	1	1	2	1
Age	ns	ns	3	ns
Performance status	—	ns	—	—
Cisplatin	ns	—	—	ns

From Friedlander et al., ref. 43; Rodenberg et al., ref. 50; Blumenfeld et al., ref. 12; Kallioniemi et al., ref. 59.
ns, not statistically significant.

tes, and therapy. None have been sufficiently compelling or simple enough to arouse wide interest, and only one (21) has been verified on an alternative data base.

Among the newer prognostic variables only ploidy/DNA index has been evaluated to any extent in multivariate fashion (12,43,50,59). Table 3 summarizes a number of these studies. Among the traditional variables, performance status and ascites are not well represented. However, the combined studies suggest ploidy is a powerful prognostic factor, displacing residual disease in these analyses. Stage is the only other prognostic factor of note in the table. At least one study (50) found residual disease and ploidy to be strongly correlated (e.g., residual disease less than 2.0 cm was associated with diploidy). These studies are small, and some traditional prognostic factors are not represented. However, the evidence is strong enough to suggest that ploidy should be considered in future analyses. It is well to remember that both ploidy and S-phase fraction have not lived up to expectations as prognostic factors in breast carcinoma.

Estrogen/progesterone receptor status (24,76) and rate of CA-125 fall (2,7) have also been considered in small multivariate analyses and found to be of importance. However, the data is sparse, and it is too early to make much comment on these factors.

CONCLUSION

Though controversy over prognostic factors continues, we have adequate information for our present purposes. We can distinguish stage Ia/b, well-differentiated cancers as being adequately treated by surgery and poorly differentiated, stage I cancers as requiring additional therapy. The nature of the additional therapy remains controversial, but the need for it does not. Prognosis for stage I, moderately well differentiated cancers and the various subcategories that comprise stage Ic is a bit less clear; perhaps newer factors such as ploidy will prove useful in recommending additional therapy in these groups.

However, the vast majority of ovarian cancers are advanced, and the need for treatment beyond surgery is not controversial. Nor is additional treatment so effective that we need argue about immediate versus salvage therapy, as is the case in many testicular cancers in which most recurrences after surgery can be effectively cured by chemotherapy (89). We do need prognostic factors for stratifying therapeutic trials, but the traditional factors of residual disease, stage, age, grade, and performance status are adequate, and newer factors such as ploidy are being explored.

There is a fatalistic argument that some patients, such as those with bulky residual or stage IV disease, fare so poorly that no further treatment is indicated. This would require a more accurate prognosis, but standard chemotherapy with drugs such as cyclophosphamide and carboplatin is well tolerated, and few physicians would be comfortable withholding therapy. Newer therapies are, however, becoming more intensive and toxic. If they prove more effective, there will be greater impetus to identify potentially curable patients. The imprecision of our present prognostic factors will be more acutely felt, though the appearance of newer molecular factors and the increasing use of multivariate analysis in most major studies will likely remedy this situation.

ACKNOWLEDGMENT

This work was supported in part by the Avon Program for Ovarian Cancer and NCI CA5826-23.

REFERENCES

1. Omura G, Brady M, Homesley H, Yordan E, Major F, Buchsbaum H, Park R. Long-term follow-up and prognostic factor analysis in advanced ovarian carcinoma: the Gynecologic Oncology Group Experience. *J Clin Oncol* 1991;9:1138–1150.
2. Rustin G, Gennings J, Nelstrop A, Covarrubias H, Lambert H, Bagshawe K for the North Thames Cooperative Group. Use of CA125 to predict survival of patients with ovarian carcinoma. *J Clin Oncol* 1989;7:1667–1671.
3. Carmichael J, Shelley W, Brown L, et al. A predictive index of cure versus no cure in advanced ovarian carcinoma patients—replacement of second-look laparotomy as a diagnostic test. *Gynecol Oncol* 1987;27:269–278.
4. Rubin S, Hoskins W, Saigo P, et al. Prognostic factors for recurrence following negative second-look laparotomy in ovarian cancer patients treated with platinum-based chemotherapy. *Gynecol Oncol* 1991;42:137–141.
5. Sevelda P, Vavra N, Schemper M, Salzer H. Prognostic factors for survival in Stage I epithelial ovarian carcinoma. *Cancer* 1990; 65:2349–2352.
6. Gynaecological Group, Clinical Oncology Society of Australia, and the Sydney Branch, Ludwig Institute for Cancer Research. Chemotherapy of advanced ovarian adenocarcinoma: a randomized comparison of combination versus sequential therapy using chlorambucil and cisplatin. *Gynecol Oncol* 1986;23:1–13.
7. Sevelda P, Schemper M, Spona J. CA 125 as an independent prognostic factor for survival in patients with epithelial ovarian cancer. *Am J Obstet Gynecol* 1989;161:1213–1216.
8. International Federation of Gynecology and Obstetrics. Changes in definitions of clinical staging for carcinoma of the cervix and ovary. *Am J Obstet Gynecol* 1987;156:236–241.
9. Pettersson F, Coppleson M, Creasman W, Ludwig H, Shepherd J. Annual report on the results of treatment in gynecologic cancer. *International Federation of Gynecology and Obstetrics*, vol 20. Stockholm, Sweden: 1988.
10. Redman J, Petroni G, Saigo P, Geller N, Hakes TB. Prognostic factors in advanced ovarian carcinoma. *J Clin Oncol* 1986;4: 515–523.
11. van Houwelingen J, ten Bokkel Huinink W, van der Burg M, van Ooosterom AT, Neijt JP. Predictability of the survival of patients with advanced ovarian cancer. *J Clin Oncol* 1989;7: 769–773.
12. Blumenfeld D, Braly P, Ben-Ezra J, Klevecz R. Tumor DNA content as a prognostic feature in advanced epithelial ovarian carcinoma. *Gynecol Oncol* 1987;27:389–398.
13. Webb MJ, Decker D, Mussey E, Williams TJ. Factors influencing survival in stage I ovarian cancer. *Am J Obstet Gynecol* 1973; 116:222–226.
14. Einhorn N, Nilsson B, Sjovall K. Factors influencing survival in carcinoma of the ovary: study from a well defined Swedish population. *Cancer* 1985;55:2019–2025.
15. Petterson F, Kolstad P, Ludwig H, Ulfelder H. Annual report on the results of treatment in gynecological cancer. *International Federation of Gynecology and Obstetrics*, vol 19. Stockholm, Sweden: 1985.
16. Swenerton K, Hislop T, Spinelli J, LeRiche J, Yang N, Boyes D. Ovarian carcinoma: a multivariate analysis of prognostic factors. *Obstet Gynecol* 1985;65:264–269.
17. Dembo A, Davy M, Stenwig A, Berle E, Bush R, Kjorstad K. Prognostic factors in patients with stage I epithelial ovarian carcinoma. *Obstet Gynecol* 1990;75:263–273.
18. Piver MS, Barlow JJ, Lele SB. Incidence of subclinical metastasis in stage I and II ovarian carcinoma. *Obstet Gynecol* 1978; 52:100–104.
19. Young R, Decker D, Wharton JT, Piver MS, Sindelar W, Edwards B, Smith J. Staging laparotomy in early ovarian cancer. *JAMA* 1983;250:3072–3076.
20. McGowan L, Lesher L, Norris H, Barnett M. Misstaging of ovarian cancer. *Obstet Gynecol* 1985;65:568–572.
21. Dembo A, Bush R. Choice of postoperative therapy based on prognostic factors. *Int J Radiation Oncol Biol Phys* 1982;8: 893–897.
22. Schray M, Martinez A, Cox R, Ballon S. Radiotherapy in epithelial ovarian cancer: analysis of prognostic factors based on long-term experience. *Obstet Gynecol* 1983;62:373–382.
23. Wils J, van Geuns H, Baak J. Proposal for therapeutic approach based on prognostic factors including morphometric and flow-cytometric features in stage III-IV ovarian cancer. *Cancer* 1988; 61:1920–1925.
24. Slotman B, Nauta J, Rao BR. Survival of patients with ovarian cancer. *Cancer* 1990;66:740–744.
25. Munnel EW, Taylor HC. Ovarian carcinoma. A review of 200 primary and 51 secondary cases. *Am J Obstet Gynecol* 1949;58: 943.
26. Gallager HS. Prognostic importance of histologic type in ovarian carcinoma. *Natl Cancer Inst Monogr* 1975;42:13–14.
27. Day TG, Gallager HS, Rutledge FN. Epithelial carcinoma of the ovary: prognostic importance of histologic grade. *Natl Cancer Inst Monogr* 1975;42:15–18.
28. Decker DG, Malkasian GD, Taylor WF. Prognostic importance of histologic grading in ovarian carcinoma. *Natl Cancer Inst Monogr* 1975;42:9–11.
29. Omura G, Bundy B, Berek J, Curry S, Delgado G, Mortel R. Randomized trial of cyclophosphamide plus cisplatin with or without doxorubicin in ovarian carcinoma: a Gynecologic Oncology Group Study. *J Clin Oncol* 1989;7:457–465.
30. Baak JP, Langley FA, Talerman A, et al. Interpathologist and intrapathologist disagreement in ovarian tumor grading and typing. *Analyt Quant Cytol Histol* 1986;8:354–357.
31. Hernandez E, Bhagavan BS, Parmley TH, et al. Interobserver variability in the interpretation of epithelial ovarian cancer. *Gynecol Oncol* 1984;17:117–123.
32. Van Orden DE, McAllister WB, Zerne SRM, Morris JM. Ovarian carcinoma. The problems of staging and grading. *Am J Obstet Gynecol* 1966;94:195–202.
33. Ozols RF, Garvin AJ, Costa J, Simon RM, Young RC. Advanced ovarian cancer. Correlation of histologic grade with response to therapy and survival. *Cancer* 1980;45:572–581.
34. Broders AC. Carcinoma: grading and practical application. *Arch Pathol* 1926;2:376–380.
35. Czernobilsky B. Common epithelial tumors of the ovary. In: *Pathology of the female genital tract*. Berlin: Springer-Verlag, 1984;511–560.
36. Russel P. The pathological assessment of ovarian neoplasms. III: The malignant epithelial tumors. *Pathology* 1979;11: 493–532.
37. Sorbe B, Frankendal B, Veress B. Importance of histologic grading in the prognosis of epithelial ovarian carcinoma. *Obstet Gynecol* 1982;59:576–582.
38. Serov SF, Scully RE, Sobin LH. *Histological typing of ovarian tumors*. Geneva: World Health Organization; 1973;9:17.
39. Jacobs AJ, Deligdisch L, Deppe G, Cohen CJ. Histologic correlates of virulence in ovarian adenocarcinoma. I. Effect of differentiation. *Am J Obstet Gynecol* 1982;143:574–580.
40. Kuhn W, Kaufmann M, Feichter GE, Rummel HH, Schmid H, Heberling D. DNA flow cytometry, clinical and morphological parameters as prognostic factors for advanced malignant and borderline ovarian tumors. *Gyn Oncol* 1989;33:360–367.
41. Marsoni S, Torri V, Valsecchi MG, et al. Prognostic factors in advanced epithelial ovarian cancer. *Br J Cancer* 1990;61: 444–450.
42. Gruppo Interegionale Cooperativo Oncologico Ginecologia.

Randomized comparison of cisplatin with cyclophosphamide; cisplatin and with cyclophosphamide/doxorubicin/cisplatin in advanced ovarian cancer. *Lancet* 1987;2:353–359.
43. Friedlander M, Hedley D, Swanson C, Russell P for the Gynecologic Oncology Group of the Clinical Oncology Society of Australia. Prediction of long-term survival by flow cytometric analysis of cellular DNA content in patients with advanced ovarian cancer. *J Clin Oncol* 1988;6:282–290.
44. Barber HRK, Sommers SC, Snyder R, et al. Histologic and nuclear grading, and stromal reactions as indices for prognosis in ovarian cancer. *Am J Obstet Gynecol* 1975;121:795–807.
45. Deligdisch L, Jacobs A, Cohen CJ. Histologic correlates of virulence in ovarian adenocarcinoma II. Morphologic correlates of host response. *Am J Obstet Gynecol* 1982;144:885–889.
46. Jacobs AJ, Deligdisch L, Deppe G, et al. Histologic correlates of virulence in ovarian adenocarcinoma I. Effect of differentiation. *Am J Obstet Gynecol* 1982;143:574–580.
47. Dyson JL, Beilby JOW, Steele SJ. Factors influencing survival in carcinoma of the ovary. *Br J Cancer* 1971;25:237–249.
48. Haapsalo H, Collan Y, Atkin NB. Major prognostic factors in ovarian carcinomas. *Int J Gynecol Cancer* 1991;1:155–162.
49. Baak JPA, Wisse-Brekelmans ECM, Langley FA, Talerman A, Delemarre JFM. Morphometric data to FIGO stage and histological type and grade for prognosis of ovarian tumors. *J Clin Pathol* 1986;39:1340–1346.
50. Rodenburg C, Cornelisse C, Heintz P, Hermans J, Jan Fleuren G. Tumor ploidy as a major prognostic factor in advanced ovarian cancer. *Cancer* 1987;59:317–323.
51. Griffiths TC. Surgical resection of tumor bulk in the primary treatment of ovarian carcinoma. *Natl Cancer Inst Monogr* 1975; 42:101–104.
52. Creasman W, Omura G, Brady M, Yordan E, DiSaia P, Beecham J. A randomized trial of cyclophosphamide, doxorubicin, and cisplatin with or without Bacillus Calmette-Guerin in patients with suboptimal stage III and IV ovarian cancer: a Gynecologic Oncology Group Study. *Gynecol Oncol* 1990;39:239–243.
53. Mangioni C, Bolis G, Pecorelli S, et al. Randomized trial in advanced ovarian cancer comparing cisplatin and carboplatin. *J Natl Cancer Inst* 1989;81:1464–1471.
54. Edmonson JH, Fleming TR, Decker DG, et al. Different chemotherapeutic sensitivities and host factors affecting prognosis in advanced ovarian carcinoma versus minimal disease. *Cancer Treat Rep* 1979;63:241–247.
55. Pruett KM, Gordon AN, Estrada R, Lynch GR. Small-cell carcinoma of the ovary: an aggressive epithelial cancer occurring in young patients. *Gynecol Oncol* 1988;29:365–369.
56. DeVita VT, Hellman S, Rosenberg SA. *Cancer: Principles and Practice of Oncology*, 3rd ed. Philadelphia: JB Lippincott Company; 1989.
57. Oken MM, Cuech RH, Tormey DC, et al. Toxicity and response criteria of the Eastern Co-operative Oncology Group. *Am J Clin Oncol* 1982;5:649–653.
58. Bjorkholm E, Pettersson F, Einhorn N, Krebs I, Nilsson B, Tjernberg B. Long-term follow-up and prognostic factors in ovarian carcinoma. *Acta Radiologica Oncol* 1982;21:413–419.
59. Kallioniemi O, Punnonen R, Mattila J, Lehtinen M, Koivula T. Prognostic significance of DNA index, multiploidy and S-phase fraction in ovarian cancer. *Cancer* 1988;61:334–339.
60. Atkin NB. Modal DNA value and chromosome number in ovarian neoplasia: a clinical and histopathological assessment. *Cancer* 1971;27:1064–1073.
61. Hedley DW, Friedlander ML, Taylor IW, Rugg CA, Musgrove EA. Method for analysis of cellular DNA content of paraffin-embedded pathological material using flow cytometry. *J Histochem Cytochem* 1983;11:1333–1335.
62. Friedlander ML, Taylor IW, Russell P, Tattersall MHN. Cellular DNA content—a stable feature in epithelial ovarian cancer. *Br J Cancer* 1984;49:173–179.
63. Iversen O-E. Prognostic value of the flow cytometric DNA index in human ovarian carcinoma. *Cancer* 1988;61:971–975.
64. Christov K, Vassilev N. Flow cytometric analysis of DNA and cell proliferation in ovarian tumors. *Cancer* 1987;60:121–125.
65. Volm M, Bruggemann A, Gunther M, Kleine W, Pfleiderer A, Vogt-Schaden M. Prognostic relevance of ploidy, proliferation and resistance-predictive tests in ovarian carcinoma. *Cancer Res* 1985;45:5180–5185.
66. Conte PF, Alama A, Rubagotti A, et al. Cell kinetics in ovarian cancer. Relationship to clinicopathologic features, responsiveness to chemotherapy and survival. *Cancer* 1989;64:1188–1191.
67. Ozols RF, Wilson JKV, Grotzinger KR, Young RC. Cloning of human ovarian cancer cells in soft agar from malignant effusions and peritoneal washings. *Cancer Res* 1980;40:2743–2747.
68. Von Hoff DD, Dronmal R, Salmon SE, et al. A Southwest Oncology Group study on the use of a human tumor cloning assay for predicting response in patients with ovarian cancer. *Cancer* 1991;67:20–27.
69. Dittrich C, Dittrich E, Sevelda P, Hudec M, Salzer H, Grunt T, Eliason J. Clonogenic growth in vitro: an independent biologic prognostic factor in ovarian carcinoma. *J Clin Oncol* 1991;9:381–388.
70. Brescia R, Barakat R, Beller U, Frederickson G, Suhrland M, Dubin N, Demopoulos R. The prognostic significance of nuclear DNA content in malignant epithelial tumors of the ovary. *Cancer* 1990;65:141–147.
71. Murray K, Hopwood L, Volk D, Wilson JF. Cytofluorometric analysis of the DNA content in ovarian carcinoma and its relationship to patient survival. *Cancer* 1989;63:2456–2460.
72. Iversen O-E, Skaarland E. Ploidy assessment of benign malignant ovarian tumors by flow cytometry. *Cancer* 1987;60:82–87.
73. Bast RC Jr, Klug TL, St John E, et al. A radioimmunoassay using a monoclonal antibody to monitor the course of epithelial ovarian cancer. *N Engl J Med* 1983;309:883–887.
74. van der Burg ME, Lammes FB, van Putten WL, Stoter G. Ovarian cancer: the prognostic value of the serum half-life of CA 125 during induction chemotherapy. *Gynecol Oncol* 1988;30:307–312.
75. Friedlander M, Quinn M, Fortune D, Foo MS, Toppila M, Hudson CN, Russell P. The relationship of steroid receptor expression to nuclear DNA distribution and clinicopathological characteristics in epithelial ovarian tumors. *Gynecol Oncol* 1989;32:184–190.
76. Bizzi A, Codegoni AM, Landoni F, et al. Steroid receptors in epithelial ovarian carcinoma: Relation to clinical parameters and survival. *Cancer Res* 1988;48:6222–6226.
77. Galli MC, DeGiovanni C, Nicoletti G, et al. The occurrence of multiple steroid hormone receptors in disease-free and neoplastic human ovary. *Cancer* 1981;47:1297–1302.
78. Palmer DC, Muir IM, Alexander AI, Cauchi M, Bennett RC, Quinn MA. The prognostic importance of steroid receptors in endometrial carcinoma. *Obstet Gynecol* 1988;72:388–393.
79. Quinn MA, Pearce P, Fortune DW, Koh SH, Hsieh C, Cauchi M. Correlation between cytoplasmic steroid receptors and tumor differentiation and invasion in endometrial carcinoma. *Br J Obstet Gynaecol* 1985;92:399–406.
80. Slamon D, Godolphin W, Jones L, et al. Studies of the HER-2/neu proto-oncogene in human breast and ovarian cancer. *Science* 1989;244:709–712.
81. Berry JM, Swensen RE, Brophy NA, Scudder SA, Sikic BI. Increased expression of the multidrug resistance gene MDR1 in ovarian cancers. *Proc Am Assoc Cancer Res* 1989;30:146.
82. Bourhis J, Goldstein LF, Riou G, Pastan I, Gottesman MM, Benard J. Expression of a human multidrug resistance gene in ovarian carcinomas. *Cancer Res* 1989;49:5062–5065.
83. Rubin S, Finstad C, Hoskins W, et al. Expression of P-glycoprotein in epithelial ovarian cancer: evaluation as a marker of multidrug resistance. *Am J Obstet Gynecol* 1990;163:69–73.
84. Levin L, Hryniuk WM. Dose intensity analysis of chemotherapy regimens in ovarian carcinoma. *J Clin Oncol* 1987;5:756–767.
85. Rubin SC, Hoskins WJ, Hakes TB, Markman M, Cain JM, Lewis JL. Recurrence after negative second-look laparotomy for ovarian cancer: analysis of risk factors. *Am J Obstet Gynecol* 1988;159:1094–1098.
86. Lippman SM, Alberts DS, Slymen DJ, et al. Second-look laparotomy in epithelial ovarian carcinoma. Prognostic factors associated with survival duration. *Cancer* 1988;61:2571–2577.

87. Podratz KC, Malkasian GJ, Wieand HS, Cha SS, Lee RA, Stanhope CR, Williams TJ. Recurrent disease after negative second-look laparotomy in stages III and IV ovarian carcinoma. *Gynecol Oncol* 1988;29:274–282.
88. Voest E, Van Houwelingen J, Neijt J. A meta-analysis of prognostic factors in advanced ovarian cancer with median survival and overall survival [measured with the log (relative risk)] as main objectives. *Eur J Cancer Clin Oncol* 1989;27:711–720.
89. Einhorn LH, Crawford ED, Shipley WU, Loehrer PJ, Williams SD. Testicular cancer. In: DeVita VT, Hellman S, Rosenberg SA, eds. *Cancer: Principles and Practice of Oncology*, 3rd ed. Philadelphia: JB Lippincott; 1989;1071–1089.

CHAPTER 8

Early Diagnosis of Epithelial Ovarian Cancer

J. R. van Nagell, Jr. and P. D. DePriest

Ovarian cancer remains the leading cause of death from gynecologic cancer in the United States. This year, over 20,000 new patients will be detected with ovarian cancer, and over 12,000 will die of the disease (1). Although significant advances have been made in the treatment of epithelial ovarian cancer, most patients still present with advanced stage disease in which prognosis is poor. According to SEER data, the five-year survival of patients with ovarian cancer increased from 36% in 1975 to only 39% in 1990 (1). These statistics are particularly disturbing when the excellent survival rate for patients with stage I ovarian cancer is considered (2–4). Clearly, if we are to make a significant impact on mortality, we must develop methods to detect ovarian cancer in an early stage when it is highly curable.

Because early stage ovarian cancer produces no symptoms, detection must focus on the screening of asymptomatic women. In order for patients to receive a maximum benefit from screening, a disease should be a significant cause of mortality, have a reasonably high prevalence in the screened population, have a preclinical phase that can be detected by screening, and be amenable to therapy so that the survival of patients with early stage disease is significantly higher than that of patients with advanced disease (5). Ovarian cancer fulfills all of these criteria. Ovarian cancer is generally agreed to be a major cause of mortality in our population. The incidence of ovarian cancer in the United States continues to rise, and it is the cause of more deaths than all other gynecologic cancers combined. The prevalence of ovarian cancer is approximately 50 per 100,000 in women over the age of 50, a rate which may increase in women with a documented family history of the disease. Bourne and coworkers (6) reported that in England, the prevalence of ovarian cancer increased from 0.4 per 1,000 in the general population to 3.9 per 1,000 in women with a documented history of ovarian cancer in a primary or secondary relative. Although the exact duration of the preclinical phase in ovarian cancer remains unknown, increasing evidence indicates that such a phase does exist. Statistical analysis of screening data indicates that benign epithelial ovarian tumors are more common in women with a documented family history of ovarian cancer (6), and transition from benign to borderline or malignant epithelium has been documented in serous ovarian neoplasms (7). If molecular genetic studies confirm that certain benign epithelial ovarian tumors have malignant potential, the surgical removal of these tumors should prevent the subsequent development of ovarian malignancy in the screened population. Finally, early stage ovarian cancer is significantly more curable than advanced stage disease. The five-year survival of patients with stage I ovarian cancer is 90% as compared to 10 to 15% in patients with stage III or stage IV disease (1).

Statistical definitions that are used in ovarian cancer screening are illustrated in Table 1. For screening purposes, a true negative is defined as the absence of ovarian cancer for one year after a negative test (8). This definition is important because it is impossible to perform surgery on all patients with negative screenings. A true positive is defined as the presence of histologically documented ovarian cancer in a patient with a positive screening. An optimal screening test should be safe, easy to perform, time efficient, and acceptable to patients. It should also have high sensitivity, high specificity, and positive predictive value (9). With these criteria, the two most promising screening methods for ovarian cancer are transvaginal ultrasound (TVS) and serum CA-125.

J. R. van Nagel, Jr. and P. D. DePriest: Division of Gynecologic Oncology, Department of Obstetrics and Gynecology, University of Kentucky Medical Center, Lexington, Kentucky 40536

TABLE 1. *Statistical definitions in ovarian cancer screening*

Term	Screen	Findings
True Positive (TP)	Positive	Ovarian cancer
False Positive (FP)	Positive	No ovarian cancer
True Negative (TN)	Negative	Absence of ovarian cancer for 1 year. Confirmed by annual TVS examination.
False Negative (FN)	Negative	Ovarian cancer

Sensitivity, TP/TP + FN; specificity, TN/TN + FP; Positive Predictive Value, TP/TP + FP; Negative Predictive Value, TN/TN + FN.

TRANSVAGINAL SONOGRAPHY

The use of abdominal ultrasound as a screening method for ovarian cancer was first proposed by Campbell and co-workers (10). These investigators reported a high correlation between actual and sonographically determined ovarian volume measurements, and they established criteria for normal ovarian size and morphology in postmenopausal women. Approximately 5,500 asymptomatic women were screened, and five primary ovarian cancers were detected. All patients had stage I disease and are presently alive and well after conventional therapy. Although abdominal ultrasound was effective in detecting most ovarian tumors, it is not an ideal screening method. Abdominal ultrasound requires a full bladder for proper visualization of pelvic structures, and bladder filling is often uncomfortable and time-consuming. In addition, the excessive distance between the abdominal transducer and the pelvis makes accurate visualization of the ovaries impossible in certain patients.

The use of transvaginal sonography for ovarian cancer screening was initiated at the University of Kentucky Medical Center in 1986 (11,12). Screening was initially performed using a 5 mHz vaginal transducer from a Phillips SDR unit. Asymptomatic women over the age of 40 with no known ovarian tumors were eligible for the investigation. Interobserver variation in ultrasound-generated ovarian dimensions was minimal (13), and a high correlation was seen between actual ovarian volume and the volume predicted by TVS. In premenopausal women, ovarian volume fluctuated markedly throughout the menstrual cycle. In addition, two-thirds of ovarian tumors detected by TVS in premenopausal women spontaneously disappeared. As a result of these findings, it was recommended that subsequent TVS screening trials be limited to postmenopausal women in whom the prevalence of ovarian cancer is highest and cyclic fluctuation of ovarian volume can be avoided.

Recently, the efficacy of TVS screening in postmenopausal women has been evaluated (14). Screening was performed on 1,300 asymptomatic postmenopausal patients with no known pelvic abnormalities. Ovarian volume was calculated using the prolate ellipsoid formula (width × height × thickness × 0.523), and ovarian volume in excess of 8 cm^3 was defined as abnormal. This value was two standard deviations above that of the normal postmenopausal ovary, as reported by Goswamy and co-workers (15). Patients with an abnormal ovarian volume on ultrasound had a repeat sonogram in 4 weeks. If the repeat screen indicated a persistent ovarian tumor, an exploratory laparotomy was recommended. With this protocol, ovarian tumors were detected in 33 patients (2.5%), and 27 underwent surgery. Only one-third of these patients had an ovarian abnormality that was palpable on clinical examination. Fourteen women were found to have ovarian serous cystadenomas, and three had ovarian carcinomas. One patient had a metastatic ovarian tumor from an occult colon carcinoma, and two patients had primary ovarian cancers. The two patients with primary ovarian cancers had stage IA disease, and both had normal pelvic examinations and serum CA-125 values. These patients are presently alive and well approximately 3 years after treatment. With the statistical definitions presented in Table 1, TVS had a sensitivity of 1.000, a specificity of 0.981, and a positive predictive value of 0.111. One of the major concerns about TVS screening is that it may cause a significant amount of unnecessary surgery. In this investigation, over 60% of women undergoing exploratory laparotomy for a persistent abnormality on sonography had either a serous cystadenoma or an ovarian carcinoma.

Two adjunctive methods currently being investigated to improve the specificity of TVS are the morphology index and the color flow Doppler. The risk for malignancy in ovarian tumors can be correlated with specific sonographic patterns (16). Unilocular cystic ovarian tumors, independent of size, have been shown to have a very low risk for malignancy. In contrast, ovarian tumors with internal papillations or a complex morphologic pattern have a significantly higher risk for malignancy. With this data, a morphology index can be constructed to predict risk for malignancy in sonographically detected tumors. The number of small ovarian tumors (<5 cm diameter) that have been studied using this methodology is minimal. Preliminary evidence suggests that morphologic criteria alone may be unable to distinguish benign from malignant ovarian tumors in approximately 10% of cases (17). Nevertheless, the use of a morphologic index should improve the overall specificity of TVS.

The use of color flow Doppler to differentiate benign from malignant ovarian lesions is based on observed changes in tissue vascularity. During malignant transformation, vascular endothelial cell growth is stimu-

TABLE 2. *Summary of screening sonography for ovarian cancer*

Author	Type ultrasound	Number of patients	Ovarian cancers detected	Stage of disease
Campbell et al. (1989)	TAS	5,500	5	Stage I (5)
van Nagell et al. (1991)	TVS	1,300	2	Stage I (2)
Bourne et al. (1991)	TVS	776	3	Stage I (3)

TAS, transabdominal sonography; TVS, transvaginal sonography.

lated, and tumor angiogenesis occurs (18). Transvaginal color Doppler can be used to study the flow patterns within ovarian and pelvic vessels. A pulsed Doppler range gate allows quantitative analysis of flow velocity wave forms in these vessels. Using this technology, Bourne and colleagues (19) reported that ovarian carcinomas could be distinguished from benign ovarian tumors. Ovarian malignancies had a significantly lower pulsatility index than corresponding benign lesions, particularly in postmenopausal patients. Although these preliminary data are encouraging, Doppler flow sonography needs to be evaluated in a large number of patients with stage I ovarian cancers to determine if objective vascular changes are identifiable in the earliest malignant lesions.

Two criteria that have been used to evaluate the efficacy of a screening test are its ability to lower the stage at detection and its effect on case-specific mortality. To date, approximately 8,000 asymptomatic women have been screened by sonography (Table 2). Ten primary ovarian cancers have been detected, and all patients have had stage I tumors. All women are presently alive with no evidence of disease after conventional therapy, and the case-specific mortality is 0%.

A final and most important characteristic of an effective screening test is the requirement that it produce a statistically significant reduction in site-specific ovarian cancer mortality in the screened population. Evaluation of this parameter will require a carefully designed multi-institutional trial comparing TVS to pelvic examination as a screening method for ovarian cancer in large numbers of women.

SERUM CA-125

The serum marker that has been most extensively evaluated as a screening test for ovarian cancer is CA-125. CA-125 is an antigenic determinant on a high molecular weight glycoprotein that is recognized by the monoclonal antibody OC-125 (20). CA-125 is expressed by epithelial ovarian malignancies, and immunohistochemical staining studies indicate that antigen concentration is greatest on the tumor cell surface (21). Serum levels of this marker have been reported to be elevated (>30 u/ml) in over 80% of ovarian cancer patients. The frequency of elevated serum CA-125 is related directly to stage of disease. It varies from 50% in patients with stage I disease to over 90% in patients with stage III and IV tumors (22). CA-125 levels are also increased in the sera of patients with a number of benign gynecologic diagnoses, including pelvic inflammatory disease and endometriosis. However, most of these benign conditions occur in premenopausal women.

Two major prospective studies have investigated the value of CA-125 as a primary screening method for ovarian cancer. Jacobs and co-workers (8) evaluated the screening specificity of CA-125 in 1,010 asymptomatic postmenopausal women. In this investigation, a CA-125 value ≥30u/ml was defined as abnormal. The definition of specificity was the same as that presented in Table 1. When used alone, serum CA-125 had a specificity of 0.970. However, the combination of CA-125 and ultrasound had a specificity of 0.998. In a more recent prospective investigation, Einhorn and co-workers (23) presented the results of CA-125 screening in 5,550 apparently healthy women. Serum CA-125 was elevated (≥30 u/ml) in 175 women (3.1%). These women underwent intensive surveillance with repeat CA-125 determinations, abdominal sonograms, and pelvic examinations every 3 months. On the basis of clinical or ultrasound findings, laparotomies were performed on 12 women over 50 years of age. Six ovarian cancers were discovered. Two of these patients had stage I disease, and four had stage II or III disease. In this age group, the specificity of CA-125 was 0.970.

A major problem with serum CA-125 as a screening method for ovarian cancer is its lack of sensitivity. As mentioned previously, only 50% of patients with clinically detectable stage I ovarian cancers have elevated serum CA-125 levels, and this percentage is even lower in patients with sonographically detected tumors. Consequently, serum CA-125 seems to be least effective in detecting patients with the most curable ovarian cancers.

TRIAL DESIGN FOR OVARIAN CANCER SCREENING

Analysis of available data suggests that the most effective method for primary ovarian cancer screening is TVS. Vaginal sonography is extremely sensitive in the detection of small ovarian tumors, but its specificity and positive predictive value are only moderate. For this reason, other adjunctive modalities such as a morphology index, Doppler flow sonography, or serum markers must be evaluated in large numbers of patients to determine if they can increase the specificity of TVS. As mentioned previously, confirmation of malignant potential in certain benign or borderline epithelial ovarian tumors would increase the specificity of TVS as a screening method.

A final issue is the choice of the population to be screened. TVS is most effective as a screening method in postmenopausal patients, in whom physiologic changes in ovarian volume do not occur (12). Also, the prevalence of ovarian cancer is highest in women over the age of 50, and the criteria for normal ovarian volumes have been more clearly defined for postmenopausal women. Most investigators agree that a persistent ovarian tumor with volume of ≥ 10 cm^3 in a postmenopausal woman is abnormal and should be removed surgically.

A second group who would benefit from screening is the group of women with a documented history of ovarian cancer in a primary or secondary relative. Lynch and co-workers (24) have emphasized that women with a strong family history of ovarian cancer are at high risk to develop the disease. In certain cases, this risk may approach 50%. Interestingly, women with a family history of ovarian cancer, the breast cancer–ovarian cancer syndrome, or the Lynch Type II syndrome tend to develop ovarian cancer at a significantly younger age than those without genetic predisposition. Bourne and co-workers (6) reported the results of ovarian cancer screening in 776 women with a documented family history of the disease. Three cases of primary ovarian cancer were detected, and one patient developed a serous cystadenocarcinoma at the age of 38. It is our present recommendation that women with a positive family history of ovarian cancer enter screening protocols at the age of 30.

Although preliminary results of ovarian cancer screening by TVS are encouraging, a properly designed multi-institutional trial must be instituted. From an epidemiological viewpoint, an optimal study would consist of a randomized controlled trial (RCT) comparing the efficacy of TVS to pelvic examination as a screening method for ovarian cancer (9). Women in the screening arm would receive annual TVS and, if the first screening were abnormal, would have a repeat sonogram in 4–6 weeks. If the repeat TVS were abnormal, exploratory laparotomy would be recommended. Adjunctive studies before laparotomy might include a morphologic index, serum marker determinations, and Doppler flow sonography. Women in the control arm would receive an annual pelvic examination and, if this were abnormal, would have a repeat pelvic examination in 4–6 weeks. Exploratory laparotomy would be recommended in patients with a persistent abnormality on pelvic examination. Such a trial would consist of annual screening for 3–4 years followed by a observation period of 6 years. Asymptomatic postmenopausal women, or women over the age of 30 with a documented family history of ovarian cancer, would be eligible for participation in this trial. Standardized criteria for abnormality should be specified both for TVS and pelvic examination and should differ for premenopausal and postmenopausal patients. End results criteria for this RCT would be stage of ovarian cancer at detection, case-specific death rate, and site-specific mortality in each arm of the trial. Although the study design of an RCT is theoretically optimal, patient accrual in the control arm might be difficult. Another trial option might consist of a single TVS screening arm in which a pelvic examination would serve as an internal control. The end results criteria of this study would be the same as those of the RCT. Until the results of such a trial are available, TVS and other screening modalities should be considered as experimental methods, and their use should be limited to institutions participating in controlled clinical research studies. Once the efficacy of a screening method for ovarian cancer has been confirmed, the issue of cost effectiveness and optimal eligibility requirements for those to be screened can be addressed.

REFERENCES

1. Boring C, Squires T, Tong T. Cancer statistics 1991. *CA Cancer J Clin* 1991;41:19–36.
2. Gallion H, van Nagell JR, Donaldson ES, Higgins RV, Powell DE, Kryscio RJ. Adjuvant oral alkylating agent chemotherapy in patients with stage I epithelial ovarian cancer. *Cancer* 1989;63:1070–1073.
3. Piver MS, Malfetano J, Baker TR, Lele SB, Marchetti DL. Adjuvant cisplatin-based chemotherapy for stage I ovarian adenocarcinoma: a preliminary report. *Gynecol Oncol* 1989;35:69–72.
4. Young RC, Walton LA, Ellenberg SS, et al. Adjuvant therapy in stage I and stage II epithelial ovarian cancer. *N Engl J Med* 1990;311:1021–1027.
5. Hulka BS. Cancer screening: degrees of proof and practical application. *Cancer* 1988;62:1776–1789.
6. Bourne TH, Whitehead M, Campbell S, Royston P, Bhan V, Collins WP. Ultrasound screening for familial ovarian cancer. *Gynecol* Oncol [*in press*].
7. Stenback F. Benign, borderline, and malignant serous cystadenomas of the ovary. *Pathol Res Pract* 1981;172:58–72.
8. Jacobs I, Bridges J, Reynolds C, et al. Multimodal approach to screening for ovarian cancer. *Lancet* 1988;2:268–271.
9. Prorok PC. Evaluation of screening programs for the early detection of cancer. *Statistical Textbooks Monographs* 1984;51:267–328.
10. Campbell S, Bhan V, Royston P, Whitehead M, Collins W. Transabdominal ultrasound screening for early ovarian cancer. *BMJ* 1989;299:1363–1367.
11. Higgins RV, van Nagell JR, Donaldson ES, et al. Transvaginal sonography as a screening method for ovarian cancer. *Gynecol Oncol* 1989;34:402–406.
12. van Nagell JR, Higgins RV, Donaldson ES, et al. Transvaginal sonography as a screening method for ovarian cancer: a report of the first 1000 cases screened. *Cancer* 1990;65:573–577.

13. Higgins RV, van Nagell JR, Woods CH, Thompson EA, Kryscio RK. Interobserver variation in ovarian measurements using transvaginal sonography. *Gynecol Oncol* 1990;39:69–71.
14. van Nagell JR, DePriest PD, Puls LE, et al. Ovarian cancer screening in asymptomatic postmenopausal women by transvaginal sonography. *Cancer* 1991;68:458–462.
15. Goswamy RK, Campbell S, Whitehead MI. Screening for ovarian cancer. *Clin Obstet Gynecol* 1983;10:621–643.
16. Granberg S, Wikland M, Jansson I. Macroscopic characterization of ovarian tumors and the relation to histologic diagnosis: criteria to be used for ultrasound evaluation. *Gynecol Oncol* 1989;35:139–144.
17. Luxman D, Bergman A, Sagi J, David M. The postmenopausal adnexal mass: correlation between ultrasonic and pathologic findings. *Obstet Gynecol* 1991;77:726–731.
18. Folkman J, Watson K, Ingber D, Hanahan D. Induction of angiogenesis during transition from hyperplasia to neoplasia. *Nature* 1989;339:58–61.
19. Bourne TH, Campbell S, Steer CV, Whitehead MI, Collins WP. Transvaginal colour flow imaging: a possible new screening test for ovarian cancer. *BMJ* 1989;229:1367–1370.
20. Bast RC, Feeney M, Lazarus H, Nadler LM, Colvin RB, Knapp RC. Reactivity of a monoclonal antibody with human ovarian carcinoma. *J Clin Invest* 1981;68:1331–1337.
21. Kabawat SE, Bast RC, Bhan AK, Welch WR, Knapp RC, Colvin RB. Tissue distribution of a coelomic epithelium-related antigen recognized by the monoclonal antibody OC125. *Lab Invest* 1983;48:42a (abst).
22. Jacobs I, Bast RC. The CA-125 tumour-associated antigen: a review of the literature. *Hum Reprod* 1989;4:1–12.
23. Einhorn N, Sjovall K, Knapp R, et al. Prospective evaluation of the specificity of serum CA-125 levels for detection of ovarian cancer in a normal population. *Obstet Gynecol* [*in press*].
24. Lynch HT, Watson P, Bewtra TA, et al. Hereditary ovarian cancer. Heterogeneity in age at diagnosis. *Cancer* 1991;67:1460–1466.

CHAPTER 9

Radiologic Evaluation of Ovarian Cancer

D. David Dershaw and David M. Panicek

The radiologic evaluation of ovarian cancer involves a wide spectrum of imaging techniques based on a variety of physical principles. Plain film studies allow characterization of tissues on the basis of their atomic number and can readily differentiate air, fat, water or soft tissue, and metal densities. The information available on plain film images can be increased by the administration of contrast materials. Barium agents can be used to opacify the gastrointestinal tract lumen, and intravenous iodinated agents can be used to opacify the urinary tract. Opacification of pelvic and retroperitoneal lymph nodes by means of bipedal lymphangiography can aid in studying the status of these lymph nodes.

The roles of these examinations in assessing the disease process have been dramatically augmented by the advent of sectional imaging techniques. Computed tomography (CT) refines the differentiation of various tissues on the basis of x-ray attenuation. The administration of oral and intravenous contrast agents further improves anatomic definition and tissue characterization. Sonography images tissues on the basis of density, which determines the speed at which sound travels through them, and on the presence of acoustic interfaces. This imaging technique is best utilized in the differentiation of solid from fluid-filled structures. The advent of Doppler sonography also allows the study of vascular flow. Most recently, magnetic resonance imaging (MRI) has enabled the radiologist to image on the basis of proton density and relaxation times.

Each modality has advantages and disadvantages for studying women with ovarian cancer. The efficacy of the techniques noted in this chapter depends partially on the equipment that is used and the experience and expertise of the examiner. The level of skill in performing and interpreting these studies will vary. The determination of which technique should be used in studying any individual patient will also depend on the availability of equipment and on considerations of cost, radiation exposure, and risk to the patient.

PLAIN FILM STUDIES

The plain film of the abdomen may be capable of confirming the presence of a pelvic mass by showing displacement of bowel loops. Characterization of the mass is often limited. However, the presence of fat or calcium in a dermoid may permit its diagnosis on plain film. Psammomatous calcification in primary or metastatic ovarian carcinoma is sometimes visible. In the clinical evaluation of bowel obstruction, the plain abdominal film is often adequate to determine the presence or absence of obstruction. Characteristic patterns may also be seen with serosal implants of bowel loops and with ascites.

The presence of secondary chest disease is rare in women with early ovarian carcinoma, but chest radiography is valuable for monitoring later involvement. Owing to the rarity of preliminary involvement without extensive abdominal disease, routine chest CT is not indicated in women with early stage ovarian cancer and a negative chest radiograph.

INTRAVENOUS PYELOGRAPHY

The significance of intravenous pyelography in the preoperative staging of ovarian carcinoma may be related more to habit than to clinical utility. Hillman (1) found a true positive rate of 7% with a sensitivity of 33% for intravenous pyelography in determining the extension of gynecologic tumors. Sectional imaging

D. D. Dershaw and D. M. Panicek: Department of Radiology, Memorial Sloan-Kettering Cancer Center, New York, New York 10021

techniques are superior in determining this information and also add information about the primary tumor. These techniques can assess the presence or absence of urinary tract obstruction, and CT can evaluate the presence or absence of duplicated collecting systems and follow the course of the ureters. Therefore, despite its frequent use, intravenous pyelography is rarely necessary in evaluating women with ovarian cancer.

BARIUM STUDIES

The spread of intra-abdominal tumor relates to the patterns of flow of ascitic fluid, as described by Meyers and McSweeney (2,3). The most common sites of metastatic disease are the pouch of Douglas, the right lower quadrant, the sigmoid colon, and the right paracolic gutter. The small bowel may be more frequently involved than the large bowel. In a review of 284 women with gynecologic tumors, all women with small bowel abnormalities and ovarian cancer had metastatic disease to the small bowel (4). Small bowel disease may be manifested by masses with associated desmoplastic reaction, kinking, and obstruction. In women with small bowel obstruction who have had pelvic irradiation, the site of obstruction may be helpful in differentiating the etiology. Yuhasz and colleagues found that all obstructions caused by radiation were at the ileum, whereas the jejunum or the duodenum were the site of 58% of obstructions owing to metastatic disease (4).

Metastatic involvement of the bowel is manifested on barium studies by patterns of fixation and angulation of bowel loops and the identification of a mass (Fig. 1). Although characteristic of tumor involvement, the pattern is not pathognomonic of malignancy (5).

Evidence of direct involvement of the bowel may be readily identified, but omental tumor may be difficult to diagnose. Contiguous spread from the greater omentum to the transverse colon is evident when the superior margin of the transverse colon is altered by mass effect, tethering, nodularity, or even circumferential narrowing. Omental disease is only indirectly imaged by barium study, and CT is more appropriate for imaging tumor at this site (6).

LYMPHANGIOGRAPHY

The injection of iodinated fatty contrast material into dorsal pedal lymphatics leads to the opacification and visualization of lymphatic vessels in the lower extremities, pelvis, and retroperitoneum. Tumor involvement is manifested by altered dynamics of flow in the lymphatic vessels and by enlargement and/or aberrant internal architecture of the lymph nodes (Fig. 2). Failure to diagnose metastatic disease is due to metastases too small to be visualized, failure to opacify involved nodes, and complete nodal replacement by metastatic disease. The most reliable sign of metastatic disease is a filling defect within an involved node, which is caused by a metastatic focus that grows within a node and destroys normal nodal tissue. In this situation, metastases as small as 5 mm can be visualized (7).

Bipedal lymphangiography allows only limited opacification of the lymph nodes. Hypogastric and presacral nodes are usually not opacified, and abdominal lymph nodes are not visible. Retroperitoneal lymph nodes above the level of the cisterna chyli are also not studied with this technique.

The lymphatic drainage of the ovaries is usually to paraaortic nodes extending from the aortic bifurcation cephalad to the renal hilus. External and common iliac nodal groups may also be involved. Anastomoses between ovarian lymph vessels and those of the uterus and fallopian tubes may result in alternate drainage pathways. Additionally, tumor involvement of the ovarian capsule can result in iliac and inguinal nodal disease. Despite this variable pattern, the utilization of lymphangiography along with CT can lead to the detection of over 90% of nodal metastases (7).

The presence of paraaortic nodal metastases has been demonstrated by lymphangiography in 18–70% of patients with ovarian cancer (8–11). In one study of 72 lymphangiograms, metastatic nodal disease was present in 33 (46%), with nodal disease found in paraaortic nodes in 23, iliac nodes in 19, inguinal nodes in 9, and supraclavicular nodes in 2. Metastatic disease confined to paraaortic nodes was found in 14 and confined to iliac nodes in 4 (8). The distribution of nodal metastases may relate to the histology of the primary ovarian tumor. Germ cell tumors have been found to metastasize to paraaortic nodes in 90% of cases with metastases and to iliac nodes in less than one-third of cases. Epithelial ovarian cancers, however, metastasize to iliac nodes in over 40% of cases (11). This may be due to a greater propensity for epithelial tumors to involve the ovarian capsules and adjacent pelvic organs, leading to pelvic nodal disease. Germ cell tumors are more likely to be confined by the capsule and spread by anatomic drainage pathways.

SONOGRAPHY

The sonographic evaluation of the pelvis can be performed using a variety of techniques. Routine examination entails distention of the urinary bladder to displace gas-filled loops of small bowel out of the pelvis. Gas within these loops disrupts the passage of sound waves. The patient is scanned with the transducer placed on the anterior abdominal wall, and gynecologic structures are visualized behind the distended bladder.

Because resolution in sonography is inversely re-

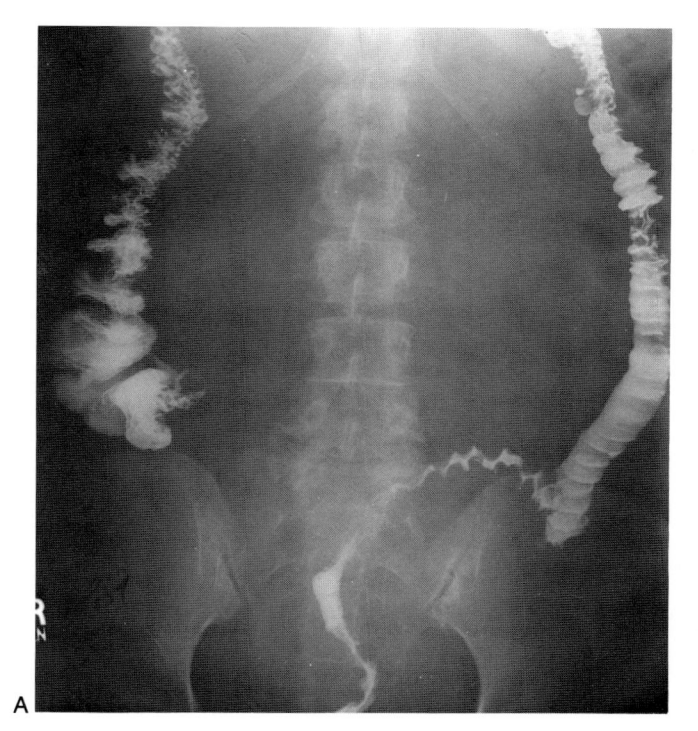

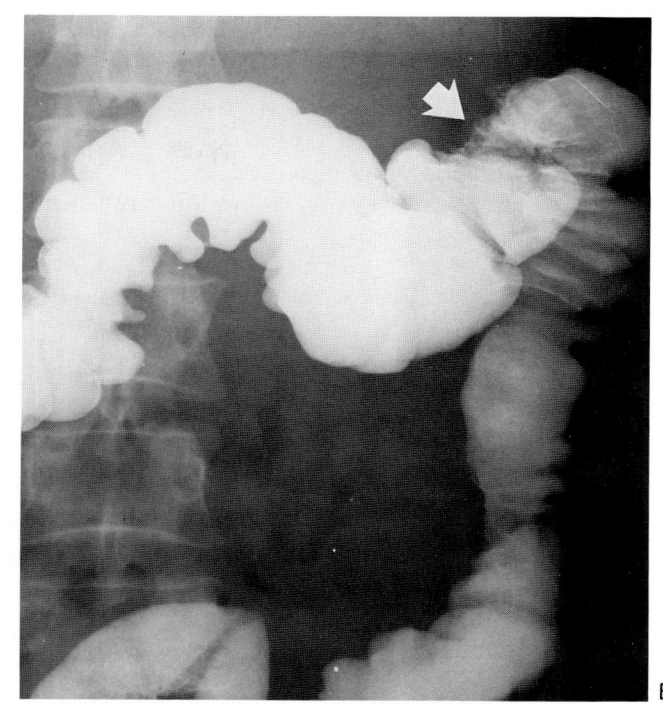

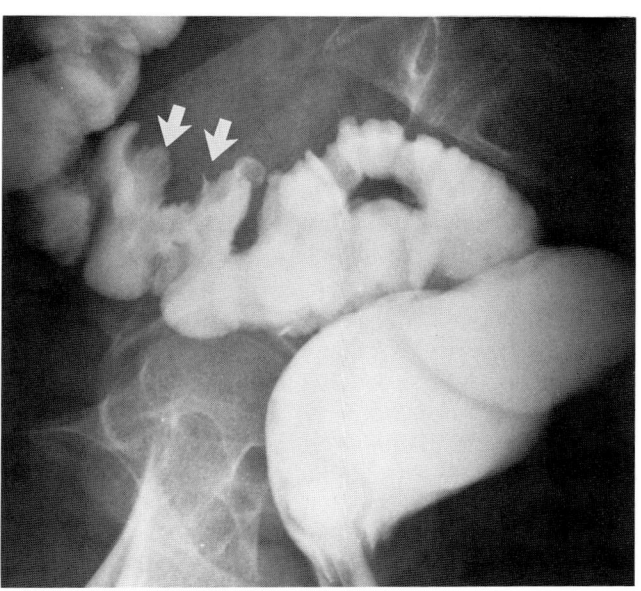

FIG. 1. Barium enema manifestations of intra-abdominal ovarian cancer with increasing involvement of the large bowel. **(A)** Postevacuation film from a barium enema shows elevation of the sigmoid colon secondary to an adjacent, large ovarian tumor. Generalized haziness throughout the abdomen and some slight displacement of the opacified colon away from the flank walls is also present and is due to extensive ascites. **(B)** In the distal transverse colon at the splenic flexure, irregularity (*arrow*) is secondary to serosal implantation of metastatic ovarian cancer at this site. **(C)** Spot lateral radiograph of the rectum shows direct tumor invasion of the rectosigmoid (*arrows*) by local ovarian cancer.

lated to the distance sound must travel to image tissue, better definition of structures and pathology is possible when the transducer can be positioned close to the uterus and ovaries. Transvaginal scanning is designed to take advantage of this principle. Closer approximation of the transducer to gynecologic structures allows for greatly improved detail (Fig. 3) and permits the examination to be performed without the discomfort of urinary bladder distention. However, the high-frequency sound waves utilized in endovaginal scanning cannot penetrate deeply into the pelvis, and, therefore, a somewhat limited area may be visualized. Additional information may be gained with the use of Doppler scanning, which enables blood flow to be imaged.

The normal adult ovary has a variable size but can measure up to 5 cm in one dimension, with tridimensional measurements usually varying from $1 \times 2 \times 3$ cm to $2 \times 3 \times 4$ cm. Ovarian size diminishes with the end of ovulation and menstruation. Postmenopausal ovaries may be difficult to image sonographically.

The ability of sonography to detect the presence of a pelvic mass is great, but this is often a nonspecific finding. Not only is the histology of the mass usually not identifiable sonographically, but the site of origin

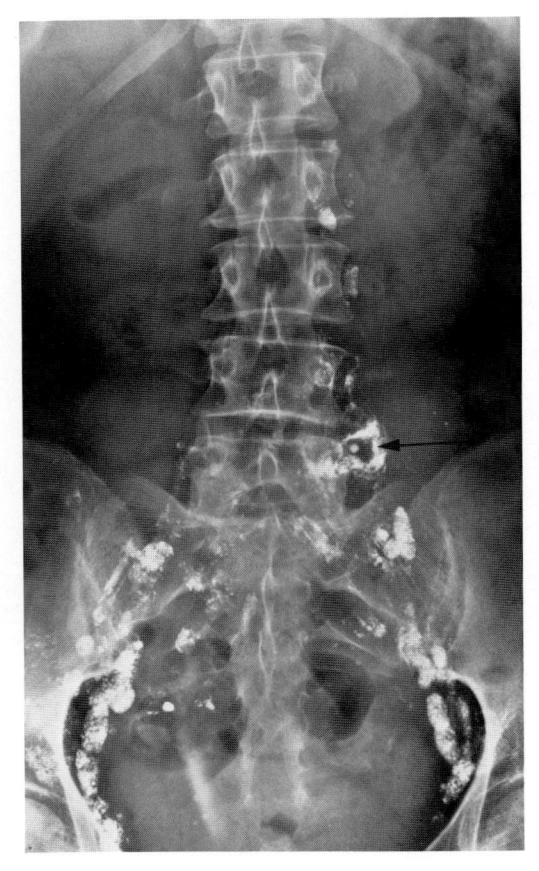

FIG. 2. Bipedal lymphangiogram demonstrates generalized enlargement of pelvic nodes bilaterally, as well as a filling defect in a retroperitoneal node (*arrow*) due to metastatic involvement by ovarian cancer.

may also not be determined by ultrasound. Quinn studied the pattern of cystic ovarian teratomas (12). One was purely cystic, but the remaining 12 all contained at least one dermoid plug or mural nodule. Mural nodules varied from 1.5 to 4.0 cm in diameter, and 13 of 15 were hyperechoic. This pattern was thought to be characteristic for this tumor (Fig. 4). Although simple ovarian cysts and dermoid cysts may be diagnosed sonographically, the pattern of other lesions is nonspecific.

Goldstein et al. found that postmenopausal women with single, unilocular adnexal cysts up to 5 cm in diameter all had benign pathology (13). Of 42 women studied, 26 underwent surgery, and the remaining 16 were followed. No malignant tissue was found in unilocular postmenopausal cysts. Granberg found one malignancy in 296 unilocular ovarian cysts (0.3%) (14). Sixty percent of the women who had unilocular cysts were over age 40. Multilocular cysts were malignant in 8% of cases (20 of 229), 70% (147 of 209) of multilocular solid tumors were malignant, and 39% (31 of 80) of solid tumors were malignant. In the evaluation of cystic masses, papillary vegetation on the cyst wall was most frequent in malignant tumors, but neither the thickness of the cyst wall nor that of septae correlated with malignancy. Simple cysts up to 10 cm in diameter were benign. In another study of 65 epithelial ovarian carcinomas, characteristics of malignant tumors were irregular borders and association with ascites or peritoneal growths (15). The diagnosis of malignancy had a sensitivity and specificity of 84.7% and 92.3%, respectively. Hurmann found sonographic evidence of malignancy in only 38 of the 52 (73%) women with malignant ovarian masses (16). Another series of 100 women undergoing surgery for ovarian masses found that ultrasound predicted a correct pathologic diagnosis in only 68% of cases, and sonography was frankly misleading in 15% of cases (17). Ovarian malignancy was correctly identified in 24 of 30 women, for a sensitivity of 80%. The positive and negative predictive values for adnexal malignancy were 73% and 91%, respectively. Another study noted that patterns of internal consistency, septae, papillary projections, and tumor borders are nonspecific (18). Although a dermoid tumor may be reliably diagnosed, other adnexal tumors are indistinguishable. However, loss of wall definition (Fig. 5), omental involvement, and ascites were again noted to suggest malignancy in the study. Also, as tumor echogenicity increases, the likelihood of malignancy increases (19). This is due to increasing amounts of solid material within these masses. The exceptions are an echogenic plug within a dermoid cyst or masses that are almost totally echogenic or solid.

Although the sonographic pattern of tumors is nonspecific (Fig. 6), usual patterns exist for many ovarian neoplasms. Serous tumors are cystic, cystadenomas usually large, thin-walled, possibly septated masses with few internal echoes. Serous cystadenocarcinomas show more internal architecture, with multiple septae and papillary projections. Focal areas of mural thickening may also be present. Ascites may be associated with either, but it is more common with the malignant type (20) (Fig. 7). Mucinous tumors are also largely cystic, and a similar pattern is seen in benign and malignant types, although mucinous cystadenocarcinoma often contains more solid elements than its benign counterpart. As with serous tumors, the presence of fixation to surrounding structures and increasing mural irregularity suggest malignancy.

Solid ovarian neoplasms may also be found. They have been described with some germ cell tumors and in Brenner tumors of the ovary (7,21). The latter have been described sonographically as a hypoechoic solid mass, often with peripheral calcification. They cannot be reliably differentiated from other solid, benign adnexal tumors such as fibromas, thecomas, or exophytic uterine leiomyomas.

The differential for the usual, complex pattern of primary ovarian neoplasms includes a variety of other disease processes. Metastases to the adnexa can pres-

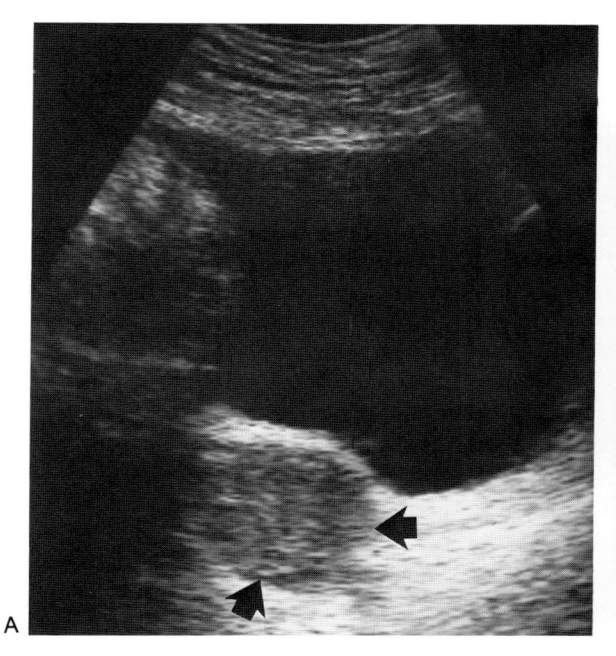

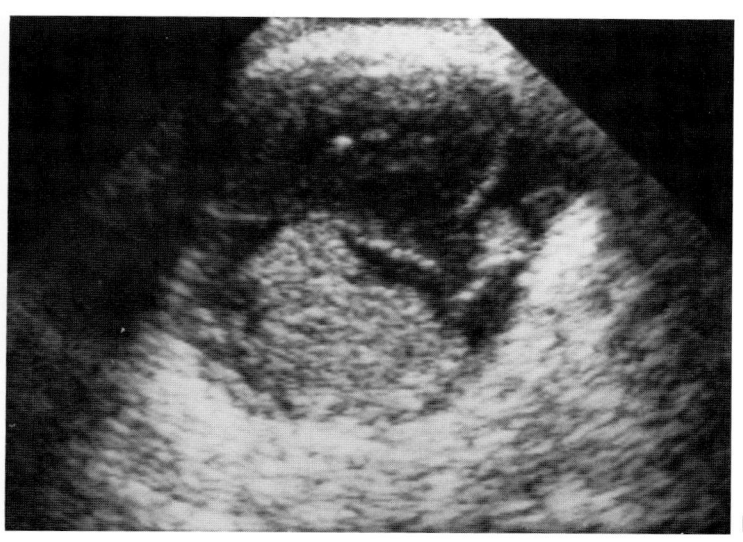

FIG. 3. Recurrent ovarian cancer scanned transabdominally **(A)** and transvaginally **(B)**. Transabdominal scanning shows the presence of a solid mass (*arrows*) at the vaginal apex. Internal texture is poorly defined. Transvaginal scanning shows the heterogeneity of the internal architecture of this complex tumor mass.

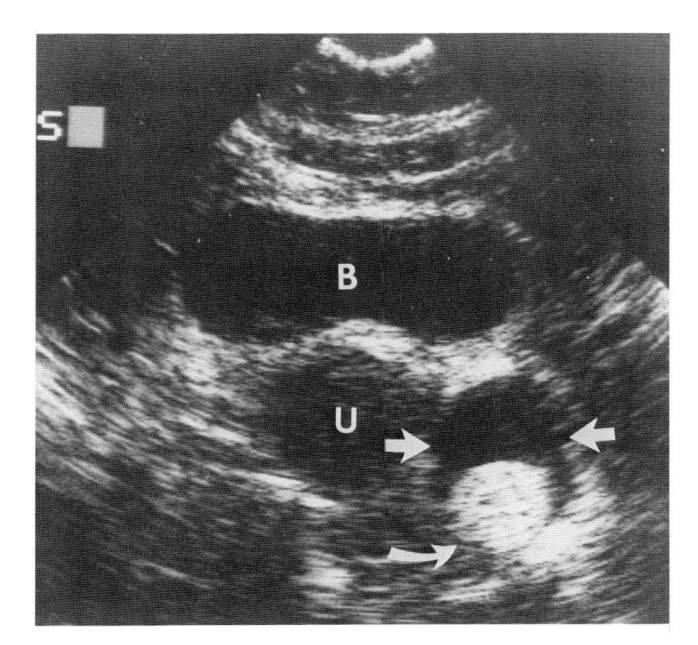

FIG. 4. Transverse transabdominal ultrasound shows a complex left adnexal mass (*arrows*) with a brightly echogenic focus (*curved arrow*). This pattern is characteristic for a dermoid cyst. (*B*, bladder; *U*, uterus).

ent an identical pattern of a complex, largely cystic mass with solid components. These metastases are usually due to primary tumors of the breast or gastrointestinal tract (22). Solid metastases are associated with leukemia and lymphoma (23). Benign, multicystic processes that mimic ovarian carcinoma sonographically include a multicystic ovary of ovarian hyperstimulation syndrome, pelvic inflammatory disease, nonadnexal inflammatory processes such as appendicitis and diverticulitis, and tumors originating in adjacent structures (24,25).

Sonography is usually more successful in localizing pelvic masses. Wu and Siegel have examined the utility of pelvic sonography in 70 girls ranging in age from neonates to 19 years (26). Although the researchers included no malignant lesions in this series, they concluded that the site of origin could be reliably determined sonographically but that the sonographic pattern of masses was nonspecific. In 10 women with androgen-secreting benign tumors, the results were more disappointing (27). However, none of these tumors were ovarian. Nonpalpable tumors—those less than 2 cm^3—could usually not be found by sonography.

Recent work has suggested that Doppler interrogation of adnexal masses may be useful in differentiating benign from malignant disease. Hata and colleagues (28) reported on Doppler studies of 105 women, of whom 8 had ovarian carcinoma. No abnormal flow was found in normal women, and only 8 of 44 women (18.2%) with benign tumors, all of which were of uter-

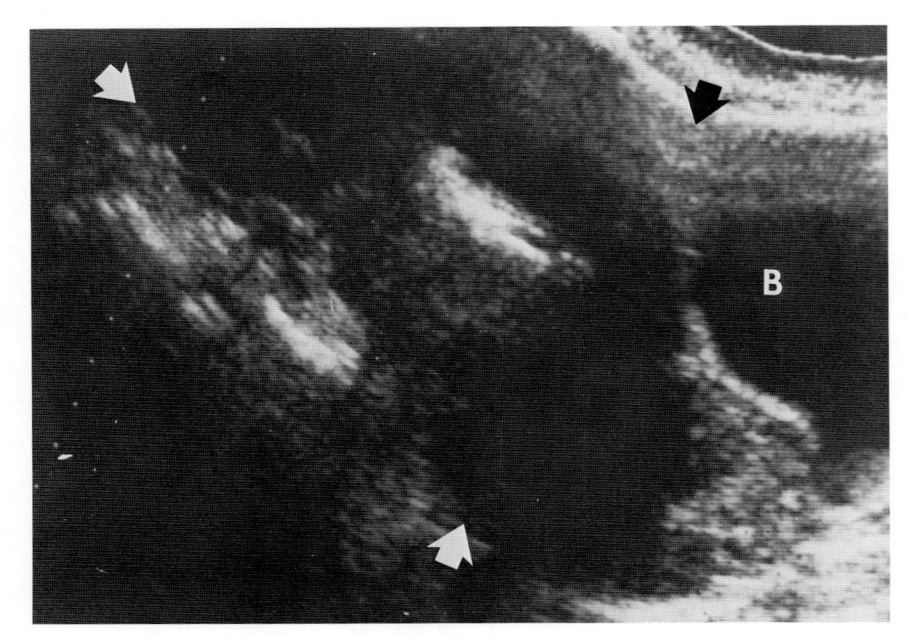

FIG. 5. Sagittal ultrasound of an ovarian leiomyosarcoma (*arrows*) shows a poorly marginated mass in a pattern characteristic for tumor which is locally invading surrounding structures. (*B*, bladder).

ine origin, were found to have abnormal flow patterns. All women with ovarian cancer, as well as all those with endometrial carcinoma and trophoblastic disease, had abnormal flow patterns. If all malignancies in this series were considered, an abnormal flow pattern had a sensitivity and specificity of 42% and 83%, respectively. However, for ovarian carcinoma, the sensitivity and specificity were 100%. Following chemotherapy, most patients also showed a decrease in tumor blood flow.

These data are supported by a more recent study by Kurjak et al. (29). Kurjak's study group contained 56 women with malignant ovarian masses, nine of which were metastatic. Abnormal Doppler signals were found in six of seven stage I ovarian cancers and 39 of 40 stage III and IV ovarian cancers. Metastatic disease to the ovary did not reliably show abnormal flow patterns, although they were often secondary to hypervascular primary tumors of the breast, thyroid, and rectum. In the entire population of 14,317 women in this study, which included 640 women with benign and malignant pelvic masses, the sensitivity and specificity for Doppler assessment of adnexal masses were 96.4% and 99.8%, respectively, with a positive predictive value of 98.2%.

In addition to its use in evaluating the primary tumor, ultrasound is useful in the further work-up of the patient with ovarian cancer. The ability to image hepatic metastases (Fig. 8) and hydronephrosis helps in staging disease. Ascites is readily imaged, and peritoneal implants are also sometimes visible. As with other imaging techniques, the absence of findings may be a less accurate indication of the extent of disease. Lund and colleagues studied 50 women with CT and ultrasound before second- and third-look laparotomy to determine if these modalities could preclude this surgery (30). Only metastases larger than 2 cm could be detected by either modality. If undetected microscopic disease was included as a false negative result, then the negative predictive values for ultrasound and CT were 47% and 45%, respectively. If microscopic disease is not included, then these values were 60% for both modalities. Lund's group concluded that neither modality was sensitive enough to replace second-look laparotomy.

Other researchers have found similar disappointing results. Murolo found that ultrasound was negative before second-look laparotomy in 94 of 129 women and positive in 35. At surgery, 57 were in complete pathologic remission, 16 had microscopic residual disease, 23 had macroscopic disease less than 2 cm in diameter, and 33 had macroscopic disease greater than 2 cm (31). Sonography was able to reliably identify women with no residual disease, with a 92.2% correlation with surgical results. However, women with microscopic disease or macroscopic disease less than 2 cm could not be identified by sonography.

The ability of sonography to identify residual or recurrent disease in the peritoneal cavity may depend on the site of disease. In 98 women undergoing follow-up laparotomy after chemotherapy, 94% of disease in the pelvis could be sonographically detected (32). This was more sensitive than physical examination. Only sheet-like lesions were undetectable. In the liver, 91% of metastases were identified. However, tumor within the

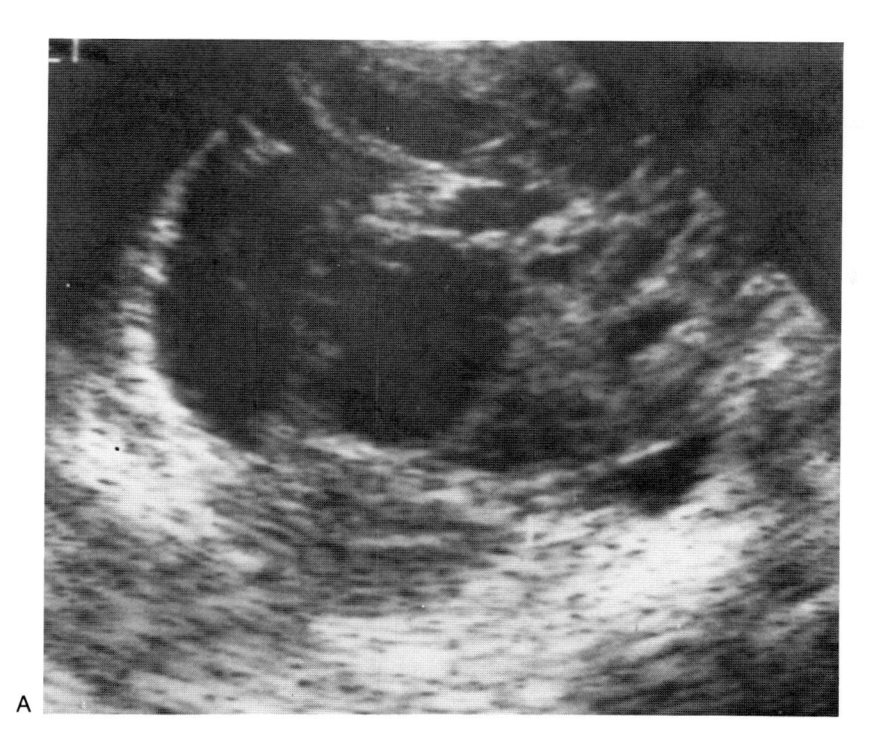

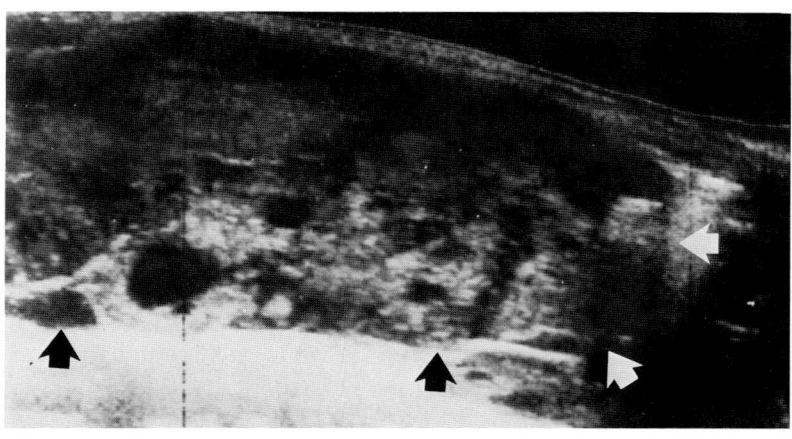

FIG. 6. (A) Transvaginal sonogram of an endodermal sinus tumor shows a complex mass containing large elements of fluid within this ovarian cancer. (B) Sagittal scan of the lower abdomen shows a large ovarian cancer (arrows) extending from the pelvis into the lower abdomen. This tumor is largely solid, containing a paucity of fluid elements.

peritoneal cavity was not readily detected, with even large tumors being missed.

Recent work has demonstrated that, in the sonographic work-up of suspected recurrence of pelvic disease, transrectal sonography is superior to routine transabdominal sonography. In a series of 52 women with signs or symptoms of pelvic recurrence, of whom 18 had ovarian cancer, transrectal sonography was performed in 50 (33). One woman was not studied because of a rectovaginal fistula, and discomfort precluded examination in another. Transrectal sonography was able to define recurrence in the vaginal cuff region, the bladder, presacrally, and at the pelvic sidewalls. Tumors as small as 1.2 cm in their shortest diameter and 2.3 cm in greatest diameter could be visualized. No disease beyond the true pelvis could be seen with this technique. In comparison to transabdominal sonography, transrectal studies gave additional information in the central pelvis in 19%, at the pelvic sidewalls in 25%, and in the presacral region in 33%. Transrectal sonography was shown to be superior to CT in all areas.

Another series of 21 women with clinically suspected pelvic recurrence included 3 women with ovarian cancer (34). Criteria for recurrence included increased anteroposterior diameter of the vaginal cuff measuring greater than 2.2 cm, presence of a mass at the vaginal cuff, structural alteration of the vaginal cuff, or infiltration of the rectovaginal septum, bladder, or parametria. Transrectal sonography had true positive and true negative findings for recurrence in 9 and 10 cases, respectively, with 2 false positive studies. Transabdominal scanning had true positive and true negative studies in 3 and 7 cases, respectively, with 2 false positive and 3 false negative studies. Transrectal examination had

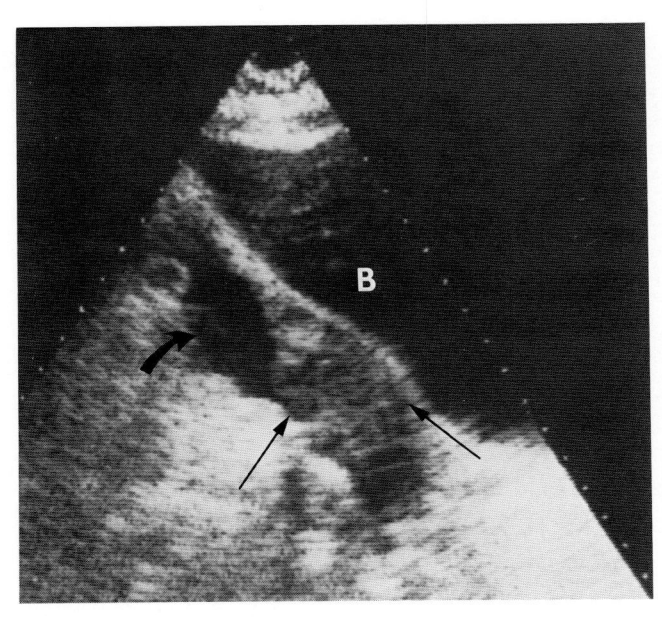

FIG. 7. Sagittal scan through the pelvis shows a papillary adenocarcinoma (*arrows*) with an associated small volume of ascites (*curved arrow*). (*B*, bladder).

a sensitivity of 100%, a specificity of 83.3%, and an overall accuracy of 90.5%. Its superiority to routine transabdominal scanning in this setting seems clear.

Interest has grown recently in the utilization of sonography to screen asymptomatic women for ovarian cancer. Abnormal ovarian size or morphology signals tumor; in women undergoing serial examination, change in ovarian volume on follow-up scan can also indicate the presence of tumor (35). Campbell et al. used transabdominal sonography in a prospective study of 5,479 asymptomatic women (36). They reported five cases of ovarian cancer, including four stage IA and one stage IB. No evidence that any cases of ovarian cancer were missed was reported. The false positive rate was 2.3%. Transabdominal screening was also attempted (37) in another group of 115 women who were at high risk for ovarian cancer. No cancers were found. However, in postmenopausal women, sonography was capable of identifying 87% of ovaries, whereas at gynecologic examination only 30% could be palpated. In premenopausal women, sonography detected 92% of ovaries. This suggests an advantage to examining these asymptomatic women by sonography.

Other evidence supports the idea that transvaginal sonography improves the ability to detect early ovarian cancers. Fleischer et al. reported on the transvaginal

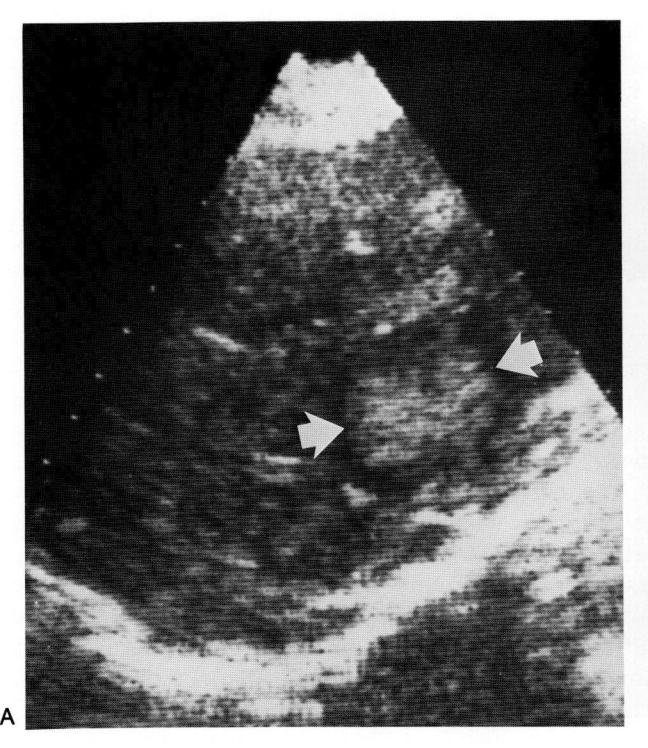

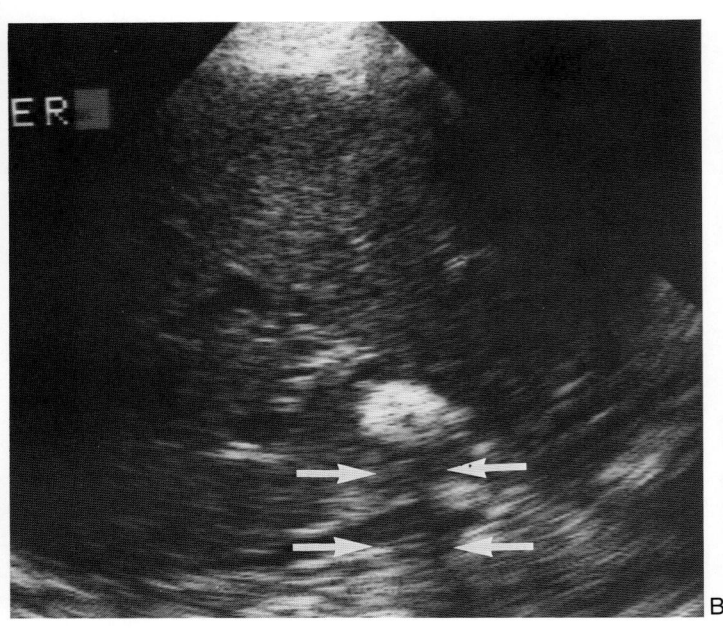

FIG. 8. (**A**) A solitary hepatic metastasis is demonstrated sonographically by disruption of the normal liver echotexture owing to the increased echogenicity of this metastatic focus (*arrows*). (**B**) Calcified, metastatic disease to the liver demonstrates a characteristic pattern of very bright echogenicity within the metastatic tumor accompanied by absence of echoes behind the tumor; that is, acoustic shadowing (*arrows*).

sonography of 67 ovaries in 34 postmenopausal women (38). Sixty percent of ovaries could be imaged. Normal postmenopausal ovaries measured 2.2 ± 0.7 cm by 1.2 ± 0.3 cm by 1.1 ± 0.6 cm, with an average volume of 2.6 ± 2.0 cm^3. The average size of nonvisualized ovaries at pathology was 0.7 × 0.4 cm, and five of six were atrophic on pathologic examinations. Four tumors, all benign, were missed and ranged in size from 0.5 cm to 6.0 cm. None were palpable. Nine adnexal lesions were detected, including three serous cystadenomas and one tubal carcinoma. In this study, the positive predictive value for detection of an ovarian lesion was 94%, and the negative predictive value for exclusion of an ovarian mass was 92%.

Transvaginal sonography was used in another study of 1,000 asymptomatic women 40 years old or older (39). For premenopausal ovaries, the upper limit for normal ovarian volume was 18 cm^3, and in postmenopausal women this was 8 cm^3. Of 31 women with abnormal scans, 24 underwent laparotomy. All tumors were identical in size to the dimensions seen on sonography. One adenocarcinoma was found, and all other tumors were benign, including eight serous cystadenomas. All normal patients have been rescreened, and there was no evidence that disease was missed in any of these women.

The use of color Doppler with transvaginal sonography has been suggested to improve the specificity of screening for ovarian cancer. Boune has examined the efficacy of using abnormal color patterns, which are caused by increased blood flow owing to neovascularity, as well as an abnormal pulsatility index (i.e., altered impedance to blood flow) as an indication of malignancy in women with abnormal-appearing ovaries on transvaginal sonography (40). In women with abnormal ovarian morphology, 9 of 10 with benign masses showed no alteration in color flow or pulsatility index, but 7 women with ovarian cancer showed alterations in both of these parameters. One woman with a small ovarian cystadenocarcinoma failed to demonstrate any change. This small study indicated that color flow imaging may be useful in decreasing the false positive rate of transvaginal sonography for ovarian carcinoma.

Not all researchers have found sonography to be a worthwhile technique for screening for ovarian cancer. In a study of 801 women 40 years old or older who were at high risk for ovarian cancer, 163 women had abnormal scans, and 3 were found to have significant tumors (41). These included two cases of endometrial carcinoma and one borderline malignant ovarian tumor. The authors believed that the uterine tumors would become clinically apparent within a short period and that sonography was not efficacious as a screening modality for ovarian cancer. However, the Ultrasonography Task Force of the American Medical Association has concluded that "transvaginal sonography, coupled with Doppler technology, may be of value in the early diagnosis of ovarian cancer, particularly when used in conjunction with other clinical data, such as tumor markers" (42).

COMPUTED TOMOGRAPHY

CT is advantageous in studying women with ovarian cancer because of its ability to image not only the true pelvis, but also the upper abdomen and hypogastrium, including areas not readily accessible to sonography. Additionally, when indicated, evaluation of the chest and skeleton are possible.

Proper examination requires the administration of both oral and intravenous contrast material. Limiting factors include a paucity of fat, which especially increases the difficulty of evaluating the retroperitoneum. As with sonography, CT patterns are often nonspecific. The identification of small retroperitoneal lymph nodes is nondiagnostic and may represent either reactive or neoplastic adenopathy.

No appreciable difference in the ability of CT versus sonography to demonstrate pelvic masses has been shown. In a prospective study of 74 patients, CT was able to detect 96% of pelvic masses as compared to a 91% detection rate by sonography (43). In the staging of recurrent disease, both modalities had an equivalent accuracy of 81%, although CT was superior in staging newly diagnosed tumors. This study group included cervical and endometrial carcinomas as well as benign masses. In a recent series of 130 women with 170 epithelial ovarian tumors, CT was able to detect 87% of tumors, and sonography could detect 86% (44). Benign serous cystadenomas were characterized with a sensitivity of 69% by CT and 70% by ultrasound; benign mucinous cystadenomas were characterized with a sensitivity of 62% by CT and 50% by sonography. In 14 borderline tumors, CT suggested malignancy in 64% and sonography in 36%. The overall accuracy of identifying malignant disease was 94% by CT and 80% by sonography. The sensitivity of CT was superior, but no difference in the specificity of the two modalities was found.

Normand et al. found CT and sonography complementary in evaluating women with ovarian cancer (45). Their retrospective study of 184 patients with ovarian tumors demonstrated superiority of sonography for the detection of pelvic masses, hepatic metastases, and urinary tract obstruction. CT was superior in detecting adenopathy as well as peritoneal and gastrointestinal involvement.

In characterizing benign versus malignant disease by CT, Rhode and Steinbrich reported an 81% accuracy (46). In their study, criteria for benign ovarian neoplasms included thin walls, smooth borders, homogeneous density, no hypervascularity, and no evidence of metastatic disease. Ascites was not uniformly considered a malignant finding. For malignant disease, the criteria were irregular mural thickening, irregular borders, inhomogeneous density, nodular internal architecture, irregular calcification, increased vascularity, and evidence of metastatic disease. The failure to accurately characterize 19% of tumors with these criteria points out the limitations of CT characterization. The authors were also unable to characterize granulosa cell tumors or dysgerminomas that presented as solid masses, unless metastatic disease was present.

Although not pathognomonic for various histologic types of tumor, there are some characteristic CT patterns. Epithelial tumors account for 90% of ovarian tumors and, when well-differentiated, are predominantly cystic, fluid-filled structures (47). On CT these can vary from a purely fluid-filled mass to a mixed solid and cystic mass or even appear solid in poorly differentiated neoplasms (Fig. 9). Irregular mural thickening and nodularity and the presence of septations are characteristic findings. Extracapsular extension is manifested by poor definition of margins (46). Poorly defined, irregular calcifications may also be present

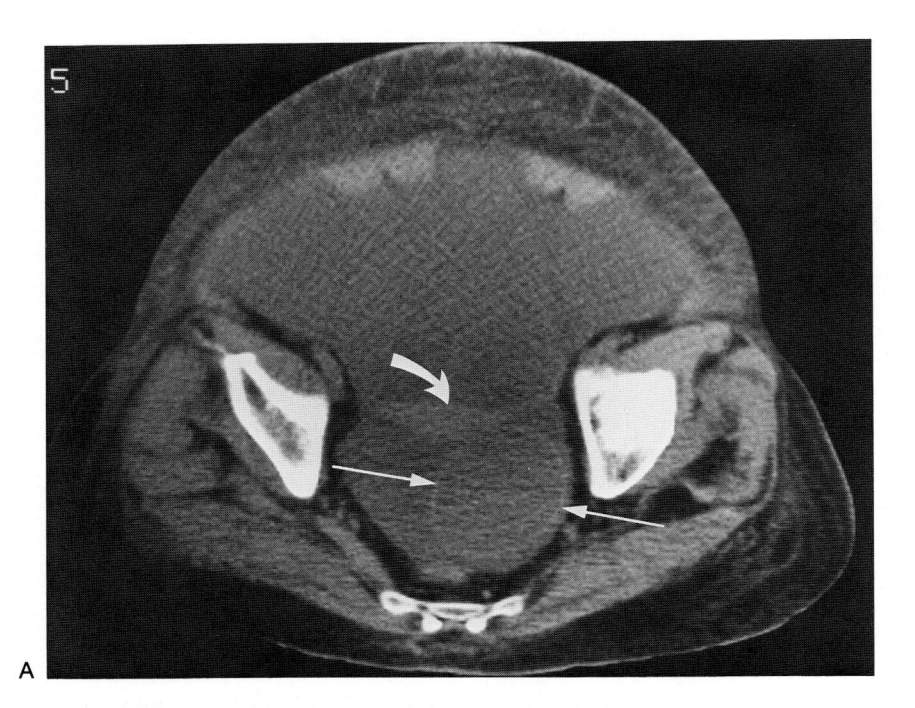

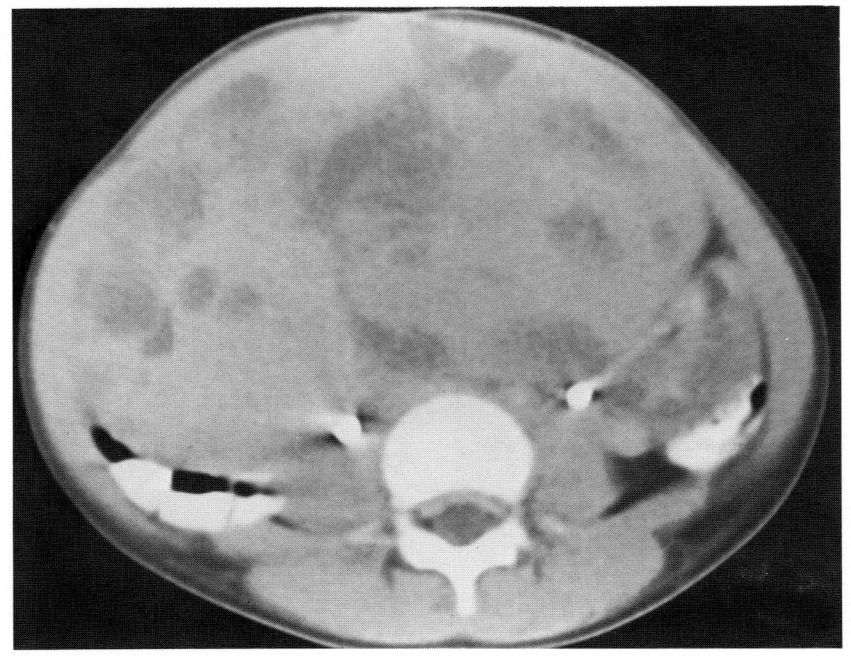

FIG. 9. CT scans of primary ovarian cancers. The primary neoplasm can vary in appearance from a purely cystic mass with a thin wall **(A)** to a predominantly solid mass containing cystic areas which was a granulosa theca cell tumor **(B)**. Note the presence of ascites in (A), outlining the primary mass (*arrows*) and uterus (*curved arrow*).

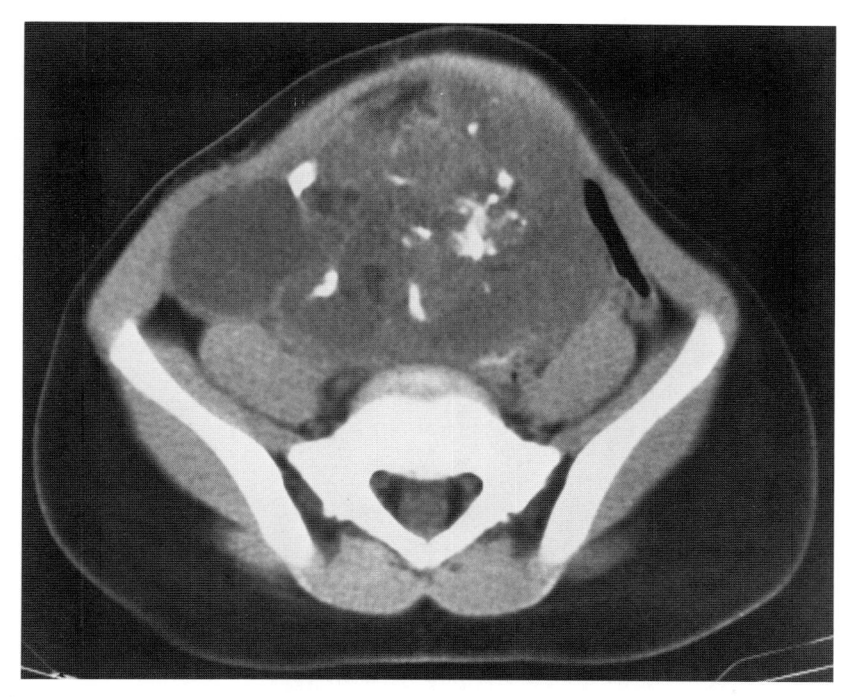

FIG. 10. CT of malignant teratoma in an 8-year-old girl. The bulky mass contains solid and cystic areas as well as multiple irregular and amorphous calcifications.

(Fig. 10). Intravenous contrast material should be given by bolus technique and can demonstrate enhancement owing to tumor neovascularity. This enhancement may not be evident when contrast has been administered by drip infusion (48). A similar CT pattern may be found with inflammatory processes, and these may not be easily differentiated from tumors. Solid primary malignancy may also be mimicked by metastatic disease (49). Clinical history usually makes the appropriate diagnosis obvious in this setting. A characteristic CT pattern is present in an adnexal mass containing a focal calcification, fat-fluid level, and a solid mass projecting inside the lesion; the diagnosis of dermoid cyst is possible in this setting (50). However, malignant change in these lesions cannot be diagnosed without evidence of metastatic spread.

Although it is valuable for evaluating masses in the adnexae, CT is most important in determining whether disease has spread beyond the ovary. Peritoneal deposits are often present (Fig. 11) and frequently measure 1 cm or smaller. These smaller lesions usually are not resolvable by CT. The common occurrence of metastatic seeding to the diaphragm and hepatic capsule requires that these areas be included on studies for staging of ovarian cancer (48). Calcification within these implants, when this pattern is present, makes them more easily identifiable (Fig. 12). Otherwise, thin CT sections may be necessary to evaluate for their presence.

As with sonography, ascites is readily detected by CT (Fig. 13). Small volumes accumulating in the cul-de-sac or flanks can be diagnosed (51). The presence of ascites also facilitates the diagnosis of peritoneal implants, especially when smaller than 1 cm (52). These implants are usually difficult to define by CT. Buy et al. found that CT diagnosed metastatic seeding in 17 of 27 women (63%) and in 63 of 104 biopsy sites (61%) (53). The sites most commonly involved were the right subphrenic region, the pouch of Douglas, and the greater omentum. Another study of metastases from serous carcinomas of the ovary noted that, although peritoneal metastases are often difficult to discover by CT, calcifications are not unusual in peritoneal or nodal metastases (Fig. 14) from this tumor and can make the identification of metastatic sites easy (54).

Giunta et al. described a technique for improving the visualization of peritoneal metastases (55). In 33 women with known ovarian cancer but without CT evidence of metastases or ascites, 3000 cc of 2.4% nonionic contrast material was injected intraperitoneally. With this technique, a diagnosis of peritoneal seeding was made in 22 women. Of these 22 diagnoses, 19 were true positives, and 3 were false positives. Metastases smaller than 1 cm could be visualized. Compartmentalization of the peritoneal cavity was apparent, and whether lesions were intraperitoneal or extraperitoneal could be determined. These data were important in determining whether to utilize intraperitoneal chemother-

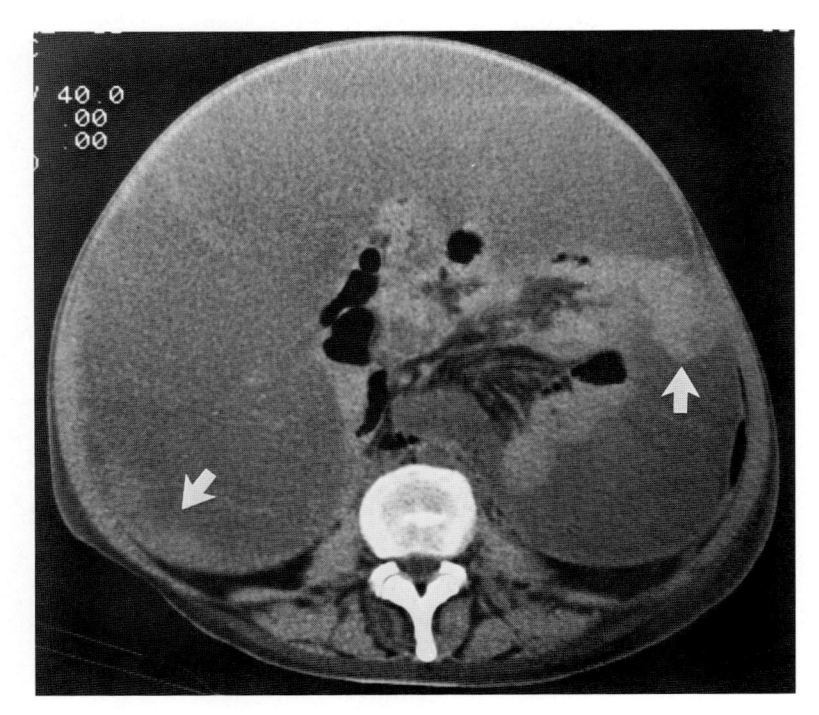

FIG. 11. CT image demonstrates the presence of tense ascites, which displaces small bowel loops and mesentery centrally, allowing identification of peritoneal deposits (*arrows*).

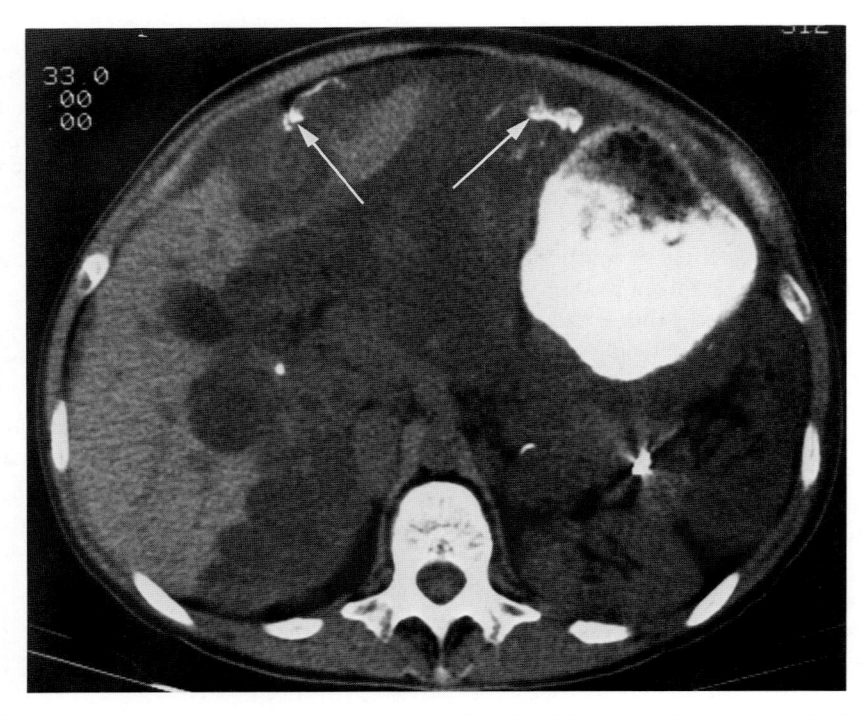

FIG. 12. CT image demonstrates pseudomyxoma peritonei, which contains a characteristic pattern of amorphous, curvilinear calcifications (*arrows*).

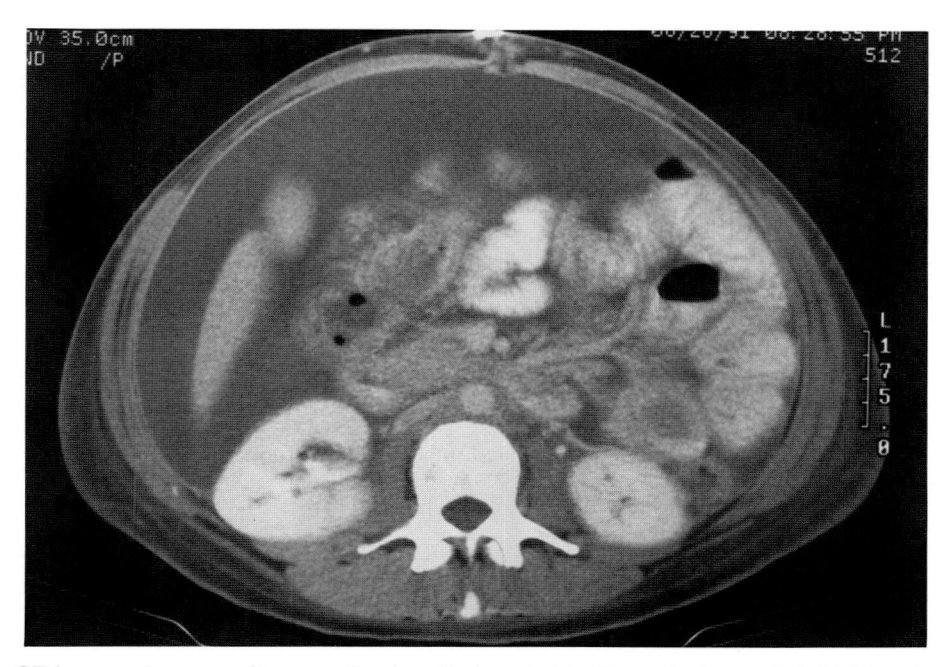

FIG. 13. CT image shows ascites, predominantly located in the anterior and right lateral portions of the abdomen.

apy. It was not possible to diagnose small omental lesions.

Mesenteric and omental metastases (Fig. 15) may be visualized by CT. Their patterns include rounded masses, cakelike masses, poorly defined masses, and stellate masses (56). In a study of 52 women, Whitley found that CT was 100% sensitive in identifying peritoneal, omental, and mesenteric disease, but the specificity of CT was low for disease in peritoneum (64%) and omentum (67%) and higher for mesenteric metastases (88%) (56). In patients with a small amount of intraperitoneal fat or with disease in continuity with the primary tumor, these masses may be difficult to appreciate.

CT scanning through the abdomen and pelvis allows evaluation of the nodal groups at risk for metastatic disease from ovarian cancers. Unlike lymphangiography, CT can visualize upper paraaortic and retrocrural nodes. Hypogastric nodes, which may not be opacified

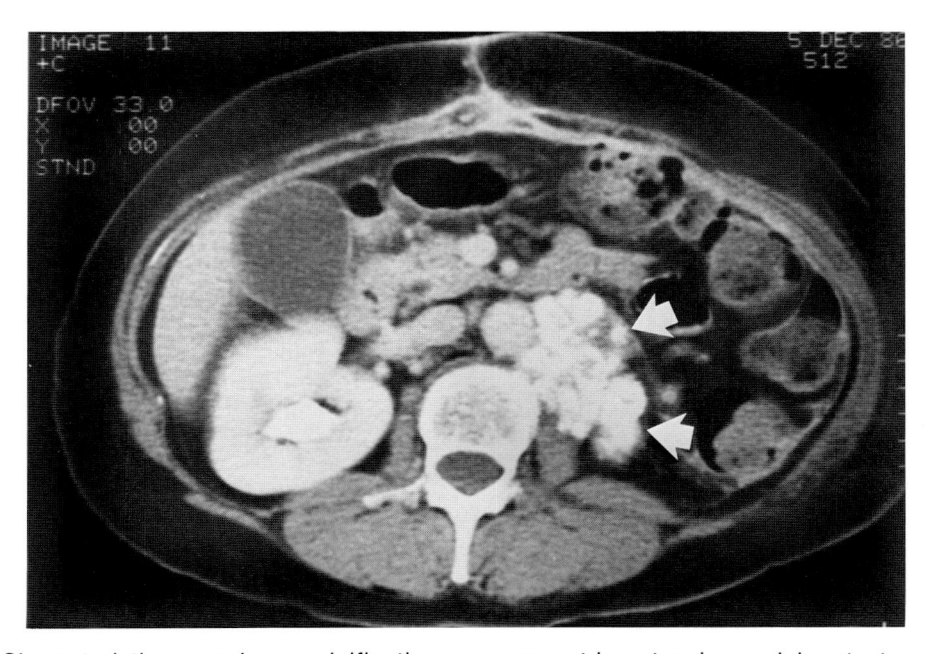

FIG. 14. Characteristic amorphous calcifications are present in extensive nodal metastases (*arrows*) from ovarian cancer. The left kidney is absent.

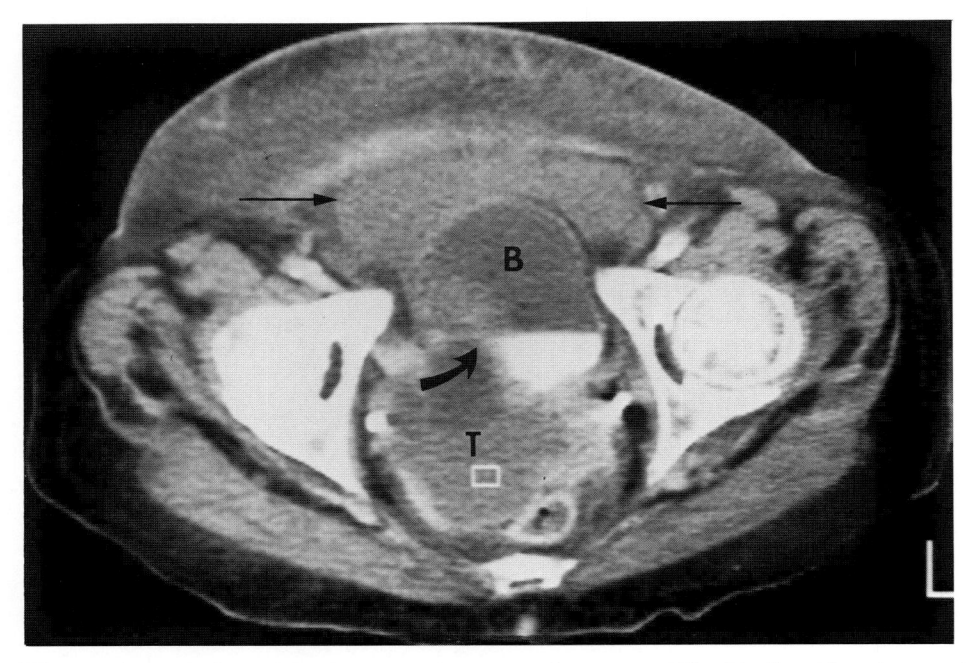

FIG. 15. CT scan through the pelvis shows a primary ovarian tumor (*T*) with direct involvement (*curved arrow*) of the adjacent bladder (*B*). Additionally, tumor caking along the anterior pelvic wall (*arrows*) is also present.

during lymphangiography, are also included on CT studies. CT manifests lymphadenopathy by the presence of nodal enlargement. Nodes that contain metastatic deposits but remain small, especially if smaller than 1 cm, will not be defined as abnormal by CT. Disruption of the internal architecture of these nodes can be diagnosed only by lymphangiography. In a comparison of CT findings with pathologic examination of nodes removed at second-look laparotomy, Goldhirsch and co-workers found a CT sensitivity of 83% in 26 patients whose nodes were removed if they were palpable and larger than 1 cm (57).

Other sites of disease can also be assessed by CT; renal (Fig. 16) and biliary obstruction, for example, are readily assessed. Involvement of the bowel is better imaged by barium study than with CT. However, CT findings of bowel involvement may be present. Oral contrast administration is mandatory to evaluate the gastrointestinal tract. CT may be superior to surgical exploration in assessing uterine involvement. In one report of seven women who had no evidence of uterine involvement intraoperatively, CT suggested uterine disease, and involvement of the uterus was confirmed at repeat surgery (58). Amendola reported a similar experience (48).

CT is also advantageous in the evaluation of more distant disease (Fig. 17). Pulmonary metastases and pleural effusions may be readily evident on chest CT but not seen on routine chest radiographs (Fig. 18). They may contain characteristic calcifications (59).

Cerebral metastases, although rare in ovarian cancer, are also amenable to CT diagnosis. In 14 women in whom cerebral metastases were identified, all lesions were enhanced with intravenous contrast and were located in the cerebral hemispheres (60). Nine of these patients had single lesions. This study suggested that early diagnosis and resection of these metastases may improve overall survival in some patients.

The ability of CT or any other radiologic technique to replace second- or third-look laparotomy has not been demonstrated. When measurable disease is present, these findings are accurate, but a negative CT study is not reliable for excluding abdominal or pelvic disease. Brenner examined 52 women with CT who were undergoing second-look laparotomy (61) and found that 42% of patients with a negative scan had residual tumor found at surgery. Many of these patients, however, had microscopic disease discovered only on peritoneal washings. Goldhirsch et al. conducted a similar study on 26 women (57). CT was negative in five women who had tumor larger than 1 cm. CT best evaluated nodal disease, of which 83% was detected. Sixty-three percent of residual pelvic tumor was detected; 50% of omental tumor was seen, but only 11% of disease at other locations could be identified preoperatively. Calkins found that in 57 patients on whom CT scans were performed before second-look laparotomy, only 9 of 25 women (36%) in whom disease was found surgically had disease that was visible on CT (62). Peritoneal seeding was present in the other 16

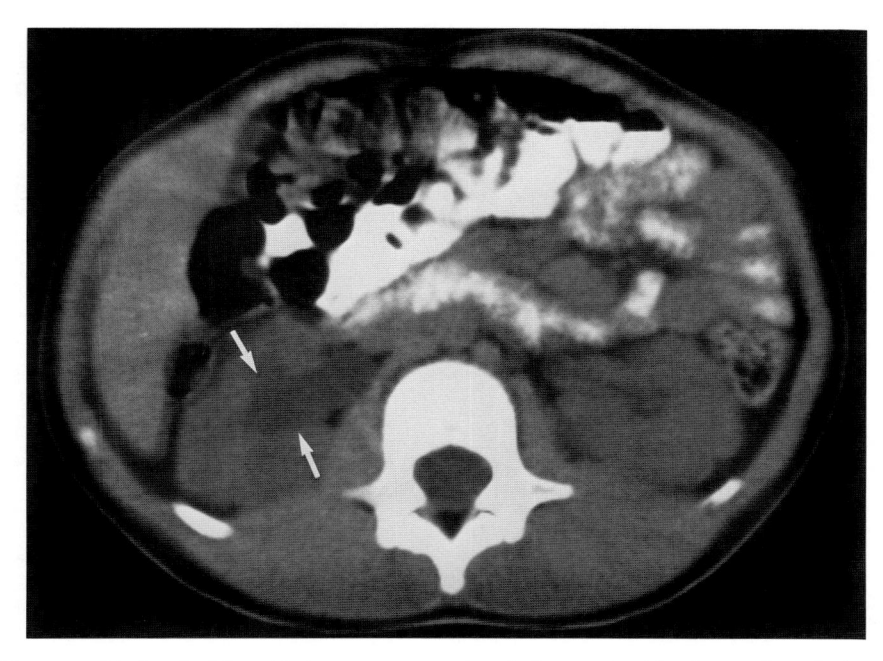

FIG. 16. CT image obtained without intravenous contrast shows right hydronephrosis (*arrows*), which is caused by a large pelvic ovarian tumor.

patients but could not be detected by CT. This failure to detect small, residual disease was also reported by Silverman et al. (63). In this study of 55 patients, CT correctly identified residual or recurrent pelvic disease in 85% (17 of 20) and 75% (3 of 4) of bulky abdominal disease, respectively. In women with carcinomatosis due to small tumor implants, disease was recognized on CT in only 2 of 24 cases (8%). For 280 surgical findings present, CT had a sensitivity of 40% and a specificity of 99%. Somewhat more encouraging results were reported in a study of 35 women with epithelial ovarian cancer (64). Surgical and CT findings were in agreement in 86% of cases.

One study has indicated efficacy for CT in evaluating

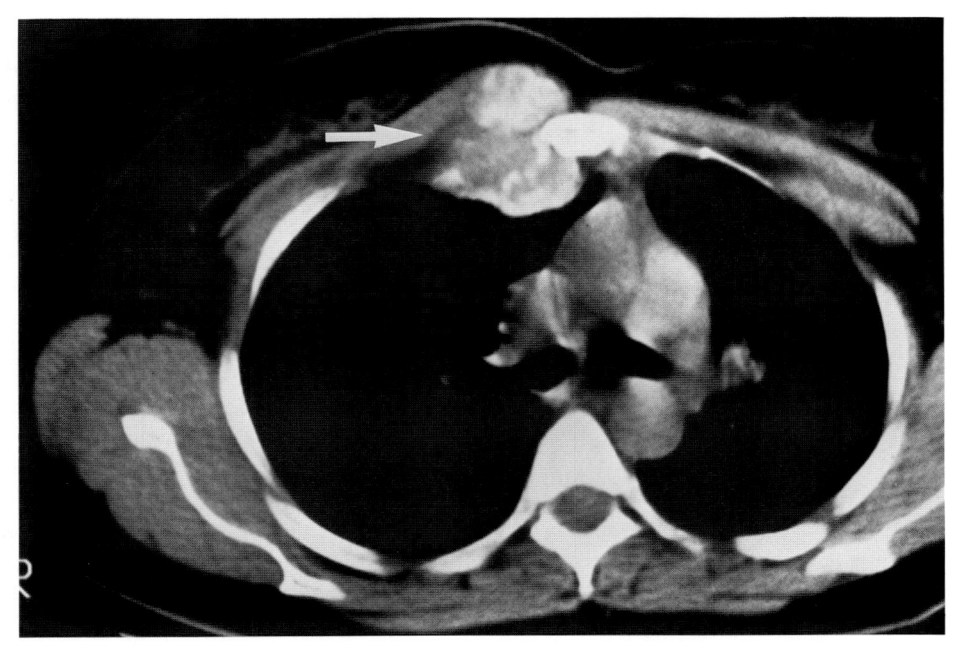

FIG. 17. CT scan through the mid chest shows a large, partially calcified ovarian cancer metastasis in the right anterior chest wall (*arrow*).

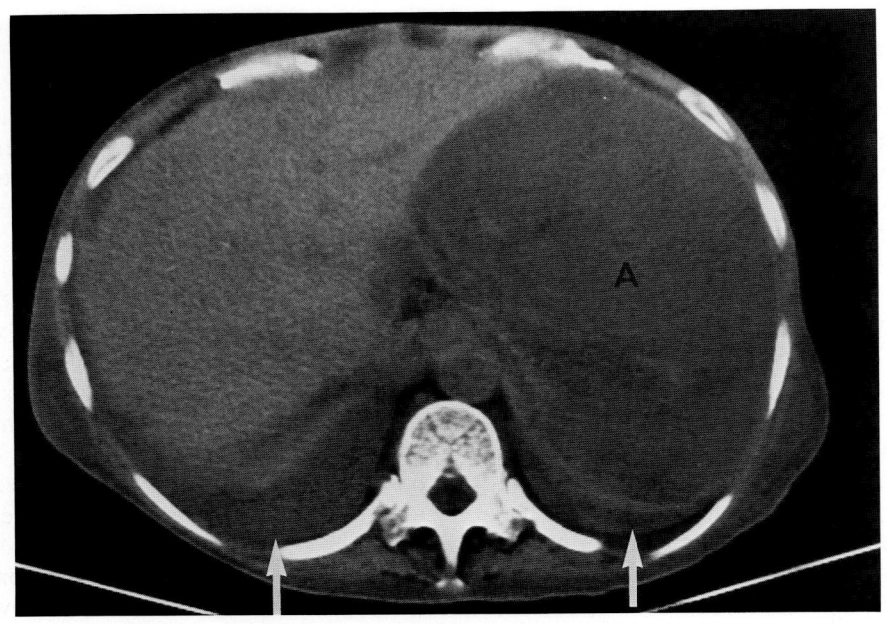

FIG. 18. CT scan through the lower chest demonstrates bilateral posterior fluid collection (*arrows*), which are in the pleural space and represent pleural effusion. In addition, a large septated collection of ascites (*A*) is present in the left upper quadrant of the abdomen.

response to therapy of known tumor (65). CT scans were done of 105 women with known disease to evaluate the effect of therapy. CT was capable of evaluating therapeutic response but was not reliable in determining complete remission or possible recurrence.

MAGNETIC RESONANCE IMAGING (MRI)

Although MR imaging has been in clinical use for less than a decade, the technique already has had a profound influence on the diagnosis, staging, and follow-up of many types of neoplasms throughout the body. In patients with ovarian cancer, however, its contributions and role relative to those of other imaging modalities have yet to be defined; indeed, as recently as 1990, McCarthy stated that "there is no particular role for MRI in the work-up of ovarian cancer" (66). Nevertheless, MR imaging can make important contributions in the work-up of some patients with ovarian tumors in certain circumstances.

MR imaging provides excellent contrast between different types of soft tissues, including normal and cancerous tissues, without the use of ionizing radiation. A complex interaction of carefully controlled radiowaves and magnetic fields allows images of startling clarity to be obtained. By selecting appropriate technical parameters, the radiologist can accentuate or minimize the brightness of various substances on the image, such as tumorous tissue, fat, water, or blood. The resulting images can not only depict the location and anatomic relationships of an ovarian mass but can also help characterize the composition and structure of the mass (66–82).

The entire abdomen and pelvis can be included on an MRI study, allowing assessment for distant metastatic disease in addition to local staging of an ovarian neoplasm. One current limitation in such an assessment is the lack of a suitable oral contrast agent to be administered during MR imaging; as a result, bowel loops may be indistinguishable from tumor deposits or normal adnexa.

MR images can be produced in any spatial plane desired; axial and coronal planes generally provide the most useful information in patients with ovarian neoplasms (72,75,78). Owing to the combination of its multiplanar capabilities and high soft-tissue contrast, MR imaging is very accurate in distinguishing adnexal from uterine masses; this ability is particularly valuable in cases that are indeterminate by sonography (66,72, 74–76,78,81). For example, MR imaging can differentiate a subserosal or pedunculated leiomyoma that has low signal intensity on all images from an ovarian malignancy that has increased signal intensity on T2-weighted images.

Most MR imaging examinations of patients with ovarian neoplasms are performed without administration of any intravenous contrast material. Gadolinium-DTPA (Gd-DTPA) is currently the only MRI contrast agent commercially available in the United States. One report has suggested that use of an intravenous contrast agent (Gd-DOTA, an analogue of Gd-DTPA) may improve tumor delineation and the depiction of internal structure of an ovarian mass, aiding in differential diagnosis; however, the degree of enhancement did not facilitate the distinction between benign and malignant masses (68). Nevertheless, studies involving large numbers of women with adnexal masses will need to be performed to define any benefit to the administration of MRI contrast materials.

Certain patients—those who harbor metallic aneurysm clips, cardiac pacemakers, metallic intraocular foreign bodies, or cochlear implants—cannot undergo MR imaging. Very large patients (generally those weighing more than 250 lb) may be unable to fit inside the magnet. Additionally, a small fraction of patients cannot tolerate the MRI examination, which may take more than 1 hour to complete, due to a claustrophobia-like reaction to being inside the MR imager; such patients may subsequently be able to complete the examination after receiving anxietolytic medication.

Infants and children younger than 6 years generally require sedation and very careful monitoring, often by an anesthesiologist, during an MRI examination. Pregnant patients can safely undergo MR imaging for further evaluation of suspected pelvic masses (79,82).

A normal ovary is seen as a relatively homogeneous, oval structure with low signal intensity similar to that of muscle on T1-weighted MR images; distinction between adnexa and adjacent bowel may be difficult on such images (66,68,75,78). On T2-weighted images, however, the normal ovary becomes brighter, similar to, or greater than the signal from fat. By contrast, the signal from the myometrium of the uterus is relatively low, similar to that of skeletal muscle, on T1- or T2-weighted images.

In one study, both normal adnexa were shown by MR imaging in 13 of 15 (87%) women of reproductive age, using contiguous 10-mm thick sections (75).

Follicles and nonhemorrhagic physiologic cysts within the ovary are hypointense relative to muscle on T1-weighted images, and they become quite intense on T2-weighted images; their signal intensity is similar to that of urine in the bladder on all types of images (66,69, 71,72,75).

Several studies involving small numbers of patients have shown relatively little specificity for the MR imaging appearance of ovarian masses, with the exception of cystic teratomas, hemorrhagic cysts, and endometriomas (71,75,77,80,81). A solid ovarian mass (benign or malignant) typically will be larger than a normal ovary and will have signal similar to that of skeletal muscle on T1-weighted images. On T2-weighted images, a solid mass will generally be less intense than urine but as intense as or brighter than fat. Areas of old hemorrhage within a mass will be bright on both T1- and T2-weighted images (77,78). A cystic ovarian mass, or the cystic component of a complex ovarian mass, may have signal intensity similar to that of urine on all images (75). If the fluid within the cystic mass has a high protein content or contains old blood, its signal intensity will be increased on T1-weighted images (75).

A cystic teratoma typically contains fat or sebum whose signal intensity remains similar to that of subcutaneous fat on all MR images (Fig. 19); additionally, the presence of fat produces a characteristic "chemical shift" artifact (66,80). Other common findings of cystic teratomas on MR imaging include gravity-dependent layering or floating debris, frond-like or nodular protrusions (plugs) from the cyst wall, or fat-fluid levels (80).

Masses with high signal intensity on both T1- and T2-weighted MR images often represent endometrio-

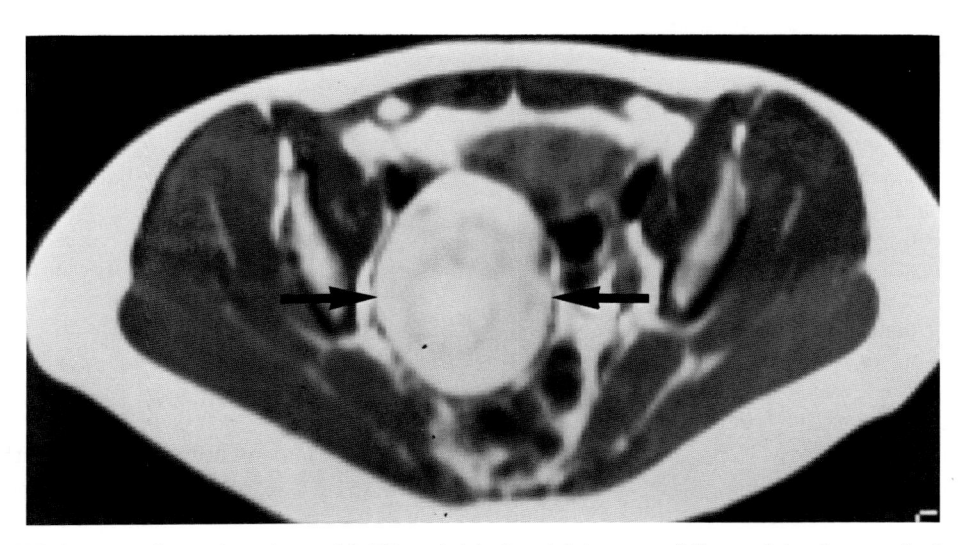

FIG. 19. MR image of ovarian dermoid. T1-weighted axial image of the pelvis demonstrates a right pelvic mass (*arrows*), the predominant signal intensity of which is identical to that of subcutaneous fat. This finding is characteristic of dermoid tissue.

mas or hemorrhagic cysts, although a hemorrhagic malignancy may have a similar appearance (75,77,78,81).

Any ability of MR imaging to differentiate benign from malignant ovarian masses is based more on the morphologic characteristics of a mass than on the MRI signal pattern; masses with thick septae, internal nodularity, or considerable soft-tissue components are very suspicious for representing malignancy (66). Experience with benign and malignant tumors elsewhere in the body strongly suggests that MR imaging is unlikely to obviate the need for biopsy of a suspect adnexal mass.

MR imaging can demonstrate evidence of metastatic disease from an ovarian malignancy, such as ascites, peritoneal deposits, lymphadenopathy, or liver metastases (Fig. 20). However, ascites is shown easily by sonography or CT, and peritoneal deposits generally are more evident on CT than MR imaging because of the lack of an MRI bowel contrast material. MR imaging may demonstrate subtle pelvic lymphadenopathy or liver metastases better than CT, although such superiority has yet to be reported specifically for patients with ovarian cancer.

SUMMARY

Imaging techniques can add important information to the diagnosis and management of women with ovarian cancer. Plain film studies may help confirm the presence of a mass or ascites, and patterns of calcification may narrow diagnostic considerations. Bowel gas patterns are useful to evaluate for the possibility of obstruction and may indicate the presence of carcinomatosis. Information traditionally obtained by intravenous pyelography can be readily ascertained with sectional imaging techniques, and this test is therefore rarely necessary in evaluating these patients. Barium

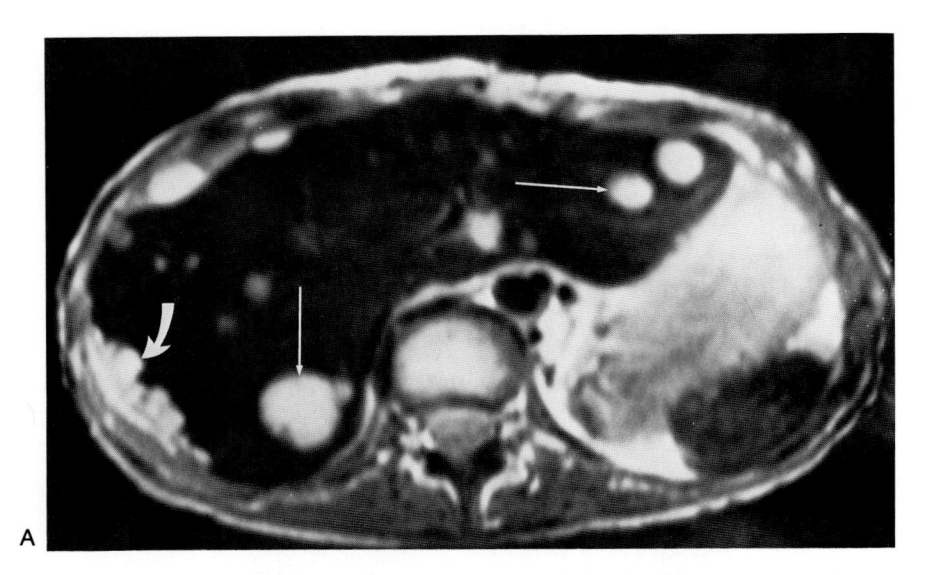

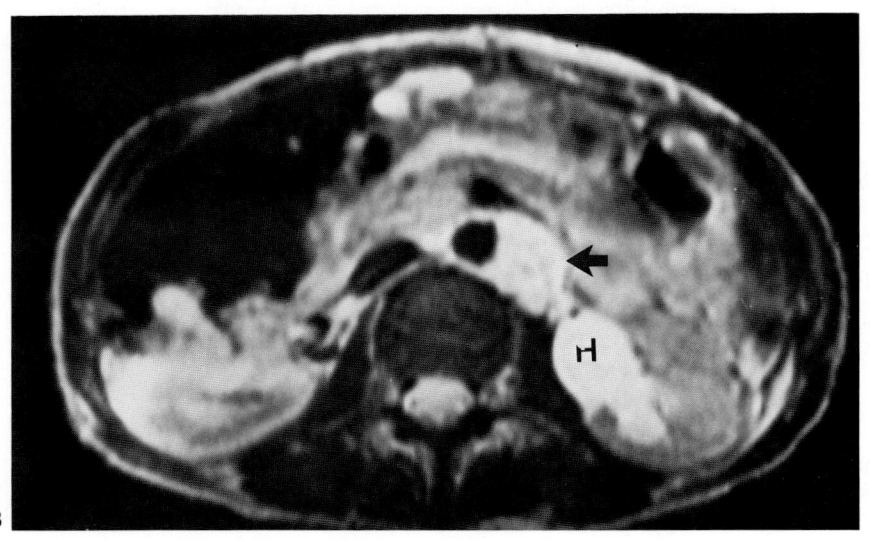

FIG. 20. T2-weighted MR images of metastatic ovarian cancer. **(A)** High signal intensity areas are present in the liver (*arrows*) as well as on the liver capsule (*curved arrow*) due to metastatic ovarian cancer. **(B)** Metastases are also evident in the paraaortic lymph nodes (*arrow*), causing left hydronephrosis (*H*).

studies, however, are the most sensitive in determining large and small bowel involvement by tumor. When available, lymphangiography can demonstrate small space-occupying nodal metastases within some pelvic and retroperitoneal lymph nodes. These nodal metastases, when they do not enlarge the node, cannot be diagnosed by any other modality.

Sectional imaging techniques, especially sonography and CT, are basic techniques in diagnosing, staging, and following women with ovarian cancer. The efficacy of MR imaging is less certain in this setting. These modalities can confirm the presence of an adnexal mass, although a pathologic diagnosis is rarely possible on the basis of the images that are produced. Sonography, especially when performed transvaginally and with Doppler, may be capable of effectively screening asymptomatic women at risk for ovarian cancer. Both CT and sonography can identify small volumes of ascites and large metastatic tumors. Sonography is less effective in the hypogastrium and in studying lymph nodes, and neither technique is very accurate in detecting small omental and mesenteric tumor seeding. Peritoneal implants are not reliably diagnosed, and microscopic disease cannot be detected. CT and sonography are reliable in following measurable disease in women being treated for known tumor, but negative scans do not preclude the presence of pelvic or abdominal disease. Therefore, when results of these studies are normal, CT and sonography do not eliminate the need for surgical exploration to restage women with known tumor.

REFERENCES

1. Hillman BJ, Clark RL, Babbit G. Efficacy of the excretory urogram in the staging of gynecologic malignancies. *Am J Roentgenol* 1984;143:997–999.
2. Meyers MA, McSweeney J. Secondary neoplasms of the bowel. *Radiology* 1972;105:1–11.
3. Meyers MA. Distribution of intra-abdominal malignant seeding: dependency on dynamics of flow of ascitic fluid. *Am J Roentgenol* 1973;119:198–206.
4. Yuhasz, Laufer I, Sutton G, Herlinger H, Caroline DF. Radiography of the small bowel in patients with gynecologic malignancies. *Am J Roentgenol* 1985;144:303–307.
5. Gedgaudas RK, Kelvin FM, Thompson WM, Rice RP. The value of preoperative barium-enema examination in the assessment of pelvic masses. *Radiology* 1983;146:609–613.
6. Ruebesin SE, Levine MS. Omental cakes: colonic involvement by omental metastases. *Radiology* 1985;154:593–596.
7. Lewis E, Wallace S. Radiologic diagnosis of ovarian cancer. In: Piver MS, ed. *Ovarian malignancies. Diagnostic and therapeutic advances*. Edinburgh: Churchill Livingstone 1987;59–80.
8. Athey PA, Wallace SA, Jing BS, et al. Lymphangiography in ovarian cancer. *Am J Roentgenol* 1975;123:106–113.
9. Fuchs WA. Malignant tumors of the ovary. In: Fuchs WA, Davidson JW, Fischer HW, eds. *Recent results in cancer research—lymphangiography in cancer*. New York: Springer-Verlag, 1969;119–123.
10. Douglas B, McDonald JS, Baker JW. Lymphangiography in carcinoma of the ovary. *Proc R Soc Med* 1971;54:400.
11. Musumeci F, Banfi A, Bolis G. Lymphangiography in patients with ovarian epithelial cancer: an evaluation of 289 consecutive cases. *Cancer* 1977;40:1444–1449.
12. Quinn SF, Erickson S, Black WC. Cystic ovarian teratomas: the sonographic appearance of the dermoid plug. *Radiology* 1985;155:477–478.
13. Goldstein SR, Subramanyam B, Synder JRT, et al. The postmenopausal cystic adnexal mass: the potential role of ultrasound in conservative management. *Obstet Gynecol* 1989;73:8–10.
14. Granberg S, Wikland M, Jansson I. Macroscopic characterization of ovarian tumors and the relation to the histologic diagnosis: criteria to be used for ultrasound evaluation. *Gynecol Oncol* 1989;35:139–144.
15. Conte M, Guariglia L, Benedetti Panici PL, et al. Ovarian carcinoma: an ultrasound study. *Eur J Gynaecol Oncol* 1990;11:33–36.
16. Hurmann UJ Jr, Locher GW, Goldhirsch A. Sonographic patterns of ovarian malignancy. *Obstet Gynecol* 1987;69:777–781.
17. Benacerraf BR, Finkler NJ, Wojciechoski C, Knapp RC. Sonographic accuracy in the diagnosis of ovarian masses. *J Reprod Med* 1990;35:491–495.
18. Achiron R, Schejter E, Malinger G, Zakut H. Observations on the ultrasound diagnosis of ovarian neoplasms. *Arch Gynecol Obstet* 1987;241:183–190.
19. Moyle JW, Rochester D, Sidler L, et al. Sonography of ovarian tumors: predictability of tumor type. *Am J Roentgenol* 1983;141:985–991.
20. Czernobilsky B. Primary epithelial tumors of the ovary. In: Blaustein A, ed. *Pathology of the female genital tract*. New York: Springer-Verlag, 1982;511–560.
21. Athey PA, Siegal MF. Sonographic features of Brenner tumor of the ovary. *J Ultrasound Med* 1987;6:367–372.
22. Rochester D, Levin B, Bowie JD, Kunzman A. Ultrasonic appearance of the Krukenberg tumor. *Am J Roentgenol* 1977;129:919–920.
23. Bickers GH, Siebert JJ, Anderson JC, et al. Sonography of ovarian involvement in childhood acute lymphocytic leukemia. *Am J Roentgenol* 1981;137:399–401.
24. Rankin RN, Hutton LC. Ultrasound in ovarian hyperstimulation syndrome. *J Clin Ultrasound* 1981;9:473–476.
25. Fleicher AC, James AE Jr, Millis JB, Julian C. Differential diagnosis of pelvic masses by gray scale sonography. *Am J Roentgenol* 1978;131:469–476.
26. Wu A, Siegel MJ. Sonography of pelvic masses in children: diagnostic predictability. *Am J Roentgenol* 1987;148:1199–1202.
27. Surrey ES, de Ziegler D, Gambone JC, Judd HL. Preoperative localization of androgen-secreting tumors: clinical, endocrinologic and radiologic evaluation of ten patients. *Am J Obstet Gyn* 1988;158:1313–1322.
28. Hata T, Hata K, Senoh D, et al. Doppler ultrasound assessment of tumor vascularity in gynecologic disorders. *J Ultrasound Med* 1989;8:309–314.
29. Kurjak A, Zalud I, Alfirevic Z. Evaluation of adnexal masses with transvaginal color ultrasound. *J Ultrasound Med* 1991;10:295–297.
30. Lund B, Jacobson K, Rasch L, et al. Correlation of abdominal ultrasound and computed tomography scans with second- or third-look laparotomy in patients with ovarian carcinoma. *Gynecol Oncol* 1990;37:279–283.
31. Murolo C, Costantini S, Foglia G, et al. Ultrasound examination in ovarian cancer patients. A comparison with second look laparotomy. *J Ultrasound Med* 1989;8:441–443.
32. Khan O, Cosgrove DO, Fried AM, Savage PE. Ovarian carcinoma follow-up: US versus laparotomy. *Radiology* 1986;159:111–113.
33. Meanwell CA, Rolfe EB, Blackledge G, et al. Recurrent female pelvic cancer: assessment with transrectal ultrasonography. *Radiology* 1987;162:278–281.
34. Squillaci E, Salzani MC, Grandinetti ML, et al. Recurrence of ovarian and uterine neoplasms: diagnosis with transrectal US. *Radiology* 1988;169:355–358.
35. Campbell S, Collins WP, Royston P, et al. Developments in ultrasound screening for early ovarian cancer. In: Sharp F, Mason WP, Leake RE, eds. *Ovarian cancer. Biologic and therapeutic challenges*. New York: WW Norton, 1990;217–227.

36. Campbell S, Royston P, Bhan V, et al. Novel screening strategies for early ovarian cancer by transabdominal ultrasonography. *Br J Obstet Gynaecol* 1990;97:304–311.
37. Granberg S, Wikland M. A comparison between ultrasound and gynecologic examination for detection of enlarged ovaries in a group of women at risk for ovarian carcinoma. *J Ultrasound Med* 1988;7:59–64.
38. Fleischer AC, McKee MS, Gordon AN, et al. Transvaginal sonography of postmenopausal ovaries with pathologic correlation. *J Ultrasound Med* 1990;9:637–644.
39. van Nagell JR Jr, Higgins RV, Donaldson ES, et al. Transvaginal sonography as a screening method for ovarian cancer. A report of the first 1000 cases screened. *Cancer* 1990;65:573–577.
40. Boune T, Campbell S, Steer C, et al. Transvaginal color flow imaging: a possible new screening technique for ovarian cancer. *BMJ* 1989;299:1367–1370.
41. Anolf E, Jorgensen C, Astedt B. Ultrasound examination for detection of ovarian carcinoma in risk groups. *Obstet Gynecol* 1990;75:106–109.
42. Council on Scientific Affairs, American Medical Association. Gynecologic Sonography. Report of the Ultrasonography Task Force. *JAMA* 1991;265:2851–2855.
43. Sanders RC, McNeil BJ, Finberg HJ, et al. A prospective study of computed tomography and ultrasound in the detection and staging of pelvic masses. *Radiology* 1983;146:430–442.
44. Buy JN, Ghossain MA, Sciot C, et al. Epithelial tumors of the ovary: CT findings and correlation with US. *Radiology* 1991; 178:811–818.
45. Normand F, Bruneton JN, Vigne E, et al. Comparison of echography and x-ray computed tomography in cancer of the ovary. *Bull Cancer* (*Paris*) 1988;75:889–893.
46. Rhode U, Steinbrich W. Differential diagnosis of ovarian benign and malignant tumors by CT. *J Belge Radiol* 1983;66:9.
47. Scully RE. Tumors of the ovary and maldeveloped gonads. In: *Atlas of tumor pathology*, 2nd ser, fascicle 16. Armed Forces Institute of Pathology 1979, Washington, DC.
48. Amendola MA. The role of CT in the evaluation of ovarian malignancy. *Crit Rev Diagn Imaging* 1985;24:329–368.
49. Gross BH, Moss AA, Mihara K, et al. Review: computed tomography of gynecologic disease. *Am J Roentgenol* 1983;141: 765–773.
50. Skane P, Huebner KG. Computed tomography of cystic ovarian teratomas with gravity-dependent layering. *J Comput Assist Tomogr* 1983;7:837–841.
51. Jolles H, Coulam CM. CT of ascites: differential diagnosis. *Am J Roentgenol* 1980;135:315–322.
52. Kalavidouris A, Gouliamos A, Ponifex G, et al. Computed tomography of ovarian carcinoma. *Acta Radiol Diagn* 1984;25: 203–208.
53. Buy JN, Moss AA, Ghossain MA, et al. Peritoneal implants from ovarian tumors: CT findings. *Radiology* 1988;169:691–694.
54. Mitchell DG, Hill MC, Hill S, Zaloudek C. Serous carcinoma of the ovary: CT identification of metastatic calcified implants. *Radiology* 1986;158:649–652.
55. Ginata S, Tipaldi L, Diotellevi F, et al. CT demonstration of peritoneal metastases after intraperitoneal injection of contrast material. *Clin Imaging* 1990;14:31–34.
56. Whitley NO, Boheman ME, Baker LP. CT patterns of mesenteric disease. *J Comput Assist Tomogr* 1982;6:490–496.
57. Goldhirsch A, Triller JK, Greiner R, et al. Computed tomography prior to second-look operation in advanced ovarian cancer. *Obstet Gynecol* 1983;62:630–634.
58. Johnson RJ, Blackledge G, Eddleston B, Crowther D. Abdomino-pelvic computed tomography in the management of ovarian carcinoma. *Radiology* 1983;146:447–452.
59. Franchi M, LaFianza A, Babilonti L, et al. Serous carcinoma of the ovary: value of computed tomography in detection of calcified pleural and pulmonary metastatic implants. *Gynecol Oncol* 1990;39:85–88.
60. LeRoux PD, Berger MS, Elliott JP, Tamini HK. Cerebral metastases from ovarian carcinoma. *Cancer* 1991;67:2194–2199.
61. Brenner DE, Shaff MI, Jones HW, et al. Abdominopelvic computed tomography: evaluation in patients undergoing second-look laparotomy for ovarian carcinoma. *Obstet Gynecol* 1985; 65:715–719.
62. Calkins AR, Stehman FB, Wass JL, et al. Pitfalls in the interpretation of computed tomography prior to second-look laparotomy in patients with ovarian cancer. *Br J Radiol* 1987;60:975–979.
63. Silverman PM, Osborne M, Dunnick NR, Brandy LC. CT prior to second-look operation in ovarian cancer. *Am J Roentgenol* 1988;150:829–832.
64. Reuter KL, Griffin T, Hunter TE. Comparison of abdominopelvic computed tomography results and findings at second-look laparotomy in ovarian carcinoma patients. *Cancer* 1989;63: 1123–1128.
65. Thorvinger B, Samuelsson L, Skjaerris J. Computed tomography of malignant ovarian disease. *Acta Radiol* 1987;28:739–742.
66. McCarthy S. Gynecologic applications of MRI. *Crit Rev Diagn Imaging* 1990;31:263–281.
67. Surratt JT, Siegel MJ. Imaging of pediatric ovarian masses. *Radiographics* 1991;11:533–548.
68. Thurnher S, Hodler J, Baer S, Marincek B, vonSchulthess GK. Gadolinium-DOTA enhanced MR imaging of adnexal tumors. *J Comput Assist Tomogr* 1990;14:939–949.
69. Shapiro I, Lanir A, Sherf M, Clouse ME, Lee RG. Magnetic resonance imaging of gynecologic masses. *Gynecol Oncol* 1987; 28:186–200.
70. Lewis E. The use and abuse of imaging in gynecologic cancer. *Cancer* 1987;60:1993–2009.
71. Mawhinney RR, Powell MC, Worthington BS, Symonds EM. Magnetic resonance imaging of benign ovarian masses. *Br J Radiol* 1988;61:179–186.
72. Mitchell DG, Mintz MC, Spritzer CE, et al. Adnexal masses: MR imaging observations at 1.5T, with US and CT correlation. *Radiology* 1987;162:319–324.
73. Mitchell DG. Magnetic resonance imaging of the adnexa. *Semin Ultrasound CT MR* 1988;9:143–157.
74. Weinreb JC, Barkoff ND, Megibow A, Demopoulos R. The value of MR imaging in distinguishing leiomyomas from other solid pelvic masses when sonography is indeterminate. *Am J Roentgenol* 1990;154:295–299.
75. Dooms GC, Hricak H, Tscholakoff D. Adnexal structures: MR imaging. *Radiology* 1986;158:639–646.
76. Powell MC, Worthington BS, Symonds EM. The application of magnetic resonance imaging (MRI) to ovarian carcinoma. In: Sharp F, Soutter WP, eds. *Ovarian cancer—the way ahead*. Chichester: John Wiley & Sons, 1987;141–158.
77. Hamlin DJ, Fitzsimmons JR, Pettersson H, Riggall FC, Morgan L, Wilkinson EJ. Magnetic resonance imaging of the pelvis: evaluation of ovarian masses at 0.15 T. *Am J Roentgenol* 1985; 145:585–590.
78. Hricak H. MRI of the female pelvis: a review. *Am J Roentgenol* 1986;146:1115–1122.
79. Weinreb JC, Brown CE, Lowe TW, et al. Pelvic masses in pregnant patients: MR and US imaging. *Radiology* 1986;159: 717–724.
80. Togashi K, Nishimura K, Itoh K, et al. Ovarian cystic teratomas: MR imaging. *Radiology* 1987;162:669–673.
81. Riccio TJ, Adams HG, Munzing DE, Mattrey RF. Magnetic resonance imaging as an adjunct to sonography in the evaluation of the female pelvis. *Magn Reson Imaging* 1990;8:699–704.
82. Kier R, McCarthy SM, Scoutt LM, et al. Pelvic masses in pregnancy: MR imaging. *Radiology* 1990;176:709–713.

CHAPTER 10

Diagnosis and Staging of Epithelial Ovarian Cancer

John P. Curtin

Surgical intervention plays a key role in the management of ovarian neoplasms. The surgeon who performs an initial laparotomy for ovarian cancer should confirm the diagnosis, establish the extent and stage of disease, and maximally debulk any extraovarian tumor.

Thorough preoperative evaluation of the patient provides essential information that allows the surgeon to obtain informed consent from the patient, to discuss the planned extent of surgery, and to review options regarding preservation of normal function. Additional information will assist in determining proper preoperative preparation (i.e., bowel prep) and intraoperative positioning of the patient.

DIAGNOSIS

Evaluation of Presumed Ovarian Neoplasm

An asymptomatic adnexal mass is a common clinical problem in gynecology. Most of these masses prove to be either functional cysts or benign neoplasms, depending primarily on the age of the patient. Ovarian malignancies are rarely detected on routine examination. Patients with ovarian cancer usually present with symptoms of advanced disease (Table 1); only 2% of patients with ovarian cancer are asymptomatic at the time of diagnosis (1). Epithelial ovarian cancer is predominantly a disease of women over age 40 (2) (Fig. 1).

The evaluation of a patient with possible ovarian cancer requires a complete health and family history and a careful physical examination. Important questions about healthy history include menstrual status,

J. P. Curtin: Gynecology Service, Memorial Sloan-Kettering Cancer Center, New York, New York 10021

bowel or bladder symptoms, weight loss, breast symptoms, and general well-being. Questions about family history should focus on familial ovarian cancer, with an emphasis on first-degree relatives with cancer.

Age and menstrual status are relatively accurate in predicting the possibility of malignancy and, to some extent, histologic subtype. In a 10-year study of 861 women who underwent laparotomy for a primary ovarian neoplasm, the risk of malignancy was 13% in premenopausal women and 45% in postmenopausal women. The risk of malignancy increased by 12-fold from ages 20 to 29 to ages 60 to 69 (3) (Fig. 2).

The physical examination must be thorough. The physician should investigate common sites of ovarian cancer metastasis and should look for either second primary tumors (especially of the breast) or primary tumors at other sites that have metastasized to the ovaries. Clinical examination can sometimes provide indications of malignancy, especially in cases of advanced, extraovarian disease. Suspicious findings (e.g., ascites) are noted most commonly on the abdominal and pelvic examination. Ascites, as evidenced by a distended abdomen with a fluid wave, can have several

TABLE 1. *Distribution by stage for carcinoma of the ovary as reported by the FIGO annual report (includes LMP and invasive cancers)*

Stage	Patients	Percent
I	2,230	26.1%
II	1,313	15.4%
III	3,339	39.1%
IV	1,391	16.3%
No stage	268	3.1%
Total	8,541	100.0%

From Pettersson, ref. 2.

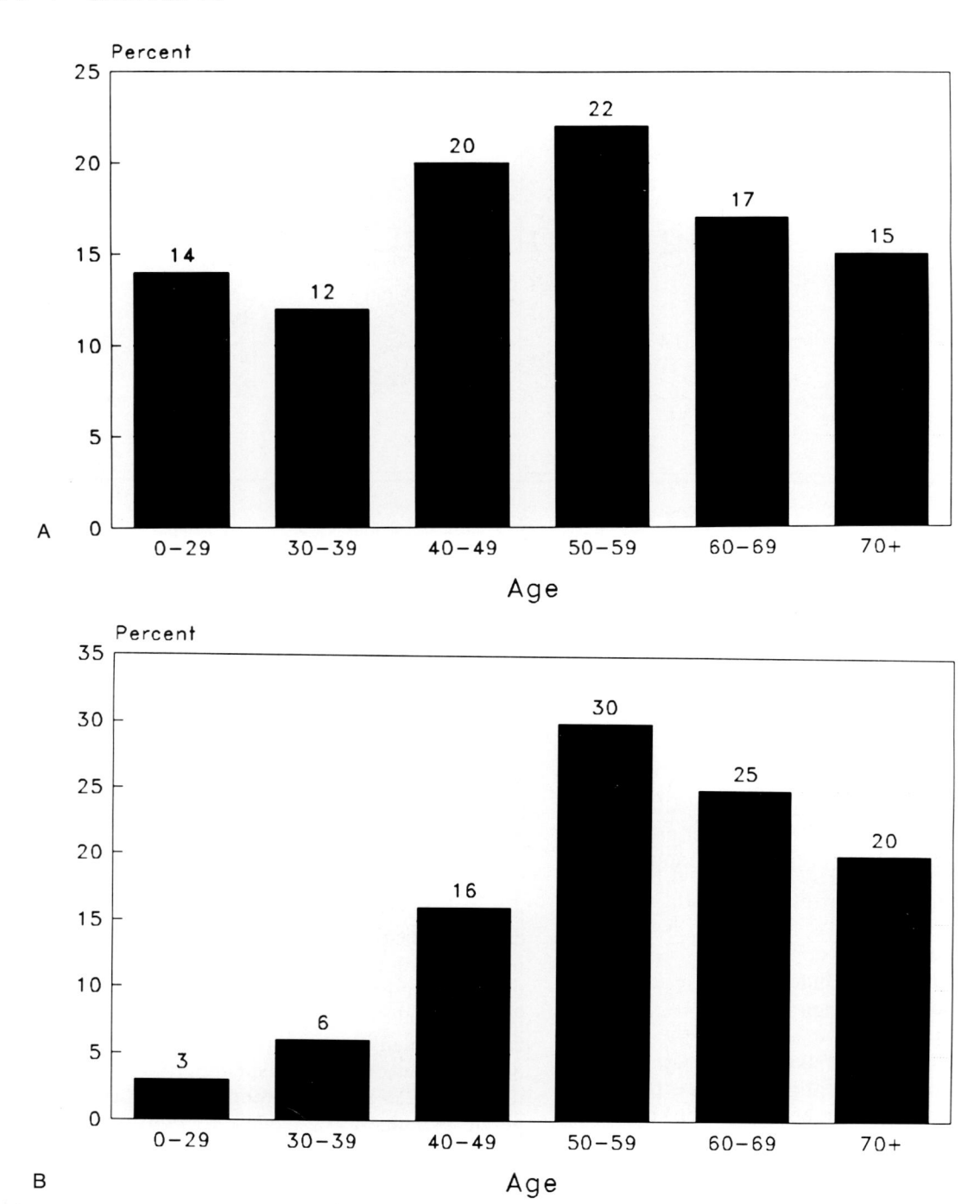

FIG. 1. Annual report of ovarian carcinoma of low malignant potential **(A)** and of obviously malignant ovarian carcinoma **(B)**, FIGO 1988.

different sources. However, in the absence of intrinsic liver disease or significant congestive heart failure, ascites must be considered a malignant process. In women, the most common cause of malignant ascites is ovarian cancer. Other suspicious findings that are common in ovarian cancer include palpable omental masses, often large and irregular. Occasionally, periumbilical metastases (Sister Mary Joseph's node) may be noted or misidentified as an umbilical hernia. Inguinal lymph nodes are rarely a site of clinical metastases in ovarian cancer.

The pelvic examination should note the presence or absence of estrogen effects, especially in postmenopausal women. A Pap smear of the cervix should be obtained, and any suspicious lesion must be biopsied. The initial bimanual examination should also note the

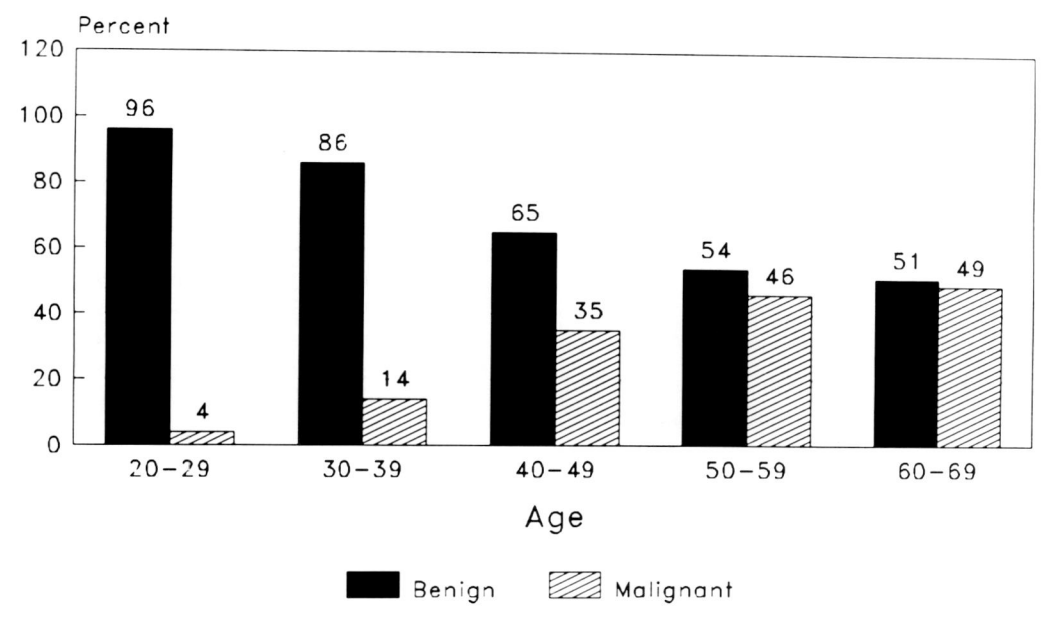

FIG. 2. Rate of benign versus malignant findings, by age, in patients with ovarian neoplasms.

size and mobility of the uterus and the presence of adnexal masses. If an adnexal mass is present, its attachment to the uterus and pelvic side walls and its consistency can provide clues as to whether or not it is malignant.

The rectovaginal examination is the most important part of the physical examination for a patient with possible ovarian cancer. A firm or solid adnexal mass, cul-de-sac bulging due to ascites, and cul-de-sac nodularity represent a possible ovarian malignancy that requires surgical confirmation. Conversely, a smooth, mobile, cystic mass is more likely to be a benign or low-malignant-potential tumor of the ovary.

The rectal examination includes screening for colorectal cancer, which may present with a pelvic mass, and evaluation of possible compromise of the rectum by local extension of an ovarian tumor. Stool, if present, should be tested for occult blood. If a rectal mass or polyp is palpated (approximately one-third of colorectal cancers can be detected by digital exam), an appropriate work-up should be obtained before surgery. Discrimination between a primary ovarian cancer and a primary colorectal cancer may not be possible preoperatively, but knowledge of mucosal involvement, narrowing of the rectal lumen, and the possible need for low anterior resection during surgery can be obtained by careful preoperative examination.

Serum Tumor Markers

Serum measurement of the antigen CA-125 is the most commonly used serum tumor marker in epithelial ovarian carcinoma. First described by Bast and colleagues (4), CA-125 is elevated in 80% of patients with ovarian cancer. It may also be elevated in the presence of malignancies at other sites (e.g., pancreas, breast, colon). Approximately 1% of the patients at an obstetrics and gynecology clinic were found to have a serum CA-125 level of greater than 65 u/mL; none of these patients had ovarian cancer. Common causes of elevated CA-125 in patients with benign gynecologic disease include pregnancy (first trimester), leiomyoma, endometriosis, and pelvic inflammatory disease (5).

The role of serum CA-125 in the management of ovarian cancer continues to evolve. Despite its high sensitivity, serum CA-125 has not been useful in screening for occult ovarian carcinoma. As described by Jacobs and colleagues, an excess of false positive tests will be reported in any large screening project because of the low annual incidence of ovarian cancer (6). Preliminary results have confirmed the low yield of mass screening (7). This issue is further complicated by recent reports stating that only one-half of patients with early disease will have an elevated CA-125 (8,9). This group of patients with early disease must be the focus of any screening project if the intention is to improve overall survival.

Serum CA-125 is helpful in the preoperative evaluation of patients with adnexal masses and suspected ovarian cancer. Vasilev and colleagues reviewed the predictive value of preoperative serum CA-125 levels for 180 patients with an adnexal mass scheduled for exploratory laparotomy (10). Of those whose serum CA-125 was elevated preoperatively ($n=52$), 25% were found to have a malignancy. The majority of these malignancies were epithelial ovarian cancers. Only 4

TABLE 2. *Preoperative CA-125 in patients with an adnexal mass*

	Benign		Malignant	
	≤35[a]	>35	≤35[a]	>35
Vasilev (10), n = 182	128	36	4	14
Malkasian (11), n = 158	72	18	15	53
Total	200	54	19	67

[a] CA-125 levels measured in u/ml.

of 128 patients with an adnexal mass and a normal serum CA-125 level before surgery had malignant neoplasms. Malkasian and colleagues reported similar findings (11). The higher percentage of malignancies reported by Malkasian's group probably relates to a predominant referral population (Table 2).

Imaging Studies of Suspected Ovarian Neoplasm

Pelvic ultrasound, in combination with serum tumor marker levels and clinical examination, adds slightly to the specificity of preoperative diagnosis. In the presence of a palpable adnexal mass or a mass detected by ultrasound, serum CA-125 levels further improve sensitivity and specificity, especially in the postmenopausal patient. Serum CA-125 levels (either normal or elevated) significantly increase the positive and negative predictive values when combined with clinical examination and ultrasound in postmenopausal women (12). Ultrasound is a relatively cost-effective imaging technique, and for patients with an uncertain clinical diagnosis, transabdominal and transvaginal ultrasound are probably the most valuable diagnostic studies for distinguishing benign from malignant adnexal masses.

Patients with obvious malignant processes (e.g., ascites, palpable abdominal masses, cul-de-sac mass with nodularity, elevated CA-125) probably do not require imaging studies beyond the standard radiograph evaluation.

Computed tomography (CT) scans and magnetic resonance imaging (MRI) scans provide information about pelvic, intraabdominal, and retroperitoneal structures. CT and MRI scans are most accurate when a significant amount of disease is present (i.e., intraabdominal metastases are ≥2 cm in size, with or without ascites). The following additional information can be obtained from CT or MRI scans: views of the liver, gallbladder, and pancreas, all of which are possible sites of an occult primary tumor presenting as an adnexal mass; retroperitoneal lymphadenopathy; and views of the lower thorax, which may reveal small pleural effusions. An MRI scan can also provide reasonably accurate details of tissue planes in the pelvis, which are particularly important when the differential diagnosis is uterine leiomyoma versus ovarian neoplasm. The MRI scan may be useful for an asymptomatic young patient with presumed uterine leiomyoma who desires future fertility (13).

After the diagnostic evaluation of an adnexal mass, the physician has the information to predict with accuracy whether the patient is likely to have a benign or malignant neoplasm (Table 3). In a few instances, some authors have suggested that surgery can be avoided if certain criteria are met, even in a postmenopausal woman (14). However, most patients with a persistent adnexal mass will require laparoscopy, laparotomy, or both (15). Using the diagnostic information obtained from physical examination, serum tumor markers, and imaging studies, the surgeon can properly counsel the patient about the diagnosis and extent of surgery. This information is helpful for all patients, but it is particularly important for young patients who desire preservation of fertility and ovarian function.

PREOPERATIVE PREPARATION OF THE PATIENT WITH AN ADNEXAL MASS

Laboratory Studies

Baseline preoperative laboratory studies should include a complete blood count (with differential), serum electrolytes, liver function studies, and urinalysis. Additional studies may include coagulation screening studies (partial thromboplastin time and protime).

Complete blood count information can provide additional clues as to whether the tumor is benign or malignant and, if malignant, whether it is likely to be ovarian in origin. If the patient is not anemic and if sufficient time exists before surgery, autologous blood donation should be considered. Patients with ovarian cancer commonly have normocytic anemia or chronic disease. Patients who present with microcytic anemia and iron deficiency anemia without an obvious source of blood loss (i.e., vaginal bleeding) should be suspected of a gastrointestinal tumor until proven otherwise. Ovarian tumors are rarely associated with leukocytosis. Patients with thrombocytosis, especially when associated with elevated serum CA-125, are likely to have an ovarian malignancy. The mechanism of this association of thrombocytosis and malignancy may be related to the production of IL-6 by ovarian malignancies. IL-6 is a potent growth factor for megakaryocytes. Another possible cause of thrombocytosis is corrected iron deficiency anemia.

Serum electrolytes are unlikely to provide clues about the etiology of an adnexal mass. However, they are part of the normal preoperative work-up. Liver function tests (LFTs) occasionally yield elevated results; if so they must be evaluated prior to surgery. If

TABLE 3. *Adnexal mass—predictive factors*

	Benign	Indeterminate	Malignant
Age	≤35 years	35–50	>50
Exam	Smooth mobile	Bilateral	Fixed cul-de-sac nodules
Ultrasound	Simple, thin-walled cyst	Septated 5–10 cm	Solid areas, ascites, >10 cm
Serum Ca-125	Less than 35 mIu/ml	35–65 mIu/ml	>65 mIu/ml
History	Regular menses, multiparous, oral contraceptive use		Infertility, nulligravida

no medical explanation for elevated LFTs is found (e.g., hepatitis, alcohol abuse, cholelithiasis), liver metastasis should be suspected, even if the elevation is mild. Documentation of liver metastasis by ultrasound or CT scan should be done preoperatively. If the patient has liver metastasis and an adnexal mass, this author's anecdotal experience indicates that these patients are more likely to have gastrointestinal cancer than ovarian cancer.

As previously discussed, the standard serum tumor marker for the preoperative evaluation of patients with an adnexal mass is CA-125. Additional tumor markers may be elevated when the CA-125 level is normal, or they may point toward another primary tumor. A markedly elevated carcinoembryonic antigen (CEA) and a normal serum CA-125 favor primary gastrointestinal cancer. However, combinations of serum tumor markers, such as LASA and NB-70k, usually add more to patient expense than to sensitivity and specificity (Table 3).

Radiographic Studies

A two-view chest x-ray is the one radiographic test that should be done for all patients suspected of having ovarian cancer. Only 5 to 10% of all patients with an ovarian malignancy will have an abnormal preoperative chest x-ray, but the findings can significantly affect staging of the cancer and clinical management (16). Discrete pulmonary nodules, consistent with metastatic disease, are unusual in primary ovarian cancer. Pleural effusions are the most common abnormality noted on preoperative chest x-rays. They are the most common reason for additional studies, and they occasionally require therapeutic intervention. A pleural effusion noted on x-ray is indicative of at least 150 to 200 cc of fluid in the pleural cavity; smaller volumes may be detected by CT scan. Pleural effusions often represent transdiaphragmatic flow of ascitic fluid. Small effusions are unlikely to affect the safe administration of anesthesia, but a thoracentesis is necessary for staging. A pleural effusion that is positive for malignant cells indicates a stage IV ovarian malignancy; 70% of patients with an ovarian malignancy and pleural effusions will have malignant cells in the pleural fluid. Preferably, the thoracentesis should be done a day or more before surgery, rather than in the immediate preoperative period. The risks caused by a small pneumothorax are minimal in a patient who does not undergo immediate surgery. Conversely, a small pneumothorax may expand rapidly after anesthesia induction, particularly when nitrous oxide is used as an anesthetic.

Larger effusions (greater than one-third of pleural space) should be drained preoperatively, as both a diagnostic procedure and a therapeutic measure. The most direct method for draining effusions is placement of a chest tube, which can be done under local anesthesia. Drainage of effusions maximizes respiratory reserve during surgery. If the chest tube is left in place, it will allow continuous drainage intraoperatively and postoperatively. It may also alleviate the need for repeated thoracentesis and allow scarification of the pleura when drainage is reduced.

Additional preoperative studies for the patient with few or no symptoms and a pelvic mass depend on the patient's age, family history, and symptoms, particularly if these symptoms are related to the gastrointestinal tract. A barium enema should be strongly considered for all patients who are suspected of having epithelial ovarian cancer, with the possible exception of young patients with no symptoms, negative stool guaiac, and a negative family history. A normal barium enema can aid in intraoperative decision making, and an abnormal study occasionally reveals a primary colorectal tumor or metastases with mucosal ulceration. An upper gastrointestinal series may be indicated for patients with symptoms suggestive of a primary stomach cancer.

An intravenous pyelogram (IVP) may also be obtained preoperatively. However, if the patient has had a CT scan with contrast, little additional information can be obtained from an IVP. In the Gynecologic Oncology Group ovarian cancer staging study, the IVP was the radiologic test that was most commonly abnormal; 45% of IVPs done preoperatively demonstrated abnormalities that were most often related to displacement of the ureters by pelvic masses (16).

Lymphangiography has also been suggested as a preoperative study for patients suspected of having an ovarian malignancy (13). However, although abnormal findings have high sensitivity and specificity, normal reports do not (17). Because the findings of lymphangiography are unlikely to alter the surgical approach, this study is rarely indicated for patients with suspected ovarian cancer.

Preoperative preparation of the patient includes both mechanical and antibiotic bowel preparation. Immediately preoperatively, a dose of prophylactic antibiotics is administered. At the Memorial Sloan-Kettering Cancer Center, Ancef is given unless the patient has a significant allergic history.

As prophylaxis against thrombosis and subsequent thromboembolism, 5,000 units of subcutaneous heparin are given preoperatively to all patients suspected of having an ovarian malignancy. Low-dose heparin is continued during the postoperative period until the patient is ambulatory. Ovarian cancer patients are considered to be at high risk for deep venous thrombosis. The role of prophylactic heparin in prevention of deep-vein thrombosis in patients with gynecologic malignancies has been debated. One group reported that subcutaneous heparin is not an effective prophylactic against deep-vein thrombosis and pulmonary embolism (18,19), but a review of a large number of randomized trials of prophylactic subcutaneous heparin demonstrated a significant decrease in both deep-vein thrombosis and pulmonary embolism (20). Alternatives to subcutaneous heparin are compression stockings or a combination of heparin and compression stockings (21).

INTRAOPERATIVE MANAGEMENT

Prelaparotomy Procedures

After induction of anesthesia, the patient is placed in the lithotomy position and examined. In patients thought to have an early ovarian malignancy (i.e., unilateral cysts, no ascites, possibly elevated CA-125), care must be taken to avoid rupturing the mass by a too-vigorous bimanual examination. After examination under anesthesia, most patients undergo proctosigmoidoscopy. This procedure is particularly important for the patient with an advanced, bulky pelvic tumor, in whom optimal debulking is likely to require resection of the rectosigmoid. Confirmation of the length of intact rectal mucosa may aid in the decision to attempt primary anastomosis after resection versus colostomy. In the Gynecologic Oncology Group study of early ovarian cancers, 10% of preoperative proctosigmoidoscopies were abnormal (16).

After these "nonsterile" procedures, the perineum and vagina are prepared, and cystoscopy is performed. If necessary, ureteral stents may be placed to aid in the identification of the ureters during the dissection of the ovarian mass. After cystoscopy, an endometrial sampling may be performed, depending on the patient's age and operative symptoms and the planned procedure. For postmenopausal women with an adnexal mass and no postmenopausal bleeding, the planned procedure should include a hysterectomy, and the results of an endometrial biopsy will have little influence on this choice. However, in young patients with a potential early ovarian malignancy for whom preservation of the uterus is being considered, an endometrial biopsy must be done to rule out a concomitant endometrial pathology such as hyperplasia or adenocarcinoma.

Laparotomy

After the patient is properly positioned and draped, the surgeon always proceeds with a midline incision if ovarian carcinoma is suspected. After the peritoneal cavity is opened, the presence or absence of ascites should be documented. If ascites is present, the estimated volume is noted, and a sample is sent for cytologic evaluation. If no ascites is noted, peritoneal washings with saline are done for cytologic evaluation. The practice at Memorial Sloan-Kettering Cancer Center is to send three specimens when washings are obtained; one is sent from the pelvis, and one each is sent from the paracolic gutters. Evidence of malignant cells is a determinant used in staging patients with ovarian carcinoma (stages I and II). In addition to staging requirements, the presence or absence of malignant cells in either ascites or washings in stage I or II disease probably has prognostic significance (22), as does the volume of ascites (23). The prognostic value of peritoneal cytology in patients with advanced disease is questionable, although by convention a single specimen is usually obtained.

Next, the pelvis is closely examined, and the size of the primary tumor mass or masses is noted. Adhesions and contiguous invasion of the tumor should be recorded; dense adhesions may have significant prognostic implications in early stage ovarian cancer (23). The abdomen should then be thoroughly explored. The presence or absence of tumor on the peritoneal surfaces, diaphragm, liver, spleen, gallbladder, and large and small bowel must be carefully documented. Inspection should be both visual and tactile, because small tumor implants are often evidenced only by surface irregularities. The retroperitoneal structures should be palpated.

In the case of early disease, the initial surgical step is usually an adnexectomy, with rapid frozen section review. If the patient is young and has an apparently encapsulated lesion, cystectomy is preferred. The argument against cystectomy in a patient with possible ovarian cancer and clinical stage I disease is fear of rupturing the cyst. If the histology confirms a malignancy, rupture of the cyst would change the stage to IC. Although the stage is upgraded in this situation, the effect on outcome is uncertain. Initial reviews of patients with stage I disease reported a worse prognosis for patients with ruptured ovarian capsules, as compared to patients with an intact capsule (24). However, more recent series have reported that capsule rupture is not an adverse factor in terms of prognosis (23,25). Depending on the report of the frozen section, additional surgical procedures including omentectomy, peritoneal and diaphragm biopsies, and lymph node sampling may be performed to more accurately stage the disease according to International Federation of Gynecology and Obstetrics (FIGO) criteria for staging of ovarian malignancies (Table 4).

Recently, Buchsbaum and associates reported on the Gynecologic Oncology Group (GOG) prospective surgical staging study of patients with stage I, stage II, and optimal (tumor metastasis ≤1 cm) stage III ovarian cancer (16). Overall, 9 of 97 patients thought to have stage I disease and 15 of 43 patients thought to have stage II disease were upstaged by biopsy results. Buchsbaum and associates also reviewed the morbidity associated with the staging procedure: They noted 74 complications in 154 patients. The most common complications—injuries of the bowel, bladder, and ureter—were associated with tumor debulking.

The value of reexploration of patients with an inadequate staging operation as their initial procedure is well described. Early reports that 20 to 45% of patients referred for early ovarian cancer had more advanced disease at restaging laparotomy (26–28) were confirmed in the GOG staging study. In the group of patients who initially underwent complete staging by a gynecologic oncologist, only 11 of 129 (8.5%) were upstaged by surgical findings. However, in the group of patients who were referred from outside hospitals and underwent a second laparotomy for staging, 13 of 58 (22.5%) were upstaged at reexploration (16).

Once the diagnosis of an early ovarian cancer is confirmed by frozen section, the surgeon should proceed with surgical staging. Suspicious nodules or plaques larger than 2 cm should be excised and sent for frozen section. Establishment of a stage IIIC tumor by frozen section changes the focus of the operative procedure. Once the diagnosis of stage III is confirmed, the surgeon should concentrate on debulking any remaining tumor.

If obvious macroscopic tumor is not present, biopsies of peritoneal surfaces and an infracolic omentectomy follow the excision of the primary tumor. The majority of these peritoneal biopsies should be from the pelvis and should include both pelvic sidewalls, the cul-de-sac, and the vesical peritoneum. Outside the pelvis, the paracolic peritoneal surface, any thickening and/or adhesions of the bowel mesentery should be biopsied. The diaphragms are biopsied also; various techniques have been reported. The most direct technique is to grasp the peritoneal surface of the diaphragm with a long Allis clamp and to excise the tented portion of the peritoneum. Other methods include scraping or curetting the diaphragm with Kevorkian curettes or wooden blades; these specimens are usually sent for cytology rather than histopathology. Because these methods sample a greater area of the diaphragm,

TABLE 4. *FIGO staging of primary ovarian cancer*

Stage I	Growth limited to the ovaries
Stage IA	Growth limited to one ovary; no ascites; no tumor on the external surface; capsule intact
Stage IB	Growth limited to both ovaries; no ascites; no tumor on the external surfaces; capsules intact
Stage IC[a]	Tumor either stage IA or IB, but with tumor on surface of one or both ovaries; or with capsule ruptured; or with ascites present containing malignant cells or with positive peritoneal washings
Stage II	Growth involving one or both ovaries with pelvic extension
Stage IIA	Extension and/or metastases to the uterus and/or tubes
Stage IIB	Extension to other pelvic tissues
Stage IIC[a]	Tumor either stage IIA or IIB, but with tumor on surface of one or both ovaries; or with capsule(s) ruptured; or with ascites present containing malignant cells or with positive peritoneal washings
Stage III	Tumor involving one or both ovaries with peritoneal implants outside the pelvis and/or positive retroperitoneal or inguinal nodes. Superficial liver metastasis equals stage III
	Tumor is limited to the true pelvis but with histologically proven malignant extension to small bowel or omentum
Stage IIIA	Tumor grossly limited to the true pelvis with negative nodes but with histologically confirmed microscopic seeding of abdominal peritoneal surfaces
Stage IIIB	Tumor involving one or both ovaries with histologically confirmed implants of abdominal peritoneal surfaces, none exceeding 2 cm in diameter. Nodes are negative
Stage IIIC	Abdominal implants greater than 2 cm in diameter and/or positive retroperitoneal or inguinal nodes
Stage IV	Growth involving one or both ovaries with distant metastases. With pleural effusion, there must be positive cytology to allot a case to stage IV
	Parenchymal liver metastasis equals stage IV

the yield of cytologic sampling may be higher than biopsy (29).

Particular attention should be given to inspection of the appendix, if it is present. If the preliminary pathology review demonstrates a mucinous tumor, an appendectomy should be performed. The decision of whether to do an appendectomy in other cases of early stage ovarian cancer is made on an individual basis. Metastasis to the appendix is relatively uncommon in early stage ovarian cancer. Rose and colleagues found only 2 of 47 (4.3%) patients with metastatic lesions (30). Other factors that can influence the surgeon are indications for incidental appendectomy regardless of the diagnosis of ovarian malignancy (31). Generally, patients under 30 years of age are likely to benefit the most from a prophylactic appendectomy.

Lymph Node Sampling in Early Ovarian Cancer

The role of lymph node sampling in the staging of epithelial ovarian cancer has been the topic of considerable debate. Knapp and Friedman, in a report of 26 patients with stage I ovarian cancer, were among the first authors to describe the importance of aortic lymph node sampling in early stage disease. Five of 26 patients reported had aortic lymph node metastases, and, as expected, these patients had a significantly lower survival rate (32). Subsequent reports, usually of relatively small numbers of patients whose charts were analyzed retrospectively, found that the incidence of lymph node metastases in stage I and II ovarian cancer ranged from 10% to 30% (33–35). European studies (36) often reported a very high incidence of lymph node metastases, which has often been attributed to the more thorough, complete pelvic and paraaortic lymphadenectomy championed by Burghardt and associates (Table 5). The GOG conducted the largest study, which was reported by Buchsbaum and associates. It is the only prospective study that proscribes the surgical extent of lymph node sampling. Buchsbaum and associates found that only 4 of 97 patients with stage I ovarian cancer had aortic lymph node metastasis. For patients with stage II disease, 8 of 41 (19.5%) had aortic lymph node metastasis (16).

Based partly on the GOG surgical staging results, pelvic and aortic lymph nodes are sampled as part of the complete staging in clinically early ovarian cancer. The fat pad obtained from the paraaortic area must be in close proximity to the renal vessels and ovarian vessels (39).

SURGERY IN ADVANCED OVARIAN CANCER

Patients with obviously advanced malignancies require a different surgical approach. The initial biopsy may come from the most accessible tumor (omentum, anterior abdominal wall, or pelvic mass). After biopsy is obtained for tissue diagnosis, the surgeon must determine the extent of disease and the resectability of the tumor. The judgment regarding resectability is based on many factors, including the age and general health of the patient, the site of the tumor, the surgeon's capability and experience, and preoperative preparation. All specimens that are resected should be clearly identified. The information from pathologic review may seriously influence staging and treatment decisions. At the completion of the operation, the surgeon must carefully dictate the operative findings, including the size of the initial disease, the amount of tumor that was removed, and the size and site of residual disease. Information about residual disease will be an important guide to the surgeon if the patient requires a second-look laparotomy.

In patients with ovarian cancer that is greater than stage I or II, lymph node metastasis can have an impact on staging only when the intraperitoneal disease is either microscopic (stage IIIA) or less than 2 cm in diameter (stage IIIB). A positive lymph node biopsy would increase the stage to IIIC. This subgroup of patients, though uncommon, should undergo sampling of both pelvic and aortic lymph nodes. The issue of lymph node biopsy becomes problematic when diffuse, bulky intraabdominal disease is encountered. For these patients, the added risk and morbidity of lymph node sampling is not indicated unless intraabdominal disease can be successfully debulked. Occasionally, excision of large retroperitoneal lymph nodes is part of the debulking procedure.

Burghardt has suggested that pelvic and paraaortic lymphadenectomy (not sampling) has a significant impact on patient survival (40–42). Patients who undergo this lymph node resection, even those with bulky intraabdominal disease, are reported to have improved survival. These studies, though interesting, are retrospective reviews and may reflect only the biologic potential of the tumor; patients with less aggressive tumors may

TABLE 5. *Early stage ovarian cancer—incidence of lymph node metastasis*

Authors	Stage I	Stage II
Knapp (32)	5/26 (19%)	—
DiRe (37)	16/134 (12%)	—
Chen (33)	2/11 (18%)	2/10 (20%)
Averette (38)	1/11 (9%)	5/17 (29%)
Pickel (36)	7/28 (23%)	4/13 (31%)
Buschbaum (16)	4/95 (4%)	8/41 (19.5%)
Total	35/305 (11.5%)	19/81 (23.4%)

be more likely to undergo the complete surgical procedure, including lymphadenectomy.

Patients with advanced malignant epithelial ovarian neoplasms are not candidates for conservative, fertility-sparing surgery. The extent of tumor debulking depends on the patient's general medical status, the surgeon's ability, and the location of the tumor. At the end of the debulking and staging procedure, patients are generally classified into one of three categories: no residual disease, optimally debulked disease (residual 1–2 cm), or suboptimally debulked disease (gross residual >2 cm). Approximately 70% of patients with malignant epithelial neoplasms are classified as having no residual disease or as being optimally debulked after surgery.

For patients with stage I (no ascites, no dense adhesions), grade I malignant epithelial neoplasms, no further therapy is indicated. Follow-up and prognosis are similar to those for neoplasms of low malignant potential (LMP). Patients with stage IA, grade 1 tumors with dense adhesions, or grades 2 and 3 tumors, require adjuvant therapy. Patients with more advanced disease require combination chemotherapy that usually consists of cisplatin, cytoxan, and, in some instances, doxorubicin. The clinical response of advanced disease is excellent. Sixty percent to 70% of patients have no measurable residual disease as determined by physical examination or radiographic methods.

PROBLEMS WITH FROZEN SECTION

An intraoperative frozen section histologic diagnosis should resolve three primary issues for the surgeon. First, it should reveal whether the lesion is benign or malignant. In the management of epithelial ovarian neoplasms, this distinction may be clouded by the difficulty of differentiating between a tumor of low malignant potential and a grade 1 tumor. However, this differentiation should not be an issue for the surgeon. The staging is the same regardless of whether final permanent sections demonstrate a low malignant potential (LMP) or a grade 1 adenocarcinoma. For a higher grade lesion (grades 2 and 3), lymph node sampling should be performed.

The second issue to be resolved by the pathologist is whether the cell type is adenocarcinoma, germ cell, or stromal. The rare clinical situation in which this differentiation is important is in evaluation of a young patient with advanced disease (stage III or IV) who desires to maintain fertility. In this setting, preservation of the contralateral ovary may be possible only if the tumor is a germ cell malignancy. If it is an adenocarcinoma, a bilateral salpingo-oophorectomy is standard therapy. Definitive therapy may have to be postponed if the diagnosis cannot be made on frozen section.

The third important fact obtained by frozen section review is the likely site of origin of the tumor, identifying it as either a primary ovarian cancer or as metastatic cancer from another site. The organs most commonly associated with metastasis to the ovary include the endometrium, breast, colon, and stomach (see Chapter 29). If the pathologist suspects a primary bowel cancer that has metastasized to the ovary, a careful search is necessary. A negative preoperative barium study of the gastrointestinal tract can be reassuring, although it is not totally reliable. An elevated CEA level is also suspicious, but this finding occurs in 10% of primary ovarian tumors.

Clinically, a primary bowel or stomach cancer can be very similar in appearance to an advanced ovarian cancer. Surgical findings may include ascites, extensive intraperitoneal carcinomatosis, and an omental cake of tumor. However, the natural history and prognosis of these two diseases is very different. Debulking surgery and chemotherapy have little impact on survival in patients with advanced, metastatic gastrointestinal primary adenocarcinoma. In contrast, responses to chemotherapy and survival after optimal surgical debulking have improved in patients with ovarian carcinoma.

If the frozen section report reveals a primary gastrointestinal site, the surgeon's goal changes from debulking to palliation. Palliative surgical procedures should attempt to resect the presumed primary tumor and bypass potential areas of bowel obstruction. Colostomy will occasionally be required.

FERTILITY-SPARING SURGERY

Rarely, a patient with invasive epithelial cancer may undergo removal of only the involved ovary if she has unilateral disease and expresses a strong desire for preservation of fertility. Cystectomy, which may be sufficient therapy for a tumor of low malignant potential, is inadequate for an invasive tumor; unilateral adnexectomy is the minimum procedure. Complete surgical staging should be carried out. Biopsy of the contralateral ovary is certainly indicated if an abnormality is present. The value of a wedge or sliver biopsy of a normal-appearing contralateral ovary is questionable, especially considering the potential for adhesion formation. The surgeon's first priority is to rule out an occult, more advanced stage tumor. Care must also be taken to minimize the potential for adhesion formation when the uterus and ovary are retained for fertility. Whether or not a biopsy of the remaining ovary is done, placement of an absorbable adhesion barrier over the ovary is prudent after meticulous control of bleeding.

REFERENCES

1. Flam F, Einhorn N, Sjovall K. Symptomatology of ovarian cancer. *Eur J Obstet Gynecol Reprod Biol* 1988;27:53–57.
2. Pettersson F. Annual report of the results of treatment in gynecologic cancer. International Federation of Gynecology and Obstetrics (FIGO), 1988.
3. Jacobs I, Oram D, Fairbanks J, Turner J, Frost C, Grudzinskas JG. A risk of malignancy index incorporating CA-125, ultrasound, and menopausal status for the accurate preoperative diagnosis of ovarian cancer. *Br J Obstet Gynaecol* 1990;97:922–999.
4. Bast RC, Klug TL, St John E, et al. A radioimmunoassay using a monoclonal antibody to monitor the course of epithelial ovarian cancer. *N Engl J Med* 1983;309:883–887.
5. Niloff JM, Knapp RC, Shcaetzl E, Reynolds C, Bast RC. CA-125 levels in obstetric and gynecologic patients. *Obstet Gynecol* 1984;64:703–707.
6. Jacobs IJ, Stabile I, Budges J, et al. Multimodal approach to screening for ovarian cancer. *Lancet* 1988;I:268–271.
7. Zurawski VR, Sjovall K, Schoenfeld DA, et al. Prospective evaluation of serum CA-125 levels in a normal population, phase I: the specificities of single and serial determinations in testing for ovarian cancer. *Gynecol Oncol* 1990;36:299–305.
8. Zurawski VR, Knapp RC, Einhorn N, et al. An initial analysis of preoperative serum CA-125 levels in patients with early stage ovarian carcinoma. *Gynecol Oncol* 1988;30:7–14.
9. VanNagell JR. Ovarian cancer screening. [Editorial]. *Cancer* 1991;68:679–680.
10. Vasilev SA, Schlaerth JB, Campeau J, Morrow CP. Serum CA-125 levels in preoperative evaluation of pelvic masses. *Obstet Gynecol* 1988;71:751–756.
11. Malkasian GD, Knapp RC, Lavin RT, et al. Preoperative evaluation of serum CA-125 levels in premenopausal and postmenopausal women patients with pelvic masses: discrimination of benign from malignant disease. *Am J Obstet* 1988;159:341–346.
12. Finkler NK, Benacerraf B, Lavin PT, Wojcrechowski C, Knapp RC. Comparison of serum CA-125, clinical impression, and ultrasound in preoperative evaluation of ovarian masses. *Obstet Gynecol* 1988;72:659–683.
13. Binkovitz LA, King BF, Corfman RS. Advances in gynecologic imaging and intervention. *Mayo Clin Proc* 1991;66:1133–1151.
14. Goldstein SR, Subramanyam B, Snyder JR, Beller U, Raghavendra BN, Beckman EM. The postmenopausal cystic adnexal mass: the potential role of ultrasound in conservative management. *Obstet Gynecol* 1989;73:8–10.
15. Parker WH, Berek JS. Management of selected cystic adnexal masses in postmenopausal women by operative laparoscopy: a pilot study. *Am J Obstet Gynecol* 1990;163:1574–1577.
16. Buchsbaum HJ, Brady MF, Delgado G, et al. Surgical staging of carcinoma of the ovaries. *Surg Gynecol Obstet* 1989;169:226–232.
17. Musumeci R, DePalo G, Kenda R, et al. Retroperitoneal metastases from ovarian carcinoma: reassessment of 365 patients studied with lymphography. *Am J Roentgenol* 1980;134:449–452.
18. Clarke-Pearson DL, DeLong ER, Synan IS, Creasman WT. Complications of low-dose heparin prophylaxis in gynecologic oncology. *Obstet Gynecol* 1984;64:689–694.
19. Clarke-Pearson DL, Olt G. Thromboembolism in patients with gynecologic tumors: risk factors, natural history, and prophylaxis. *Oncology* 1989;3:39–45.
20. Collins R, Scrimgeour A, Yusuf S, Petro R. Reduction in fatal pulmonary embolism and venous thrombosis by perioperative administration of subcutaneous heparin. *N Engl J Med* 1988;318:1162–1173.
21. Consensus Conference. Prevention of venous thrombosis and pulmonary embolism. *JAMA* 1986;256:744–749.
22. Yoshimura S, Scully RE, Taft PD, Herrington JB. Peritoneal fluid cytology in patients with ovarian cancer. *Gynecol Oncol* 1984;17:161–167.
23. Dembo AJ, Davy M, Steenwig AE, Berle EJ, Bush RS, Kjorstad K. Prognostic factors in patients with stage I epithelial ovarian cancer. *Obstet Gynecol* 1990;75:263–273.
24. Webb MJ, Decker DG, Mussey E, Williams TJ. Factors influencing survival in stage I ovarian cancer. *Am J Obstet Gynecol* 1973;116:222–226.
25. Sevelda P, Dittrich C, Salzer H. Prognostic value of the rupture of the capsule in stage I epithelial ovarian carcinoma. *Gynecol Oncol* 1989;35:321–322.
26. Piver MS, Barlow JJ, Lele SB. Incidence of subclinical metastasis in stage I and II ovarian carcinoma. *Obstet Gynecol* 1978;52:100–104.
27. Young RC, Decker DG, Wharton JT, et al. Staging laparotomy in early ovarian cancer. *JAMA* 1983;250:3072–3076.
28. Guthrie D, Davy MLJ, Philips PR. A study of 656 patients with early ovarian cancer. *Gynecol Oncol* 1984;17:363–369.
29. Jadhon ME, Morgan MA, Kelsten ML, Carlson JA, Mikuta JJ. Cytologic smears of peritoneal surfaces as a sampling technique in epithelial ovarian carcinoma. *Obstet Gynecol* 1990;75:102–106.
30. Rose PG, Reale FR, Fisher A, Hunter RE. Appendectomy in primary and secondary staging operations for ovarian malignancy. *Obstet Gynecol* 1991;77:116–118.
31. Fisher KS, Ross DS. Guidelines for therapeutic decision in incidental appendectomy. *Surg Gynecol Obstet* 1990;171:95–98.
32. Knapp RC, Friedman EA. Aortic lymph node metastases in early ovarian cancer. *Am J Obstet Gynecol* 1974;119:1013–1017.
33. Chen SS, Lee L. Incidence of para-aortic and pelvic lymph node metastases in epithelial carcinoma of the ovary. *Gynecol Oncol* 1983;16:95–100.
34. Chen SS, Lee L. Prognostic significance of morphology of tumor and retroperitoneal lymph nodes in epithelial carcinoma of the ovary. I. Correlation with lymph node metastasis. *Gynecol Oncol* 1984;18:87–93.
35. Burghardt E, Pickel H, Lahoussen M, Stettner H. Pelvic lymphadenectomy in operative treatment of ovarian cancer. *Am J Obstet Gynecol* 1986;155:315–319.
36. Pickel H, Lahoussen M, Stettner H, Girardi F. The spread of ovarian cancer. *Baillieres Clin Obstet Gynaecol* 1989;3:3–12.
37. DiRe F, Fontanelli R, Raspagliesi, DiRe EM. The value of lymphadenectomy in the management of ovarian cancer. In: Sharp CF, Mason WP, Leake R, eds. *Ovarian cancer: biologic and therapeutic challenges.* London: Chapman and Hall, 1990.
38. Averette HE, Lovecchio JL, Townsend PA, Sevin BU, Gurtanner RE. Retroperitoneal lymphatic involvement by ovarian carcinoma. In: Grundmann, ed. *Cancer campaign: carcinoma of the ovary.* Stuttgart: Gustav Fischer Verlag, 1983.
39. Belenson JL, Goldberg MI, Averette HE. Para-aortic lymphadenectomy in gynecologic cancer. *Gynecol Oncol* 1979;7:188–198.
40. Burghardt E, Lahoussen M, Stettner H. The significance of pelvic and para-aortic lymphadenectomy in the operative treatment of ovarian cancer. *Baillieres Clin Obstet Gynaecol* 1989;3:157–165.
41. Burghardt E, Girardi F, Lahoussen M, Tamussino K, Stettner H. Patterns of pelvic and paraaortic lymph node involvement in ovarian cancer. *Gynecol Oncol* 1991;40:103–106.
42. Chen SS, Lee L. Prognostic significance of morphology of tumor and retroperitoneal lymph nodes in epithelial carcinoma of the ovary. II. Correlation with survival. *Gynecol Oncol* 1984;18:94–99.

CHAPTER 11

Primary Cytoreduction

William J. Hoskins

Surgery plays a unique role in the treatment of ovarian cancer. It is the most important facet of therapy for this disease, but only rarely does it produce a cure without the aid of another modality. Because surgery must be combined with other types of therapy, the physician, or team of physicians, must be aware of the interactions between the various types of treatment.

This chapter focuses on the use of surgery as initial therapy for ovarian cancer. Additional aspects of the surgical treatment of ovarian cancer are discussed in other chapters of this book.

HISTORICAL PERSPECTIVE OF CYTOREDUCTION

The first report of cytoreductive surgery for an ovarian tumor was also the first report of an abdominal operation in the United States. Efraim McDowel, in 1809, removed a 22-pound ovarian tumor from a woman in Kentucky (1).

"Ovariotomists" in the late 18th and early 19th centuries advocated the resection of primary tumors. In 1916 several gynecologic surgeons, including Bonney, Graves, and Lynch, began to recommend the removal of primary ovarian cancers, even when metastases were unresectable (2). Munnel, in 1968, performed a retrospective review of patients with ovarian cancer who had been treated with radiation therapy (3) and reported improved survival in patients who had undergone omentectomy. Improved survival was also seen in patients who had had partial removal of tumor in addition to laparotomy and biopsy. Delcos and Quinlan reported in 1969 that patients with nonpalpable ovarian cancer survived longer than patients with palpable ovarian cancer (4). These authors demonstrated four-year survivals of 72% and 25%, respectively, for stages II and III nonpalpable disease as compared to only 33% and 9%, respectively, for stages II and III palpable disease.

In 1975 Griffiths reported on a series of patients who underwent primary cytoreductive surgery followed by single alkylating agent chemotherapy (5). Because the chemotherapy treatments were similar in all the patients, survivals with regard to the amount of residual disease at the beginning of chemotherapy could be effectively compared. Median survival was directly related to the diameter of residual disease (measured in centimeters). The results of this report are summarized in Table I. Griffiths' report is particularly significant because he was the first investigator to attempt to quantify residual disease and its effect on a measurable end point such as survival.

Since Griffiths' report, multiple studies have demonstrated the importance of primary cytoreductive surgery in ovarian cancer. These studies are discussed in more detail in subsequent sections of this chapter.

THEORETICAL BASIS OF PRIMARY CYTOREDUCTION

Basic information about tumor growth kinetics is essential to an understanding of the theoretical basis of cytoreductive surgery. This same information about tumor growth kinetics provides us with related knowledge about the mechanisms by which chemotherapy eradicates tumors. Interestingly, successful therapy for ovarian cancer almost always involves a combination of surgery and chemotherapy, and growth kinetics must be considered in relation to both of these modalities.

Cells in any living tissue, including human cancers, are considered to be in either the growth fraction or the nonproliferating fraction. The growth fraction includes

---

W. J. Hoskins: Gynecology Service, Memorial Sloan-Kettering Cancer Center, New York, New York, 10021

TABLE 1. *The influence of residual disease on survival in ovarian cancer*

Residual disease	Survival in months
0 Residual	39
0–0.5 cm	29
0.6–1.5 cm	18
>1.5 cm	11

Adapted from Griffiths, ref. 5.

the active cell cycle and consists of the senthesis (S) phase, the premitotic (G2) phase, and the mitotic (M) phase. The resting, or nonproliferating, phase is the G0 phase. Tissues that constantly divide to replenish themselves (e.g., hair, gastrointestinal mucosa, bone marrow) are referred to as renewal tissues. Tissues that are not constantly dividing (e.g., muscles, nerves) are nonrenewal tissues.

Even in renewal tissues, only a portion of the cells are in the growth fraction. Most cells are in the resting phase. Cancers are like renewal tissues, with active growth fractions; as with other renewal tissues, only a portion of the cancer cells are in an active growth phase. The significant difference between cancers and renewal tissues is the lack of control exhibited by cancers. Cancers continue to grow without regulation and eventually kill their host through disruption of normal body functions.

The growth rate of cancer varies with the type and differentiation of the cancer. However, most cancers appear to have an exponential growth rate (a straight line when plotted on a logarithmic scale against time on a linear scale). The smallest tumor that can usually be detected is about 1 cm (1 gm). This particle represents about 10^8 to 10^9 tumor cells and usually represents about 30 doublings of the tumor. If a tumor this small continues to grow, it will reach 1 kg in another 10 doublings (6). A tumor size of 1 kg is usually considered to be potentially lethal.

The actual growth of solid tumors is marked by an increase in the duration of the doubling time as tumors become larger. This slowing process results in a flattening of the growth curve that has been shown mathematically by the Gompertz equation. The simulated growth curve of solid tumors is usually called a gompertzian growth curve (Fig. 1). One theoretical explanation for this flattening growth curve holds that tumors tend to outgrow their nutrients, with a resulting increase in doubling time. It has also been postulated that a high percentage of these large tumors are in a resting, or nondividing, phase of the cell cycle.

Mutation characteristically occurs in tumors. These alterations result in cell lines that are resistant to chemotherapeutic agents. Paradoxically, although an increase in the number of cells that are actively dividing may render more cells chemosensitive, this rapid divi-

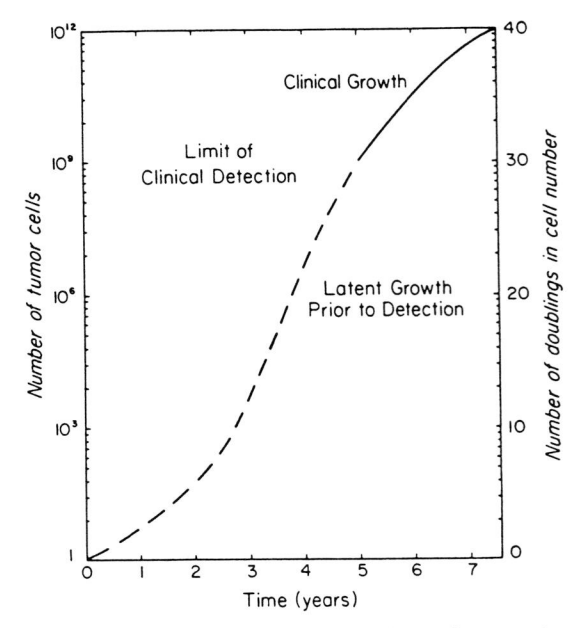

FIG. 1. Hypothetical growth curve for a human tumor. Note that the tumor grows for five years before attaining a size of ~1 g (~10^9 cells), when it can first be clinically detected. Thereafter, despite some slowing of growth, it attains a lethal mass of ~1 kg (~10^{12} cells) in a further 2.5 years. (From ref. 6, with permission.)

sion may also cause a greater likelihood of cell mutation and subsequent resistance to chemotherapy.

Another important characteristic of tumors is their ability to metastasize and grow at distant sites. Metastasis is a complex process in which a tumor cell invades a blood vessel or lymphatic channel and, after transportation to another site, leaves the vessel and begins to establish a new tumor separate from the primary tumor. Experimental data indicate that only a small percentage of tumor cells are able to metastasize, and only the hardiest cells survive the process. In ovarian cancer, blood-borne metastasis is rare, but transperitoneal metastasis is common. The bloodstream is a hostile environment for free tumor cells. Most cells that enter the circulatory system do not survive to implant as metastatic disease. The peritoneal cavity, whether it contains normal peritoneal fluid or ascitic fluid, does not appear to be a hostile environment. Intraperitoneal dissemination of metastases is not inhibited. Ovarian cancers also metastasize frequently via the lymphatic system. These tumors vary in their ability to metastasize early in the disease process. Borderline and well-differentiated cancers metastasize late, whereas poorly differentiated cancers metastasize early.

This information about tumor growth kinetics provides the groundwork for a discussion of the theoretical basis for cytoreductive surgery. Griffiths (2) states that the rationale for cytoreduction can be divided into three components: (1) a direct effect whereby the host benefits from the mechanical effect of cytoreduction; (2) the concept of first-order kinetics in which the removal of tumor bulk decreases the tumor burden exponentially and leaves less residual tumor to be eradicated by chemotherapy; and (3) the excision of large tumor masses that results in residual tumor aggregates that are more sensitive to chemotherapy.

Because of the silent spread of ovarian cancer by direct peritoneal implantation of cancer cells, patients with ovarian cancer often have significant tumor burdens at diagnosis. The tumor can also involve the surfaces of the intestinal tract. Although ovarian cancer usually does not invade deeply into the viscera, surface spread may involve much of the gastrointestinal tract, with a devastating effect on function. As a result, patients diagnosed with advanced ovarian cancer often have significant metabolic deficiencies (7). The removal of large tumor masses in the abdomen can result in an immediate improvement in the functioning of the gastrointestinal tract and in the patient's sense of wellbeing. However, cytoreduction benefits some patients more than others. A patient with a partial small bowel obstruction will experience immediate relief of the obstruction, but a patient with small tumor implants on the surface of most of the intestine may feel less of a benefit from surgical cytoreduction.

Perhaps an even more important effect of the mechanical debulking of large tumor masses is the removal of tumor masses that do not have a good blood supply. Removal of these masses eliminates tumors that are unlikely to achieve a significant level of circulating chemotherapy. Cytoreduction may also remove portions of a tumor with few cells in the active growth portion of the cell cycle.

The concept that states, by first-order kinetics, that removal of tumor results in an exponential decrease in tumor and thus results in less cancer for the chemotherapy to destroy has been proposed by many authors as the most important result of cytoreductive surgery. In reality, this effect is probably the least important, especially in primary therapy. As described previously, the reduction of 1 kg of tumor to 1 gm represents the effect of only 10 tumor doublings, and an additional seven three-log kills would be necessary to eradicate the last cell (2). Most surgeons who treat ovarian cancer are aware that cytoreduction from 1 kg to 1 gm is rarely possible; usually a much greater amount of tumor remains. Studies have shown that although cytoreduction to nodules of 1 cm does provide some benefit, the greatest improvement in survival is seen in patients in whom all gross tumor can be removed. Residual disease in these latter cases is often less than 1 gm. Additionally, in the absence of miliary disease, successful surgical cytoreduction may produce its greatest benefit by the theory of first-order kinetics.

The theory that surgical cytoreduction results in residual tumor that is more sensitive to chemotherapy is probably the most important aspect of primary cytoreductive surgery. Schabel, in 1969, discussed the relationship of growth kinetics to the therapy of solid tumors (8). He pointed out that the growth curve of experimental tumors can be explained by the gompertzian equation in which the doubling time of tumors increases as the tumors become larger. This increase is due to a smaller portion of cells in the active growth fraction. Griffiths has pointed out that the removal of large tumor masses by cytoreduction causes a high percentage of cells to enter the pool of actively dividing cells that are most sensitive to chemotherapy (2). Small tumor implants of between 0.1 mg and 5.0 mg have virtually 100% of their cells in the dividing pool. Although it is impossible to extrapolate directly from experimental tumor systems to solid tumors in humans, this theory does offer a plausible explanation for the clinical data that document improved survival in patients with small residual disease. On the other hand, as pointed out by Goldie and Coldman in 1979, the more cells in the active growth fraction, the greater the number of mutations and the greater the opportunity for the development of drug resistant clones (9). When the overall improved survival in patients with small residual disease is considered, however, the advantages of cytoreduction appear to outweigh the disadvantages. Drug resistant clones are perhaps most likely to occur in poorly differentiated tumors, which have overall decreased cure rates in spite of their good response to chemotherapy.

In summary, although the theoretical benefits of primary cytoreductive surgery appear to fit the indirect clinical data, extrapolated data and indirect evidence of benefits are always indications for caution. Other factors may have been overlooked, and only a prospective trial will be able to prove the value of primary cytoreduction.

THE TECHNIQUE OF PRIMARY CYTOREDUCTIVE SURGERY

Few operations call for as much skill and surgical judgment as the primary operation for ovarian cancer. Knowledge of the natural history and patterns of spread of the disease, a complete histologic diagnosis, an understanding of the patient's desires related to quality of life and childbearing, and an accurate preoperative assessment of medical status are all essential to a successful procedure. The surgeon must also be aware of the potential effects the surgical procedure may have on subsequent therapy.

In the case of a malignant germ cell tumor, the issue of conservation of reproductive capacity is significant. In general, any reproductive organ that is not directly involved by the tumor should be preserved. Because these tumors are very sensitive to chemotherapy and yield high relapse-free survival rates, even patients with advanced disease can retain reproductive function. Extensive cytoreductive surgical procedures, with preservation of an uninvolved uterus and adnexa, are indicated. Patients with complete cytoreduction of a malignant germ cell tumor have a much better chance for cure than patients with residual disease.

When ovarian cancer is confined to one ovary and the patient desires further childbearing, removal of the affected adnexa and a full staging operation are the surgical procedures of choice. The details of the staging procedure are discussed in Chapter 10. A complete evaluation of the entire abdomen, including thorough sampling of lymph nodes, is required. Patients with early disease who do not desire further childbearing should undergo total abdominal hysterectomy and bilateral salpingo-oophorectomy. They should also have a complete staging operation.

In patients with advanced disease, a procedure that includes total abdominal hysterectomy, bilateral salpingo-oophorectomy, omentectomy, and resection of all gross disease is ideal. Unfortunately, this ideal is achievable in only a minority of cases. In the Gynecologic Oncology Group (GOG) studies, approximately 40% of patients were left with disease of 1 cm or less, and, in this group, only 28% had all gross disease removed (10). Only 28% of the 40% (11%) of patients with stages III and IV disease were left with no gross residual disease.

One of the characteristics of ovarian cancer that allows some success in surgical removal is the tendency for the disease to remain on the surface of intraabdominal structures. The careful surgeon often can dissect tumor from the surface of the intestine without the need for resection. A tumor-bearing omentum can usually be removed in its entirety. If only the infracolic omentum is involved, it can usually be separated at the edge of the transverse colon. If the supracolic omentum is involved, the omentum should be separated from the transverse colon to expose the lesser sac. The entire omentum can then be resected along the greater curvature of the stomach. Care must be taken to ligate the gastroepiploic vessels on either side and to ligate the small gastric vessels from the gastroepiploic arcade.

Dissection in the pelvis is facilitated by a retroperitoneal approach that allows identification of the blood supply to the pelvic viscera (infundibulopelvic ligament and uterine artery) and to the structures to be preserved (iliac vessel, ureter, and obturator nerve) (Figs. 2 and 3). With complete visualization of the retroperitoneum, the surgeon can mobilize the uterus and

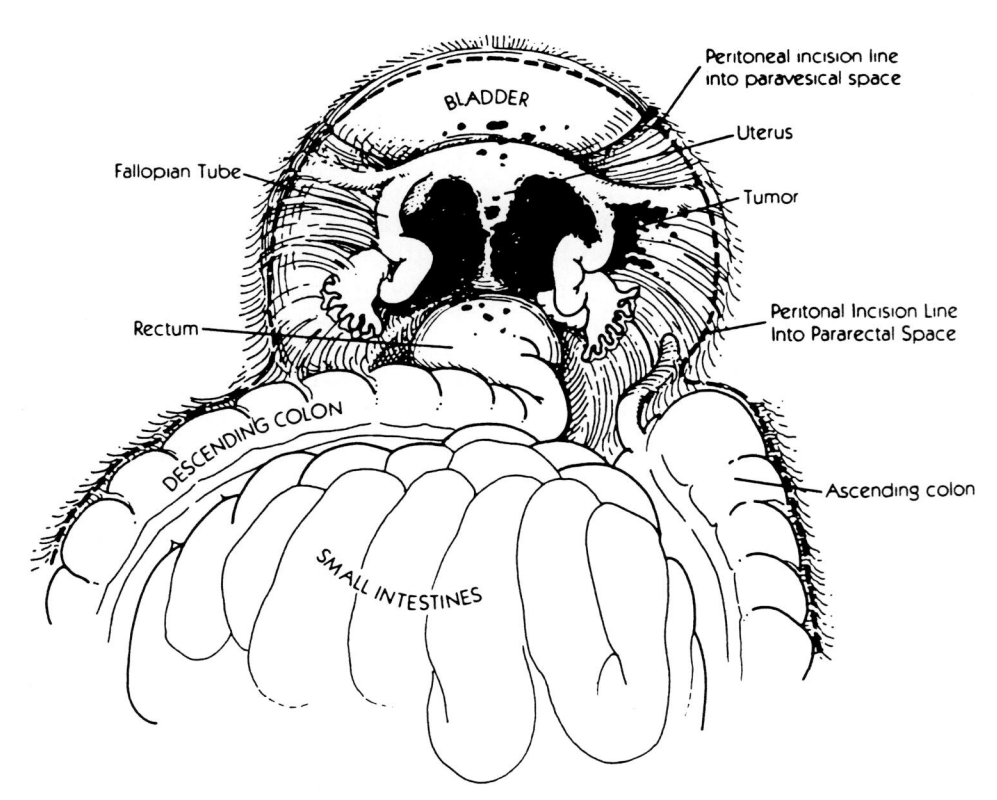

FIG. 2. Retroperitoneal approach for advanced ovarian cancer. (Reproduced from PPO Updated 1(2), Feb. 1987, with permission.)

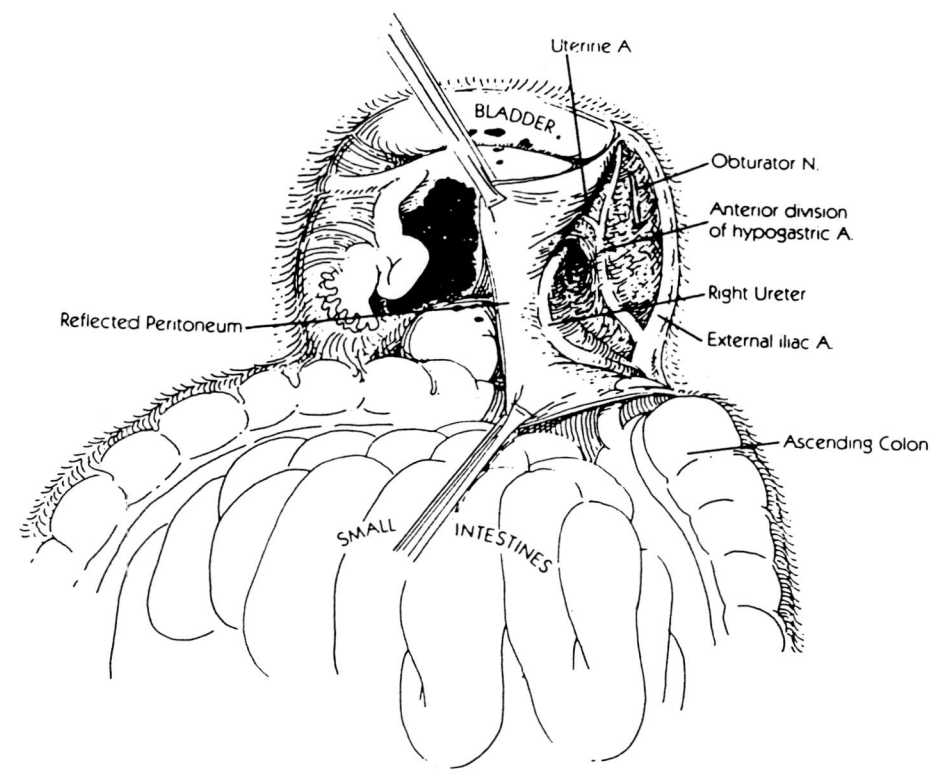

FIG. 3. Retroperitoneal approach for advanced ovarian cancer. (Reproduced from PPO Updated 1(2), Feb. 1987, with permission.)

adnexa medially. If the anterior cul-de-sac is involved by tumor, it can be removed by stripping the peritoneum from the bladder muscularis. Opening the bladder to facilitate dissection and avoid injury to the base of the bladder is occasionally helpful. The management of the ureter depends on the degree to which the parametrium is involved by tumor. The ureter usually can be mobilized to the parametrium for an extrafascial hysterectomy. However, sometimes the ureter must be dissected through the parametrium to the bladder so that involved parametrial tissue can be resected.

If the posterior cul-de-sac is obliterated by tumor, a retrograde hysterectomy as described by Hudson may be required (11). In this procedure, the vagina is entered anteriorly. The uterus is freed from the cardinal and uterosacral ligaments, and the entire cul-de-sac and attached rectum can then be lifted up and out of the pelvis by stretching of the distal rectum. This procedure often facilitates dissection of the cul-de-sac tumor from the surface of the rectum. When the tumor has invaded into the rectal wall, the rectum is divided with a right-angled stapler, and the entire specimen can be mobilized. The proximal sigmoid colon is severed, and continuity is reestablished with a transanal stapled anastomosis.

The decision to perform one or more bowel resections in order to achieve cytoreduction requires the judgment of the surgeon. A good starting point is an evaluation of whether such resections would render the patient disease-free or nearly disease-free. Bowel resections are not logical options in patients who have other unresectable disease, unless symptomatic obstruction is present. Intestine should be resected only if the procedure relieves a symptomatic obstruction or allows optimal cytoreduction. In these cases, the surgeon should not hesitate to perform the resection.

Some tumors that are attached to peritoneal surfaces are easily removed. An example is tumors on the anterior or lateral abdominal peritoneum. Other tumors, such as those involving the diaphragm (with plaque-like growth), are much more difficult to remove. Resection of isolated diaphragmatic metastases may be indicated in a patient who would then be disease-free. Unfortunately, this procedure is not always feasible.

Resection of other organs such as the spleen should be performed only in cases in which the resection would leave the patient free of gross disease. The same is true for lymphadenectomy. If a patient has enlarged pelvic and/or paraaortic lymph nodes and if all or most intraabdominal disease is resected, therapeutic lymphadenectomy may be performed. However, such cases are infrequent.

Decisions during the primary operation for ovarian cancer are often difficult, and they require a great deal of judgment and experience. Even an experienced surgeon is not always able to determine resectability without a significant amount of dissection. As the surgery proceeds, the surgeon must keep the final objective in mind. He or she should not hesitate to call a halt to the procedure or to continue once the findings indicate what would be best for the patient.

EFFECT OF PRIMARY CYTOREDUCTION ON RESPONSE, SURVIVAL, PROGRESSION-FREE INTERVAL, AND SECOND LOOK

A substantial body of literature provides indirect evidence of the benefit of primary cytoreductive surgery. End points that can be used in the evaluation of these studies include response rates, survival, progression-free intervals, and second-look results. Direct evidence for the efficacy of primary cytoreductive surgery would require a randomized trial in which patients receive either cytoreductive surgery or only biopsy (by either laparoscopy or needle biopsy) and then receive a standard chemotherapeutic regimen. The end points could be either progression-free interval or survival. However, the problem with such a study is the belief by many physicians that the indirect evidence of the benefit of cytoreductive surgery is sufficient to make such a study unethical. The GOG actually designed a study to evaluate cytoreductive surgery but closed it because of lack of accrual.

The criterion that is usually used to denote residual disease after primary cytoreductive surgery is the diameter of the largest residual mass. Other factors that may be important are total volume of residual disease and number of residual lesions. In 1986, Redman and associates compared total volume of residual disease, estimated in cubic centemeters, to the volume of the largest residual mass in cubic centemeters (12). Using overall median response rate and survival, they found essentially no difference between the volume of the largest residual mass and total residual volume. The results of their analysis are shown in Table 2.

Gall and co-workers (13) reported on a GOG study in which all patients had less than 3 cm of residual disease. They found improved survival in patients with only one lesion as compared to patients with multiple lesions. Few investigators have evaluated number of lesions as a prognostic factor, but this report by Gall and associates raises an issue that should be evaluated by other investigators.

Response Rate

Table 3 lists several articles that report response rates in relation to residual disease after primary cytoreductive surgery. As shown, patients with less than 2 cm of residual disease (in all cases, diameter of largest mass) have an improved overall response rate and a better complete response rate. This improvement is more pronounced in patients treated with multidrug regimens than in those treated with single alkylating agents. In another study, Young and colleagues (14) noted a 100% complete response rate in patients with <2 cm residual disease treated with HexaCAF compared to an 18% complete response rate in patients with <2 cm residual disease treated with L-PAM. Griffiths (2) has suggested that these results represent the Goldie-Coldman effect in that small residual tumors with a high growth fraction respond better to multidrug regimens.

Survival

The ultimate test of any prognostic factor or any therapy is its effect on survival. Table 4 reviews selected studies that provide information on the survival of patients with advanced ovarian cancer in relation to the amount of residual disease left after the primary operation. Median survival in 388 patients with "optimal" disease was 36.7 months, compared to survival of 16.6 months in 537 patients with suboptimal disease. In most of these series, the patients received platinum-based, multidrug chemotherapy. Figure 4 illustrates an example of one study in which the end point was survival (22).

TABLE 2. *Relation of the largest residual mass with total residual disease in advanced ovarian cancer*

Variable	Volume (cm³)	Number	Median response (in months)	p value	Median survival (in months)	p value
Largest mass	<10	34	23	.003	38	.0085
	10–80	21	26		36	
	>80	31	9		19	
Total Disease	<40	28	34	.007	43	.00068
	40–200	29	20		27	
	>200	29	8		17	

Adapted from Redman JR, et al., ref. 12.

TABLE 3. *Effect of residual disease after primary cytoreductive surgery on response rate in advanced ovarian cancer*

Author (ref.)	Year	Rx	Number	Residual	Response (%) Complete	Response (%) Total
Young et al. (14)	1978	HexaCAF v. L-PAM	19	<2 cm		84
			58	>2 cm		53
Ehrlich et al. (15)	1979	PAC	14	<3 cm	46	78
			25	>3 cm	32	54
Wharton and Herson (16)	1981	L-PAM	45	<2 cm	12	29
			59	>2 cm	8	24
Conte et al. (17)	1986	CAP v. CP	37	<2 cm	70	76
			38	>2 cm	32	82
Total/Mean			115	Optimal	42.7	66.8
			180	Suboptimal	24.0	53.3

HexaCAF, Hexamethylmelamine, cyclophosphamide, amethopterin, 5-flourouracil; PAC, Cisplatin, adriamycin, cyclophosphamide; L-PAM, Melphalan; CAP v. CP, Cisplatin, adriamycin, cyclophosphamide versus cisplatin, cyclophosphamide.

Progression-Free Interval

Progression-free interval is a better indicator of disease control than response rate, but it is less informative than survival rate. It is often used as a surrogate end point in randomized trials so that future studies can be planned before survival end points are ready for evaluation. Table 5 shows the effect of primary cytoreductive surgery on progression-free interval.

Second-Look Surgical Reassessment

After survival, the second most reliable end point used to measure the success of therapy for patients

TABLE 4. *The effect of residual disease at the conclusion of primary cytoreductive surgery on survival*

Author (ref.)	Year	Rx	Residual (in cm)	Number	Survival (in months)
Griffiths (5)	1975	L-PAM	0	29	39
			0–0.5	28	29
			0.6–1.5	16	18
			>1.5	29	11
Hacker et al. (18)	1983	varied	<0.5	7	40
			0.6–1.5	24	18
			>1.5	16	6
Vogl et al. (19)	1983	CHAP	<2	32	>40
			>2	68	16
Pohl et al. (20)	1984	varied	<2	37	45
			>2	57	16
Delgado et al. (21)	1984	varied	<2	21	45
			>2	54	16
Redman et al. (12)	1986	CAP	<3	34	38
			>3	51	26
Conte et al. (17)	1986	CAP V CP	<2	37	>40
			>2	38	16
Neijt et al. (22)	1987	CHAP V CP	<1	88	40
			>1	219	21
Piver et al. (23)	1988	PAC	<2	35	48
			>2	5	21
Total/Mean			Optimal	388	36.7
			Suboptimal	537	16.6

L-PAM, Melphalan; CHAP, Cyclophosphamide, hexamethylmelamine, adriamycin, cisplatin; CAP, Cisplatin, adriamycin, cyclophosphamide; CP, Cisplatin, cyclophosphamide; PAC, Cisplatin, adriamycin, cyclophosphamide.

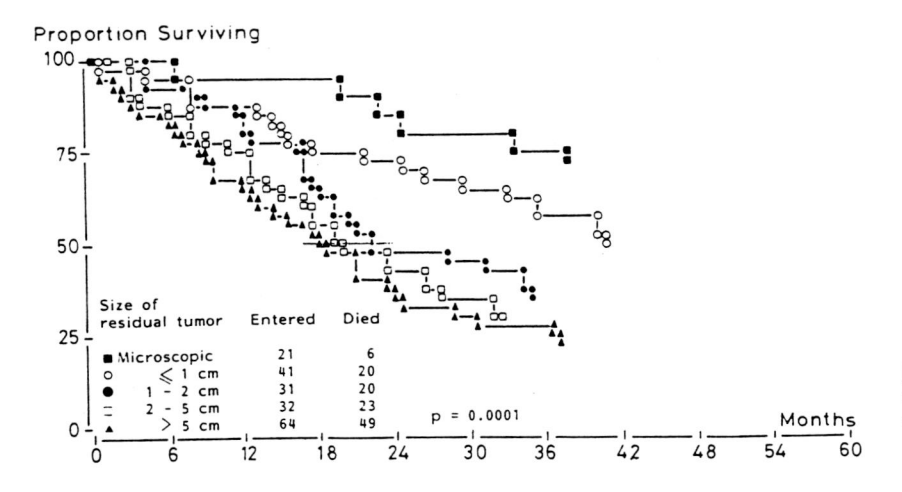

FIG. 4. Survival of patients in relation to the largest cross-sectional tumor diameter before the initiation of chemotherapy. From Neijt et al., ref. 43.

with advanced ovarian cancer is second-look surgical reassessment. This procedure is the most accurate method of assessing response to therapy. The information it yields also provides a reliable prediction of survival. Several studies have demonstrated that the recurrence rate of patients with stages III and IV ovarian cancer ranges from 35% to 50%, and prediction of ultimate survival must be modified to that extent. A literature review in Table 6 demonstrates the effect of primary cytoreductive surgery on the results of second-look surgical reassessment. As can be seen in this review of over 1,000 patients, a direct relationship exists between the amount of residual disease at the conclusion of primary cytoreduction and the likelihood of a negative second-look surgical reassessment. Unfortunately, these figures are not corrected for stage and grade, and the "no residual" group includes patients with early stage disease.

In a recent report from the GOG, Creasman and coworkers (36) reviewed the long-term survival of patients treated on a protocol that evaluated whether melphalan plus corynebacterium parvum was better than melphalan alone in patients with stage III ovarian cancer and residual disease of 3 cm or less after primary cytoreduction. Because no difference existed between the two treatment arms, the entire population was considered as a single group. In a multivariant analysis, patient age, histologic grade of tumor, and the amount of residual disease at the conclusion of primary cytoreductive surgery were statistically important prognostic factors. Because the influence of other prognostic factors was corrected in this analysis, the finding of significance for residual disease is even more striking than in previous studies.

THE CASE AGAINST THE BENEFITS OF PRIMARY CYTOREDUCTIVE SURGERY

Although many potential criticisms of primary cytoreductive surgery can be made, they usually fall into two categories: disadvantages related to the procedure itself and questions about the scientific validity of the studies that demonstrate a benefit.

TABLE 5. *The effect of primary cytoreductive surgery on progression-free interval (PFI) in advanced ovarian cancer*

Author (ref.)	Year	Rx	Residual (in cm)	Number	Median PFI
Vogl et al. (19)	1983	CHAP	<2	32	38
			>2	68	12
Redman et al. (12)	1986	CAP	<3	34	23
			>3	51	14
Piver et al. (23)	1988	PAC	<2	35	25
			>2	5	13
Omura et al. (10)	1989	CAP v. CP	<1	99	48
			>1	250	21
Total/Mean			Optimal	200	33.5
			Suboptimal	374	15.0

CHAP, Cyclophosphamide, hexamethylmelamine, adriamycin, cisplatin; CAP, Cisplatin, adriamycin, cyclophosphamide; PAC, Cisplatin, adriamycin, cyclophosphamide; CP, Cisplatin, cyclophosphamide.

TABLE 6. *The effect of primary cytoreductive surgery on the result of second look surgical reassessment in ovarian cancer*

Author (ref.)	Year	Number	Percent negative		
			None	Optimal	Suboptimal
Curry (24)	1981	27	76	33	33
Webb (25)	1982	59	95	36	20
Cohen (26)	1983	73	73	35	34
Barnhill (27)	1984	96	67	61	14
Podratz (28)	1985	135	82	44	39
Smirtz (29)	1985	88	75	37	19
Cain (30)	1986	177	76	50	28
Dauplat (31)	1986	51	85	73	19
Gallup (32)	1987	65	71	63	13
Carmichael (33)	1987	146	62	30	25
Lund (34)	1990	131	77	55	25
Ayhan (35)	1991	49	92	61	15
Total/Mean		1,097	77.6	48.2	23.7

To address the first category of criticisms, the following disadvantages have been cited: (1) morbidity of the procedure, (2) decrease in quality of life as a result of the radical operation, and (3) delay of chemotherapy. Several authors have addressed the issue of unacceptable morbidity. Chen and Bochner (37) reviewed 60 patients who underwent optimal cytoreduction for stages III and IV epithelial ovarian cancer. They reported a 1.7% postoperative mortality and a 5% incidence of serious postoperative morbidity. The mean operating time was 3.6 hours, and the mean blood loss was 1,644 cc. The patients had an average postoperative stay of 16 days (including the first course of chemotherapy). Heintz and co-workers (38) reported on 70 patients who underwent initial cytoreductive surgery. These patients demonstrated a serious morbidity rate of 26%, but this rate decreased to 10% in the latter period of the study. The decrease in morbidity was attributed to improved cardiovascular monitoring and increased use of hyperalimentation.

Blythe and Wahl (39) addressed the issue of quality of life after cytoreductive surgery. They compared 19 patients who had undergone extensive cytoreductive operations (to residual disease of 2 cm or less) to 17 patients who were not cytoreduced. Quality of life was good or good to fair in 74% of the patients who were successfully cytoreduced. A similar quality of life was reported in only 18% of the suboptimally debulked group. Thirty-three "adverse quality of life" events were reported in the optimally cytoreduced group, and 40 such events were reported in the suboptimal group. The investigators concluded that the optimally cytoreduced patients had a better overall quality of life, despite postoperative recovery for the more extensive operation.

Hacker (40) has stated that although delaying chemotherapy for two weeks is not significant, long delays because of serious postoperative complications may have an adverse effect. In actual fact, few or no data exist about when chemotherapy should be started or whether there is an optimal "window" for starting chemotherapy.

A much more difficult issue is whether the survival benefit of initial cytoreductive surgery relates to the surgery or to the disease process itself. In other words, do some patients survive longer because of cytoreductive surgery or because of differences in the biology of the disease? Potter and co-workers (41) studied 163 patients with stages III or IV epithelial ovarian cancer and evaluated patients by both residual disease and extent of surgery. They found a direct correlation between the volume of residual disease and survival. However, patients who required extensive operations (peritoneal stripping or bowel resection) to achieve disease-free status had a lower survival rate than patients who were rendered disease-free by less extensive operations.

Recently, Hoskins and associates (42) reviewed a GOG study in which 324 patients were entered on an optimal (<1 cm) disease protocol for stage III epithelial ovarian cancer. Patients were randomized to receive cisplatin and cyclophosphamide, with or without doxorubicin. The treatment arms were the same with regard to progression-free interval and survival. The investigators proposed the theory that if patients with abdominal disease of 1 cm or less had the same progression-free interval and survival as patients with bulky disease who were cytoreduced to 1 cm or less, then cytoreductive surgery was the single most important factor influencing their survival. However, a statistically significant difference in survival was seen between these two groups of patients, and the investigators concluded that cytoreductive surgery alone was not the only determining factor.

Does the patient who is optimally cytoreduced have a different disease process than the patient who cannot be cytoreduced? The patient who cannot be cytoreduced (assuming equal attempts by equally qualified surgeons) may indeed have more aggressive disease than the patient who can be cytoreduced. The differences in survival seen by single surgeons, with optimal and suboptimal patients exhibiting different survival rates, do seem to substantiate an inherent difference in the type or extent of disease. However, these observations are difficult to quantify in scientific units.

CONCLUSION

Compelling theoretical reasons support the use of primary cytoreductive surgery for patients with epithelial ovarian cancer. The advent of effective, multidrug therapy has made reduction of tumor residuum more important than ever.

In selected patients with early disease, surgery alone may be curative. In patients with advanced disease, however, a variety of mechanisms combine to provide a survival benefit to patients with minimal residual disease. Clear evidence indicates that the amount of residual disease is directly related to survival, and the patient with the least disease appears to receive the greatest benefit. Patients with no gross residual disease have a much better chance of prolonged survival than patients with any residual disease. The ideal dividing line between optimal and suboptimal disease in patients with residual cancer is probably quite low, in the range of 1–1.5 cm. For patients with larger residual disease, some differences exist with regard to the size of the residuum, but these differences are small.

Patients who undergo radical cytoreductive surgery do not seem to suffer from a decrease in quality of life. In fact, quality of life can be significantly improved if surgery is successful. The mortality rate for cytoreduction is acceptably low, and the morbidity rate is reasonable.

Surgical cytoreduction is not an isolated prognostic factor, however. Studies such as those of Potter and co-workers and Hoskins and associates indicate the involvement of other factors. Neither of these studies imply that primary cytoreduction is not beneficial; they merely point out that other factors are also important. In view of our limited knowledge, these factors are best described as the biology of the tumor.

Finally, what is the future of primary cytoreductive surgery? Technical advances are unlikely to change the success rate of the operation to any substantial degree. However, many patients would benefit from having a trained oncologic surgeon perform the initial surgery for ovarian cancer.

An interesting concept is chemosurgical (or interval) cytoreduction. To date, several small, uncontrolled studies have not been promising. However, new drugs and ideas may renew interest in this concept. If taxol and some of the other new drugs under investigation continue to exhibit high response rates, the combination of initial chemotherapy, interval debulking, and a course of therapy with an entirely different regimen may hold promise. Also, some investigators are evaluating diagnosis by laparoscopy followed by brief, intensive chemotherapy and interval debulking. The results of these preliminary investigations may change the way we think about surgery for ovarian cancer.

REFERENCES

1. Hoskins WJ. Surgical principles in gynecologic oncology. In: Hoskins WJ, Perez CA, Young RC, eds. *Principles and practice of gynecologic oncology*. Philadelphia: JB Lippincott, 1992, pp. 188–189.
2. Griffiths CT. Surgery at the time of diagnosis in ovarian cancer. In: Blackledge G, Chan KK, eds. *Management of ovarian cancer*. London: Butterworths, 1986;60.
3. Munnell EW. The changing prognosis and treatment in cancer of the ovary: a report of 235 patients with primary ovarian cancer 1952–1961. *Am J Obstet Gynecol* 1968;100:790.
4. Delclos L, Quinlan EJ. Malignant tumors of the ovary managed with postoperative megavoltage irradiation. *Radiology* 1969;93:567.
5. Griffiths CT. Surgical resection of tumor bulk in the primary treatment of ovarian cancer. *Natl Cancer Inst Monograph* 1975;42:101.
6. Tannock IF. Principles of cell proliferation: cell kinetics. In: Devita VT, Hellman S, Rosenberg SA, eds. *Cancer, principles and practice of oncology*. 3rd ed. Philadelphia: JB Lippincott, 1989;2–5.
7. Fuller AF, Griffiths CT. Ovarian cancer cachexia-surgical interactions. *Gynecol Oncol* 1979;8:301.
8. Shabel FM Jr. The use of tumor growth kinetics in planning "curative" chemotherapy of advanced solid tumors. *Cancer Research* 1969;29:2384.
9. Goldie JH, Coldman JA. A mathematical model for relating the drug sensitivity of tumors to their spontaneous mutation rate. *Cancer Treatment Rep* 1979;63:1727.
10. Omura GA, Bundy BN, Berek JS, Currey S, Delgado G, Mortel R. Randomized trial of cyclophosphamide plus cisplatin with or without doxorubicin in ovarian carcinoma: a Gynecologic Oncology Group study. *J Clin Oncol* 1989;7:457.
11. Hudson CN. Surgical treatment of ovarian cancer. *Gynecol Oncol* 1973;1:370.
12. Redman JR, Petroni GR, Saigo PE, Geller NL, Hakes TB. Prognostic factors in advanced ovarian cancer. *J Clin Oncol* 1986;4:515.
13. Gall S, Bundy BN, Beecham J, et al. Therapy of stage III (optimal) epithelial carcinoma of the ovary with melphalan or melphalan plus cornyebacterium parvum (a Gynecologic Oncology Group study). *Gynecol Oncol* 1986;25:26.
14. Young RC, Chabner BA, Hubbard SP, et al. Advanced ovarian adenocarcinoma: a prospective clinical trial of melphalan (L-PAM) versus combination chemotherapy. *N Engl J Med* 1978;299:1261.
15. Ehrlich CE, Einhorn L, Williams SD, et al. Chemotherapy for stage III–IV epithelial ovarian cancer with cisdichlorodiamineplatinum (II), adriamycin, and cyclophosphamide: a preliminary report. *Cancer Treat Rep* 1979;63:281.
16. Wharton JT, Herson J. Surgery for common epithelial tumors of the ovary. *Cancer* 1981;48:582.
17. Conte PF, Bruzzone M, Chiaro S, et al. A randomized trial comparing cisplatin plus cyclophosphamide versus cisplatin, doxo-

rubicin and cyclophosphamide in advanced ovarian cancer. *J Clin Oncol* 1986;4:965.
18. Hacker NF, Berek JS, Lagasse LD, et al. Primary cytoreductive surgery for epithelial ovarian cancer. *Obstet Gynecol* 1983;61:413.
19. Vogl SE, Pagano M, Kaplan BH, et al. Cisplatin based combination chemotherapy for advanced ovarian cancer: high overall response rate with curative potential only in women with small tumor burdens. *Cancer* 1983;51:2024.
20. Pohl R, Dallenback-Hellweg G, Plugge T, et al. Prognostic parameters in patients with advanced malignant ovarian tumors. *Eur J Gynaecol Oncol* 1984;3:160.
21. Delgado G, Oram D, Petrilli ES. Stage III ovarian cancer: the role of maximal surgical reduction. *Gynecol Oncol* 1984;18:293.
22. Neijt JP, van der Burg MEL, Vriesendorp R, et al. Randomized trial comparing two combination chemotherapy regimens (Hexa-CAF vs CHAP-5) in advanced ovarian carcinoma. *Lancet* 1984;2:549.
23. Piver MS, Lele SB, Marchetti DL, et al. The impact of aggressive debulking surgery and cisplatin chemotherapy on progression-free survival in stage III and IV ovarian carcinomas. *J Clin Obstet Gynecol* 1988;6:983.
24. Curry S, Zembo M, Nahhas W, et al. Second-look laparotomy for ovarian cancer. *Gynecol Oncol* 1981;11:114.
25. Webb MJ, Snyder JJ, Williams TJ, Decker DG. Second-look laparotomy in the management of gynecologic malignancy. *Gynecol Oncol* 1982;13:345.
26. Cohen CJ, Goldberg JD, Holland JF, et al. Improved therapy with cisplatin regimens for patients with ovarian carcinoma (FIGO stages III and IV) as measured by surgical end-staging (second-look operation). *Am J Obstet Gynecol* 1983;145:955.
27. Barnhill DR, Hoskins WJ, Heller PB, Park RC. The second-look surgical reassessment for epithelial ovarian carcinoma. *Gynecol Oncol* 1984;19:148.
28. Podratz KC, Malkasian G Jr, Hilton JF, Harris EA, Gaffey TA. Second-look laparotomy in ovarian cancer: evaluation of pathologic variables. *Am J Obstet Gynecol* 1985;152:230.
29. Smirtz LR, Stehman FB, Ulbright TM, Sutton GP, Ehrlich CE. Second-look laparotomy after chemotherapy in the management of ovarian malignancy. *Am J Obstet Gynecol* 1985;20:152–661.
30. Cain J, Saigo P, Pierce V, et al. A review of second-look laparotomy for ovarian cancer. *Gynecol Oncol* 1986;23:14.
31. Dauplat J, Ferriere JP, Gorbinet M, et al. Second-look laparotomy in managing epithelial ovarian carcinoma. *Cancer* 1986;57:1627.
32. Gallup DG, Talledo OE, Dudzinski MR, Brown KW. Another look at the second-assessment procedure for ovarian epithelial carcinoma. *Am J Obstet Gynecol* 1987;157:590.
33. Carmichael JA, Shelley WE, Brown LB, et al. A predictive index of cure versus no cure in advanced ovarian carcinoma patients—replacement of second-look laparotomy as a diagnostic test. *Gynecol Oncol* 1987;27:269.
34. Lund B, Jacobsen K, Rasch L, Jensen F, Olesen K, Feldt RK. Correlation of abdominal ultrasound and computed tomography scans with second- or third-look laparotomy in patients with ovarian carcinoma. *Gynecol Oncol* 1990;37:279.
35. Ayhan A, Yarali H, Develioglu O, Uren A, Ozyilimaz F. Prognosticators of second-look laparotomy findings in patients with epithelial ovarian cancer. *J Surg Oncol* 1991;46:222.
36. Creasman WT, Gall S, Bundy BN, Beecham J, Mortel R, Homesley HD. Second-look laparotomy in the patient with minimal residual stage III ovarian cancer (a Gynecologic Oncology Group study). *Gynecol Oncol* 1989;35:378.
37. Chen SS, Bochner R. Assessment of morbidity and mortality in primary cytoreductive surgery for advanced ovarian cancer. *Gynecol Oncol* 1985;20:190.
38. Heintz APM, Hacker NF, Berek JS, et al. Cytoreductive surgery in ovarian carcinoma: feasibility and morbidity. *Obstet Gynecol* 1986;67:783.
39. Blythe JG, Wahl TP. Debulking surgery: does it increase the quality of survival? *Gynecol Oncol* 1982;14:396.
40. Hacker NF. Controversial aspects of cytoreductive surgery in epithelial ovarian cancer. *Baillieres Clin Obstet Gynaecol* 1989;3:49.
41. Potter ME, Partridge EE, Hatch KD, Soong S, Austin JM, Shingleton HM. Primary surgical therapy of ovarian cancer: how much and when. *Gynecol Oncol* 1991;40:195.
42. Hoskins WJ, Thigpen JT, Bundy BN, et al. The influence of initial surgery on progression-free interval and survival in optimal (<1 cm) stage III epithelial ovarian cancer. *Gynecol Oncol* [*in press*].
43. Neijt JP, ten Bokkel Huinink WW, van der Burg MEL, et al. Randomized trial comparing two combination chemotherapy regimens (CHAP-5 v. CP) in advanced ovarian carcinoma. *J Clin Oncol* 1987;5:1157–1168.

CHAPTER 12

Second-Look Laparotomy in Ovarian Cancer

Stephen C. Rubin

HISTORICAL ASPECTS

The concept of a secondary surgical exploration to assess tumor status after treatment for an intraabdominal malignancy was developed in the department of surgery at the University of Minnesota during the late 1940s and early 1950s (1,2). Patients who had undergone primary surgical treatment for gastrointestinal malignancies were systematically reexplored in an attempt to identify recurrent tumor before the development of clinical symptoms. In a 1957 publication, Arhelger et al. set forth the following rationale and technique (3):

> This concept of reoperation in the absence of symptoms and clinically detectable recurrence offers new hope in the treatment of some advanced malignancies. Additionally, it has provided a unique opportunity to study the biology of the spread of residual visceral cancer and has permitted objective observations of the limitations of conventional primary operations. . . . Approximately six months after the original excision and while the patients are asymptomatic and without evidence of residual cancer, they are reoperated upon. A thorough search for any residual is made; any suspicious nodule is removed, together with any remaining lymph node bearing tissue near the primary site of operation. Residual cancer, if found, is removed, unless the situation is obviously out of hand. If cancer is found at this second-look operation, subsequent exploratory operations called third, fourth, and so on, looks are carried out at similar intervals of time until no cancer is found. Once a patient has undergone a negative exploration . . . no more surgery is recommended unless clinical evidence of a recurrence becomes apparent. . . .
>
> At the time of re-exploration, systematic examination of the entire abdominal cavity and the contained viscera is performed. This has included an examination of both the intraperitoneal and extraperitoneal areas insofar as possible. A detailed identification and tabulation as to location of the residuals by the surgeon and the pathologist have been made; the specimens for histologic examination have been meticulously examined, using multiple and, in some cases, serial sections. It has been common to study as many as 30 specimens from a single case.
>
> Because false negatives can occur either by failure of the surgeon to recognize residual cancer or through failure of the pathologist to find small areas of cancer in tissues removed, every effort has been made to reoperate thoroughly, removing, if possible, all suspicious tissues.

The results of these interesting early studies are reminiscent of contemporary studies in ovarian cancer. About one-half of the patients undergoing reexploration had tumor identified, the morbidity of the surgery was minimal, and the lives of some patients with residual disease were salvaged by further therapy.

In the early literature on reoperation for cancer of the ovary, the term *second-look laparotomy* was used with a variety of meanings. As early as 1945, it was noted that certain cases of ovarian cancer that were unresectable on initial surgery might become operable after treatment (in this case, radiotherapy) (4). The phenomenon was noted by Kottmeier (5), and various authors have described such operations as "second-look" operations (6–8). Many authors have also used the term to describe operations performed for relief of symptoms, including intestinal obstruction, or for resection of known progressive or recurrent cancer (9–11). Other reports, including some relatively recent series, have included asymptomatic patients thought on the basis of preoperative evaluation to have persistent cancer (12–14).

A consensus gradually evolved that the term *second-look laparotomy* should refer only to a systematic surgical reexploration in asymptomatic patients who have completed a planned program of treatment, usually chemotherapy, after initial surgery for ovarian cancer. Patients thought to have tumor present based on preoperative evaluation including physical examination and

S. C. Rubin: Gynecology Service, Memorial Sloan-Kettering Cancer Center, New York, New York 10021

radiographic imaging should not be included in reports on second-look laparotomy.

In the 1960s alkylating agent chemotherapy was found to produce responses in patients with ovarian cancer. In a landmark 1966 report from the M. D. Anderson Hospital, Rutledge and Burns noted that "there has been some reluctance to accept this form of treatment for advanced ovarian cancer because of the variable response which is difficult to evaluate and the fear of toxicity" (15). They went on to ask several questions relevant to the issue of second-look surgery, including "should laparotomy be used more often when a patient has an unusually good response to determine if the drug can be discontinued?" and "is chemotherapy capable of totally eradicating advanced ovarian cancer?" In this report on 288 patients with "advanced inoperable" ovarian cancer treated with melphalan either alone or in combination with irradiation, 28 patients underwent reexploration to determine if therapy could be discontinued. Twelve of these patients had no tumor identified after receiving from 4 to 35 months of chemotherapy. Two patients had recurrence of tumor during the period of observation. The authors noted that "a good response to the drug is reason for laparotomy" and went on to say that "when the status of disease remains unknown after a long period of drug therapy, laparotomy may be the only method of evaluation." They noted that the absence of detectable cancer at the time of reexploration is not proof of cure, and they suggested that the pelvic and aortic lymph nodes may be sites of occult metastases. Subsequent reports from M. D. Anderson provided long-term follow-up on what was by then referred to as second-look surgery in ovarian cancer. These reports provided important information about patient selection, duration of chemotherapy, and further management after second-look surgery (12,16).

In the 1970s two events led the way to the widespread use of second-look laparotomy in the management of ovarian cancer. The first was the recognition that the long-term use of alkylating agents could result in the development of acute leukemia (17,18), which provided an impetus for attempting to determine the latest point to which chemotherapy could be safely continued. The second was the recognition of cisplatin as a highly active agent in the treatment of ovarian cancer (19,20) and the development of combination chemotherapy regimens that included platinum. Platinum-based regimens produced higher overall response rates than nonplatinum regimens. The majority of patients, particularly those with small-volume residual tumor, achieved a complete clinical response and became candidates for second-look laparotomy.

RATIONALE FOR SECOND-LOOK LAPAROTOMY

Epithelial ovarian cancer lends itself to reassessment by laparotomy. Although the general concept of ovarian cancer as a disease that remains confined to the peritoneal cavity and retroperitoneal lymphatics is not entirely accurate, these areas are almost always involved. According to data on 8,451 ovarian cancer patients reported to the International Federation of Gynecology and Obstetrics and published in their 1988 annual report (21), only 16.3% of these patients had stage IV disease, which indicates that clinically detectable distant metastases are unusual at the time of diagnosis. Later in the course of the disease, distant metastases may occur more frequently. For example, in an autopsy series of 86 patients who died from ovarian cancer, Bergman reported liver or lung metastases in about one-third of cases, bone metastases in 14%, and spleen, kidney, adrenal, or skin metastases in 6% to 8% (22). However, distant metastases in the absence of disease in the peritoneal cavity or retroperitoneal lymphatics would be extremely unusual. With the natural history and patterns of spread of ovarian cancer, laparotomy is a reasonable means of searching for clinically occult residual disease.

Most ovarian cancer patients will have no clinically detectable disease at the completion of primary chemotherapy. Although it is still controversial, aggressive primary cytoreductive surgery in advanced ovarian cancer has been accepted as valuable by most gynecologic oncologists (23). In reports from many authors (24–32), "optimal" cytoreduction appears to be possible in about one-third of patients with bulky advanced ovarian cancer. The large majority of such patients, when treated with platinum-based chemotherapy, will have no clinical evidence of disease at the completion of treatment. Although patients who are suboptimally cytoreduced do not fare as well, a significant proportion will be rendered free of clinically detectable disease by chemotherapy. When these two groups are combined with patients initially found to have small-volume advanced disease and those with early stage disease, we can estimate that some 50% to 60% of all ovarian cancer patients will be without clinical evidence of disease at the completion of primary chemotherapy.

There is no accurate, noninvasive means of detecting clinically occult residual disease. A variety of methods have attempted to determine disease status in ovarian cancer patients treated with chemotherapy. Cytologic analysis of peritoneal fluid obtained by culdocentesis may be useful in detecting residual ovarian cancer (33, 34). Although the unequivocal presence of cancer cells in this fluid is clear evidence that cancer is still present, the accuracy of peritoneal cytology in detecting residual tumor is quite low. In a recent report from Memorial Sloan-Kettering, Rubin et al. reported on 96 women undergoing secondary operations for ovarian cancer who had multiple cytologic washings taken with the abdomen open (35). Among patients with gross intraperitoneal disease, only 34% had positive cytology; in patients with microscopic disease, 28% had positive washings.

A number of authors have investigated the use of laparoscopy as a means of evaluating ovarian cancer patients and possibly avoiding second-look laparotomy (36–39). Laparoscopy, including open techniques, is likely to carry significant hazard for the group of patients who have had extensive intraabdominal tumor and prior major abdominal surgery, a group that includes most ovarian cancer patients. In one of the early studies, Berek and colleagues reported on 119 laparoscopic evaluations performed in 57 ovarian cancer patients to determine disease status during or after chemotherapy (36). Fourteen percent of these patients had major complications requiring laparotomy, most of which involved intestinal perforation. In Berek's experience, adhesions will preclude adequate assessment of the peritoneal cavity by laparoscopy in at least 25% of patients (37). Adhesions also limit the ability to detect cancer. In a series in which 22 patients with no tumor found on laparoscopy underwent immediate laparotomy, Ozols and co-workers found tumor in 12 (55%) (40). In view of the risk, the unreliability of a negative laparoscopy, and the limitations in assessment of the retroperitoneum and resection of gross residual disease, laparoscopy has not gained a significant role in the reevaluation of ovarian cancer.

Cross-sectional imaging, using techniques such as computerized tomography (CT), ultrasound, and magnetic resonance, has been evaluated in the detection of intraperitoneal ovarian cancer. In some cases, these techniques have been compared directly to second-look laparotomy. In general, they have not been useful in the detection of tumor masses in the clinically important size range of <2 cm. In some cases, they may in fact miss much larger masses. In one series that compared CT with surgical exploration in 52 ovarian cancer patients, CT failed to detect pelvic and abdominal masses up to 3 cm as well as large omental cakes. The overall diagnostic accuracy was only 58% (41). Evaluation of results reported by several other authors supports the conclusion that CT lacks sufficient diagnostic accuracy to be a substitute for second-look laparotomy (42–48).

Results of studies comparing sonography to second-look laparotomy indicate that sonography is also inadequate to preclude laparotomy (49–51). In a series of 129 patients with ovarian cancer who underwent sonography prior to second-look, Murolo et al. (50) reported a sensitivity of only 8.6% for residual tumor masses smaller than 2 cm in diameter. Khan et al. reported on sonographic findings in 98 ovarian cancer patients who underwent surgical reexploration and concluded that accuracy for the peritoneal cavity in general was very low, with even large masses escaping detection (49).

According to individuals who are experienced with the use of magnetic resonance imaging (MRI) in ovarian cancer, this modality also lacks sufficient accuracy to replace laparotomy (52). Newer imaging modalities such as positron emission tomography with radiolabeled antitumor monoclonal antibodies are under investigation at a number of centers, including Memorial Sloan-Kettering. However, external imaging techniques are unlikely to approach the accuracy of exploratory laparotomy in detecting residual ovarian cancer in the near future.

Serum tumor markers, most notably CA-125, have been studied as a possible means of avoiding second-look laparotomy for disease reassessment in ovarian cancer patients. After the initial report by Bast et al. (53), which indicated that serial measurement of serum CA-125 reflected disease activity, numerous authors reported on CA-125 levels and surgical findings at the time of second-look laparotomy (54–58). In general, an elevated CA-125 level is a reliable indicator of persistent disease, although occasional false positives do occur. However, patients with normal CA-125 levels will often be found to have tumor present at exploration. Rubin et al. (59) reported on CA-125 levels at the time of secondary surgery in 96 ovarian cancer patients who had previously had an elevated level at a time when tumor was known to be present, and who were thus considered "marker positive." Among patients who had a normal CA-125 level at the time of surgery, 62% were found to have tumor. Not all of the patients in this series were clinically free of disease before surgery. Some were found to have large tumor masses despite a normal CA-125 level, although the accuracy of the CA-125 level did vary with the size of the tumor masses present.

A normal serum CA-125 level is thus a very poor predictor of the absence of disease at the time of second-look laparotomy. An elevated level reliably predicts the presence of tumor. However, with the likely benefits of secondary cytoreduction (discussed later) and the importance of assessing the condition of the peritoneal cavity for possible subsequent intraperitoneal therapy, an elevated CA-125 does not necessarily obviate laparotomy.

Treatment of residual tumor identified at the time of second-look laparotomy can be effective. A major component of the argument against second-look laparotomy has traditionally related to the supposed ineffectiveness of all forms of secondary therapy for epithelial ovarian cancer. Clearly, if further therapy has no benefit, the early detection of residual disease can have little importance, especially when an invasive procedure is involved. This excessively nihilistic position has been rebutted in recent years by a number of important findings from studies of second-line therapy. Patients with a good initial response to platinum-based therapy have a significant likelihood of a second response, particularly if dose intensification can be achieved by intraperitoneal drug delivery. A study from Memorial Sloan-Kettering reported by Markman et al. (60) evaluated the influence of a prior response to intravenous cisplatin on responses to second-line intraperitoneal platinum regimens. Among 89 evaluable patients, the surgically documented overall and complete response rates were 56% and 33%, respectively, among patients with a prior response to platinum, compared with 11% and 3% among prior nonresponders. Most patients who reach the point of second-look laparotomy will fall into the prior responder category. It is also clear that patients with small-volume disease respond better to second-line intraperitoneal treatment (61), which further supports the argument for second-look laparotomy for early detection of residual tumor. Preliminary evidence from Memorial Sloan-Kettering indicates that responders to second-line treatment live longer than nonresponders.

Other developments in second-line therapy also support the use of second-look laparotomy. Recent reports indicate that intravenous ifosfamide and intraperitoneal mitoxantrone have activity in ovarian cancer patients who have been refractory to platinum (62,63). Taxol, a new drug with a novel mechanism of action that has activity in platinum-refractory patients (64), has entered intraperitoneal trials (65). The use of techniques to ameliorate myelosuppression—including autologous marrow transplantation, peripheral stem cell harvest and reinfusion, and colony-stimulating factors—are likely to further increase the efficacy of secondary therapy and the importance of second-look laparotomy.

Secondary cytoreduction at the time of second-look laparotomy is often possible and may improve response rates and survival following second-line treatment. About one-half of all patients who undergo second-look laparotomy will have tumor identified. Because about 80% of patients with a positive second-look operation will have gross tumor present, approximately 40% of all patients undergoing the operation may be candidates for secondary cytoreduction. Experienced gynecologic cancer surgeons can accomplish optimal cytoreduction in a significant proportion of these patients. Reported success rates range from 24% to 84% (10–12,66–68); the variation is probably due to differences in patient selection, surgical aggressiveness, and the definition of "optimal."

As previously noted, patients with small-volume residual tumor appear to have an increased rate of response to secondary therapy as compared to those with large-volume residual. This advantage appears to pertain whether patients are found to have small-volume disease or whether they can be cytoreduced to small-volume residual disease. Studies of the effect of secondary cytoreduction on survival have often included patients treated by a variety of second-line chemotherapeutic regimens, which hampers interpretation. In a series reported by Chambers et al. (69), which compared 23 patients with microscopic residual disease and 6 with gross residual disease, secondary cytoreduction did not appear to influence survival. Other researchers have reported similar findings (11). On the other hand, Podratz et al. studied 116 patients with a positive second-look laparotomy and found a four-year survival of 55% in patients with microscopic residual disease, compared with 19% in patients with gross residual disease (70). In a recent study by Hoskins et al. on 67 patients found to have tumor at second-look, patients cytoreduced to microscopic residual disease had a five-year survival of 51%, which is similar to that of patients found to have only microscopic disease and is significantly better than the less-than-10% survival in patients left with gross residual disease (71). Lippman et al. have also reported that patients who underwent optimal resection (less than 2 cm residual tumor) at the time of second-look had a significantly better survival than those who underwent suboptimal resection (72).

As second-line treatment regimens evolve and long-term follow-up accrues, the improvement in response rates seen in patients with small-volume residual disease is likely to translate into an improvement in long-term survival, which lends support to the proponents of cytoreduction at the time of second-look laparotomy.

TECHNIQUE OF SECOND-LOOK LAPAROTOMY

Second-look laparotomy is intended to be a meticulous surgical evaluation of the entire peritoneal cavity and selected retroperitoneal areas to maximize the possibility of detecting residual ovarian cancer. Surgeons should review the operative reports from the patient's initial ovarian cancer operation to familiarize themselves with the extent and location of areas of tumor remaining at the end of the first operation. The patient must have a clear understanding of the purposes of the operation, both diagnostic and therapeutic, and of the way in which subsequent treatment will depend on the outcome of the surgery. Issues such as intestinal resection, removal of remaining internal reproductive organs, and the placement of an intraperitoneal port and catheter system should be discussed if appropriate.

A careful pelvic examination should be performed in the operating room under anesthesia. Cytoscopy and proctoscopy should be considered, particularly if they were not performed at the time of the patient's initial surgery. When the uterus is still present, a dilatation and currettage should be performed. The abdomen should be entered through a generous vertical incision to allow complete access to the upper abdomen. Peritoneal washings for cytologic evaluation should be obtained from multiples areas, usually including the pelvis, both paracolic gutters, and the undersurfaces of both hemidiaphragms. If the initial abdominal exploration reveals obvious gross tumor, frozen section confirmation should be obtained. After complete assessment of the peritoneal cavity and retroperitoneal lymph nodes, involved areas should be resected if optimal cytoreduction appears possible. Careful note should be made of the size and location of residual tumor, both before and after cytoreduction. These observations will be essential in assessing the patient's response to first-line chemotherapy and in selecting the most appropriate second-line treatment.

If no tumor is identified at the initial exploration, the surgeon must begin a careful search for areas of occult disease, focusing attention on areas of known prior residual tumor and areas of frequent spread. The undersurfaces of both hemidiaphragms should be examined and sampled histologically or cytologically. A sterile proctoscope or laparoscope may be used to aid in the visualization of these areas. The remaining omentum, if any, should be removed. Intestinal adhesions should be carefully lysed and portions submitted for pathologic evaluation. The intestines should be closely examined, including both the serosal and the mesenteric aspects. Random biopsies may be taken from the paracolic gutters. The pelvic viscera should be carefully examined and biopsies taken from the surfaces of the bladder, rectum, and cul-de-sac. Surgical pedicles from the initial operation should be identified and sampled, especially the stumps of the infundibulopelvic ligaments. Any internal reproductive organs still present should generally be removed. The aortic lymph nodes should be thoroughly sampled. Because recent reports indicate that the majority of patients with advanced ovarian cancer have metastatic disease in the pelvic lymph nodes, both at the time of primary surgery and at second-look (73,74), these nodes should be sampled as well. When no gross tumor is identified, a properly performed second-look operation may take several hours and produce 20 and 30 individual histologic and cytologic specimens.

CLINICAL CORRELATES OF SECOND-LOOK LAPAROTOMY FINDINGS

Over the years, many authors and institutions have published series on second-look laparotomy. Table 1 presents data compiled from 29 reports, including 2,309 patients, published between 1981 and 1990 (14,69,72, 75–101). Series in which not all patients were clinically free of disease at the time of exploration were excluded; this information is limited to the current definition of second-look laparotomy. The weighted means show that 54% of patients had disease detected at second-look laparotomy, whereas 46% did not. There is no discernable difference in the proportion of patients with disease detected from the early publications to the more recent, although the time period that was reviewed spans the transition from alkylating-agent therapy to platinum-based therapy. Differences in results among the various series are probably explainable based on variation in patient population.

As shown in Table 2 (13,69,75,77,78,80–82,85,

TABLE 1. Results of second-look laparotomy

First author (ref.)	Year	Total patients	Percent negative	Percent positive
Curry (75)	1981	27	63	37
Webster (76)	1981	22	73	27
Roberts (77)	1982	63	57	43
Webb (78)	1982	59	46	54
Cohen (79)	1983	73	41	59
Phibbs (80)	1983	42	40	60
Ballon (81)	1984	25	44	56
Barnhill (82)	1984	96	50	50
Berek (83)	1984	56	32	68
Milstead (84)	1984	22	55	45
Rocereto (85)	1984	36	64	36
Gershenson (86)	1985	246	34	66
Podratz (87)	1985	135	47	53
Smirz (88)	1985	88	40	60
Cain (89)	1986	177	59	41
Dauplat (14)	1986	51	47	53
Miller (90)	1986	88	43	57
Carmichael (91)	1987	173	31	69
Gallup (92)	1987	65	52	48
Ho (93)	1987	39	44	56
McCusker (94)	1987	42	48	52
Podczaski (95)	1987	94	52	48
Chambers (69)	1988	67	43	57
Lippman (72)	1988	70	30	70
Sonnendecker (96)	1988	39	72	28
de Gramont (97)	1989	86	37	63
Ghatage (93)	1990	155	50	50
Kamura (99)	1990	42	76	24
Lund (100)	1990	131	55	45
Ayhan (101)	1991	49	57	43
Total		2,358		
Weighted mean			46	54

TABLE 2. Percent negative at second-look laparotomy by stage of disease

First author (ref.)	Year	Total patients	Stage I percent negative	Stage II percent negative	Stage III percent negative	Stage IV percent negative
Schwartz (13)	1980	186	67	45	16	39
Curry (75)	1981	27	100	83	50	0
Roberts (77)	1982	63	86	75	30[a]	—
Webb (78)	1982	59	80	60	34[a]	—
Phibbs (80)	1983	42	100	80	19	33
Ballon (81)	1984	25	50	50	41	50
Barnhill (82)	1984	96	74	71	34	25
Rocereto (85)	1984	36	100	100	37	0
Podratz (87)	1985	135	86	77	38[a]	—
Smirz (88)	1985	88	60	86	26	55
Cain (89)	1986	177	79	68	48	45
Carmichael (91)	1987	173			32	22
Gallup (92)	1987	65	86	60	38	50
Podczaski (95)	1987	94	81	92	42	0
McCusker (94)	1987	42	100	71	48	0
Chambers (69)	1988	67	100	85	30	0
Sonnendecker (96)	1988	39	92	100	56	63
Kamura (99)	1990	42	89	63	58	100
Lund (100)	1990	109		71	33	27
Ayhan (101)	1991	49	100	80	50	29
Total		1,428				
Weighted Mean			85	75	37	34

[a] Includes some stage IV patients.

87–89,91,92,94–96,99–101), the stage of disease strongly influences the likelihood of finding disease at the time of second-look laparotomy. In stages III and IV, more than 60% of patients will have cancer detected at second-look. Stage II patients fare considerably better, and, in stage I, only some 15% are found to have residual tumor. Many of the series reviewed probably included patients who did not have complete surgical staging as stage I. In a group of rigorously staged stage I patients, the proportion with a positive second-look should be considerably lower than 15%, which represents only those patients whose occult microscopic disease is primarily platinum-resistant.

The significance of histologic tumor grade as a prognostic factor in ovarian cancer is unclear. Early reports have indicated that tumor grade (as distinct from cell type) has important prognostic significance (102). More recent reports of patients treated with platinum-based regimens have suggested less importance to tumor grade (79). Many publications have reported on the results of second-look laparotomy as related to the histologic grade of the tumor. As indicated in Table 3 (77–80,82,87,88,91,92,99–101), there does seem to be a trend toward an increased proportion of positive operations in patients with higher grade tumors. No report has used a multivariate analysis, however, to determine whether tumor grade is an independent predictor of second-look outcome apart from the effects of stage and residual tumor.

The amount of residual tumor following the primary cytoreductive operation is a strong predictor of second-look findings. Table 4 (14,44,72,75,78–80,82,83, 87–89,91,92,101) summarizes 15 reports including 1,262 patients. In patients with no residual tumor, 77% had no tumor detected at second-look, compared with 47% in patients with optimal residual and only 22% in patients with suboptimal residual. These data are skewed, however, by the fact that many authors have included stage I patients among the "no residual" group. Comparison of the optimal and suboptimal groups, comprised only of patients with metastatic disease, also shows a strong effect of the amount of residual tumor on second-look findings. Although the predictive effect of residual tumor seems clear, the extent to which this is due to the beneficial effects of primary cytoreduction versus the basic biology of the tumor continues to generate controversy.

COMPLICATIONS OF SECOND-LOOK LAPAROTOMY

Significant morbidity might be expected in an extensive surgical exploration in patients who are elderly, have an advanced malignancy, have recently had intensive chemotherapy, or have had prior extensive abdominal surgery. Fortunately, this is not the case. When performed by experienced surgeons in tertiary

TABLE 3. Percent negative at second-look laparotomy by histologic grade of tumor

First author (ref.)	Year	Total patients	Grade 1 percent negative	Grade 2 percent negative	Grade 3 percent negative
Roberts (77)	1982	63	76	52	47
Webb (78)	1982	59	71	57	38
Cohen (79)	1983	73	46	35	42
Phibbs (80)	1983	42	29	71	17
Barnhill (82)	1984	96	59	50	32
Podratz (87)	1985	135	73	61	49
Smirz (88)	1985	88	37	33	46
Carmichael (91)	1987	146	27	15	41
Gallup (92)	1987	56	80	63	37
Kamura (99)	1990	42	83	83	58
Lund (100)	1990	90	23	39	43
Ayhan (101)	1991	49	53	71	38
Total		939			
Weighted Mean			59	47	42

care centers, second-look laparotomy is associated with relatively little serious morbidity. In a review that included seven major series published since 1980, no deaths were reported in 682 operations (103). Infections were the most common complications, including those of the surgical wound (6.3%), urinary tract (5.6%), and lungs (2.8%). A 1.6% incidence of gastrointestinal injury was reported as well as a 0.4% incidence of postoperative intestinal obstruction.

PROGNOSTIC SIGNIFICANCE OF SECOND-LOOK LAPAROTOMY FINDINGS

The amount of tumor detected at second-look laparotomy holds major prognostic significance. Patients with gross tumor detected at second-look have a poor outlook, particularly if optimal cytoreduction cannot be accomplished (as discussed earlier in this chapter). In series in which long-term survival is reported separately for patients with gross residual disease, three-year survival following second-look is approximately 20% (13,87). Hoskins et al. (71) reported a five-year survival of only 10% in patients left with gross residual tumor following second-look. With the development of second-line chemotherapy regimens that may produce responses in platinum refractory patients (62–65), these figures may improve.

For the approximately 10% of patients undergoing second-look laparotomy who are found to have microscopic disease, the outlook is considerably better.

TABLE 4. Percent negative at second-look laparotomy by residual tumor at initial laparotomy

First author (ref.)	Year	Total patients	No residual percent negative	Optimal residual percent negative	Suboptimal residual percent negative
Curry (75)	1981	27	76	33	33
Webb (78)	1982	59	95	36	20
Cohen (79)	1983	73	73	35	34
Phibbs (80)	1983	42		48	11
Barnhill (82)	1984	96	67	61	14
Berek (83)	1984	56		41	12
Podratz (87)	1985	135	82	44	39
Smirz (88)	1985	88	75	37	19
Cain (89)	1986	177	76	50	28
Dauplat (14)	1986	51	85	73	19
Gallup (92)	1987	65	71	63	13
Carmichael (91)	1987	146	62	30	25
Lippman (72)	1988	67		49	7
Lund (44)	1990	131	77	55	25
Ayhan (101)	1991	49	92	61	15
Total		1,262			
Weighted Mean			77	47	22

Copeland et al. (104), reporting from M. D. Anderson on the long-term outcome of 50 patients with microscopic disease found at second-look, noted survival rates of 96% and 71% at two years and five years, respectively. These figures are likely to improve, and long-term cures may even be possible, given the promising results reported with second-line intraperitoneal chemotherapy in patients with small-volume residual disease (60,105,106).

Our understanding of the prognostic significance of a negative second-look laparotomy has evolved considerably in recent years. It has been known since the early days of second-look surgery that even the most carefully performed operation may fail to detect areas of tumor. In addition, ovarian cancer may on occasion spread beyond the areas examined at second-look surgery. In many published reports, the true incidence of recurrence following negative second-look laparotomy has been substantially underestimated. Table 5 (13,14, 72,75,78,81–83,86–92,94–96,98,107–113) summarizes information on recurrence after negative second-look laparotomy from 27 reports including 1,232 patients. The combined incidence of recurrence in these reports is a misleadingly low 17%. This low figure results from a number of factors, most importantly the limited follow-up available in many of the studies. In reports from Memorial Sloan-Kettering, Rubin et al. (110,113) have attempted to define more accurately the chance of recurrence following negative second-look laparotomy and to define risk factors for recurrence. In a 1988 publication (110), they established the importance of the type and duration of chemotherapy on the rate of recurrence, reporting for the first time that patients treated for shorter periods with platinum-based regimens had a much higher risk of recurrence than patients treated for long periods of time with nonplatinum-based regimens. This difference is attributable primarily to the facts that more patients will achieve a complete clinical response with platinum-based regimens and that they are required to maintain this disease-free state for a relatively brief period to become eligible for second-look. Patients treated with alkylating-agent regimens had to be clinically free of disease for 18 to 24 months prior to second-look, so many patients with early recurrences were screened out of the pool of patients eligible for second-look. Although these findings do not detract from the fact that platinum-based therapy has been a major improvement, they do indicate that older studies of recurrence following second-look that included patients treated with nonplatinum regimens may not be applicable to present therapy. In a more recent publication, Rubin et al. (113) have shown that the risk of recurrence after a negative second-look laparotomy in platinum-treated patients is approximately 50% overall, with more than one-half the recurrences first noted outside the peritoneal cavity. Multivariate analysis showed the risk of recurrence to be related to stage, histologic grade, and the amount of residual tumor following primary cytoreduction. These results highlight the need for trials of consolidation therapy to decrease the risk of recurrence in patients achieving negative second-look laparotomy.

CONCLUSIONS

As part of a comprehensive program for the management of ovarian cancer, second-look laparotomy is a valuable and safe technique for assessing response to chemotherapy. Information obtained from the operation can be important in clinical decision making. Although it is true that the benefit of second-look laparotomy to the individual patient has never been tested in a prospective clinical trial, the widespread use of surgical reassessment has contributed immeasurably to our understanding of the biologic behavior of ovarian cancer and to the development of effective chemotherapy for this disease. The continued evolution of both primary and secondary treatment regimens for ovarian

TABLE 5. *Recurrence following negative second-look laparotomy*

First author (ref.)	Year	Total patients	Percent recurrence
Schwartz (13)	1980	58	28
Curry (75)	1981	17	18
Roberts (77)	1982	36	17
Webb (78)	1982	32	12
Ballon (81)	1984	11	9
Barnhill (82)	1984	48	13
Berek (83)	1984	18	22
Gershenson (86)	1985	85	24
Podratz (87)	1985	77	16
Smirz (88)	1985	30	27
Cain (89)	1986	94	14
Copeland (107)	1986	79	40
Dauplat (14)	1986	24	17
Miller (90)	1986	38	21
Potkul (108)	1986	34	6
Carmichael (91)	1987	53	57
Gallup (92)	1987	34	24
McCusker (94)	1987	20	5
Podczaski (95)	1987	49	14
Lippman (72)	1988	21	24
Podratz (109)	1988	50	30
Rubin (110)	1988	83	25
Sonnendecker (96)	1988	28	18
Luesly (111)	1989	21	43
Ayhan (112)	1990	24	17
Ghatage (98)	1990	77	19
Rubin (113)	1991	91	44
Total		1,232	
Weighted Mean			17

cancer will be greatly facilitated by the appropriate use of second-look laparotomy.

REFERENCES

1. Wangensteen O. Cancer of the colon and rectum with special reference to (1) earlier recognition of alimentary tract malignancy; (2) secondary delayed re-entry of the abdomen in patients exhibiting lymph node involvement; (3) subtotal excision of the colon; (4) operation in obstruction. *Wis Med J* 1949;48:591–597.
2. Wangensteen O, Lewis F, Tongen L. The "second-look" in cancer surgery. *Lancet* 1951;71.
3. Arhelger S, Jenson C, Wangensteen O. Experiences with the "second-look" procedure in the management of cancer of the colon and rectum. *Lancet* 1957;2:412–417.
4. Parks T. Carcinoma of the ovary treated preoperatively with deep X-ray. *Am J Obstet Gynecol* 1945;49:676.
5. Kottmeier H. Radiotherapy in the treatment of ovarian carcinoma. *Clin Obstet Gynecol* 1961;4:865.
6. Wallach R, Blinick G. The second-look operation for carcinoma of the ovary. *Surg Gynecol Obstet* 1970;131:1086.
7. Tepper E, Sanfilippo LJ, Gray J, Romney SL. Second look surgery after radiation therapy for advanced stages of cancer of the ovary. *Am J Roentgenol* 1971;112:755–759.
8. Wallach RC, Kabakow B, Jerez E, Blinick G. The importance of second-look surgical procedures in the staging and treatment of ovarian carcinoma. *Semin Oncol* 1975;2:243–246.
9. Stuart GC, Jeffries M, Stuart JL, Anderson RJ. The changing role of "second-look" laparotomy in the management of epithelial carcinoma of the ovary. *Am J Obstet Gynecol* 1982;612–616.
10. Raju KS, McKinna JA, Barker GH, Wiltshaw E, Jones JM. Second-look operations in the planned management of advanced ovarian carcinoma. *Am J Obstet Gynecol* 1982;144:650–654.
11. Luesley DM, Chan KK, Fielding JW, Hurlow R, Blackledge GR, Jordon JA. Second-look laparotomy in the management of epithelial ovarian carcinoma: an evaluation of fifty cases. *Obstet Gynecol* 1984;64:421–426.
12. Smith JP, Delgado G, Rutledge F. Second-look operation in ovarian carcinoma: postchemotherapy. *Cancer* 1976;38:1438–1442.
13. Schwartz PE, Smith JP. Second-look operations in ovarian cancer. *Am J Obstet Gynecol* 1980;138:1124–1130.
14. Dauplat J, Ferriere JP, Gorbinet M, et al. Second-look laparotomy in managing epithelial ovarian carcinoma. *Cancer* 1986;57:1627–1631.
15. Rutledge F, Burns B. Chemotherapy for advanced ovarian cancer. *Am J Obstet Gynecol* 1966;96:761.
16. Smith J, Rutledge F. Chemotherapy in the treatment of cancer of the ovary. *Obstet Gynecol* 1970;107:691–703.
17. Kaslow R, Wisch N, Glass J. Acute leukemia following cytotoxic chemotherapy. *JAMA* 1972;219:75–76.
18. Reimer R, Hoover R, Fraumeni JJ, Young R. Acute leukemia after alkylating-agent therapy of ovarian cancer. *N Engl J Med* 1977;297:177–181.
19. Wiltshaw E, Kroner T. Phase II study of cis-dichlorodiamine-platinum in advanced adenocarcinoma of the ovary. *Cancer Treat Rep* 1976;60:55.
20. Bruckner H, Cohen C, Gusberg S, et al. Chemotherapy of ovarian cancer with adriamycin and cis-platinum. *Proc Am Soc Clin Oncol* 1976;17:287.
21. Pettersson F. *Annual report on the results of treatment in gynecological cancer.* Stockholm: International Federation of Gynecology and Obstetrics, 1988.
22. Bergman F. Carcinoma of the ovary. A clinicopathological study of 86 autopsied cases with special reference to mode of spread. *Acta Obstet Gynecol Scand* 1966;45:211–231.
23. Rubin S, Lewis JJ. Surgery for ovarian cancer. In: Nichols D, ed. *Gynecologic and obstetric surgery.* St. Louis: Mosby, 1992.
24. Young R, Chabner B, Hubbard S, et al. Advanced ovarian adenocarcinoma: a prospective clinical trial of melphalan (L-PAM) versus combination chemotherapy. *N Engl J Med* 1978;299:1261–1266.
25. Smith J, Day T. Review of ovarian cancer at the University of Texas System Cancer Center, M. D. Anderson Hospital and Tumor Institute. *Am J Obstet Gynecol* 1979;135:984–992.
26. Delgado G, Oram DH, Petrilli ES. Stage III epithelial ovarian cancer: the role of maximal surgical reduction. *Gynecol Oncol* 1984;18:293–298.
27. Neijt J, ten Bokkel Huinink W, van der Berg M, et al. Randomized trial comparing two combination chemotherapy regimens (Hexa-CAF vs CHAP-5) in advanced ovarian carcinoma. *Lancet* 1984;2:594–600.
28. Wharton J, Edwards C. Cytoreductive surgery for common epithelial tumors of the ovary. *Clin Obstet Gynecol* 1984;10:235–244.
29. Redman JR, Petroni GR, Saigo PE, Geller NL, Hakes TB. Prognostic factors in advanced ovarian carcinoma. *J Clin Oncol* 1986;4:515–523.
30. Heintz AP, Hacker NF, Berek JS, Rose TP, Munoz AK, Lagasse LD. Cytoreductive surgery in ovarian carcinoma: feasibility and morbidity. *Obstet Gynecol* 1986;67:783–788.
31. Neijt J, ten Bokkel Huinink W, van der Burg M, et al. Randomized trial comparing two combination chemotherapy regimens (CHAP-5 vs CP) in advanced ovarian carcinoma. *J Clin Oncol* 1987;5:1157–1168.
32. Piver MS, Lele SB, Marchetti DL, Baker TR, Tsukada Y, Emrich LJ. The impact of aggressive debulking surgery and cisplatin-based chemotherapy on progression-free survival in stage III and IV ovarian carcinoma. *J Clin Oncol* 1988;6:983–989.
33. McGowan L, Bunnag B. The evaluation of therapy for ovarian cancer. *Gynecol Oncol* 1976;4:375.
34. Goldberg G, Learmonth G, Bloch B, Levin W. Role of cul-de-sac aspiration cytology in the management and follow-up of patients with ovarian carcinoma. A preliminary report. *J Reprod Med* 1985;30:867–870.
35. Rubin SC, Dulaney ED, Markman M, Hoskins WJ, Saigo PE, Lewis JJ. Peritoneal cytology as an indicator of disease in patients with residual ovarian carcinoma [see comments]. *Obstet Gynecol* 1988;851–853.
36. Berek JS, Griffiths CT, Leventhal JM. Laparoscopy for second-look evaluation in ovarian cancer. *Obstet Gynecol* 1981;58:192–198.
37. Berek JS, Hacker NF. Laparoscopy in the management of patients with ovarian carcinoma. *Clin Obstet Gynaecol* 1983;10:213–222.
38. Lele SB, Piver MS. Interval laparoscopy as predictor of response to chemotherapy in ovarian carcinoma. *Obstet Gynecol* 1986;68:345–347.
39. Piver MS, Lele SB, Barlow JJ, Gamarra M. Second-look laparoscopy prior to proposed second-look laparotomy. *Obstet Gynecol* 1980;55:571–573.
40. Ozols RF, Fisher RI, Anderson T, Makuch R, Young RC. Peritoneoscopy in the management of ovarian cancer. *Am J Obstet Gynecol* 1981;140:611–619.
41. Brenner DE, Shaff MI, Jones HW, Grosh WW, Greco FA, Burnett LS. Abdominopelvic computed tomography: evaluation in patients undergoing second-look laparotomy for ovarian carcinoma. *Obstet Gynecol* 1985;65:715–719.
42. Megibow AJ, Bosniak MA, Ho AG, Beller U, Hulnick DH, Beckman EM. Accuracy of CT in detection of persistent or recurrent ovarian carcinoma: correlation with second-look laparotomy. *Radiology* 1988;166:341–345.
43. Calkins AR, Stehman FB, Wass JL, Smirz LR, Ellis JH. Pitfalls in interpretation of computed tomography prior to second-look laparotomy in patients with ovarian cancer. *Br J Radiol* 1987;60:975–979.
44. Lund B, Jacobsen K, Rasch L, Jensen F, Olesen K, Feldt RK. Correlation of abdominal ultrasound and computed tomography scans with second- or third-look laparotomy in patients with ovarian carcinoma. *Gynecol Oncol* 1990;37:279–283.
45. Reuter KL, Griffin T, Hunter RE. Comparison of abdominopelvic computed tomography results and findings at second-look

laparotomy in ovarian carcinoma patients. *Cancer* 1989;63:1123–1128.
46. Goldhirsch A, Triller JK, Greiner R, Dreher E, Davis BW. Computed tomography prior to second-look operation in advanced ovarian cancer. *Obstet Gynecol* 1983;62:630–634.
47. Clarke-Pearson D, Bandy LC, Dudzinski M, Heaston D, Creasman WT. Computed tomography in evaluation of patients with ovarian carcinoma in complete clinical remission. Correlation with surgical-pathologic findings. *JAMA* 1986;255:627–630.
48. Stehman FB, Calkins AR, Wass JL, Smirz LR, Sutton GP, Ehrlich CE. A comparison of findings at second-look laparotomy with preoperative computed tomography in patients with ovarian cancer. *Gynecol Oncol* 1988;29:37–42.
49. Khan O, Cosgrove DO, Fried AM, Savage PE. Ovarian carcinoma follow-up: US versus laparotomy. *Radiology* 1986;159:111–113.
50. Murolo C, Constantini S, Foglia G, et al. Ultrasound examination in ovarian cancer patients. A comparison with second look laparotomy. *J Ultrasound Med* 1989;8:441–443.
51. Nardelli GB, Onnis GL, Lamaina V, Petrillo MR. Ultrasound evaluation in the follow-up of ovarian cancer today. *Clin Exp Obstet Gynecol* 1987;14:174–178.
52. Fishman-Javitt M, Stein H, Lovecchio J. *Imaging of the pelvis: MRI with correlations to CT and ultrasound.* Boston: Little, Brown, 1990.
53. Bast RJ, Klug T, St. John E, et al. A radioimmunoassay using a monoclonal antibody to monitor the course of epithelial ovarian cancer. *N Engl J Med* 1983;309:883.
54. Niloff JM, Bast RJ, Schaetzl EM, Knapp RC. Predictive value of CA 125 antigen levels in second-look procedures for ovarian cancer. *Am J Obstet Gynecol* 1985;151:981–986.
55. Berek JS, Knapp RC, Malkasian GD, et al. CA 125 serum levels correlated with second-look operations among ovarian cancer patients. *Obstet Gynecol* 1986;67:685–689.
56. Atack DB, Nisker JA, Allen HH, Tustanoff ER, Levin L. CA 125 surveillance and second-look laparotomy in ovarian carcinoma. *Am J Obstet Gynecol* 1986;154:287–289.
57. Potter ME, Moradi M, To AC, Hatch KD, Shingleton HM. Value of serum CA-125 levels: does the result preclude second look? *Gynecol Oncol* 1989;33:201–203.
58. Meier W, Stieber P, Eiermann W, Schneider A, Fateh MA, Hepp H. Serum levels of CA 125 and histological findings at second-look laparotomy in ovarian carcinoma. *Gynecol Oncol* 1989;35:44–46.
59. Rubin SC, Hoskins WJ, Hakes TB, et al. Serum CA 125 levels and surgical findings in patients undergoing secondary operations for epithelial ovarian cancer. *Am J Obstet Gynecol* 1989;160:667–671.
60. Markman M, Reichman B, Hakes T, et al. Responses to second-line cisplatin-based intraperitoneal therapy in ovarian cancer: influence of a prior response to systemic cisplatin. *J Clin Oncol* 1991;9:1801–1805.
61. Markman M, Reichman B, Hakes T, et al. Intraperitoneal chemotherapy as treatment for ovarian carcinoma and gastrointestinal malignancies: the Memorial Sloan-Kettering Cancer Center experience. *Acta Med Austriaca* 1989;16:65–67.
62. Markman M, Hakes T, Reichman B, et al. Single agent ifosfamide therapy of ovarian cancer previously treated with cisplatin. *Gynecol Oncol* 1991;40:2.
63. Markman M, Hakes T, Reichman B, et al. Phase II trial of weekly or biweekly intraperitoneal mitoxantrone in epithelial ovarian cancer. *J Clin Oncol* 1991;9:978–982.
64. McGuire W, Rowinsky E, Rosenshein N, et al. Taxol: a unique antineoplastic agent with significant activity in advanced ovarian epithelial neoplasms. *Ann Intern Med* 1989;111:273–279.
65. Markman M, Rowinsky E, Hakes T, et al. Phase I trial of taxol administered by the intraperitoneal route: a Gynecologic Oncology Group study. *J Clin Oncol* 1992;10:1485–1491.
66. Berek JS, Hacker NF, Lagasse LD, Nieberg RK, Elashoff RM. Survival of patients following secondary cytoreductive surgery in ovarian cancer. *Obstet Gynecol* 1983;61:189–193.
67. Griffiths CT, Parker LM, Fuller AJ. Role of cytoreductive surgical treatment in the management of advanced ovarian cancer. *Cancer Treat Rep* 1979;63:235–240.
68. Maggino T, Tredese F, Valente S, et al. Role of second look laparotomy in multidisciplinary treatment and in the follow up of advanced ovarian cancer. *Eur J Gynaecol Oncol* 1983;4:26–29.
69. Chambers SK, Chambers JT, Kohorn EI, Lawrence R, Schwartz PE. Evaluation of the role of second-look surgery in ovarian cancer. *Obstet Gynecol* 1988;72:404–408.
70. Podratz KC, Schray MF, Wieand HS, et al. Evaluation of treatment and survival after positive second-look laparotomy. *Gynecol Oncol* 1988;31:9–24.
71. Hoskins WJ, Rubin SC, Dulaney E, et al. Influence of secondary cytoreduction at the time of second-look laparotomy on the survival of patients with epithelial ovarian carcinoma. *Gynecol Oncol* 1989;34:365–371.
72. Lippman SM, Alberts DS, Slymen DJ, et al. Second-look laparotomy in epithelial ovarian carcinoma. Prognostic factors associated with survival duration. *Cancer* 1988;61:2571–2577.
73. Burghardt E, Winter R. The effect of chemotherapy on lymph node metastases in ovarian cancer. *Baillieres Clin Obstet Gynaecol* 1989;3:167–171.
74. Burghardt E, Girardi F, Lahousen M, Tamussino K, Stettner H. Patterns of pelvic and paraaortic lymph node involvement in ovarian cancer. *Gynecol Oncol* 1991;40:103–106.
75. Curry S, Zembo M, Nahhas W, Jahshan A. Second-look laparotomy for ovarian cancer. *Gynecol Oncol* 1981;11:114.
76. Webster KD, Ballard LJ. Ovarian carcinoma; second-look laparotomy postchemotherapy. Preliminary report. *Cleve Clin Q* 1981;48:365–371.
77. Roberts WS, Hodel K, Rich WM, DiSaia PJ. Second-look laparotomy in the management of gynecologic malignancy. *Gynecol Oncol* 1982;13:345–355.
78. Webb MJ, Snyder JJ, Williams TJ, Decker DG. Second-look laparotomy in ovarian cancer. *Gynecol Oncol* 1982;14:285–293.
79. Cohen CJ, Goldberg JD, Holland JF, et al. Improved therapy with cisplatin regimens for patients with ovarian carcinoma (FIGO stages III and IV) as measured by surgical end-staging (second-look operation). *Am J Obstet Gynecol* 1983;145:955–967.
80. Phibbs GD, Smith JP, Stanhope CR. Analysis of sites of persistent cancer at "second-look" laparotomy in patients with ovarian cancer. *Am J Obstet Gynecol* 1983;147:611–617.
81. Ballon SC, Portnuff JC, Sikic BI, Turbow MM, Teng NN, Soriero OM. Second-look laparotomy in epithelial ovarian carcinoma: precise definition, sensitivity, and specificity of the operative procedure. *Gynecol Oncol* 1984;17:154–160.
82. Barnhill DR, Hoskins WJ, Heller PB, Park RC. The second-look surgical reassessment for epithelial ovarian carcinoma. *Gynecol Oncol* 1984;19:148–154.
83. Berek JS, Hacker NF, Lagasse LD, Poth T, Resnick B, Nieberg RK. Second-look laparotomy in stage III epithelial ovarian cancer: clinical variables associated with disease status. *Obstet Gynecol* 1984;64:207–212.
84. Milsted R, Sangster G, Kaye S, et al. Treatment of advanced ovarian cancer with combination chemotherapy using cyclophosphamide, adriamycin and cis-platinum. *Br J Obstet Gynaecol* 1984;91:927–931.
85. Rocereto TF, Mangan CE, Giuntoli RL, Sedlacek TV, Ball HJ, Mikuta JJ. The second-look celiotomy in ovarian cancer. *Gynecol Oncol* 1984;19:34–45.
86. Gershenson DM, Copeland LJ, Wharton JT, et al. Prognosis of surgically determined complete responders in advanced ovarian cancer. *Cancer* 1985;55:1129–1135.
87. Podratz KC, Malkasian G Jr, Hilton JF, Harris EA, Gaffey TA. Second-look laparotomy in ovarian cancer: evaluation of pathologic variables. *Am J Obstet Gynecol* 1985;152:230–238.
88. Smirz LR, Stehman FB, Ulbright TM, Sutton GP, Ehrlich CE. Second-look laparotomy after chemotherapy in the management of ovarian malignancy. *Am J Obstet Gynecol* 1985; 661–668.
89. Cain J, Saigo P, Pierce V, et al. A review of second-look laparotomy for ovarian cancer. *Gynecol Oncol* 1986;23:14.
90. Miller DS, Ballon SC, Teng NN, Seifer DB, Soriero OM. A critical reassessment of second-look laparotomy in epithelial ovarian carcinoma. *Cancer* 1986;57:530–535.

91. Carmichael JA, Shelley WE, Brown LB, et al. A predictive index of cure versus no cure in advanced ovarian carcinoma patients—replacement of second-look laparotomy as a diagnostic test. *Gynecol Oncol* 1987;27:269–281.
92. Gallup DG, Talledo OE, Dudzinski MR, Brown KW. Another look at the second-assessment procedure for ovarian epithelial carcinoma. *Am J Obstet Gynecol* 1987;157:590–596.
93. Ho AG, Beller U, Speyer JL, Colombo N, Wernz J, Beckman EM. A reassessment of the role of second-look laparotomy in advanced ovarian cancer. *J Clin Oncol* 1987;5:1316–1321.
94. McCusker MC, Hoffman JS, Curry SL, Koulos JP, Gondos B. The role of second-look laparotomy in treatment of epithelial ovarian cancer. *Gynecol Oncol* 1987;28:83–88.
95. Podczaski ES, Stevens CJ, Manetta A, Whitney CW, Larson JE, Mortel R. Use of second-look laparotomy in the management of patients with ovarian epithelial malignancies. *Gynecol Oncol* 1987;28:205–214.
96. Sonnendecker EW. Is routine second-look laparotomy for ovarian cancer justified? *Gynecol Oncol* 1988;31:249–255.
97. de Gramont A, Drolet Y, Varette C, et al. Survival after second-look laparotomy in advanced ovarian epithelial cancer. Study of 86 patients. *Eur J Cancer Clin Oncol* 1989;25:451–457.
98. Ghatage P, Krepart GV, Lotocki R. Factor analysis of false-negative second-look laparotomy. *Gynecol Oncol* 1990;36:172–175.
99. Kamura T, Tsukamoto N, Saito T, Kaku T, Matsuyama T, Nakano H. Efficacy of second-look laparotomy for patients with epithelial ovarian carcinoma. *Int J Gynaecol Obstet* 1990;33:141–147.
100. Lund B, Williamson P. Prognostic factors for outcome of and survival after second-look laparotomy in patients with advanced ovarian carcinoma. *Obstet Gynecol* 1990;76:617–622.
101. Ayhan A, Yarali H, Develioglu O, Uren A, Ozyilmaz F. Prognosticators of second-look laparotomy findings in patients with epithelial ovarian cancer. *J Surg Oncol* 1991;46:222–225.
102. Decker D, Malkasian G, Taylor W. Prognostic importance of histologic grading in ovarian carcinoma. *Natl Cancer Inst Monogr* 1975;42:9.
103. Rubin SC, Lewis JJ. Second-look surgery in ovarian carcinoma. *Crit Rev Oncol Hematol* 1988;8:75–91.
104. Copeland LJ, Gershenson DM, Wharton JT, et al. Microscopic disease at second-look laparotomy in advanced ovarian cancer. *Cancer* 1985;55:472–478.
105. Markman M, Hakes T, Reichman B, et al. Intraperitoneal therapy in the management of ovarian carcinoma. *Yale J Biol Med* 1989;62:393–403.
106. Reichman B, Markman M, Hakes T, et al. Phase I trial of concurrent intraperitoneal and continuous intravenous infusion of fluorouracil in patients with refractory cancer. *J Clin Oncol* 1988;6:158–162.
107. Copeland LJ, Gershenson DM. Ovarian cancer recurrences in patients with no macroscopic tumor at second-look laparotomy. *Obstet Gynecol* 1986;68:873–874.
108. Potkul RK, Delgado G, Petrilli ES, Yageric A. Ovarian carcinoma. The significance of restaging laparotomies with negative outcomes. *Arch Surg* 1986;121:1262–1264.
109. Podratz KC, Malkasian GJ, Wieand HS, et al. Recurrent disease after negative second-look laparotomy in stages III and IV ovarian carcinoma. *Gynecol Oncol* 1988;29:274–282.
110. Rubin SC, Hoskins WJ, Hakes TB, Markman M, Cain JM, Lewis JJ. Recurrence after negative second-look laparotomy for ovarian cancer: analysis of risk factors. *Am J Obstet Gynecol* 1988;159:1094–1098.
111. Luesley DM, Chan KK, Lawton FG, Blackledge GR, Mould JM. Survival after negative second-look laparotomy. *Eur J Surg Oncol* 1989;15:205–210.
112. Ayhan A, Urman B, Yarali H, Yuce K, Ayhan A. Predictors of recurrent disease after negative second-look laparotomy for epithelial ovarian cancer. *J Surg Oncol* 1990;44:119–121.
113. Rubin SC, Hoskins WJ, Saigo PE, et al. Prognostic factors for recurrence following negative second-look laparotomy in ovarian cancer patients treated with platinum-based chemotherapy. *Gynecol Oncol* 1991;42:137–141.

CHAPTER 13

Secondary Cytoreduction of Ovarian Malignancies

Laura L. Williams

Ovarian cancer ranks fourth among causes of cancer death in women and is the leading cause of death from gynecologic malignancies. For all stages and cell types combined, the five-year survival has increased from 36% prior to 1979 to 38% during the years 1979 through 1984 (1). This small increase may reflect more aggressive surgical cytoreduction and improvements in adjunctive treatment modalities. Nevertheless, it was estimated that in 1991, over 20,700 women were diagnosed with ovarian cancer and that approximately 12,500 women died from the disease (1). Clearly, improvements in current therapeutic modalities and new and aggressive treatment strategies are needed to affect the prognosis of women with this disease.

The initial approach to the ovarian cancer patient is surgical. The purpose of the initial surgical procedure is to define the extent of disease by thorough exploration, to establish the histology and grade of the tumor, and to cytoreduce tumor bulk (2). Subsequent therapy is determined by these findings and by the amount of disease remaining after cytoreduction. Despite aggressive surgical cytoreduction and subsequent treatment with multiagent chemotherapy, approximately 75% of women with epithelial ovarian carcinoma will have persistent or recurrent tumor and will thus be candidates for secondary surgical debulking procedures. In contrast, improvements in combination chemotherapy regimens have markedly improved the long-term outlook of patients with germ cell malignancies; however, a significant number of young women undergo secondary surgical procedures for recurrence after initial conservative surgery designed to conserve fertility. Finally, recurrent stromal tumors of the ovary, although rare, have been amenable to secondary cytoreduction by virtue of slow growth and late recurrences confined to the peritoneal cavity. This chapter explores the role of secondary surgical cytoreduction in the management of patients with ovarian cancer.

EPITHELIAL OVARIAN CARCINOMA

Concepts of Surgical Cytoreduction

Approximately 20% of patients with epithelial ovarian cancer are diagnosed with disease confined to the ovary (3). For these women, meticulous surgical staging establishes the absence of occult metastases and the histology and grade of the tumor. When properly staged, over 90% of patients with well-differentiated tumors confined to the ovary are cured by surgery alone (4). The majority of women, however, present with extraovarian spread; indeed, more than 60% of patients with epithelial ovarian cancer have evidence of intraabdominal metastases at staging laparotomy (5). For these patients, therapeutic success depends on an aggressive, comprehensive multimodal treatment approach.

The importance of initial surgical cytoreduction in the outcome of patients with advanced disease is clear. In theory, surgical reduction of tumor bulk removes devascularized, necrotic tissue, thereby increasing the proportion of cells in the growth phase of the cell cycle. Well-vascularized, actively dividing tumor is more susceptible to the cytotoxic effects of multiagent chemotherapy. In addition, according to the Goldie-Coldman hypothesis, the probability of eliminating tumor is greatest when tumor volume is small and when chemotherapeutic agents with independent modes of action are employed (6).

L. L. Williams: Department of Obstetrics and Gynecology, Vanderbilt University Medical Center, Nashville, Tennessee 37232-2516

The clinical relevance of these theoretic considerations is apparent in studies analyzing the impact of optimal initial cytoreduction on outcome in patients with advanced disease. In a 1991 review (2), Hoskins and Rubin summarized the effect of optimal initial cytoreduction on 1,494 patients reported in 13 series. Optimal residual disease, defined by the author of each series, ranged from ≤.5 cm to ≤3 cm. Patients with optimally cytoreduced tumor had substantially higher complete clinical response rates to first-line chemotherapy, prolonged progression-free intervals, and longer median survival than did patients left with bulky tumor following initial surgical debulking. Nevertheless, although substantial benefit appears possible from aggressive primary cytoreductive surgery that results in optimal residual disease, the majority of patients are left with bulky tumor following the initial surgical procedure. Hoskins reviewed seven series which describe the technical feasibility of cytoreduction at staging laparotomy and found that only 33% of patients were left with tumor nodules <2 cm in size (7). The majority of patients with advanced ovarian cancer, therefore, begin first-line chemotherapy with bulky disease.

With the addition of cisplatin and its analogue carboplatin to multiagent chemotherapy regimens, 50–70% of patients with advanced disease will be clinically disease-free following first-line chemotherapy (8). Only one-half of complete clinical responders, however, will be disease-free at second-look laparotomy. In addition, long-term follow-up of surgically documented complete responders to cisplatin-based chemotherapy has shown relapse rates of almost 50% (9). Therefore, approximately three-fourths of patients with advanced ovarian cancer treated with cisplatin-based chemotherapy regimens will have persistent or recurrent tumor following initial treatment and may be candidates for secondary surgical cytoreduction.

Although the benefit of aggressive primary cytoreduction has been established, the value of secondary cytoreduction in the management of advanced epithelial ovarian cancer is unclear. Patients who undergo secondary cytoreductive surgery at second-look laparotomy report technical success rates, complications, and survival different from those reported for patients who undergo secondary cytoreduction as an interval procedure or at reexploration after a prolonged disease-free interval and for patients who progress on first-line cisplatin-based chemotherapy. In addition, many reports include patients treated with a variety of first-line regimens in whom clinical disease status and response to first-line chemotherapy is unknown. At present, patients with epithelial malignancies who undergo secondary cytoreductive surgery may be classified as those clinically free of disease after a planned regimen of first-line chemotherapy who are found to have macroscopic tumor at second-look laparotomy; patients found to have bulky, unresectable tumor at initial surgery who undergo interval cytoreduction as part of a planned chemosurgical treatment approach; those with recurrent disease after a prolonged disease-free interval; and patients who progress on first-line therapy.

Secondary Cytoreduction at Second-Look Laparotomy

The surgical assessment of disease status following the successful completion of a planned chemotherapy regimen has become an important part of the management of advanced ovarian cancer. The purpose of the second-look surgical procedure, as applied to ovarian cancer patients by Rutledge and Burns in the mid-1960s (10), was to identify complete responders to first-line chemotherapy who may benefit from discontinuation of treatment. With the introduction of cisplatin to combination chemotherapy regimens and the improvement in second-line treatment, other potential benefits of the procedure have been defined. Presently, theoretical benefits of second-look laparotomy, defined as the systematic exploration of clinically disease-free patients after a planned program of first-line therapy, include the following: the identification of patients with small-volume disease, who may benefit from the early and more effective institution of second-line therapy; the termination of therapy in patients found to be disease-free; and the identification of disease-free patients determined to be at substantial risk for relapse who may benefit from the administration of consolidation therapy.

Some authors have proposed that the debulking of macroscopic tumor found at second-look laparotomy offers a fourth potential benefit to the procedure. Experience with second-look laparotomy after cisplatin-based first-line chemotherapy indicates that approximately one-half of patients in complete clinical remission have persistent tumor at surgery (11) and that the majority of these patients will have macroscopic disease (12). Table 1 illustrates the surgical findings in 431

TABLE 1. *Findings in patients with persistent disease at second-look laparotomy*

	Patients with macroscopic tumor[a]	Patients with microscopic tumor
Podczaski et al. (17)	38	15
Luesley et al. (23)	45	8
Chambers et al. (21)	22	10
Podratz et al. (16)	90	26
Hoskins et al. (18)	50	17
Creasman et al. (78)	38	5
Ballon et al. (74)	8	6
Smirz et al. (75)	37	16
Total	328 (76%)	103 (24%)

[a] Tumor nodules ≥5 mm in diameter.

TABLE 2. *Cytoreduction achieved at second-look laparotomy*

Author	Number of patients	Residual disease after secondary cytoreduction					
		Microscopic	Optimal[a]	Suboptimal[a]	Bulky	Unknown
Schwartz and Smith (13)	112	39 (35%)	36 (32%)	23 (21%)	14 (12%)	
Dauplat et al. (19)	27	13 (48%)			5 (19%)	9 (33%)
Lippman et al. (15)	27		14 (52%)	13 (48%)		
Podratz et al. (16)	90		62 (69%)	28 (31%)		
Chambers et al. (21)	22	16 (74%)	3 (13%)	3 (13%)		
Luesley et al (23)	45	15 (33%)	14 (31%)	16 (36%)		
Hoskins et al. (18)	50	16 (32%)	27 (34%)	7 (14%)		
Podczaski et al. (17)	19		1 (5%)	18 (95%)		
Bertelsen (14)	92		35 (38%)	57 (62%)		

[a] Defined by the author.

patients with persistent disease at second-look surgery. All patients were in complete clinical remission following first-line treatment, and over 90% of the first-line chemotherapy regimens contained cisplatin. Of 431 operations in which tumor was found, 24% had microscopic disease in random biopsy specimens or cell washings, whereas 76% had macroscopic tumor ≥5 mm in diameter. Therefore, of those patients found to have tumor at second-look laparotomy, approximately 75% may be candidates for secondary cytoreduction.

Success Rates of Secondary Cytoreduction

Reported success rates of cytoreduction at second-look surgery vary widely. Nine series which report a detailed analysis of the cytoreduction of macroscopic disease at second-look laparotomy are listed in Table 2. Over 25% of these patients were treated with melphalan or combination regimens not containing cisplatin. Three-quarters of patients were clinically disease-free prior to surgery; in the remaining one-fourth, disease status is unknown. Optimal cytoreduction, defined by the author of each series, was achieved in 290 of 484 (60%) patients (range 5% to 69%). Suboptimal cytoreduction was accomplished in 193 of 484 (40%) patients (range 14% to 95%). In 256 patients, a residual disease category of "microscopic" was specified; cytoreduction to microscopic residual occurred in 99 (39%) patients. This large range in technical success rates may reflect small numbers of patients in some series, lack of homogeneous first-line treatment, and variations in clinical disease status prior to surgery. To address these considerations, 234 clinically disease-free patients treated with cisplatin-based chemotherapy are detailed in Table 3. Of these patients, 71% achieved optimal cytoreduction, whereas 29% achieved suboptimal debulking. Forty-seven of 117 (40%) patients' disease were cytoreduced to microscopic residual. From these data, it appears that approximately 30% of patients found to have macroscopic disease at second-look laparotomy will be left with macroscopic small-volume disease after secondary cytoreduction, 30% will have bulky tumor remaining, and 40% will be left with microscopic residual disease.

Impact on Survival

Few authors have addressed the impact of secondary cytoreductive surgery on survival. In 1980, Schwartz and Smith (13) were the first to report survival after

TABLE 3. *Secondary cytoreduction at second-look laparotomy in patients treated with first-line cisplatin-based chemotherapy*

Author	Amount of residual disease following secondary cytoreduction				
	Number of patients	Microscopic	≤5 mm	<2 cm	≥5 mm	>2 cm
Lippman et al. (15)	27			14		13
Podratz et al. (16)	90		62		28	
Chambers et al. (21)	22	16		3		3
Luesley et al. (23)	45	15		14		16
Hoskins et al. (18)	50	16		26		7
Optimal		166 (71%)				
Suboptimal		67 (29%)				

second-look laparotomy relative to maximum diameter of the largest residual tumor mass after completion of the operation. In this report, 186 patients with epithelial tumors underwent second-look surgery after staging laparotomy and treatment with first-line single-agent chemotherapy, primarily melphalan. Second-look surgery initially was performed as an interval debulking procedure in patients with evidence of response to treatment, subsequently in patients with prolonged marrow suppression who could not tolerate additional chemotherapy, and finally only in patients who had received 12 or more cycles of chemotherapy. Although the first group had bulky disease prior to the second-look surgery, clinical disease status of the latter two groups is unknown. The two-year and five-year survival rates for complete removal of tumor were 47.5% and 27%, respectively. If partial cytoreduction was accomplished and tumor nodules <2 cm were left, the two- and five-year survival rates were 29.5% for each interval. Of patients left with >2 cm tumor, 9% lived two years. The authors concluded that laparotomy is indicated in patients who, by laparoscopy, have localized residual tumor that may be completely removed, as complete secondary cytoreduction results in improved five-year survival.

Since this initial report, other studies have described the effects of secondary cytoreduction at second-look laparotomy on survival, but not all authors have reached similar conclusions. Some authors have reported improved survival in patients who achieve optimal secondary debulking (14–17); others have reported survival benefit only for those who are completely cytoreduced and thus are presumed to be left with microscopic residual (18,19). These reports are reviewed with attention to first-line chemotherapy treatment, clinical disease status prior to surgery, and residual disease categories following secondary cytoreduction.

In a report from Hershey Medical Center, Podczaski and associates (17) described 38 clinically disease-free patients found to have macroscopic disease at second-look surgery. Approximately two-thirds received cisplatin-containing first-line chemotherapy regimens, and one-third were treated with melphalan and combination regimens not containing cisplatin. Five-year actuarial survival for patients cytoreduced to <2 cm nodules was 31% compared with 6% for patients with >2 cm residual. Forty-seven percent of patients with microscopic disease were alive five years from surgery, but the authors do not analyze survival in those found to have microscopic disease versus those completely cytoreduced at surgery. Bertelsen (14) describes secondary cytoreduction in 92 cisplatin-treated patients; clinical disease status prior to surgery is unknown. A statistically significant survival advantage was found for those who underwent secondary debulking of macroscopic tumor to <1 cm residual. Twenty-five percent of patients with <1 cm residual survived four years compared with 4% of those left with >1 cm tumor. Patients cytoreduced to microscopic residual are included in the former group. Lippman et al. (15), reporting on 27 clinically disease-free patients, found a 49% three-year actuarial survival rate for the group of patients with microscopic and <2 cm residual disease and a 29% rate for those left with >2 cm disease. A report from the Mayo Clinic (16) describes secondary cytoreduction of macroscopic tumor in 90 cisplatin-treated patients. All patients were clinically disease-free prior to surgery. The projected four-year survival for patients with microscopic disease was 55% compared with 21% and 14% for patients with lesions ≤5 mm and >5 mm, respectively ($p < .01$). The survival of patients found to have microscopic disease versus those completely cytoreduced was not analyzed. Analysis of survival among the two subgroups with macroscopic disease suggests prolonged survival for the patients with smaller residua, but this difference was not statistically significant. Dauplat and associates (19) analyzed the effect of complete removal of tumor in 27 patients undergoing second-look surgery after first-line cisplatin-based chemotherapy. Approximately 50% of these patient had clinical evidence of disease prior to surgery. The authors found a statistically significant improvement in survival at two years when complete secondary cytoreduction was accomplished. Berek et al. (20), analyzing secondary cytoreduction in 11 complete clinical responders to first-line non–cisplatin-containing therapy, found a median survival of 22 months for six patients optimally debulked compared to 10 months for the five patients with suboptimal debulking.

In 1989 Hoskins and associates (18) reported a detailed analysis of the effects of secondary cytoreduction at second-look laparotomy on survival in a group of patients treated at Memorial Sloan-Kettering Cancer Center. Sixty-seven patients with epithelial ovarian cancer achieved clinical disease-free status after first-line chemotherapy. Sixty-one patients received cisplatin-based combination chemotherapy, one patient received a noncisplatin chemotherapy regimen, and five patients were treated with single alkylating agent therapy. Median follow-up from time of the second-look laparotomy was 28 months. Table 4 compares the size of the largest lesion found at the time of second-look laparotomy versus the size of the largest tumor nodule left at the conclusion of secondary cytoreduction. Seventeen patients were found to have microscopic disease at surgical exploration; an additional 16 patients underwent 100% cytoreduction of macroscopic tumor to leave 33 patients with microscopic residual at the conclusion of the procedure. The degree to which secondary cytoreduction was possible is illustrated in Table 5. Five-year survival in the 16 patients who were

TABLE 4. *Diameter of the largest tumor nodule found at second-look laparotomy versus the diameter of the largest tumor nodule left after secondary cytoreductive surgery[a]*

Size of largest tumor nodule	Largest mass found		Largest mass left	
	Number of patients	%	Number of patients	%
Microscopic disease	17	25	33	49
Less than 2 cm	28	42	26	39
Greater than 2 cm	22	33	7	10
Not stated	—	—	1	2
Total	67	100	67	100

[a] Reprinted with permission.

TABLE 5. *Success of secondary cytoreductive surgery at the time of second-look laparotomy[a]*

% Cytoreduction	Number of patients	%
Microscopic disease found[b]	17	25
Complete cytoreduction (100%)[c]	16	24
75–99	11	16
50–74	2	3
25–49	2	3
0–24	12	18
Not stated	7	11
Total	67	100

[a] Reprinted by permission.
[b] Surgical negative second-look laparotomy, but random biopsies or cell washings revealed microscopic disease.
[c] All gross disease removed, but patient presumed to have microscopic residual disease.

completely debulked was 51% and was not statistically different from the 62% 5-year survival of the 17 patients found to have microscopic disease at exploration (Fig. 1). Furthermore, patients with gross residual disease, regardless of size, had 5-year survivals of less than 10% compared with all patients with microscopic residual. Analysis of the percent cytoreduction accomplished demonstrated that patients cytoreduced 75–99% had a median survival of 24.2 months compared with a median survival of only 12 months in the patients cytoreduced less than 75%. The authors conclude that a significant survival benefit exists for those patients who are able to be secondarily cytoreduced to microscopic residual at second-look laparotomy. Although less sig-

```
□   MICRO DISEASE    MEDIAN=63.80 MONTHS    ( 17 PTS.   10 CENSORED)
+   0 RESIDUAL       MEDIAN NOT REACHED     ( 16 PTS.    9 CENSORED)
△   <= 2 CM RESIDUAL MEDIAN=20.73 MONTHS    ( 26 PTS.    6 CENSORED)
☆   >  2 CM RESIDUAL MEDIAN=16.66 MONTHS    (  7 PTS.    1 CENSORED)
```

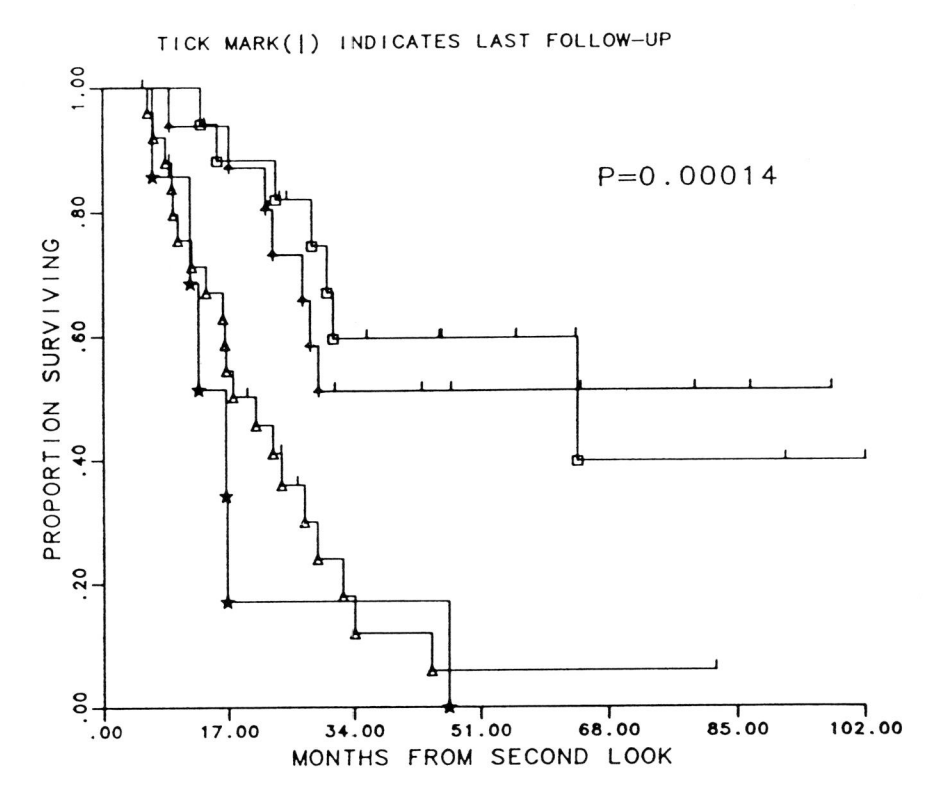

$P = 0.00014$

FIG. 1. Relationship of the diameter of the largest tumor nodule remaining after secondary cytoreductive surgery to survival. Reprinted with permission.

nificant, 75% secondary cytoreduction in tumor bulk offers survival advantage. The authors point out that whether this improved survival is the result of the secondary cytoreductive surgery or merely reflects the biological properties of the tumor that allow cytoreduction remains unanswered.

Other researchers, however, have found that secondary cytoreduction at second-look laparotomy offers no survival advantage. Chambers and colleagues (21), reporting on 22 clinically disease-free patients, found that size of residual disease at the end of second-look surgery had no bearing on survival. The details of cytoreduction and the size of residual tumor nodules are not stated. Hainsworth and associates (22) from Vanderbilt University reported the long-term results of a first-line chemotherapy regimen consisting of hexamethylmelamine, cyclophosphamide, doxorubicin, and cisplatin (H-CAP) in patients with advanced disease. In this series, forty-seven clinically disease-free patients underwent second-look laparotomy. The probability of survival relative to residual disease following second-look surgery is illustrated in Fig. 2. Median survival for patients who achieved partial response (macroscopic residual) was 22 months compared with 28 months for those who had surgically induced complete response, but this difference was not statistically significant. In an analysis of the survival benefit of second-look laparotomy, the West Midlands Ovarian Cancer Group (23) randomized patients with advanced epithelial ovarian cancer into three treatment arms. All patients received first-line cisplatin-based chemotherapy, and patients in two of the three arms underwent second-look laparotomy if no clinical evidence of progression of disease remained. Analysis of 24 patients left with microscopic residual and 29 patients with <2 cm residual revealed no significant difference in survival. The authors conclude that second-look laparotomy should not be routinely performed for the purpose of debulking.

Complications of Secondary Cytoreduction

In a 1988 report (11), Rubin and Lewis detailed the complications experienced by 682 patients undergoing second-look laparotomy. The authors noted that wound, urinary tract, pulmonary, and gastrointestinal tract complications were all seen at low rates, a tribute to modern surgical and anesthetic techniques. Similarly, analysis of complications in patients undergoing aggressive attempts at secondary cytoreduction at second-look surgery revealed acceptable, although slightly higher, rates of postoperative ileus, hemorrhage, and infections of the urinary tract, wound, and lungs. A review of six series that published complications following secondary cytoreductive surgery at second-look laparotomy revealed acceptable morbidity and one postoperative death. Table 6 illustrates these findings.

In summary, the incorporation of cisplatin into first-line chemotherapy regimens has resulted in improved complete clinical response rates; indeed, over 70% of patients with advanced disease will be clinically disease-free at the completion of first-line treatment. However, approximately 50% of these complete clinical responders will have disease present at second-look laparotomy, and over 75% of these patients will have macroscopic disease. Thus, of 100 patients undergoing second-look laparotomy after cisplatin-based chemotherapy, approximately 38 will be candidates for secondary cytoreductive surgery. Attempts to cytoreduce macroscopic disease have been moderately successful; approximately 40% of patients with macroscopic tumor undergo 100% cytoreduction resulting in microscopic residual, 30% are partially debulked and left with optimal residual disease, and 30% are left with bulky tumor. It is encouraging to note that aggressive later attempts at debulking in these patients who are undergoing repeat laparotomy after first-line chemotherapy have not resulted in excessive morbidity.

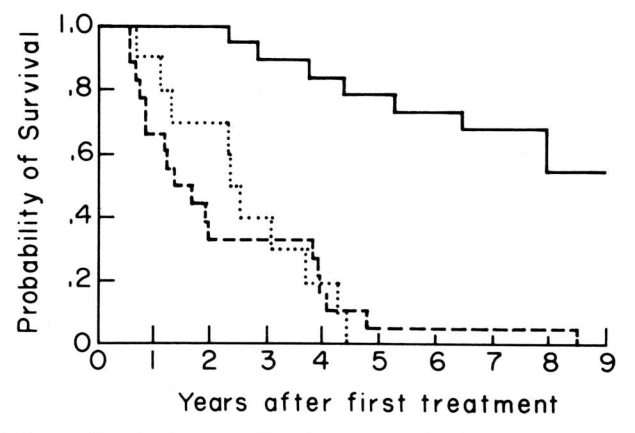

FIG. 2. Survival according to surgically documented response in the 47 patients who had second-look laparotomy. Pathologic complete response shown by solid line; surgically induced complete response shown by dotted line; partial or no response shown by dashed line. Reprinted with permission.

TABLE 6. *Complications of secondary cytoreduction at second-look laparotomy in 385 patients*

Complication	# Patients	% Patients
Ileus	107	28
Hemorrhage >500 cc	55	14
Urinary Tract Infection	31	8
Wound Infection	31	8
Pulmonary	10	3
Deaths[a]	1	.3

[a] Cerebrovascular accident.

Although the prognosis of those left with bulky tumor after second-look is uniformly poor, the benefit of secondary cytoreduction to microscopic or optimal residual remains unproven. Indeed, investigators who analyzed patients treated in a uniform fashion have reported dissimilar results. Nevertheless, long-term follow-up indicates that a survival benefit may exist for patients left with microscopic disease after secondary cytoreduction; patients left with small-volume macroscopic disease have 5-year survivals in some series approaching those left with bulky tumor after second-look surgery. Whether this survival benefit of complete secondary cytoreduction is a function of the surgical debulking or a reflection of properties of the tumor that permit cytoreduction is unknown.

Thus, complete secondary cytoreduction at second-look laparotomy following first-line cisplatin-based chemotherapy remains a potential benefit to the procedure. Its ultimate impact on the outcome of advanced ovarian cancer patients will depend on the effectiveness of salvage agents for the treatment of persistent disease. Salvage therapies such as intraperitoneal chemotherapy, biological response modifiers, whole abdominal radiation therapy, and intraperitoneal chemotherapy are effective only in patients with small-volume disease. Increasing availability and effectiveness of these agents may ultimately establish the role of aggressive secondary cytoreductive surgery at second-look laparotomy.

Secondary Cytoreduction as an Interval Procedure

Definition

In a 1989 report (7), Hoskins reviewed the rate of success in achieving optimal cytoreduction at the initial surgical procedure in 1,777 patients with Stage III and IV epithelial ovarian cancer. Only 33% of patients reported in seven series were left with tumor nodules <2 cm. The majority of patients with advanced disease, therefore, begin first-line chemotherapy with bulky intraabdominal tumor. With intent to improve the outcome of these patients, some investigators have attempted a second surgical debulking procedure as part of a planned treatment approach in patients who show clinical response to first-line chemotherapy. The purpose of this interval debulking procedure is to accomplish optimal cytoreduction after initial treatment with chemotherapy has enhanced the likelihood of resection. Subsequent therapy would be administered, hopefully, before the emergence of drug-resistant cell lines. Interval cytoreductive surgery has been attempted after two to three cycles of chemotherapy, after 5 to 10 cycles of cisplatin-based therapy, and after neoadjuvant, high-intensity drug regimens.

Success Rates of Interval Cytoreductive Surgery

Although the number of studies assessing the technical feasibility of interval debulking is small, the majority of investigators have reported success rates in excess of 50% (24–30). A review of seven series that report the feasibility of interval cytoreduction is presented in Table 7. In four of these studies (24–26,29), patients underwent interval cytoreductive surgery as part of a planned management program after first-line chemotherapy for patients with bulky residual disease after primary surgery. In two series (27,28), interval debulking was employed after first-line treatment with neoadjuvant cisplatin-based chemotherapy. In one report (30) the initial diagnosis of ovarian cancer was made by fine-needle aspiration; prior to debulking surgery, patients underwent first-line treatment with radiotherapy, chemotherapy, or both. Optimal residual disease, defined by the author of each series, ranged from 1 to 2 cm, with the exception of the residual reported by Raju et al. (25). In this study, the size of a gross residual tumor is not specified. These seven reports defined optimal interval cytoreduction as the complete removal of existing tumor. Success rates of interval cytoreduction ranged from 8% in the small series reported by Vogl and associates (24) to 96% in a group of patients treated at the Sidney Farber Cancer Institute (26). Of the 286 patients undergoing interval

TABLE 7. Technical success of interval cytoreduction

Author	# Patients undergoing interval debulking	# Patients with optimal cytoreduction[a]	% Patients with optimal cytoreduction
Raju et al. (25)	49	9	18
Parker et al. (26)	23	22	96
Vogl et al. (24)	12	1	8
Einhorn (30)	102	55	54
Neijt et al. (29)	47	30	63
Lawton et al. (28)	28	25	89
Ng et al. (27)	25	17	68
Total	286	159	56

[a] Defined by the author of each series.

cytoreductive surgery, 159 (56%) were left with optimal residual disease.

Impact on Survival

Despite the apparent technical success of interval cytoreduction of tumor, there appears to be little evidence to suggest a favorable impact on survival in patients who receive conventional cisplatin-based combination chemotherapy prior to a second cytoreductive surgery. A report from the Royal Marsden Hospital in London (25) describes the incorporation of the "second-look operation" to carry out further debulking in patients responding to 5 to 10 cycles of cisplatin-based chemotherapy. All patients had incomplete initial surgery. At interval surgery, 38 patients were found to have macroscopic tumor, and 9 of these had all macroscopic tumor removed. Survival of these nine patients was no better than the survival of those left with macroscopic tumor and only slightly better than patients left with bulky disease after interval surgery. The authors conclude that interval debulking surgery does not appear to be valuable in patients with persistent disease after 5–10 cycles of cisplatin-based chemotherapy, but they chose to evaluate this concept further in a subsequent group of patients.

In the follow-up publication (31), patients who had interval cytoreduction as part of a planned treatment program after first-line chemotherapy were compared with patients having the same chemotherapy, and the same response to chemotherapy, but who had not undergone interval surgery. All patients underwent initial surgery with varying degrees of cytoreduction and received five cycles of cisplatin-based combination chemotherapy. Patients in group A underwent a second surgical procedure with intent to further debulk tumor. Patients in group B did not undergo a second operation but continued chemotherapy based on the clinical assessment of response to first-line treatment. Analysis of survival curves of the two groups indicates that in the case of partial responders to first-line treatment, the group that had interval debulking surgery had marginally prolonged survival compared with those who had no further cytoreductive surgery (25% alive at 42 months compared with 10%). This effect was limited to patients who had less than a hysterectomy and oophorectomy but more than a biopsy at first surgery. The overall survival of all responding patients, with or without interval surgery and regardless of the extent of the initial cytoreduction, was not statistically significant. The investigators concluded that secondary cytoreductive surgery has a limited role as part of a planned program for the treatment of advanced ovarian cancer outside of a clinical research setting.

Four reports have described the results of interval debulking surgery attempted early in the course of first-line treatment (26,29,32,33). Parker and associates (26) treated 72 women with advanced disease with five courses of cisplatin-based chemotherapy. Twenty-three of 35 women with >2 cm residual tumor after initial cytoreductive surgery underwent secondary cytoreductive surgery after one to two cycles of treatment. Optimal interval cytoreduction, defined as residual tumor <2 cm, was accomplished in 22 of these women (96%). Chemotherapy was then completed, and all patients underwent reevaluation of disease status. Patients who achieved optimal residual disease after the interval procedure had a median survival of 22 months, whereas the median survival of those optimally debulked after the initial surgical procedure had not been reached at follow-up. Median survival of patients who were disease-free at interval laparotomy was comparable to that of patients who had achieved disease-free status after optimal initial cytoreduction. In these patients, interval cytoreductive surgery readily resulted in tumor size <2 cm, but only those who easily became clinically disease-free after chemotherapy had long median survival after the second operation.

The West Midlands Ovarian Cancer Group (32,33) attempted early cytoreductive surgery after initial treatment with cisplatin-based chemotherapy in 28 patients with >2 cm disease after first surgery. Survival of the patients debulked at interval surgery to <2 cm was compared to the survival of 195 consecutive patients treated at the same institution with chemotherapy without early second surgery. The latter group was divided into patients who were initially debulked to <2 cm and those with >2 cm disease after primary surgery. The group of patients with <2 cm disease after initial cytoreductive surgery had significantly prolonged survival compared with those left with >2 cm after initial surgery or those optimally debulked at interval surgery. The authors concluded that early secondary debulking surgery does not appear to alter prognosis.

Wils and associates (33) described the treatment of 88 patients with advanced disease after initial surgery and chemotherapy with cyclophosphamide, adriamycin, and cisplatin. Twenty-four patients who had undergone suboptimal initial surgery underwent interval cytoreductive surgery after a median of three courses of chemotherapy. Median survival of 42 months among 38 patients undergoing primary optimal debulking surgery (residual <1.5 cm) was similar to that of 18 patients achieving optimal secondary cytoreduction. The authors point out that although the results of this comparison suggest a role for intervention surgery in the management of patients with bulky disease, flaws in the comparison of the two groups should not be overlooked. First, patients with delayed cytoreduction were operated on only after demonstrating sufficient chemosensitivity to make debulking feasible; patients who underwent initial optimal surgery were not preselected in this fashion. Second, many patients in the delayed debulking group presented with large, bulky intraabdominal tumor. Conversion of unresectable to resectable tumor after chemotherapy may reflect inherent biological properties of the tumor that allow more effective chemo- or surgical cytoreduction. The authors suggest that these considerations can be addressed only in a randomized trial comparing chemotherapy with chemotherapy plus early secondary surgery in patients with unresectable tumor at presentation.

A report from the Netherlands Cancer Institute (29) deserves special note. In this study, 191 patients with advanced ovarian cancer were randomized to receive first-line treatment with cyclophosphamide, hexamethylmelamine, adriamycin, and cisplatin (CHAP-5), or with cisplatin and cytoxan after initial surgery. Response to chemotherapy and toxicity of the two regimens were assessed. In addition, in those patients in whom initial debulking was not performed, interval cytoreductive surgery was performed as soon as chemotherapy rendered the tumor masses resectable. The impact of this interval debulking procedure is illustrated in Fig. 3. Cytoreduction to tumor nodules ≤1 cm did not lead to longer survival compared with patients with nodules >1 cm. Furthermore, patients with tumor diameters smaller than 1 cm prior to the initiation of chemotherapy had significantly longer survival than did those left with 1 cm after interval cytoreduction (Fig. 4). The authors conclude that a second surgical attempt after initiation of chemotherapy is unlikely to alter the outcome of patients initially suboptimally debulked.

Two additional reports have evaluated interval debulking following neoadjuvant, intensive cisplatin-based chemotherapy (27,28). In the first study (28), twenty-eight patients with incompletely resected ovarian cancer (>2 cm residual) were treated with two to four cycles of cisplatin-based chemotherapy. The cisplatin dose ranged from 75–100 mg/m^2 and was administered at three-week intervals. Interval cytoreductive surgery was carried out at a median interval of 12.7 weeks after the first surgery. After interval surgery, 16 patients had no macroscopic disease, 5 patients had less than 1 cm residual, 4 had less than 2 cm residual, and 3 had bulky residual. Therefore, before restarting chemotherapy, 25 of 28 patients (89%) had less than 2 cm residual, and 57% had microscopic residual disease. Morbidity of the second surgical resection was acceptable. In these patients, this combined intense chemotherapy-interval debulking treatment approach was technically feasible, was associated with minimal morbidity, and left the majority of patients (81%) with microscopic disease. The authors propose that in theory, further chemotherapy may be administered at a point when residual tumor burden is minimal, thus enhancing the likelihood of response. The investigators have initiated a randomized trial to evaluate the impact of this treatment plan on survival.

The second study to analyze the technical success of repeat cytoreductive surgery following neoadjuvant

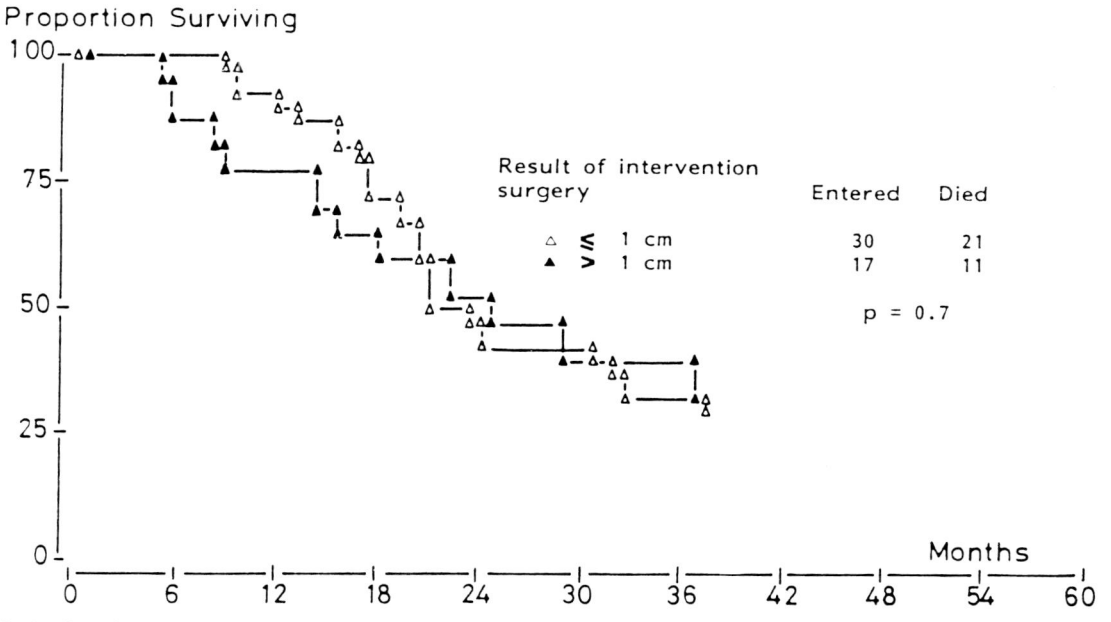

FIG. 3. Survival after successful intervention surgery (<1 cm) or attempted intervention surgery without successful removal of tumor (>1 cm). Reprinted with permission.

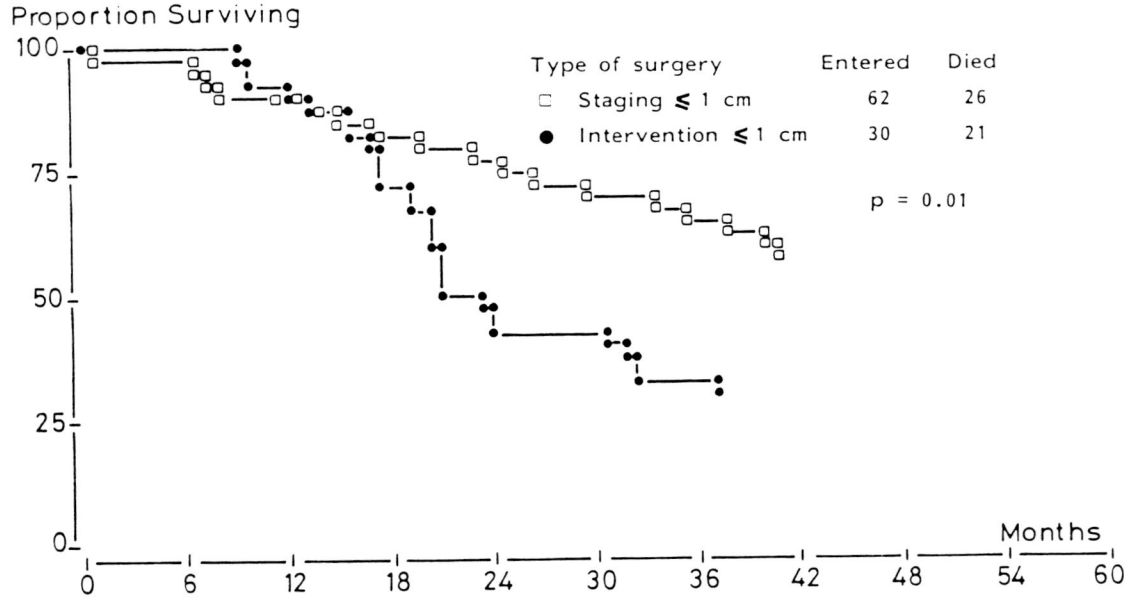

FIG. 4. Survival after cytoreductive surgery leading to tumor residuals of <1 cm at the staging laparotomy (staging) or during chemotherapy (intervention cytoreductive surgery). Reprinted with permission.

chemotherapy was conducted at Memorial Sloan-Kettering Cancer Center (27). Forty-three patients with advanced disease underwent initial cytoreductive surgery and two courses of first-line chemotherapy with cytoxan 1,000 mg/m^2 and cisplatin 160 mg/m^2 (40 mg/m^2 for 5 days). Repeat cytoreductive surgery was carried out 6 weeks after the second course of chemotherapy. All patients were then treated with four courses of intraperitoneal cisplatin-based chemotherapy. Results of this chemosurgical debulking program are depicted in Fig. 5. Twenty-five patients had >1 cm residual tumor following the initial surgical procedure. After chemotherapy, 7 of the 25 patients were found to have <1 cm tumor at interval laparotomy, and 18 were found to have >1 cm tumor. Of these 18 patients, 12 (67%) were secondarily cytoreduced to <1 cm tumor at interval surgery. Thus, of 25 patients initially suboptimally debulked, 19 (76%) had <1 cm tumor prior to the initiation of intraperitoneal chemotherapy. Analysis of the impact of this treatment regimen on survival is ongoing.

The technical success rates reported with interval debulking surgery following first-line chemotherapy treatment are high. Bulky tumors responsive to chemotherapy may have inherent biological properties that permit cytoreduction both by chemotherapeutic and surgical means. Yet, it seems unlikely that interval debulking surgery after first-line chemotherapy with conventional cisplatin-based regimens will significantly affect the outcome of patients who undergo suboptimal initial cytoreduction. The Goldie-Coldman hypothesis suggests that larger tumor bulk implies greater probability of spontaneous mutation to resistant cell lines (6). This theory may explain the lack of impact on survival of interval cytoreduction surgery after prolonged first-line chemotherapy treatment; even after successful secondary debulking to small-volume residual, chemotherapy-resistant tumor cells persist. Unfortunately, attempts to decrease the number of drug-resistant cell lines by early incorporation of the interval procedure into the treatment plan have not resulted in substantial improvement in survival, which may reflect lack of effective salvage regimens for patients with persistent, chemotherapy-resistant disease. Although early experience with neoadjuvant, intense first-line regimens indicates that the majority of patients can achieve marked cytoreduction of tumor bulk, the impact of this treatment approach on survival is unclear.

Secondary Cytoreduction of Recurrent Disease

Several reports have examined the role of secondary cytoreductive surgery in patients who relapse after achieving disease-free status after primary treatment. One report, from M. D. Anderson Cancer Center (34), reviewed 30 patients who underwent secondary cytoreductive surgery after a disease-free interval of at least 6 months following initial treatment. Seven patients were treated with cisplatin-based first-line chemotherapy, 11 with a combination regimen not containing cisplatin, and 12 with melphalan alone. The amount of residual disease following secondary cytoreductive surgery was as follows: nine patients with microscopic

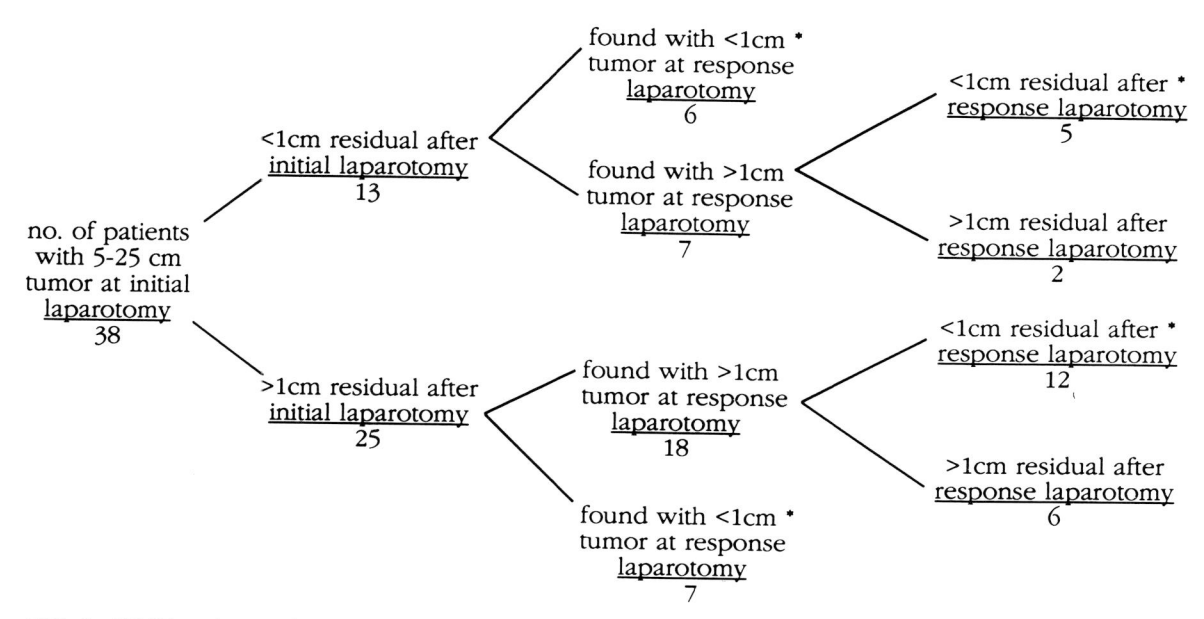

```
                                    found with <1cm *
                                  / tumor at response
                                /   laparotomy              <1cm residual after *
                              /        6                  / response laparotomy
              <1cm residual after <                      /        5
            / initial laparotomy  \  found with >1cm  <
          /         13              \ tumor at response \
        /                             laparotomy         \ >1cm residual after
no. of patients                           7                response laparotomy
with 5-25 cm                                                      2
tumor at initial
laparotomy                                                  <1cm residual after *
    38        \                        found with >1cm   / response laparotomy
                \                    / tumor at response /        12
                  >1cm residual after  laparotomy       <
                  initial laparotomy       18            \ >1cm residual after
                          25         \                     response laparotomy
                                       \ found with <1cm *         6
                                         tumor at response
                                         laparotomy
                                              7
```

FIG. 5. Of 25 patients with >1 cm tumor after initial surgery, 19 patients were reduced to >1 cm tumor by neoadjuvant chemotherapy alone (7) or neoadjuvant chemotherapy and secondary cytoreduction (12).

disease, four patients with <1 cm macroscopic tumor, four patients with ≥1 cm but <2 cm tumor, six patients with ≥2 cm disease, and seven patients with large residual plaques. Optimal debulking, defined by the authors as residual tumor <2 cm, occurred in 57% of patients who underwent secondary cytoreduction.

The apparent technical success of the procedure did not result in significantly prolonged survival. Although median survival for the entire group was 62 months, median survival from the time of secondary cytoreduction was only 16.3 months. Patients who had residual tumor <2 cm after secondary cytoreduction survived a median of 18 months, whereas patients with residual tumor >2 cm had median survival of 13.3 months. When the interval between first and second operations was >18 months, patients survived a median of 19 months after the second surgery; when the interval was less than 18 months, patients survived 13.5 months. The authors attributed these results to lack of response to salvage regimens, noting that only 9% of patients had partial response to subsequent treatment, whereas 68% had progressive disease. Of the 13 patients receiving salvage cisplatin-based chemotherapy, only one patient had a partial response. The authors concluded that although technically feasible, any potential benefit derived from secondary cytoreductive surgery was negated by lack of effective salvage agents.

Investigators from Memorial Sloan-Kettering Cancer Center reached somewhat different conclusions regarding the efficacy of salvage treatment in patients who undergo reexploration after relapse. In a 1989 report (35), the authors reviewed 57 evaluable patients with refractory or recurrent ovarian cancer who were treated with intraperitoneal etoposide and cisplatin after reexploration laparotomy. Thirteen patients who had a treatment-free interval of >1 year were considered to have recurrent disease; 44 patients with a treatment-free interval <1 year were considered to have refractory disease. All patients were treated with first-line cisplatin-based chemotherapy regimens, and each patient underwent laparotomy to debulk tumor and to document disease status prior to the initiation of intraperitoneal chemotherapy. Of the 13 patients with recurrent disease, 5 had surgically documented complete responses to intraperitoneal chemotherapy, and 3 had partial responses for a combined response rate of 62%. Responses to intraperitoneal chemotherapy were seen in patients with microscopic tumor as well as in patients with disease up to 2 cm in size. Follow-up is ongoing to determine the impact of this treatment on survival. These data suggest, however, that further evaluation of salvage regimens known to be effective in patients with small-volume disease is warranted, because these agents may enhance the value of secondary cytoreductive surgery after relapse.

Secondary Cytoreduction in Nonresponders to First-Line Therapy

Experience with first-line cisplatin-based chemotherapy regimens indicates that patients who progress prior to the completion of first-line treatment rarely respond to salvage regimens and rapidly die of progressive disease (36–38). Perhaps because of the uniformly poor prognosis of patients who show early resistance to chemotherapy or because of the lack of effective salvage agents in cisplatin nonresponders, few institutions have attempted secondary cytoreduction in patients who progress on first-line therapy. As indicated in the studies by Michel et al. (39) and Morris et al. (34), secondary cytoreduction of tumor bulk appears to offer little substantial benefit in terms of survival or meaningful palliation to first-line therapy nonresponders.

In a 1989 report (39), Michel and associates from the Institut Gustave-Roussy evaluated the role of secondary cytoreductive surgery in 77 patients who had clinical evidence of failure to first-line treatment. Over 85% of patients received first-line cisplatin-based chemotherapy. Second-look surgery was performed before the end of the planned treatment regimen in all cases. Thirty-two of the 77 patients underwent optimal (<2 cm) cytoreduction, whereas 45 patients had suboptimal (>2 cm) resection. After the second surgery, patients received salvage treatment consisting of chemotherapy or radiation therapy. The median survival of both groups was 12 months. The authors concluded that secondary cytoreductive surgery does little to alter the uniformly poor prognosis of patients with progressive disease on first-line treatment.

The report from M. D. Anderson Cancer Center (34) analyzed 31 patients with progressive disease and 2 patients with stable disease who underwent secondary cytoreduction before the completion of a planned course of chemotherapy. In contrast to the group of patients reported by Michel et al. (39), only seven (21%) of the patients treated at M. D. Anderson received first-line cisplatin-based regimens. Cytoreductive surgery, when technically feasible, was often radical; 17 patients had segmental colon resection, 10 underwent small bowel resection, and 1 patient each underwent exenteration and splenectomy. Although there were no intraoperative complications and no mortalities related to surgery, morbidity was substantial. Seven patients had prolonged ileus, seven patients had serious infections requiring antibiotic therapy, and one patient experienced disseminated intravascular coagulation and gastrointestinal bleeding. In this report, survival following secondary cytoreductive surgery was significantly improved only if patients were left with <1 cm residual tumor. For the 18 patients with microscopic residual disease or disease <2 cm following secondary cytoreduction, median survival from the time of second surgery (12 months) was not significantly different from the survival of the 15 patients with residual disease >2 cm (7.8 months). However, for patients with <1 cm tumor following second surgery, median survival was 19 months compared with 8.3 months for patients with >1 cm residual ($p < .004$). These patients with <1 cm residual after secondary cytoreductive surgery constituted 21% of the entire group.

Response to salvage treatment was poor. Twenty-nine of 31 evaluable patients progressed on second-line therapy, including 13 of 14 patients treated with cisplatin-based regimens following first-line treatment with alkylating agents. In this series, the aggressive surgical effort offered a significant survival advantage only to patients with <1 cm residual disease following secondary cytoreduction, and these patients accounted for only a small portion of the total group (21%). Furthermore, patients who had a short interval between primary and secondary surgery, regardless of the amount of residual disease, had increased morbidity and shorter survival, suggesting that the biology of the tumor, rather than aggressive surgical debulking, may play a significant role in the behavior of these tumors. With the lack of effective salvage therapy after first-line chemotherapy failure and the substantial morbidity incurred by the procedure, there is little evidence that secondary cytoreduction offers any substantial benefit to patients who progress on first-line therapy.

EPITHELIAL TUMORS OF LOW MALIGNANT POTENTIAL

Histology and Behavior

Carcinomas of low malignant potential comprise approximately 10–15% of epithelial ovarian neoplasms (40). Histologically, these tumors are characterized by the stratification of neoplastic epithelial cells with detachment of cellular clusters from their sites of origin, nuclear atypia, mitotic activity, and the absence of stromal invasion (41). The diagnosis is most frequently made in the fifth decade of life, although these tumors have been reported in patients 6 to 86 years of age (41). Women of childbearing age are more frequently affected by borderline than by frank ovarian malignancies. In contrast to malignant ovarian carcinomas, in which the majority of patients present with widespread intraabdominal metastases, from 39% to 84% of serous borderline tumors and 65% to 100% of mucinous borderline neoplasms present with disease confined to the ovary (42).

Tumors of low malignant potential are distinguished from ovarian carcinomas by their indolent clinical course and delayed recurrences. The vast majority of patients with disease confined to the ovary are cured by surgery alone (41–44), although occasional relapse and death from recurrent disease have been described (44,45). In patients with advanced stage disease, however, wide variations in response to treatment and ultimate outcome have been reported. Because the natural history of extraovarian spread of these tumors has not been established, the role of adjuvant therapy in these patients has not been clearly defined. Nevertheless, the five-year survival of patients with borderline tumors, regardless of stage or postoperative treatment, is approximately 85% (44). In some of these patients, secondary cytoreduction of recurrent tumor plays a major therapeutic role.

Secondary Cytoreduction of Borderline Malignancies

Stage I Tumors

Initial surgery consisting of total abdominal hysterectomy and bilateral salpingo-oophorectomy cures over 95% of patients with disease confined to the ovary (43,44,46), and adjuvant therapy does not seem to affect these results (44). Many women, however, are diagnosed with borderline ovarian malignancies during the reproductive years when conservation of fertility is an important concern. For this reason, investigators have performed conservative initial operations such as ovarian cystectomy and unilateral salpingo-oophorectomy with or without contralateral wedge biopsy in patients who appear to have disease confined to the ovary. After conservative surgery, relapse rates of 12% to 21% (41,43,47) have been reported, and the majority of women with relapses have undergone reexploration with secondary surgical cytoreduction.

Reports from three institutions have analyzed the role of conservative surgery in patients with stage I borderline tumors. Tazelaar and colleagues (43) reported 20 patients who underwent ovarian cystectomy or unilateral salpingo-oophorectomy for stage IA borderline tumors. Three patients (15%) suffered recurrence in the contralateral ovary at intervals of 29, 31, and 37 months. Secondary cytoreductive surgery consisted of total abdominal hysterectomy and unilateral salpingo-oophorectomy in two patients and unilateral salpingo-oophorectomy and wedge biopsy in the third patient. Each patient remained clinically disease-free after an average follow-up of 37 months. Soo and associates (41) treated 31 patients with stage I disease with ovarian cystectomy and found persistence or recurrence in 4 (13%). After secondary surgery consisting of total abdominal hysterectomy and bilateral salpingo-oophorectomy in three patients and unilateral salpingo-oophorectomy in one, each patient remained disease-free at 5, 6, 6, and 10 years after the second surgery. Bostwick and associates (47) reported four recurrences among 14 women who underwent initial conservative surgery for stage I tumors. Following subsequent definitive surgery, each was clinically disease-free after 23 to 42 months. Because of these results, the authors of these studies suggest that patients who wish to retain fertility may benefit from conservative surgery for borderline malignancies confined to the ovary. The majority of women will be adequately treated with less than extirpative surgery, but even if relapse occurs, definitive secondary surgery offers a chance for cure.

Advanced Stage Tumors

In an attempt to define response to treatment, some institutions have performed second-look surgery in patients with advanced borderline malignancies (48–51). The surgical assessment of disease status has shown that tumors of low malignant potential do not uniformly respond to cytotoxic treatment. Indeed, following first-line cytotoxic therapy, the rate of persistent disease documented at second-look surgery ranges from 20% to 100% (50,51). These series contain small numbers of patients treated with a variety of first-line and salvage agents, and no clearly superior treatment regimen has emerged. Perhaps because of the paucity of data regarding the effectiveness of salvage therapy or lack of information concerning the natural history of patients with advanced disease, there has been little enthusiasm for evaluating the role of secondary cytoreductive surgery at second-look laparotomy.

The role of secondary cytoreduction in patients with advanced ovarian tumors of low malignant potential is currently limited to the treatment of recurrent disease. Table 8 illustrates the results of secondary surgical cytoreduction and subsequent salvage treatment in 27 patients who relapsed after initial treatment for advanced disease. Residual tumor size following the second surgical procedure is unknown. Of the 10 patients treated by surgery alone, 2 have no evidence of disease at follow-up, and 5 of the 17 patients who received adjuvant therapy after surgery are clinically disease-free. The disease-free survival of some patients may be enhanced by the second surgery and subsequent adjunctive therapy, but owing to the small numbers of patients and the variety of treatment regimens employed, the relative contribution of the treatment modalities cannot be assessed.

STROMAL TUMORS

The World Health Organization classification of ovarian tumors of stromal origin includes the following histologic types: granulosa cell, theca-fibroma cell, Sertoli and Leydig cell, gynandroblastoma, and sex cord (52). Taken together, these tumors of stromal origin comprise approximately 7% of all ovarian malignancies (53). Because of their rarity and lack of uniform surgical staging and subsequent treatment, and because of the propensity for indolent behavior and late recurrence, our understanding of the natural history of these tumors is limited. Nevertheless, it appears that

TABLE 8. *Secondary cytoreduction of advanced stage tumors of low malignant potential*

Author	Number of patients	Number of recurrences	Treatment of recurrence	Disease status	Follow-up (in months)[a]
Chambers et al. (21)	21	2	Surgery + chemotherapy	NED	38–96
Julian and Woodruff (76)	26	8	Surgery	4 DOD[b] 3 AWD[c] 4 DID[d]	>60
Tasker and Langley (77)	20	6	Surgery + chemotherapy	6 DOD	
Bostwick et al. (47)	22	9	Surgery + chemotherapy or radiation therapy	2 DOD 1 DID 1 AWD	6–53
Soo et al. (41)	2	2	Surgery	2 NED	54

[a] From time of secondary cytoreduction.
[b] Dead of disease.
[c] Alive with disease.
[d] Dead of intercurrent disease.

the vast majority of patients with stromal tumors present with disease confined to the ovary (54–56). Recurrences are unusual, often occurring years after initial treatment (55,57). With the exception of the granulosa cell tumor, which accounts for 70% of stromal malignancies (53), few series report the details of the treatment of recurrent disease; thus, the value of secondary surgical procedures and salvage therapy in these tumors is unknown.

Granulosa Cell Tumors

Our knowledge of the patterns and mode of spread of granulosa cell tumors is limited by lack of comprehensive surgical staging in most published reports. In two large series (55,56), retrospective staging identified 78% and 91% of patients to have disease confined to the ovary. Lack of uniformity of both the initial surgical approach and subsequent therapy in these patients limits the interpretation of survival data, but it appears that from 80% to 90% of patients with disease confined to the ovary had long-term disease-free survival with or without adjuvant treatment following initial surgery (55,56). Others have described recurrence rates of 24% to 25% (58,59), but in these reports, little information is provided regarding the stage at presentation or the details of adjunctive therapy.

Only two reports (55,57) have detailed the treatment of recurrent granulosa cell tumors. The first, from Columbia University (57), describes the treatment of late recurrences in five women who underwent initial conservative surgery for granulosa cell tumor. Two patients had single resectable intraabdominal recurrences 5 and 17 years after initial surgery. One of these is clinically well 7 years after complete resection of the recurrence with no additional postoperative treatment. The other undergoes treatment for advanced Hodgkin's disease. Three patients experienced recurrences at multiple sites within the abdomen. One of these three underwent incomplete secondary cytoreduction of a massive intraabdominal recurrence on two separate occasions within a 9-year period; each surgical procedure was followed by postoperative radiotherapy, and she is clinically without evidence of disease 5 years from the second surgery. One patient is clinically well 3 years following the second debulking of recurrent abdominal and pelvic tumor; no adjuvant treatment was employed. The fifth patient underwent secondary cytoreduction of sigmoid metastases followed by adjunctive pelvic radiation therapy 1 year after initial surgery for granulosa cell tumors. Eighteen years later a larger intraabdominal recurrence was completely resected, and she remains disease-free 1 year following the completion of alkeran chemotherapy. The second report (55), from the Mayo Clinic, describes the treatment of 22 women with recurrent granulosa cell tumor. The average interval to first recurrence was 6 years. Treatment methods included surgery with or without radiation or chemotherapy, with radiation alone, with chemotherapy alone, or without treatment. The details of secondary cytoreduction are unknown. Sixteen (73%) of the 22 patients died of disease, including 7 of 10 patients who underwent secondary surgery with or without additional treatment. The average survival after recurrence was 5.6 years. From these limited data and the observation that these tumors grow slowly and tend to remain confined to the peritoneal cavity, it appears that the secondary cytoreduction of recurrent disease may offer substantial palliation for prolonged periods; the benefit of salvage radiation or chemotherapy remains unproven.

GERM CELL MALIGNANCIES

Dysgerminoma

Dysgerminoma, the most common malignant germ cell tumor, comprises approximately 40% of all ovarian germ cell malignancies and accounts for 1–3% of all ovarian cancers (60). Relative to epithelial tumors, dysgerminomas occur more often in women in their reproductive years; indeed, over 85% of dysgerminomas occur in women less than 29 years of age (61). For this reason, conservation of fertility has played an important role in the treatment of the disease. Recent advances in chemotherapeutic techniques coupled with a better understanding of the role of thorough surgical staging has led to marked improvement in both the prognosis and quality of life of young women affected by this disease.

In contrast to epithelial malignancies, approximately 75% of patients with dysgerminoma are diagnosed with disease confined to the ovary (62). Much of the information regarding the extent of disease at initial presentation comes from primary surgical procedures performed prior to the current practice of meticulous surgical staging. Nevertheless, analysis of survival in 145 patients reported in three series (63–65), some of whom may have been understaged, indicates that over 90% of patients with stage I dysgerminoma are alive 10 years after diagnosis. Moreover, in these three series combined, 23 (65%) of 35 patients who relapsed after initial conservative treatment were successfully salvaged (61). Although the majority of these patients underwent secondary cytoreductive surgery followed by radiotherapy, in some cases, secondary cytoreductive surgery alone resulted in long-term disease-free survival (64).

For stages Ib, II, and III, initial cytoreductive surgery followed by whole pelvic and abdominal radiation therapy resulted in 5-year survival rates of 63–83% (61,64,65). Recent experience with combination chemotherapy regimens for the treatment of advanced disease has yielded promising results both in terms of cure and preservation of fertility, although the optimal choice of drugs and the duration of therapy have not been clearly established (62,66,67). In addition, in contrast to epithelial malignancies, response rates to salvage agents for the treatment of recurrent disease are high (62), even among patients with bulky, intraabdominal, and retroperitoneal recurrences (66). For these patients, secondary cytoreduction of recurrent disease, either prior to or following salvage chemotherapy, may offer a chance for long-term cure. As experience with these chemotherapeutic regimens accumulates, the role of secondary cytoreduction of recurrent disease will be defined.

Nondysgerminomatous Germ Cell Malignancies

Before the use of multiagent chemotherapy, the outlook for women with nondysgerminomatous germ cell tumors was dismal; indeed, 87% of all patients with endodermal sinus tumors (68), 67% of patients with stage I grade 3 immature teratomas (69), and 54% of women with mixed germ cell malignancies (70) died of disease despite surgery with or without additional radiotherapy. With the incorporation of effective combination chemotherapy regimens into the treatment of both early and advanced stage disease, survival has dramatically improved (69,71–73). In two series that have evaluated the use of cisplatin, bleomycin, and vinblastine chemotherapy for all stages of nondysgerminomatous germ cell tumors, 22 of 22 evaluable patients remain disease-free 7 months to 8 years following diagnosis (69,73). Nevertheless, a group of patients with nondysgerminomatous germ cell malignancies demonstrate resistance to both primary and salvage treatment (71). In these women, the availability and effectiveness of new salvage agents will establish the role of secondary cytoreductive surgery.

REFERENCES

1. Boring C, Squires T, Tong T. Cancer statistics, 1991. *CA Cancer* 1991;41:19–36.
2. Hoskins W, Rubin S. Surgery in the treatment of patients with advanced ovarian cancer. *Semin Oncol* 1991;18:213–221.
3. Silverberg E, Boring C, Squires T. Cancer statistics, 1990. *CA Cancer J Clin* 1990;40:9–26.
4. Young R, Walton L, Ellenberg S, et al. Adjuvant therapy in stage I and II epithelial ovarian cancer. *N Engl J Med* 1990;322:1022–1027.
5. Young R, Fuks Z, Hoskins W. Cancer of the ovary. De Vita VT, Hellman S, Rosenberg SA, eds. *Cancer: principles and practice of oncology* (3rd ed.). Philadelphia: JB Lippincott, 1989:1162–1196.
6. Goldie J, Coldman A. The somatic mutation theory of drug resistance: the "Goldie-Coldman" hypothesis revisited. *PPO* 1989;3:3–6.
7. Hoskins WJ. The influence of cytoreductive surgery on progression-free interval and survival in epithelial ovarian cancer. *Baillieres Clin Obstet Gynaecol* 1989;3:59–71.
8. Ozols R, Young R. Chemotherapy of ovarian cancer. *Semin Oncol* 1991;18:222–232.
9. Rubin S, Hoskins W, Saigo P, et al. Prognostic factors for recurrence following negative second-look laparotomy in ovarian cancer patients treated with platinum-based chemotherapy. *Gynecol Oncol* 1991;42:137.
10. Rutledge F, Burns B. Chemotherapy for advanced ovarian cancer. *Am J Obstet Gynecol* 1966;96:761.
11. Rubin SC, Lewis JJ. Second-look surgery in ovarian carcinoma. *Crit Rev Oncol Hematol* 1988;8:75–91.
12. Williams L, Hoskins W. Can cytoreductive surgery aid ovarian cancer survival? *Contemp OB/GYN* 1990;13–24.
13. Schwartz PE, Smith JP. Second-look operations in ovarian cancer. *Am J Obstet Gynecol* 1980;138:1124–1130.
14. Bertelsen K. Tumor reduction surgery and long-term survival in advanced ovarian cancer: a DACOVA study. *Gynecol Oncol* 1990;38:203–209.
15. Lippman S, Alberts D, Slymen D, et al. Second-look laparotomy in epithelial ovarian carcinoma. *Cancer* 1988;61:2571–2577.
16. Podratz K, Schray M, Wieand H, et al. Evaluation of treatment and survival after positive second-look laparotomy. *Gynecol Oncol* 1988;31:9–21.
17. Podczaski E, Manetta A, Kaminski P, et al. Survival of patients with ovarian epithelial carcinomas after second-look laparotomy. *Gynecol Oncol* 1990;36:43–97.
18. Hoskins W, Rubin S, Dulaney E, et al. Influence of secondary cytoreduction on the survival of patients with epithelial ovarian carcinoma. *Gynecol Oncol* 1989;34:365–371.
19. Dauplat J, Ferriere J, Gorbinet M, et al. Second-look laparotomy

in managing epithelial ovarian carcinoma. *Cancer* 1986;57: 1627–1631.
20. Berek JS, Hacker NF, Lagasse LD, Nieberg RK, Elashoff RM. Survival of patients following secondary cytoreductive surgery in ovarian cancer. *Obstet Gynecol* 1983;61:189–193.
21. Chambers SK, Chambers JT, Kohorn EI, Lawrence R, Schwartz PE. Evaluation of the role of second-look surgery in ovarian cancer. *Obstet Gynecol* 1988;404–408.
22. Hainsworth J, Grosh W, Burnett L, Jones H III, Wolff S, Greco F. Advanced ovarian cancer: long-term results of treatment with intensive cisplatin-based chemotherapy of short duration. *Ann Intern Med* 1988;108:165–170.
23. Luesley DM, Chan KK, Lawton FG, Blackledge GR, Mould JM. Survival after negative second-look laparotomy. *Eur J Surg Oncol* 1989;15:205–210.
24. Vogl S, Seltzer V, Calanog A, et al. "Second-effort" surgical resection for bulky ovarian cancer. *Cancer* 1984;54:2220–2225.
25. Raju K, McKinna J, Barker G, Wiltshaw E, Jones M. Second-look operations in the planned management of ovarian carcinoma. *Am J Obstet Gynecol* 1982;144:650–654.
26. Parker L, Griffiths C, Janis D, et al. Advanced ovarian carcinoma: Integration of surgical treatment and chemotherapy with cyclophosphamide (C), adriamycin (A), and cis-diamminedichloroplatinum (P). *ASCO Abstracts* 1983.
27. Ng L, Rubin S, Hoskins W, et al. Aggressive chemosurgical debulking in patients with advanced ovarian cancer. *Gynecol Oncol* 1990;38:358–363.
28. Lawton FG, Redman CW, Luesley DM, Chan KK, Blackledge G. Neoadjuvant (cytoreductive) chemotherapy combined with intervention debulking surgery in advanced, unresected epithelial ovarian cancer. *Obstet Gynecol* 1989;73:61–65.
29. Neijt JP, Aartsen EJ, Bouma J, Heintz AP, vanLent M, vanLindert A. Cytoreductive surgery with or without preceding chemotherapy in ovarian cancer. *Prog Clin Biol Res* 1985;201: 217–223.
30. Einhorn N, Nilsson B, Sjovall K. Chemotherapy preceding surgery or irradiation in carcinoma of the ovaries. *Prog Clin Biol Res* 1985;201:207–211.
31. Wiltshaw E, Raju KS, Dawson I. The role of cytoreductive surgery in advanced carcinoma of the ovary: an analysis of primary and second surgery. *Br J Obstet Gynaecol* 1985;92:522–527.
32. Redman CW, Blackledge G, Lawton FG, Varma R, Luesley DM, Chan KK. Early second surgery in ovarian cancer—improving the potential for cure or another unnecessary operation? *Eur J Surg Oncol* 1990;16:426–429.
33. Wils J, Blijham G, Naus A, et al. Primary or delayed debulking surgery and chemotherapy consisting of cisplatin, doxorubicin, and cyclophosphamide in stage III-IV epithelial ovarian carcinoma. *J Clin Oncol* 1986;4:1068–1073.
34. Morris M, Gershenson D, Wharton J, Copeland L, Edwards C, Stringer A. Secondary cytoreductive surgery for recurrent epithelial ovarian cancer. *Gynecol Oncol* 1988;34:334–338.
35. Reichman B, Markman M, Hakes T, et al. Intraperitoneal cisplatin and etoposide in the treatment of refractory/recurrent ovarian carcinoma. *J Clin Oncol* 1989;7:1327–1332.
36. Chambers S, Chambers J, Kohorn E, Schwartz P. Etoposide (VP-16-213) plus cis-Diamminedichloroplatinum as salvage therapy in advanced epithelial ovarian cancer. *Gynecol Oncol* 1987; 27:233–240.
37. Pater J, Carmichael J, Krepart G, et al. Second-line chemotherapy of stage III-IV ovarian carcinoma: a randomized comparison of melphalan to melphalan and hexamethylmelamine in patients with persistent disease after doxorubicin and cisplatin. *Cancer Treat Rep* 1987;71:277–281.
38. Sessa C, D'Incalci M, Valente I, Bolis G, Colombo N, Mangioni C. Hexamethylmelamine-CAF (cyclophosphamide, methotrexate, and 5-FU) and cisplatin-CAF in refractory ovarian cancer. *Cancer Treat Rep* 1982;66:1233–1234.
39. Michel G, Zarca D, Castaigne D, Prade M. Secondary cytoreductive surgery in ovarian cancer. *Eur J Surg Oncol* 1989;15: 201–204.
40. Rutgers J, Scully R. Ovarian mullerian mucinous papillary cystadenomas of borderline malignancy. *Cancer* 1988;61:340–348.
41. Soo Kim L, Cajigas H, Scully R. Ovarian cystectomy for serous borderline tumors: a follow-up study of 35 cases. *Obstet Gynecol* 1988;72:775.
42. Snider D, Stuart G, Nation J, Robertson I. Evaluation of surgical staging in stage I low malignant potential ovarian tumors. *Gynecol Oncol* 1990;40:129–132.
43. Tazelaar H, Bostwick D, Ballon S, Hendrickson M, Kempson R. Conservative treatment of borderline ovarian tumors. *Obstet Gynecol* 1985;66:417.
44. Creasman W, Park R, Norris H, DiSaia P, Morrow C, Hreshshyshyn M. Stage I borderline ovarian tumors. *Obstet Gynecol* 1982;59:93.
45. Gershensen D, Sylvia E. Serous ovarian tumors of low malignant potential. *Cancer* 1990;65:578–585.
46. Rice L, Berkowitz R, Mark S, Yavner D, Lage J. Epithelial ovarian tumors of borderline malignancy. *Gynecol Oncol* 1990; 39:195.
47. Bostwick D, Tazelaar H, Ballon S, Hendrickson M, Kempson R. Ovarian epithelial tumors of borderline malignancy. *Cancer* 1986;58:2052–2065.
48. Nation J, Krepart G. Ovarian carcinoma of low malignant potential: staging and treatment. *Am J Obstet Gynecol* 1986;154: 290–293.
49. Barnhill D, Heller P, Brzozowski P, et al. Epithelial ovarian carcinoma of low malignant potential. *Obstet Gynecol* 1985;65: 53–59.
50. Fort G, Pierce V, Saigo P, Hoskins W, Lewis J. Evidence for the efficacy of adjuvant therapy in epithelial ovarian tumors of low malignant potential. *Gynecol Oncol* 1988;32:269–272.
51. O'Quinn A, Hannigan E. Epithelial ovarian neoplasms of low malignant potential. *Gynecol Oncol* 1985;21:177–185.
52. Young R, Scully R. Sex cord-stromal, steroid cell, and other ovarian tumors with endocrine, paraendocrine, and paraneoplastic manifestations. In: Coppleson M, ed. *Blaustein's pathology of the female genital tract*, 3rd ed. New York: Springer-Verlag, 1987;607–658.
53. Hoskins W, Rubin S. Malignant gonadal stromal of the ovary: clinical features and management. In: Coppleson M, ed. *Gynecologic oncology*, 2nd ed. London: Churchill Livingstone, 1991; 963–972.
54. Roth L, Anderson M, Govan A, Langley F, Gowing N, Woodcock A. Sertoli-Leydig cell tumors. *Cancer* 1981;187–191.
55. Evans A, Gaffey T, Malkasian G, Annegers J. Clinicopathologic review of 118 granulosa and 82 theca cell tumors. *Obstet Gynecol* 1980;55:231–238.
56. Bjorkholm E, Silfversward C. Prognostic factors in granulosa-cell tumors. *Gynecol Oncol* 1980;11:261–274.
57. Simmons R, Sciarra J. Treatment of late recurrent granulosa cell tumors of the ovary. *Surg Gynecol Obstet* 1967;124:65–70.
58. Fox H, Agrawal K, Langley F. A clinicopathologic study of 92 cases of granulosa cell tumor of the ovary with special reference to the factors influencing prognosis. *Cancer* 1974;35:231–241.
59. Norris H, Taylor H. Prognosis of granulosa-theca cell tumors of the ovary. *Cancer* 1968;21:255–263.
60. Berek J. Nonepithelial ovarian and tubal cancers. In: Berek S, Hacker N, eds. *Practical gynecologic oncology*, 1st ed. Baltimore: Williams and Wilkins, 1989;365–390.
61. Thomas G, Dembo A, Hacker N, DePetrillo A. Current therapy for dysgerminoma of the ovary. *Obstet Gynecol* 1987;70:268.
62. Creasman W, Soper J. Assessment of the contemporary management of germ cell malignancies of the ovary. *Am J Obstet Gynecol* 1985;153:828–834.
63. Malkasian G, Symmonds R. Treatment of unilateral encapsulated ovarian dysgerminomas. *Am J Obstet Gynecol* 1964;90: 379.
64. Gordon A, Lipton D, Woodruff J. Dysgerminoma: a review of 158 cases from the Evil Novak Tumor Registry. *Obstet Gynecol* 1981;58:497.
65. Asadourian L, Taylor H. Dysgerminoma: an analysis of 105 cases. *Obstet Gynecol* 1969;33:370.
66. Gershensen D, Wharton J, Kline R, Larson D, Kavanagh J, Rutledge F. Chemotherapeutic complete remission in patients with metastatic ovarian dysgerminoma. *Cancer* 1986;58: 2594–2599.
67. Jacobs A, Harris M, Deppe G, DasGupta I, Cohen C. Treatment

of recurrent and persistent germ cell tumors with cisplatin, vinblastine, and bleomycin. *Obstet Gynecol* 1982;59:129.
68. Kurman R, Norris H. Endodermal sinus tumor of the ovary: a clinical and pathologic analysis of 71 cases. *Cancer* 1976;38:2404–2419.
69. Carlson R, Sikic B, Turbow M, Ballon S. Combination cisplatin, vinblastine, and bleomycin chemotherapy (PVB) for malignant germ-cell tumors of the ovary. *J Clin Oncol* 1983;1:645–651.
70. Kurman R, Norris H. Malignant mixed germ cell tumors of the ovary; a clinical and pathologic analysis of 30 cases. *Obstet Gynecol* 1976;48:579.
71. Gershenson D, Del Junco G, Copeland L, Rutledge F. Mixed germ cell tumors of the ovary. *Obstet Gynecol* 1984;64:200.
72. Slayton R, Park R, Silverberg S, Shingleton H, Creasman W, Blessing J. Vincristine, dactinomycin, and cyclophosphamide in the treatment of malignant germ cell tumors of the ovary. *Cancer* 1985;56:243–248.
73. Taylor M, Depetrillo A, Turner R. Vinblastine, bleomycin, and cisplatin in malignant germ cell tumors of the ovary. *Cancer* 1985;56:1341–1349.
74. Ballon S, Portnuff J, Sikic B, Turbow M, Teng N, Soriero O. Second-look laparotomy in epithelial ovarian carcinoma: precise definition, sensitivity, and specifity of the operative procedure. *Obstet Gynecol* 1982;17:154–160.
75. Smirz L, Stehman F, Ulbright T, Sutton G, Ehrlich C. Second-look laparotomy after chemotherapy in the management of ovarian malignancy. *Obstet Gynecol* 1985;152:661–668.
76. Julian C, Woodruff D. The biologic behavior of low-grade papillary serous carcinoma of the ovary. *Obstet Gynecol* 1972;40:860–867.
77. Tasker M, Langley F. The outlook for women with borderline epithelial tumors of the ovary. *Brit J Obstet Gynecol* 1985;92:969–973.
78. Creasman WT, Gall S, Bundy BN, Beecham J, Mortel R, Homesley HD. Second-look laparotomy in the patient with minimal residual stage III ovarian cancer (a Gynecologic Oncology Group study). *Gynecol Oncol* 1989;35:378–382.

CHAPTER 14

Central Venous and Intraperitoneal Access in Patients with Ovarian Cancer

Luis Vaccarello and William J. Hoskins

Patients with epithelial ovarian carcinoma will receive multiple courses of chemotherapy, frequently with several different regimens. At Memorial Sloan-Kettering Cancer Center, the primary route of chemotherapy administration has been intravenous. A significant number of patients receive chemotherapeutic agents intraperitoneally in cases of small-volume disease.

The successful administration of chemotherapy depends partly on a reliable route into the patient's circulation. For patients with poor peripheral vascular access, chemotherapy has taken the form of semipermanent catheters and ports. Intraperitoneal administration of chemotherapy is achieved largely through the use of Tenckhoff catheters or semipermanent ports.

The rationale, techniques, and complications of central venous and intraperitoneal access are discussed in this chapter.

VENOUS ACCESS

Patients with ovarian carcinoma frequently encounter problems because of poor intravenous access. These difficulties may be obvious at the time of presentation or may develop over the course of multiple chemotherapeutic treatments. As peripheral venous access becomes more difficult, patients suffer undue physical and psychological trauma that is indirectly related to their cancer. Multiple, painful attempts at venipuncture, infiltration of intravenous catheters with extravasation of vesicant drugs, and potential delays in the administration of chemotherapy may occur.

Central venous access, for short-term or long-term use, is often beneficial in the management of the cancer patient. Central lines can be used for drawing blood samples and for the administration of various intravenous solutions that include crystalloids, blood products, parenteral nutrition, and chemotherapy. For some patients, central venous access is the only way that required treatments can be administered. Cancer patients may also feel less anxiety if they know that a central catheter or port is in place and that peripheral sticks will not be required.

Long-term venous access can be provided by right atrial catheters that exit externally through the skin. These catheters were originally described by Broviac and colleagues in 1973 and were later modified by Hickman et al. in 1979 (1,2). Newer technology has allowed the development of totally implantable devices (ports) that can be accessed through the skin (3,4). Device selection and placement are dictated by the patient's needs and the operator's experience and preference.

Device/Catheter Selection

Patients with ovarian carcinoma may present with multiple medical problems, including overt ascites, symptoms of bowel obstruction, and other conditions that require central monitoring and access for rapid fluid infusion during the initial debulking laparotomy. A polyurethane multilumen catheter can be placed by a subclavian or internal jugular approach to meet short-term perioperative needs.

After initial surgery, patients with ovarian carcinoma usually require multiple courses of chemotherapy and are at risk for the complications associated with these treatments. The peripheral administration

---

L. Vaccarello and W. J. Hoskins: Gynecology Service, Memorial Sloan-Kettering Cancer Center, New York, New York 10021

of cytotoxic chemotherapy and needle punctures for laboratory tests can contribute to peripheral vein sclerosis. Prolonged admissions for persistent emesis (requiring intravenous fluids), transfusion for anemia, and antibiotic administration for nadir fever are commonly encountered in heavily treated ovarian cancer patients. When long-term central access is being considered, the needs of each individual patient must be assessed in relation to the condition of peripheral veins. Some patients require central access for administration of total parenteral nutrition; others become candidates for central venous access because they cannot physically and/or emotionally tolerate repeated venipunctures.

Central venous access makes use of either an external catheter or an implantable port. Both of these devices are available with single or multiple lumens and are made with a silicone rubber (silastic) catheter. The external catheters (Fig. 1) are designed so that a portion is tunneled in the subcutaneous tissue before the skin is exited. The catheter is anchored by a Dacron cuff that allows fibroblastic infiltration and scar formation to prevent dislodgment (1). Some catheters have a silver-impregnated cuff that is intended to decrease infectious complications (5,6).

The implantable port (Fig. 2) is designed so that the intravenous catheter is attached to a reservoir that is placed in a subcutaneous pocket. The reservoir is accessed by a noncoring (Huber) needle through a self-sealing silicone septum.

Selection of the access device should be based on the patient's needs and the advantages and limitations of the device (Tables 1,2). Most ovarian cancer patients require intermittent long-term central venous access for chemotherapy, phlebotomy, fluid replacement, and blood product replacement. The implantable port is well-suited for intermittent access and has an obvious cosmetic advantage over the external catheter. It also has a lower infection rate and requires less overall maintenance care.

Patients who require daily access through catheters (e.g., nutritional support with TPN) are better served by an external catheter. External catheters provide easier access for both the health care staff and the patient, who may require TPN or other intravenous support at home.

Device Insertion Technique

The insertion of central venous catheters or implantable ports can be performed by direct cut-down to the vessel or by a percutaneous technique (7–10). The percutaneous approach employs a sheathed dilator that is inserted into a central vein by a modified Seldinger technique. The catheter is threaded through the sheath, which pulls apart as it is removed from the skin.

The vessels that are most commonly used to gain access to the right atrium are the external and internal jugular veins, the subclavian veins, and the cephalic veins. If these veins cannot be accessed because of anatomical limitations or the disease process, alternative veins can be found in the lower extremities or the abdominal wall (11–13).

The placement of catheters and ports should be performed under strict sterile conditions, preferably in an operating room with intravenous sedation and local anesthetics. The use of fluoroscopy aids in the final localization of the catheter and helps to prevent some of

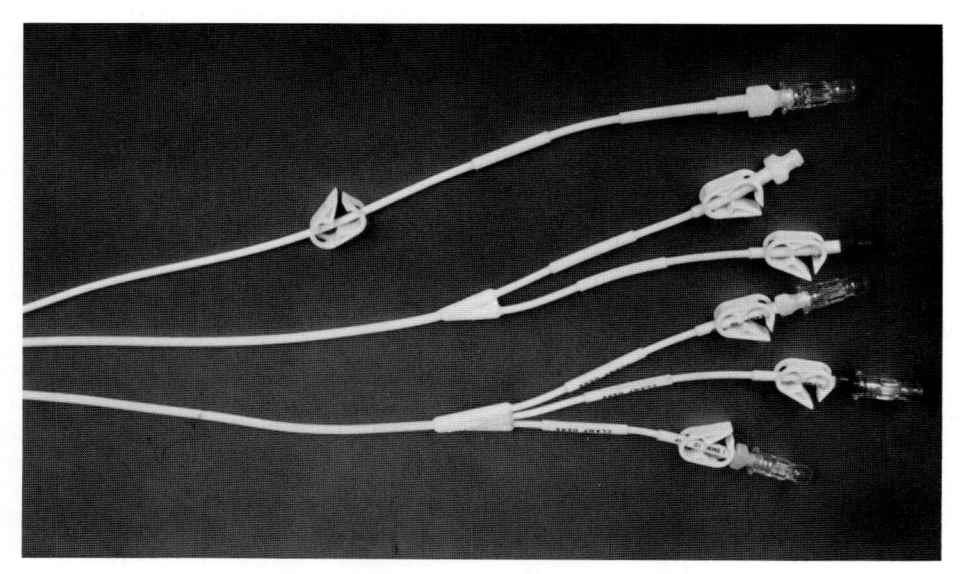

FIG. 1. Single-, double-, and triple-lumen catheters. Distal Dacron cuff and proximal silver-impregnated Vitacuff and shown.

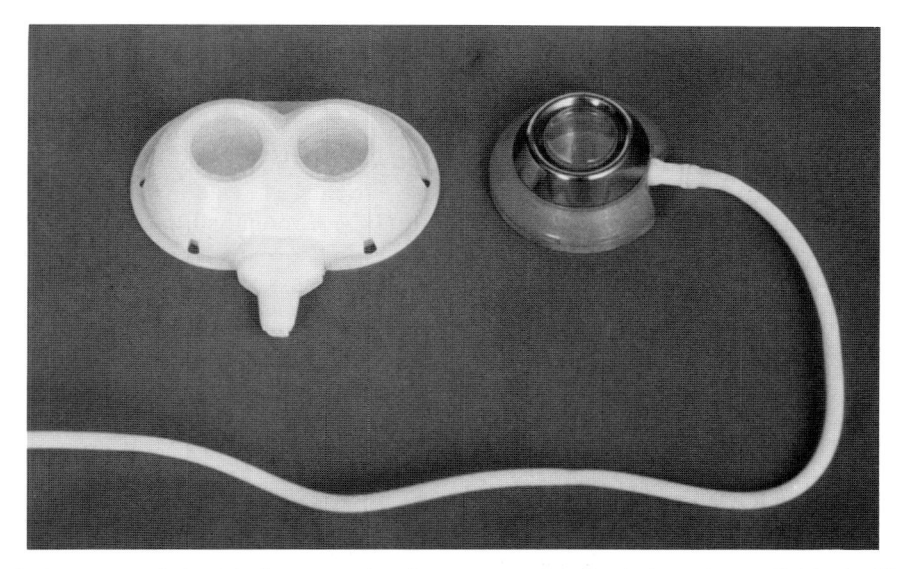

FIG. 2. Single-lumen and double-lumen subcutaneous ports. Each type is available in titanium and plastic.

the complications of catheter placement, especially in patients with anomalous anatomy (14). Bedside insertions of a catheter using a percutaneous technique have been reported, with acceptable rates of complication (15,16). Three of 113 insertions resulted in malposition of the catheter tip and had to be changed.

As previously mentioned, catheters and ports can be inserted by a percutaneous approach utilizing the pull-apart sheath over vein dilator introducer. These sets are available from most manufacturers. This method is best suited to insertion into the subclavian or internal jugular veins. A needle is inserted into the lumen of the vein until blood returns easily. A guidewire is passed through the needle, and its location in the superior vena cava is confirmed by fluoroscopy (17). Any kinks or loops must be corrected before proceeding. The patient may complain of ipsilateral neck discomfort if the wire has traveled into the internal jugular vein (18). In the monitored setting, cardiac arrhythmias can be seen when the wire tip is in the right atrium (19).

The catheter should be measured to estimate the location of the tip at the junction of the superior vena cava and right atrium (20,21). A subcutaneous tunnel is created along the lateral sternal border for external catheters or to the reservoir site for ports. Creating the tunnel before the catheter is inserted may be easier and may prevent inadvertant dislodgment after insertion. After the needle is removed, the combination vein dilator and pull-apart sheath is guided over the wire until the sheath is within the vessel lumen. The guidewire is withdrawn, and blood return from the dilator is confirmed before removal from the sheath. The catheter is then threaded through the sheath into the lumen of the vein. The sheath is withdrawn and pulled apart for removal while the catheter is held in place. Fluoroscopy should again be used to confirm location.

The Dacron cuff of an external catheter should be several centimeters within the tunnel. Secure anchoring from fibroblast infiltration takes 4 to 6 weeks. During this time, the catheter is sutured to the skin with permanent suture.

For subcutaneous ports (Fig. 3), the reservoir pocket is usually created in the infraclavicular fossa and cov-

TABLE 1. *Advantages and disadvantages of central venous catheters*

Advantages	Disadvantages
Ease of insertion	Cosmetically unaesthetic
Ease of access for daily use	Higher infection rate
No risk of extravasation	More maintenance (time and expense)
Low device cost	Risk of pulling out
Repairable catheter	More physically limiting

TABLE 2. *Advantages and disadvantages of implantable ports*

Advantages	Disadvantages
Cosmetically aesthetic	Accesed by skilled professional
Low maintenance	Risk of needle dislodgment
Reduced infections	Noncoring needle required
Lower long-term cost	Flow limited to 19-gauge Huber needle
No physical restrictions	More involved insertion
	Higher device cost

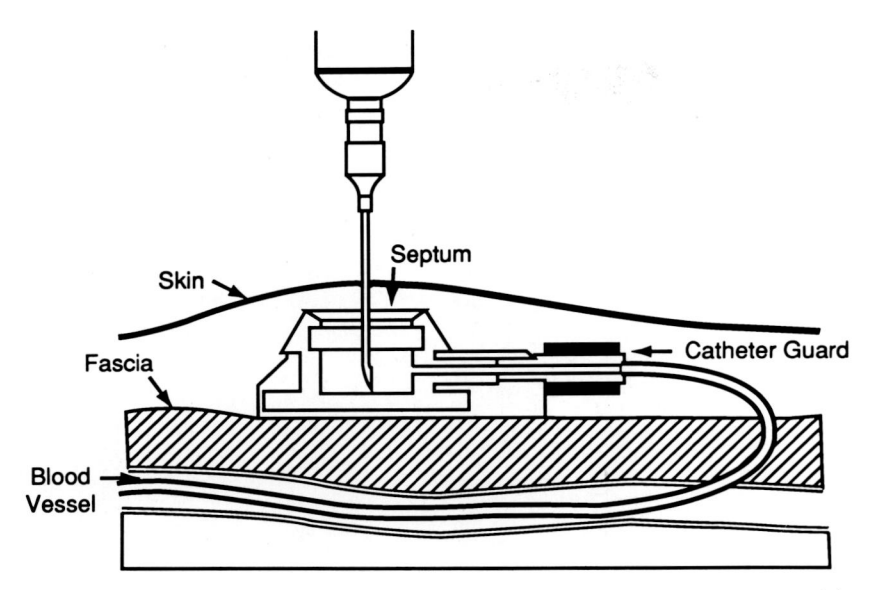

FIG. 3. Subcutaneous location of implantable port, similar for both intravenous and intraperitoneal access. The peritoneal catheter has circumferential openings in the intraperitoneal portion.

ered by a recommended 0.5 cm to 2.0 cm thickness of tissue. If the pocket is too deep, needle dislodgment and difficulty in localizing the port may become problems. A covering that is too thin may lead to erosion of the port through the skin. Several permanent sutures are placed through the port into fascia to prevent movement or actual flipping of the port. After blood return is confirmed, the catheter or port is flushed with heparinized saline and is ready for immediate use. A chest x-ray should be performed to rule out a pneumothorax and to confirm placement.

The percutaneous insertion technique can be performed with less operative time than the cut-down method, with comparable rates of complication when evaluated retrospectively (7,22). In thrombocytopenic patients, percutaneous insertion has up to an 11% association with hemorrhagic morbidity (23). A cut-down to the cephalic or external jugular vein is a preferred method that is relatively safe in this population (24,25). Patients who are at high risk for pneumonothorax because of chronic lung disease, prior pneumonectomy, or other anatomic abnormalities may also benefit from this method of insertion (26).

A popular method is a cut-down to the cephalic vein in the deltopectoral groove (2,25,27,28). Through this incision, the vein can be localized, and the reservoir pocket can be created medially over the chest wall. When the cephalic vein is too small to accept a catheter, a modified Seldinger technique described by Coit and Turnbull (25) will often be successful. The external and internal jugular veins are also readily accessible for a cut-down insertion.

When the vein has been isolated, two absorbable sutures are passed below it. The vein is ligated distally with one, and the other is held proximally. The reservoir pocket is created, and the system is flushed with heparinized saline. The catheter can be cut to an estimated length at this time or after fluoroscopic confirmation of catheter tip location. A venotomy is made, and, with the aid of an introducer, the catheter is passed centrally and confirmed by fluoroscopy. The second suture is ligated proximally, with care not to occlude the lumen. The remainder of the procedure is similar to that described for a percutaneous insertion.

Complications

Complications associated with central venous devices can be divided into two categories: early complications, mainly related to insertion, and late complications encountered during standard use (Table 3). Early complications such as pneumothorax or vascular injury are more commonly associated with the percutaneous insertion technique (7,14,26). According to re-

TABLE 3. *Complications of central venous access devices*

Early	Late
• Pneumothorax	• Infection
• Hemothorax/hydrothorax	• Vein thrombosis
• Mediastinal hematoma	• Catheter occlusion
• Arterial laceration	• Retrograde flow
• Thoracic duct injury	• Needle dislodgment
• Nerve injury	• Tip erosion
• Air embolism	• Catheter migration, evulsion
• Catheter/guidewire embolism	

ports from Food and Drug Administration (FDA) records, insertion injury is the most common cause of operative death and is directly related to the health care professional (14). Operator experience is a key factor and is inversely related to complications from percutaneous insertion techniques (29,30).

The incidence of pneumothorax at the time of catheter insertion has been reported to be <5% (3,7,15,27). Patients who are symptomatic or have significant or expanding pneumothoraxes on serial chest x-ray require placement of a chest tube. Small (<15%), asymptomatic pneumothoraxes can be managed expectantly with follow-up radiographs (26). Insertion with fluoroscopy may aid in the early recognition and management of this complication.

Infection

Infectious morbidity from the long-term use of ports and catheters is the most common late complication and the most significant reason for device removal (24). Several nonrandomized studies have reported significantly less infectious complications in patients with ports than in patients with external catheters (31–33). Selection bias, such as the preferential use of catheters in patients with hematologic malignancies and ports in patients with solid tumors (24), may have influenced the incidence of infection. However, studies of comparable populations receiving ports and catheters also show a significant difference in favor of ports (31,32). The incidences of infection with catheters and ports were reported as 45% and 7%, respectively, in a group of patients prospectively followed at Memorial Hospital (33). The rate of infection in a pediatric series was 0.06 per 100 days for ports and 0.13 per 100 days for catheters (32).

Infections can occur at the exit site of catheters, in the reservoir pocket for ports, and along the subcutaneous tract of the catheter (tunnel infection). Septicemia can be present in association with one of the preceding infections or alone. Antibiotic therapy, however, allows a significant number of devices to be preserved (34,35), even in the neutropenic patient (36).

The most common pathogens that have been isolated in port-related or catheter-related infections are coagulase-negative staphylococci and *S. aureus* (which account for >70% of isolates), followed by gram-negative enteric bacilli and Candida species (34,36–39). The spectrum of recovered organisms points to the skin and gut as possible sources of infection. Migration of skin flora along the catheter tract or its introduction during catheter use or port access using poor sterile technique could account for the high incidence of staph species. Gram-negative enteric organisms can seed the catheter after entrance into the circulatory system through an altered mucosal barrier, especially during periods of neutropenia (36,40).

Exit site infections (e.g., erythema, induration, tenderness, and/or purulence within 2 cm of the catheter exit from the skin [33]) account for 25–45% of device-related infections (34,36). Systemic antibiotics and local care can successfully treat 70–85% of these episodes, allowing preservation of the catheter (34,36). For patients who no longer need the catheter, removal without antibiotics is sufficient treatment if neutropenia is not a problem (36).

Catheter tunnel infections present with similar signs and symptoms along the catheter tract but do not involve the exit site (36). Port pocket infections are placed in this category because their clinical behavior is similar to that of tunnel infections. The incidence of tunnel infections is less than 20% of the total infections in most series. They are the most difficult to cure, and device preservation is possible in only 25–30% of cases (34,36). In the series by Benezra from Memorial Hospital, 12 of 15 catheters requiring removal for tunnel infection were culture-positive for *Pseudomonas* species. Prompt removal of the device was recommended upon detection of *Pseudomonas* (34). Port pocket infections are equally difficult to cure without removal. The organism most frequently isolated from port pocket infections at Memorial Hospital is *S. aureus* (24).

Catheter-related sepsis without tunnel or exit involvement is the most common infectious complication from central venous access devices. Catheter-related sepsis is defined by positive blood culture through the device, with a ≥10-fold colony count from peripherally drawn cultures (34). If peripherally drawn cultures are unavailable, a minimum of 10^3 colony-forming units of bacteria from the catheter is sensitive and specific for the diagnosis (24,38). When broad spectrum antibiotics are run through the device, 60–70% of patients respond to treatment without removal of the catheter or port (35,41).

The decision to remove a catheter or port because of infection should be made on an individual basis, but certain guidelines can be followed (Table 4).

TABLE 4. *Conditions for device removal*

1. Unresolved bacteremia after 48 to 72 hours of antibiotics, especially if *S. aureus* is involved (42–44)
2. Bacteremia with *Xanthomonas* and *Pseudomonas* species in the compromised host (45)
3. Persistent tunnel infection in the presence of *Pseudomonas* (34)
4. Persistent pocket infection in the presence of *S. aureus* (24)
5. Fungemia (46,47)
6. Septic thrombophlebitis

Thrombosis

Deep venous thrombosis (DVT) of the upper extremities and large veins of the thorax is being diagnosed with increased frequency (48–52). A recent review by Horattas et al. found a twofold increase in upper extremity DVT, which makes up approximately 4% of all DVTs (48). Approximately 40% of these upper extremity DVTs were related to central venous catheters.

The incidence of thrombosis associated with central venous catheters varies from 3% to 38% in the literature (48–52). This variation depends greatly on the method used for diagnosis and whether the population was studied prospectively or retrospectively. Primary cancer diagnosis and the reason for catheter usage in a study population can also affect the incidence of thrombosis. Horattas' group's review of prospective studies found a 28% incidence of venous thrombosis, of which 12% were associated with pulmonary emboli (48). Anderson and associates found a similar incidence of pulmonary emboli, with two of three patients in the series dying as a result of this condition (50).

Factors such as Virchow's triad of endothelial injury, hypercoagulability, and altered blood flow predispose patients to thrombosis. When catheters are used, these predisposing factors are affected by the catheter size, type of catheter material, duration of use, type of infusate, and location of catheter tip (48,50).

The diagnosis of vein thrombosis is usually made from clinical signs and symptoms, including ipsilateral area swelling, increased superficial vascular pattern, head and neck venous engorgement, swelling of the face, and pain in the arm, neck, or shoulder. Venography of the extremity or through the catheter can be used to document the clot. Because the use of dye can exacerbate thrombosis in some patients, techniques such as digital subtraction angiography can be equally effective and carry less risk because of the reduced amount of dye that is used. Duplex ultrasound is also very effective in the neck, where it is not impeded by the bony structures of the chest.

Unlike spontaneous axillary or subclavian vein thrombosis, catheter-related thrombosis does not appear to lead to symptoms of chronic obstruction, even in the case of untreated or undissolved thrombi (52). Lack of sufficient numbers for comparative studies in any one institution leaves this medical problem without a standardized approach, but most authors agree that treatment can be initiated with the catheter in place and should include anticoagulation with heparin followed by Coumadin (48–50,52). Moss et al. (49) and Horattas et al. (48) recommend usage of fibrinolytic therapy only through a clotted catheter in order to restore function. Resolution of symptoms and preservation of catheter function can be achieved in 70–100% of patients (49,50,52). The catheter can be removed if it is no longer needed, if it no longer functions, or if thrombosis or infection persists. Reinsertion of central venous catheters in these patients does not appear to carry increased risk. In Moss's series, 9 patients had 11 catheters reinserted without any complications or subsequent thrombosis (49).

The use of materials such as silicone elastomer for catheters has decreased thrombosis over catheters made of polyvinyl chloride or polyurethane. Still, even the perfect material cannot eliminate the risk of thrombosis.

Reduction in the incidence of catheter thrombosis from 37% to 9.5% was accomplished in one prospective study by the use of low-dose warfarin, at 1 mg per day (51). No bleeding complications occurred, and no changes in the coagulation parameters studied could explain warfarin's protective effect. If these findings are confirmed by larger studies, low-dose warfarin will be an acceptable safe means of thrombosis prophylaxis.

Catheter Care and Maintenance

The implanted port has the advantage of requiring no home care on the part of the patient. Port access should be accomplished by trained health care personnel in a sterile fashion, using noncoring Huber needles. These needles are specially made to prevent damage to the silicone diaphragm of the port, which can be accessed 1,000 to 2,000 times using 19- or 22-gauge needles, respectively. Huber needles of different lengths are available with a 90° turn, allowing the accessed site to be covered during long infusions. A transparent occlusive dressing is recommended, because it gives protection while allowing visibility to check needle position and skin condition.

Blood return should be confirmed from the port or catheter prior to use. Occasionally a saline flush will be required, but if resistance is met, forceful irrigation should be avoided. If a clotted catheter is suspected, an attempt at clearance can be made using fibrolytic agents such as urokinase, as per manufacturer's recommendations. The position of the catheter tip in the proper place must be ascertained radiographically.

Irrigation with saline followed by heparinized solution must be performed after every use of the port or catheter. Heparin concentrations of 100 USP u/ml are recommended by manufacturers, but concentrations of 10–1,000 USP u/ml have also been used effectively. Ports should be flushed once every 4 weeks if they are not in use. A Groshong catheter used with a port does not require flushing between uses because of its patented valve system.

The care of a percutaneous catheter is significantly more involved. Routine maintenance includes catheter flushes, exit site skin care and dressing changes, and luer-lock cap changes. The patient and family must be instructed in this care, and assistance can be provided by visiting health care professionals. Routine maintenance schedules recommended by the manufacturer should be followed unless an institutional guideline exists.

INTRAPERITONEAL ACCESS

Dedrick and colleagues described the pharmacokinetic rationale for the intraperitoneal delivery of chemotherapeutic agents in 1978 (53). Since this report, interest in intraperitoneal treatment for patients with epithelial ovarian cancer has been intense. Ovarian cancer, which tends to remain confined to the peritoneal cavity and is responsive to chemotherapy, seems ideal for this modality of therapy. In the last decade, many investigators have attempted to define the role of intraperitoneal therapy in ovarian cancer (54–58).

Although few of these reports have assessed delivery systems in detail, the delivery and distribution of intraperitoneal agents hold primary importance. Any system that is used should have the following characteristics: easy initial insertion; easy removal after therapy; simplicity for nursing personnel; low rate of malfunction; low complication rate; and good patient acceptance.

Methods

Methods of access for intraperitoneal therapy fall into three main categories: (A) repeated paracentesis, which requires insertion of a catheter for each course of therapy and removal when therapy is completed; (B) a semipermanent catheter into the peritoneal cavity, which has an external fitting that allows catheter access for repeated administrations of therapy; and (C) a semipermanent intraperitoneal catheter with a subcutaneous port that can be accessed by a percutaneous needle for administration of the therapeutic agent. Both of the semipermanent catheter systems use a modification of the Tenckhoff catheter for the intraperitoneal portion. The modified Tenckhoff catheter is simply a silastic catheter 4.88 mm in diameter and of variable length (usually 31–48 cm), with multiple circumferential openings 1 mm in diameter for a length of 5–10 cm and a 2.64 mm opening at the distal end. The classic Tenckhoff catheter has a section of nonperforated tubing, approximately 7–10 cm in length, that is designed to be tunneled subcutaneously to a separate site where it exits the body. This end is fitted with an attachment suitable for connection to a syringe or intravenous tubing for instillation of the infusate. In a totally implanted system, the section of nonperforated tubing can be cut to the desired length and fitted to an implantable port. Both the classic and the modified Tenckhoff catheters can have one or more fixed Dacron cuffs. A single cuff is usually located in the subcutaneous tissue where the catheter exits the skin. In a totally implanted system, the cuff is located in the subcutaneous tissue where the catheter exits the abdominal cavity. If the catheter has two cuffs, one is located in the subcutaneous tissue where the catheter exits the abdominal cavity, and the other is either where the catheter exits the skin or, in the case of a totally implanted system, near the connection to the port. Totally implantable systems, which have recently been made without cuffs, are preferred at the Memorial Sloan-Kettering Cancer Center.

The type of port for totally implantable catheter systems varies depending on the manufacturer, but all ports are metal or plastic devices with a penetrable, self-sealing, silicone septum that prevents extravasation of injected material when the needle is withdrawn (similar to the single port in Fig. 2). All of the devices can be fixed to the underlying tissues with suture. The means of attachment vary from four attached rings to plastic-covered metal flanges with perforations for sutures. All of these devices must be accessed with a noncoring needle to prevent injury of the port septum. Figure 3 shows an implantable port and the noncoring needle.

Devices for one-time access to the peritoneal cavity can be composed of virtually any type of needle and catheter system. In all cases, a needle is used for entry into the peritoneal cavity, and a catheter is threaded through the needle into the cavity. The needle can be withdrawn once the catheter is inside the peritoneal cavity. Several commercially available paracentesis kits can be used for the administration of therapeutic agents into the peritoneal cavity.

Surgical Considerations

Access to the peritoneal cavity by separate paracentesis with each treatment course avoids the need to place a semipermanent catheter either at the time of a planned operation or as a separate procedure. The technique involves percussion of the abdomen to avoid underlying fixed loops of bowel, sterile preparation of the skin, and injection of a local anesthetic. In patients with ascites, withdrawal of peritoneal fluid indicates the proper position of the needle. In patients without ascites, entrance into the cavity can usually be felt, and fluid in a syringe flows easily without back pressure. Aspiration should be performed to rule out inadvertent entry into a bowel loop. The catheter should pass easily through the needle, without resistance. Entry into the peritoneal cavity can be confirmed by the injection of a water-soluble radiopaque dye or a radioactive material suitable for external imaging. Injection of one of these agents also allows confirmation of distribution within the peritoneal cavity. An alternate method of placing the intraperitoneal catheter is the use of ultrasound to localize the cavity and to guide the insertion of the catheter. However, this technique does not document even distribution within the peritoneal cavity.

The major disadvantages of paracentesis for intraperitoneal access are the repeated procedures and the cumulative risk of infection. Development of adhesions from previous surgery or from the effects of the therapeutic agent can also cause successive paracentesis to become progressively more difficult. Other disadvantages may include the patient's reluctance to undergo repeated procedures and the labor-intensive demands on the physician, who must place the catheter before each course of treatment. The advantages of this method are the absence of either an external or internal semipermanent device and the decreased risk of intestinal complications from a semipermanent catheter. Also, when therapy is completed, no semipermanent catheter has to be removed, and no abdominal scars remain.

The technique for placement of a semipermanent catheter is the same for the intraabdominal portion of the procedure. If placement is to be performed during a laparotomy, no additional incision is needed to place the catheter into the abdominal cavity. The catheter can be placed anywhere in the abdominal cavity, but we usually choose a location 3 cm to 6 cm lateral to the midline incision in the mid-abdomen (at the level of the umbilicus). Uniform location of the catheter entry point into the abdomen facilitates location of the catheter if malfunction requires corrective procedures. If the catheter has a Dacron cuff at the point of exit from the abdominal cavity, uniform location of the catheter facilitates location of the incision for removal. In addition, location of the entry point at 3 cm to 6 cm lateral to the abdominal incision avoids inadvertent injury to the catheter when the abdomen is closed.

For the external type of catheter, a subcutaneous tunnel at least 6 cm in length is made, and the catheter is brought out through the skin. The Dacron cuff should be located in the subcutaneous tissue below the exit site of the catheter. A suture of monofilament nylon anchors the catheter until the Dacron cuff becomes fixed in the subcutaneous tissue (usually 4 to 6 weeks). In addition to providing an anchoring mechanism that prevents migration of the catheter, the Dacron cuff may aid in the prevention of retrograde infection. Care must be taken to ensure that the cuff is well below the skin surface so that it does not erode through the skin at the entry site.

For the totally implanted catheter and port system, the catheter is tunneled to an appropriate site for port placement. The port should ideally be placed over a firm surface to allow easy access to the system. Ports in the abdominal wall are difficult to stabilize during access of the port. In obese patients, access may be impossible in this location. Some surgeons prefer the inguinal area just inferior to the iliac crest, where the inguinal ligament and dense fascia of the lower abdominal wall can be used as support structures for the port. Unfortunately, this location is unsatisfactory for obese patients, and it may show under the clothes of slender patients. At the Memorial Sloan-Kettering Cancer Center, we prefer to place the port on the lower, lateral rib cage. The underlying rib cage provides an excellent surface for stabilization of the port during access, and the port is readily accessible, even in very obese patients. Placement of the port should avoid the bra line so that clothes are not uncomfortable for the patient. A more lateral position is sometimes necessary in women with large breasts. We have found this location to be comfortable for our patients and easily accessible for nurses. If a patient sleeps habitually on one side, the port should be placed on the opposite side if possible.

Fixation of the port with permanent sutures is very important because migration, and even rotation of the port, can occur in improperly fixed devices. We use monofilament nylon suture and fix the port at three or four points. The skin is closed with a subcuticular closure, and we avoid using the port until the skin begins to heal well (usually 5 to 10 days). In very obese patients, a little fat tissue can be removed from the site over the port to allow easy identification and access.

Complications

A growing body of literature has addressed the complications of intraperitoneal therapy. These complications include failure to function, complications related to surgical placement, infectious complications, and intestinal complications.

Failure to Function

Original studies of intraperitoneal therapy administered a quantity of infusate into the peritoneal cavity and allowed a "dwell" of several hours, followed by removal of the fluid. In most cases, removal of the fluid was difficult. Early investigators were often plagued by episodes of "outflow" obstruction. As intraperitoneal chemotherapy became more common, most investigators abandoned attempts to remove the therapeutic agents. There is little reason to remove any of the modern intraperitoneal therapeutic agents after treatment. Therefore, the only significant obstruction to flow is inflow obstruction, or obstruction of the catheter that prevents infusion of the therapeutic agent.

In the paracentesis method of administering intraperitoneal therapy, inflow obstruction is caused either

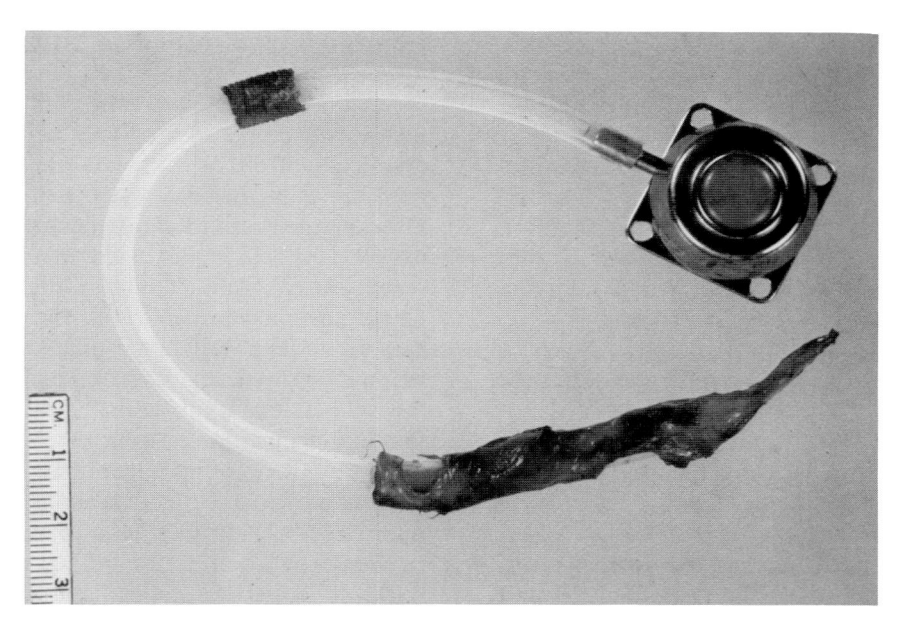

FIG. 4. Subcutaneous port system occluded by fibrinous sheath surrounding the intraperitoneal portion of the catheter.

by failure to obtain access or by placement of the catheter in an area of the cavity that does not allow access to enough of the cavity to hold the entire volume of the infusate. In the case of semipermanent catheters, inflow obstruction is the inability to repeatedly infuse the therapeutic agent or to infuse the desired amount.

Obstructions are usually caused by intraabdominal adhesions and portend badly for continued intraperitoneal therapy. On occasion, the formation of localized adhesions around the catheter results in catheter malfunction that can be relieved by a limited surgical procedure. These localized adhesions cause a sheath around the catheter to form (Fig. 4), which should be removed to allow continued functioning.

Table 5 demonstrates four reports that provide information about the incidence of inflow obstruction. The incidence of inflow obstruction is remarkably consistent between the four studies. Davidson and associates (58) reported on 11 patients whose catheters had to be replaced because of inflow obstruction. Of these 11 patients, 3 (27.3%) developed a second complication.

In two cases, inflow obstruction recurred, and in one case, an infection occurred. Thus, some cases of inflow obstruction can be corrected, but the incidence of recurrent obstruction (2 of 11, or 18%) is more than double that for primary catheters. Davidson and associates also reported that in 15 patients in whom the cause of inflow obstruction was determined, 12 obstructions were caused by the development of a fibrous sheath around the catheter. In two patients the catheter lumen became obstructed, and in one patient the port rotated 180° and could not be accessed.

Surgical Complications

The reported incidence of surgical complications related to the insertion or use of intraperitoneal catheters is quite low. In a review of 400 cases from four series, Davidson and colleagues reported only one case of bowel obstruction related to an intraperitoneal catheter. In addition, intestinal and vascular injury from the

TABLE 5. *Inflow obstruction with implanted port and catheter systems*

Author (ref.)	Year	Number of patients	Number of inflow obstructions	Percent inflow obstructions
Pfeifle et al. (59)	1984	54	3	5.6
Piccart et al. (60)	1985	145	3	2.1
Braly et al. (61)	1986	33	2	6.1
Davidson et al. (58)	1991	227	20	8.8
Total		459	28	6.1*

* Overall percent (28 of 459)

insertion of semipermanent catheter does not appear to be a significant risk, although it can occur. The occasional cases of intestinal perforation during paracentesis rarely lead to infection.

Infectious Complications

Table 6 presents a review of the infectious complications reported in four series of patients with semipermanent catheter and port systems. In these 459 patients, the mean incidence of infectious complications was 8.9%, with a low incidence of 5.6% and a high incidence of 18.2%. The complications included peritonitis, port infections, and superficial cellulitis. Davidson and colleagues reported that in 8 of 20 cases of infection, perforation of the intestine had occurred. Of the 12 infections that were not associated with bowel perforation, 6 were treated with intravenous antibiotics, and 1 was treated with oral antibiotics. In all cases therapy was unsuccessful, and the catheters were removed. For the remaining patients with infections, the catheters were removed without any attempt to salvage them with antibiotic therapy. In 8 of the 12 patients, purulence was noted at the port site when the system was finally removed. In their series of 227 patients, Davidson and associates reported only two cases (0.9%) of peritonitis.

When Davidson et al. evaluated the patients who had had a second catheter placed after an infectious complication, they found that 50% of those patients had further catheter complications. One-half of these further complications were infectious, and one-half were obstructive.

Braly and associates (61) found no increase in the rate of infectious complications in patients who had catheters placed at the time of large bowel resection. Davidson and colleagues reported a trend towards a higher infection rate in patients whose catheters were placed at the time of bowel surgery, but the trend was not statistically significant. Although most surgeons are concerned about placement of an intraperitoneal catheter at the time of bowel resection, no definite evidence has associated it with an increased infection rate.

Intestinal Complications

Several authors have reported the erosion of semipermanent catheters into the large or small intestine (58,61–63). Both Davidson et al. and Wakefield et al. reported this erosion at the site of an intestinal anastomosis. Other authors (including Davidson and colleagues) reported intestinal perforation in patients who did not have an intestinal anastomosis. The incidence of intestinal perforation varies from 0% to 3.5% in most series. Usually, when the diagnosis of perforation is made by x-ray dye studies, the catheter has been removed without exploratory laparotomy. The sheath that builds up around the catheter probably acts to seal off the perforation and to prevent leakage. When the diagnosis is made at laparotomy, most authors recommend oversewing the area of perforation.

CONCLUSION

The establishment of intraperitoneal and intravenous access has become an important aspect in the management of patients with ovarian cancer. The continued utilization of intensive intravenous chemotherapy for the primary treatment of patients with ovarian cancer often requires the utilization of semipermanent establishment of central venous access. Recent experimental protocols utilizing the reinfusion of autologous stem cells will make establishment of central venous access even more important.

The apparent success of intraperitoneal chemotherapy in the management of selected patients with ovarian cancer requires the establishment and maintenance of semipermanent access devices into the peritoneal cavity. For selected patients, intraperitoneal chemotherapy appears to be the best option for salvage treatment. Repeated paracentesis do not appear feasible or acceptable for most patients.

Finally, evidence to date indicates that the implementation of semipermanent devices totally beneath the skin results in significantly less infection than that seen with semipermanent catheters exiting through the skin. This decrease in the infection rate, combined with the more aesthetic placement of all devices beneath the

TABLE 6. *Infectious complications with implanted port and catheter systems*

Author (ref.)	Year	Number of patients	Number of infectious complications	Percent infectious complications
Pfeifle et al. (59)	1984	54	3	5.6
Piccart et al. (60)	1985	145	12	8.3
Braly et al. (61)	1986	33	6	18.2
Davidson et al. (58)	1991	227	20	8.8
Total		459	41	8.9

skin, results in greater utility of the devices and better patient acceptance.

REFERENCES

1. Broviac JW, Cole JJ, Scribner GH. A silicone rubber atrial catheter for prolonged parenteral alimentation. *Surg Gynecol Obstet* 1973;136:602.
2. Hickman RO, Buckner CD, Clift RA, et al. A modified right atrial catheter for access to the venous system in marrow transplant recipients. *Surg Gynecol Obstet* 1979;148:871.
3. Niederhuber JE, Ensminger W, Gyves JW, et al. Totally implanted venous and arterial access system to replace external catheters in cancer treatment. *Surgery* 1982;92:706.
4. Gyves J, Ensminger W, Niederhuber J, et al. Totally implanted system for intravenous chemotherapy in patients with cancer. *Am J Med* 1982;73:841–845.
5. Maki DG, Cobb L, Garman JK, et al. An attachable silver-impregnated cuff for prevention of infection with central venous catheters: a prospective randomized multicenter trial. *Am J Med* 1988;85:307.
6. Flowers RH, Schwenzer J, Kopel RF, et al. Efficacy of an attachable subcutaneous cuff for the prevention of intravascular catheter-related infection: a randomized, controlled trial. *JAMA* 1989;261:878.
7. Jansen RFM, Wiggers T, vanGeel BN, et al. Assessment of insertion techniques and complication rates of dual lumen central venous catheters in patients with hematological malignancies. *World J Surg* 1990;14:101.
8. Heimbach DM, Ivey TD. Technique for placement of a permanent home hyperalimentation catheter. *Surg Gynecol Obstet* 1976;143:635–636.
9. Kondi ES, Pietrafitta JJ, Barriola JA. Technique for placement of a totally implantable venous access device. *J Surg Oncol* 1988;37:272–277.
10. Lechner P, Anderhuber F, Tesch NP. Anatomical bases for a safe method of subclavian venipuncture: clinical experience in 350 cases. *Surg Radiol Anat* 1989;11:91–95.
11. Stenzel JP, Green TP, Fuhrman BP, et al. Percutaneous femoral venous catheterizations: a prospective study of complications. *J Pediatr* 1989;114:411–415.
12. Pokorny WJ, McGill CW, Harburg FJ. Use of azygous vein for central catheter insertion. *Surgery* 1985;97:362.
13. Krog M, Gerdin B. Techniques, materials, and devices. An alternative placement of implantable central venous access systems. *J Parenter Enteral Nutr* 1989;13:666.
14. Scott WL. Complications associated with central venous catheters: a survey. *Chest* 1988;94:1221–1224.
15. Malviya VK, Deppe G, Gove N, Maline JMJ. Vascular access in gynecologic cancer using the Groshong right atrial catheter. *Gynecol Oncol* 1989;33:313–316.
16. Delmore JE, Horbelt DV, Jack BL, Roberts DK. Experience with the Groshong long-term central catheter. *Gynecol Oncol* 1989;34:216–218.
17. Robertson LJ, Mauro MA, Jaques PF. Radiologic placement of Hickman catheters. *Radiology* 1989;170:1007–1009.
18. Selby JB, Tegtmeyer CJ, Amodeo C, et al. Insertion of subclavian hemodialysis catheters in difficult cases: value of fluoroscopy and angiographic techniques. *AJR Am J Roentgenol* 1989;152:641–643.
19. Luks FI, Picard DL, Pizzi WF. Electrocardiographic guidance for percutaneous placement of central venous catheters. *Surg Gynecol Obstet* 1989;169:157–158.
20. Bottino J, McCredie RB, Groschel DA, et al. Long-term intravenous therapy with peripherally inserted silicone elastomer central venous catheters in patients with malignant disease. *Cancer* 1979;43:1937.
21. Stanislav GV, Fitzgibbons RJJ, Bailey RTJ, et al. Reliability of implantable central venous access devices in patients with cancer. *Arch Surg* 1987;122:1280.
22. Davis SJ, Thompson JS, Edney JA. Insertion of Hickman catheters: a comparison of cutdown and percutaneous techniques. *Am Surg* 1984;50:673–676.
23. Stellato TA, Gauderer MW, Lazarus HM, Herzig RH. Percutaneous silastic catheter insertion in patients with thrombocytopenia. *Cancer* 1985;56:2691–2693.
24. Groeger JS, Lucas AB, Coit D. Venous access in the cancer patient. In: Devita VT Jr, Hellman S, Rosenberg SA, eds. *Principles and practice of oncology updates*, vol 5, no 3. Philadelphia: JB Lippincott, 1991.
25. Coit D, Turnbull AD. A safe technique for the placement of implantable vascular access devices in thrombocytopenic patients. *Surg Gynecol Obstet* 1988;167:429.
26. Hickman RD, Romsey PG, Tapper D. Central venous access. In: Greer BE, Berek JS, eds. *Gynecologic oncology, treatment rationale and techniques*. New York: Elsevier Science Publishing, 1991 pp. 285–308.
27. Brincker H, Sacter G. Fifty-five patient years' experience with totally implanted system for intravenous chemotherapy. *Cancer* 1986;57:1124.
28. Heimbach DM, Ivey TD. Technique for placement of a permanent home hyperalimentation catheter. *Surg Gynecol Obstet* 1976;143:635–636.
29. Fares LG, Block PH, Feldman SD. Improved house staff results with subclavian cannulation. *Am Surg* 1986;52:101.
30. Bernard RW, Stohl WM. Subclavian vein catheterization: a prospective study. *Am Surg* 1971;191:174–184.
31. Greene FL, Moore W, Strickland G, McFarland J. Comparisons of a totally implantable access device for chemotherapy (Port-A-Cath) and long term percutaneous catheterization (Broviac). *South Med J* 1988;8:580–583.
32. Ross MN, Haase GM, Poole MA, et al. Comparison of totally implanted reservoirs with external catheters as venous access devices in pediatric oncology patients. *Surg Gynecol Obstet* 1988;167:141.
33. Groeger JS, Lucas A, Brown A. Venous access device infections in adult cancer patients: catheters vs. port. *28th Interscience Conference on Antimicrobial Agents and Chemotherapy (ICAAC)* 1988;158.
34. Benezra D, Kiehn T, Gold JWM, et al. Prospective study of infections in indwelling central venous catheters using quantitative blood cultures. *Am J Med* 1988;85:495.
35. Raaf J. Results from use of 826 vascular access devices in cancer patients. *Cancer* 1985;55:1312.
36. Press OW, Ramsey PG, Larson EB, et al. Hickman catheter infections in patients with malignancies. *Medicine* 1984;63:189–200.
37. Cercenado E, Rodriguez-Creixems EJ, et al. A conservative procedure for the diagnosis of catheter-related infections. *Arch Intern Med* 1990;140:1417.
38. Brun-Buisson C, Abrouk F, Legrand P, et al. Diagnosis of central venous catheter related-sepsis. *Arch Intern Med* 1987;147:873.
39. Kappers-Klunne MC, Degener JE, Stijnen T, et al. Complications from long-term indwelling central venous catheters in hematologic patients with special reference to infection. *Cancer* 1989;64:1747.
40. Tancrede CH, Andremont AO. Bacterial translocation and gram negative bacteremia in patients having hematological malignancies. *J Infect Dis* 1985;15:99.
41. Mirro JJ, Rao BS, Stokes DC, et al. A comparison of placement techniques and complications of externalized catheters and implantable port use in children with cancer. *J Pediatr Surg* 1990;25:120.
42. Hartman GE, Shochat SJ. Management of septic complications associated with silastic catheters in childhood malignancy. *Pediatr Infect Dis J* 1987;6:1042.
43. Dugdale DC, Ramsey PG. Staphylococcus aureus bacteremia in patients with Hickman catheters. *Am J Med* 1990;89:137–141.
44. Raviglione MC, Battan R, Pablos-Mendez A, et al. Infections associated with Hickman catheters in patients with the acquired immunodeficiency syndrome. *Am J Med* 1989;86:780–786.
45. Elting LS, Bodey GP. Septicemia due to xanthomonas species and non-aeruginosa pseudomonas species: increasing incidence of catheter-related infections. *Medicine* 1990;5:296.

46. Eppes SC, Troutman JL, Gutman LT. Outcome of treatment of candidemia in children whose central catheters were removed or retained. *Pediatr Infect Dis J* 1989;8:99.
47. Dato VM, Dajani AS. Candidemia in children with central venous catheters: role of catheter removal and amphotericin B therapy. *Pediatr Infect Dis J* 1990;5:309.
48. Horattas MC, Wright DJ, Fenton AH, et al. Changing concepts of deep venous thrombosis of the upper extremity: report of a series and review of the literature. *Surgery* 1988;104:561.
49. Moss JD, Wagman LD, Riihimaki DC, et al. Central venous thrombosis related to the silastic Hickman-Broviac catheter in an oncologic population. *J Parenter Enteral Nutr* 1989;13:397.
50. Anderson AJ, Krasnow SH, Boyer MW, et al. The major Hickman catheter complication in patients with solid tumor. *Chest* 1989;95:71–75.
51. Bern MM, Lokich JJ, Wallach SR, et al. Very low doses of warfarin can prevent thrombosis in central venous catheters. A randomized prospective trial. *Ann Intern Med* 1990;112:423.
52. Haire WD, Lieberman RP, Edney J, et al. Hickman catheter-induced thoracic vein thrombosis: frequency and long-term sequelae in patients receiving high-dose chemotherapy and marrow transplantation. *Cancer* 1990;66:900.
53. Dedrick RL, Myers CE, Bungay PM, DeVita VTJ. Pharmacokinetic rationale for peritoneal drug administration in the treatment of ovarian cancer. *Cancer Treat Rep* 1978;62:1.
54. Myers CE, Collins JM. Pharmacology of intraperitoneal chemotherapy. *Cancer Invest* 1983;1:395.
55. Markman M. Intraperitoneal antineoplastic agents for tumors principally confined to the peritoneal cavity. *Cancer Treat Rev* 1986;13:219.
56. Reichman B, Markman M, Hakes T, et al. Intraperitoneal cisplatin and etoposide in the treatment of refractory/recurrent ovarian carcinoma. *J Clin Oncol* 1989;7:43.
57. ten Bokkel Huinink WW, Dubbelman R, Aartsen E, et al. Experimental and clinical results with intraperitoneal cisplatin. *Semin Oncol* 1985;12:43.
58. Davidson SA, Rubin SC, Markman M, et al. Intraperitoneal chemotherapy: analysis of complications with an implanted subcutaneous port and catheter system. *Gynecol Oncol* 1991;41:101.
59. Pfeifle CE, Howell SB, Markman M, Lucas WE. Totally implantable system for peritoneal access. *J Clin Oncol* 1984;2:1277.
60. Piccart MJ, Speyer JL, Markman M, et al. Intraperitoneal chemotherapy: technical experience at five institutions. *Semin Oncol* 1985;12:90.
61. Braly P, Doroshow J, Hoff S. Technical aspects of intraperitoneal chemotherapy in abdominal carcinomatosis. *Gynecol Oncol* 1986;25:319.
62. Varney RR, Goel R, van Sonnenberg E, Lucas WE, Casola G. Delayed erosion of intraperitoneal chemotherapy catheters into the bowel. *Cancer* 1989;64:762.
63. Kourie TB, Botha JR. Erosion of the caecum by a Tenckhoff catheter: a case report. *S Afr J Surg* 1985;23:117.

CHAPTER 15

Palliative Surgery in Ovarian Cancer

Carol L. Brown and John L. Lewis, Jr.

Surgery is an integral part of the initial therapy for ovarian cancer both for establishing the diagnosis and for carrying out maximal cytoreduction. It is also important for accurately assessing response after chemotherapy, and it plays a major role in the palliative therapy of ovarian cancer. Palliative surgery can be defined as any procedure whose purpose is to relieve symptoms caused by recurrent or progressive cancer without direct antitumor effect—that is, "to ease without cure" (1). This chapter focuses on surgical procedures carried out to relieve symptoms and complications of recurrent ovarian cancer. The goals of palliative surgery in patients with ovarian cancer should be to relieve discomfort, improve quality of life, and prolong life in those who will ultimately die of their disease. In selected patients, another goal of palliative surgery may be to correct a mechanical or physiologic derangement caused by progressive tumor (such as ureteral obstruction), thus enabling the patient to receive further antineoplastic therapy given with the hope of response. Palliative surgery should not be performed in patients whose death is imminent, which distinguishes it from terminal care.

Over 12,000 women die each year from ovarian cancer (2), the majority with symptoms from progressive intraabdominal tumor that is no longer responding to chemotherapy. For these patients, surgical procedures may be the only possible means of easing their discomfort. Thus, for any physician caring for patients with advanced ovarian cancer, familiarity with palliative surgical options is essential. The relative importance of palliative surgery to the overall care of patients with ovarian cancer is illustrated by the fact that of 427 laparotomies performed on patients with ovarian cancer at Memorial Sloan-Kettering Cancer Center between January 1989 and December 1990, 9% were considered palliative, performed solely for the purpose of relieving symptoms of progressive or recurrent cancer (Table 1). The majority of these laparotomies were performed to relieve intestinal obstruction, but as Table 2 illustrates, symptoms from pleural effusions and ureteral obstruction are also common indications for palliative surgical procedures in this group of patients. This chapter will review the indications for palliative surgery, the available techniques, and the success and complication rates in relation to intestinal obstruction, intestinal fistula, ascites, pleural effusions, and ureteral obstruction.

INTESTINAL OBSTRUCTION

Between 5% and 50% of women with ovarian cancer will develop symptoms of intestinal obstruction during the course of their illness (3–6). For the majority of these patients, the etiology of intestinal obstruction is not adhesions from prior surgery or radiation therapy, but progressive intraabdominal tumor (3,7,8). Bowel obstruction is frequently the terminal event in ovarian cancer patients and represents the most frequent indication for palliative surgery.

Clinical Presentation/Diagnostic Studies

The pattern of intraperitoneal spread of ovarian cancer typically results in diffuse carcinomatosis involving the intestine in patients with advanced or recurrent disease, producing symptoms more suggestive of chronic, intermittent intestinal obstruction than acute bowel obstruction (4). These symptoms include abdominal pain, nausea, vomiting, and obstipation. This clinical picture allows time for obtaining appropriate diagnostic studies to localize the site of obstruction and guide plans for

---

C. L. Brown and J. L. Lewis, Jr.: Gynecology Service, Department of Surgery, Memorial Sloan-Kettering Cancer Center, New York, New York 10021

TABLE 1. *Laparotomies in ovarian cancer patients, Memorial Sloan-Kettering Cancer Center, January 1989 to December 1990[a]*

Year	Total Laparotomies	Purpose	
		Treatment[b]	Palliation[c]
1989	199	177	22 (11%)
1990	228	211	17 (7%)
Total	427	388	39 (9%)

[a] Patients with epithelial ovarian cancer.
[b] Includes primary staging/cytoreduction, laparotomies to assess response to treatment, laparotomies for recurrence.
[c] Includes laparotomies for intestinal obstruction, intestinal fistula, hemorrhage, and abscess.

further management. Upright and flat plate abdominal radiographs are usually the first studies obtained, and they may reveal multiple dilated loops of intestine and differential air fluid levels, which typically characterize small bowel obstruction (Figs. 1 and 2). The site of obstruction is often not confined to the small intestine, as illustrated by data from studies of ovarian cancer patients explored for intestinal obstruction (Table 3). Since as many as 45% of ovarian cancer patients presenting with intestinal obstruction have some component of colonic obstruction, diagnostic evaluation should include a barium enema in most cases. This study may reveal that what appeared as only small bowel obstruction on abdominal radiographs is actually a combination of small and large bowel obstruction (Fig. 3), a fact that may alter plans for surgical management. When a bypass procedure is planned, it is important to know how much of the colon is free of obstruction so that the site of anastomosis will be distal to the affected area.

TABLE 2. *Palliative surgical procedures in ovarian cancer patients, Memorial Sloan-Kettering Cancer Center, January 1989 to December 1990[a]*

Procedure	Number performed
Laparotomy for intestinal obstruction	32
Laparotomy for intestinal fistula	6
Laparotomy for abscess	1
PEG placement[b]	16
Chest tube placement/sclerosis	16
Pleurectomy	2
PCN placement[c]	2
Retrograde ureteral stent placement	2
Total	77

[a] Paracentesis not included in tabulations.
[b] Percutaneous endoscopic gastrostomy.
[c] Percutaneous nephrostomy.

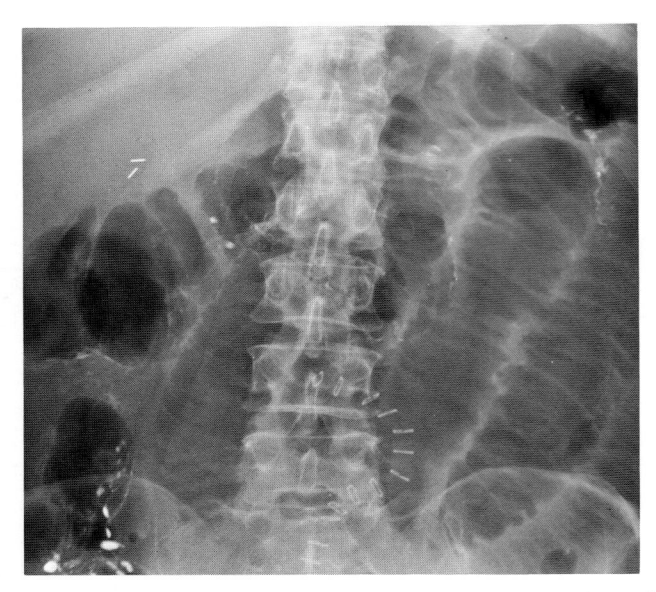

FIG. 1. Flat plate radiograph of patient with small bowel obstruction.

Upper gastrointestinal (GI) series with small bowel follow-through is useful for localizing the site of obstruction in proximal or distal bowel and for distinguishing partial from complete obstruction. Choice of contrast medium for studies of the upper GI tract is debated in the literature. The use of gastrografin, a water soluble agent, avoids the hazards of barium im-

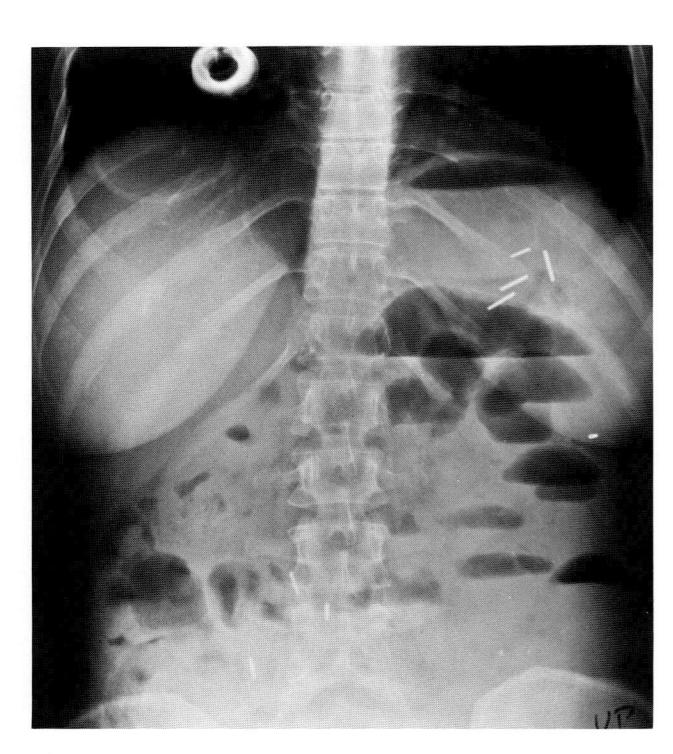

FIG. 2. Upright radiograph of patient with small bowel obstruction.

TABLE 3. Sites of intestinal obstruction in ovarian cancer[a]

Author (ref.)	Number of patients	SBO (number)[b]	LBO (number)[c]	Both (number)
Rubin et al. (22)	54	24	18	12
Clarke-Pearson et al. (7)	49	30	16	3
Krebs et al. (24)	104	64	25	15
Tunca et al. (4)	126	66	41	19
Total	333	184	100	49

[a] 55% small bowel obstruction, 30% large bowel obstruction, 15% combined small bowel and large bowel obstruction.
[b] Small bowel obstruction.
[c] Large bowel obstruction.

paction or extravasation, but its hyperosmolarity rapidly draws fluid into the intestinal lumen, limiting the radiologist's ability to visualize distal small intestine. The yield of a gastrografin study may be increased by administering the contrast through an intestinal tube that has passed into the small bowel just proximal to the obstructed area. If there is no evidence of large bowel obstruction, upper tract studies with barium are probably most useful in the diagnostic evaluation of ovarian cancer patients (9). If a patient has symptoms of obstruction but normal abdominal films, an upper GI series may diagnose gastric outlet obstruction (Fig. 4). The etiology may be tumor obstructing the gastric outlet (10) or ascitic fluid trapped in the lesser sac. A computed tomography (CT) scan or ultrasound is usually required to diagnose the latter condition, which can be successfully palliated by paracentesis (11,12).

Nonoperative Management of Bowel Obstruction

When intestinal obstruction is suspected in a patient with ovarian cancer, replacement of volume losses and correction of electrolyte imbalances by administration of intravenous fluids is the first step in management. After appropriate diagnostic studies have been obtained, the next step should be decompression of the obstructed bowel by intestinal intubation. Whether long or short tubes are more appropriate for intestinal decompression in management of bowel obstruction is debated. Review of studies in the surgical literature of both benign- and malignancy-associated small bowel obstruction reveals no advantage of Miller-Abbott or Cantor tubes over nasogastric tubes with regard to relieving obstruction (13–16). However, many authors in

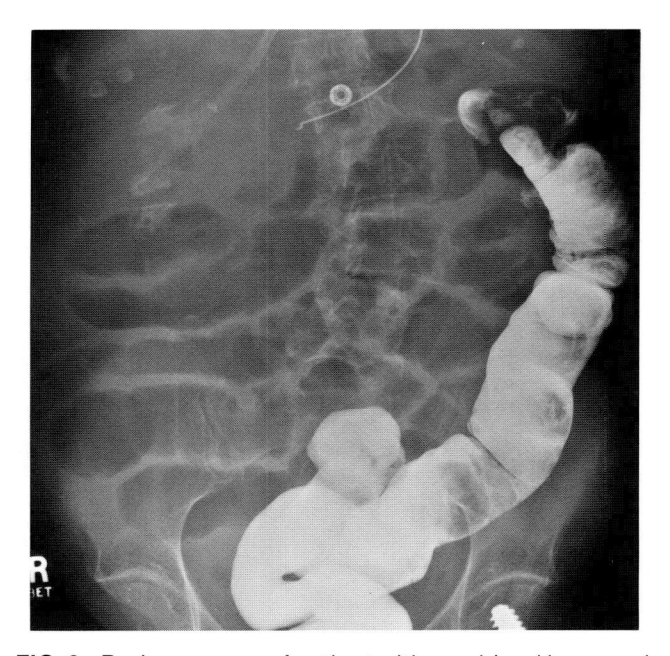

FIG. 3. Barium enema of patient with combined large and small bowel obstruction.

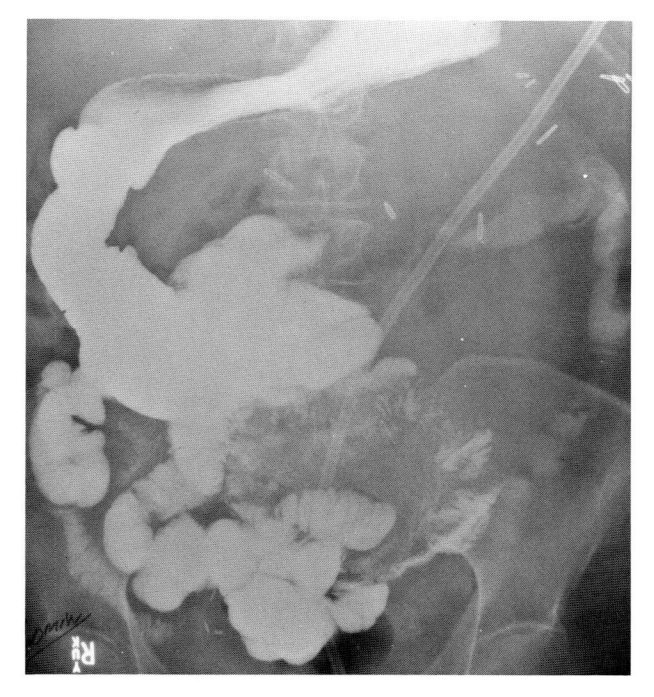

FIG. 4. Upper GI series in patient with gastric outlet obstruction secondary to ascites trapped in lesser sac.

the gynecologic literature favor the use of long tubes, particularly in patients with obstruction secondary to progressive intraabdominal ovarian cancer (9,17–21). The diffuse carcinomatosis frequently found intraoperatively in these patients makes distinguishing bowel proximal and distal to the site of obstruction difficult. The presence of a Miller-Abbott or Cantor tube in the proximal small bowel lumen aids the surgeon in making this distinction and in avoiding extensive dissection of cancer-coated loops of bowel. The placement of long intestinal tubes can be accomplished only in patients who have evidence of peristaltic activity to ensure passage of the tube to the site of obstruction.

The chronic nature of symptoms in ovarian cancer patients with bowel obstruction often allows for a prolonged trial of intravenous hydration, intestinal intubation, and parenteral nutritional support as nonoperative management. Strangulation is rarely a complication of malignancy-associated intestinal obstruction, reported in only 1–3% of such cases compared to 10% of cases of benign mechanical bowel obstruction (13,14,16). In the studies of intestinal obstruction in patients with advanced ovarian cancer, operative findings of strangulation or ischemic bowel are rarely, if ever, reported (4,5,7,17,22–25). Krebs and Goplerud (17) found no difference in operative mortality between ovarian cancer patients undergoing >48 hours versus <48 hours of tube decompression preoperatively as long as effective decompression was established within 48 hours of admission. The median duration of nonoperative management (intravenous hydration and intestinal intubation) reported in patients with ovarian cancer ranges from 6 to 11.3 days without adverse effect. This confirms the safety of such an approach in these patients (3,7,19) and contradicts the adage that a surgeon should "never let the sun set or rise on a bowel obstruction."

Despite the demonstrated safety of a prolonged trial of intestinal decompression, intravenous fluids, and nutritional support in the management of bowel obstruction in patients with ovarian cancer, nonoperative therapy is usually ineffective. Obstruction due to malignant intraabdominal tumor was relieved by such measures in fewer than 30% of cases reported in the surgical literature (13,14,16). Helmkamp and Kimmel found that only 32% of ovarian cancer patients with small bowel obstruction had restoration of bowel function for at least 30 days after tube drainage and IV hydration (19). Krebs and Goplerud (17) found only 10% of similar cases resolved with tube decompression alone, and of these patients, the majority were readmitted with recurrent obstruction within 4 weeks. Although a trial of nonoperative management is warranted in all ovarian cancer patients with bowel obstruction to avoid the risks of surgery (exceptions are obstruction of the colon and gastric outlet), it is clear that most patients with progressive intraabdominal tumor will fail this trial and must be considered candidates for palliative surgery.

Preoperative Preparation and Intraoperative Techniques

In addition to correction of fluid and electrolyte imbalances and decompression of dilated bowel by intubation, preoperative management of intestinal obstruction in patients with advanced ovarian cancer should include attempted mechanical bowel preparation if feasible. For patients with small bowel obstruction, cathartics from above, such as magnesium citrate, should not be given. However, the colon should be evacuated with enemas. In order to reduce complications, oral antibiotics—typically neomycin and erythromycin—may be administered on the day prior to surgery if there is still some bowel function present. An intravenous antibiotic with coverage including anaerobic and gram-negative organisms should be given on call to surgery (26). A variety of surgical techniques for intestinal resection and bypass have been described (20,22). The advantages of intestinal stapling techniques in reducing operative time, blood loss, and improved blood flow to the anastomosis have also been reported (27–29). Bypass, resection, and colostomies are performed with approximately equal frequency when ovarian cancer patients are explored for bowel obstruction (4,5, 7,22–24). Although some authors suggest that bypass is faster and safer for these patients who often have edematous bowel and multiple adhesions, no evidence in the literature suggests that bypass versus resection affects survival or postoperative morbidity (4,23). In approximately 20% of patients undergoing exploration, surgical correction is not possible (4,22–24).

Survival and Efficacy of Palliative Surgery for Bowel Obstruction

Deciding whether to operate on a patient with intestinal obstruction due to progressive ovarian cancer is difficult. A review of the published studies of surgery in these patients reveals data on the effectiveness and risks of such procedures (Tables 4–6). The median survival after surgery for intestinal obstruction is uniformly short (<8 months in all series). Little difference is evident when comparison of survival among those who underwent actual bypass or resection versus those who had "open and close" procedures is possible (Table 4). Median survival among patients who were not considered surgical candidates, and therefore were managed by hydration and tube decompression alone, is reported as 2 to 3 months (4,8,25,30). Thus, there

TABLE 4. *Survival after palliative surgery for intestinal obstruction*

Author (ref.)	Number of patients	Median survival[a]	Exploration only[b]
Castaldo (5)	23	17% at 1 yr; 80% at 2 mo	—
Tunca (4)	90	7.0 mo	2.0 mo
Piver (23)	60	2.5 mo	2.0 mo
Krebs (24)	98	4.2 mo	<1.0 mo
Clarke-Pearson (7)	49	4.6 mo	—
Larson (8)	19	3.4 mo	3.0 mo
Rubin (22)	52	6.8 mo	1.8 mo
Lund (3)	25	2.3 mo	1.0 mo

[a] Survival in patients undergoing surgical correction of obstruction.
[b] Survival in patients undergoing exploration only.

TABLE 6. *Mortality of palliative surgery for intestinal obstruction*

Author (ref.)	Number of procedures	Operative Mortality[a]	
		Number of deaths	Rate
Castaldo (5)	25	3	12%
Tunca (4)	90	13	14%
Piver (23)	60	10	17%
Krebs (24)	118	26	22%
Clarke-Pearson (7)	49	7	14%
Larson (8)	19	3	16%
Lund (3)	25	8	32%
Rubin (22)	54	9	17%
Total	440	79	18%

[a] Defined as deaths <30 days after surgery. All except Piver (23) and Rubin (22) include patients who died from progressive tumor unrelated to surgical procedure.

is little evidence in the literature that surgery alone increases length of survival in these patients with bowel obstruction.

Perhaps more important to the patient with bowel obstruction is whether palliative surgery improves the quality of remaining life by restoring gastrointestinal function. In most studies the success of surgery is measured by length of survival, but in one report the specifics of restoring GI function are addressed. Rubin et al. (22) report that 79% of 43 patients with ovarian cancer undergoing a definitive procedure to correct intestinal obstruction left the hospital tolerating a regular or low-residue diet.

Complications of Palliative Surgery for Bowel Obstruction

By whatever means the effectiveness of palliative surgery for bowel obstruction is measured, it is achieved at considerable cost to the patient in terms of complications. The morbidity and mortality associated with surgery for bowel obstruction in patients with progressive ovarian cancer is substantial. Combined data from several studies show an overall major complication rate of 32% and operative mortality of 18% (Tables 5 and 6). Common complications include fistulas and anastomotic leaks, 12% and 4%, respectively, as well as infections. The operative mortality data are difficult to interpret, because many studies do not separate patients who died of progressive tumor within 30 days of surgery from those who died as a result of surgery. The incidence of recurrent obstruction, reported in only a few studies, ranges from 17% to 26% (4,5,7,24).

Selecting Patients for Surgical Palliation

With the significant risks of attempted surgical correction of bowel obstruction, criteria that predict successful outcome would aid the surgeon in preoperative selection of candidates for surgical palliation. Several authors have attempted to identify factors prognostic for successful outcome in patients with advanced ovarian cancer who undergo palliative surgery for intestinal obstruction. Krebs and Goplerud (24) found age, nutritional status, tumor burden, ascites, and prior radiation therapy correlated with prognosis as measured by "im-

TABLE 5. *Morbidity of palliative surgery for intestinal obstruction*

Author (ref.)	Number of procedures	Number of fistulas	Number of anastomotic leaks	Total complications[a]	Rate of complications[a]
Castaldo (5)	25	3	2	10	40%
Piver (23)	60	4	2	19	32%
Clarke-Pearson (7)	49	9	3	24	49%
Rubin (22)	54	6	0	9	15%
Total	188	22	7	61	32%

[a] Includes pneumonia, wound infection, urinary tract infection, sepsis, pulmonary embolus, and myocardial infarction.

proved health and survival for 8 weeks." By assigning a risk score of 0 to 2 to each factor, they describe a system that may be used to select which patients are likely to benefit from surgery. Other authors confirm the validity of this scoring system (8). Clarke-Pearson et al. (31), using logistic regression analysis, identified preoperative tumor burden and serum albumin level as variables significantly associated with postoperative survival. Rubin et al. (22) found no correlation between survival or operability and age, prior radiotherapy, or number of previous surgeries. Piver et al. (23) found that survival was predicted by response to chemotherapy that followed the surgical procedure. Because no reliable, objective method exists for predicting which patients will benefit, deciding who should undergo palliative surgery for obstruction must be based on the patient's performance status, medical contraindications to general anesthesia, the availability and feasibility of postoperative chemotherapy, and the wishes of the patient and her family.

Percutaneous Endoscopic Gastrostomy

The management of patients who are not candidates for exploration or whose obstructions are not corrected by surgery has been made easier by the availability of percutaneous endoscopic gastrostomy (PEG). Before the development of this technique, gastrostomy was performed at the time of laparotomy for obstruction or as a separate procedure to allow prolonged decompression of the GI tract, thus avoiding complications of prolonged use of a nasogastric tube, such as nasal or gastric erosion and bleeding (32,33). Modification of the technique utilizing endoscopy allows percutaneous placement of gastrostomy or jejunostomy with intravenous sedation in an ambulatory surgical setting (34–37). Stellato and Gauderer reported successful placement of a PEG in two patients with advanced ovarian cancer (38). Malone et al. (39) describe the M. D. Anderson experience in 10 patients with bowel obstruction from advanced ovarian cancer, all of whom had successful PEG placement and survived an average of 5 weeks post procedure with minimal morbidity and no operative mortality. The largest series to date is that of Herman et al. (34) from Memorial Sloan-Kettering Cancer Center; Herman's group successfully placed PEGs in 23 of 26 patients with intestinal obstruction secondary to progressive ovarian cancer who had either failed nonoperative management or could not be palliated at laparotomy. Eighty-one percent of these patients had tumor on the anterior abdominal well, and 58% had moderate to severe ascites, factors that had previously been considered relative contraindications to PEG placement. Complications in this series were few and were limited to tube blockage and leaking around the tube site. No procedure-related deaths occurred, and 88% of the patients (none of whom tolerated enteral intake before the procedure) were able to ingest full liquids or soft foods because of the use of large-caliber tubes for drainage, thus improving their quality of life.

Clearly, the use of the PEG technique can successfully palliate intestinal obstruction and improve quality of life without the morbidity and mortality of laparotomy. PEG should be the procedure of choice in ovarian cancer patients who fail a trial of intestinal intubation but are not considered surgical candidates, or for those in whom surgery is unsuccessful.

The Role of Total Parenteral Nutrition

Defining the role of total parenteral nutrition (TPN) in the palliation of intestinal obstruction is a problem commonly encountered in the care of patients with advanced ovarian cancer. The benefit of TPN in cancer patients receiving chemotherapy in terms of response to treatment or survival is controversial (40–42), and trials of TPN in surgical cancer patients yield conflicting results (43). A reduction in postoperative morbidity was demonstrated in a randomized trial of patients with upper GI tract cancers (44), and decreased operative morbidity and mortality was shown by a metaanalysis of 18 surgical trials (45). Data regarding the impact of TPN in the management of patients with gynecologic cancer, and specifically with intestinal obstruction owing to ovarian cancer, are scarce. Krebs and Goplerud (24) found 25% mortality at 8 weeks postoperatively in patients receiving perioperative TPN, and 44% mortality in those not receiving TPN. Rubin et al. (22) found no correlation between use of TPN and ability to correct obstruction surgically. It is clear that a large percentage of ovarian cancer patients with intestinal obstruction are malnourished. In a prospective study of patients admitted to the gynecology service at Memorial Sloan-Kettering Center, Sclafani and Brennan (43) found that 29% of the ovarian cancer patients met criteria for severe malnutrition and suffered greater surgical morbidity than those with mild or no malnutrition.

The use of home TPN in the management of patients with inoperable bowel obstruction from advanced malignancies is advocated by some authors (46–49). August et al. (46) describe nine patients with ovarian cancer and bowel obstruction who were managed with home TPN as part of a larger group of patients. Forty-four percent of the patients lived >40 days, but in 44% of cases, the staff evaluating the patients felt no benefit was derived from TPN in regards to improving quality of life. Chapman et al. (47) describe a single ovarian cancer patient with bowel obstruction managed with home TPN, PEG, and epidural morphine for pain. Although these authors reported that her quality of life was greatly improved, she developed rectovaginal and vesicovaginal fistulas two months into her nine months of survival and required multiple hospitalizations for treatment of urosepsis. Acknowledged by most of these authors are the negative aspects of home TPN: infections, thrombotic complications, and expense. Some suggest strict criteria regarding life expectancy and performance status be used in selecting patients appropriate for such therapy (48). An alternative to home TPN consisting of management with PEG, intravenous fluids, and administration of systemic narcotics for pain has been shown to be effective and well tolerated by patients, families, and physicians (50,51). Because of the incidence of complications, significant expense, and the theoretical danger of TPN accelerating tumor growth (shown in animal models) (52), TPN should be used only in patients with intestinal obstruction who are concurrently receiving and have the possibility of responding to chemotherapy. Although withdrawing TPN may be difficult for all involved, patients and their families must understand that such therapy is inappropriate for the preceding reasons in those who are no longer responding to therapy.

INTESTINAL FISTULA

Clinical Presentation/Incidence/Etiology

Although the majority of intestinal fistulas encountered by the gynecologic oncologist are the result of late effects of radiation therapy in patients with cervical or corpus cancer (53,54), fistulas are seen in patients with ovarian cancer. They are second to obstruction as the most common indication for palliative intestinal surgery in these patients (55, Table 2). Common causes of intestinal fistulas in ovarian cancer patients are recurrent or progressive tumor and prior operations for cytoreduction or intestinal obstruction complicated by inadvertent enterotomy or anastomotic breakdown (56). According to the data in Table 5, 12% of palliative procedures for intestinal obstruction are subsequently complicated by fistulas. Radiation therapy alone almost never results in an intestinal fistula in patients with ovarian cancer. However, the vascular damage and adhesions caused by radiation therapy certainly increase the risk of fistulas after subsequent operations. In Piver and Lele's series (56), 25% of 43 enteric fistulas seen over an 18-year period occurred in patients with ovarian cancer, and none were radiation induced. Rubin et al. (55) reported that in 36 major operations performed for intestinal fistula or perforation over a 3-year period, 17% were in patients with ovarian cancer, only one of whom had received radiation therapy. Enterocutaneous fistula is the most common type seen in patients with ovarian cancer, but rectovaginal, enterovaginal, and vesicovaginal fistulas are also encountered, especially in patients with bulky pelvic recurrence after prior bowel surgery or radiation therapy. The most common presenting symptom of intestinal fistula is drainage of bowel contents through skin, vagina, or bladder. Development of enterocutaneous fistulas in postoperative patients or those with tumor perforation of intestine may be heralded by appearance of an area of erythema and induration on the skin of the abdomen.

Diagnosis/Management

The initial steps in management of intestinal fistulas in patients with ovarian cancer are similar to those of intestinal obstruction: intravenous hydration to replace fluids and electrolytes, antibiotics in cases of abscess or sepsis, complete bowel rest by prohibiting oral intake, and the use of nasogastric or long tube decompression (9,20,53). Critical to managing intestinal fistulas is protection of the skin surrounding the fistula site from the ulcerative effects of bowel contents by using stoma adhesive, a collecting bag, and sump drainage of fistulas when needed (9,20,56). TPN should be used in most ovarian cancer patients with intestinal fistulas in an effort to increase the chances of spontaneous closure (9,20,54). For fistulas caused by progressive, inoperable abdominal tumor or for those occurring postoperatively in a patient failing surgical palliation of obstruction owing to progressive tumor, TPN is usually not appropriate. Without the hope of a response to chemotherapy, TPN provides nutrition to the tumor and thus may serve only to prolong the patient's suffering. As in intestinal obstruction, a trial of nonoperative therapy is warranted because some fistulas will close spontaneously, but this is unlikely if the cause is progressive tumor or if distal obstruction is present (9,20,53,55,56). Attempted surgical correction of intestinal fistula has significant morbidity and limited success, and thus it is inappropriate for some patients with progressive tumor. The decision to operate must be made by the surgeon, patient, and family and must take into account the likelihood of success, performance status, and life expectancy.

If surgical correction is to be attempted, preoperative localization of the fistula site and detection of multiple fistulas are critical. Piver and Lele (56) found that a fistulogram—injection of a water soluble contrast medium such as Gastrografin through the fistula tract—was most often successful as a single test for preoperative diagnosis. Gastrografin enema is also indicated to exclude an associated colonic fistula (9).

For small bowel fistulas, important features of intraoperative management are using meticulous dissection to avoid enterotomies and completely isolating the involved loop of bowel from the intestinal stream. If the loop cannot be resected, the proximal end should be brought as a mucous fistula and the distal end closed (9,53–55). Piver and Lele (56) observed 28% operative mortality in patients who did not have isolation of the involved bowel loop versus none in those in whom isolation was achieved. Overall, they reported a 38% major complication rate and 17% operative mortality for enteric fistulas. In patients with colonic fistulas, a diverting colostomy, the procedure of choice, can often be accomplished with minimal operative time and morbidity. Data regarding the efficacy and recurrence risk of palliative surgery for intestinal fistula is sparse, but in Rubin's series (55), 2 of 36 patients (including nonovarian cancer patients) had recurrent fistula as a postoperative complication. For patients who fail surgical correction or are not candidates for laparotomy, PEG drainage and IV fluids are probably the best palliative option for high-output fistulas. In low-output fistulas, a collection device and meticulous skin care may be the only therapy needed.

MALIGNANT EFFUSIONS

In patients with ovarian cancer, the accumulation of clinically significant effusions can present diagnostic and therapeutic problems in three body cavities: the abdominal cavity, pleural space, and the pericardial sac.

Ascites

Ascites is frequently seen in patients with advanced ovarian cancer at time of initial diagnosis, but it usually disappears after one or two cycles of chemotherapy (57). In only a small number of patients is ascites refractory to chemotherapy or recurrent in amounts large enough in latter stages of the illness to cause symptoms such as abdominal pain or respiratory distress requiring intervention.

Paracentesis is the technique most commonly used to palliate symptoms of ascites. Studies reveal a distinct pathophysiology of ascites formation in patients with ovarian cancer as compared to patients with hepatic cirrhosis or portal hypertension (58–61). But, as in the latter group of patients, when performing paracentesis in patients with ovarian cancer, adequate volume replacement must be provided in order to maintain hemodynamic stability when large amounts of fluid are removed during one procedure (25). In patients who have had multiple prior laparotomies or previous intraperitoneal chemotherapy, ascites may be loculated, and ultrasonography or CT scan can aid in localizing the appropriate site for paracentesis (62). If paracentesis is not effective, few options are available. Intraperitoneal bleomycin has been reported to control ascites in patients with ovarian cancer, but experience is limited to a small number of patients (63,64). Peritoneovenous shunts have been used in ovarian cancer patients with refractory ascites with limited success and high complication rates (65–68). Souter et al. (66) described 11 patients with ovarian carcinoma who had recurrent ascites despite systemic and intracavitary chemotherapy and were treated with a peritoneovenous shunt procedure. Each patient achieved temporary relief of symptomatic ascites, but blockage of the shunt complicated 50% of the cases, and autopsies of 11 of 12 patients exhibited thrombotic or embolic complications related to the shunt. Edney et al. (67) placed shunts in eight patients with ovarian cancer who survived an average of 71 weeks, with 75% having relief of symptoms. However, most of these patients probably received cytotoxic chemotherapy after the procedure, so how much successful palliation can be attributed to the shunt is questionable.

Pleural Effusions

Recurrent pleural effusions often cause debilitating symptoms that require palliative therapy in patients with advanced ovarian cancer. Studies of the extraabdominal spread of ovarian cancer reveal that 25–33% of ovarian cancer patients develop pleural effusions, most as a manifestation of recurrent or refractory disease rather than as part of initial diagnosis (69,70). In a review of cytology from malignant pleural effusions in 472 patients, ovarian cancer was the second most common cause of effusion in women after breast cancer (71). The pathophysiology of pleural effusions in ovarian cancer is unclear, but up to 25% in one series were cytologically negative for malignancy (70). Patients requiring palliative intervention for pleural effusion commonly present with symptoms of dyspnea, pleuritic chest pain, or cough. Diagnosis is easily confirmed by chest radiograph, which should include decubitus views to distinguish loculated from free-flowing fluid. If the fluid does not layer on x-ray, ultrasonography or CT scan are indicated to localize the largest pocket of fluid.

The first step in management of pleural effusions in ovarian cancer patients is thoracentesis. Thoracentesis is a technically simple procedure that provides rapid relief of symptoms and is rarely associated with morbidity, which can include pneumothorax and reexpansion pulmonary edema if too much fluid is removed rapidly (72,73). Although it is highly effective, the symptomatic relief provided by thoracentesis is often temporary. Anderson et al. found 97% of malignant effusions reaccumulated at a mean of 4.2 days after thoracentesis (74). With repeated taps, the risk of complications as well as the risk of loculation increase, limiting the therapeutic usefulness to those requiring urgent but temporary relief of symptoms.

Two methods of treatment have been shown to prevent recurrence of symptomatic pleural effusions in patients with ovarian cancer. Fourteen of 20 patients receiving cisplatin-based chemotherapy had radiographic resolution of their effusions for at least six months in one report (75). In the majority of patients, however, symptomatic pleural effusion signals progression or recurrence of tumor previously treated with cytotoxic chemotherapy, and for these individuals successful palliation is best achieved by thoracostomy tube drainage and sclerosis. Drainage of the effusion by placement of a thoracostomy tube alone can produce 36–55% complete responses (71,76). Several studies have demonstrated improved responses by instilling sclerosing agents into the pleural space after drainage (72,76–79). A variety of agents have been utilized, including bleomycin, tetracycline, and talc. All of these agents produce fibrosis and obliteration of the pleural space, thus preventing reaccumulation of fluid (72). Ten to 15% of patients may experience side effects from chest tube sclerosis, which commonly include low-grade fever and mild to moderate pleuritic chest pain, depending on the agent used (63,64,73–77,79). Bleomycin can be administered without chest tube drainage and is reportedly less painful, but its cost limits its usefulness (63), leaving talc and tetracycline as the most frequently utilized agents in practice. Complete response rates with this technique of pleurodesis are reported between 65% and 100% (72), but most studies include only a few patients with effusions from ovarian cancer. Jones et al. (75) report 52% complete responses in patients with ovarian cancer undergoing tetracycline sclerosis at the start of cytotoxic chemotherapy and 41% in those developing effusions after completing primary chemotherapy. Contraindications to this technique are presence of empyema, entrapped lung, or bleeding diathesis (72).

For patients whose pleural effusions are refractory to chest tube sclerosis or patients who are not candidates for this technique, other management options include pleurectomy and thoracoscopic pleurodesis. In a series of 106 patients, only 1 of whom had ovarian cancer, control of effusion was obtained by pleurectomy in all patients; 27% operative mortality in patients with extrathoracic primary cancers other than breast, however, makes the palliative benefit in this group questionable (80). Thoracoscopy with lysis of any loculations, complete drainage of fluid, and administration of sclerosing agent may be an alternative with significantly less morbidity (81).

Pericardial Effusions

Pericardial effusion is an uncommon complication of advanced ovarian cancer reported as occurring in only 2.4% of patients in a large series describing sites of distant metastases (69). In 50% of these patients the diagnosis was made at autopsy, so the true incidence may be underestimated by this study. For the symptomatic patient with pericardial effusion, diagnosis is usually suggested by chest x-ray and confirmed by cardiac echo. In the nonemergent setting, treatment options include drainage of the pericardial sac via ultrasound-guided needle placement or creation of a pericardial window. In suitable patients, radiation therapy or chemotherapy may be subsequently given in an attempt to prevent recurrence. For patients exhibiting cardiovascular collapse from tamponade, bedside pericardiocentesis is the only option, although it is usually ineffective (69).

URETERAL OBSTRUCTION

Although recurrent ovarian cancer tends to spread intraperitoneally, obstruction of the ureters, which are completely retroperitoneal, does occur with surprising frequency in patients with progressive disease. Lewis et al. (25) found at least 16% of patients admitted with advanced ovarian cancer had ureteral obstruction. In an autopsy study of 117 patients, ureteral obstruction was found in 28% of cases, making it the second most common manifestation of tumor-related morbidity after intestinal obstruction (82). In a review of multiple studies of malignant ureteral obstruction, ovarian cancer was the fourth most common primary tumor site producing clinically significant blockage, comprising 8% of over 500 cases (83). An ovarian cancer patient with ureteral obstruction may exhibit oliguria or anuria, dehydration, azotemia, and marked electrolyte imbalances. Diagnostic evaluation in such a patient should include renal ultrasound, CT scan, or both. Marked thinning of the renal cortex noted in these studies indicates long duration of obstruction and significant parenchymal damage, making palliative intervention a less attractive option.

Just as the development of the PEG technique has changed management of patients with inoperable bowel obstruction, the advances in endoscopic urologic technology and interventional radiology have altered the management of patients with malignant ureteral obstruction. Percutaneous nephrostomy (PCN) and endoscopic retrograde ureteral stent placement are the procedures of choice for patients with this complication of advanced ovarian cancer. Use of PCN for palliation of malignant ureteral obstruction is well described in the urologic literature, with success rates approaching 80–90%. Complications consist primarily of dislodgement and urinary infection and range from 20% to 40% (83–85). Multiple studies in the gynecologic literature confirm these results and include several patients with obstruction secondary to advanced ovarian cancer (86–93). Pellman et al. (87) and Zadra et al. (83) report a 60% success rate for endoscopic retrograde stent placement in ovarian cancer patients, and Zadra comments that the retrograde technique was easiest in the ovarian cancer patients compared with others in that series (83,87).

The relative ease and safety of these techniques for relieving malignant ureteral obstruction have made them attractive options, but most authors caution against liberal use of palliative urinary diversion in patients with recurrent malignancy. Soper and colleagues (90) note that although life may be significantly prolonged by PCN, the quality of life was uniformly poor in patients with recurrent cancer. Carter et al. (91) acknowledge that the use of these techniques as palliation is controversial: One may be avoiding a peaceful death due to uremia and substituting a painful death due to progressive tumor. Feuer et al. (93) used the presence of any one of five poor prognostic criteria, including lack of any further effective antitumor therapy, to screen patients for appropriateness of PCN placement and found that patients with adverse prognostic criteria derived little survival or "quality of life" benefit from the procedure (93). Most authors agree that palliative urinary diversion with PCN or retrograde stents should be reserved for patients with recurrent malignancy for whom further antineoplastic therapy is available.

REFERENCES

1. Gove PB, ed. *Webster's third new international dictionary of the English languge, unabridged.* Springfield, MA: Miriam Webster, 1986;1625.
2. Boring CC, Squires TS. Cancer statistics. 1991. *Cancer J Clin* 1991;41:19–35.
3. Lund B, Hansen M, Lundvall F, Nielsen NC, Sorensen BI, Hansen HH. Intestinal obstruction in patients with advanced carcinoma of the ovaries treated with combination chemotherapy. *Surg Gynecol Obstet* 1989;169:213–218.
4. Tunca JC, Buchler DA, Mack EA, Ruzicka FF, Crowley JJ, Carr WF. The management of ovarian cancer caused bowel obstruction. *Gynecol Oncol* 1981;12:186–192.
5. Castaldo TW, Petrilli ES, Ballon SC, Lagasse LD. Intestinal operations in patients with ovarian carcinoma. *Am J Obstet Gynecol* 1981;139:80–84.
6. Krebs HB, Helmkamp F. Management of intestinal obstruction in ovarian cancer. *Oncology* 1989;3:25–36.
7. Clarke-Pearson DL, Chin N, DeLong ER, Rice R, Creasman WT. Surgical management of intestinal obstruction in ovarian cancer. *Gynecol Oncol* 1987;26:11–18.
8. Larson JE, Podczaski ES, Manetta A, Whitney CW, Mortel R. Bowel obstruction in patients with ovarian carcinoma: analysis of prognostic factors. *Gynecol Oncol* 1989;35:61–65.
9. Hacker NF, Berek JS, Lagasse LD. Gastrointestinal operations in gynecologic oncology. In: Knapp RC, Berkowitz RS, eds. *Gynecologic oncology*, New York: Macmillan, 1986;471–491.
10. Katz LB, Frankel A, Cohen C, Slater G. Ovarian carcinoma complicated by gastric outlet obstruction. *J Surg Oncol* 1981;18:261–264.
11. Mann WJ, Calayag PT, Muffoletto JP, Ross F, Chalas E, Deitch J. Management of gastric outlet obstruction caused by ovarian cancer. *Gynecol Oncol* 1991;40:277–279.
12. Krebs HB, Walsh J, Goplerud DR. Gastric outlet obstruction caused by ascitic fluid entrapment in the lesser sac, a complication of advanced ovarian cancer: report of two cases. *Gynecol Oncol* 1982;14:105–111.
13. Ketcham AS, Hoye RC, Pilch YH, Morton DL. Delayed intestinal obstruction following treatment for cancer. *Cancer* 1970;25:406–410.
14. Osteen RT, Guyton S, Stelle G, Wilson RE. Malignant intestinal obstruction. *Surgery* 1980;87:611–615.
15. Brolin RE. Partial small bowel obstruction. *Surgery* 1984;95:145–149.
16. Bizer LS, Liebling RW, Delany HM, Gliedman ML. Small bowel obstruction. *Surgery* 1981;89:407–413.
17. Krebs HB, Goplerud DR. The role of intestine intubation in obstruction of the small intestine due to carcinoma of the ovary. *Surg Gynecol Obstet* 1984;158:467–471.
18. Krebs HB, Goplerud DR. Mechanical intestinal obstruction in patients with gynecologic disease: a review of 368 patients. *Am J Obstet Gynecol* 1987;157:577–583.
19. Helmkamp BF, Kimmel J. Conservative management of small bowel obstruction. *Am J Obstet Gynecol* 1985;152:677–679.
20. Carey L, Fabri P. The intestinal tract in relation to gynecology. In: Thompson JD, Rock JA, eds. *Te Lindes operative gynecology*. Philadelphia: JB Lippincott, 1992;1017–1047.
21. Berek JS. General surgical operations. In: Berek JS, Hacker N, eds. *Practical gynecologic oncology*. Baltimore: Williams and Wilkins, 1989;521–523.
22. Rubin SC, Hoskins WJ, Benjamin I, Lewis JL Jr. Palliative surgery for intestinal obstruction in advanced ovarian cancer. *Gynecol Oncol* 1989;34:16–19.
23. Piver MS, Barlow JJ, Lele SB, Frank A. Survival after ovarian cancer induced intestinal obstruction. *Gynecol Oncol* 1982;13:44–49.
24. Krebs HB, Goplerud DR. Surgical management of bowel obstruction in advanced ovarian carcinoma. *Gynecol Oncol* 1983;61:327–330.
25. Lewis JL Jr. Palliative therapy of advanced ovarian cancer. *Clin Obstet Gynecol* 1969;12:1038–1049.
26. Donato D, Angelides A, Irani H, Penalver M, Averette H. Infectious complications after gastrointestinal surgery in patients with ovarian cancer and malignant ascites. *Gynecol Oncol* 1992;44:40–47.
27. Penalver M, Averette H, Sevin B, Lichtinger M, Girtanner R. Gastrointestinal surgery in gynecologic oncology: evaluation of surgical techniques. *Gynecol Oncol* 1987;28:74–82.
28. Chalas E, Mann WJ, Westermann CP, Patsner B. Morbidity and mortality of stapled anastomoses on a gynecologic oncology service: a retrospective review. *Gynecol Oncol* 1990;37:82–86.
29. Wheeless CR Jr, Smith JJ. A comparison of the flow of iodine 125 through three different intestinal anastomoses: standard, Gambee, and stapler. *Obstet Oncol Gynecol* 1983;5:25–36.
30. Fernandes JR, Seymour RJ, Suissa S. Bowel obstruction in patients with ovarian cancer: a research for prognostic factors. *Am J Obstet Gynecol* 1988;158:244–249.
31. Clarke-Pearson DL, DeLong ER, Chin N, Rice R, Creasman WT. Intestinal obstruction in patients with ovarian cancer variables associated with surgical complications and survival. *Arch Surg* 1988;123:42–45.
32. Greene JF, Sawicki MC, Doyle WF. Gastric ulceration: a complication of double lumen nasogastric tubes. *JAMA* 1973;224:338–339.
33. Ghahremani GG, Turner MA, Port RB. Iatrogenic injuries of the upper gastrointestinal tract in adults. *Gastrointest Radiol* 1980;5:1–10.
34. Herman LL, Hoskins WJ, Shike M. Percutaneous endoscopic

gastrostomy for decompression of the stomach and small bowel. *Gynecol Oncol* [in press].
35. Gauderer MW, Ponsky JL. A simplified technique for constructing a tube feeding gastrostomy. *Surg Gynecol Obstet* 1981;152:83–85.
36. Sangster W, Cuddington GD, Bachulis BL. Percutaneous endoscopic gastrostomy. *Am J Surg* 1988;155:677–679.
37. Grant JP. Comparison of percutaneous endoscopic gastrostomy with Stamm gastrostomy. *Ann Surg* 1988;207:598–602.
38. Stellato TA, Gauderer MW. Percutaneous endoscopic gastrostomy for gastrointestinal decompression. *Ann Surg* 1987;205:119–122.
39. Malone JM, Koonce T, Larson DM, Freedman RS, Carrasco CH, Saul PB. Palliation of small bowel obstruction by percutaneous gastrostomy in patients with progressive ovarian carcinoma. *Obstet Oncol Gynecol* 1986;68:431–433.
40. Klein S, Simes J, Blackburn GL. Total parenteral nutrition and cancer clinical trials. *Cancer* 1986;58:1378–1386.
41. Brennan MF. Total parenteral nutrition in the cancer patient. *N Engl J Med* 1981;305:375–381.
42. Burt ME, Gorschboth CM, Brennan MF. A controlled, prospective randomized trial evaluating the metabolic effects of enteral and parenteral nutrition in the cancer patient. *Cancer* 1982;49:1092–1105.
43. Sclafani LM, Brennan MF. Nutritional support of the gynecologic oncology patient. In: Hoskins WJ, Perez CA, Young RC, eds. *Principles and practice of gynecologic oncology*. Philadelphia: JB Lippincott, 1992;417–429.
44. Muller JM, Brenner V, Dienst C, et al. Preoperative parenteral feeding in patients with gastrointestinal carcinoma. *Lancet* 1982;1:79.
45. Detsky AS, Baker JP, O'Rourke K, et al. Perioperative parenteral nutrition: a meta-analysis. *Ann Intern Med* 1987;107:195.
46. August DA, Thorn D, Fisher RL, Welchek CM. Home parenteral nutrition for patients with inoperable malignant bowel obstruction. *JPEN J Parenter Enteral Nutr* 1991;15:323–327.
47. Chapman C, Bosscher J, Remmenga S, Park R, Barnhill D. A technique for managing terminally ill ovarian carcinoma patients. *Gynecol Oncol* 1991;41:88–91.
48. Weiss SM, Worthington PH, Prioleau MA, Rosato F. Home total parenteral nutrition in cancer patients. *Cancer* 1982;50:1210–1213.
49. Moley JF, August D, Norton JA, Sugarbaker PH. Home parenteral nutrition for patients with advanced intraperitoneal cancers and gastrointestinal dysfunction. *J Surg Oncol* 1986;33:186–189.
50. Gemlo B, Rayner AA, Lewis B, et al. Home support of patients with end-stage malignant bowel obstruction using hydration and venting gastrostomy. *Am J Surg* 1986;152:100–104.
51. Baines M, Oliver DJ, Carter RL. Medical management of intestinal obstruction in patients with advanced malignant disease. *Lancet* 1985;990–993.
52. Popp MB, Wagner SC, Brito OJ. Host and tumor responses to increasing levels of intravenous nutritional support. *Surgery* 1983;94:300–307.
53. Smith DH, Pierce VK, Lewis JL Jr. Enteric fistulas encountered on a gynecologic oncology service from 1969 through 1980. *Surg Gynecol Obstet* 1984;158:71.
54. Rubin SC, Markman M, Nori D. Management of late effects of treatment. In: Hoskins WJ, Perez CJ, Young RC, eds. *Principles and practice of gynecologic oncology*. Philadelphia: JB Lippincott, 1992;417–429.
55. Rubin SC, Benjamin I, Hoskins WJ, Pierce VK, Lewis JL Jr. Intestinal surgery in gynecologic oncology. *Gynecol Oncol* 1989;34:30–33.
56. Piver MS, Lele S. Enterovaginal and enterocutaneous fistulae in women with gynecologic malignancies. *Gynecol Oncol* 1976;48:560–563.
57. Ozols RF, Rubin SC, Dembo AJ, Robboy S. Epithelial ovarian cancer. In: Hoskins WJ, Perez CA, Young RC, eds. *Principles and practice of gynecologic oncology*. Philadelphia: JB Lippincott, 1992;731–781.
58. Cruikshank DP, Buchsbaum HJ. Effects of rapid paracentesis. Cardiovascular dynamics and body fluid composition. *JAMA* 1973;225:1361–1382.
59. Halpin TF, McCann TO. Dynamics of body fluids following the rapid removal of large volumes of ascites. *Am J Obstet Gynecol* 1971;110:103–106.
60. Hirabayashi K, Graham J. Genesis of ascites in ovarian cancer. *Am J Obstet Gynecol* 1970;106:492–497.
61. Lifshitz S, Buchsbaum HJ. The effect of paracentesis on serum proteins. *Gynecol Oncol* 1976;4:347–353.
62. Ross GJ, Kessler HB, Clain MR, Galenby RA, Hartz WH, Ross LV. Sonographically guided paracentesis for palliation of symptomatic malignant ascites. *Am J Roentgenol* 1989;153:1309–1311.
63. Paladine W, Cunningham TJ, Sponzo R, Donavan M, Olson K, Horton J. Intracavitary bleomycin in the managment of malignant effusions. *Cancer* 1976;38:1903–1908.
64. Ostrowski MJ. An assessment of the long-term results of controlling the reaccumulation of malignant effusions using intracavitary bleomycin. *Cancer* 1986;57:721–727.
65. Cheung DK, Raaf JH. Selection of patients with malignant ascites for a peritoneovenous shunt. *Cancer* 1982;50:1204–1209.
66. Souter RG, Wells C, Tarin D, Kettlewell MG. Surgical and pathologic complications associated with peritoneovenous shunts in management of malignant ascites. *Cancer* 1985;55:1973–1975.
67. Edney JA, Hill A, Armstrong D. Peritoneovenous shunts palliate malignant ascites. *Am J Surg* 1989;158:598–601.
68. Lacy JH, Wieman TJ, Shively EH. Management of malignant ascites. *Surg Gynecol Obstet* 1984;159:397–412.
69. Dauplat J, Hacker NF, Berek JS, Rose TP, Sagae S. Distant metastases in epithelial ovarian carcinoma. *Cancer* 1987;60:1561–1566.
70. Kerr VE, Cadman E. Pulmonary metastases in ovarian cancer. *Cancer* 1985;56:1209–1213.
71. Johnston NW. The malignant pleural effusion: a review of the cytopathologic diagnosis of 584 specimens from 472 consecutive patients. *Cancer* 1985;56:905–910.
72. Austin EH, Flye MW. The treatment of recurrent malignant pleural effusion. *Ann Thorac Surg* 1979;28:190–203.
73. Olopade OI, Ultmann JE. Malignant effusions. *CA Cancer J Clin* 1991;41:166–179.
74. Anderson CB, Philpott GW, Ferguson TB. The treatment of malignant pleural effusions. *Cancer* 1979;33:918–922.
75. Jones CM, Rubin SC, Berchuck A, Lewis JL Jr. Management of pleural effusions in patients with epithelial ovarian cancer. *Gynecol Oncol* 1989;32:108–109 (abst).
76. O'Neill W, Spurr C, Muss H, Richards R, White D, Coper MR. A prospective study of chest tube drainage and tetracycline sclerosis versus chest tube drainage in treatment of malignant pleural effusion. *Proc ASCO* 1980;21:349.
77. Sherman S, Grady KJ, Seidman JC. Clinical experience with tetracycline pleurodesis of malignant pleural effusions. *South Med J* 1987;80:716–719.
78. Johnson LP, Rivkin SE, Weber EL. Palliation in malignant pleural effusion. *Am Surg* 1975;41:529–534.
79. Zaloznik AJ, Oswald SG, Langin M. Intrapleural tetracycline in malignant pleural effusions. *Cancer* 1983;51:752–755.
80. Martini N, Bains MS, Beattie EJ. Indications for pleurectomy in malignant effusion. *Cancer* 1975;35:734–738.
81. Boutin C, Viallat J, Cargnino F, Farisse P. Thoracoscopy in malignant pleural effusions. *Am Rev Respir Dis* 1981;124:588–592.
82. Dvoretsky PM, Richard KA, Angel C, Rabinowitz L, Beecham JB, Bonfiglio TA. Survival time, cause of death and tumor/treatment related morbidity in 100 women with ovarian cancer. *Hum Pathol* 1988;19:1273–1279.
83. Zadra JA, Jewett MA, Keresteci AG, et al. Nonoperative urinary diversion for malignant ureteral obstruction. *Cancer* 1987;60:1353–1357.
84. Culkin DJ, Wheeler JS Jr, Marsan RE, Nam SI, Canning JR. Percutaneous nephrostomy for palliation of metastatic ureteral obstruction. *Urology* 1987;30:229–231.
85. Perinetti E, Catalona WJ, Manley CB, Geise G, Fair WR. Percutaneous nephrostomy: indications, complications and clinical usefulness. *J Urol* 1978;120:156–158.

86. Mann WJ, Jander P, Orr JW, Taylor PT, Hatch KD, Shingleton HM. The use of percutaneous nephrostomy in gynecologic oncology. *Gynecol Oncol* 1980;10:343–349.
87. Pellman C, Sall S, Canalog A. The relief of ureteral obstruction by internal ureteral stent in patients with gynecologic malignancy. *Gynecol Oncol* 1977;5:152–160.
88. Coddington CC, Thomas JR, Hoskins WJ. Percutaneous nephrostomy for ureteral obstruction in patients with gynecologic malignancy. *Gynecol Oncol* 1984;18:334–348.
89. Baker VV, Dudzinski MR, Fowler WC, Currie JL, Walton LA. Percutaneous nephrostomy in gynecologic oncology. *Am J Obstet Gynecol* 1984;149:772–774.
90. Soper JT, Blaszczyk TM, Oke E, Clarke-Pearson D, Creasman WT. Percutaneous nephrostomy in gynecologic oncology patients. *Am J Obstet Gynecol* 1988;158:1126–1131.
91. Carter J, Ramirez C, et al. Percutaneous urinary diversion in gynecologic oncology. *Gynecol Oncol* 1991;40:248–252.
92. Dudley BS, Gershenson DM, Kavanagh JJ, Copeland LJ, Carrasco CH, Rutledge FN. Percutaneous nephrostomy catheter use in gynecologic malignancy: M. D. Anderson hospital experience. *Gynecol Oncol* 1986;24:273–278.
93. Feuer FA, Furchter R, Seruri E, Maiman M, Remy JC, Boyce JG. Selection for percutaneous nephrostomy in gynecologic cancer patients. *Gynecol Oncol* 1991;42:60–63.

CHAPTER 16

The Role of Radiotherapy in the Management of Epithelial Ovarian Cancer

Borys R. Mychalczak and Zvi Fuks

Although numerous reports have been published over the last two decades indicating that radiation is capable of eradicating and permanently controlling ovarian tumor masses, its role in the management of ovarian carcinoma remains a controversial subject. Long-term remissions in eight patients with advanced ovarian carcinoma using "x-ray therapy" was first reported by Eymer (1) in 1912. Further advances in the treatment of ovarian carcinoma during the orthovoltage radiotherapy era were limited owing to the poor penetration of available beams and the inability to treat deep-seated tumors without excessive skin doses. Because of this limitation, it was concluded by Rubin (2) in 1962 that any major improvement in the treatment of this disease would come from earlier detection rather than from improvement in existing radiotherapeutic techniques. However, this outlook has changed with the introduction of supervoltage radiotherapy and the feasibility of utilizing large-shaped treatment fields to deliver high doses of radiation to deep-seated tumors (3). Much of the earlier success was seen in patients with stage II disease. In a report by Fuks and Bagshaw (4), 16 stage IIB patients with documented residual disease in the pelvis after initial surgery were treated with lower abdominal radiation to doses of 5,000 to 6,000 cGy, resulting in a 46% 5-year disease-free survival rate.

Although this and similar studies have shown that high-dose radiation can permanently eradicate ovarian tumor masses, the long-term results of radiation therapy have, in general, been disappointing. For patients in early stage disease, 5-year and 10-year survival ranges from 60% to 80%, and for advanced stage patients, who comprise 75% of the patient population, 5- and 10-year survival ranges from only 7% to 20% (5–7). These frustrating results have led to a reevaluation of the role of radiotherapy in the management of ovarian carcinoma. This review discusses the results and techniques of radiotherapy used to treat patients with ovarian carcinoma, with an emphasis on the reasons behind the apparent failure of radiotherapy to cure many patients, and suggests several new strategies to help improve future results.

SELECTION OF RADIATION DOSE AND TREATMENT FIELDS

As has been shown in other disease sites, the total dose of radiation needed to control tumor deposits increases with the size of the tumor mass (8). Similar data from Schray et al. (9) suggest that in ovarian carcinoma the tumoricidal dose is also tumor size dependent. In this report, patients with early stage disease and known residual pelvic tumors were treated with external beam radiation therapy to a total of 5,000–6,000 cGy to the lower abdomen. A pelvic relapse rate of 45% (9 of 20 patients) was seen in patients with tumor residual larger than 2 cm, in contrast to only 8% (2 of 26) of patients with minimal residual disease less than 2 cm in size. Similarly, Dembo et al. (5,10,11) treated stage I, II, and IIIA patients with 4,500 cGy to the pelvis and 2,250 cGy to the upper abdomen. The actuarial 5-year survival was 19% in 26 patients with residua larger than 2 cm and 78% in a group of 50 patients with small (<2 cm) or no residual tumors. These data suggest that doses in excess of 5,000–6,000 cGy are probably necessary to control tumor masses larger than 2 cm, but that for smaller tumors (<2 cm) doses may be in the range of 4,500–5,000 cGy.

B. R. Mychalczak and Z. Fuks: Department of Radiation Oncology, Memorial Sloan-Kettering Cancer Center, New York, New York 10021

In general, it is thought that a dose on the order of 5,000 cGy is necessary to control microscopic deposits of tumor. However, several studies utilizing lower doses of external beam radiation therapy in epithelial ovarian carcinoma have shown that this dose may be even lower. In the studies by Dembo (5,10,11), stage I–III patients with completely resected tumors were randomized to receive either pelvic irradiation (4,500 cGy) or abdominopelvic irradiation (4,500 cGy to pelvis and 2,250 cGy to the upper abdomen by the moving strip technique). The 5-year actuarial survival in the patients receiving abdominopelvic radiation was 78%, as compared to 51% for the patients treated to the pelvis alone. This survival advantage was attributed to a 30% increase in the control of occult upper abdominal metastases in the group that received 2,250 cGy to the upper abdomen. Similarly, Delclos and Smith (12) reported a 49% 5-year disease-free survival rate in 71 stage II patients treated to the pelvis plus 2,600–2,800 cGy to the upper abdomen by the moving strip technique; they reported only a 17% rate (3 of 18) of stage II patients treated with 5,000–5,500 cGy to the pelvis only. In addition, Perez et al. (13) reported a 16% 5-year survival in six stage II patients treated with 5,000 cGy to the pelvis only, as compared with a 57% rate (four of seven patients) for patients treated to the pelvis plus 2,500–3,000 cGy to the upper abdomen by the moving strip technique. Although complete surgical staging was not routinely performed in all of these patients, these studies indicate that abdominopelvic radiotherapy is superior to pelvic radiotherapy alone, and that doses of 2,250–3,000 cGy may be sufficient to eradicate and permanently control microscopic deposits of ovarian carcinoma.

The probability of tumor sterilization depends not only on the availability of tumoricidal doses but also on the feasibility of delivering such doses to all sites of disease without significant injury to normal organs included in the treatment fields. According to Rubin et al. (14), the tolerance of critical normal organs, especially the liver and kidneys, is significantly less than the dose needed to control any gross residual disease and limits the total dose of whole abdominal irradiation that can be safely delivered. The somewhat higher tolerance of the small intestines, rectum, and bladder allows for the delivery of potentially tumoricidal doses to tumors not exceeding 2 cm in size. For this reason, only patients with either minimal or microscopic residual disease (depending on their location) are candidates for cure by a radiotherapeutic approach.

TREATMENT TECHNIQUES

Two classic techniques have traditionally been used in patients with ovarian carcinoma: the open field technique (15) and the moving strip technique (16–18). The open field technique involves irradiation through two large fixed portals (anterior and posterior) shaped to encompass the peritoneal cavity. In general, the entire abdominopelvic contents are irradiated to a total of 3,000 cGy in 20 fractions. Shielding limits the dose to the kidneys and liver to approximately 2,000 cGy to protect these organs from radiation damage. The lower abdomen is then boosted to a total of 4,500–5,500 cGy in 8 to 14 fractions. In some patients with stage I or II disease, radiation has historically been restricted to the pelvic peritoneum (1,3,4,11,12,16,19–21), and in some patients the pelvic fields have been extended to include the paraaortic region in order to encompass nodes with lymphographic evidence of disease (22–24). Although the usual fractionation scheme with the open field technique entails the delivery of one daily fraction of 150–180 cGy, two recent studies have described the use of hyperfractionated dose schedules to improve the tolerance of whole abdominal irradiation (25,26). This technique utilizes the difference in cell kinetics between normal and tumor cells and their differential repair capacity of sublethal or potentially lethal radiation damage (27). By employing low dose per fraction (80–125 cGy) given at intervals of 6 hours two or three times daily, this technique yields less damage to the late-responding normal tissues without compromising the lethal effects of the rapidly growing tumor cells (27).

A modification of the open field approach has been described by Martinez et al. (6). This group's technique is designed to cover the areas known to be at high risk for microscopic metastases and involves a design of treatment fields and dose fractionation schemes that improves the tolerance over that of whole abdominal irradiation. The treatment is initiated with the delivery of 900 cGy to the true pelvis via anterior- and posterior-opposed portals at daily fractions of 150–180 cGy, continues with 3,000 cGy whole abdominal irradiation, and is completed with 1,200 cGy to a "T-shaped" field that includes the paraaortic and medial diaphragmatic regions as well as the pelvis. Shielding of the kidneys and liver limits the dose of radiation to levels below tolerance. Reports on the use of this technique have demonstrated it to be well tolerated (6).

In another modification of the open field technique, the "delayed-split technique," the upper and lower abdomen are treated through separate portals separated by a time interval in an attempt to improve the tolerance over that of whole abdominal irradiation (28).

The design of the moving strip technique involves the division of the peritoneal cavity into equal horizontal segments (16). Treatment starts with irradiation of the lowest four segments of the pelvis. On consecutive days, the irradiated volume is moved cephalad from one segment to the adjacent segment in an orderly fashion until the entire abdomen has been treated. The total dose to each point in the peritoneal cavity is usually 3,000 cGy delivered in 10 fractions over 12 days. The kidneys and liver are usually shielded by partial-thickness lead blocks designed to permit the delivery of 50% of the dose. An additional dose of 2,000 cGy in 20 fractions over 12 days is usually delivered to the pelvis by an open field technique to increase the pelvic dose.

The nominal standard dose (NSD) method of Ellis (29) calculates the doses employed by this technique to be equivalent to those delivered by the open field technique. In a randomized trial comparing the open field technique and the moving strip technique, Dembo et al. (30) showed similar 5-year survivals. A recent report by Fyles et al. (31) demonstrated that patients treated with the moving strip technique had a significantly greater risk of developing chronic diarrhea, pneumonitis, and hepatic enzyme elevation than did patients treated with the open field technique.

ACUTE MORBIDITY AND LONG-TERM COMPLICATIONS

Acute toxicity, although dose dependent, consists usually of gastrointestinal symptoms and suppression of bone marrow activity. The incidence of diarrhea, vomiting, and weight loss during the course of treatment in a series of 167 patients receiving high radiation doses (4,500–6,000 cGy) to the lower abdomen was 78% (4). In most patients, the gastrointestinal symptoms subsided within a few weeks after the completion of treatment. However, in 29% of the patients, diarrhea with or without gastrointestinal bleeding persisted over a period of a few months after treatment. In 24 of the 167 patients (14%), severe bowel stenosis and bleeding developed that required surgical intervention. Similar rates of acute and chronic radiation-induced enteritis have been reported by other investigators using the moving strip technique (16,19,32).

Although the moving strip technique was designed to decrease the morbidity of whole abdominal irradiation observed with the open field technique, the NSD (29) doses and the time, dose, fractionation (TDF) (33) values for the two techniques show similar values for both techniques (3). Because the NSD doses and the TDF values provide an estimate of the normal tissue tolerances for fractionated radiation programs, nearly identical values imply biologically equivalent programs. Indeed, recent studies comparing the open field and moving strip techniques have shown that the rates of acute morbidity and survival in patients treated with either technique are similar (4,11,19,30,34). However, as mentioned in a report by Fyles et al. (31), patients treated with the moving strip technique had a significantly higher number of late complications.

Some reduction in the peripheral blood counts almost always occurs during the course of radiation (4). Although counts usually return to normal shortly after cessation of treatment, evidence shows that the activity of the irradiated bone marrow remains impaired to a certain degree for extended periods after radiation therapy (35). Radiation-induced hepatitis and nephritis may occur with radiation doses exceeding 2,500 cGy (12,16–18,32,36–38). More recently, however, these symptoms have not commonly been observed owing to careful application of appropriate protection to the liver and kidneys.

RESULTS OF PRIMARY TREATMENT WITH EXTERNAL BEAM RADIOTHERAPY

Although the FIGO staging classification (39) has been used to report the results of treatment in ovarian carcinoma, many recent studies have shown that the size of the tumor residuum after initial surgery is more powerful than the FIGO stage in predicting the outcome in patients treated with either chemotherapy or radiation; these studies show that prognosis is significantly improved when the diameter of the largest residual tumor mass does not exceed 2 cm (20,21,40–44). Therefore, many investigators have recently suggested use of this parameter rather than the FIGO stage as a reference for comparison of outcome data.

In patients with stage I disease, not all patients who undergo a complete tumor resection are at risk of relapse after surgery. Two prospectively randomized studies have addressed this issue. Dembo (11) reported on a group of 54 stage IA patients randomized after initial surgery between observation and pelvic irradiation. There were only nine relapses, and all of these occurred in patients with moderately poor or poorly differentiated tumors. No relapses occurred in 24 patients with well-differentiated tumors, regardless of whether postoperative treatment was given or not. A similar result was found in a study by the Gynecology Oncology Group (GOG) (45), which randomized stage IA or IB patients with well- or moderately differentiated tumors, intact capsules, no ascites, and negative peritoneal washings to either intermittent oral melphalan chemotherapy or no postoperative treatment. No difference was shown in the overall 5-year survival rate (94% for the observation and 98% for the melphalan-treated group), and the rate of relapses in both groups was similar. This finding has recently been reconfirmed in a report by Dembo et al. (46), which demonstrated in a group of 642 stage I patients that, in addition to the degree of differentiation, other tumor variables that predicted for a high probability of relapse after complete tumor removal were the presence of dense adhesions between the tumor and pelvic organs and the presence of extensive ascites. When the effects of these factors were accounted for, no other covariates were significant in predicting the outcome, including tumor bilaterality, tumor cyst rupture, capsular penetration, tumor size, histologic subtypes, patient's age, and the type of postoperative therapy. On the basis of these observations, researchers have suggested that stage IA and IB patients with well- or moderately differentiated tumors, and without positive peritoneal cytology or densely adherent tumors, require no postoperative therapy.

Postoperative treatment is generally recommended for patients with adverse tumor prognostic factors, although there are no randomized trials comparing whole abdominal irradiation to no treatment in this group of patients. In general, the best long-term results of radiotherapy have been reported in patients who successfully underwent a complete resection of all visible tumor masses at the time of initial surgery. As mentioned previously, when radiation is used as the primary modality of treatment, whole abdominal irradiation is regarded as the technique of choice. This approach is based on the patterns of failure after radiotherapy (Table 1). In the study by the GOG (47), 57% (four of seven) of the relapses occurred in the upper abdomen in a group of 23 stage IA and IB patients randomized to receive pelvic irradiation only. Schray (9) reported that of 19 relapses observed in 61 stage I and II patients treated with pelvic irradiation, only 5 were in the pelvis. The other 14 (74%) were detected in the upper abdomen. Dembo (11) showed a similar high rate of upper abdominal relapse in stage IA patients who received pelvic irradiation only (Table 1). On the other hand, treatment with whole abdominal fields reduces the rate of upper abdominal relapse. The Princess Margaret group in Toronto (5,10,11) randomized patients with stage IB, II, and III disease without tumor residual after initial surgery between pelvic and abdominopelvic radiotherapy. Of the 11 relapses observed in the 50 patients receiving abdominopelvic irradiation, none occurred in the upper abdomen. This finding contrasts the 21 out of 39 (54%) upper abdominal relapses observed in the patients randomized to receive pelvic irradiation (Table 1). As mentioned previously, the decrease in upper abdominal relapse in this study translated into an improved 5-year survival of 78% for patients receiving whole abdominal irradiation as compared to 51% of the patients receiving pelvic irradiation with or without chlorambucil. Similar findings were noted by Delclos and Smith (12) and by Fuller et al. (49), who observed a 40% 10-year survival in 64 patients treated with pelvic irradiation with or without paraaortic irradiation as compared with a 71% rate in 42 patients receiving abdominopelvic irradiation. Similar results in patients treated with whole abdominal irradiation have been reported by many other investigators (7,50–52) (Table 2).

Although it has been shown that postoperative radiotherapy can permanently eradicate small residual tumors (<2 cm) in the pelvis after initial surgery, long-term disease-free survival has been observed in less than 50% of these patients (Table 2). Dembo (5,11) reported that the 5-year survival rate for these patients was only 58% for stage II and 43% for stage III. A 54% 5-year survival in 42 stage II and III patients was noted by Martinez (6). Weiser (7) observed a 42% survival rate at 10 years in 24 patients. The prognosis of patients treated with radiotherapy for large residual tumors (>2 cm) has been extremely poor (Table 2). Fuks (53) accumulated data from 13 series in a review of the old literature and calculated a mean of 10% (range 0–15%) for published 5-year survival data in 1,020 stage III patients. Data in more recent series appears to be quite consistent. Dembo (5) reported 5- and 10-year surviv-

TABLE 1. *Correlation of sites of relapse with treatment fields in early stage ovarian carcinoma patients treated with external beam radiotherapy*

Author (ref.)	Year published	Stage	Treatment	Total relapses	Sites of relapse	
					Pelvic ± upper abdomen	Upper abdomen ± distant
Hreshchyshyn et al. (47)	1980	IA+IB	Pelvic	7/23 (30%)	3/7	4/7
Schray et al. (9)	1983	I+II	Pelvic	19/61 (31%)	5/19	14/19
Dembo (11)	1984	IA	Pelvic	5/27 (18%)	1/5	4/5
		IB+II+III0	Pelvic+CHB	39/82 (47%)	19/39	21/39
					28/70 (40%)	43/70 (61%)
Dembo (11)	1984	IB+II+III0	WAR	11/50 (22%)	11/11	0/11
Macbeth et al. (48)	1988	I+II+IIIA	WAR	25/57 (44%)	14/25	11/25
					25/36 (69%)	11/36 (30%)

WAR, whole abdominal radiotherapy.
CHB, chlorambucil.

TABLE 2. *Long-term (5–10 year) survival in ovarian carcinoma patients treated with whole abdominal irradiation: correlation of survival with the size of tumor remaining after initial surgery*

Author (ref.)	Year	Number with residual tumor: percent surviving	Number with minimal residual tumors: percent surviving	Number with large residual tumor: percent surviving
Dembo (5)	1985	46(48%)	55(43%)	71(18%)
Martinez et al. (6)	1985	30(68%)	42(54%)	54(20%)
Fuller et al. (49)	1987	20(77%)	12(62%)	10(0%)
Macbeth et al. (48)	1988	57(57%)		
Goldberg and Peschel (50)	1988	60(77%)	14(7%)	
van Bunningen et al. (51)	1988	85(75%)		
Weiser (7)	1988	37(59%)	24(42%)	23(10%)
Lindner et al. (52)	1990	63(65%)	10(40%)	
Survival (mean)		65%	41%	12%

als of 18% and 17%, respectively, for 71 patients with stage III disease and large residual tumors. A similar 20% survival at 5 years was noted in 54 patients reported by Martinez (6). Weiser (7) showed a 10% survival at 10 years in 20 patients (Table 2). Therefore, treatment of these patients with radiotherapy alone is not regarded as the treatment of choice.

RESULTS OF TREATMENT WITH INTRAPERITONEAL COLLOIDAL RADIOISOTOPES

Intraperitoneal radioactive colloids have been used in the management of malignant ascites and intraabdominal malignancies for over four decades. Radioactive gold (^{198}Au) was initially the most popular isotope (54). However, over the last 30 years, colloidal radioactive phosphorous (^{32}P) has become the agent of choice (55) for several reasons. As a pure beta emitter, ^{32}P has a higher average beta energy of 0.69 MeV as compared to 0.32 for ^{198}Au, which offers improved tumor penetration in the range of 1.5 mm to 3.0 mm. The longer half-life of 14.3 days as compared to 2.69 for ^{198}Au permits a relatively long shelf life, and the absence of gamma radiation offers improved radiation safety to the treating staff. The standard dose of ^{32}P is 10–15 mCi when given in a single intraperitoneal application. Recently, Boye et al. (56) reported that dose calculations based on the uniform distribution of ^{32}P in a capillary layer covering the intraperitoneal surface gave an estimated tissue surface dose of about 3,000 cGy per 10 mCi of ^{32}P administered. However, the exact uptake and distribution of ^{32}P in the peritoneal cavity is unknown, and significant degrees of inhomogeneity exist (57–59). The abdominal distribution results from adsorption to the mesothelial cells and absorption by the macrophages of the peritoneal surface. The radioactive colloid particles appear to become fixed to the peritoneal surface within 24 hours. Therefore, frequent changes of position for several hours after its administration appear to prevent accumulation in the gravity-dependent portion of the peritoneum (59). The distribution of ^{32}P appears to improve with its instillation in large volumes of fluid. Despite such manipulations, the highest concentrations of the colloid particles are usually found on the peritoneum of the diaphragm, liver, and omentum and on the anterior abdominal wall of the pelvic region; only a relatively low and nontherapeutic dose is delivered to the paraaortic and pelvic lymph nodes (56–59).

The use of intraperitoneal ^{32}P appears to be safe and well tolerated if the ^{32}P is administered carefully and distributed adequately within the abdomen. In a recent review, the toxicity of intraperitoneal ^{32}P was assessed in a group of 69 patients who were entered onto a Gynecologic Oncology Group protocol that randomized patients to intraperitoneal ^{32}P versus melphalan for early stage ovarian carcinoma (60). Although 11 patients had mild to moderate abdominal pain requiring minimal medication, 2 had severe pain caused by needle entry into the colon. Only six patients had severe gastrointestinal symptoms, with one suffering a small bowel perforation 20 months after ^{32}P treatment. Three required surgery for small bowel obstruction. No patients had suppression of marrow activity as manifested by a low white blood count or low platelet count. No deaths were attributable to treatment with ^{32}P.

Because the effective depth of irradiation (1.5–3.0 mm) is limited by the average energy of the emitted beta particles (0.69 MeV) of ^{32}P, most studies reporting the use of intraperitoneal ^{32}P were limited to patients with early stage disease or those with minimal or no residual disease remaining after surgery. Hilaris et al. (61) compared the results in 26 patients with stage I disease treated with postoperative intraperitoneal ^{32}P with 31 patients who did not receive the isotope. At 5 years, 92% of the patients receiving ^{32}P were alive, as compared with 64% of the surgery group. Pelvic radiation was given to 32% of the surgery patients and 35% of the ^{32}P patients. Most of the patients in this study were not completely staged. Piver et al. (62) reported on 25 stage IA to IC patients without evidence of microscopic disease at laparoscopy who received 15 mCi of colloidal ^{32}P intraperitoneally. Seventy-two percent had a complete TAH/BSO, and only 28% had an omentectomy. Twelve percent of the patients had grade III tumors, with 21% being clear cell. The 5- and 10-year disease-free and overall survival rates were 84% and 75%, respectively. Similarly, Soper (63) reported that the overall 5-year survival among 49 stage I and II patients were 84% and 86%, respectively, with disease-free survival rates of 79% and 57%, respectively. Only 29% of these patients had a complete TAH/BSO, and only 71% had an omentectomy. Nine of the 12 recurrences involved extraperitoneal sites, including 42% with a component of failure in the pelvic or paraaortic lymph nodes, indicating the need for careful staging and the inability of ^{32}P to sterilize microscopic disease in retroperitoneal nodal sites. Although retrospective reports on cure rates in patients with early stage disease completely resected utilizing ^{32}P appear to be comparable to those treated with whole abdominal irradiation, a direct comparison is impossible because of the influence of multiple prognostic factors and patient selection bias. No randomized trials have compared the use of ^{32}P against a completely staged high-risk group with no adjuvant treatment, but two recent randomized trials have tested its use against other forms of therapy in patients with early stage disease. In a recent study by the GOG (45), 141 patients with poorly differentiated stage I tumors or patients with stage II tumors were randomly allocated to treatment with either intermittent oral melphalan chemotherapy or with a single intraperitoneal instillation of 15 mCi of ^{32}P at the time of initial surgery. With a median follow-up of 6 years, the 5-year survival rates of the ^{32}P group (78%) and for the melphalan group (81%) were within the range reported for whole abdominal irradiation. Another study by the Clinical Trials Group of the National Cancer Institute of Canada (64) randomized 157 stage I to III patients to whole abdominal irradiation, pelvic irradiation followed by intermittent oral melphalan chemotherapy, or pelvic irradiation and a single intraperitoneal dose of 10–20 mCi of ^{32}P. The 5-year survival rates (62%, 61%, and 66% for the three groups, respectively) were also within the range reported for whole abdominal irradiation. A significant complication rate of 29% was seen in the group receiving pelvic radiation and intraperitoneal ^{32}P, as compared to 11% rates for the patients receiving the other treatments.

Intraperitoneal instillation of ^{32}P has also been recently employed in stage III patients who were treated initially with cisplatin-based combinations and who had minimal or no tumor residua after second-look laparotomy. In patients proven to be in pathologic complete remission at second-look laparotomy, Spencer et al. (65) reported no recurrences among 14 patients treated with ^{32}P as compared to 4 out of 17 receiving no further treatment ($p = 0.076$). Although there was a trend of improved survival, the numbers of patients were small, and the grade of the tumors was not stated. Varia et al. (66) reported that the 4-year survival in 43 patients with no evidence of disease at second-look laparotomy receiving ^{32}P was 89%, as compared to 51% for 14 receiving no other treatment. Only 2 of 34 patients recurred if the original tumor had been grade 1 or stage I. In contrast, 7 of 18 patients with both tumor grade greater than one and stage greater than one relapsed. In a follow-up study with larger patient numbers and longer follow-up, Rogers (67) reported a 5-year disease-free survival of 86% and 67%, respectively, for those receiving and not receiving ^{32}P ($p = 0.05$).

In patients with a positive second-look laparotomy, recurrence and survival appear to be related to the volume of residual disease left at second-look laparotomy (Table 3). Reddy (68) reported that 61% of 13 patients with microscopic or less than 3 mm residual disease after second-look laparotomy were disease-free with a median follow-up of 28.5 months. The five patients who recurred all had one or more of the following high-risk features: high-grade tumor, advanced stage disease, or gross residual tumor. Similarly, Soper et al. (69) reported results in 23 patients who received intraperitoneal ^{32}P salvage therapy after second- or third-look laparotomy. The overall 4-year survival rates for second-look and third-look were 75% and 57%, respectively, with disease-free survival of 56% and 27%, respectively. Patients with microscopic residual or those completely resected during surgery had a 36% disease-free survival at 4 years. All five patients with residual macroscopic disease developed a recurrence and died of disease within 3 years.

Potter et al. (70) reported similar findings in a group of 32 patients treated secondarily after recurrence or after a positive second-look laparotomy. All four patients with macroscopic residual tumors after the second operative intervention were dead of disease within 3 years. Patients with microscopic disease or those completely resected had similar relapse rates of 54% and 53%, respectively. The findings of Varia et al. (66) differ somewhat from the previous reports in that only one of seven patients treated with minimal residual disease, defined as less than 2 cm in size after second-look laparotomy, recurred after treatment with ^{32}P alone. It is not clear from this report how many of these patients actually had microscopic residual disease. In summary, although use of intraperitoneal ^{32}P seems to be

TABLE 3. *Ovarian carcinoma patients treated with intraperitoneal ^{32}P after second- or third-look laparotomy: number of patients free of recurrence at 2–5 years according to findings after surgery*

			Positive second-look		
Author (ref.)	Year	Negative second look	Microscopic or <3 mm tumors	>3 mm tumors completely resected	Residual tumors (>3 mm)
Soper et al. (69)[a]	1987		6/10	4/8	0/5
Varia et al. (66)	1988	38/43			6/7[b]
Spencer et al. (65)	1989	14/14			
Potter et al. (70)	1989		6/13	7/15	0/4
Total		52/57(91%)	14/23(61%)	11/23(48%)	6/16(38%)

[a] Five patients treated after third-look laparotomy.
[b] Patients defined as having minimal disease <2 cm at second-look laparotomy.

valuable in patients with pathologic complete remission and in those with only microscopic tumor residua after second-look laparotomy, its use in patients with larger residua is not indicated.

RESULTS OF COMBINED MODALITY TREATMENT

With the introduction of cisplatin-based combination chemotherapy and the finding that 41% to 76% of patients with advanced stage disease can attain a complete clinical remission (CR), it was hoped that an improvement in 5-year survival rates would follow. Unfortunately, published series have shown the 5-year survival rates to range only between 14% and 30% (42,43,53,71–80), representing only a small improvement over the results obtained with whole abdominal irradiation alone (Table 2). This is due in part to the finding that only 50% of the patients obtaining a complete clinical remission are confirmed to be in pathologic complete remission (81). Of these patients, up to 50% will ultimately develop a recurrence with the likelihood of a recurrence depending on the initial stage, grade, amount of residual disease after initial staging operation, and type of chemotherapy used (82). In an attempt to improve upon these results, consolidation with whole abdominal irradiation has been proposed (83). As seen previously, the best long-term results of radiotherapy have been reported in patients with small residual disease (5,11). Fortunately, recent experience with second-look laparotomy has shown that the residual tumors found after chemotherapy are frequently small and that a complete or near complete resection is achievable in approximately 40% of the patients (84,85). In an attempt to further improve upon these results, Ng et al. (78) have recently reported on a series of advanced stage patients treated at Memorial Sloan-Kettering Cancer Center in New York with a program of maximal chemosurgical debulking. After initial surgery and debulking, patients received two courses of cisplatin (160 mg/m^2) and cyclophosphamide (1,000 mg/m^2) and were then subjected to a second surgical cytoreductive attempt. Whereas only 34% (13 of 38) of the patients had been optimally debulked to residual tumors of less than 1 cm after the first operation, the rate of optimal debulking increased to 79% (30 of 38) at the completion of the second operation.

Most sequential chemosurgical protocols have used a trimodality design consisting of an initial phase of tumor mass reduction by sequential surgery, cisplatin-based combination chemotherapy, and a second-look cytoreductive effort followed by a definitive curative attempt with tumoricidal doses of whole abdominal irradiation. In early reports of the experience, this approach had utilized whole abdominal irradiation primarily as salvage therapy in patients who had failed previous curative attempts with first- and second-line chemotherapy (22,86–89). Most of these patients were heavily pretreated with chemotherapy, and the moving strip technique was most often employed. For these reasons, the radiation was poorly tolerated; it resulted in early discontinuation of treatment owing to marrow toxicity in 30% to 53% of patients and caused chronic radiation enteritis requiring surgery in 27% to 63% of those surviving long enough to develop this complication (22,86–89). Most subsequent studies have attempted to improve the tolerance of radiotherapy by utilizing the open-field technique and treating patients with low dose per fraction (90–98), although even with these changes, moderate toxicity was still encountered (83).

As mentioned previously, in an attempt to further improve tolerance, researchers have suggested the use of a hyperfractionated whole abdominal irradiation approach (25,26). Kong et al. (25) treated 23 patients with cisplatin-cyclophosphamide chemotherapy and a second cytoreductive operation, followed by hyperfractionated whole abdominal irradiation delivered by two fractions of 100 cGy daily to a total dose of 3,000 cGy. Six patients with gross residual pelvic disease received an additional pelvic boost to 1,500 cGy in 15 fractions. Only one patient failed to complete treatment, and another patient developed tumor-related bowel obstruction without evidence of recurrent disease. Similar results were reported by Morgan et al. (26) in 15 patients treated with whole abdominal irradiation in fractions of 80 cGy delivered twice per day to a total of 2,600–3,060 cGy. A pelvic boost of 1,500–1,920 cGy was delivered to nine patients with gross residual disease in the pelvis. All patients were treated with cisplatin-based combination chemotherapy and a second cytoreductive surgery prior to treatment with radiotherapy. All patients completed the course of radiotherapy, and no episodes of chronic radiation enteritis requiring surgical intervention were reported.

One phase II study was specifically designed to test the basic hypothesis of the combined modality approach. Fuks et al. (83) reported the results in 38 stage III patients induced with 3 to 14 courses of the CHAD combination chemotherapy given for tumor mass reduction, followed by a second cytoreductive laparotomy and consolidation with whole abdominal irradiation. After the second cytoreductive operation, 76% of the patients had no gross residual tumors. The consolidation phase, consisting of whole abdominal irradiation, was relatively well tolerated. However, the actuarial 5-year survival and disease-free survival rates for the whole group were 27% and 17%, respectively. These results are similar to those observed in a historical series of patients treated with CAP chemotherapy (42) or those treated with CHAP-5 combination chemotherapy (74) without the use of whole abdominal irradiation. Despite numerous recent publications on the topic (Table 4), only one has addressed the issue in a prospective randomized phase III study (102). In this study, 41 patients with advanced epithelial ovarian cancer with pathologic complete response or minimal residual disease at second-look laparotomy after three courses of cisplatin-based chemotherapy were randomized to either three more courses of the same chemotherapy or whole abdominal irradiation utilizing an open field technique. The treatment was tolerated relatively well with only one bowel obstruction occurring in a patient receiving radiotherapy. At a median follow-up of 22 months, 11 of 20 patients in the radiotherapy arm progressed with 9 dying, as compared with 6 of 21 in the chemotherapy arm with 3 dying of disease.

These and similar disappointing results have been observed in other studies published recently. As seen in Table 4, the combined modality approach appears to have no value in patients with gross residual tumors greater than 1 cm in diameter prior to radiotherapy. Whether there are any true benefits in patients with microscopic or no residual tumors is an open question. Although approximately 50% of the patients in this group have remained disease free at 2 to 5 years after completing radiotherapy, similar results are seen in patients with microscopic residua treated with systemic (103) or intraperitoneal (104) chemotherapy instead of whole abdominal irradiation. Although some nonrandomized studies (93,96) have reported an improvement in survival for patients in pathologic complete remission after cisplatin-based chemotherapy and consolidation with whole abdominal irradiation, the information derived from these studies has limited value because

TABLE 4. *Stage III ovarian carcinoma treated with combination chemotherapy, second cytoreductive surgery, and whole abdominal irradiation: number of patients surviving without evidence of progressing disease 2–5 years after completion of treatment according to size of the largest tumor mass remaining at the completion of the second cytoreductive operation*

		Number surviving without progressing disease		
Author (ref.)	Year	Microscopic or no residual tumors	Minimal residual tumors (<1 cm)	Large residual tumors (>1 cm)
Hainsworth et al. (87)	1983	3/11	0/5	0/1
Hacker et al. (22)	1985	4/16	2/6	0/18
Peters et al. (89)	1986	2/9	0/7	0/6
Solomon et al. (90)	1988	4/12	2/2	0/4
Falcone et al. (91)	1988	5/6	4/10	
Green et al. (92)	1988	9/10	7/10	0/3
Schray et al. (94)	1988	8/22	6/31	
Kersh et al. (96)	1988	4/7	7/10	1/4
Kong et al. (25)	1988	7/12	1/2	1/9
Morgan (26)	1988	5/5	1/9	
Fuks et al. (83)	1988	1/3	1/10	0/6
Reddy et al. (99)	1989	9/16	4/14	
Kucera et al. (100)	1990	2/10	0/6	
Bolis et al. (101)	1990	6/18	0/8	
Total		69/157 (44%)	35/130 (27%)	2/51 (4%)

the studies have entailed few and selected patients for only short periods of time. It is already apparent that the current approach to the application of combined modality therapy offers little benefit. This lack of efficacy is frustrating, especially regarding patients with only microscopic disease after the second cytoreduction, where the doses of radiation employed could be expected to control such deposits. The reasons for the disappointing outcome are not well understood.

A possible explanation relates to the emergence of acquired pleiotropic drug resistance. Acquired resistance to cisplatin has been demonstrated clinically in several studies in which tumor specimens obtained from patients before and after cisplatin therapy were tested for their level of sensitivity to this drug (105–107). Furthermore, Louie et al. (108) has shown in in vitro experiments that ovarian tumor cell lines refractory to cisplatin exhibited a cross-resistance to irradiation as well. In addition, when cisplatin-sensitive human ovarian carcinoma cells are transplanted into nude mice, resistant clones have developed rapidly after short course treatments with the drug (109). It is possible, then, that exposure to these or similar drugs could lead to a pleiotropic resistance involving both a multidrug resistance and a cross-resistance to irradiation (105–108,110,111). Although recent studies have demonstrated a direct correlation between the chemotherapy dose intensity and initial response in advanced stage disease (112), thereby making more patients candidates for potentially tumoricidal treatment with whole abdominal irradiation, this correlation is unlikely to affect the sensitivity of microscopic tumors to the effects of radiation, even if a second surgical cytoreductive attempt results in an increase in the number of patients with microscopic residua. Several mechanisms have been implied in the induction of resistance to cisplatin. The intracellular levels of glutathione (GSH) have been shown to correlate with the degree of sensitivity of mammalian cells to the effects of ionizing radiation (113), and other experiments have indicated that it may be associated with enhanced repair of DNA damage (114). One study has shown that a likely mechanism of induction of resistance to cisplatin involves the overexpression of several enzymes that are involved in the metabolism of GSH and which bind and metabolize cytotoxic drugs, making them less toxic (115). This mechanism, if it is indeed the basis of the unexpected radiation resistance, may have significant clinical implications: Most patients treated by the combined modality approach have received numerous courses of chemotherapy, which prolongs the exposure of the surviving cells to the effects of the drugs, thereby increasing the likelihood of the development of resistant clones and the possibility of cross-resistance to radiation.

SUMMARY AND FUTURE STRATEGIES

Stage I patients with tumor grades 2 and 3, positive peritoneal cytology, or ascites and those with densely adherent tumors should be considered for postoperative treatment, because even in these early stage patients the risk of relapse can approach 45% (46). There are no randomized trials in this group of patients to indicate that any treatment would be beneficial over observation alone. However, because the salvage of failing patients is extremely difficult by any means, it is prudent to recommend treatment in these patients even if only a small portion of them may be potentially cured. The choice of postoperative treatment is open to debate. Radiotherapy should include treatment of the entire peritoneal contents because this is the main route of dissemination of ovarian cancer. An open field technique is preferable because complications can be kept to a minimum (31). Alternately, these patients can be treated with intraperitoneal colloidal ^{32}P if good distribution of the isotope is possible. Results similar to findings for patients treated with whole abdominal irradiation have been achieved and in a randomized trial have been shown to be as effective as single agent chemotherapy (45).

In patients with advanced stage or large tumor residua (>2 cm), the 5-year survivals in patients treated with whole abdominal irradiation are extremely poor (Table 2). These patients should therefore not be considered for treatment with this modality. The remaining patients, namely those with small tumor residua (<2 cm), are candidates for treatment with whole abdominal irradiation. However, depending on the amount of residual disease and the tumor grade, survivals will range from 40% to 75% (Table 2). Despite impressive responses with cisplatin-based chemotherapy, the long-term survival rates reported thus far are perhaps only slightly better than the rates for those treated with whole abdominal irradiation alone (42,43,53,71–80). Furthermore, there have been no randomized phase III trials comparing these two modalities in this somewhat "favorable" group of patients.

The consolidation or salvage of advanced stage patients with whole abdominal irradiation after chemotherapy is of limited value at present, benefiting perhaps only those with microscopic tumor residua (Table 4). If the reason for this ineffectiveness is the emergence of pleiotropic drug resistance with cross-resistance to radiation, then strategies to reverse these processes or to prevent them from occurring should be exploited.

One such suggestion is use of short, intense courses of chemotherapy rather than prolonged treatments; these courses are sufficient to cause effective cytoreduction but are perhaps not enough to confer drug/radiation resistance. Many protocols are currently utilizing such a scheme (55), but consolidation has usually been employed with intraperitoneal chemotherapy rather than with whole abdominal irradiation (116). This short-course chemotherapy hypothesis is presently being tested in a Gynecologic Oncology Group (GOG) phase II study.

Another possible circumvention of the problem is the use of new drugs that do not confer resistance to radiation. Two possible candidates are taxol (117) and tetraplatin (118). These drugs have been shown to be effective in patients with ovarian carcinoma refractory to treatment with cisplatin (119,120), but their pattern of cross-resistance with radiation, if any, is unknown.

Because cisplatin resistance has been associated with elevated levels of GSH (110), its depletion could enhance the cytotoxicity of platinum compounds. Studies with buthionine sulfoximine (BSO), a specific inhibitor of gamma-glutamylcysteine synthetase, have demonstrated this in vitro (111,114). This drug has recently been used in a clinical trial with an alkylating agent in patients with refractory ovarian carcinoma (121). Other studies have shown that similar results can be obtained with the use of compounds such as aphidicolin, which inhibit the capacity of cells to repair DNA damage, a phenomenon commonly seen in patients with resistance to cisplatin (114,122,123).

Radiosensitizing agents have recently been used in an attempt to improve upon current results. Because the escalation of dose with external beam whole abdominal irradiation beyond 3,000 cGy is impossible owing to excessive toxicity, this type of approach seems logical. King et al. (124) have recently treated a group of 11 patients with concomitant whole abdominal irradiation and intraperitoneal cisplatin. The results were similar to those found in the literature for cisplatin-based chemotherapy alone, and toxicity was high. Similarly, Lichter et al. (125) treated 28 patients with sequential chemotherapy and whole abdominal irradiation with intraperitoneal misonidazole, a hypoxic cell sensitizer. Only five patients (18%) achieved a pathologic complete response, and again, toxicity was moderately severe. Unfortunately, although the treatment perhaps sensitized tumor cells, it also enhanced normal organ toxicity. The use of targeted radiotherapy with monoclonal antibodies against a variety of ovarian carcinoma cell lines has recently been used to circumvent this problem (126). Results in transplanted human ovarian carcinoma growing in nude mice have been encouraging (126). However, clinical experience with such agents has been limited because of the chemical instability of the conjugates and loss of chelation, leading to toxicities from deposition of the free isotope in normal tissues. Advances in chelation chemistry should decrease this type of toxicity and facilitate the clinical use of monoclonal antibody radioconjugates.

The recent outcome of the combined modality approach has been extremely frustrating, but with a better understanding of the mechanisms involved in pleiotropic drug resistance and the development of new drugs such as taxol, the prospects for the future are encouraging.

REFERENCES

1. Eymer H. Beeinflussug von Proliferierenden Ovarialtumoren Durch Roentgenstrahlen. *Strahlen* 1912;1:358–361.
2. Rubin P, Griese JW, Terry R. Has postoperative irradiation proved itself? *Am J Roentgenol* 1962;89:849–866.
3. Fuks Z. External radiotherapy of ovarian cancer: standard approaches and new frontiers. *Semin Oncol* 1975;2:253–266.
4. Fuks Z, Bagshaw MA. The rationale for curative radiotherapy for advanced ovarian carcinoma. *Int J Radiat Oncol Biol Phys* 1975;1:21–32.
5. Dembo AJ. Abdominopelvic radiotherapy in ovarian carcinoma. A 10-year experience. *Cancer* 1985;55:2285–2290.
6. Martinez A, Schray MF, Howes AE, Bagshaw MA. Postoperative radiation therapy for epithelial ovarian cancer: the curative role based on a 24-year experience. *J Clin Oncol* 1985;3:901–911.
7. Weiser EB, Burke TW, Heller PB, Woodward J, Hoskins WJ, Park RC. Determinants of survival of patients with epithelial ovarian carcinoma following whole abdomen irradiation (WAR). *Gynecol Oncol* 1988;30:201–208.
8. Fletcher GH. Basic clinical parameters. In: Fletcher GH, ed. *Textbook of radiotherapy*, 3rd ed. Philadelphia: Lea & Febiger, 1980;180–216.
9. Schray MF, Cox RS, Martinez A. Lower abdominal radiotherapy for Stages I, II and selected III epithelial ovarian cancer. 20 years experience. *Gynecol Oncol* 1983;15:78–87.
10. Dembo AJ, Bush RS, Beale FA. Ovarian carcinoma: improved survival following abdominopelvic irradiation in patients with a completed pelvic operation. *Am J Obstet Gynecol* 1979;134:793–800.
11. Dembo AJ. Radiotherapeutic management of ovarian cancer. *Semin Oncol* 1984;11:238–250.
12. Delclos L, Smith JP. Tumors of the ovary. In: Fletcher G, ed. *Textbook of Radiotherapy*, 2nd ed. Philadelphia: Lea and Febiger, 1973;690–702.
13. Perez CA, Walz BZ, Jacobson PL. Radiation therapy in management of carcinoma of the ovary. *Natl Cancer Inst Monogr* 1975;42:119–125.
14. Rubin P, Cooper R, Phillip TL, eds. *Radiation biology and radiation pathology syllabus*. Chicago: American College of Radiology, 1974.
15. Hanks G, Bagshaw MA. Megavoltage radiation therapy and lymphangiography in ovarian cancer. *Radiology* 1969;93:649–654.
16. Delclos L, Barun EJ, Herrera JER, Sampiere VA, Van Rossenbeek E. Whole abdominal irradiation by cobalt-60 moving strip technique. *Radiology* 1963;81:632–641.
17. Dembo AJ, Bush RS, Beale FA, et al. The Princess Margaret study of ovarian cancer stages I, II, and asymptomatic III presentations. *Cancer Treat Rep* 1979;63:249–254.
18. Perez CA, Korba A, Zivnusk F, Prasad S, Katz-einstein AK. Cobalt 60 moving strip technique in the management of carcinoma of the ovary: analysis of tumor control and morbidity. *Int J Radiat Oncol Biol Phys* 1978;4:379–388.
19. Dembo AJ, VanDyk J, Japp B, et al. Whole abdominal irradiation by a moving strip technique for patients with ovarian cancer. *Int J Radiat Oncol Biol Phys* 1979;5:1933–1942.
20. Dembo AJ, Bush RS. Choice of postoperative therapy based on prognostic factors. *Int J Radiat Oncol Biol Phys* 1982;8:893–897.
21. Einhorn N, Nilsson B, Sjoval K. Factors influencing survival in carcinoma of the ovary. Study from a well-defined Swedish population. *Cancer* 1985;55:2019–2025.
22. Hacker NF, Berek JS, Burnison CM, Heintz PM, Juillard GH,

Lagasse LD. Whole abdominal radiation as salvage therapy for epithelial ovarian cancer. *Obstet Gynecol* 1985;65:60–66.
23. Mesumeci R, Depalo G, Kenda R, et al. Retro-peritoneal metastases from ovarian carcinoma: reassessment of 365 patients studied with lymphography. *Am J Roentgenol* 1980;134:449–452.
24. Parker BR, Castellin RA, Fuks Z, Bagshaw MA. The role of lymphography in patients with ovarian cancer. *Cancer* 1974;34:100–105.
25. Kong JS, Peters LJ, Wharton JT, et al. Hyperfractionated split-course whole abdominal radiotherapy for ovarian carcinoma: tolerance and toxicity. *Int J Radiat Oncol Biol Phys* 1988;14:1–7.
26. Morgan L, Chafe W, Mendenhall W, et al. Hyperfractionation of whole-abdomen radiation therapy: salvage treatment of persistent ovarian carcinoma following chemotherapy. *Gynecol Oncol* 1988;31:122–134.
27. Peters LJ, Ang KK. Unconventional fractionation schemes in radiotherapy. *Important Adv Oncol* 1986;269–286.
28. Order SE, Rosenshein NB, Klein JL, et al. New methods applied to the analysis and treatment of ovarian cancer. *Int J Radiat Oncol Biol Phys* 1979;5:861–873.
29. Ellis F. Dose-time fractionation. A clinical hypothesis. *Clin Radiol* 1969;20:1–7.
30. Dembo AJ, Bush RS, Beale FA, et al. A randomized clinical trial of moving strip versus open field whole abdominal irradiation in patients with invasive epithelial cancer of the ovary. *Int J Radiat Oncol Biol Phys* 1983;9:97(abst).
31. Fyles AW, Dembo AJ, Bush RS, et al. Analysis of complications in patients treated with abdominopelvic radiation therapy for ovarian carcinoma. *Int J Radiat Oncol Biol Phys* 1992;22:847–851.
32. Wharton JT, Delclos L, Gallagher S, Smith JP. Radiation hepatitis induced by abdominal irradiation with the cobalt 60 moving strip technique. *Am J Roentgenol* 1973;117:73–80.
33. Orton CG, Ellis F. A simplification in the use of the NSD concept in practical radiotherapy. *Br J Radiol* 1973;46:529–537.
34. Fazekas JT, Maier JF. Irradiation of the ovarian carcinoma. A prospective comparison of the open field and moving strip techniques. *Am J Roentgenol* 1974;120:118–123.
35. Kjellgren O, Johsson L. Bone marrow depression in the pelvis after megavoltage irradiation for ovarian cancer. *Obstet Gynecol* 1969;105:849–855.
36. Hintz BL, Fuks Z, Kempson RL, et al. Results of postoperative megavoltage radiotherapy of malignant surface epithelial tumors of the ovary. *Radiology* 1975;114:695–700.
37. Ingold JA, Reed GB, Kaplan HS, et al. Radiation hepatitis. *Am J Roentgenol* 1965;93:200–205.
38. Luxton R. Radiation nephritis. *Q J Med* 1953;22:215–242.
39. International Federation of Gynecology and Obstetrics. Changes in definitions of clinical staging for carcinoma of the cervix and ovary. *Am J Obstet Gynecol* 1986;156:263–264.
40. Bjorkhom E, Petterson F, Einhorn N, Krebs I, Nilsson B, Tjernberg B. Long-term follow up and prognostic factors in ovarian carcinoma: the Radiumhemmet series 1958–1973. *Acta Radiat Oncol* 1982;21:413–419.
41. Swenerton KD, Hislop TG, Spinelli J, LeRiche JC, Yang N, Boyes DA. Ovarian carcinoma: a multivariate analysis of prognostic factors. *Obstet Gynecol* 1985;65:264–270.
42. Redman JR, Petroni GR, Saigo PE, Geller L, Hakes TB. Prognostic factors in advanced ovarian carcinoma. *J Clin Oncol* 1986;4:515–523.
43. Krag KJ, Canellos GP, Griffiths CT, et al. Predictive factors for long-term survival in patients with advanced ovarian cancer. *Gynecol Oncol* 1989;34:88–93.
44. Friedlander ML, Dembo AJ. Prognostic factors in ovarian cancer. *Semin Oncol* 1991;18:205–212.
45. Young RC, Walton LA, Ellenberg SS, et al. Adjuvant therapy in stage I and stage II epithelial ovarian cancer. Results of two prospective randomized trials. *N Engl J Med* 1990;22:1021–1927.
46. Dembo AJ, Davy M, Stenwig AE. Prognostic factors in patients with stage I epithelial ovarian cancer. *Obstet Gynecol* 1990;75:263–273.
47. Hreshchyshyn MM, Park RC, Blessing JA, et al. The role of adjuvant therapy in stage I ovarian cancer. *Am J Obstet Gynecol* 1980;138:139–145.
48. Macbeth FR, Macdonald H, Williams CJ. Abdominal and pelvic radiotherapy in the management of early stage ovarian carcinoma. *Int J Radiat Oncol Biol Phys* 1988;15:353–358.
49. Fuller DB, Sause WT, Plenk HP, et al. Analysis of postoperative radiation therapy in stage I through III epithelial ovarian carcinoma. *J Clin Oncol* 1987;5:897–905.
50. Goldberg N, Peschel RE. Postoperative abdominopelvic radiation therapy for ovarian cancer. *Int J Radiat Oncol Biol Phys* 1988;14:425–429.
51. Van Bunningen B, Bouma J, Kooijman C, et al. Total abdominal irradiation in stage I and II carcinoma of the ovary. *Radiother Oncol* 1988;11:305–310.
52. Lindner H, Willich H, Atzinger A. Primary adjuvant whole abdominal irradiation in ovarian carcinoma. *Int J Radiat Oncol Biol Phys* 1990;19:1203–1206.
53. Fuks Z. The role of radiation therapy in the management for ovarian carcinoma. *Ins J Med Sci* 1977;8:815–828.
54. Decker DG, Webb MJ, Holbrook MA. Radiogold treatment of epithelial cancer of the ovary. *Am J Obstet Gynecol* 1973;115:751–756.
55. Rosenshein NB, Leichner PK, Vogelsang G. Radiocolloids in the treatment of ovarian cancer. *Obstet Gynecol Surv* 1979;34:708–719.
56. Boye E, Lindegaard MW, Paus E, Skretting A, Davy M, Jakobsen E. Whole-body distribution of radioactivity after intraperitoneal administration of ^{32}P colloids. *Br J Radiol* 1984;57:395–402.
57. Leichner PK, Rosenshein NB, Leibel SA, Order SE. Distribution and tissue dose of intraperitoneally administered radioactive chromic phosphate ^{32}P in New England white rabbits. *Radiology* 1980;134:729–734.
58. Currie JL, Bagne F, Harris C, et al. Radioactive chromic phosphate suspension: studies on distribution, dose absorption, and effective therapeutic radiation in phantoms, dogs and patients. *Gynecol Oncol* 1981;12:193–218.
59. Sullivan DC, Harris CC, Currie JL, Wilkinson RH, Creasman WT. Observations on the intraperitoneal distribution of chromic phosphate (^{32}P) suspension for intraperitoneal therapy. *Radiology* 1983;146:539–541.
60. Walton LA, Yadusky A, Rubinstein L. Intraperitoneal radioactive phosphate in early ovarian carcinoma: an analysis of complications. *Int J Radiat Oncol Biol Phys* 1991;20:939–944.
61. Hilaris BC, Clark DGC. The value of postoperative intraperitoneal injection of radiocolloids in early cancer of the ovary. *Am J Roentgenol* 1971;112:749–754.
62. Piver MS, Lele SB, Bakshi S, Parthasarathy KL, Emrich LY. Five- and ten-year estimated survival and disease-free rates after intraperitoneal chromic phosphate: stage I ovarian adenocarcinoma. *Am J Clin Oncol* 1988;11:515–519.
63. Soper JT, Berchuk A, Clarke-Pearson DL. Adjuvant intraperitoneal chromic phosphate therapy for women with apparent early ovarian carcinoma who have not undergone comprehensive surgical staging. *Cancer* 1991;68:725–729.
64. Klaassen D, Shelly W, Starreveld A, et al. Early stage ovarian cancer: a randomized clinical trial comparing whole abdominal radiotherapy, melphalan, and intraperitoneal chromic phosphate: a National Cancer Institute of Canada clinical trials group report. *J Clin Oncol* 1988;6:1254–1263.
65. Spencer TR, Marks RD, Fenn JO, Jenrette JM, Lutz MH. Intraperitoneal ^{32}P after negative second-look laparotomy in ovarian carcinoma. *Cancer* 1989;63:2434–2437.
66. Varia M, Rosenman J, Venkatraman S, et al. Intraperitoneal chromic phosphate therapy after second-look laparotomy for ovarian cancer. *Cancer* 1988;61:919–927.
67. Rogers L, Varia M, Halle J, Freddo J, O'Keefe T, Fowler W Jr. P32 following second-look laparotomy for epithelial ovarian cancer. *Int J Radiat Oncol Biol Phys* 1990;19(1):167–168 (Abst).
68. Reddy S, Sutton GP, Stehman FB, Hornback NB, Ehrlich CE. Ovarian carcinoma: adjuvant treatment with P-32. *Radiology* 1987;165:275–278.

69. Soper TS, Wilkinson RH Jr, Bandy LC, Clarke-Pearson DL, Creasman WT. Intraperitoneal chromic phosphate P-32 as salvage therapy for persistent carcinoma of the ovary after surgical restaging. *Am J Obstet Gynecol* 1987;156:1153–1158.
70. Potter ME, Partridge EE, Shingleton HM, et al. Intraperitoneal chromic phosphate in ovarian cancer: risks and benefits. *Gynecol Oncol* 1989;32:314–318.
71. Ozols RF, Young RC. Ovarian cancer. *Curr Probl Cancer* 1987; 1:59–122.
72. Ozols RF, Young RC. Chemotherapy of ovarian cancer. *Semin Oncol* 1991;18:222–232.
73. Louie KG, Ozols RF, Myers CE, et al. Long-term results of a cisplatin-containing combination chemotherapy regimen for the treatment of advanced ovarian carcinoma. *J Clin Oncol* 1986; 4:1579–1585.
74. Neijt JP, ten Bokkel Huinink WW, van der Berg ME, et al. Randomized trial comparing two combination chemotherapy regiments (CHAP 5 v CP) in advanced ovarian carcinoma. *J Clin Oncol* 1987;5:1157–1168.
75. Beilinson JL, Lee KR, Jarell MA, McClure M. Management of epithelial ovarian neoplasms using platinum-based regimen: a ten year experience. *Gyn Oncol* 1990;37:66–73.
76. Omura GA, Bundy BN, Berek JS, Curry S, Delgado G, Mortel R. Randomized trial of cyclophosphamide plus cisplatin with or without doxorubicin in ovarian carcinoma: a Gynecologic Oncology Group study. *J Clin Oncol* 1989;7:457–465.
77. Sutton GP, Stehman FB, Einhorn LH, Roth LM, Blessing JA, Ehrlich CE. Ten-year follow-up of patients receiving cisplatin doxorubicin, and cyclosphosphamide chemotherapy for advanced epithelial ovarian carcinoma. *J Clin Oncol* 1989;7: 223–229.
78. Ng LW, Rubin SC, Hoskins WJ, et al. Aggressive chemosurgical debulking in patients with advanced ovarian cancer. *Gynecol Oncol* 1990;38:358–363.
79. Williams CJ, Mead GM, Macbeth FR, et al. Cisplatin combination chemotherapy versus chlorambucil in advanced ovarian carcinoma: mature results of a randomized trial. *J Clin Oncol* 1985;3:1455–1462.
80. Wiltshaw E, Evans B, Rustin G, Gilbey E, Baker J, Barker G. A prospective randomized trial comparing high-dose cisplatin with low-dose cisplatin and chlorambucil in advanced ovarian carcinoma. *J Clin Oncol* 1986;4:722–729.
81. Rubin SC, Lewis JL Jr. Second-look surgery in ovarian carcinoma. *Crit Rev Oncol Hematol* 1988;8:75.
82. Rubin SC, Hoskins WT, Hakes TB, et al. Recurrence after negative second-look laparotomy for ovarian cancer: analysis of risk factors. *Am J Obstet Gynecol* 1988;158:1094.
83. Fuks Z, Rizel S, Biran S. Chemotherapeutic and surgical induction of pathological complete remission and whole abdominal irradiation for consolidation does not enhance the cure of stage III ovarian carcinoma. *J Clin Oncol* 1988;6:509–516.
84. Hoskins WJ. The influence of cytoreductive surgery on progression-free interval and survival in epithelial ovarian cancer. *Bailliere Clin Obstet Gynaecol* 1989;3:59–71.
85. Hoskins WJ, Rubin SC, Dulaney E, et al. Influence of secondary cytoreduction at the time of second-look laparotomy on the survival of patients with epithelial ovarian carcinoma. *Gynecol Oncol* 1989;34:365–371.
86. Piver MS, Barlow JJ, Lee FT, Vongtama V. Sequential therapy for advanced ovarian adenocarcinoma: operation, chemotherapy, second-look laparotomy and radiation therapy. *Am J Obstet Gynecol* 1975;122:355–357.
87. Hainsworth JD, Malcolm A, Johnson DH, Burnett LS, Jones HW, Greco FA. Advanced minimal residual ovarian carcinoma; abdominopelvic irradiation following combination chemotherapy. *Obstet Gynecol* 1983;61:619–623.
88. Hoskins WJ, Lichter AS, Whillington R, Artman LE, Bibro MC, Park RC. Whole abdominal and pelvic irradiation in patients with minimal disease at second-look surgical reassessment for ovarian carcinoma. *Gynecol Oncol* 1985;20:271–280.
89. Peters WA III, Blaski JC, Bagley CM Jr, Rudolph RH, Smith MR, Rivkin SE. Salvage therapy with whole-abdominal irradiation in patients with advanced carcinoma of the ovary previously treated by combination chemotherapy. *Cancer* 1986;58: 880–882.
90. Solomon HJ, Atkinson KH, Coppleson JVM, et al. Ovarian carcinoma: abdominopelvic irradiation following reexploration. *Gynecol Oncol* 1988;31:396–401.
91. Falcone A, Chiara S, Franzone P, et al. Moving strip abdominopelvic radiotherapy after cis-platinum–based chemotherapy and second-look operation: a feasibility study in advanced ovarian cancer. *Am J Clin Oncol* 1988;11:16–20.
92. Green JA, Warenius HM, Errington RD, Myint S, Spearing G, Slater AJ. Sequential cisplatin/cyclophosphamide chemotherapy and abdominopelvic radiotherapy in the management of advanced ovarian cancer. *Br J Cancer* 1988;58:635–639.
93. Goldhirsch A, Griener R, Dreher E, et al. Treatment of advanced ovarian cancer with surgery, chemotherapy, and consolidation of response by whole-abdominal radiotherapy. *Cancer* 1988;62:40–47.
94. Schray MF, Martinez A, Howes AE, et al. Advanced epithelial ovarian cancer: salvage whole abdominal irradiation for patients with recurrent or persistent disease after combination chemotherapy. *J Clin Oncol* 1988;6:1433–1439.
95. Menczer J, Modan M, Brenner J, Ben-Baruch G, Brenner H. Abdominopelvic irradiation for Stage II–IV ovarian carcinoma patients with limited or no residual disease at second-look laparotomy after completion of cisplatinum-based combination chemotherapy. *Gynecol Oncol* 1986;24:149–154.
96. Kersh CR, Randall ME, Constable WC, et al. Whole abdominal radiotherapy following cytoreductive surgery and chemotherapy in ovarian carcinoma. *Gynecol Oncol* 1988;31:113–120.
97. Cheung AYC. Salvage radiotherapy for carcinoma of the ovary following chemotherapy. *Gynecol Oncol* 1988;30:15–20.
98. Cain JM, Russell AH, Greer BE, Tamimi HK, Figge DC. Whole abdominal radiation for minimal residual epithelial ovarian carcinoma after surgical resection and maximal first-line chemotherapy. *Gynecol Oncol* 1988;29:168–175.
99. Reddy S, Hartsell W, Graham J, et al. Whole abdomen radiation therapy in ovarian carcinoma: its role as a salvage therapeutic modality. *Gynecol Oncol* 1989;35:307–313.
100. Kucera PR, Berman ML, Treadwell P, et al. Whole-abdominal radiotherapy for patients with minimal residual epithelial ovarian cancer. *Gynecol Oncol* 1990;36:338–342.
101. Bolis G, Zanaboni F, Vanoli P, et al. The impact of whole-abdomen radiotherapy on survival in advanced ovarian cancer patients with minimal residual disease after chemotherapy. *Gynecol Oncol* 1990;39:150–154.
102. Bruzzone M, Repetto L, Chiara S, et al. Chemotherapy versus radiotherapy in the management of ovarian cancer patients with pathological complete response or minimal residual disease at second look. *Gynecol Oncol* 1990;38:392–395.
103. Copeland LI, Gershenson DM, Wharton JT, Atkinson EN. Microscopic disease at second-look laparotomy in advanced ovarian cancer. *Cancer* 1985;55:472–478.
104. Howell SB, Zimm S, Markman M, et al. Long-term survival of advanced refractory ovarian carcinoma patients with small-volume disease treated with intraperitoneal chemotherapy. *J Clin Oncol* 1987;5:1607–1612.
105. Wolf CR, Hayward IP, Lawrie SS, et al. Cellular heterogeneity and drug resistance in two ovarian adenocarcinoma cell lines derived from a single patient. *Int J Cancer* 1987;39:696–701.
106. Inoue K, Mukaiyama T, Mitsui I, Ogawa M. In vitro evaluation of anticancer drugs in relation to development of drug resistance in the human tumor clonogenic assay. *Cancer Chemother Pharmacol* 1985;15:208–213.
107. Simmonds AP, McDonald EC. Ovarian carcinoma cells in culture: assessment of drug sensitivity by clonogenic assay. *Br J Cancer* 1984;50:317–326.
108. Louie KG, Behrens BC, Kinsella TJ, et al. Radiation survival parameters of antineoplastic drug-sensitive and resistant human ovarian cancer cell lines and their modification by buthionine sulfoximine. *Cancer Res* 1985;45:2110–2115.
109. Andrews PA, Jones JA, Varki NM, Howell SB. Rapid emergency of acquired cis-diamminedichloroplatinum (II) resistance in an in vivo model of human ovarian carcinoma. *Cancer Commun* 1990;2:93–100.

110. Behrens BC, Hamilton TC, Masuda H, et al. Characterization of a cis-diamminedichloroplatinum (II) resistant human ovarian cancer cell line and its use in evaluation of platinum analogs. *Cancer Res* 1987;47:414–418.
111. Hamilton TC, Winker MA, Louie KG, et al. Augmentation of adriamycin, melphalan and cisplatin cytotoxicity in drug-resistant and sensitive human ovarian carcinoma cell lines by buthionine sulfoximine mediated glutathione depletion. *Biochem Pharmacol* 1985;34:2583–2586.
112. Levin L, Hryniuk WM. Dose intensity analysis of chemotherapy regimens in ovarian carcinoma. *J Clin Oncol* 1987;5:756–767.
113. Biaglow JE, Varnes ME, Epp ER, Clark EP, Tuttle SW, Held KD. Role of glutathione in the aerobic radiation response. *Int J Radiat Oncol Biol Phys* 1989;16:1311–1319.
114. Lai G-M, Ozols RF, Young RC, Hamilton TC. Effect of glutathione on DNA repair in cisplatin-resistant human ovarian cancer cell lines. *J Natl Cancer Inst* 1989;81:535–539.
115. Fairchild CR, Cowan KH. Keynote address: multidrug resistance: a pleiotropic response to cytoxic drugs. *Int J Radiat Oncol Biol Phys* 1990;20:361–367.
116. Hakes TB, Markman M, Reichman BS, et al. Pilot study of intravenous (IV) cyclophosphamide/cisplatin (CTX/CDDP) and intraperitoneal CDDP for advanced ovarian cancer (AOC): a preliminary report. *Proc Am Soc Clin Oncol* 1989;8:152.
117. Rowinsky EK, Casenave LA, Donehower RC. Taxol: a noel investigational antimicrotubul agent. *J Natl Cancer Inst* 1990;82:1247–1259.
118. Perez RP, O'Dwyer PJ, Handel LM, Ozols RF, Hamilton TC. Comparative cytotoxicity of CI-973, cisplatin, carboplatin and tetraplatin in human ovarian carcinoma cell lines. *Int J Cancer* 1991;48:265–269.
119. Thigpen T, Blessing J, Ball H, Hummrel S, Barret R. Phase II trial of taxol as a second line-therapy for ovarian carcinoma. *Proc Am Soc Clin Oncol* 1990;9:156.
120. Teicher BA, Holden SA, Herman TS, et al. Characteristics of five human tumor cell lines and sublines resistant to cis-diamminechloroplatinum (II). *Int J Cancer* 1991;47:252–260.
121. Hamilton T, O'Dwyer P, Young R, Tew K, Padavic K, Comis R, Ozols R. Phase I trial of buthionine sulfoximine (BSO) plus melphalan (L-PAM) in patients with advanced cancer. *Proc Am Soc Clin Oncol* 1990;9:73.
122. Perrino FW, Loeb LA. Animal cell DNA polymerases in DNA repair. *Mutat Res* 1990;236:289–300.
123. Katz EJ, Andrews PA, Howell SB. The effect of DNA polymerase inhibitors on the cytotoxicity of cisplatin in human ovarian carcinoma cells. *Cancer Commun* 1990;2:159–164.
124. King LA, Downey GO, Potish RA, et al. Concomitant whole-abdominal radiation and intraperitoneal chemotherapy in advanced ovarian carcinoma. *Cancer* 1991;67:2867–2871.
125. Lichter AS, Ozols RF, Myers CC, et al. The treatment of advanced stage ovarian carcinoma with a combination of chemotherapy, radiotherapy and radio-sensitizer: report of a pilot study from the National Cancer Institute. *Int J Radiat Oncol Biol Phys* 1987;13:1225–1231.
126. Bookman MA, Bast RC. The immunobiology and immunotherapy of ovarian cancer. *Semin Oncol* 1991;18:270–291.

CHAPTER 17

In Vitro Evaluation of Chemotherapeutic Agents

Charles E. Welander

New information concerning human ovarian cancers falls into two broad categories. The first and largest category is descriptive information concerning tumor incidence, precise determination of extent of disease, and host factors, including molecular studies of tumor cells, all of which can be associated with responses to standard therapy. None of these parameters can be changed; they are the "given" part brought by each new patient. The other category of new information relates to treatment choices, over which clinicians may have some control. Surgical skills applied to ovarian cancer therapy, the choice of cytotoxic drugs, and the use of immunotherapy are examples of the second category of new modalities. Ultimate success in clinical oncology comes when physicians are able to match the given parameters with the most appropriate treatment options.

The impact of individual drugs on tumor cell growth can be measured. Reports of chemosensitivity testing published during the past 30 years have included papers that propose or attempt to justify new technical methodology and papers that describe applications of chemosensitivity screening to individualized patient treatment planning. This chapter presents a summary of recent papers describing various methods for drug sensitivity testing and discusses three ways that the technology of chemosensitivity testing can be applied to human ovarian cancer studies. The first application is preclinical, in which ovarian cancer cells are used to screen new investigational drugs for antitumor activity. A second area of preclinical investigation involves more detailed pharmacologic studies of active cytotoxic drugs. A third and very different application is an effort to screen primary ovarian cancers from surgical specimens of patients who are likely to undergo chemotherapy. Testing a patient's tumor cells with a panel of drugs will often identify which drugs are the most active and thereby allow individualized treatment planning. However, the end point here is a patient's response to therapy. Many patient factors that are unchangeable, such as performance status, bulk of tumor, and molecular prognostic indicators, may have more bearing on the ultimate outcome than the chemosensitivity information from the laboratory.

METHODOLOGY OF CHEMOSENSITIVITY TESTING

A certain repetitiveness exists in medical sciences: Ideas appear, then disappear, and are later resurrected. Since the 1950s, there has been laboratory interest in chemosensitivity studies of human cancers. The proceedings of a 1970 symposium held in Williamsburg, Virginia, were published as a National Cancer Institute Monograph in 1971 (1). Most of the work up to that time involved only preclinical laboratory data, which made very few clinical correlations. Established human tumor cell lines were generally chosen for this work. In the late 1970s, investigators adapted techniques previously used to culture bone marrow cells for the in vitro growth of solid tumor cells (2). A concept of cell renewal was proposed, suggesting that solid malignancies contained cells with self-renewal capabilities as well as terminally differentiated cells. Cells capable of self-renewal and of clonal expansion have been referred to as stem cells or clonogenic cells. These cells are responsible for regrowth of the primary tumor after inadequate resection and/or tumor metastases. The drug sensitivity of these clonogenic cells theo-

---

C. E. Welander: Department of Gynecology/Oncology, Medical Center Hospital of Vermont, Burlington, Vermont 05401

retically should correlate with clinical responses to chemotherapy (3). Colony-forming assays in soft agar selectively allow cells with self-renewal capacities to form cell aggregates, while inhibiting benign stromal cell growth. Von Hoff published a review article in 1990, summarizing in vitro and in vivo correlations reported by 35 institutions over 12 years (4). Approximately 2,300 correlations have been reported, with 69% positive predictive value and 91% negative predictive value of such assays. Variations of clonogenic assay techniques have included a thymidine incorporation assay (5), a capillary tube cloning system (6), and cultures using a cellular adhesive matrix (7). Clonogenic assays theoretically are an excellent way to study primary human tumors, where a portion of the specimen will include benign connective tissue elements mixed in with tumor cells. The technology chosen must inhibit growth of these benign cells in order to identify correctly the drug sensitivity pattern of the cells having self-renewal capabilities.

Alternative methods are continuously proposed by cell biologists for predictive drug testing. Many of these are short-term assays, requiring only a few hours to perhaps a few days for interpretation. Cellular damage caused by cytotoxic drugs can be measured by vital dye exclusion (8), changes in thymidine incorporation (short-term assay) (9), bioluminescence for adenosine triphosphate (10), and fluorescence viability staining (11). These assays do not necessarily discriminate between tumor and stromal cells, nor are clonogenic cells identifiable as a distinct subpopulation. Fewer studies have been published that demonstrate correlations between these alternative in vitro methods and in vivo responses. Outside of documented clinical applicability, all chemosensitivity data exist in a vacuum, having no useful point of reference.

The majority of in vitro data and clinical response information presented in this chapter is derived from clonogenic assays and various modifications of that basic system. The ability to grow ovarian cancers in vitro exceeds that of many other human cancers. The inherent sensitivity of ovarian tumors to chemotherapy also helps to identify active drugs rather than simply to identify drug resistance.

CHEMOSENSITIVITY TESTING TO SCREEN NEW DRUGS

Drug development has been a major effort of the National Cancer Institute for almost 40 years (12). Screening new compounds for potential antitumor activity has been traditionally done with *in vivo* models, specifically two murine leukemias, L1210 and P388. Human tumor xenografts have been added for further screening of active drugs. In 1980, the National Cancer Institute began a parallel screening program, testing certain new drugs in vitro, with clonogenic assay techniques (13). Studies were done to compare drug doses in the murine models with concentrations used in the colony-forming assays. Of 28 widely used conventional cytotoxic agents, good correlation was shown between mouse LD_{50}s and clinically achievable peak plasma levels (14). One of the questions posed by the National Cancer Institute was whether any drugs found to be inactive in the murine tumor screening panel might actually have cytotoxic activity in human tumors. Of approximately 300 compounds that were inactive in the murine screening panel, 81 have shown some cytotoxic activity against human tumor cells (15). Further studies have been done to determine the degree of clinical activity of these particular compounds. An evaluation of the National Cancer Institute–sponsored large-scale drug screening program suggests that clonogenic assays using primary human tumor cells can be helpful but are not cost-effective. Primary screening can be done with reduced costs if established human tumor cell lines are selected rather than primary tumor specimens. Assay methodology can be simplified to test multiple concentrations of each drug quickly and at reasonable cost (16).

As an example of new drug evaluation, analogues of conventional cytotoxic agents have been created in the hope of reducing toxicity and/or increasing efficacy. Knowing the activity of doxorubicin in the treatment of ovarian cancers, researchers tested three analogues for similar activity with cell lines from ovarian cancers using clonogenic assay techniques (17). Each of the analogues tested showed greater inhibition of tumor colony growth than did the parent compound. Whether human toxicities of each of the new analogues are different can be tested only with actual clinical trials. Another example of drug analogue testing has been demonstrated with the vinca alkaloid group of drugs (18). Other analogues of the platinum compounds have likewise been screened in vitro for alterations of antitumor effect (19).

IN VITRO PHARMACOLOGIC STUDIES OF ACTIVE DRUGS

Once drugs have been found to have cytotoxic activity, many additional questions need to be answered. What are the optimal drug concentrations? Is prolonged intravenous infusion superior to intravenous bolus administration of a drug? Experiments evaluating new drugs are commonly done using many drug concentrations at intervals above and below an established peak plasma level. It is possible to set up paired experiments that measure the differences between brief exposure of tumor cells to a drug and prolonged exposure over hours or days (20). Clues from these data can be used to design patient treatment regimens.

New applications of chemosensitivity data are being reported. The concept of extreme drug resistance has been proposed as a characteristic possessed by certain tumor cells (21). Independent factors associated with drug resistance are detailed in other chapters of this book. However, there probably are multiple factors correlated with inherent cellular resistance to chemotherapeutic drugs (22,23). Although specific resistance pathways may vary for each drug, a combination of p-glycoprotein expression, DNA repair mechanisms, glutathione transferase activity, drug uptake or efflux, and so on can collectively affect antiproliferative effects of drugs on tumor cells. A biologic assay measuring cell division as an end point will include the combined effects of any of these significant factors. Even though measurement of one of the preceding parameters may be simpler than culturing cells in vitro, correlation with clinical outcome remains the ultimate evaluation point for all predictive tests.

To demonstrate extreme drug resistance, cultures of ovarian tumor cells are exposed to concentrations of drug for which the product of concentration and time is 100-fold greater than that clinically achievable. Clinical correlations with 450 patients whose tumors showed extreme drug resistance resulted in greater than 99% specificity for identifying nonresponders (21). Careful laboratory attention to detail is required if specificity is to remain high. Appropriate positive and negative controls are essential for each assay.

Use of extreme drug resistance data can be applied in a general fashion to the design of treatment protocols by providing negative information. Tumor types that show high percentages of specimens with extreme drug resistance to a certain drug will have such a drug deleted from protocol choices. Application of extreme drug resistance data to individual treatment planning is discussed later.

Chemosensitivity data are also being used to plan high-dose chemotherapy regimens. Increased toxicity will be noted whether high-dose levels of chemotherapy are achieved by systemic drug administration or by regional therapy (e.g., intraperitoneal or intraarterial administration). The ability to predict with more than random accuracy whether higher concentrations of potentially life-threatening therapy will be helpful is clearly beneficial. Extreme drug resistance makes this point even clearer. If up to 100 times the maximal peak plasma level does not yield any significant antiproliferative activity, then the technology of high-dose therapy will predictably fail.

Von Hoff and colleagues have published results from a series of tumor types tested with eight separate chemotherapeutic agents (24). This drug panel tested 298 evaluable ovarian tumor specimens tested at at least

TABLE 1. *Slopes for dose response lines by drug: Ovarian cancers—298 specimens[a]*

Agent	Slope ± SE[b]
Melphalan	0.637 ± 0.643
Cisplatin	0.544 ± 0.197
Ara-C	0.419 ± 0.053
Bisantrene	0.274 ± 0.124
Vinblastine	0.240 ± 0.369
Mitoxantrone	0.213 ± 0.015
Interferon	0.152 ± 0.020
Vinzolidine	0.005 ± 0.003
Median slope	0.257

[a] From ref. 24.
[b] SE, standard error.

five different concentrations. A slope of the dose response curve was determined, as shown in Table 1. Extrapolation of this dose response slope suggests that high concentrations of melphalan would predictably have the greatest probability for benefit when administered by some novel schema. As predicted by preclinical studies, high concentrations of drugs such as vinblastine, mitoxantrone, or vinzolidine would be much less likely to show increased clinical benefit.

Intraperitoneal therapy for ovarian cancer is an additional way to achieve significantly elevated local/regional drug concentrations. Drug transit across the peritoneal surface is controlled by molecular factors including molecular weight of the drug and degree of lipid solubility. Drugs having high molecular weight and low lipid solubility have slow peritoneal clearance (25). Based on pharmacokinetic parameters, which determine the area under the curve between the peritoneal cavity and plasma, cisplatin, 5-fluorouracil, and cytarabine are examples of drugs that have theoretical advantages when given by intraperitoneal routes (26).

An entirely different question is whether increasing concentrations of a drug beyond peak plasma levels makes any difference in terms of tumor cell kill. Does the increased potential toxicity of higher drug concentrations net a desired increase in antiproliferative effects on tumor cells? Data summarized by Von Hoff et al. in Table 1 suggest that ovarian cancer cells are much more likely to respond to higher concentrations of cisplatin or cytarabine than to mitoxantrone or vinblastine (24). Pharmacokinetic studies clearly can predict which drugs are feasible for intraperitoneal therapy. Preclinical chemosensitivity testing can determine whether feasible drugs are likely to be beneficial.

Combinations of drugs for the treatment of ovarian cancer have become the standard of therapy. Design of new clinical protocol regimens has been accomplished in the past by theoretical considerations of drug toxicities, mechanisms of antiproliferative effects, and historical results from clinical trials. In addition to such information, in vitro antitumor activity from single drugs and combinations of drugs can be generated with clonogenic assays (27). Statistical methods to evaluate drug interactions in vitro have been published (28,29). In vitro combined drug interactions can be identified that result in additive, synergistic, or antagonistic antiproliferative effects on tumor cells. As an example, ovarian cancer cells have been used in vitro to study the antiproliferative effects of certain biologic response modifiers, alpha and gamma interferon. Interferons in high concentrations can demonstrate some tumor cell growth inhibition but tend to have increased therapeutic benefit when used in lower concentrations together with certain cytotoxic agents (30,31). In vitro experiments that involved the screening of eight cytotoxic drugs with interferon alpha have been published. Variations of drug and/or interferon alpha concentrations were tested, with varied exposure time of tumor cells to the drugs and varied sequencing of the drug with interferon alpha. The most active combination was interferon alpha and either doxorubicin or cisplatin. Exposure of cells to interferon alpha prior to doxorubicin increased the degree of antiproliferative effect recorded (27). The mechanism of this observed drug interaction is unknown, but many intriguing possibilities exist for future study.

INDIVIDUALIZED PATIENT CHEMOSENSITIVITY TESTING

The third and best known application of in vitro clonogenic assays is individualized chemosensitivity testing for patients. When ovarian cancer cells are removed through surgery, by excisional biopsy, or by the draining of malignant effusions, they can be grown *in vitro* and tested with cytotoxic drugs. Either combinations of drugs or single agents can be screened. Dose response curves to individual drugs can be generated if novel methods of high-dose therapy are a possible treatment consideration. Extreme drug resistance can be predicted if appropriately high concentrations of drugs are tested. Correlations between the predictive tests and the clinical outcome can then be noted.

Most of the publications recording clinical correlations between chemosensitivity testing and clinical responses came from the early 1980s (4). A degree of enthusiasm was common then, as clinical oncologists sent tumors to the laboratory for culture and sensitivity testing. The most easily interpreted results were those in which drugs were screened *in vitro* as single agents, and the patient's treatment was then administered using only a single drug. Much more complicated is the situation in which drugs were tested individually but the patients were treated with two or three drugs in combination. A total of 185 clinical trials of ovarian cancers were reported by Alberts et al. (1980) (32), Natale and Kushner (1981) (33), Wilson and Neal (1981) (34), Welander et al. (1983) (35), and Arbuck et al. (1985) (36), showing a positive predictive accuracy of 72.8% and a negative predictive accuracy of 95.2%.

Two problems become obvious. One is the fact that single agent therapy is rarely used in the United States for ovarian cancer treatment, except in certain cases of recurrent disease. Drug combinations are used for most primary therapy and also for much secondary treatment. For predictive chemosensitivity assays to be clinically useful, there must be some means to evaluate combinations of drugs. The other problem concerns the fact that positive predictive accuracy is in the 70% range in most published studies. Usually a false positive result occurs when the laboratory predicts drug activity, but no significant patient response is later noted. Tumor cells having inherent sensitivity to a particular drug is only the first link in a chain of events. Drug delivery to the tumor cells in concentrations similar to those seen in vitro is required. A patient's performance status must be adequate to tolerate drug doses equivalent to those tested in vitro. Tumor bulk, as in ovarian cancer, must be an order of magnitude that will make it possible for chemotherapy to reduce cell numbers by logarithmic amounts. It comes as no surprise that positive predictors, based solely on in vitro data, often fail to correlate well with observed clinical responses. It is therefore necessary to include patient factors in any predictive equation, if positive responses are expected. Conversely, predictions of clinical nonresponsiveness are easier to make. If tumor cells show inherent resistance to a drug, then the other host factors do not matter, and nonresponsiveness to treatment will result. Extreme drug resistance is an extension of the inherent drug resistance observation, when resistance is still apparent when drugs are tested at levels up to 100 times the achievable peak plasma level (21).

Application of chemosensitivity testing to ovarian cancer therapy has been done in several institutions. A protocol was designed at Bowman Gray School of Medicine to enroll patients with advanced ovarian cancers who had not received any prior chemotherapy. Tumor was sent to the laboratory at the time of initial debulking surgery. A panel of ten drugs, each tested individually, was used to screen the tumor cells. When the assay results were available, patients were randomized to receive either standard cyclophosphamide, doxorubicin, cisplatin (CAP) therapy or the best three drugs determined by the chemosensitivity test results. Dose intensity was adjusted for each patient, in an attempt to equalize potential toxicity among the patients receiving CAP versus those receiving the "best three drugs." Patient accrual to the study was slower than desired, and the study was closed before the desired number of patients had been entered. Sixty-five patients were finally evaluable: 34 were randomized to receive CAP, and 31 received the best three drugs. The combined complete response plus partial response rates for CAP was 68% and for the best three drugs was 81% (not a statistically significant difference). The median survival duration for CAP was 17 months and for the best three drugs was 30 months ($p < .05$) (37). In order to separate out the impact of individual patient factors on responses and survival duration, much larger sample sizes would be required. Certainly, patients who have individualized drug selection fare no worse than those who have empiric protocol therapy. Whether there is enough benefit to warrant the costs of chemosensitivity testing for every patient is not yet clear.

A group of investigators in San Antonio, Texas, published their experience with results of drug selection by chemosensitivity testing versus clinicians' choice of drugs (38). Their series enrolled 133 patients with advanced and/or recurrent solid tumors of many types, including 6 who had ovarian cancers. They were divided randomly into two groups, 65 patients to receive the clinicians' choice of chemotherapy and 68 to receive the best drug based on chemosensitivity testing. Owing to the advanced nature of these patients' tumors, only 36 of the 65 patients randomized to receive clinicians' choice actually got any chemotherapy. One of the 36 had a partial response noted (3% response rate). Of the 68 patients randomized to receive the best drug from the in vitro assay, only 19 ever received any chemotherapy, 4 of whom had partial responses (21% response rate). Survival durations calculated for the two groups showed no significant difference. The advanced stage of these patients and the fact that well over one-half of the patients were unable to receive any therapy make the group a difficult one for evaluation of a predictive chemosensitivity assay (38).

Limited numbers of laboratories have the capability to perform accurate and reproducible chemosensitivity assays. Is it logistically possible to use centralized laboratories and to transport tumors to such facilities for testing? The Southwest Oncology Group (SWOG) has published a study of the results of using centralized laboratories for cell cloning studies in Tucson, Arizona, and San Antonio, Texas (39). Thirty-three institutions collaborated by shipping tumor samples from 211 patients who had advanced and/or recurrent ovarian cancers. One hundred sixty-eight of these patients had failed extensive prior chemotherapy. If the tumor sample grew in culture and did show sensitivity to one or more chemotherapeutic agents, the patient was treated according to the laboratory guidance. Of 23 such patients, 4 experienced complete responses, and 1 a partial response (total 28% complete plus partial response). The group of 101 patients whose tumors either did not form colonies in vitro or did not have any identifiable active drugs had the clinicians' choice for therapy. In this group, three patients experienced a complete response, and seven a partial response (total 11% complete plus partial response). Median survival was not different between the two groups, reported at 6.25 months versus 7 months. Of note is the fact that 44 patients of the 168 never received any chemotherapy because of rapid deterioration of their physical condition.

A separate group of 43 patients reported in this study had not received any chemotherapy prior to the cloning assay. Only 17 of this group had evaluable cloning assays. All received standard combination chemotherapy with cisplatin-based regimens. Correlations with laboratory predictions and clinical responses were 100% prediction of positive responses and 100% prediction of negative responses (39).

CURRENT STATUS OF IN VITRO DRUG TESTING

What can we conclude concerning in vitro cloning assays and the usefulness of these techniques in clinical oncology? Interest in in vitro testing of chemotherapeutic agents goes back more than 30 years, yet there still is neither widespread acceptance of a superior method nor agreement that such tests are useful at all. One area that is generally accepted as useful is the new drug development area. Reports of preclinical drug screening continue to be published, mostly using established cell lines rather than primary tumor specimens. Future application of this technology to new drug evaluation seems certain.

What about clinical application of *in vitro* testing to protocol design, to the selection of phase II drugs, or to individualized treatment planning for patients? At least three problems become obvious in the review of published literature.

1. Technical problems with the assay have prevented growth of some specimens. The SWOG trial had only 44% of specimens with evaluable *in vitro* growth. This may be related in part to the fact that most of these specimens were transported by overnight delivery from hospitals remote from the two central laboratories (39). Technical problems such as this are being addressed. The growth rate of ovarian tumor specimens in some laboratories has recently been increased to a range of 70% to 85% (40). Such an increase in predictable growth rate makes performance of clinical studies much more attractive.

2. A lack of effective chemotherapeutic drugs for recurrent solid tumors makes chemosensitivity testing difficult. If it were likely that an effective drug could be identified for each patient whose tumor

cells were tested in vitro, great interest in testing every patient's tumor would be forthcoming. However, historical clinical experience suggests that most drugs used as salvage chemotherapy for recurrent ovarian cancer will result in less than 20% response probability. With the low activity of available drugs, clinical nonresponsiveness is more likely to be predicted than response. From a practical standpoint, do clinical oncologists want to know predictions of sensitivity or of resistance? Both predictions are useful, but knowing what drug might work is better than knowing what drugs to avoid. The prediction of resistance to drugs, even to the point of extreme drug resistance, is more accurate than the prediction of sensitivity. Until better chemotherapeutic agents are available, the probability of identifying effective chemotherapeutic drugs will not increase.

3. Interpretation of most clinically related studies must include an appreciation of the type of patients entered. For example, in the SWOG multi-institutional study of 168 patients with recurrent ovarian cancers, 44 patients never received any chemotherapy because of their rapidly deteriorating physical conditions. Median survival of the responding patients was only 6 to 7 months (39). In Von Hoff and colleagues' study comparing drug selection by clinicians' choice versus the cloning assay data, only 55 of 133 patients were ever treated as per protocol design (38). For many reasons, the patients who were chosen to test the hypothesis that chemosensitivity testing may be beneficial were not the optimal ones.

FUTURE DIRECTIONS

Investigation that defines prognostic indicators or predictive tests goes forward on the premise that such information will permit therapeutic intervention that will make a difference in ultimate responses to therapy. When we evaluate clinical applications of chemosensitivity testing, perhaps an improved response rate can be observed. However, most of the clinical trials have shown statistically insignificant changes in survival duration when therapy based on cloning assays is compared to empirically selected drugs.

Where then, is the place of predictive cloning assays in clinical oncology? Perhaps there is some clinical usefulness to predicting extreme drug resistance, certainly for those patients who are considering high-dose therapy. Otherwise, the definitive study—comparing a standard multidrug regimen with a multidrug regimen selected by individualized cloning assays—still remains to be done. Until that study is available, the technology of in vitro drug testing will probably best be left to preclinical areas such as evaluating new drugs for antitumor activity.

The idea of predictive drug screening is remarkably persistent. This suggests that the concept is logical, but still plagued by technical problems and the lack of effective drugs to test. Work will undoubtedly continue in many laboratories toward improving the technology and demonstrating the clinical usefulness of the tests. It is hoped that improved drug development in the future will result in better in vitro and in vivo results.

REFERENCES

1. Hall TC. *Prediction of response in cancer therapy*. National Cancer Institute Monograph 34; 1971.
2. Salmon SE, Hamburger AW, Soehnlen B, Durie BGM, Alberts DS, Moon TE. Quantitation of differential sensitivity of human tumor stem cells to anticancer drugs. *N Engl J Med* 1978;298:1321–1327.
3. Selby P, Buick RN, Tannock I. A critical appraisal of the "human tumor stem-cell assay." *N Engl J Med* 1988;308:129–134.
4. Von Hoff DD. He's not going to talk about in vitro predictive assays again, is he? *J Natl Cancer Inst* 1990;82:96–101.
5. Sondak VK, Bertelsen CA, Tanigawa N, et al. Clinical correlation with chemosensitivities measured in a rapid thymidine incorporation assay. *Cancer Res* 1984;44:1725–1728.
6. Von Hoff DD, Forseth BJ, Huong M, et al. Improved plating efficiencies for human tumors cloned in capillary tubes versus petri dishes. *Cancer Res* 1986;46:4012–4017.
7. Baker FL, Spitzer G, Agani JA, et al. Drug and radiation sensitivity measurements of successful primary monolayer culturing of human tumor cells using cell-adhesive matrix and supplemental medium. *Cancer Res* 1986;46:1263–1274.
8. Weisenthal LM, Dill PL, Kurnick NB, et al. Comparison of dye exclusion assay with a clonogenic assay in the determination of drug-induced cytotoxicity. *Cancer Res* 1983;43:258–264.
9. Khoo SK, Hurst T, Webb MJ, Mackay EV. Short-term in vitro chemosensitivity testing of tumours of the ovary, cervix and uterus. *Aust N Z J Obstet Gynaecol* 1986;26:288–294.
10. Garewal HS, Ahmann FR, Schifman RB, et al. ATP assay: ability to distinguish cytostatic from cytocidal anticancer drug effects. *J Natl Cancer Inst* 1986;77:1039–1045.
11. Rotman B, Teplitz C, Dickinson K, Cozzolino JP. Individual human tumors in short-term micro-organ cultures: chemosensitivity testing by fluorescent cytoprinting. *In Vitro Cell Dev Biol* 1988;24:1137–1146.
12. DeVita VT, Oliverio VT, Muggia FM, et al. The drug development and clinical trials programs of the Division of Cancer Treatment, National Cancer Institute. *Cancer Clin Trials* 1979;2:195–216.
13. Shoemaker RH, Wolpert-DeFilippes MK, Kern DH, et al. Application of a human tumor colony-forming assay to new drug screening. *Cancer Res* 1985;45:2145–2153.
14. Sheithauser W, Clark GM, Salmon SE, Dorda W, Shoemaker RH, Von Hoff DD. Model for estimation of clinically achievable plasma concentrations for investigational anticancer drugs in man. *Cancer Treat Rep* 1986;70:1379–1382.
15. Marsh JC, Shoemaker RH, Salmon SE, Kern DH, Venditti JM. Relationship between in vitro tumor stem cell assay and in vivo antitumor activity using the P388 leukemia. *Int J Cell Cloning* 1988;6:60–68.
16. Taetle R, Abramson I. Drug screening and biological systems. *J Natl Cancer Inst* 1988;80:720–721.
17. Berens ME, Saito T, Welander CE, Modest EJ. Antitumor activity of new anthracycline analogues in combination with interferon alfa. *Cancer Chemother Pharmacol* 1987;19:301–306.
18. Takasugi BJ, Salmon SE, Nelson RL, Young L, Liu RM. Antitumor activity of vinzolidine in the human tumor clonogenic assay

and comparison with vinblastine. *Invest New Drugs* 1984;2:49–53.
19. Ridgway H, Stewart DP, Michaelis N, Guthrie MJ, Speer RJ. Successful screening of platinum complexes as potential antitumor agents with an L1210 clonogenic assay. *J Clin Hematol Oncol* 1984;14(1):1–7.
20. Alberts DS, Salmon SE, Chen H-SG, Moon TE, Young L, Surwit EA. Pharmacologic studies of anticancer drugs with the human tumor stem cell assay. *Cancer Chemother Pharmacol* 1981;6:253–264.
21. Kern DH, Weisenthal LM. Highly specific prediction of antineoplastic drug resistance with an in vitro assay using suprapharmacologic drug exposures. *J Natl Cancer Inst* 1990;82:582–588.
22. Deffie AM, Alam T, Senevirante C, et al. Multifactorial resistance to Adriamycin: relationship of DNA repair, glutathione transferase activity, drug efflux and *p*-glycoprotein in cloned cell lines of Adriamycin-sensitive and resistant P-388 leukemia. *Cancer Res* 1988;48:3595–3602.
23. Keizer HG, Schuurhuis GJ, Broxterman HJ, et al. Correlation of multidrug resistance with decreased drug accumulation, altered subcellular drug distribution, and increased *p*-glycoprotein expression in cultured SW-1573 human lung tumor cells. *Cancer Res* 1989;49:2988–2993.
24. Von Hoff DD, Clark GM, Weiss GR, et al. Use of in vitro dose response effects to select antineoplastics for high-dose or regional administration regimens. *J Clin Oncol* 1986;4:1827–1834.
25. Jones RB, Myers CE, Guarino AM, Dedrick RL, Hubbard SM, DeVita VT. High volume intraperitoneal chemotherapy ("belly bath") for ovarian cancer. *Cancer Chemother Pharmacol* 1978;1:161–166.
26. Markman M. Intraperitoneal chemotherapy as treatment of ovarian carcinoma: why, how, and when? *Obstet Gynecol Surv* 1987;42:533–539.
27. Welander CE, Morgan TM, Homesley HD, Trotta PP, Spiegel RJ. Combined recombinant human interferon alpha$_2$ and cytotoxic agents studied in a clonogenic assay. *Int J Cancer* 1985;35:721–729.
28. Valeriote F, Lin H. Synergistic interaction of anticancer agents: a cellular perspective. *Cancer Chemother Rep* 1975;59:895–900.
29. Momparler RL. In vitro systems for evaluation of combination chemotherapy. *Pharmacol Ther* 1980;8:21–35.
30. Saito T, Berens ME, Welander CE. Interferon-gamma and cytotoxic agents studied in combination using a soft agarose human tumor clonogenic assay. *Cancer Chemother Pharmacol* 1987;19:233–239.
31. Higashihara J, Saito T, Berens ME, Welander CE. Effects of scheduling and ascites-associated macrophages on combined antiproliferative activity of alpha-2b interferon and gamma-interferon in a clonogenic assay. *Cancer Chemother Pharmacol* 1988;22:215–222.
32. Alberts DS, Chen H-SG, Soehnlen B, Salmon S, Surwit EA, Young L. In vitro clonogenic assay for predicting response of ovarian cancer to chemotherapy. *Lancet* 1980;2:340–342.
33. Natale RB, Kushner B. Applications of the human tumor cloning assay to ovarian cancer. *Proc Amer Assoc Cancer Res* 1981;22:156.
34. Wilson AP, Neal FE. In vitro sensitivity of human ovarian tumors to chemotherapeutic agents. *Br J Cancer* 1981;44:189–200.
35. Welander CE, Homesley HD, Jobson VW. In vitro chemotherapy testing of gynecologic tumors: basis for planning therapy? *Am J Obstet Gynecol* 1983;147:188–195.
36. Arbuck SG, Pavelic ZP, Piver MS, et al. Limitations of drug sensitivity testing in soft agar for clinical management of patients with ovarian carcinoma. *Obstet Gynecol* 1985;66:115–120.
37. Welander CE. Predicting response to chemotherapy with a clonogenic assay. In: Sharp F, Soutter WP, eds. *Ovarian cancer—the way ahead*. London: The Chameleon Press Ltd, 1987;175–186.
38. Von Hoff DD, Sandbach JF, Clark GM, et al. Selection of cancer chemotherapy for a patient by an in vitro assay versus a clinician. *J Natl Cancer Inst* 1990;82(2):110–124.
39. Von Hoff DD, Kronmal R, Salmon SE, et al. A Southwest Oncology Group study on the use of a human tumor cloning assay for predicting response in patients with ovarian cancer. *Cancer* 1991;67:20–27.
40. Welander CE. The human tumor clonogenic assay used to study ovarian cancers. In: Alberts DS, Surwit EA, eds. *Ovarian cancers*. Boston: Martinis Nijhoff, 1985;37–52.

CHAPTER 18

Dose Intensity in the Treatment of Ovarian Carcinoma

Leslie Levin

Basic pharmacological and biological principles imply that the dose of chemotherapy delivered per unit time is likely to be an important consideration in determining treatment outcome. This is implied because maximum cell-kill is a function of adequate drug dose (1) and the interval between treatments to prevent cell regrowth. The term *dose intensity* (DI) is used to define drug dose delivered per unit time and is expressed as mg/m^2 body surface area per week. This concept has been intuitively applied to most chemotherapy regimens in which sequential courses are often administered as close together as drug-induced toxicity allows. Although drug dose is unquestionably important in determining the response to chemotherapy (1), the impact of dose intensity has only recently been analyzed for a number of tumor sites (2–7).

THE CALCULATION OF DOSE INTENSITY

A standard regimen is first selected for calculating DI. The DI of a drug in a particular regimen is expressed as a fraction of the DI for the same drug in the standard regimen; this fraction is called the *relative dose intensity* (RDI) for that particular drug (i.e., relative to the DI of the same drug in the standard regimen). The sum of the RDIs of the drugs in the regimen being analyzed, divided by the number of drugs in the standard regimen, is referred to as the *average dose intensity* (ADI) for the entire regimen. Regimens incorporating only one or more of the drugs used in the standard regimen can be analyzed within this type of metaanalysis. Furthermore, for the purpose of calculating the ADI of a regimen containing less than the number of drugs in a standard regimen, the missing drugs are assigned an RDI of 0.

Table 1 provides an example of the calculation of RDIs and ADIs for drug regimens using one or more of the following drugs: cyclophosphamide (C), hexamethylmelamine (H), doxorubicin (A), and cisplatin (P). The DI for each drug appears in the first column and for the standard regimen in the second column. The RDI for each drug appears in the third column and is obtained by dividing the DI for the drug in the regimen being analyzed by the DI for the same drug in the standard regimen. If one of the drugs in the regimen being analyzed is missing, a DI of 0 is assigned to that particular drug so that the RDI also becomes 0. The ADI for the regimen is calculated as the sum of the RDIs divided by the number of drugs in the standard regimen (in this case, 4).

PROJECTED VERSUS RECEIVED DI

Many of the earlier DI analyses were retrospective and therefore evaluated the effect of *projected* DI (i.e., drug dose called for in the protocol) as opposed to the *received* DI (i.e., drug dose actually received by the patients). Because of the variation in *received* DI owing to the unpredictability of toxic side effects requiring dose adjustments, a poor correlation between *projected* DI and outcome is anticipated. Therefore, a statistically significant correlation between *projected* DI and outcome would probably give rise to a more highly significant correlation between *received* DI and outcome.

The calculation of *received* DI is slightly different from that of *projected* DI (8) because it entails a summation and averaging of *each patient's* RDI and takes

---

L. Levin: Department of Oncology, University of Western Ontario, and London Regional Cancer Centre, Canada. Ontario, Canada N6A 4L6

TABLE 1. Calculation of relative and average dose intensity

	Dose intensity (DI) of drug regimen being analyzed (mg/m²/week)[a]	Dose intensity (DI) of standard regimen (mg/m²/week)	Relative dose intensity (RDI)
C[b]	a	a'	a/a'
H	b	b'	b/b'
A	c	c'	c/c'
P	d	d'	d/d'

$$\text{Average dose intensity (ADI)} = \frac{\frac{a}{a'} + \frac{b}{b'} + \frac{c}{c'} + \frac{d}{d'}}{4}$$

[a] Where a drug is missing from the regimen, a DI of 0 is assigned to the drug.
[b] C, cyclophosphamide; H, hexamethylmelamine; A, doxorubicin; P, cisplatin.

treatment delays into account. Individual RDIs are then averaged for the entire study population. A minimum number of received cycles of chemotherapy for each patient analyzed is established so that patients who receive fewer than the acceptable number of cycles are excluded from analysis.

METHODOLOGICAL CONSIDERATIONS OF RETROSPECTIVE ANALYSIS

In an analysis of retrospective studies, it is important to characterize clearly those studies which are eligible for analysis so that known prognostic variables are kept as constant as possible. Ideally, prospectively randomized studies should be analyzed, to minimize investigator bias within reported studies.

DOSE INTENSITY CONSIDERATIONS IN OVARIAN CARCINOMA

Ovarian carcinoma is a moderately chemosensitive tumor and has therefore been the focus of many studies to optimize treatment outcome. The plethora of clinical trials has produced diverse results and, especially with the introduction of drugs such as cisplatin, which have debilitating toxicities, has polarized treatment strategies. For many years, single alkylating agent chemotherapy was the mainstay of treatment for advanced ovarian carcinoma, with overall response rates of 60% but with little impact on median survival time (average 10 months) because of the short duration of response. Nevertheless, treatment was easy to administer and well tolerated, interfering minimally with the patient's quality of life. The first evidence that cisplatin was effective in the treatment of advanced ovarian carcinoma gave rise to a spate of clinical trials incorporating low-dose and high-dose cisplatin with and without other drugs such as cyclophosphamide, doxorubicin, and hexamethylmelamine. Although doses used ranged between 20 mg/m² and 200 mg/m² every 3 to 4 weeks, it is important to note that the effective dose of cisplatin for other disease sites was established at 100 mg/m² every 3 to 4 weeks; few, if any, deviated from this dose whether it was used alone or in combination with other drugs. Overviews and intertrial comparisons in ovarian carcinoma often ignored these dose differences, so neither prognostic variables nor drug doses were standardized for the purpose of these comparisons. It is therefore not surprising that intertrial comparisons have often given rise to inconsistent conclusions.

It was against this background that Levin and Hryniuk (5,7) attempted to evaluate the contribution of various drugs to clinical response and survival in advanced ovarian carcinoma, employing dose intensity calculations in a metaanalysis of published prospective randomized studies incorporating one or more of the drugs cyclophosphamide, hexamethylmelamine, doxorubicin, and cisplatin (CHAP) and no other drugs. Their analysis enabled an evaluation of the contribution of each drug to outcome through intergroup analysis, while attempting to keep prognostic variables constant.

THE OVARIAN CANCER DI ANALYSIS

The RDIs and ADIs for studies fulfilling criteria set out in the following paragraph were calculated using a standard CHAP regimen described by Greco et al. (5,9). For this analysis, all alkylating agent doses were converted to cyclophosphamide equivalents (5) and are referred to here as *cyclophosphamide*.

Selection of Studies for DI Analysis

Prognostic variables were kept as constant as possible in this DI analysis. Only those studies that fit the following criteria were analyzed: (A) Only one or more of the drugs cyclophosphamide, hexamethylmelamine, doxorubicin, and cisplatin had been used; (B) patients had been prospectively randomized between two or more treatment arms; (C) only stage III and IV ovarian carcinomas of epithelial origin had been treated; (D) no patients had had previous chemotherapy; (E) no more than 20% of patients had received previous radiotherapy; and (F) more than 65% of patients had ≥2 cm residual disease at the beginning of treatment. Histologic grade was ≥2 in 70% of patients in 48 study groups in which this was reported.

Results of the DI Analysis

Average DI correlated with clinical response (Fig. 1) and median survival time. The received DI from an NCIC clinical trial evaluating the efficacy of cisplatin and doxorubicin is also shown as asterisks in Fig. 1 and lies on the left shoulder of the curve. Received DI lies on the left shoulder of the projected DI curve because the plot of projected DI overestimates the amount of drug that is actually received by the patient; dose reductions are required for toxicity, so the received DI is less than the projected DI for a given response.

Performance status was described in 11 of the studies analyzed and in each, all patients were ECOG level 0–2. A plot of ADI versus median survival for these 11 studies with comparable performance status is shown in Fig. 2—the correlation is still significant, indicating that differences in performance status could not account for correlations found between DI and clinical response rates or survival in the larger analysis.

Although a significant correlation has been found between RDI for single agent cyclophosphamide and clinical response (10), this correlation was not significant for cyclophosphamide within multiagent regimens (5). Data were insufficient to evaluate the correlation between the RDI for single agent doxorubicin and clinical response, but the RDI for doxorubicin within multiagent regimens failed to correlate with clinical response (5). Unlike the RDIs for cyclophosphamide and doxorubicin, however, the RDI for cisplatin, when used as a single agent or within multiagent regimens, correlated significantly with clinical response (Fig. 3) and median survival time. Furthermore, this correlation was also significant when cisplatin was employed as a second-line single agent; the ADI for cisplatin-containing multiagent second-line regimens also showed a significant correlation with clinical response (7) (Fig. 4).

A disproportionate contribution of cisplatin to outcome may have distorted any correlation between RDI and outcome for cyclophosphamide or doxorubicin within multiagent regimens. However, other possible reasons for the latter observation are discussed in the section dealing with ideal dosing of drugs active in ovarian carcinoma. *The DI analysis did not support the notion that adding cyclophosphamide, doxorubicin, or hexamethylmelamine to cisplatin was unnecessary.* Indeed, for any fixed RDI for cisplatin, clinical response is greater when other drugs are added to cisplatin than when cisplatin is used as a single agent (10). This is substantiated by a large prospective randomized study

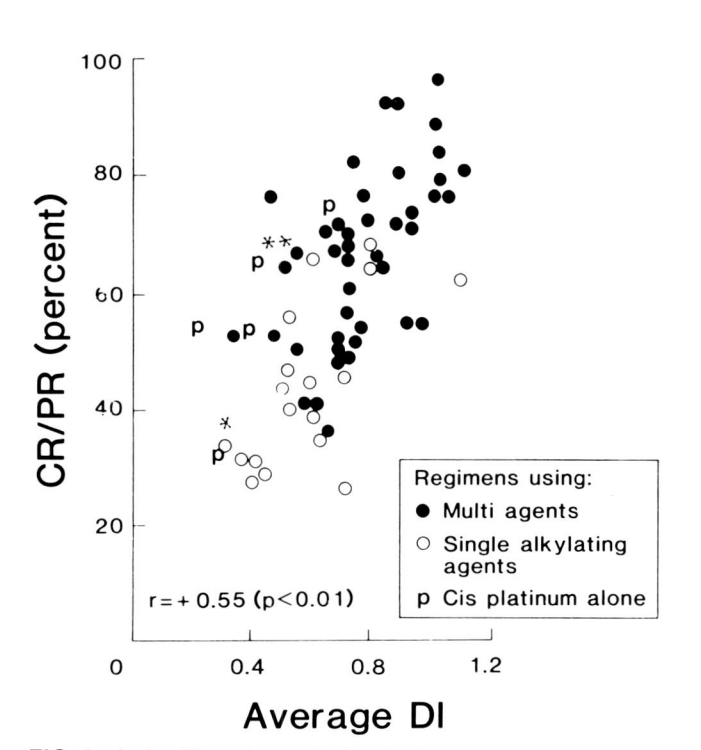

FIG. 1. A significant correlation is demonstrated between average DI and overall clinical response rates. Asterisks represent three ranges for *received* DI in a prospective NCIC study. Reprinted with permission of the W. B. Saunders Company.

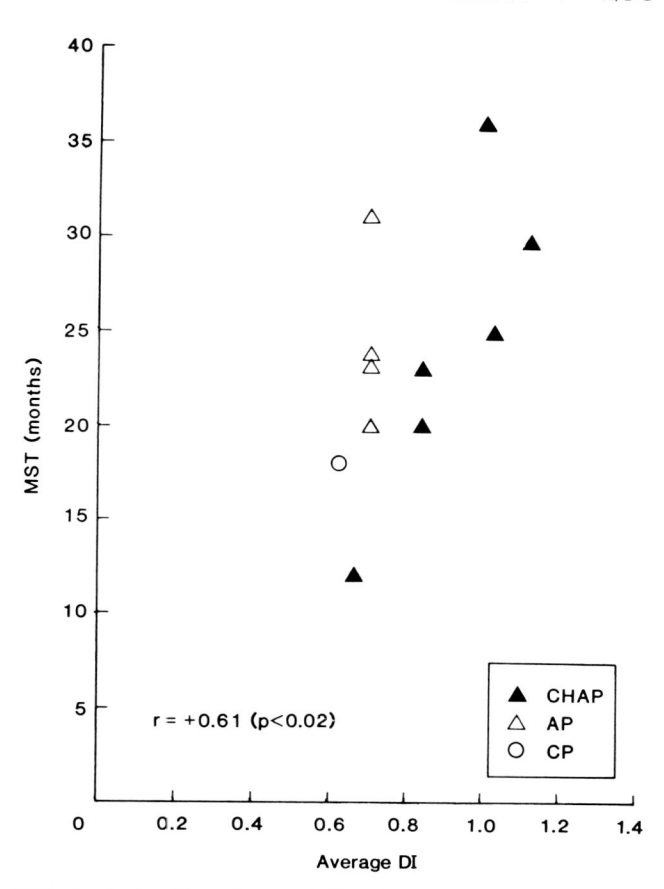

FIG. 2. A significant correlation between average DI and median survival is demonstrated for studies in which it was possible to standardize for performance status. Reprinted with permission of the W. B. Saunders Company.

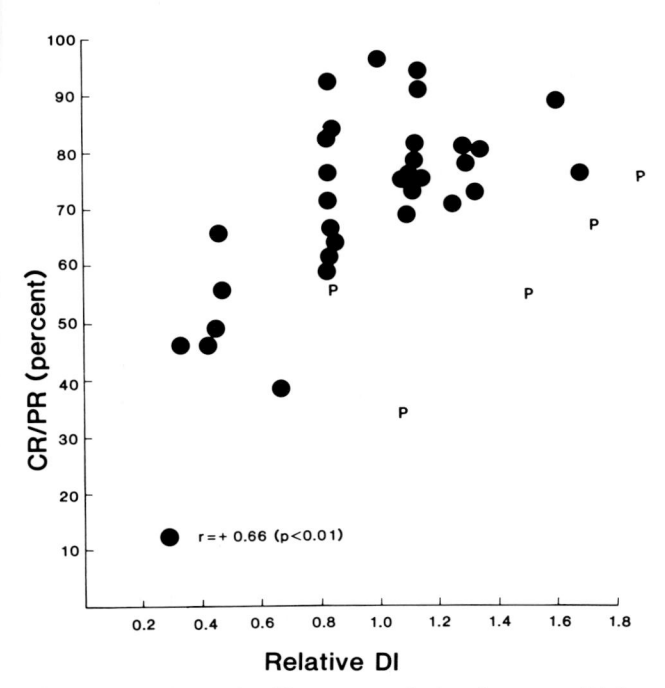

FIG. 3. There is a significant correlation between DI for cisplatin, (P) within multiagent regimens or when used alone. These data indicate that a higher relative DI for P is required to achieve a clinical response if P is used as a single agent rather than with a multiagent regimen. Reprinted with permission of the W. B. Saunders Company.

(11) in which the clinical response was significantly improved when cyclophosphamide and doxorubicin were added to cisplatin. In this study, the dose of cisplatin was fixed in all three arms.

From these observations it appears that within the limits of the RDIs so far tested, the ideal chemotherapy regimen in ovarian carcinoma is one that incorporates at least cyclophosphamide, doxorubicin, and cisplatin, with special consideration given to the RDI for cisplatin. Another important finding from the DI analysis was the observation that clinical response rates and median survival times were superior for cisplatin-containing multiagent regimens than for non–cisplatin-containing multiagent regimens or single alkylating agents in low, intermediate, and high ADI ranges (Fig. 5).

THE IDEAL DOSE OF DRUGS ACTIVE IN OVARIAN CARCINOMA

Cisplatin

An extrapolation of the curve in Fig. 3 through the zero point supports the notion that the maximal contribution of RDI for cisplatin occurs between 0 and 1.0, if it is assumed that an RDI of 0 $mg/m^2/wk$ for cisplatin produces a clinical response of 0%. However, although the curve appears to be less steep for an RDI > 1.0, there is no evidence that the curve plateaus beyond this point.

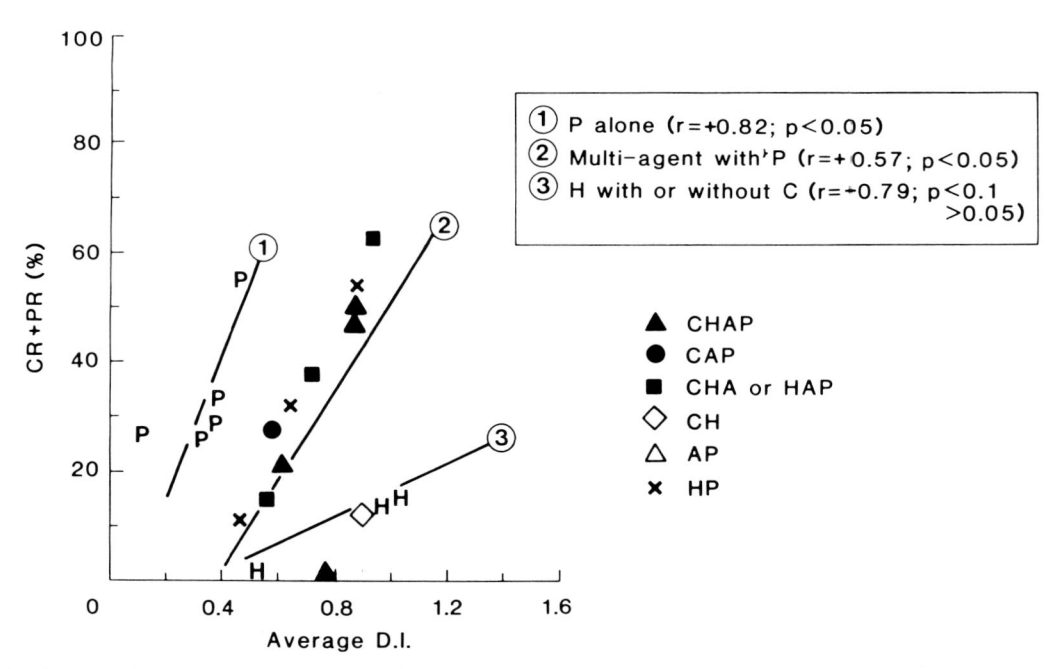

FIG. 4. A correlation between average DI and response was present only in cisplatin-containing regimens, probably reflecting the important contribution of RDI for cisplatin on outcome. Reprinted with permission of the W. B. Saunders Company.

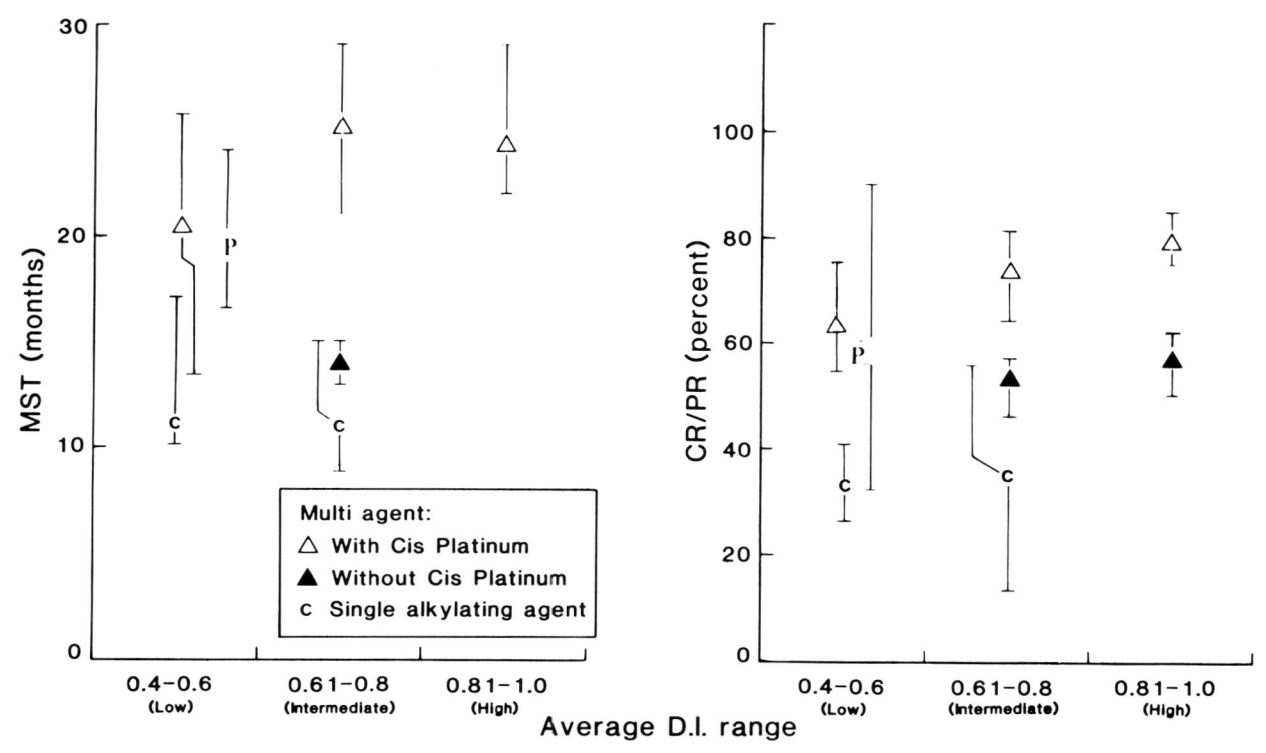

FIG. 5. For all ranges, median survival MST and complete response/partial response CR/PR were superior for cisplatin regimens than for noncisplatin regimens. Reprinted with permission of the W. B. Saunders Company.

Many studies have attempted to use cisplatin and carboplatin at very high doses. The DI analysis predicts lower efficacy, however, at doses on the shallow slope of the DI curve. Nevertheless, very high dose cisplatin and carboplatin used in refractory ovarian cancer patients have demonstrated benefit (12,13). The use of hypertonic saline to reduce cisplatin-associated nephrotoxicity (14), the use of an ACTH analogue to limit cisplatin-induced neurotoxicity (15), and the more effective control of emesis have enabled higher doses of cisplatin to be used in clinical trials.

A realistic and reasonable received dose of cisplatin within multiagent regimens is probably predicated upon schedule and total dose delivered. Appropriate scheduling for cisplatin is important if it reduces toxicity (16) and, in doing so, increases the *received* DI. However, certain drug-related toxicities appear to be independent of schedule; for example, the relationship between total dose of cisplatin may be more important than schedule in producing cisplatin-induced neurotoxicity (17).

Given the preceding considerations, an ideal RDI for cisplatin within multiagent regimens should be taken from the steep segment of the DI curve shown in Fig. 3. For multiagent regimens, an RDI for cisplatin 25 mg/m^2/week would be a reasonable upper limit to test in the first instance. The DI analysis demonstrates the desirability of adding other active drugs to platinum agents, so it is important to select a dose of cisplatin at the upper limit of the *steep portion* of the DI curve, which would maximize response and allow for incorporation of other drugs at higher RDIs than could be achieved if higher, less effective RDIs for cisplatin were used.

Carboplatin

Evidence shows that carboplatin is as effective as cisplatin when used as a front-line drug in the treatment of ovarian carcinoma (18). One of the limiting factors in the use of carboplatin within multiagent regimens, however, is its potent myelosuppressive effect. Therefore, if drugs such as doxorubicin, cyclophosphamide, hexamethylmelamine, and/or taxol are to be employed in front-line multiagent regimens in ovarian carcinoma, cisplatin is preferable at a dose unlikely to produce significant myelosuppression. Carboplatin should then be reserved as a second line single agent.

Relatively low dose carboplatin has also been used in combination with lower doses of cisplatin in front-line regimens to maximize the dose of platinum while reducing toxicity. Maximizing the efficacy of carboplatin by taking the area under the curve into account, adjusted for by measuring the glomerular filtration rate (19), is a refinement on drug delivery as defined by dose intensity.

The use of autologous bone marrow transplantation and/or biological response modifiers may allow for the use of high-dose carboplatin with other myelosuppressive drugs, but the cost of this approach would limit its routine application.

Cyclophosphamide and Other Alkylating Agents

The DI analysis for multiagent regimens in ovarian carcinoma provided no evidence to support a relationship between the RDI for cyclophosphamide and outcome. There are two possible explanations for this. First, cisplatin may have contributed disproportionately to outcome when compared to cyclophosphamide (or doxorubicin or hexamethylmelamine), possibly obscuring the DI effect for the latter drugs. Second, although RDIs for cisplatin within multiagent regimens were similar to the RDIs for cisplatin used as a single agent, this was not true for alkylating agents. Doses of single agent cyclophosphamide that produced a 30–60% clinical response rate (RDI > 2.0) have rarely been used with cisplatin-containing multiagent regimens. It is therefore possible that within multiagent regimens, *the RDI range for cyclophosphamide was not wide enough and the doses of cyclophosphamide were not high enough to test for the relationship between RDI for cyclophosphamide and clinical response*. This concept of threshold dose intensity is discussed elsewhere (20) as it relates to the DI for vincristine within multiagent regimens in breast cancer.

Doxorubicin

Although the RDI for doxorubicin within multiagent regimens does not correlate with outcome, doses used in most studies were within the lower dose echelons for this drug, and the RDI range tested was small. The dose of doxorubicin used in multiagent regimens may therefore not have exceeded the threshold DI for this drug, beyond which a relationship between RDI and outcome might have become apparent.

Hexamethylmelamine

No comment can be made regarding the efficacy of this drug within multiagent regimens based on the DI analysis because there was almost no variation in the dose within studies that incorporated this drug.

Taxol and Other New Drugs

The DI analysis demonstrates the need to establish the most effective dose that can be administered per unit time for drugs with established efficacy in ovarian carcinoma. The same concern holds true for drugs undergoing phase I and II testing; an evaluation for a threshold DI within multiagent regimens is an important consideration when designing trials. A reduction in the effective dose of new drugs incorporated in multiagent regimens is usually necessary to reduce overlapping toxicities. However, there is an inherent risk of reducing any advantage for new drugs incorporated in multiagent regimens if the DI for the drug within regimens is not adequately tested.

CONFOUNDING ISSUES IN DI ANALYSIS

The Effect of Scheduling

As alluded to earlier in this chapter, scheduling may be important as it affects received DI, because schedules producing less toxicity are likely to result in higher received DIs. For example, whereas it was previously reported that scheduling of methotrexate on L1210 leukemia in mice affected outcome (21), further analysis revealed that the twice weekly schedule was better tolerated by the mice than the daily schedule. As a result, a fourfold greater DI could be administered (22). This effect of scheduling also seems to apply to humans. For example, administering cisplatin at 40 $mg/m^2/day$ for 5 consecutive days produced more toxicity than a schedule of 100 mg/m^2 on days 1 and 8 of each cycle, possibly owing to less accumulation of the ultrafiltrable plasma platinum when the latter regimen was employed (16). Administering lower doses of doxorubicin and cisplatin at more frequent intervals may also produce less toxicity than administering single large doses at less frequent intervals (22,23).

The effect of scheduling and circadian rhythms on outcome has been reported (24–26). Although it is claimed that circadian rhythms may influence activation, distribution and disposition of drugs, and sensitivity of normal tissues (24), no controlled studies have investigated this phenomenon, and its application should therefore be regarded as investigational at this time. Nevertheless, if it is established that doxorubicin and cisplatin produce different toxicities at the same DI when circadian rhythm is taken into account, this would affect *received* DI and total dose of drug delivered.

The Effect of Total Dose

Dose intensity analysis cannot differentiate between the relative effect of total dose delivered and drug dose delivery per unit time, especially because studies using higher DIs are likely to be associated with higher total doses of drugs delivered. The importance of distin-

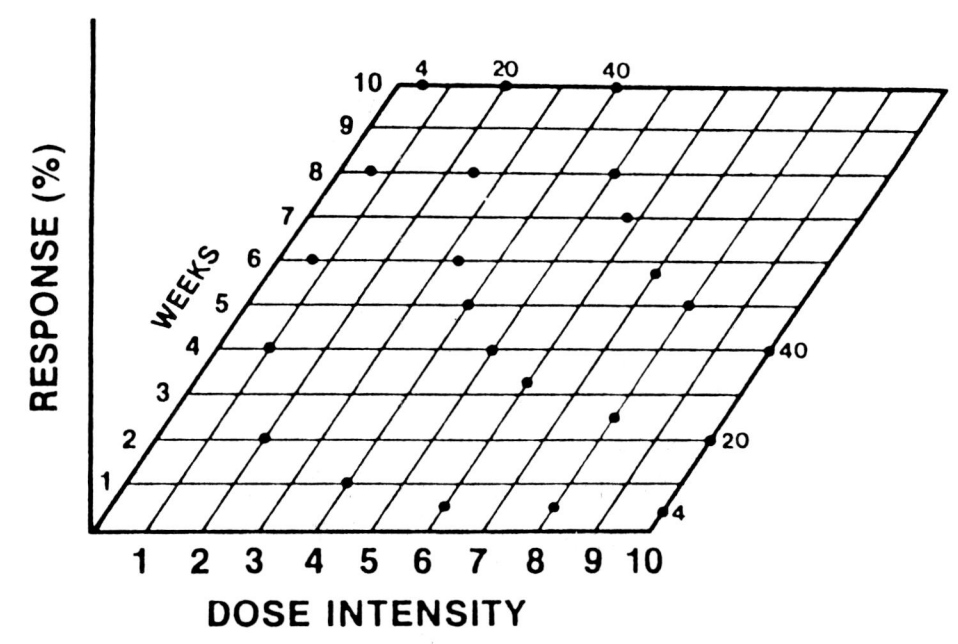

FIG. 6. Each point represents a fixed total dose for drug X of 4, 20, or 40 units but at different schedules. Reprinted with permission of the J. B. Lippincott Company.

guishing between the relative impact of total dose versus dose per unit time on outcome has been discussed hypothetically by Hryniuk (20) as shown in Figs. 6, 7, and 8. In Fig. 6, the total dose of drug X is 4, 20, or 40 units. This total dose can be administered over variable times but for the same total dose, thereby producing a different range of DIs for each total dose.

If total dose alone is the key factor in determining outcome, the same percentage response will be anticipated irrespective of the duration over which the total

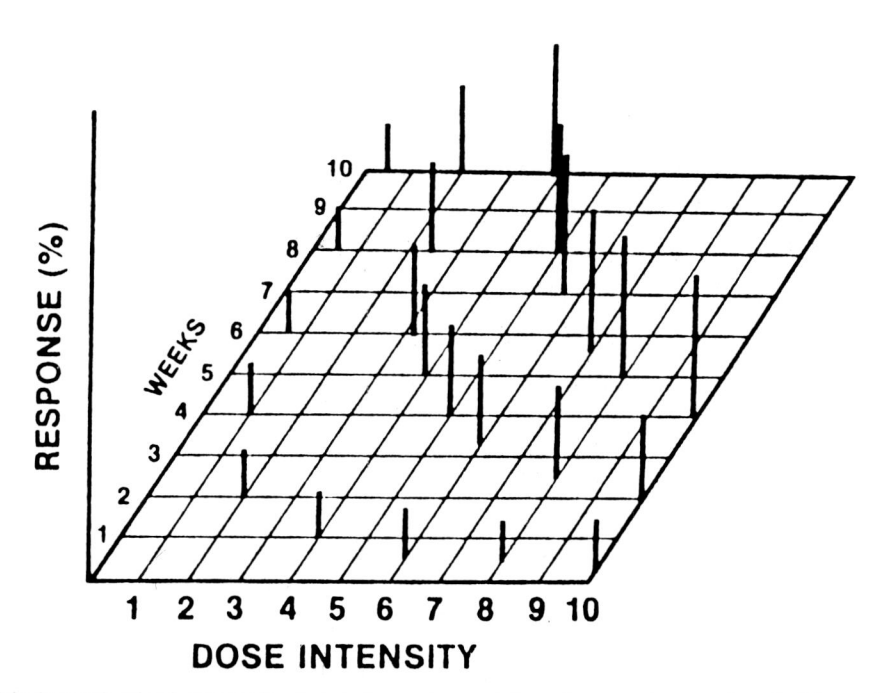

FIG. 7. In this hypothetical example, *total dose* alone determines outcome for 4, 20, or 40 units: the higher the total dose, the better the response. Of note, if response is read for points along the x-axis, it *appears* that dose intensity is responsible for improved responses, whereas in fact total dose is. Reprinted with permission of the J. B. Lippincott Company.

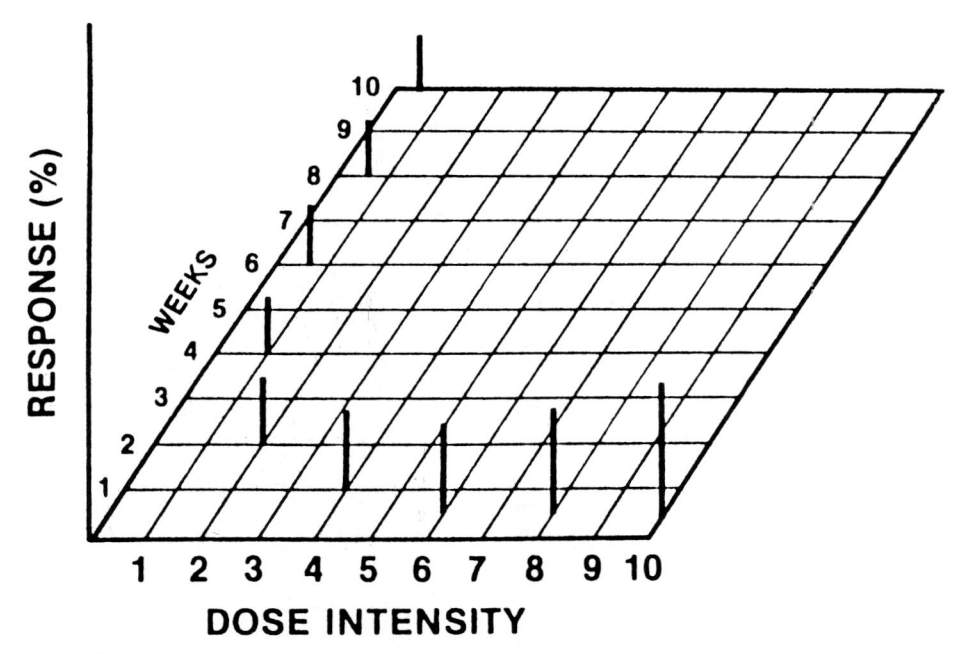

FIG. 8. In this hypothetical example, *dose intensity* determines outcome for a fixed total dose of drug X—here shown only for 4 units. Reprinted with permission of the J. B. Lippincott Company.

dose is delivered, as shown in Fig. 7. In this same figure, it appears that, in reading across the DI axis for any fixed duration of treatment, there is an increase in response rate. However, because the total dose for each point is different, this apparent increase in percentage response is merely fortuitous, and in this hypothetical example it is the total dose that governs the response.

If the duration over which a fixed total dose of chemotherapy is administered is the key factor determining outcome, an increase in response rate will be expected as the DI increases, despite maintaining a fixed total dose. This relationship is demonstrated in Fig. 8, in which only data for drug X in a total dose of 4 units are shown.

Number of Cycles of Chemotherapy Administered

The log cell-kill per cycle of chemotherapy delivered is predicated on the level of the tumor's chemosensitivity. In the case of exquisitely chemosensitive tumors, such as certain types of testicular cancer, only 4 cycles of chemotherapy may be required to eliminate all tumor cells, almost regardless of tumor size. Most oncologists regard ovarian carcinoma as only moderately chemosensitive to known cytotoxic drugs, and it seems unlikely that each cycle of effective chemotherapy will achieve more than a 2 log cell-kill. A 2 cm tumor nodule represents 10^8 to 10^9 cells, so in an ideal situation, 4 to 5 cycles of chemotherapy will be required to eliminate all tumor cells. Allowing for cell regrowth between cycles and treatment delays, one would expect at least 6 cycles of chemotherapy to be appropriate. Although the latter rule is conjectural, it emphasizes the importance of minimizing differences in numbers of cycles administered between two arms of studies when testing the validity of DI curves.

Apparent Versus True Drug Resistance

Drug resistance can be broadly divided into two types—apparent and true (27).

Apparent Drug Resistance

Apparent drug resistance applies to the impaired delivery of sufficient amounts of drugs to kill tumor cells effectively. Extracellular factors such as reduced blood supply (28) and hypoxemia (29) may interfere with the delivery of drugs to the tumor cells and cytotoxic efficacy. However, *inadequate drug concentration as a result of inadequate drug dosing is likely to be an important factor giving rise to apparent drug resistance.* This is the area of greatest concern in which DI may be operative.

True Drug Resistance

There are numerous examples of true drug resistance (27). *There are limits to dose intensification, beyond which no further benefits will occur because of cellular resistance to cytotoxic drugs*. The DI analysis can be used as a tool to define the relative contributions of various drugs within multiagent regimens and to identify the upper dose limits for drugs effectiveness. Beyond these points, true drug resistance is operative, or higher doses of drug are not possible because of unacceptable toxicity; other approaches to treatment need to be explored.

TESTING FOR DOSE INTENSITY

An argument could be made that because the DI analysis is a summary of numerous trials, validation of the analysis by prospectively testing DI response curves is not required. However, with the pitfalls of retrospective analysis and especially intertrial differences in hidden variables, prospective studies should be encouraged (A) to test the linear relationship between DI and outcome and (B) to define the range of doses to optimize outcome within acceptable limits of toxicity.

The relative contribution of total dose versus DI on outcome should be addressed in a three-arm study to test a DI response curve prospectively. In such a study, the RDIs and the ADIs should vary between two arms, but the number of cycles should remain fixed. This setup would test the original DI-response curve. In order to test whether differences between the two arms are due to differences in total dose delivered or to DI, a third arm would need to be introduced in which RDIs and the ADIs are the same as in the lower DI arm but the number of cycles is increased to produce the same total dose delivered as in the higher DI arm. If there are no differences between the high DI arm and the third arm in which total dose is the same, it may be concluded that *total* dose, and not DI, is responsible for any differences between the first two arms. However, if the high DI arm produces an improved outcome, it may indicate that *DI*, and not total dose, is responsible for differences between the first two arms.

Studies aimed at testing the DI-response curve should ensure that RDI and ADI levels selected fall within the limits of the original analysis. High DI arms should ideally be tested in a pilot study to ensure a close approximation between received and projected DIs by evaluating toxicity. Step-wise increments in RDIs and ADIs would hopefully identify the most effective chemotherapy combination.

CONCLUSIONS

Dose intensity metaanalysis is a useful tool for intertrial comparisons with respect to drug doses and the relative efficacy of individual drugs within multiagent regimens, as long as other known prognostic variables are evenly matched between studies. This type of analysis cannot differentiate between the relative contributions of DI and total dose delivered, however; the relative contributions can be tested only in appropriately designed clinical trials.

The ovarian carcinoma DI analysis supports the use of multiagent platinum-based chemotherapy with attention to an adequate RDI for platinum but with the realization that a threshold DI effect needs to be tested for cyclophosphamide and doxorubicin within these multiagent regimens.

REFERENCES

1. Frei E, Canellos GP. Dose: a critical factor in cancer chemotherapy. *Am J Med* 1980;69:585–593.
2. Hryniuk W, Bush H. The importance of dose intensity in chemotherapy of metastatic breast cancer. *J Clin Oncol* 1984;2:1281–1288.
3. Hryniuk W, Levine MN. Analysis of dose intensity for adjuvant chemotherapy trials in stage II breast cancer. *J Clin Oncol* 1986;4:1162–1170.
4. Hryniuk W, Levine MN, Levin L. Analysis of dose intensity for chemotherapy in early (stage II) and advanced breast cancer. *Natl Cancer Inst Monogr* 1986;1:87–94.
5. Levin L, Hryniuk W. Dose intensity analysis of chemotherapy regimens in ovarian carcinoma. *J Clin Oncol* 1987;5:756–767.
6. Hryniuk WM, Figueredo A, Goodyear M. Application of dose intensity to problems in chemotherapy of breast and colorectal cancer. *Semin Oncol* 1987;14(4):3–11(suppl 4).
7. Levin L, Hryniuk W. The application of dose intensity to problems in chemotherapy of ovarian and endometrial cancer. *Semin Oncol* 1987;14(4):12–19(suppl 4).
8. Hryniuk W, Goodyear M. The calculation of received dose intensity. *J Clin Oncol* 1990;8:1935–1937.
9. Greco FA, Julian CG, Richardson RL, Burnett L, Hande KR, Oldham RK. Advanced ovarian cancer: brief intensive combination chemotherapy in second-look operation. *Obstet Gynecol* 1981;58:200–205.
10. Levin L, Simon R, Hryniuk W. Dose intensity analysis in ovarian carcinoma revisited [submitted for publication].
11. Gruppo Interegionale Cooperativo Oncologico Ginecologia. Randomised comparison of cisplatin with cyclophosphamide/cisplatin and with cyclophosphamide/doxorubicin/cisplatin in advanced ovarian cancer. *Lancet* 1987;2:353–359.
12. Ozols RF, Ostchega Y, Myers CE, Young RC. High dose cisplatin in hypertonic saline in refractory ovarian cancer. *J Clin Oncol* 1985;3:1246–1250.
13. Ozols RF, Ostchega Y, Curt G, Young RC. High dose carboplatin in refractory ovarian cancer patients. *J Clin Oncol* 1987;5:197–201.
14. Ozols RF, Corden BJ, Jacobs J, Wesley MN, Ostchega Y, Young RC. High-dose cisplatin in hypertonic saline. *Ann Intern Med* 1984;100:19–24.
15. van der Hoop RG, Vecht CJ, van der Burg MEL, et al. Prevention of cisplatin neurotoxicity with an ACTH (4–9) analogue in patients with ovarian cancer. *N Engl J Med* 1990;322:89–94.
16. Gandara DR, Degregorio MW, Wold H. High dose cisplatin in hypertonic saline: reduced toxicity of a modified dose schedule and correlation with plasma pharmacokinetics. *J Clin Oncol* 1986;4:1787–1793.
17. Piccart MJ, Speyer JL, Wernz JL, et al. Advanced ovarian cancer: three year results of a 6–8 month, 2 drug cisplatin-containing regimen. *Eur J Clin Oncol* 1987;23:631–641.

18. Alberts D, Green S, Hannigen E, et al. Improved efficacy of carboplatin/cyclophosphamide vs cisplatin/cyclophosphamide: preliminary report of a phase III, randomized trial in stages III-IV, suboptimal ovarian cancer. *Proc Amer Soc Clin Oncol* 1989;8:151.
19. Calvert AH, Newell DR, Gumbrell LA. Carboplatin dosage: prospective evaluation of a simple formula based on renal function. *J Clin Oncol* 1989;7:1748–1756.
20. Hryniuk W. The importance of dose intensity in the outcome of chemotherapy. In: De Vita VT, Hellman S, Rosenberg SA, eds. *Important advances in oncology.* New York: JB Lippincott, 1988;121–141.
21. Goldin A, Venditti JM, Humphreys SR. Modification of treatment schedules in the management of advanced mouse leukemia with amethopterin. *J Natl Cancer Inst* 1956;17:203.
22. Torti FM, Bristow MR, Howes AE, et al. Reduced cardiotoxicity of doxorubicin delivered on a weekly schedule. Assessment of endomyocardial biopsy. *Ann Intern Med* 1983;99:745–749.
23. Bagley CM, Rudolph RH, Rivkin SE, Yon JL Jr. High-dose cisplatin therapy for cancer of the ovary: neurotoxicity. *Ann Intern Med* 1985;102:719.
24. Hrushesky WJM. The clinical application of chronobiology to oncology. *Am J Anat* 1983:168:519–542.
25. Hrushesky WJM. Circadian timing of cancer chemotherapy. *Science* 1985;228:73–75.
26. Roemeling RV, Langevin TR, Buchwald H, Grage T, Kennedy BJ, Hrushesky WJ. Time of day modified continuous FUDR infusion, using an implanted programmable pump, improves therapeutic index. *Proc Amer Soc Clin Oncol* 1986;5:83.
27. Levin L, Harris JF, Chambers AF. Factors in resistance to chemotherapy cure. In: Stoll BA, ed. *Pointers to cancer prognosis.* The Netherlands: Martinus Nijhoff Publishers, 1987; 156–170.
28. Folkman J. How is blood vessel growth regulated in normal and neoplastic tissue? *Cancer Res* 1986;46:467–473.
29. Tannock I. Response of aerobic and hypoxic cells in a solid tumor to adriamycin and cyclophosphamide and interaction of the drugs with radiation. *Cancer Res* 1982;42:4921–4926.

CHAPTER 19

Drug Resistance in Ovarian Cancer

Robert F. Ozols, Peter J. O'Dwyer, and Thomas C. Hamilton

Epithelial ovarian cancer is a highly drug-sensitive tumor. Approximately 60% to 80% of patients with advanced ovarian cancer will have objective responses to treatment with cisplatin-based regimens, and 50% of patients will achieve a clinical complete remission. Furthermore, 30% to 40% of patients who undergo a surgical exploration will have pathologically confirmed complete remission. Unfortunately, a complete remission is not tantamount to a cure, and approximately 30% to 50% of patients will ultimately relapse. Patients who never achieve a complete remission as well as those patients who relapse are essentially incurable. Even though second-line treatments can produce clinically meaningful responses, survival for these patients is usually less than 12 months. Overall, only 15% to 20% of all patients with advanced stage ovarian cancer are alive 5 years after diagnosis.

Thus, even though ovarian cancer is highly responsive to chemotherapy, most patients are not cured. A multiplicity of pharmacologic, biologic, and biochemical factors are likely to interact to limit the effectiveness of chemotherapy in this disease. Although an analysis of each factor will lead to an increased understanding of the individual events associated with the development of drug resistance, clinical drug resistance is undoubtedly the result of an interaction of many factors. Strategies aimed at reversing drug resistance in patients must simultaneously deal with the problems of drug delivery, intrinsic drug resistance, and dose.

RELATIVE DRUG RESISTANCE

It is intuitively obvious that cytotoxic drug levels must be achieved in the tumor in order for patients to achieve a response to therapy. Ovarian cancer remains confined to the peritoneal cavity for extended periods of time. In an effort to increase drug delivery directly to the tumor, intraperitoneal administration of chemotherapeutic agents has been extensively evaluated in the last decade. This topic is reviewed elsewhere in this text (1). Although a pharmacologic advantage has been achieved with most active drugs administered directly into the peritoneal cavity, there remains little evidence that survival advantage is achieved in any subset of patients with ovarian cancer following intraperitoneal chemotherapy compared to treatment via the intravenous route (2).

An alternative strategy to increase drug levels intracellularly in tumor cells has been to administer high-dose intravenous chemotherapy. This too is an important area in clinical research and is discussed elsewhere in this text by McGuire (3). Retrospective clinical studies have suggested a strong correlation between dose intensity and survival in patients with advanced ovarian cancer (4). However, this correlation has been weakened by the frequent inability to administer high doses of cisplatin owing to dose-limiting peripheral neuropathy (5). More recently carboplatin has been utilized in high-dose therapy studies because it is essentially devoid of neurotoxicity, nephrotoxicity, and ototoxicity (6). The dose-limiting toxicity of carboplatin is myelosuppression, and clinical trials are underway using a variety of strategies aimed at ameliorating this particular toxicity. The use of high-dose chemotherapy with autologous bone marrow transplantation and peripheral stem cell reconstitution is described by Shpall elsewhere in this text (7). In addition, trials are in progress with cytokines, which may ultimately replace the need for collection of either autologous bone marrow stem cells or circulating peripheral stem cells. Currently available cytokines such as GM-CSF and G-CSF have little if any impact upon the dose-limiting throm-

R. F. Ozols, P. J. O'Dwyer, and T. C. Hamilton: Fox Chase Cancer Center, Philadelphia, Pennsylvania 19111

bocytopenia of carboplatin, although they can decrease the neutropenic effects. A new generation of cytokines, however, is being evaluated. These include IL-1 alpha, IL-3, IL-6, and stem cell factor, which may have stimulatory effects upon thrombocytopoiesis.

As pointed out by McGuire (3) and Shpall (7), no firm evidence yet exists to prove that high-dose therapy with platinum compounds prolongs survival compared to treatment with standard doses. The lack of definitive evidence that high-dose therapy is superior may be due in part to the selection of patients for clinical trials. The initial studies with high-dose chemotherapy and autologous bone marrow transplantation were primarily focused on patients who had received prior chemotherapy and had bulky residual disease. Although high-dose chemotherapy was associated with transient responses in a significant number of these patients, most patients ultimately relapsed and were not cured by this intensive treatment approach. Prospective randomized trials of dose-intense chemotherapy in previously untreated patients with advanced ovarian cancer have included different population groups as well. In the Gynecologic Oncology Group (GOG) trial in which untreated patients were randomized to receive cisplatin at two different dose intensities, patients were eligible only if they had stage IV disease or suboptimal stage III disease (8). In this GOG trial, the initial results have failed to demonstrate any advantage for the more dose-intense therapy compared to standard therapy. In contrast, the eligibility for the Scottish Ovarian Cancer trial included patients with optimal stage III disease. In this trial patients were randomized to receive two different dose intensities as well as different total doses of cisplatin. In the preliminary analysis of this trial, a highly statistically significant survival advantage followed treatment with higher doses of cisplatin (9). It remains to be determined whether the improvement in survival occurred primarily in patients with small-volume residual disease who received the more dose-intense platinum regimen. Nevertheless, these studies are consistent with previous observations regarding the lack of efficacy of high-dose chemotherapy in other diseases, in which patients have bulky breast cancer and testicular cancer disease. Autologous bone marrow transplantation studies in breast cancer, for example, are primarily focused on patients who have small-volume disease or a clinical complete remission following induction chemotherapy (7).

In vitro studies of the cytotoxic effects of platinum compounds may have direct implication for the clinical use of these agents. Table 1 summarizes the relative resistance to cisplatin for a series of human ovarian cancer cell lines. The most sensitive cell lines (A2780 and PEO 1) were obtained from patients prior to the development of platinum resistance (10). Cell lines

TABLE 1. *In vitro sensitivities of human ovarian cancer cell lines*[a]

Cell line	Origin	IC50 (nm)	Relative resistance
A2780	Untreated patient	0.11	1
2780CP70	In vitro induction resistance to cisplatin	5.03	46
OVCAR 3	Resistant patient	0.21	2
OVCAR 4	Resistant patient	0.18	1.6
OVCAR 10	Resistant patient	7.67	70
PEO 1	Cisplatin-sensitive patient	0.07	0.7
PEO 4	Cisplatin-resistant patient	0.32	3

[a] From ref. 10.

OVCAR 3, OVCAR 4, OVCAR 10, and PEO 4 were obtained from patients while they were resistant to platinum-based chemotherapy (11). Cell line 2780CP70 was made resistant in vitro by stepwise exposure of the sensitive cell line A2780 to increasing concentrations of cisplatin (12). Marked heterogeneity was apparent in the relative degree of resistance to cisplatin in cell lines from clinically drug-resistant patients. Cell lines OVCAR 3, OVCAR 4, and PEO 4 were no more than threefold resistant to cisplatin, compared to cell lines from previously untreated patients. In contrast, OVCAR 10, also from a drug-resistant patient, had a 70-fold increase in relative resistance to cisplatin. These results suggest that some patients who become resistant to standard doses of platinum-based chemotherapy have tumors with only a moderate degree of platinum resistance; thus, the potential exists to overcome this resistance by chemotherapeutic regimens that increase the dose of cisplatin threefold or fourfold. However, some patients will have highly drug resistant tumors—even high-dose therapy will likely not be effective for them because even the most intense platinum-based chemotherapy regimens, which include bone marrow transplantation, are able to increase the dose intensity only sevenfold or eightfold (7). These laboratory results suggest that further studies aimed at overcoming relative drug resistance by increasing the dose of platinum analogues should focus on patients who have small-volume disease and who retain at least a degree of sensitivity to platinum-based therapy.

BIOCHEMICAL MECHANISMS OF RESISTANCE TO ALKYLATING AGENTS AND PLATINUM COMPOUNDS

Alkylating agents and platinum compounds have been the most active drugs used in the treatment of patients with ovarian cancer. Since platinum was introduced into clinical trial in the late 1970s, it has been associated with higher response rates and increased durations of complete remission with a modest prolongation of survival (13). Patients who have developed clinical resistance to cisplatin historically have not been successfully salvaged with second-line agents. The development of taxol appears to be changing this situation (14). The importance of platinum and classical alkylating agents in the treatment of ovarian cancer has focused research efforts toward defining biochemical pathways leading to resistance to these drugs. The broad cross-resistance that is associated with cisplatin resistance has also been the subject of experimental study. These investigations have been greatly aided by the development of relevant models of drug resistance in human ovarian cancer cells.

Drug-Resistant Ovarian Cancer Cell Lines

In the last 10 years we and others have developed a series of human ovarian cancer cell lines in which mechanisms of drug resistance have been studied (11,12,15). The cell lines we have examined can be divided into four categories: (A) cell lines established from previously untreated patients; (B) cell lines established from patients at a time they were clinically drug resistant (Fig. 1); (C) matched pairs of cell lines from the same patient prior to and after the development of drug resistance; and (D) drug-resistant ovarian cell lines produced by in vitro exposure of sensitive cell lines to alkylating agents, platinum compounds, or adriamycin. Cell lines with induced resistance in vitro to platinum also express cross-resistance to bifunctional alkylating agents such as melphalan and to irradiation (Fig. 2) (16–19). Similarly, selection for melphalan resistance produces cross-resistance to cisplatin and radiation. These patterns of cross-resistance are typical of clinical ovarian cancer and suggest that observations made in these drug-resistant cell lines will have potential clinical relevance.

Another important aspect of cell lines with in vitro–induced resistance is the fact that the levels of resistance can be selected (20). Cell lines with high levels of resistance to platinum agents have facilitated the identification of potential specific mechanisms of resistance such as DNA repair. It has been argued, however, that such high levels of resistance in these cell lines do not have clinical relevance, because most clinical resistance is of a lower magnitude. As noted, however, some patients with drug-resistant ovarian cancers will have tumors that are highly resistant to cisplatin. It should also be noted that the discovery of the *mdr*-1 gene and the involvement of dihydrofolate reductase in resistance to natural products and methotrexate was based on examination of cell lines with approximately 1,000-fold resistance to the respective drugs. Furthermore, once mechanisms of drug resistance can be identified in highly drug resistant cell lines, more careful and sensitive analysis of cell lines and tumor biopsies with a lower degree of resistance is feasible in order to establish clinical relevance of a specific mechanism.

In Vivo Models of Drug Resistance

Representative in vivo models of ovarian cancer are required in order to determine whether any potential modulation of drug resistance has clinical relevance. Although mechanisms of drug resistance in general terms can be studied in vitro and inhibitors of biochemical pathways can be identified, the potential to produce a differential effect on tumor cells versus normal cells requires evaluation in vivo. It has been postulated that once a mechanism of drug resistance is identified *in vitro*, pharmacologic agents will be capable of inhibiting those specific biochemical processes. Once resis-

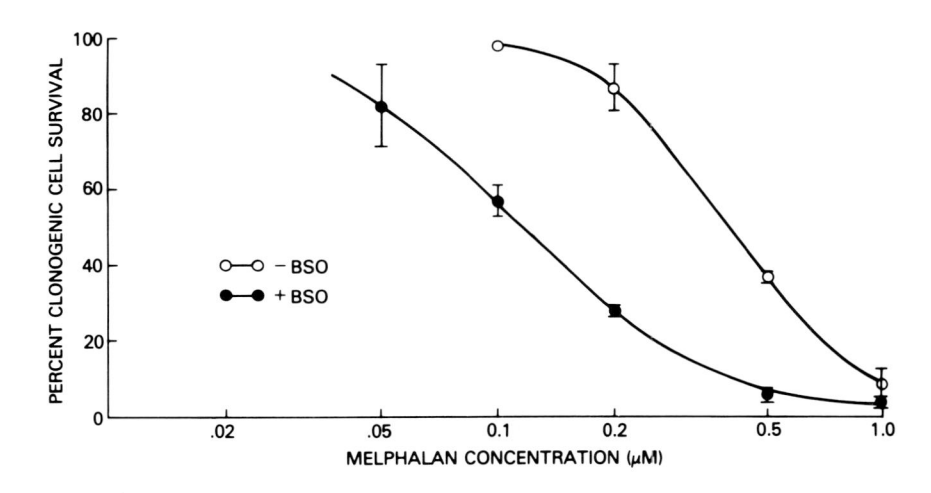

FIG. 1. Dose response curve for melphalan in OVCAR 3, a cell line established from a drug resistant patient, with and without buthionine sulfoximine (BSO) in the culture medium. From ref. 33.

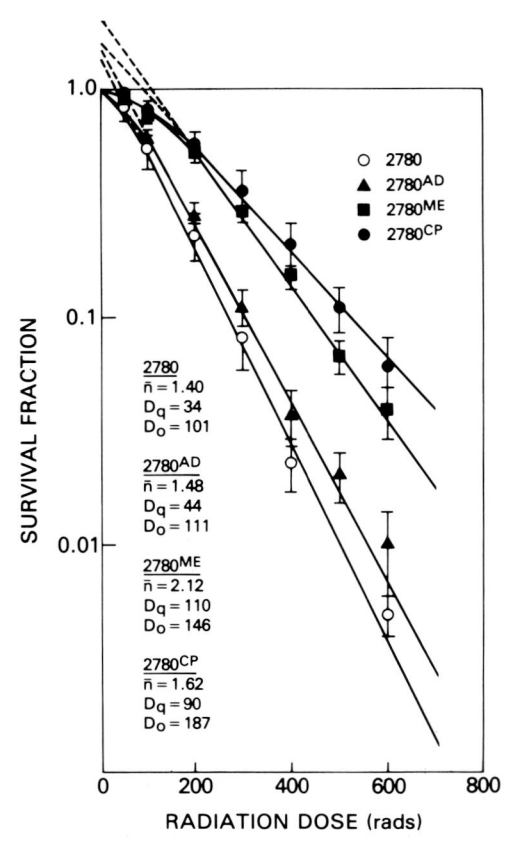

FIG. 2. Radiation survival curves for cell line 2780 and its drug-resistant variants; 2780 was a previously untreated ovarian cancer and 2780AD, 2780ME, and 2780CP were made resistant in vitro to adriamycin, melphalan, and cisplatin, respectively. 2780ME and 2780CP were relatively more resistant to radiation than 2780 and 2780AD. From ref. 19.

Curve parameters shown on figure:

2780: $\bar{n} = 1.40$, $D_q = 34$, $D_o = 101$
2780AD: $\bar{n} = 1.48$, $D_q = 44$, $D_o = 111$
2780ME: $\bar{n} = 2.12$, $D_q = 110$, $D_o = 146$
2780CP: $\bar{n} = 1.62$, $D_q = 90$, $D_o = 187$

tance is reversed in vitro, then in vivo studies will be performed to investigate potential therapeutic advantage. If advantage is possible, large-scale toxicology studies will be warranted as the next step in clinical development. Such a sequence has been followed to develop novel clinical modulators of drug resistance.

We have developed a unique model of human ovarian cancer in nude mice that has been utilized extensively for the preclinical evaluation of a novel new therapeutic approach aimed at reversing drug resistance and identifying the activity of new drugs and biological agents (21). This model was produced first by selection of the human ovarian cancer cell line OVCAR 3 for growth in vivo by subcutaneous injection into athymic nude mice (22). Tumor cells from subcutaneous nodules were subsequently selected for substrate-independent growth by suspension in agarose. These latter cells were then injected intraperitoneally into female nude athymic mice and produced ascites and intraperitoneal carcinomatosis. The animals reproducibly die from bowel obstruction or respiratory compromise secondary to massive intraabdominal disease. The tumor cells can be readily transplanted intraperitoneally into other nude mice.

BIOCHEMICAL MECHANISMS OF RESISTANCE TO ALKYLATING AGENTS AND PLATINUM COMPOUNDS

Both carrier-independent and carrier-dependent mechanisms of transport have been shown to exist for alkylating agents in different experimental systems (15). Vistica has shown that the melphalan carrier appears to be an amino acid active transport system (23). Decreased transport of melphalan has been described by Begleiter et al. (24) in some resistant murine cells. In human ovarian cancer cells with in vitro–induced resistance to melphalan, uptake differences between melphalan-resistant and melphalan-sensitive cell lines were not detected (18).

Similarly, the transport of platinum compounds in human tumor cells has not been completely characterized, and the intracellular drug level may be influenced by multiple mechanisms (12,15). Evidence supports the hypothesis that cisplatin may enter cells by both passive diffusion and by carrier-dependent transport (25). Furthermore, transport of cisplatin may be linked to the transport of neutral amino acids (26). There have been numerous reports of decreased platinum accumulation in resistant cell lines (15). However, the precise molecular defect associated with a decrease in drug accumulation and the development of platinum resistance in these cell lines has not been identified. It is also unclear whether the decreased intracellular concentration is due exclusively to reduced ability of the drug to enter the cell or to enhanced ability of the resistant cell to pump the drug out from the cytoplasm (27). A recent report notes that a membrane glycoprotein is increased in a cisplatin-resistant murine lymphoma cell line (28); however, this glycoprotein is distinct from the multidrug transporter (P-170), which is coded for by the *mdr*-1 gene and is responsible for enhanced efflux of natural products in drug-resistant tumor cells (29,30). Bourhis et al. (31), in an analysis of 50 human ovarian carcinoma specimens for *mdr*-1 expression, reported undetectable levels in tumor biopsies from previously untreated patients and very low levels of expression in three of ten patients who were previously treated with the natural products vincristine or adriamycin. No increased expression of the *mdr*-1 gene in specimens from patients resistant to cisplatin and cyclophosphamide was found. Currently, it appears that decreased cell-associated drug is a factor in cisplatin drug resistance, although it appears to be mediated by proteins distinct from the P-170 drug transporter. In addition, the relative contribution of decreased cisplatin accumulation to clinical drug resistance remains to be established.

SULFHYDRYL MOLECULES AND DRUG RESISTANCE

Glutathione (GSH) is the major nonprotein thiol, and metallothionein the primary protein sulfhydryl compound within cells. Resistance to platinum compounds and alkylating agents has been associated with alterations in metabolism and levels of both these compounds (16–18,32–35). GSH plays a critical role in normal cellular homeostasis, primarily by its function as a cofactor for a variety of enzymes and by its involvement in detoxification pathways. GSH protects the cellular environment from environmental toxins, either by binding to these agents or by facilitating their metabolism and transport (12,20).

It has now been established in several laboratories that selection/induction of resistance to cisplatin and bifunctional alkylating agents is associated with twofold to threefold increases of cellular GSH compared to levels in the relatively drug-sensitive parental cells from which resistant variants were developed. The 2780 ME and 2780 CP cell lines with induced resistance to melphalan and cisplatin, respectively, were found to have a 2.4-fold and 3.2-fold increase in GSH, respectively, compared to the parental A2780 drug-sensitive cell line from which they were derived (12,20,35,36). Studies on GSH content in human ovarian cancer cells were the result of initial observations made by Vistica's laboratory in murine L1210 leukemia cells with resistance to melphalan (32). Chemosensitivity could be restored in these cell lines by depletion of GSH. This observation became clinically relevant by the subsequent synthesis of the synthetic amino acid buthionine sulfoximine (BSO) by Miester (37). BSO irreversibly inhibits the enzyme gamma glutamyl cysteine synthetase, which leads to decreased levels of GSH. GSH levels have been measured in a series of human ovarian cancer cell lines, and higher levels were shown to be present in the OVCAR 3 and 4 cell lines that were derived from clinically drug-resistant patients. Incubating drug-resistant cell lines with BSO lowered GSH levels and partially restored sensitivity to melphalan and to platinum compounds (11,16). In addition, GSH was shown to be involved in cross-resistance to radiation between melphalan- and cisplatin-resistant cell lines. Lowering of GSH levels enhanced the sensitivity to radiation in 2780 ME and 2780 CP (19).

These in vitro studies of melphalan were followed by in vivo studies of BSO and melphalan in the OVCAR 3 transplantable tumor in nude mice (33). Treatment of mice with oral BSO (30 mM in their drinking water) reduced GSH levels in tumor cells by 90%, with a similar reduction of GSH content in the gastrointestinal mucosa and bone marrow cells. BSO treatment alone had no effect on survival of OVCAR-3 tumor–bearing mice. Melphalan alone (5 mg/kg) increased median survival from 46 days for control animals to 75 days. However, the addition of BSO to melphalan treatment resulted in further increase in survival to a median of 102 days (Fig. 3).

GSH has also been shown to bind cisplatin, which could readily influence platinum availability for DNA binding or for the quenching of DNA-platinum mono-

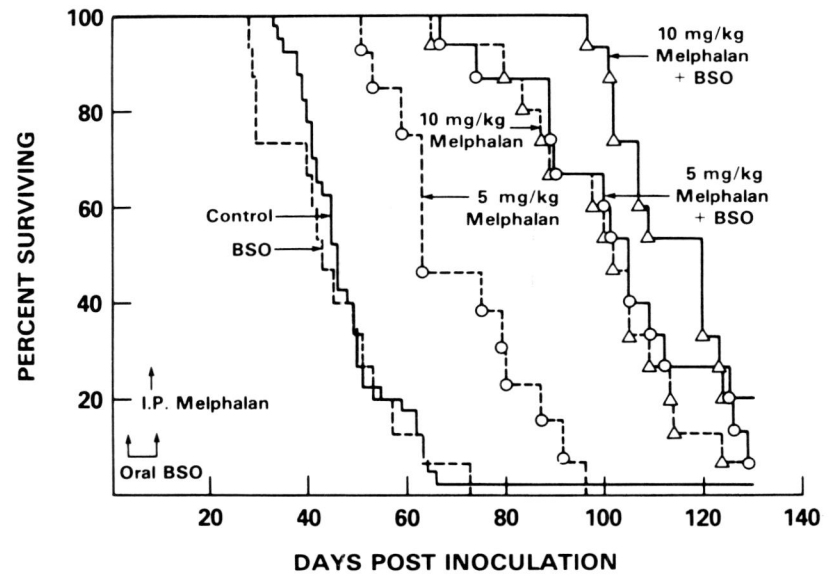

FIG. 3. Prolongation of survival of nude mice with OVCAR-3 ovarian cancer cells implanted intraperitoneally following treatment with melphalan and buthionine sulfoximine. From ref. 33.

adducts (38). Cellular GSH content is under complex regulation. Tumor cells have the capacity to increase the GSH content markedly. It has recently been shown by Godwin et al. (20) that GSH content increased approximately 12-fold in cell lines with a relatively low level of resistance (less than 30-fold) to a nearly 50-fold increase in GSH level in cell lines with greater than 1,000-fold resistance to cisplatin. A strong relationship (correlation coefficient 0.96) exists between cisplatin resistance and intracellular GSH levels. As GSH levels increase, there appears to be a constitutive increase in the steady state expression of mRNA for gamma glutamyl cysteine synthetase (gamma GCS), the enzyme involved in the first step of GSH biosynthesis (20). Furthermore, under some conditions, the steady state mRNA is increased for gamma glutamyl transpeptidase, another enzyme involved in the regulation of intracellular GSH. At low levels of resistance, stabilization of the gamma GCS enzyme may be involved in the increased levels of GSH observed (20).

Metallothioneins are a group of related proteins that bind heavy metals and trace elements (39). These small proteins are consequently thought to be important for the detoxification of heavy metals and for the availability of necessary trace elements. The key element of the drug cisplatin is atomic cisplatin, which often is loosely considered a heavy metal because of its proximity to the classical heavy metals in the periodic table. Metallothioneins may also be involved in resistance to platinum compounds. However, the relationship between metallothionein levels and cisplatin resistance remains to be determined. We have previously shown increased expression of mRNA for metallothionein II in some cell lines with in vitro–induced cisplatin resistance (40). However, we have also shown the range of expression of metallothionein II mRNA in cell lines from a series of untreated and treated ovarian cancer patients (40). There was no consistent correlation between cisplatin sensitivity and metallothionein II mRNA levels (Fig. 4). However, other studies have described an increased expression of metallothionein in association with cisplatin resistance in another tumor (41). Experimental data link metallothionein levels and resistance to alkylating agents (15). Expression vectors were used to increase cellular levels of metallothionein prior to treatment with alkylating agents, bleomycin, or radiation. Transfection of the metallothionein gene into these Chinese hamster ovary cells conferred resistance to the alkylating agents MNNG and mitomycin C but not to bleomycin or to radiation (42). At present it appears that increased levels of metallothionein are associated, under some circumstances, with resistance to alkylating agents and platinum compounds, although the causal nature of this relationship has not been established.

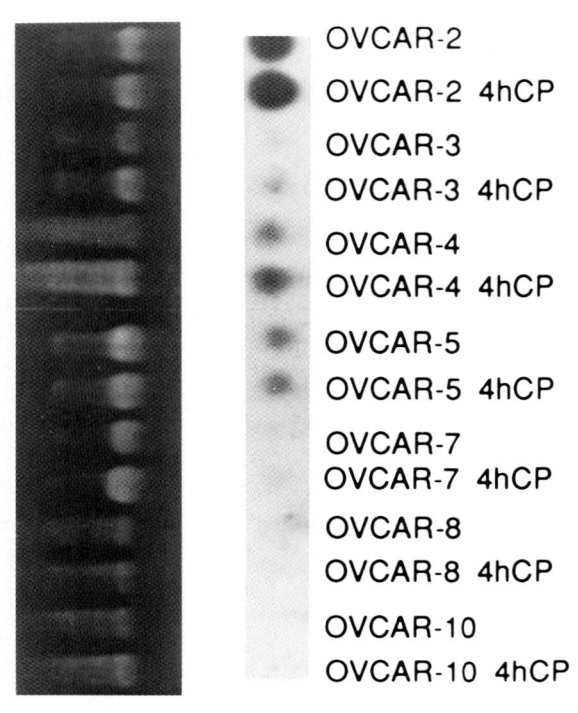

FIG. 4. Metallothionein II gene expression in cell lines derived from patients refractory to cisplatin-containing chemotherapy: paired samples with and without cisplatin. From ref. 40.

GLUTATHIONE S-TRANSFERASES AND RESISTANCE TO PLATINUM COMPOUNDS AND ALKYLATING AGENTS

The role of the glutathione S-transferase (GST) isozymes in drug resistance has been an area of intense interest in the last decade. The GST isozymes are involved in a variety of biological functions that include binding and transport of nonsubstrate ligands such as heme and bilirubin, prostaglandin and leukotriene biosynthesis, steroid isomerization, and detoxification of a number of different hydrophobic and electrophilic chemicals (43). It is in this latter regard that GST enzymes may be important in the manifestation of drug resistance by inactivating certain classes of electrophilic cytotoxic drugs, particularly alkylating agents. A diverse group of chemicals can act as substrates for GST. The initial observation that elevated expression of GST was observed in a nitrogen mustard–resistant cell line was followed by a series of other studies in which overexpression of GST isozymes was linked with acquired resistance to anticancer drugs (44). Tew and colleagues have examined GST expression in over 400 tumor biopsies including ten ovarian carcinomas (45). Preliminary results suggest that there is high alpha expression in ovarian cancer, although ovarian tumors are capable of expressing all three classes of cytosolic transferases.

Clinical interest in these enzymes stems from the work of Tew and colleagues, who described a series of tumor cell lines with acquired resistance to chlorambucil and nitrogen mustard in which the major difference between sensitive and resistant cells was the overexpression of the GST transferases (44). Furthermore, inhibition of these transferases restored sensitivity to alkylating agents. In a human colon adenocarcinoma growing subcutaneously to SCID (severe combined immunodeficiency) mice, greater tumor growth inhibition was observed by the combination of melphalan and ethacrynic acid than by treatment with either drug alone or with untreated controls (46).

In addition to resistance to alkylating agents, glutathione-dependent enzymes have also been implicated in multidrug resistance. In particular, the pi isozyme of GST has been shown to be associated with pleiotropic resistance in several models of resistance, including a multidrug resistant MCF-7 human breast cancer cell line (47). Transfection studies, however, have led to somewhat conflicting results regarding the contribution of GST pi to drug resistance. In one study, elevation of GST pi levels were produced following transfection into a drug-sensitive MCF cell line, although this did not result in multidrug resistance (48). Other investigators have transfected GST genes into monkey COS cells, which have demonstrated slight increases in resistance to alkylating agents and adriamycin (49). It has also been shown that GST pi–transfected c-Ha-ras–transformed NIH 3T3 cells developed a twofold to threefold increase of resistance at the IC37 level with a lesser effect at the IC50 level against doxorubicin (50). It remains to be established whether this gene can cause low levels of resistance that may be relevant clinically.

THE ROLE OF DNA REPAIR IN RESISTANCE TO PLATINUM AND ALKYLATING AGENTS

It is generally accepted that the cytotoxicity of alkylating agents and platinum compounds is due to the formation of lethal lesions in nuclear DNA. The alkylating agent and cisplatin adducts are thought to disrupt DNA synthesis and RAN transcription processes. In vitro studies with cisplatin and pure DNA have shown that the majority of lesions are intrastrand adducts located at the N7 position of adjacent guanine residues (Pt[GG]) or between an adenine flanked by a 3′ guanine residue (Pt[AG]) (36,51–56). The major (Pt[GG]) lesion accounts for approximately 65% of platinum bound to DNA in vitro. However, considerably fewer intrastrand adducts are found (35%) in the DNA isolated from cisplatin-treated cells in tissue culture. This apparent discrepancy may result from a slower formation of crosslinks from cisplatin-DNA monoadducts (which account for approximately 40% of the total DNA-bound platinum in cultured cells). Quenching of cisplatin-CNA monoadducts by glutathione may also occur in cells in order to prevent the formation of the more lethal crosslinks (57,58). Platinum is also capable of forming interstrand crosslinks, such as links between guanine residues on opposite strands of the DNA. Even though only 1% of the total bound platinum may be in the form of interstrand crosslinks, these lesions may be important in the cytotoxicity of platinum compounds (36,56). The possibility remains that a combination of interstrand and intrastrand adducts is responsible for the cytotoxicity observed with platinum compounds. In order for a cell to survive following formation of these adducts, it must have the capacity to repair them or to tolerate the DNA damage that they produce.

Data have been presented in support of the hypothesis that the capacity to repair damaged DNA rapidly and efficiently is a mechanism of resistance to platinum and alkylating agents. This mechanism may account in part for the primary resistance associated with exposure to alkylating agents or platinum compounds, but it also can explain the frequently observed cross-resistance present between many chemotherapeutic agents that have DNA as their target. Increased DNA repair activity has been noted in cisplatin-resistant ovarian cancer cell lines as well as other drug-resistant tumor cells (59–64). Compared to repair activity in sensitive cells, the drug-resistant tumor cells have approximately twofold to fourfold higher levels of DNA repair (Fig. 5). These studies have measured DNA repair at the level of the whole genome, even though DNA repair may preferentially occur in actively transcribed genes (65,66). This may in turn account for the lack of a direct correlation between the degree of resistance and an increase in overall DNA repair levels. A more dramatic repair rate difference may exist in specific genomic regions between sensitive and resistant cells. However, such a relationship between cisplatin resistance and increased repair activity in actively transcribed genes has not yet been established.

Several DNA repair mechanisms have been identified, primarily on the basis of studies in prokaryotes. Although the enzymes responsible for mammalian DNA repair are still incompletely characterized, it appears that the nucleotide excision repair pathway is a primary repair mechanism for DNA damage induced by cisplatin, alkylating agents, and irradiation (67–69). The first step of the repair process involves recognition of the DNA damage, which is followed by incision of DNA on either side of the lesion. A new DNA strand is generated that replaces the excised segment requiring ligation of a new segment onto the existing strand of DNA. Such a process involves the activity of endonu-

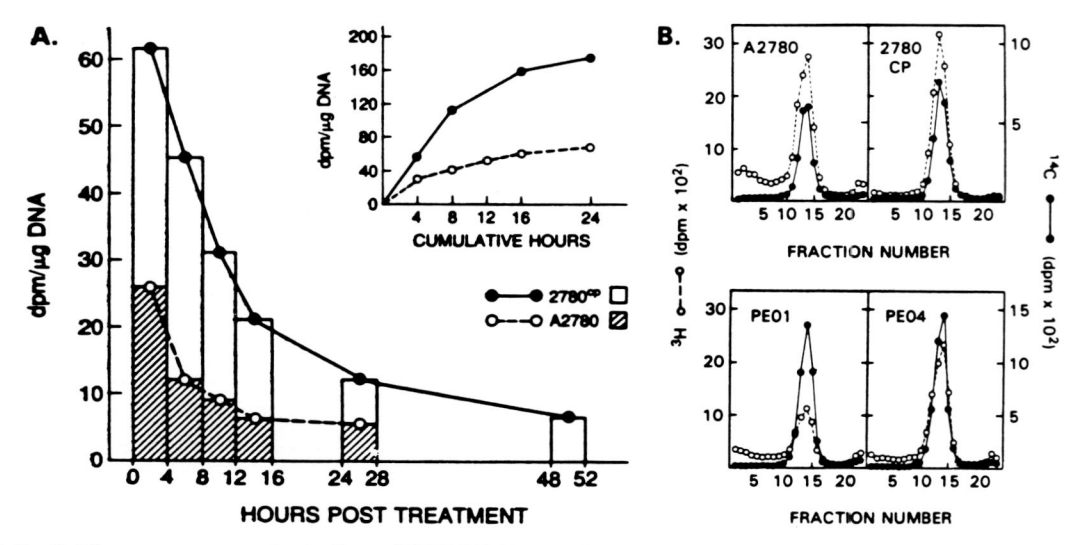

FIG. 5. A: Time course repair studies of 2780CP. The ordinate represents DNA repair capacity measured hours after exposure to cisplatin in the sensitive (2780) and resistant (2780CP) cell lines. **B:** Inducible repair synthesis in four cell lines following treatment with cisplatin. PEO 4 was established from a patient after development of drug resistance; PEO 1 was established prior to cisplatin resistance. From ref. 59.

cleases, DNA polymerases, and DNA ligases and topoisomerases.

Recently, a human excision repair gene (designated ERCC-1) with significant homology to the yeast excision repair gene RAD10 has been isolated and cloned (70). This gene also shares homology with the *E. coli* excision repair genes uvrA and uvrC (71,72). The structure and similarity between ERCC-1 and known excision repair enzymes suggests that it performs similar functions in mammalian cells. This gene has the ability to complement excision repair–defective mutant Chinese hamster ovary cells and to decrease their sensitivity to cisplatin (73).

In addition to induction of DNA repair enzymes, the cellular response to DNA damage also includes cell-cycle arrest (15). The DNA damage secondary to ultraviolet radiation, alkylating agents, and cisplatin induces transcription of many enzymes involved in DNA replication and repair, such as DNA polymerases alpha and beta, thymidylate synthetase, thymidine kinase, and dihydrofolate reductase (74–76). A protein has been recently identified that binds double-stranded DNA modified by cisplatin (51). This protein may be involved in the recognition and/or repair of cisplatin-induced damage. Further study of this and other proteins induced by DNA damage are underway.

GSH also appears to facilitate DNA repair (34). Thiols such as GSH are necessary cofactors for a variety of enzymes, including DNA polymerases. GSH is also required for synthesis of deoxyribonucleotide triphosphates, which are precursors for replicative and repair DNA synthesis. As previously noted, GSH binds to DNA crosslink precursors of bifunctional alkylating agents and cisplatin, and this quenching prevents crosslink formation, producing lesions that may be more easily repaired (58). Studies on repair inhibition following GSH depletion have also directly demonstrated a role for GSH in the DNA repair process (34). Lowering GSH levels is associated with significantly diminished repair of radiation-induced DNA-protein crosslinks as well as single-strand breaks (77). GSH depletion has also been shown to inhibit unscheduled DNA synthesis after treatment of spermatocytes and hepatocytes with 1,2-dibromoethane (78). Our laboratory has demonstrated that lowering of GSH levels by treatment of cells with BSO decreased DNA repair activity as measured by inhibition of unscheduled DNA synthesis (34). Exposure of these cells to glutathione ester increased cellular GSH level and restored DNA repair capacity (Fig. 6).

Once DNA damage is produced by alkylating agents, there is arrest of cells in G2 (15). Cell cycle arrest allows repair of potentially lethal DNA damage prior to the cells entering mitosis. Alkylating-agent treated, G2-arrested cells made to prematurely enter mitosis (by exposure to caffeine) have greater DNA damage and less viability than do cells allowed to progress normally into G2 after a period for DNA repair (79,80). Studies in RAD mutant yeasts provide further evidence for the relationship of G2 arrest with DNA repair (81,82). These mutants are hypersensitive to ultraviolet radiation and alkylating agents, are unable to arrest in G2, and have increased DNA damage and decreased viability compared to wild type RAD cells following treatment with alkylating agents or radiation. However, if entry into mitosis is delayed in these mutant

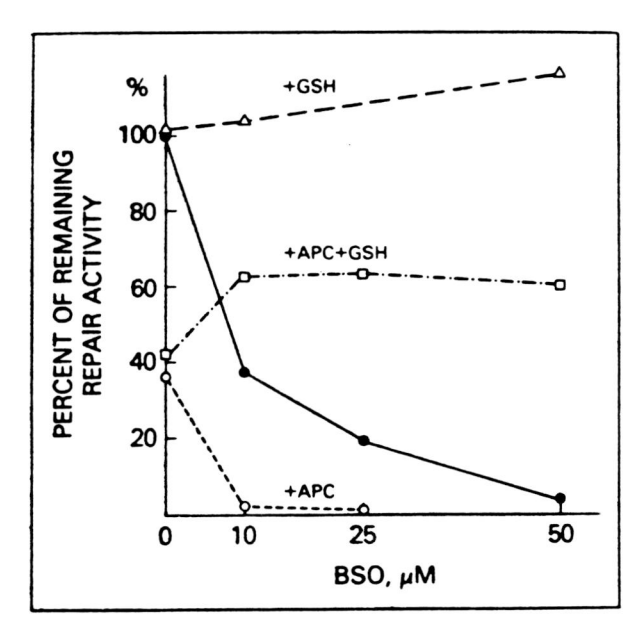

FIG. 6. Dose-dependent suppression of DNA repair by incubation with BSO (*solid line*). Total inhibition of DNA repair is observed with aphidicolin plus BSO. GSH ester completely, or partially if aphidicolin is present, restores DNA repair activity. From ref. 34.

yeasts by exposure to microtubular inhibitors, these yeasts can now repair their DNA and have similar survival compared to the wild type. These observations support a model in which mutation in the RAD gene disrupts a cell-cycle regulatory mechanism, which allows for repair of damage to DNA prior to mitosis. It has been postulated that similar regulatory genes exist in humans (15).

It has also been demonstrated that DNA repair-deficient cells are hypersensitive to alkylating agents and cisplatin (83–85), providing further evidence for the importance of DNA repair process in cytotoxicity to these agents. Furthermore, the repair of platinum-DNA adducts in growth-arrested human fibroblasts also correlates with decreased cytotoxicity (86). Sorensen and Eastman examined the G2 arrest, cytotoxicity, and cisplatin concentrations in murine L1210 leukemia cells (87). Cisplatin concentrations that cause sublethal injury produced transient cell-cycle arrest, after which cells recovered. Higher concentrations of cisplatin led to longer periods of G2 arrest and ultimately to disruption of DNA, suggesting that a threshold for DNA damage exists beyond which repair mechanisms cannot restore genomic integrity necessary for cell survival.

Our laboratory has examined the relationship between DNA repair and resistance to platinum compounds and alkylating agents in human ovarian cancer cells (59,60). The 2780CP cell line was selected by stepwise intermittent exposure of the sensitive parental A2780 cell line to cisplatin. The cisplatin-resistant cell line was fivefold resistant to cisplatin under the conditions of the DNA repair assay and was also cross-resistant to melphalan, adriamycin, and irradiation. In these cells, DNA repair synthesis was increased nearly threefold relative to A2780, following treatment of these cells with equal doses of cisplatin. Repair synthesis in both cell lines was highest during the 4-hour period following cisplatin exposure; it returned to base levels by 12 hours in the drug-sensitive cell line but remained elevated for an additional 24 hours after exposure to cisplatin in the 2780CP cells. Similar studies in the cisplatin-sensitive PEO 1 and cisplatin-resistant PEO 4 ovarian cancer cell lines, obtained from the same patient before and after onset of resistance to cisplatin, also provided evidence for the importance of DNA repair in the resistance phenotype (59). Unscheduled DNA synthesis was increased two- to threefold in the resistant PEO 4 cells relative to PEO 1 cells. In these two cell lines the degree of resistance was somewhat greater than the increased repair activity, which suggests that although DNA repair is potentially a major resistance mechanism, additional cellular factors are also involved.

Further support for the role of DNA repair in platinum resistance was obtained by Eastman and Schulte (63) in L1210 leukemia cells with resistance to cisplatin. In their systems, cisplatin resistance did not correlate as closely with increased repair as it did in our observations with the 2780CP cells and the PEO 4 cells. The relative contribution of DNA repair to the overall level of resistance to cisplatin is probably variable between cell lines and species. Further support for the importance of DNA repair in cisplatin resistance has recently been provided by Reed et al. (73), who demonstrated increased expression of the ERCC1 excision repair gene in cisplatin-resistant 2780CP cells.

The observation that cisplatin resistance is associated with DNA repair has led to numerous experimental studies exploring the relationship between cisplatin sensitivity and inhibitors of the DNA repair process. Our laboratory has examined the effects of aphidicolin, an inhibitor of DNA polymerase alpha and gamma, on unscheduled DNA synthesis following cisplatin treatment in 2780 and the resistant 2780CP cell lines (59,60). Aphidicolin inhibited repair synthesis in both cell lines in a dose-dependent manner. Repair synthesis was decreased by up to 70% in both the sensitive and resistant cell lines following exposure to aphidicolin. Cytotoxicity of cisplatin after exposure to aphidicolin was measured in these cell lines using a colony formation soft agar system. Aphidicolin in combination with cisplatin produced a 3.5-fold increase in the cytotoxicity of cisplatin in the 2780CP cells over treatment with cisplatin

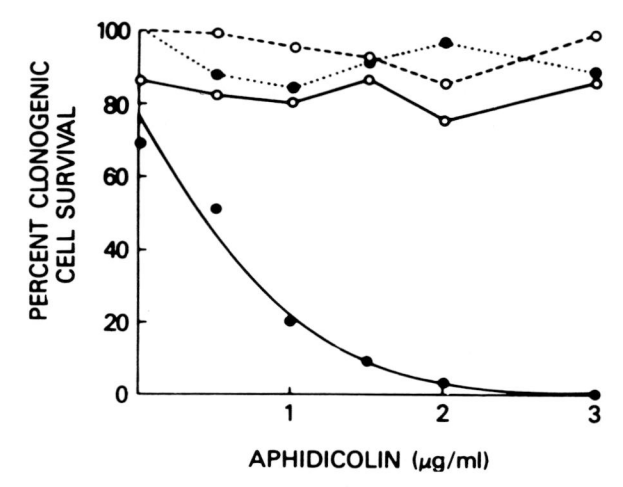

FIG. 7. Aphidicolin has no cytotoxic effect of A2780 and A2780CP (*top 2 curves*). Aphidicolin did not potentiate cytotoxicity of cisplatin in 2780 (*open circles*), but in the cisplatin-resistant cell line, aphidicolin enhanced cisplatin cytotoxicity in a dose-dependent manner. From ref. 60.

alone (Fig. 7). In the drug-sensitive A2780 cell lines, aphidicolin did not markedly increase cisplatin cytotoxicity. The partial inhibition of DNA repair with aphidicolin did not completely restore cisplatin sensitivity in the 2780CP cell lines. In these cells, almost complete inhibition of DNA repair was observed following treatment with both aphidicolin and BSO.

Katz et al. (88) have independently shown the ability of aphidicolin to enhance cisplatin cytotoxicity. In contrast, Dempke et al. (89) did not report a significantly increased effect on cisplatin cytotoxicity by aphidicolin in two other ovarian cancer cell lines, although a combination of cisplatin and high-dose aphidicolin was more effective than either drug alone. There have also been conflicting results on the effect aphidicolin has on removal of platinum from DNA. In one study, aphidicolin was shown to inhibit platinum removal from DNA (61), whereas in another study no difference in platinum levels was detected following exposure to aphidicolin (89). Johnson et al. (36) have noted that aphidicolin should not be expected to influence platinum removal from DNA. Aphidicolin inhibits DNA polymerases, which in human cells are responsible for gap filling. There is no reason to believe that the excision of damage by other enzymes should be affected by aphidicolin.

Our results with aphidicolin are also consistent with reports of cytotoxic synergy between Ara-C, another inhibitor of DNA polymerase alpha, and cisplatin (90–99). Scanlon et al. (97) have reported significantly enhanced cytotoxicity in a cisplatin-resistant human colon cancer cell line treated with cisplatin and azidothymidine (AZT). This antimetabolite also inhibits DNA polymerases beta and gamma. AZT therefore may inhibit gaps remaining in DNA strands following excision of the platinum DNA adducts, similar to the effects of aphidicolin and Ara-C. Furthermore, Perez et al. have recently observed complete inhibition of DNA repair with aphidicolin plus dideoxythymidine triphosphate, which is another inhibitor of DNA polymerase beta in a cisplatin-resistant ovarian cancer cell line (98).

More recently the effects of aphidicolin on cisplatin cytotoxicity have been studied in vivo (99). The combination of aphidicolin and cisplatin was shown to be superior in prolonging survival in a transplantable nude mice model of human ovarian cancer compared to treatment with either agent alone. These results provide further evidence that inhibition of DNA repair may be clinically useful.

In addition to aphidicolin, calmodulin inhibitors may also have potential clinical relevance owing to their ability to inhibit DNA repair and potentiate cisplatin cytotoxicity (15,100). It has been shown that calmodulin antagonists may inhibit DNA excision repair (100). Diminished repair of DNA strand breaks induced by bleomycin and other drugs suggests potential inhibition of DNA polymerases and/or DNA ligases (101). Calmodulin antagonists have been shown to potentiate the effects of cisplatin against sensitive and resistant human ovarian cancer cell lines in vitro as well as in a nude mice xenograft model (102,103). We have examined the effects of the calmodulin inhibitor trifluoperazine on cisplatin cytotoxicity in human ovarian cancer cells (104). Trifluoperazine produces a twofold enhancement of cisplatin cytotoxicity in both cisplatin-sensitive and cisplatin-resistant human ovarian cancer cell lines. Additional studies are in progress with combinations of inhibitors of DNA repair process to determine the effects on cisplatin cytotoxicity.

CISPLATIN RESISTANCE AND SIGNAL TRANSDUCTION PATHWAYS

Recent studies have implicated signal transduction pathways in cisplatin cytotoxicity and resistance. Isonishi et al. (105) have demonstrated that cisplatin sensitivity can be modulated by signal transduction pathways. Activation of protein kinase C increases the sensitivity of human ovarian cancer cell line 2.5-fold (106). Furthermore, ligand activation of the EGF receptor decreases cisplatin cytotoxicity. The c-Ha-ras oncogene is a component of the signal transduction pathway. Sklar (107) first reported that NIH 3T3 cells transformed by normal or mutant c-Ha-ras oncogene are more sensitive to cisplatin than parental cells. In contrast, researchers in Howell's laboratory have recently examined mechanisms by which increased signal transduction can lead to platinum resistance (105). They used an NIH 3T3 cell line containing a hormone-inducible form of the c-Ha-ras oncogene in their studies. Their results suggest that transcriptional activation of the mutant c-Ha-ras oncogene produces platinum resistance owing to a decrease in platinum accumulation and a concomitant increase in metallothionein. Kashaui-Sabet and colleagues have demonstrated that cyclosporine A treatment results in an increase in cisplatin cytotoxicity in the platinum-resistant 2780CP cell line (108). They have shown that this effect is due to blocking platinum–induced increases in C-fos and H-ras mRNA. Cyclosporine A has also been shown to overcome multidrug resistance in ovarian cancer and other cell lines in vitro and in vivo because of its effects on the *mdr*-1 gene product. The ability of cyclosporine A to reverse resistance to cisplatin may be due primarily to its effects on blocking expression of genes involved in signal transduction pathways.

CLINICAL TRIALS AIMED AT REVERSING PLATINUM RESISTANCE IN OVARIAN CANCER

Inhibition of Glutathione Synthesis with BSO

Investigators at Fox Chase Center were the first to evaluate the effect of BSO on alkylating agent resistance clinically (109). Drug-resistant patients received intravenous BSO every 12 hours for 6 doses, with intravenous melphalan after the fifth BSO dose. The final BSO dose was administered to allow intrastrand and interstrand crosslinks to form before recovery of GSH levels. To assess separately the toxic and biochemical effects attributable to the components of this regimen, all patients received BSO alone in the first course and received both drugs a week later. The initial dose of BSO in this study was 1500 mg/m^2 administered at 12-hour intervals for 6 doses. In the second week, the same schedule was followed, but 1 hour after the fifth dose of BSO, melphalan was administered intravenously. Cycles of BSO and melphalan were repeated at 3-week intervals. Glutathione was assayed in peripheral mononuclear cells and in tumor tissue before treatment and at intervals after treatment with BSO. The preliminary results of this study have been reported at a point when nine patients were treated with a total of 16 courses of BSO and melphalan (109). Acute toxicity following the administration of BSO alone was minimal. Neutropenia and thrombocytopenia were the most prominent side effects after combined treatment with BSO and melphalan. Anemia was initially a particular concern, because defects in GSH metabolism are known to be associated with hemolysis. However, no evidence of hemolysis was obtained during sequential routine blood tests.

GSH concentrations were measured in peripheral mononuclear cells of eight patients in an initial cycle following initiation of BSO treatment. In four patients, depletion to below 20% of control was observed by 72 hours. In an additional patient a similar degree of depletion occurred at 96 hours. A typical time course of GSH depletion is shown in Fig. 8. The rate of depletion varied considerably between patients. Recovery was observed in the majority by 120 hours. In three patients, however, no depletion of GSH was found. In four patients ovarian tumor samples were assayed for GSH. In one patient in whom the peripheral mononuclear cell GSH value did not change, those cells in the biopsy were similarly unaffected. In another patient in whom peripheral mononuclear cell GSH was 12% of control on day 3, there was also no change in the tumor. However, in two ascites samples there were pronounced effects on day 3 with depletion to 20% and 3% in malignant cells obtained in paracentesis. In this ongoing phase I study, one patient with locally extensive recurrent ovarian cancer received three courses of BSO and melphalan and achieved a partial remission after two cycles, as determined by serial CT scans. An additional three patients with ovarian cancer had disease stabilization lasting 8 or more weeks. This study demonstrates that the administration of nontoxic doses of BSO can produce GSH depletion to below 20% of control in the peripheral mononuclear cells in approximately one-half of the patients thus far treated. The relationship in humans between GSH depletion in peripheral mononuclear cells and depletion of other organs and tumor tissue is unknown. It will be important to determine if GSH depletion in tumor cells can be predicted from the examination of GSH levels in peripheral mononuclear cells.

The variable time course of GSH depletion observed in patients treated in this study supports the schedule selection: A period of treatment ranging from 1 to 3 days is needed to markedly deplete peripheral mononuclear cells of GSH in approximately 50% of patients. The variability and the extent and the time required for GSH depletion with this regimen may be related to multiple factors, including polymorphisms in the target enzyme, individual variability in the pharmacokinetics of BSO, differences in the rates of GSH metabolism. Recovery of GSH levels to baseline values in the peripheral mononuclear cells takes place within 48 hours of the last dose of BSO. This time course is consistent with murine data in which recovery by 48 hours was observed in all organs and defines a period during which time patients may be at risk from xenobiotics that depend on GSH for their detoxification.

This clinical trial demonstrated that depletion of cellular GSH levels may be achieved by the administration of an inhibitor of GSH synthesis and that such a treatment does not produce untoward nonhematologic

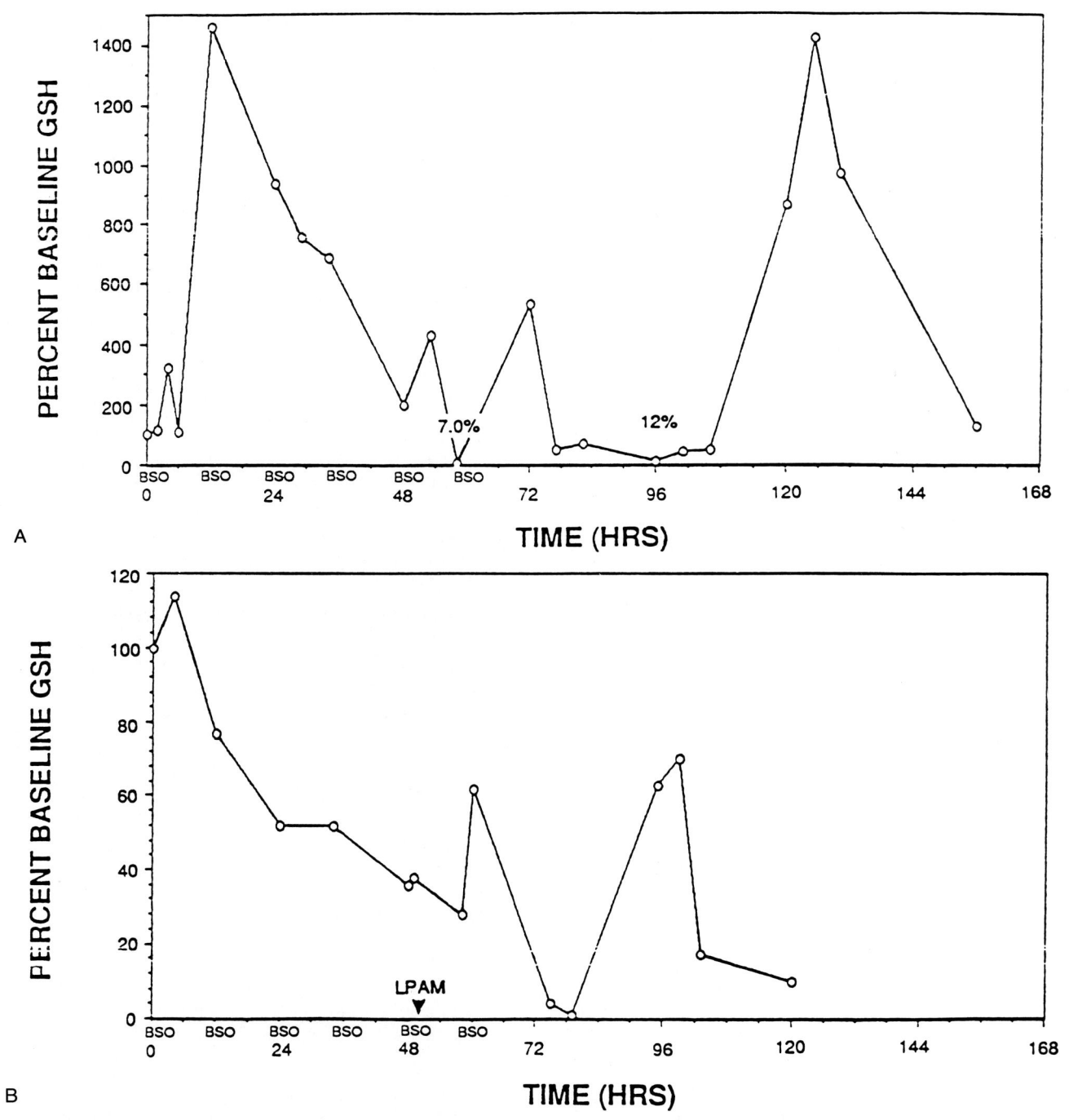

FIG. 8. A and B. Typical time course of GSH depletion in peripheral mononuclear cells following treatment with BSO. From ref. 109.

toxicity. Thus, a biochemical endpoint of altering a potentially frequent mechanism of clinical resistance to alkylating agents has been achieved. Future trials involving a large number of patients will demonstrate if this approach will increase the effectiveness of melphalan.

Trials will soon be initiated with BSO plus carboplatin. BSO plus cisplatin will not be evaluated because of the increased nephrotoxicity observed following kidney depletion of GSH.

INHIBITION OF GLUTATHIONE S-TRANSFERASE

Investigators at Fox Chase have recently reported on a phase I study of thiotepa in combination with a glutathione transferase inhibitor ethacrynic acid (110). Previous laboratory studies have demonstrated that ethacrynic acid inhibits the isozymes of GSH transferase with 50% inhibitory concentration values ranging from 0.3 μM to 6.0 μM, which restores sensitivity to alkylating agents in drug-resistant animal tumor models. A clinical trial was performed in 27 previously treated patients with advanced cancer. In this study ethacrynic acid (25–75 mg/m^2 p.o. every 6 hours for three doses) and thiotepa (30–55 mg/m^2 I.V. 1 hour after the second dose of ethacrynic acid) were administered and the major toxicity of ethacrynic acid was diuresis, which was observed at every dose level. In addition, several metabolic abnormalities occurred at 75 mg/m^2. At 50 mg/m^2, the diuretic effects of ethacrynic acid were manageable, and myelosuppression was the most important effect of the combination. Two of seven courses of ethacrynic acid (50 mg/m^2) and thiotepa (55 mg/m^2) were associated with grade 3 or 4 neutropenia and/or thrombocytopenia. Nausea and vomiting was observed to be clinically significant in 16% of patients. GSH transferase activity was assayed spectrophotometrically in the peripheral mononuclear cells of all patients. At each dose level, activity decreased following ethacrynic acid administration with recovery at 6 hours. Administration of ethacrynic acid at 50 mg/m^2 resulted in a mean nadir of transferase activity to 37% of control. These data suggest that ethacrynic acid inhibits enzymes involved in the metabolic disposition of thiotepa, including its oxidative desulfuration to tepa. The combination of thiotepa and ethacrynic acid will now be further tested in phase II trials. In addition, preclinical studies are in progress to develop more effective inhibitors of GST than ethacrynic acid.

INHIBITION OF DNA REPAIR

Reversal of Resistance with Aphidicolin

Clinical trials of aphidicolin and platinum compounds will soon be initiated in the United States. A phase I and clinical pharmacologic evaluation of aphidicolin was recently performed in Europe (111). It is significant that the dose was escalated from 12 mg/m^2 to the maximum tolerated dose of 2250 mg/m^2 with the development of local toxicity as a dose-limiting factor. Similarly, in a 24-hour continuous infusion study, the dose was escalated from 435 mg/m^2 to the maximum tolerated dose of 4500 mg/m^2. A steady state level of 3 μg/ml was achieved at doses greater than or equal to 3,000 mg/m^2, and a 24-hour continuous infusion was recommended for further clinical evaluation. These levels of aphidicolin approximate what is necessary for the potentiation of platinum toxicity in drug-resistant cell lines.

OTHER MODULATORS OF PLATINUM RESISTANCE

A clinical trial is in progress by the GOG with cyclosporine together with cisplatin in drug-resistant patients. As previously noted, the exact mechanism for the potentiation of cisplatin cytotoxicity by cyclosporine remains to be accurately defined, although it may relate to inhibition of signal transduction pathways.

THE ROLE OF *MDR* IN DRUG RESISTANCE IN OVARIAN CANCER

As previously noted, *mdr*-1 gene expression has not been shown to be elevated in ovarian cancer patients unless they have had prior exposure to natural products. Furthermore, until recently, natural products have not been a significant part of most induction regimens for previously untreated patients with advanced disease. Consequently, there has been only modest recent interest in the clinical development of modulators of drug resistance for natural products in ovarian cancer patients. However, with the identification of taxol as a highly active agent in ovarian cancer, the modulation of drug resistance developed against natural products may again prove clinically important in ovarian cancer. Experimental drug resistance to taxol is associated in part with amplification of the P-glycoprotein (*mdr*-1 gene product). However, it has not been determined if patients who develop clinical resistance to taxol express increased *mdr*-1 gene product. Clinical activity of taxol, however, suggests that mechanisms of resistance other than those mediated by *mdr*-1 are present in some patients with resistance to natural products. In a clinical trial of taxol in previously treated breast cancer patients, responses were reported in patients who were resistant to adriamycin (112).

There also is direct experimental evidence to suggest that other mechanisms of drug resistance are associated with taxol in addition to decreased drug accumulation due to increased levels of the membrane transporter protein. Tubulin mutants have been identified that have altered alpha or beta tubulin levels following the exposure of cells to low levels of taxol (113). These mutants have impaired ability to form microtubules in the absence of taxol. In addition it has been shown that taxol-resistant cells are highly sensitive to the vinca alkaloids (114). Whether this observation has clinical relevance remains to be determined.

CONCLUSIONS

There have been major recent advances in our understanding of the mechanisms associated with antineoplastic drug-resistance in human ovarian cancer cells. Drug resistance is clearly multifactorial and most likely involves alterations in transport, increased inactivation in the cytosol, and repair of damaged DNA. Consequently multiple potential targets exist for modulation of drug resistance in ovarian cancer, and clinical trials have recently been initiated aimed at reversing alkylating agent and platinum resistance, which is associated with increased levels of GSH and an increased capacity to repair damage to DNA. Modulation of drug resistance may ultimately require a combination of agents that could potentially act synergistically by inhibiting multiple critical sites that protect tumor cells from cytotoxic effects of alkylating agents and platinum compounds.

REFERENCES

1. Markman M. Intraperitoneal therapy of ovarian cancer. In: Markman M, Hoskins W, eds. *Cancer of the ovary.* New York: Raven Press [*in press*].
2. Ozols RF. Intraperitoneal chemotherapy in ovarian cancer. *J Clin Oncol* 1991;9:197–199.
3. McGuire WP. Experimental agents (nonbiological) in ovarian cancer. In: Markman M, Hoskins W, eds. *Cancer of the ovary.* New York: Raven Press [*in press*].
4. Levin L, Hryniuk WM. Dose-intensity analysis of chemotherapeutic agents in ovarian carcinoma. *J Clin Oncol* 1987;5:756–767.
5. Rothenberg ML, Ozols RF, Glotester E, et al. Dose-intensive induction therapy with cyclophosphamide, cisplatin, and consolidative radiotherapy in advanced stage epithelial ovarian cancer [*in press*].
6. Ozols RF, Ostchega Y, Curt G, et al. High dose carboplatin in refractory ovarian cancer. *J Clin Oncol* 1987;5:197–201.
7. Schpall EJ. Bone marrow transplantation. In: Markman M, Hoskins W, eds. *Cancer of the ovary.* New York: Raven Press [*in press*].
8. McGuire WP, Hoskins WJ, Brady M, et al. A phase III trial of dose intense versus standard dose cisplatin and cyclophosphamide in advanced ovarian cancer. *Proc 3rd Int Gynecol Cancer Soc* 1991;1:35.
9. Kaye SB. High dose cisplatin ($100mg/M^2$) is more effective than low dose ($50mg/M^2$) in combination with cyclophosphamide ($750mg/M^2$) for the treatment of advanced ovarian cancer. *Proc 3rd Int Gynecol Cancer Soc* 1991;1:70.
10. Perez RP, O'Dwyer PJ, Handel L, Ozols RF, Hamilton TC. Comparative cytotoxicity of CI-973, cisplatin, carboplatin and tetraplatin in human ovarian cancer cell lines. *Int J Cancer* 1991;48:265–269.
11. Hamilton T, Young R, Ozols RF. Experimental model system of ovarian cancer: applications to the design and evaluation of new treatment approaches. *Semin Oncol* 1984;11:285–298.
12. Hamilton TC. The biology of ovarian cancer. *Curr probl cancer* [*in press*].
13. Ozols RF, Young RC. Chemotherapy of ovarian cancer. *Semin Oncol* 1991;18:222–232.
14. Ozols RF. Ovarian cancer, part II treatment. *Curr Probl Cancer* [*in press*].
15. Perez RP, Hamilton RC, Ozols RF. Resistance to alkylating agents and cisplatin. Insights from ovarian carcinoma model systems. *Pharmacol Ther* 1990;48:19–27.
16. Hamilton TC, Winker M, Louie K, et al. Augmentation of adriamycin, melphalan and cisplatin cytotoxicity in drug-resistant and -sensitive human ovarian carcinoma cell lines by buthionine sulfoximine mediated glutathione depletion. *Biochem Pharmacol* 1985;34:2583–2586.
17. Hamilton TC, Lai G, Rothenberg M, Fojo A, Young R, Ozols RF. Mechanisms of resistance to cisplatin and alkylating agents. In: Ozols R, ed. *Drug resistance in cancer therapy.* Boston: Kluwer Academic Publishers, 1989;151–169.
18. Green J, Vistica D, Young R, Rogan A, Ozols RF. Potentiation of melphalan cytotoxicity in human ovarian cancer cell lines by glutathione depletion. *Cancer Res* 1984;44:5427–5431.
19. Louie K, Behrens B, Kinsella T, et al. Radiation survival parameters of antineoplastic drug-sensitive and -resistant human ovarian cancer cell lines and their modification by buthionine sulfoximine. *Cancer Res* 1985;45:2110–2115.
20. Godwin A, Meister A, O'Dwyer PJ, Hamilton TC, Anderson ME. Acquired resistance to cisplatin in human ovarian cancer cell lines is associated with increased expression of gamma glutamyl cysteine synthetase. *Proc Natl Acad Sci USA* [*in press*].
21. Hamilton TC, Young RC, McKoy WM, et al. Characterization of a human ovarian carcinoma cell line (NIH:OVCAR-3) with androgen and estrogen receptors. *Cancer Res* 1983;43:5379–5389.
22. Hamilton TC, Young RC, Louie KG, et al. Characterization of a xenograft model of human ovarian cancer which produces ascites and intra-abdominal carcinomatosis. *Cancer Res* 1984;44:5286–5290.
23. Vistica D. Cytotoxicity as an indicator for transport mechanism: evidence that melphalan is transported by two leucine-preferring carrier systems in the L1210 murine leukemia cell. *Biochim Biophys Acta* 1979;550:309–317.
24. Begleiter A, Grover J, Froese E, Goldenberg G. Membrane transport, sulfhydryl levels, and DNA cross-linking in Chinese hamster ovary cells sensitive and resistant to melphalan. *Biochem Pharmacol* 1983;32:293–300.
25. Byfield J, Calabro-Jones P. Carrier-dependent and carrier-independent transport of anti-cancer alkylating agents. *Nature* 1981;294:281–283.
26. Shionoya S, Scanlon K. Properties of amino acid transport systems in K562 cells sensitive and resistant to cis-diamminedichloroplatinum(II). *Cancer Res* 1986;46:3445–3448.
27. Kawai K, Kamatami N, Georges G, et al. Identification of a membrane glycoprotein overexpression in murine lymphoma sublines resistant to cisplatin. *J Biol Chem* 1990;265:3137–3142.
28. Andrews P, Velury S, Mann S, Howell S. Cis-diamminedichloroplatinum(II) accumulation in sensitive and resistant human ovarian carcinoma cells. *Cancer Res* 1988;48:68–73.
29. Van der Bliek A, Baas F, Van der Velde-Koerts T, et al. Genes amplified and overexpressed in human multidrug-resistant cell lines. *Cancer Res* 1988;48:5927–5932.
30. Bradley G, Juranka P, Ling V. Mechanisms of multidrug resistance. *Biochim Biophys Acta* 1988;948:87–128.
31. Bourhis J, Goldstein L, Riou G, Pastan I, Gottesman M, Bernard J. Expression of a human multidrug resistance gene in ovarian carcinomas. *Cancer Res* 1989;49:5062–5065.
32. Suzukake K, Ptero B, Vistica D. Reduction in glutathione content of L-PAM resistant L1210 cells confers drug sensitivity. *Biochem Pharmacol* 1982;31:121–124.
33. Ozols RF, Louise K, Plowman J, et al. Enhanced melphalan cytotoxicity in human ovarian cancer in vitro and in tumor-bearing nude mice by buthionine sulfoximine depletion of glutathione. *Biochem Pharmacol* 1987;36:147–153.
34. Lai G, Ozols R, Young R, Hamilton T. Effect of glutathione on DNA repair in cisplatin-resistant human ovarian cancer cell lines. *J Natl Cancer Inst* 1989;81:535–539.
35. Behrens BC, Hamilton TC, Masuda H, et al. Characterization of a cisplatin resistant human ovarian cancer cell line and its use in evaluation of platinum analogs. *Cancer Res* 1987;47:414–418.
36. Johnson SW, Ozols RF, Hamilton TC. Mechanisms of drug resistance in ovarian cancer. *Cancer* [*in press*].
37. Meister A. Novel drugs that affect glutathione metabolism. In:

Woolley PV III, Tew KD, eds. *Mechanisms of drug resistance in neoplastic cells*. San Diego: Academic Press, 1988;99–126.
38. Eastman A. Cross-linking of glutathione to DNA by cancer chemotherapeutic platinum coordination complexes. *Chem Biol Interact* 1987;61:241–248.
39. Hamer D. Metallothionein. *Annu Rev Biochem* 1986;55:913–951.
40. Schilder R, Hall L, Monks A, et al. Metallothionein gene expression and resistance to cisplatin in human ovarian cancer. *Int J Cancer* 1990;45:416–422.
41. Kelley S, Basu A, Teicher B, Hacker M, Hamer D, Lazo J. Overexpression of metallothionein confers resistance to anticancer drugs. *Science* 1988;241:1813–1815.
42. Lohrer H, Robson T. Overexpression of metallothionein in CHO cells and its effect on cell killing by ionizing radiation and alkylating agents. *Carcinogenesis* 1989;10:2279–2284.
43. Jakoby W. The glutathione-s-transferases: a group of multifunctional detoxification proteins. *Adv Enzymol Relat Areas Mol Biol* 1978;46:383–414.
44. Tew K, Clapper M. Glutathione-s-transferases and anticancer drug resistance. In: Woolley PV III, Tew KD, eds. *Mechanisms of drug resistance in neoplastic cells*. San Diego: Academic Press, 1988;141–157.
45. Tew K. *Personal communication*.
46. Clapper MJ, Hoffman J, Tew K. Sensitization of human colon xenografts to L-phenylalanine mustard using ethacrynic acid. *J Cell Pharmacol* 1990;1:71–78.
47. Cowan KH, Batist G, Tulpule A, Sinha BK, Myers CE. Similar biochemical changes associated with multidrug resistance in human breast cancer cells and carcinogen-induced resistance to xenobiotics in rats. *Proc Natl Acad Sci USA* 1986;83:9328–9332.
48. Moscow JA, Townsend AJ, Cowan KH. Elevation of Pi-class glutathione S-transferase activity in human breast cancer cells by transfection of the GST Pi-gene and its effect on sensitivity to toxins. *Mol Pharmacol* 1989;36:222–228.
49. Puchalski RB, Fahl WE. Expression of recombinant glutathione S-transferase ", Ya, or Yb1 confers resistance to alkylating agents. *Proc Natl Acad Sci USA* 1990;87:2443–2447.
50. Nakagawa K, Saijo N, Tsuchida S, et al. Glutathione S-transferase " as a determinant of drug resistance in transfectant cell lines. *J Biol Chem* 1990;256:4296–4301.
51. Eastman A. Reevaluation in the interaction of cis-dichloro-(ethylenediamine)platinum(II) with DNA. *Biochemistry* 1986;25:3912–3915.
52. Toney J, Donahue B, Kellett P, Bruhn S, Essigmann J, Lippard S. Isolation of cDNAs encoding a human protein that binds selectively to DNA modified by the anticancer drug cis-diamminedichloroplatinum(II). *Proc Natl Acad Sci USA* 1989;86:8328–8332.
53. Eastman A. The function, isolation and characterization of DNA adducts produced by anticancer platinum complexes. *Pharmacol Ther* 1987;34:155–166.
54. Reedijk J. The mechanism of action of platinum anti-tumor drugs. *Pure Appl Chem* 1987;59:181–192.
55. Fictinger-Schepmann AMJ, van der Veer J, den Hartog JHJ, Lohman PHM, Reedijk J. Adducts of the antitumor drug cis-diamminedichloroplatinum (II) with DNA: formation, identification and quantitation. *Biochemistry* 1985;24:707–713.
56. Plooy ACM, vanDijk M, Berunds F, Lohman PHM. Formation and repair of DNA interstrand cross-links in relation to cytotoxicity and unscheduled DNA synthesis induced in control and mutant human cells treated with cis-diamminedichloroplatinum (II). *Cancer Res* 1985;45:4178–4184.
57. Micetich K, Zwelling LA, Kohn KW. Quenching of DNA: platinum (II) monoadducts as a possible mechanism of resistance to cis-diamminedichloroplatinum (II) in L1210 cells. *Cancer Res* 1983;43:3609–3613.
58. Ali-Osman F. Quenching of DNA cross-link precursors of chloroethylnitrosoureas and attenuation of DNA interstrand cross-linking by glutathione. *Cancer Res* 1989;5258–5261.
59. Lai G-M, Ozols RF, Smyth JF, Young RC, Hamilton TC. Enhanced DNA repair and resistance to cisplatin in human ovarian cancer. *Biochem Pharmacol* 1988;37:4597–4600.
60. Masuda H, Ozols RF, Lai G-M, Fojo A, Rothenberg M, Hamilton TC. Increased DNA repair as a mechanism of acquired resistance to cis-diamminedichloroplatinum (II) in human ovarian cancer cell lines. *Cancer Res* 1988;48:5713–5716.
61. Masuda H, Tanaka T, Matsuda H, Kusaka I. Increased removal of DNA-bound platinum in a human ovarian cancer cell line resistant to cis-diamminedichloroplatinum (II). *Cancer Res* 1990;50:1863–1866.
62. Parker RJ, Eastman A, Bostick-Bruton F, Reed E. Acquired cisplatin resistance in human ovarian cancer cells is associated with enhanced repair of cisplatin-DNA lesions and reduced drug accumulation. *J Clin Invest* 1991;87:772–777.
63. Eastman A, Schulte N. Enhanced DNA repair as a mechanism of resistance to cis-diamminedichloroplatinum(II). *Biochemistry* 1988;27:4730–4734.
64. Batist G, Torres-Garcia S, Demuys J-M, et al. Enhanced DNA cross-like removal: the apparent mechanism of resistance in a clinically relevant melphalan-resistant human breast cancer cell line. *Mol Pharmacol* 1989;36:224–230.
65. Bohr VA. Differential DNA repair within the genome. *Cancer Rev* 1987;7:28–55.
66. Hanawalt PC. Heterogeneity of DNA repair at the gene level. *Mutat Res* 1991;247:203–211.
67. Bohr V, Phillips D, Hanawalt P. Heterogenous DNA damage and repair in the human genome. *Cancer Res* 1987;47:6426–6436.
68. Friedberg E. The molecular biology of nucleotide excision repair of DNA: recent progress. *J Cell Sci Suppl* 1987;6:1–23.
69. Sancar A, Sancar G. DNA repair enzymes. *Annu Rev Biochem* 1988;57:29–67.
70. Van Duin M, Wit J, Odijk H, et al. Molecular characterization of the human excision repair gene ERCC-1: cDNA cloning and amino acid homology with the yeast DNA repair gene RAD10. *Cell* 1986;44:913–923.
71. Hoeijmakers J. Characterization of the genes and proteins involved in excision repair of human cells. *J Cell Sci Suppl* 1987;6:111–125.
72. Doolittle R, Johnson M, Husain I, Van Houten B, Thomas D, Sancar A. Domainal evolution of a prokaryotic DNA repair protein and its relationship to active transport proteins. *Nature* 1986;323:451–453.
73. Reed E, Ormond P, Bohr V, Budd J, Bostick-Bruton F. Expression of the human DNA repair gene ERCC-1 relates to cisplatin resistance in human ovarian cancer cells. *Proc Am Assoc Cancer Res* 1989;30:448.
74. Fornace A, Alamo I, Hollander C. DNA damage-inducible transcripts in mammalian cells. *Proc Natl Acad Sci USA* 1988;85:8800–8804.
75. Fornace A, Zmudzka B, Hollander C, Wilson S. Induction of $_2$-polymerase mRNA and DNA damaging agents in Chinese hamster ovary cells. *Molec Cell Biol* 1989;9:851–853.
76. Dijt F, Fitchtinger-Schepman A, Berends F, Reedijk J. Formation and repair of cisplatin-induced adducts to DNA in cultured normal and repair-deficient human fibroblasts. *Cancer Res* 1988;48:6058–6062.
77. Olenick N, Xue L, Friedman L, Donahue L, Blaglow J. Inhibition of radiation-induced DNA-protein cross-link repair by glutathione depletion with L-buthionine sulfoximine. *Natl Cancer Inst Monogr* 1988;6:225–229.
78. Working P, Smith O, White R, Butterworth B. Induction of DNA repair in rat spermatocytes and hepatocytes by 1,2-dibromoethane: the role of glutathione. *Carcinogenesis* 1986;7:467–472.
79. Roberts J, Sturrock J, Ward K. The enhancement by caffeine of alkylation-induced cell death, mutations and chromosomal aberrations in Chinese hamster ovary cells, as a result of inhibition of post-replication DNA repair. *Mutat Res* 1974;26:129–143.
80. Lau C, Pardee A. Mechanism by which caffeine potentiates lethality of nitrogen mustard. *Proc Natl Acad Sci USA* 1982;79:2942–2946.
81. Weinert T, Hartwell L. The RAD9 gene controls the cell cycle response to DNA damage in Saccharomyces cerevisiae. *Science* 1988;241:317–322.

82. Schiestl R, Reynolds P, Prakash S, Parkash L. Cloning and sequence analysis of the Saccharomyces cerevisiae RAD9 gene and further evidence that its product is required for cell cycle arrest induced by DNA damage. *Molec Cell Biol* 1989;9:1882–1896.
83. Fraval H, Rawlings C, Roberts J. Increased sensitivity of UV-repair–deficient human cells to DNA bound platinum products which unlike thymidine dimers are not recognized by an endonuclease extracted from micrococcus luteus. *Mutat Res* 1978;51:121–132.
84. Hoy C, Thompson L, Mooney C, Salazar E. Defective DNA crosslink removal in Chinese hamster cell mutants hypersensitive to bifunctional alkylating agents. *Cancer Res* 1985;45:1737–1743.
85. Hansson J, Wood R. Repair synthesis by human cell extracts in human cell extracts damaged by cis- and trans-diamminedichloroplatinum(II). *Nucl Acids Res* 1989;17:8073–8091.
86. Pera M, Rawlings C, Roberts J. The role of DNA repair in the recovery of human cells from cisplatin toxicity. *Chem Biol Interact* 1981;37:245–261.
87. Sorenson C, Eastman A. Mechanism of cis-diamminedichloroplatinum(II)–induced cytotoxicity: role of G2 arrest of DNA double-strand breaks. *Cancer Res* 1988;48:4484–4488.
88. Katz EJ, Andrews PA, Howell SB. The effect of DNA polymerase inhibitors on the cytotoxicity of cisplatin in human ovarian carcinoma cells. *Cancer Commun* 1990;2:159–164.
89. Dempke WCM, Shellard SA, Fichtinger-Schepman AMJ, Hill BT. Lack of significant modulation of the formation and removal of platinum DNA adducts by aphidicolin glycinates in two logarithmically-growing ovarian tumor cell lines in vitro. *Carcinogenesis* 1991;12:525–528.
90. Snyder R, Carrier W, Regan J. Application of arabinofuranosyl cytosine in the kinetic analysis and quantitation of DNA repair in human cells after ultra-violet radiation. *Biophys J* 1981;35:339–350.
91. Zittoun J, Marquet J, David J, Maniey D, Zittoun R. A study of the mechanisms of cytotoxicity of Ara-C on three human leukemic cell lines. *Cancer Chemother Pharmacol* 1989;24:251–255.
92. Bergerat J-P, Drewinko B, Corry P, Barlogie B, Ho D. Synergistic lethal effect of cis-diamminedichloroplatinum and 1-$_2$-D-arabinofuranosylcytosine. *Cancer Res* 1987;47:6426–6436.
93. Fram R, Robichaud N, Bishov S, Wilson J. Interactions of cis-diamminedichloroplatinum(II) with 1-$_2$-D-arabinofuranosylcytosine in LoVo colon carcinoma cells. *Cancer Res* 1987;47:3360–3365.
94. Kern D, Morgan C, Hilderbrand-Zanki S. In vitro pharmacodynamics of 1-$_2$-D-arabinofuranosylcytosine: synergy of antitumor activity with cis-diamminedichloroplatinum(II). *Cancer Res* 1988;48:117–121.
95. Swinnen L, Barnes D, Fisher S, Albain K, Fisher R, Erickson L. 1-$_2$-D-arabinofuranosylcytosine and hydroxyurea production of cytotoxic synergy with cis-diamminedichloroplatinum(II) and modification of platinum-induced DNA interstrand cross-linking. *Cancer Res* 1989;49:1383–1389.
96. Kingston R, Sevin B, Ramos R, et al. Synergistic effects of cisplatinum and cytosine arabinoside on ovarian carcinoma cell lines, demonstrated by dual parameter flow cytometry. *Gynecol Oncol* 1989;32:282–287.
97. Scanlon K, Kashani-Sabet M, Sowers L. Overexpression of DNA replications and repair enzymes in cisplatin resistant human colon carcinoma HCT8 cells and circumvention by azidothymidine. *Cancer Commun* 1989;1:269–275.
98. Perez R, et al. Unpublished data.
99. Harrison SD, Hamilton TC, Dykes DJ, et al. Modulation of cisplatin cytotoxicity by aphidicolin glycinade in human ovarian cancer xenografts. *Proc Am Assoc Cancer Res* 1990;31:446.
100. Charp P, Regan J. Inhibition of DNA repair by trifluoperazine. *Biochim Biophys Acta* 1985;824:34–39.
101. Chafouleas J, Bolton W, Means A. Potentiation of bleomycin lethality by anticalmodulin drugs: a role of calmodulin in DNA repair. *Science* 1984;224:1346–1348.
102. Kikuchi Y, Miyauchi M, Kizawa I, Oomori K, Kato K. Establishment of a cisplatin-resistant ovarian cancer cell line. *J Natl Cancer Inst* 1986;77:1181–1185.
103. Kikuchi Y, Oomori K, Kizawa I, et al. Enhancement of antineoplastic effects of cisplatin by calmodulin antagonists in nude mice bearing human ovarian carcinoma. *Cancer Res* 1987;47:6459–6461.
104. Perez R, Handel L, Ozols R, Hamilton T. Potentiation of cisplatin cytotoxicity by trifuloperazine, a calmodulin inhibitor [in press].
105. Isonishi S, Hom DK, Thiebaut FB, et al. Expression of the C-Ha-ras oncogene in mouse NIH 3T3 cells induces resistance to cisplatin. *Cancer Res* 1991;51:5903–5909.
106. Isonishi S, Andrews P, Howell SB. Increased sensitivity to cis-diamminedichloroplatinum(II) in human ovarian cancer cell lines in response to treatment with 12-0-tetradecanoylphorbol-113-arelole. *J Biol Chem* 1990;265:3623–3627.
107. Sklar MD. Increased resistance to cis-diamminedichloroplatinum(II) in NIH 3T3 cells transferred by the ras oncogene. *Cancer Res* 1988;48:793–797.
108. Kashaui-Sabet M, Wang W, Scanlon KJ. Cyclosporine A suppresses cisplatin-induced C-fos gene expression in ovarian carcinoma cells. *J Biol Chem* 1990;265:11285–11288.
109. O'Dwyer PJ, Hamilton TC, Young RC, et al. Depletion of glutathione in normal and malignant human cells in vivo by buthionine sulfoximine: clinical and biochemical results. *J Natl Cancer Inst* [in press].
110. O'Dwyer PJ, LaCreta F, Nash J, et al. Phase I study of thiotepa in combination with the glutathione transferase inhibitor ethacrynic acid. *Cancer Res* 1991;51:6059–6065.
111. Sessa C, Zucchetti M, Davoli E, et al. Phase I and clinical pharmacologic evaluation of aphidicolin glycinate. *J Natl Cancer Inst* 1991;83:1160–1169.
112. Holmes FA, Wallers RS, Theriault RL, et al. Phase II trial of Taxol, an active drug in the treatment of metastatic breast cancer. *J Natl Cancer Inst* 1991;83:1797–1805.
113. Cabnal F. Isolation of Chinese hamster ovary cells mutants requiring continuous presence of Taxol for cell division. *J Cell Biol* 1983;97:22–29.
114. Cabral F, Wibble L, Brenner S, et al. Taxol requiring mutant chinese hamster ovary cells with impaired mitotic spindle assembly. *J Cell Biol* 1983;97:30–39.

CHAPTER 20

Chemotherapy in the Management of Celomic Epithelial Carcinoma of the Ovary

J. Tate Thigpen

Because of its proclivity to present at an advanced stage, cancer of the ovary remains the one major cancer of the female genital tract that is not amenable to early diagnosis with currently available techniques. Systemic therapy therefore plays a significant role in the management of these patients. Knowing the results of clinical trials to date, oncologists can make recommendations as to what constitutes standard therapy. These recommendations will hinge first and foremost on the histologic type of ovarian cancer. This discussion focuses on the most common histologic type, which accounts for over 80% of all ovarian cancer: celomic epithelial carcinoma of the ovary.

GENERAL CONSIDERATIONS

Among significant factors to be considered in the selection of an appropriate systemic regimen, the extent of disease at the time of diagnosis is by far the most important. The population can be divided into advanced and limited disease groups based on this information (Table 1) (1). Within the advanced disease group, the volume of residual disease is a critical determinant of patient response to chemotherapy as well as survival. Should intraperitoneal therapy prove to be superior to intravenous chemotherapy, a contention not yet established as factual, then volume of residual disease would become a determinant of the route of administration of chemotherapy.

In regard to the group of patients with limited disease, a number of risk factors must be considered: histologic grade, intracystic versus extracystic disease, disease on the external surface of the ovary, the presence of ascites, peritoneal cytology, and extraovarian disease. On the basis of these factors, patients with limited disease can be divided into two groups—those at high risk for recurrence and those at low risk (Table 2) (2,3).

ADVANCED OR RECURRENT DISEASE

A majority of patients present with advanced (stage III or IV) disease. The initial management of these patients begins with an exploratory laparotomy, which serves to determine accurately the extent of disease and to permit aggressive surgical cytoreduction. Subsequent therapy for these patients will include systemic treatment with cytotoxic and/or biologic agents.

Single Agents

Celomic epithelial ovarian carcinomas are responsive to a number of different drugs (Table 3) (4–6). Among the 17 active single agents are 13 chemotherapeutic drugs, 2 hormonal agents, and 2 biological agents.

Response rates reported for each of the active agents vary widely, a variation that may be explained by three factors: (A) the volume of residual disease at the initiation of therapy; (B) the dose and schedule of the drug; and (C) prior cytotoxic therapy to which the neoplasm has become clinically resistant as evidenced by clinical progression during therapy. With regard to the first of these factors, the importance of volume of residual disease in determining response to therapy is amply evident from clinical trials using the same regimens in minimal residual (no nodule larger than 2 cm remaining in the abdominal cavity of patients with stage III dis-

---

J. T. Thigpen: Department of Medicine, University of Mississippi School of Medicine, Jackson, Mississippi 39216

TABLE 1. The two major groups of patients based on the FIGO staging system for ovarian cancer to be considered in decision making about the use of systemic therapy[a]

Stage	Description
Limited Disease	
I	Growth limited to the ovaries
IA	One ovary; no ascites; capsule intact; no tumor on external surface
IB	Two ovaries; no ascites; capsule intact; no tumor on external surface
IC	One or both ovaries with either surface tumor or ruptured capsule or ascites or peritoneal washings with malignant cells
II	Pelvic extension
IIA	Involvement of uterus and/or tubes
IIB	Involvement of other pelvic tissues
IIC	IIA or IIB with factors as in IC
Advanced Disease	
III	Peritoneal implants outside pelvis and/or positive retroperitoneal or inguinal nodes
IIIA	Grossly limited to true pelvis; negative nodes; microscopic seeding of abdominal peritoneum
IIIB	Implants of abdominal peritoneum 2 cm or less; nodes negative
IIIC	Abdominal implants greater than 2 cm and/or positive retroperitoneal or inguinal nodes
IV	Distant metastases

[a] From ref. 1.

TABLE 2. Criteria for assignment of patients to groups at low or high risk for recurrence[a]

Group[b]	Characteristics
Low risk	Grade 1 or 2 disease
	Intact capsule
	No tumor on external surface
	Negative peritoneal cytology
	No ascites
	Growth confined to ovaries
High risk	Grade 3 disease
	Ruptured capsule
	Tumor on external surface
	Positive peritoneal cytology
	Ascites
	Growth outside ovaries

[a] From refs. 2 and 3.
[b] If any high-risk factors are present, the patient is considered high risk.

TABLE 3. Single agents active in ovarian carcinoma[a]

Drug	Patients	Response rate (percent)
Available Agents		
Alkylating agents	1,371	33
Ifosfamide	37	22
Cisplatin	190	32
Carboplatin	82	24
Doxorubicin	102	33
5-Fluorouracil	126	29
Methotrexate	34	18
Mitomycin	49	16
Hexamethylmelamine	215	24
Progestins	176	12
Antiestrogens	42	19
Alpha interferon	21	19
Investigational Agents		
Taxol	41	36
Prednimustine	36	28
Dihydroxybusulfan	26	27
Galactitol	39	15
Gamma interferon	14	29

[a] From refs. 4–6.

ease) and bulky disease (Table 4) (7–13). This relationship may depend more on the biology of the disease than on surgical cytoreduction. Regardless of the actual reason, small-volume disease responds more frequently and is associated with longer progression-free interval and survival than bulky disease.

With regard to the second factor, a metaanalysis of ovarian carcinoma clinical trials suggests a relationship between dose intensity (a function of dose and the rate at which the cumulative dose is achieved) and both response and survival (14). The only single agent for which such a relationship could be shown is cisplatin, and the range of doses over which dose intensity appears to be important is relatively narrow (6 to 12 mg/m^2/wk).

With regard to the third factor, data from a Gynecologic Oncology Group (GOG) trial of cisplatin-based intraperitoneal chemotherapy in patients with prior cisplatin-based intravenous therapy notes virtually no responses in patients clinically resistant to the intravenous regimen in contrast to reasonable activity in those

TABLE 4. The impact of volume of disease on response to chemotherapy and survival[a]

Regimen (ref.)	Minimal	Bulky
Pathological Complete Response		
PAC (7,13)	45/137 (33%)	13/107 (12%)
PAC (8)	5/17 (30%)	5/39 (13%)
HCAP (9)	18/21 (86%)	3/29 (10%)
CHEX-UP (10)	5/14 (36%)	5/37 (14%)
Median Survival Time		
PAC (7,13)	42 mo	19 mo
L-PAM (11,12)	33 mo	13 mo

[a] From refs. 7–13.

with a previous response to the intravenous therapy (15). These data suggest that clinical resistance manifested as progression of disease while on therapy is a critical predictor of response to subsequent treatment.

This last factor is a major obstacle to the development of effective salvage therapy and to the design of truly additive combination chemotherapy. Most available drugs demonstrate cross-resistance with the platinum compounds; hence, patients who progress while on platinum-based therapy can be expected not to respond to second-line therapy with other active but cross-resistant drugs.

The following discussion of specific agents attempts to consider the preceding factors. All studies of single agents include patients with bulky ovarian carcinoma so that the impact of volume of disease is minimized. Where such information is available, differing doses and schedules are compared to determine whether dose intensity is a factor in assessing drug activity. Only the issue of clinical resistance cannot be adequately addressed, because patients in phase II trials have only recently been separated into populations sensitive and resistant to primary chemotherapy.

Platinum Analogues

The platinum analogues appear to be the most active drugs in celomic epithelial carcinoma. *Cisplatin,* the most extensively studied platinum compound, has clear-cut activity in patients with no prior chemotherapy as well as in those who have received prior alkylating agents (16,17). *Carboplatin,* the second platinum compound to undergo trials in ovarian carcinoma, offers the advantage of less neurotoxicity but more thrombocytopenia than cisplatin. The drug has clearcut activity (18) and, in three comparative single-agent trials with cisplatin as well as a metaanalysis of the three, demonstrates similar activity (Table 5) (19–22).

TABLE 5. *Metaanalysis of three comparative single agent trials of carboplatin 400 mg/m^2 versus cisplatin 100 mg/m^2[a]*

Parameter	Cisplatin	Carboplatin
Total patients	195	190
Response	71/120 (59%)	80/142 (56%)
Complete	31/120 (26%)	36/142 (25%)
Partial	40/120 (33%)	44/142 (31%)
Survival (median)	23 mo	22 mo
Adverse effects (WHO grade 2 or greater)		
Leukopenia	30/171 (18%)	57/187 (30%)
Thrombocytopenia	2/171 (1%)	40/187 (22%)
Emesis	120/173 (69%)	100/187 (53%)
Neuropathy	30/173 (17%)	1/187 (1%)
Ototoxicity	22/173 (13%)	4/187 (2%)
Azotemia	2/161 (1%)	1/178 (1%)
Hypomagnesemia	15/39 (38%)	11/32 (34%)

[a] From ref. 22.

Alkylating Agents

The mustard-type alkylating agents such as cyclophosphamide, chlorambucil, and 1-phenylalanine mustard also have clear-cut activity (4). Prior to the identification of the activity of cisplatin in 1977, standard therapy for ovarian carcinoma was a single alkylating agent such as 1-phenylalanine mustard. After the demonstration of the activity of cisplatin, combinations of cisplatin with an alkylating agent became the treatment of choice based on the superior activity of the combinations (7,12). The most commonly used alkylating agent in such combinations is cyclophosphamide. The alkylating agents appear to be cross-resistant with platinum compounds.

Anthracyclines

Doxorubicin, an anthracycline, is active in ovarian carcinoma (4). Its role as a part of combination chemotherapy regimens for previously untreated ovarian carcinoma is in question because of several randomized trials that demonstrate no significant differences between combinations of a platinum analogue and alkylating agent with or without doxorubicin (13,23–25). Doxorubicin appears to be cross-resistant with the alkylating agents and with the platinum compounds.

Taxol

A diterpenoid from the bark of the western yew tree (taxus brevifolia), taxol acts by a unique mechanism to enhance tubulin polymerization and microtubule stability with consequent production of microtubule bundling throughout the cell (26). This action results in inhibition of the dynamic reorganization of the microtubular structure of the cell before cell division. As a consequence of this unique mechanism of action, taxol appears not to be cross-resistant with the platinum analogues in phase II trials of patients who are clinically resistant to platinum-based regimens.

Taxol had significant activity in three phase II trials in patients with prior platinum-based combination chemotherapy (Table 6) (6,27,28). Responses were

TABLE 6. *Phase II trials of taxol in patients with previously treated ovarian carcinoma*

Investigator (ref.)	Patients	Response
McGuire et al. (27)	40	1 CR + 11 PR (30%)[a]
Sensitive	15	6 (40%)
Resistant	25	6 (24%)
GOG (6)	43	6 CR + 9 PR (35%)
Sensitive	16	7 (44%)
Resistant	27	8 (30%)
Einzig et al. (28)	29	1 CR + 5 PR (21%)

[a] CR, complete response; PR, partial response.

seen in both platinum-sensitive and platinum-resistant patients. Adverse effects including myelosuppression, hypersensitivity reactions, and arrhythmias requiring continuous cardiac monitoring during therapy were frequent and severe but manageable and resulted in no deaths. The occurrence of anaphylactic episodes was reduced by the use of premedication with steroids and H_1 and H_2 blockers in the phase II trials. The dose-limiting toxicity is myelosuppression, which is severe but short in duration.

Taxol is clearly a highly active drug with a unique mechanism of action and evidence of clinical non–cross-resistance with platinum compounds. One major drawback that currently limits its use is the lack of a sufficient and reliable supply. Extraction of the drug from the bark of the western yew tree results in the destruction of the tree. Efforts are now being directed to the development of alternative methods to obtain the drug. Once available, the drug has great potential as a part of front-line combination chemotherapy as well as a salvage therapy.

Hexamethylmelamine

Hexamethylmelamine has clear-cut activity as a single agent in ovarian carcinoma in previously untreated patients (29) as well as in patients who have failed previous platinum-based chemotherapy (30,31). The major dose-limiting adverse effect is gastrointestinal toxicity manifested as nausea and vomiting. The drug is currently available for use in the salvage setting in patients who have failed platinum-based combination chemotherapy. Its activity in patients who have failed platinum-based therapy and its relative lack of myelosuppression make it potentially interesting as a part of first-line combination regimens.

Ifosfamide

Ifosfamide is chemically similar to cyclophosphamide but appears to be more active than its chemical cousin. The drug has clear-cut activity in ovarian carcinoma with responses noted in patients who were clinically resistant to platinum-cyclophosphamide combinations (5,32). The major toxicity other than myelosuppression is hemorrhagic cystitis, which is prevented by the use of mesna, a specific antidote to the urothelial effects. The other noteworthy adverse effect, particularly in a patient population that has received prior cisplatin, is central nervous system toxicity, which ranges from irritability to coma. The incidence of toxicity increases as renal function deteriorates and albumin drops, and it occurs more frequently with schedules that call for larger single doses that achieve a higher peak serum level of the drug (33–40). Patients with abnormal renal function or hypoalbuminemia should therefore be treated with a multiple-day schedule at reduced dose.

In summary, various drugs have activity against ovarian carcinoma. Most studies support the central role of the platinum analogues cisplatin and carboplatin in front-line therapy. Of these two, carboplatin appears to be the better choice because it causes less severe toxicity. Alkylating agents and doxorubicin are useful in combination with the platinum compounds, but they appear to be clinically cross-resistant with platinum agents. Three drugs of significant interest for use in combination with platinum because of their apparent lack of complete cross-resistance with platinum are taxol, hexamethylmelamine, and ifosfamide.

Combination Chemotherapy

Standard Therapy

The relatively large number of active drugs available in celomic epithelial carcinomas points to the potential for the development of effective combination chemotherapy. A plethora of trials of combination chemotherapy fills the medical literature. The most significant of these studies are seven randomized trials that lead logically to current standard therapy (7,12,13,41–44). Three of these trials, conducted by GOG, develop the use of cisplatin-based regimens with the two-drug combination of cisplatin plus cyclophosphamide (7,12,13). The other four trials compare cisplatin-based regimens to carboplatin-based regimens (41–44). The conclusions from these seven studies are supported by other trials of systemic therapy and form the basis for current practice. (45).

Successive GOG studies in patients with bulky advanced disease establish the superiority of cisplatin-based combination chemotherapy over single alkylating agent therapy (Table 7) (7,12). GOG protocol 22 compared melphalan alone to either melphalan plus hexamethylmelamine or doxorubicin plus cyclophosphamide (12). The only statistically significant difference was a greater clinical complete response rate in patients treated with doxorubicin plus cyclophosphamide as compared to those receiving melphalan alone. These results were the basis for selection of doxorubicin-cyclophosphamide as the control arm of GOG protocol 47, which compared doxorubicin plus cyclophosphamide to the same two drugs plus cisplatin (7). This study demonstrated a statistically significant improvement in clinical complete response rate, overall response rate, progression-free interval, and survival in patients treated with cisplatin-doxorubicin-cyclophosphamide.

GOG protocol 52 differed from the preceding two

TABLE 7. *The evolution of cisplatin-based combination chemotherapy through two GOG trials in patients with bulky advanced celomic epithelial carcinoma of the ovary[a]*

Parameter[b]	GOG protocol 22		GOG protocol 47	
	L-PAM[c]	AC[d]	AC[d]	PAC[e]
Patients	64	72	120	107
CR[e]	20%	32%	26%	51%
CR + PR	37%	49%	48%	76%
pCR			4/23	13/39
pCR/total			3%	12%
Duration	8 mo	10 mo	9 mo	15 mo
Median survival	12 mo	14 mo	16 mo	20 mo

[a] From refs. 7 and 12.
[b] CR, complete response; PR, partial response; pCR, pathologic complete response.
[c] Melphalan 0.2 mg/kg/day orally for 5 days every 4 to 6 weeks for 10 courses.
[d] Doxorubicin 50 mg/m^2 plus cyclophosphamide 500 mg/m^2, both IV, every 3 weeks for 8 courses.
[e] Cisplatin 50 mg/m^2 plus doxorubicin and cyclophosphamide, as in AC, all IV every 3 weeks for 8 courses.

trials in that it involved patients with minimal residual disease (defined as patients with stage III disease and no nodules larger than 1 cm in diameter). Patients were randomized to receive either the three-drug combination of cisplatin-doxorubicin-cyclophosphamide or cisplatin plus cyclophosphamide (Table 8) (13). The dose intensity of the two regimens was comparable as a result of the escalation of the dose of cyclophosphamide. The pathologic complete rate as documented at second-look laparotomy was not significantly different; nor were there any differences in progression-free interval or survival.

These three trials established the combination of cisplatin plus cyclophosphamide as standard chemotherapy for advanced or recurrent ovarian carcinoma. Four additional recently completed studies, however, must be considered in the current choice of standard therapy (41–44). These studies, conducted by the Southwest Oncology Group (SWOG), the National Cancer Institute of Canada (NCIC), the Gynaecological Cancer Cooperative Group, and a Mayo Clinic group, compare the relative efficacy of cisplatin-based versus carboplatin-based regimens (Table 9). The SWOG trial compared cyclophosphamide 600 mg/m^2 plus either cisplatin 100 mg/m^2 or carboplatin 300 mg/m^2 in patients with bulky stage III or stage IV disease (41). The study showed no significant differences between the two regimens with regard to response rate, progression-free interval, or survival. The toxicity of the two regimens differed, with the cisplatin regimen producing greater adverse effects. The NCIC trial compared essentially the same regimens with similar results (43).

The study conducted by the Gynaecological Cancer Cooperative Group for the European Organization for Research and Treatment of Cancer compared two four-drug combinations consisting of cyclophosphamide, doxorubicin, and hexamethylmelamine with either cisplatin or carboplatin (42). Again, no significant differences were noted with regard to response rate, progression-free interval, or survival.

The trial of carboplatin-based chemotherapy versus cisplatin-based therapy conducted by investigators at the Mayo Clinic is flawed by a major design problem (44). The dose intensity of carboplatin is well below that of cisplatin in the other arm. It is therefore difficult to determine whether the differences in progression-free interval and survival favoring the cisplatin regimen were related to a different platinum compound or to a lower dose intensity of the carboplatin. This study has two other distinguishing features. The number of patients in the trial is considerably lower; and, unlike the patients in the other three studies, who mostly had bulky disease, 65% of the patients had small-volume disease.

In summary, these seven randomized trials define two major concepts about the current standard chemotherapy for advanced ovarian carcinoma. First, platinum-based combination chemotherapy offers significant advantages over non–platinum-based regimens. Second, carboplatin offers certain advantages over cisplatin in terms of toxicity with no diminution in efficacy.

TABLE 8. *Platinum-based combination chemotherapy with and without doxorubicin in stage III minimal residual ovarian carcinoma[a]*

Parameter[b]	PAC[c]	PC[d]
Patients	173	176
Early recurrence	20	30
Refused second look	36	37
Residual disease	72	67
pCR (%)	45 (26%)	42 (24%)

[a] From ref. 13.
[b] pCR, pathologic complete response.
[c] Cisplatin 50 mg/m^2 plus doxorubicin 50 mg/m^2 plus cyclophosphamide 500 mg/m^2, all IV, every 3 weeks for 8 cycles.
[d] Cisplatin 50 mg/m^2 plus cyclophosphamide 1,000 mg/m^2, both IV, every 3 weeks for 8 cycles.

Evolving Concepts

Although the preceding results point to a combination of a platinum compound plus cyclophosphamide as standard chemotherapy for celomic epithelial carcinoma of the ovary, other evolving concepts should be noted: dose intensity, alternative routes of administration, and non–cross-resistant agents.

TABLE 9. Four randomized trials comparing cisplatin-based to carboplatin-based combination chemotherapy in previously untreated patients with ovarian carcinoma[a]

Study (ref.) and regimen	Response	Survival
Alberts et al. (41) ($n = 342$)		
Carboplatin 300 mg/m² q4wks	cCR = 34%[b]	20 mo
Cyclophosphamide 600 mg/m² q4wks	pCR = 12%[c]	
Cisplatin 100 mg/m² q4wks	cCR = 27%	16.8 mo
Cyclophosphamide 600 mg/m² q4wks	pCR = 7%	
ten Bokkel Huinink et al. (42) ($n = 339$)		
Cyclophosphamide 100 mg/m² po d14–28	cCR = 24%	107 wk
Hexamethylmelamine 150 mg/m² po d14–28		
Doxorubicin 35 mg/m² IV d1		
Carboplatin 350 mg/m² IV d1		
Cyclophosphamide 100 mg/m² po d14–28	cCR = 23%	108 wk
Hexamethylmelamine 150 mg/m² po d14–28		
Doxorubicin 35 mg/m² IV d1		
Cisplatin 20 mg/m² IV d1–5		
Pater (43) ($n = 447$)		21–49
Carboplatin 300 mg/m² q4wks	pCR = 13%	24 mo
Cyclophosphamide 600 mg/m² q4wks		
Cisplatin 75 mg/m² q4wks	pCR = 18%	23 mo
Cyclophosphamide 600 mg/m² q4wks		
Edmondson et al. (44) ($n = 103$)		
Carboplatin 150 mg/m² q4wks		20 mo
Cyclophosphamide 1,000 mg/m² q4wks		
Cisplatin 60 mg/m² q4wks		27 mo
Cyclophosphamide 1,000 mg/m² q4wks		

[a] From refs. 41–44.
[b] cCR, clinical complete response.
[c] pCR, pathologic complete response.

Dose intensity, expressed as dose of drug per square meter of body surface area per unit of time, has long been thought to have critical importance to the success of chemotherapy. In vitro data support the ability of increasing drug levels to enhance cell kill in cultures of ovarian cancer cells (45). In patients who have recurred after platinum-based chemotherapy for ovarian carcinoma, responses to higher doses of the same platinum compound (46) or to greater exposure as a result of intraperitoneal administration (47) suggest that enhanced dose can produce responses when lower doses have failed. The use of hypertonic saline to permit escalation of cisplatin dose to 200 mg/m²/course in combination with cyclophosphamide yields high response rates (48). Finally, metaanalyses have been reported to show a correlation between dose intensity of platinum and response (14).

These observations suggest that dose intensity is important, but certain issues need to be addressed. First, with regard to reported responses of "refractory" ovarian carcinoma to higher doses of drug, such responses are infrequent in patients who progress while on the lower dose therapy but are more common in patients who develop recurrent disease some time after completing prior therapy. For example, in a series of 30 patients with refractory ovarian carcinoma who were treated with high-dose carboplatin (800 mg/m²/35 days), eight responses were observed, none in patients who had progressive disease during prior therapy with a cisplatin-based regimen (49). Similar observations are emerging from second-line phase II studies of intraperitoneal chemotherapy.

Second, the reported high response rates with high-dose cisplatin regimens need to be placed into perspective. The GOG studies with regimens using 50 mg/m² of cisplatin yield results similar to those reported with the high-dose cisplatin regimens. In patients with minimal residual stage III disease (no nodule larger than 2 cm remaining), the high-dose regimen (cisplatin 200 mg/m² plus cyclophosphamide 1,000 mg/m² repeated every 4 weeks) yields a pathologic complete response rate of 38% (48), and the GOG regimen (cisplatin 50 mg/m² plus cyclophosphamide 1,000 mg/m² every 3 weeks) a pathologic complete response rate of 30% (13). In patients with bulky stage III or stage IV disease, the high-dose regimen (same as previously noted) yields a pathologic complete response rate of 12% (48), and the GOG regimen (cisplatin 50 mg/m² plus doxorubicin 50 mg/m² plus cyclophosphamide 500 mg/m² repeated every 3 weeks) a pathologic complete response rate of 11% (7). There is therefore no evidence that the high-dose cisplatin regimen yields a superior result, even though the dose intensity of the platinum compound as a function of dose and time is three times as high.

Third, although the dose-intensity metaanalysis of Levin and Hryniuk (14) does demonstrate a dose-response relationship for cisplatin, this relationship applies only over the range from 0.4 to 0.8 dose-intensity units. The "standard" regimen included cisplatin at a dose of 15 mg/m²/week. The dose-response relationship for cisplatin therefore extends from 6 mg/m²/week to 12 mg/m²/week. This metaanalysis thus supplies no support for the use of doses higher than those used by the GOG in their relatively low-dose cisplatin regimens.

Recent reports address the question of dose intensity in ovarian carcinoma more directly. Two randomized phase III trials were recently reported at the Third Biennial Meeting of the International Gynecologic Cancer Society. The first is a GOG study of 485 patients with suboptimal stage III or stage IV disease (Table 10) (50). These patients were randomized to receive either eight cycles or cisplatin 50 mg/m² plus cyclophosphamide 500 mg/m² every 3 weeks or four cycles of cisplatin 100 mg/m² plus cyclophosphamide 1000 mg/m² every 3 weeks with second-look laparotomy to follow 6 weeks after completion of chemotherapy. Received/projected dose intensity was 0.46/0.52 for the low-dose arm and 0.90/1.03 for the high-dose arm. The high-dose arm was thus 1.96 times as dose intense as the low-dose arm. Among the 172 patients with measurable disease, the low-dose arm yielded clinical response rates of 32% complete and 53% overall response; the high-dose arm yielded 26% complete and 45% overall. Median progression-free interval and survival were 12.2 and 23.9 months, respectively, for the low-dose arm and 13.3 and 20.7 months for the high-dose arm. Adverse effects were more common and more severe on the high-dose arm. These results suggest absolutely no advantage for the more dose-intense regimen.

In contrast, a report from the Scottish Ovarian Cancer Study Group evaluated cyclophosphamide 750 mg/m² with either low-dose cisplatin 50 mg/m² or high-dose cisplatin 100 mg/m² every 3 weeks for six cycles in 185 patients, one-half of whom had minimum residual disease (Table 11) (51). The end-point of the trial was survival. At 18 months follow-up, a greater percentage of patients on the high-dose arm were alive (73% versus 48%, $p = 0.0008$). There are two major differences between this trial and the GOG study. First, a significant proportion of the patients on this study had minimal residual disease. Second, the total dose of cisplatin prescribed was greater for the high-dose regimen than for the low-dose regimen on this study.

To understand the apparent contradictions in the preceding data, certain basic principles upon which the concept of dose intensity is based must be considered. The somatic mutation theory for drug resistance postulates that the failure to cure a patient results from either the failure to eradicate all drug-sensitive cells because of insufficient drug dose intensity or the emergence of cells resistant to the drug regimen (52). Enhanced dose intensity in theory functions in two ways to improve the likelihood of cure: by eradicating all sensitive cells and by eliminating cells likely to mutate to resistance before such mutations take place. Escalating dose should lead to greater cell kill until all sensitive cells have been eradicated. There is no evidence that further escalation, at least over the dose range achievable in clinical practice, can overcome cellular resistance. Dose intensity should thus be more likely to lead to enhanced survival in small-volume disease, which is less likely to contain large numbers of resistant cells, a perspective that could explain the cited data. Whether this explanation proves correct will be determined by further studies.

Intraperitoneal therapy is a logical approach to a disease process such as ovarian carcinoma that spreads primarily by intraperitoneal seeding and remains con-

TABLE 10. *Results of a preliminary analysis of GOG protocol 97 involving 485 patients and showing no difference between low dose intensity and high dose intensity cisplatin-cyclophosphamide in patients with bulky advanced ovarian carcinoma[a]*

	Low-dose arm[b]	High-dose arm[c]
Complete response	32%	26%
Overall response	53%	45%
Progression-free interval	12.2 mo	13.3 mo
Survival	23.9 mo	20.7 mo

[a] From ref. 48.
[b] Cisplatin 50 mg/m² + cyclophosphamide 500 mg/m², both IV, every 3 weeks for 8 cycles.
[c] Cisplatin 100 mg/m² + cyclophosphamide 1,000 mg/m², both IV, every 3 weeks for 4 cycles.

TABLE 11. *Scottish Ovarian Cancer Study Group trial of dose intensity in advanced ovarian carcinoma[a]*

	Low-dose regimen	High-dose regimen
Patients	83	82
Excluded	8	5
Eligible and evaluable	75	77
Suboptimal patients	40 (53%)	43 (56%)
Alive at 18 months	48%	73%

[a] From ref. 51, $p = 0.0008$.

fined clinically to the peritoneal cavity for a significant part of its course. Such an approach is feasible for major drugs active in ovarian carcinoma such as the platinum analogues and yields durable pathologic complete responses in previously treated patients with small-volume disease (53–57). The most frequent complications of the procedure are infection, catheter-related complications, abdominal pain, and bowel obstruction or perforation (58–60).

The fact that significantly higher drug levels can be achieved in peritoneal fluid by direct intraperitoneal administration suggests that much better exposure of neoplastic cells to drug can result. This enhanced exposure or "dose intensity" may be 20-fold to several hundred-fold greater than that achievable by the intravenous route. Despite the theoretical appeal of these facts, evidence raises doubt about actual results that can be attained. First, only patients with disease 5 mm or less in diameter can expect to achieve markedly enhanced exposure of tumor cells to drug. Second, even in such a favorable group of patients, emerging data suggest that only patients still clinically sensitive to intravenous cisplatin will respond to cisplatin and that the pharmacologic advantage of intraperitoneal administration does not overcome clinical resistance (15). Third, no randomized studies comparing intravenous to intraperitoneal therapy have been completed as yet; hence, direct clinical evidence of enhanced benefit is lacking. An intergroup study of SWOG, GOG, and the Eastern Cooperative Oncology Group is ongoing (61). Until data from a randomized trial demonstrate advantage for the intraperitoneal approach, the increased complication rate should limit intraperitoneal therapy to investigational use.

Non–cross-resistant drugs afford the best hope of improving clinical results at the present time. Three agents that appear to be non–cross-resistant with platinum analogues, at least to some extent, are taxol, hexamethylmelamine, and ifosfamide. The feasibility of administering taxol together with cisplatin in a schedule of cisplatin 75 mg/m^2 and taxol 135 mg/m^2 intravenously every 3 weeks has been demonstrated (62). GOG is currently comparing this combination to a combination of cisplatin 75 mg/m^2 plus cyclophosphamide 750 mg/m^2 every 3 weeks.

With regard to hexamethylmelamine, three studies suggest that the addition of this agent to platinum-based combination chemotherapy results in a late-emerging survival advantage. Two of these trials (63–65) were nonrandomized studies of hexamethylmelamine plus cyclophosphamide, doxorubicin, and cisplatin compared to historical controls of cyclophosphamide, doxorubicin, and cisplatin. Both showed superior survival for the four-drug combination. The third was a randomized trial of cisplatin plus cyclophosphamide versus the same two drugs plus doxorubicin and hexamethylmelamine (66). Although the patients with large-volume disease or poor performance status fared better with the two-drug combination, the four-drug combination yielded a late survival advantage in lower risk patients. This possible role for hexamethylmelamine in first-line combination chemotherapy in lower risk patients with advanced or recurrent disease requires confirmation.

The observation of responses to ifosfamide in patients resistant to platinum combinations (5) suggests that combinations of cisplatin plus ifosfamide might offer an advantage over platinum-cyclophosphamide regimens. No randomized trials have yet addressed this question.

No defined role exists for any of these three agents in front-line therapy for ovarian carcinoma at the present time. In the case of taxol, the ongoing randomized trial should define a role, if any, for this agent. At least in the United States, there are no current randomized trials evaluating the role of ifosfamide or hexamethylmelamine. Such trials are needed.

LIMITED DISEASE

The majority of patients with limited (stage I or II) disease have stage I disease, which is discovered at time of laparotomy for other reasons. The management of these patients begins with a careful staging laparotomy to determine that the patient has no microscopic disease within the peritoneal cavity. Definitive therapy is surgical resection, which should consist at least of a total abdominal hysterectomy and bilateral salpingo-oophorectomy plus omentectomy.

As noted previously, patients can be divided into groups of those at low risk and those at high risk for recurrence on the basis of the pathologic features of the primary neoplasm (Table 2) (3,67). Features of critical importance include histologic grade, capsular rupture, surface excrescences, peritoneal cytology, ascites, and extraovarian spread. Patients at low risk for recurrence have a 5-year disease-free survival that exceeds 95% with surgical resection only (Table 12) and require no adjuvant therapy (67).

TABLE 12. *OCSG/GPG protocol 7601: a randomized trial of patients at low risk for recurrence*[a]

	Observation	Melphalan
Patients	38	43
Recurrences	4	1
Deaths	4	2
Disease-free 5-year survival	91%	98%
Overall 5-year survival	94%	98%

[a] From refs. 3, 67. No significant differences between studies are noted. OCSG, Ovarian Cancer Study Group.

TABLE 13. *OCSG/GOG protocol 7602: a randomized trial of patients at high risk for recurrence[a]*

	IP P32	Melphalan
Patients	73	68
Recurrrences	14	13
Deaths	16	15
Disease-free 5-year survival	80%	80%
Overall 5-year survival	78%	81%

[a] From refs. 3, 67. No significant differences between studies are noted.

Patients at high risk for recurrence have an ultimate relapse rate that may approach 40–50% and hence should be considered for adjuvant therapy. Although no randomized trials have been conducted with a no-treatment control arm, survival with either intraperitoneal chromic phosphate or single agent melphalan appears to be better than expected (Table 13) (3). Intraperitoneal chromic phosphate produces fewer adverse effects. An ongoing intergroup study involving GOG, SWOG, and the North Central Cancer Treatment Group randomizes patients with high-risk stage I disease to either intraperitoneal chromic phosphate or three cycles of cisplatin 100 mg/m² plus cyclophosphamide 1,000 mg/m² every 3 weeks after surgical resection.

CONCLUSIONS

The use of chemotherapy in the management of celomic epithelial carcinoma of the ovary is essential to optimal treatment of the disease. Currently available results indicate that patients with advanced or recurrent disease should undergo a maximum surgical effort to cytoreduce disease and then receive a combination of a platinum compound plus cyclophosphamide. Optimum dose, schedule, and route of administration have yet to be determined. Patients with limited disease should be categorized as low risk or high risk for recurrence, and those with high-risk disease should receive adjuvant therapy in the form of either intraperitoneal chromic phosphate or a combination of a platinum compound plus cyclophosphamide.

REFERENCES

1. The new FIGO stage grouping for primary carcinoma of the ovary (1985). *Gynecol Oncol* 1986;25:383.
2. Young R, Walton L, Decker D, et al. Early stage ovarian cancer: preliminary results of randomized trials after comprehensive initial staging. *Proc ASCO* 1983;2:148.
3. Thigpen JT, Blessing JA, Vance RB, Lambuth BW. Management of patients with stage I and II ovarian carcinoma. In: *Proceedings of the Perugia International Cancer Conference II: recent advances in the treatment of testicular and ovarian cancer.* New York: LP Communications, 1990;41–49.
4. Thigpen JT. Single agent chemotherapy in the management of ovarian carcinoma. In: Alberts DS, Surwit EA, eds. *Ovarian carcinoma.* Boston: Martinus Nijhoff, 1985;115–146.
5. Sutton GP, Blessing JA, Photopoulos G, Berman ML, Homesley HD. Gynecologic Oncology Group experience with ifosfamide. *Semin Oncol* 1990;17(suppl 4):6–10.
6. Thigpen T, Blessing J, Ball H, Hummel S, Barrett R. Phase II trial of taxol as second-line therapy for ovarian carcinoma: a Gynecologic Oncology Group study. *Proc ASCO* 1990;9:156.
7. Omura G, Blessing J, Ehrlich C, et al. A randomized trial of cyclophosphamide and doxorubicin with or without cisplatin in advanced ovarian carcinoma. *Cancer* 1986;57:1725–1730.
8. Ehrlich C, Einhorn L, Williams S, et al. Chemotherapy for stage III-IV epithelial ovarian cancer with cis-dichlorodiammineplatinum (II), adriamycin, and cyclophosphamide: a preliminary report. *Cancer Treat Rep* 1979;63:281–288.
9. Greco F, Julian C, Richardson R, et al. Advanced ovarian cancer: brief intensive combination chemotherapy and second-look operation. *Obstet Gynecol* 1981;58:199–205.
10. Young R, Howser D, Myers C, et al. Combination chemotherapy (CHex-UP) with intraperitoneal maintenance in advanced ovarian adenocarcinoma. *Proc ASCO* 1981;22:465.
11. Gall S, Bundy B, Beecham J, et al. Therapy of stage III (optimal) epithelial carcinoma of the ovary with melphalan or melphalan plus Corynebacterium parvum (a Gynecologic Oncology Group study). *Gynecol Oncol* 1986;25:26–36.
12. Omura G, Morrow P, Blessing J, et al. A randomized comparison of melphalan versus melphalan plus hexamethylmelamine versus adriamycin plus cyclophosphamide in ovarian carcinoma. *Cancer* 1983;51:783–789.
13. Omura G, Bundy B, Berek J, et al. Randomized trial of cyclophosphamide plus cisplatin with or without doxorubicin in ovarian carcinoma: a Gynecologic Oncology Group study. *J Clin Oncol* 1989;7:457–465.
14. Levin L, Hryniuk W. Dose intensity analysis of chemotherapy regimens in ovarian carcinoma. *J Clin Oncol* 1987;5:756–767.
15. Berek J. *Personal communication of GOG data.*
16. Wiltshaw E, Kroner T. Phase II trial of cis-dichlorodiammineplatinum (II) (NSC-119875) in advanced adenocarcinoma of the ovary. *Cancer Treat Rep* 1976;60:55–60.
17. Thigpen T, Lagasse L, Homesley H, et al. Cisplatinum in the treatment of advanced or recurrent adenocarcinoma of the ovary: a phase II study of the Gynecologic Oncology Group. *Am J Clin Oncol* 1983;6:431–435.
18. Kjorstad K, Bertelsen K, Slevin M, et al. Phase II trial of carboplatin in ovarian cancer. *Proc ASCO* 1986;5:116.
19. Pecorelli S, Bolis G, Vassena L, et al. Randomized comparison of cisplatin and carboplatin in advanced ovarian cancer. *Proc ASCO* 1988;7:136.
20. Wiltshaw E. Ovarian trials at the Royal Marsden. *Cancer Treat Rev* 1985;12(suppl A):67–71.
21. Adams M, Kerby IJ, Unger L, et al. A comparison of first- and second-line efficacy of cisplatin and carboplatin in advanced ovarian cancer. *Sixth NCI-EORTC Symposium on New Drugs in Cancer Therapy,* 1989 (abst 315).
22. Rozencweig M, Martin A, Beltangady M, et al. Randomized trials of carboplatin versus cisplatin in advanced ovarian cancer. In: Bunn P, Canetta R, Ozols R, Rozencweig M, eds. *Carboplatin (JM-8): current perspectives and future directions.* Philadelphia: WB Saunders, 1990;175–192.
23. Sessa C. European studies with cisplatin and cisplatin analogues in advanced ovarian cancer. *Eur J Cancer Clin Oncol* 1986;22:1271–1277.
24. Gruppo Interregionale Cooperativo Oncologico Ginecologia. Long-term results of a randomized trial comparing cisplatin with cisplatin and cyclophosphamide with cisplatin, cyclophosphamide and adriamycin in advanced ovarian cancer. *J Clin Oncol* [in press].
25. Neijt JP, ten Bokkel Huinink WW, van der Burg MEL, et al. Randomized trial comparing two combination chemotherapy regimens (CHAP-5 v CP) in advanced ovarian carcinoma. *J Clin Oncol* 1987;5:1157–1168.
26. Rowinsky EK, Donehower RC, Jones RJ, Tucker RW. Microtubule changes and cytotoxicity in leukemic cell lines treated with taxol. *Cancer Res* 1988;48:4093–4100.

27. McGuire WP, Rowinsky EK, Rosenshein NB, et al. Taxol: a unique antineoplastic agent with significant activity in advanced ovarian epithelial neoplasms. *Ann Intern Med* 1989;111:273–279.
28. Einzig AI, Wiernik PH, Sasloff J, et al. Phase II study of taxol in patients with advanced ovarian cancer. *Proc AACR* 1990;31:187.
29. Blum RH, Livingston RB, Carter SK. Hexamethylmelamine—a new drug with activity in solid tumors. *Eur J Cancer* 1973;9:195–202.
30. Manetta A, MacNeill C, Lyter JA, et al. Hexamethylmelamine as a single second-line agent in ovarian cancer. *Gynecol Oncol* 1990;36:93–96.
31. Rosen GF, Lurain JR, Newton M. Hexamethylmelamine in ovarian cancer after failure of cisplatin-based multiple-agent chemotherapy. *Gynecol Oncol* 1987;27:173–179.
32. Thigpen T, Lambuth B, Vance R. Ifosfamide in the management of gynecologic cancers. *Semin Oncol* 1990;17(suppl 4):11–18.
33. Meanwell CA, Blake AE, Kelly KA, Honigsberger L, Blackledge G. Prediction of ifosfamide/mesna associated encephalopathy. *Eur J Cancer Clin Oncol* 1986;22:815–819.
34. Perren TJ, Turner RC, Smith IE. Encephalopathy with rapid infusion ifosfamide/mesna. *Lancet* 1987;1:390–391.
35. Meanwell CA, Kelly KA, Blackledge G. Avoiding ifosfamide/mesna encephalopathy. *Lancet* 1986;2:406.
36. Antman KH, Ryan L, Elias A, Sherman D, Grier HE. Response to ifosfamide and mesna: 124 previously treated patients with metastatic or unresectable sarcoma. *J Clin Oncol* 1989;7:126–131.
37. Osborne RJ, Slevin ML. Ifosfamide, mesna, and encephalopathy. *Lancet* 1985;1:1398–1399.
38. Heim ME, Fiene R, Schick E, Wolpert E, Queiber W. Central nervous system side effects following ifosfamide monotherapy of advanced renal carcinoma. *J Cancer Res Clin Oncol* 1981;100:113–116.
39. Goren MP, Wright RK, Pratt CB, Pell FE. Dechlorethylation of ifosfamide and neurotoxicity. *Lancet* 1986;2:1219–1220.
40. Cerny T, Kupfer A. Stabilization and quantitative determination of the neurotoxic metabolite chloracetaldehyde in the plasma of ifosfamide treated patients. *Proc ECCO* 1989;5:147.
41. Alberts DS, Green SJ, Hannigan EV, et al. Improved efficacy of carboplatin plus cyclophosphamide versus cisplatin plus cyclophosphamide: preliminary report by the Southwest Oncology Group of a phase III randomized trial in stages III and IV suboptimal ovarian cancer. *Proc ASCO* 1989;8:151 (abst).
42. ten Bokkel Huinink WW, van der Burg MEL, van Oosterom AT, et al. Carboplatin in combination therapy for ovarian cancer. *Cancer Treat Rev* 1988;15(suppl B):9–15.
43. Pater J. Cyclophosphamide/cisplatin versus cyclophosphamide/carboplatin in macroscopic residual ovarian cancer. Initial results of a National Cancer Institute of Canada Clinical Trials Group trial. *Proc ASCO* 1990;9:155 (abst).
44. Edmondson JH, McCormack GM, Wieand HS, et al. Cyclophosphamide-cisplatin versus cyclophosphamide-carboplatin in stage III–IV ovarian carcinoma: a comparison of equally myelosuppressive regimens. *J Natl Cancer Inst* 1989;81:1500–1504.
45. Alberts DS, Young L, Mason NL, et al. In vitro evaluation of anticancer drugs against ovarian cancer at concentrations achievable by intraperitoneal administration. *Semin Oncol* 1985;12(suppl):38–42.
46. Ozols R, Corden B, Jacob J, et al. High-dose cisplatinum in hypertonic saline. *Ann Intern Med* 1984;100:19–24.
47. Howell S, Zimm S, Markman M, et al. Long-term survival of advanced refractory ovarian carcinoma patients with small-volume disease treated with intraperitoneal chemotherapy. *J Clin Oncol* 1987;5:1607–1612.
48. Ozols R. High dose therapy with cisplatin and its analogs in ovarian cancer: current status and future studies. *Educational Booklet of ASCO*, 1987;69–70.
49. Ozols RF, Ostchega Y, Curt G, Young RC. High-dose carboplatin in refractory ovarian cancer patients. *J Clin Oncol* 1987;5:197–201.
50. McGuire WP, Hoskins WJ, Brady MS, et al. *A phase III trial of dose intense versus standard dose cisplatin and cytoxan in advanced ovarian cancer.* Presented at the Third Biennial Meeting of the International Gynecologic Cancer Society, Cairns, Australia.
51. Kaye SB. *High dose cisplatin (100 mg/m^2) is more effective than low dose (50 mg/m^2) in combination with cyclophosphamide (750 mg/m^2) for the treatment of advanced ovarian cancer.* Presented at the Third Biennial Meeting of the International Gynecologic Cancer Society, Cairns, Australia.
52. Coldman AJ, Goldie JH. Impact of dose-intense chemotherapy on the development of permanent drug resistance. *Semin Oncol* 1987;14(suppl):29–33.
53. Myers C. The use of intraperitoneal chemotherapy in the treatment of ovarian cancer. *Semin Oncol* 1984;11:275–284.
54. Howell S, Zimm S, Markman M, et al. Long-term survival of advanced refractory ovarian carcinoma patients with small-volume disease treated with intraperitoneal chemotherapy. *J Clin Oncol* 1987;5:1607–1612.
55. ten Bokkel Huinink W, et al. Experimental and clinical results with intraperitoneal cisplatin. *Semin Oncol* 1985;12:43.
56. Cohen C. Surgical considerations in ovarian cancer. *Semin Oncol* 1985;12:53.
57. Markman M, et al. IP chemotherapy employing a regimen of cisplatin, cytarabine, and bleomycin. *Cancer Treat Rep* 1986;70:755.
58. Markman M, Cleary S, Howell S, Lucas W. Complications of extensive adhesion formation after intraperitoneal chemotherapy. *Surg Gynecol Obstet* 1986;162:445–448.
59. Kaplan R, Markman M, Lucas W, et al. Infectious peritonitis in patients receiving intraperitoneal chemotherapy. *Am J Med* 1985;78:49–53.
60. Runowicz C, Dottino P, Shafir M, et al. Catheter complications associated with intraperitoneal chemotherapy. *Gynecol Oncol* 1986;24:41–50.
61. Ozols RF. Intraperitoneal therapy in ovarian cancer: time's up. *J Clin Oncol* 1991;9:197–199.
62. Rowinsky E, Gilbert M, McGuire W, et al. Sequences of taxol and cisplatin: phase I/pharmacologic study. *Proc ASCO* 1990;9:75.
63. Bruckner HW, Cohen CJ, Feuer E, Holland JF. Modulation and intensification of a cyclophosphamide, hexamethylmelamine, doxorubicin, and cisplatin ovarian cancer regimen. *Obstet Gynecol* 1989;73:349–356.
64. Hainsworth JD, Grosh WW, Barnett LS, et al. Advanced ovarian cancer: long-term results of treatment with intensive cisplatin-based chemotherapy of brief duration. *Ann Intern Med* 1988;108:165–170.
65. Hainsworth JD, Jones HW III, Burnett LS, Johnson DH, Greco FA. The role of hexamethylmelamine in the combination chemotherapy of advanced ovarian cancer: a comparison of hexamethylmelamine, cyclophosphamide, doxorubicin, and cisplatin (H-CAP) versus cyclophosphamide, doxorubicin, and cisplatin (CAP). *Am J Clin Oncol* 1990;13:410–415.
66. Edmondson JH, McCormack GW, Wieand HS. Late emerging survival differences in a comparative study of HCAP vs CP in stage III-IV ovarian carcinoma. In: Salmon S, ed. *Adjuvant therapy VI.* Orlando, Florida: Grune and Stratton, 1990;512–521.
67. Young R, Walton L, Decker D, et al. Early stage ovarian cancer: preliminary results of randomized trials after comprehensive initial staging. *Proc ASCO* 1983;2:148.

CHAPTER 21

Experimental Agents (Nonbiological) in Ovarian Cancer

William P. McGuire

Epithelial cancer of the ovary has generated a significant amount of research over the past two decades that is out of proportion to its incidence (14,000 deaths and 20,000 new cases in the United States annually). This is due to its occurrence in a population at the peak of productivity (peak age 40 to 60); its general responsiveness to therapy, suggesting curability; and, as discussed in Chapter 20, the fact that standard treatment for advanced ovarian cancer is still suboptimal in terms of long-term survival, dictating further research. Most patients with advanced disease (stages III–IV) succumb to the disease, often after an initial gratifying response followed by emergence of resistant clones and clinical progression. Fewer patients fail primary therapy at the outset, and these patients with primary drug resistance present an even greater challenge to current therapy.

Significant data suggest that drug resistance is quantitative rather than qualitative (1). Most in vitro studies suggest that acquired drug resistance can be overcome with 0.5 to 2 log increases in drug concentrations. Thus, some current experimental approaches in ovarian cancer are exploring methods to allow dose escalation of currently available agents, primarily classic alkylating agents and platinum compounds. Few if any of these approaches, however, approach the dose escalation necessary to overcome resistance predicted by in vitro studies. For the patient who fails primary therapy (and usually salvage therapy as well), the task of identifying new agents continues and should particularly focus on nonalkylating agents and agents with unique mechanisms of action, because congeners of standard drugs are frequently cross-resistant with the parent compound. Nearly every patient today with re-

fractory ovarian cancer is, by definition, resistant to cisplatin or one of its congeners; particular attention should be paid when screening new agents to selecting those with activity in cisplatin-resistant cell lines. This chapter explores new agents that may become part of the armamentarium in the treatment of ovarian cancer in the future and presents new ways some of the current agents are being utilized to improve their therapeutic efficacy.

NEW SALVAGE AGENTS WITH DOCUMENTED ACTIVITY IN OVARIAN CANCER

Ifosfamide (Ifex)

Ifosfamide was approved and released for treatment of refractory germ cell tumors in 1989 (2). It is a structural analogue of cyclophosphamide that can be administered at much higher doses because it causes less hematologic toxicity. Its toxicity to the bladder urothelium can be significantly reduced by concomitant administration of a uroprotective agent such as 2-mercaptoethane sulfonate (mesna). With the use of mesna other toxicities become dose-limiting, typically hematologic toxicity. Ifosfamide is commonly administered as a daily × 5 bolus schedule of 1.2–1.8 g/m² with 300–400 mg/m² mesna given 0, 4, and 8 hours after each ifosfamide dose. Another common schedule employs ifosfamide at 5–8 g/m² as a continuous 24-hour infusion with an overlapping continuous infusion of mesna (administered for at least 12 hours after completion of ifosfamide). Other significant toxicities include renal tubular abnormalities and a toxic encephalopathy. The toxic encephalopathy is probably underreported and appears to be more common with high-dose schedules, although others have not found a consistent relation-

W. P. McGuire: Department of Oncology, Johns Hopkins University, Baltimore, Maryland 21205

ship between central nervous system toxicity and the dose of ifosfamide, peak plasma levels, or the area under the concentration times time curve. Neurotoxicity may be more common in patients with renal dysfunction and/or hypoalbuminemia. In this regard, neurotoxicity may be more common in the patient who has received prior cisplatin therapy secondary to subclinical renal impairment, but no publication to date has prospectively evaluated the effect of prior cisplatin on ifosfamide-induced neurotoxicity.

The value of ifosfamide as a salvage therapy for ovarian cancer is difficult to assess. Most studies cannot be interpreted owing to incomplete descriptions of the patient characteristics (e.g., previous therapy) and unclear response criteria (3–5). Response rates in these early studies varied from 40% to 80%. In contemporary studies Taki et al. (5) reported a 40% response rate in 36 patients who had not received prior therapy and a 19% response rate in 21 patients who were previously treated (prior therapy not defined). A Gynecologic Oncology Group (GOG) trial (6) has also suggested that ifosfamide may be useful in the salvage setting in ovarian carcinoma. In that study there were three clinical complete responses (cCRs) and 5 clinical partial responses (cPRs) and an overall response rate of 20% in 41 evaluable patients who were either refractory to cisplatin or had relapsed after receiving cisplatin-based chemotherapy. Additionally, Hakes et al. (7) evaluated ifosfamide in 54 patients with prior cisplatin/cytoxan exposure and saw a partial response (PR) rate in 14% (13% for true cisplatin-refractory disease). He concluded that ifosfamide was modestly active and should be explored in combination with other drugs as part of initial therapy. However, results of a study of ifosfamide as primary therapy in 40 patients with bulky disease yielded a response rate of only 33% and ifosfamide was felt by the investigators to be no more active than standard alkylating agents (8) and was more difficult to administer. Additionally, in a study by Perren (9), 147 stage III patients were randomly assigned to treatment with carboplatin alone or to 3 cycles of ifosfamide followed by 3 cycles of carboplatin. Assessment after the third cycle revealed a 61% response rate for carboplatin and a 29% response rate for ifosfamide ($p < 0.005$); but after the sixth cycle, response rates were equal at 66%, suggesting salvage of ifosfamide failures with carboplatin. Thus, one must question the real value of this agent, at least as a single agent, in the initial therapy of ovarian cancer.

Two trials suggest that there may not be total cross-resistance between ifosfamide and other classical alkylating agents. In the first trial 49 patients were randomized to receive ifosfamide or cytoxan. Although the patient population was poorly described and no significant differences in response rates were apparent (64% for ifosfamide and 42% for cytoxan), three patients who demonstrated clinical resistance to cytoxan responded to ifosfamide on crossover (10). In another trial, 4 of 12 patients who were previously refractory to chlorambucil responded to ifosfamide (11). However, due to the small numbers of patients in these trials, the true degree of cross-resistance between ifosfamide and other alkylating agents remains uncertain. Nevertheless, cell lines resistant to cytoxan have been shown to be sensitive to ifosfamide. Some investigators have even suggested that ifosfamide will replace cyclophosphamide in many treatment regimens, a prediction this author thinks is very unlikely.

Ifosfamide has also been used in combination therapy in advanced ovarian cancer. A phase II trial of 20 patients—4 who had relapsed after initial therapy with oral alkylating agent and 16 who had progressed during therapy—were treated with cisplatin (60 mg/m^2 over 1 hour) followed by ifosfamide (4 m g/m^2 over 24 hours). A cCR was seen in four patients and a cPR in five patients (response rate 45%). Myelosuppression was dose-limiting, and dose reductions were required in 65% of the patients. Although this study demonstrated that cisplatin and ifosfamide could be administered together relatively safely in previously treated patients, it was unclear that this particular combination was more active than other cisplatin-based regimens in the treatment of ovarian cancer (12). In a Danish study (13), cisplatin (50 mg/m^2 days 1 and 2), carboplatin (200 mg/m^2 day 1), and ifosfamide (1,500 mg/m^2 days 1–3) were administered to 37 previously untreated patients with stage III disease (most with bulky residuals). A pathologic complete response (pCR) rate of 42% was seen (substantially higher than the 20% to 25% seen in other studies), but it was not statistically superior to other combination regimens. Toxicity was substantial (100% grade 3–4 hematologic toxicity). The investigators concluded that further evaluation in phase III trials was warranted.

The ability to administer ifosfamide in very high doses without significant nonhematologic toxicity and its apparent lack of cross-resistance with other alkylating agents has made ifosfamide a common agent for incorporation into conditioning regimens for patients undergoing autologous bone marrow transplantation.

In summary, the current role for ifosfamide in the treatment of ovarian cancer remains to be defined. The requirement for hospital admission for infusional schedules or multiple daily outpatient visits for bolus schedules as well as the significant toxicities associated with ifosfamide will require additional randomized trials to validate any role for this agent in first-line therapy. Although the majority of the data favor salvage activity of ifosfamide in patients with cisplatin-refractory tumors, the emergence of a better agent (taxol) relegates ifosfamide to third-line or fourth-line therapy. Finally, in light of the apparent flat dose-response curve produced by classical alkylating agents in ovarian carcinoma as retrospectively demonstrated by Levin and Hryniuk (14), one must question the rationale of incorporation of ifosfamide in very high dose into autologous transplant preparative regimens.

Taxol

Perhaps the most promising new agent to surface in the treatment of ovarian carcinoma in the past 15 years is taxol. Taxol, a unique antimicrotubule agent with a rare taxane ring, emerged from the screening of natural products and appears to possess promising activity in ovarian carcinoma (15). Interest in taxol dates from the late 1960s, when a crude extract of bark from the Pacific yew, *Taxus brevifolia*, was being tested by the National Cancer Institute and demonstrated cytotoxic activity against several murine tumors (16). Despite its preclinical promise, taxol's development as an antineoplastic agent has been slow and arduous owing to many problems: (A) there has been difficulty in large-scale extraction of bark; (B) poor aqueous solubility of taxol has hampered the development of a suitable clinical formulation; (C) the complexity of the molecule has defied a commercially feasible synthesis; (D) bark availability has been partially thwarted because of environmental issues; and (E) unusual toxicities (allergic reactions) have slowed the clinical development. Nevertheless, interest in taxol was sustained when its unique mechanism of cytotoxic action was appreciated (17,18). Unlike other antimicrotubule agents such as the vinca alkaloids, colchicine, and podophyllotoxin that induce the depolymerization of microtubules, taxol shifts the dynamic equilibrium between tubulin dimers and microtubules toward polymerization, inducing excessively stable and nonfunctional microtubules.

Phase I studies of taxol were begun in 1983, but a high incidence of severe acute hypersensitivity reactions (HSRs) slowed the development (19). This problem was largely solved by infusion of taxol over longer periods along with the use of medications to blunt the anaphylactic response including steroids in H_1- and H_2-histamine antagonists. These measures resulted in a dramatic reduction in the incidence of HSRs and permitted the completion of phase I studies. Unfortunately, the long infusion schedules with premedication made taxol unacceptable for outpatient administration. This issue is currently being readdressed in a randomized trial of long (24 hours) and short (4 hours) infusion schedules in patients with recurrent ovarian cancer.

Furthermore, in the phase I and early phase II studies, cardiac arrhythmias were noted, which required close monitoring of patients during treatment. Nevertheless, in a more recent phase I trial, taxol was administered over 6 hours in an outpatient setting without cardiac monitoring or any premedications. In that study only 1 of 30 patients experienced any allergic reaction, and there were no episodes of clinically apparent cardiac rhythm disturbance (20). The incidence of arrhythmias in hospitalized cancer patients who are not receiving cardiotoxic therapy is not well described. In all cases of cardiac toxicity associated with taxol as a single agent or in conjunction with cisplatin, rhythm disturbances have been asymptomatic. A randomized study of the incidence of cardiac rhythm abnormalities in taxol-based and non–taxol-based therapy in ovarian cancer is currently underway.

Neutropenia was found to be taxol's principal dose-limiting toxicity in most phase I solid tumor trials (20–23). In addition, taxol induced a dose-related, cumulative neurotoxicity that was characterized principally by neurosensory manifestations including numbness and paresthesia in a glove-and-stocking distribution (24). Further investigations of taxol in phase II trials in advanced ovarian carcinoma were begun after activity was observed in patients with cisplatin-refractory ovarian carcinoma in phase I trials.

The most exciting and reproducible antineoplastic activity observed with taxol, to date, has been in advanced ovarian epithelial neoplasms (25–27). In the phase II ovarian carcinoma trial at Johns Hopkins (26), 1 pCR, 1 PRs, and 7 minor responses (MR) of relatively long duration occurred in 40 evaluable patients. Besides demonstrating an extraordinarily high response rate in patients with advanced disease (PR + CR = 30%; CR + PR + MR = 45%), these results were particularly important for several other reasons. First, most patients, including responders, were heavily pretreated with radiation and chemotherapy (mean number of prior chemotherapy regimens per patient: 2.7; per responder: 3.0). Response is rare in such patients with any drug but was seen with taxol. Second, responses occurred in patients who were refractory to cisplatin (growth while on cisplatin or recurrence within 5 months after completion of cisplatin). Significant responses were noted in 6 of 25 (24%) patients who were refractory to cisplatin and 6 of 15 (40%) patients who did not show "clear refractoriness" to cisplatin. Third, neurotoxicity, which was initially anticipated to be very severe owing to the extent of previous cisplatin-based therapies, was mild. Finally, the doses of taxol given to most patients (110–135 mg/m^2) were significantly lower than the recommended phase II doses because of limited hematopoietic tolerance. Nevertheless, responses were noted at these low doses.

Other adverse effects noted in this and subsequent phase II studies were relatively mild. These included arthralgias, myalgias, mild mucositis, and rare cardiotoxicity.

The GOG and investigators at Einstein have also reported that taxol has significant activity in advanced and refractory ovarian carcinomas. The GOG reported an overall response rate of 37% in patients who had received only one previous cisplatin-based therapy. Responses occurred in 7 of 14 (50%) patients who were not clearly cisplatin-resistant (as previously defined) and 8 of 24 (33%) patients with clear cisplatin resistance. Six cCRs were also observed, and dose reductions from the starting dose of 175 mg/m^2 were required by the majority of patients in this multi-institutional study. No clear dose-response effect emerged. In addition, investigators at Einstein have substantiated that taxol has activity in advanced ovarian carcinoma. These investigators have recently described 6 objective responses out of 30 evaluable and previously treated patients (20% response rate), including one pCR, one cCR, and four PRs. Four of the six responders had cisplatin-resistant disease.

Although a clear dose-response relationship has not been defined in phase II ovarian cancer trials to date, possibly because of the extent of previous therapy and the inability to administer high doses, the demonstration of such a relationship in future studies in less heavily pretreated patients may serve as the rationale for the concurrent use of hematopoietic growth factors with taxol alone or in combination with cisplatin. Mucositis may preclude the escalation of taxol doses above 315 mg/m^2, however, as demonstrated in a phase I study in refractory leukemia (28). Studies utilizing taxol and cytokines to abrogate hematologic toxicity were a logical next step. Sarosy et al. (29) utilized escalating doses of taxol with granulocyte colony-stimulating factor (G-CSF) (10 ug/kg/day SQ starting on day 2 and continuing until reversal of absolute neutrophil count [ANC] nadir). Doses above 250 mg/m^2 were associated with unacceptable neurotoxicity. A response rate of 50% was observed in 14 evaluable patients who had received two or fewer prior regimens. No clear dose-response relationship was obvious in doses that ranged from 170–300 mg/m^2. A subsequent phase II trial is ongoing with a fixed taxol dose of 250 mg/m^2 and G-CSF at 10–20 ug/kg/day. A 50% response rate in 38 evaluable patients has been observed to date.

Thus, the single agent response rate with taxol in previously treated ovarian cancer is 20% to 50%. These studies indicate clearly that taxol is a very active agent in advanced ovarian cancer. The responses that have been observed with taxol in advanced and cisplatin-refractory ovarian carcinomas have been reminiscent of early studies with cisplatin in the 1970s, in which substantial response rates occurred in both drug-refractory and untreated patients (30). Although current constraints in the supply of taxol remain a limiting factor in the rapid development of the agent for widespread clinical usage, current results have generated considerable interest in defining taxol's role in first-line therapy in ovarian carcinoma.

Recently, a phase I trial of cisplatin and taxol in combination has defined doses for a phase III GOG study that is comparing the efficacy of cisplatin and taxol to cisplatin and cyclophosphamide in untreated patients with suboptimal ovarian carcinoma (31). Encouraging data from the phase I trial were a relative lack of peripheral neurotoxicity, which was a concern because each drug is neurotoxic in single agent trials. In that study the sequence of administration of taxol and cisplatin was determined to influence adverse effects. The sequence of taxol followed by cisplatin produced significantly less neutropenia and was a more active sequence against cell lines in vitro (32). The phase I trial evaluated six patients with ovarian carcinoma, and one pCR, one cCR/pPR, and three cPRs were noted. The recommended phase II/III starting doses were taxol (135–170 mg/m^2) as a 24-hour infusion to be followed by cisplatin (75 mg/m^2) by infusion at 1 mg/minute. G-CSF is also being utilized in this trial, after the maximum tolerated dose (MTD) without cytokine is reached. Using G-CSF at 5 ug/kg/day taxol in doses of 250–300 mg/m^2 can be safely combined with cisplatin at a dose of 75 mg/m^2. Neurotoxicity will likely be dose-limiting in this ongoing study (33).

Several aspects of taxol have also made it attractive for evaluation through the intraperitoneal route. Taxol is a large molecule with a very bulky conformation, making egress from the peritoneal cavity relatively difficult. Additionally, taxol is probably metabolized in large part by the liver, making it a first-pass drug and further increasing the possible concentration gradient. Finally, there is little evidence of serious cutaneous reactions when taxol has extravasated from the vein, suggesting lack of local toxicity. Markman (34) has evaluated taxol intraperitoneally in doses of 25–200 mg/m^2 every 3–4 weeks in 25 patients with significant prior therapy and nonmeasurable disease. Abdominal pain was prominent at doses >125 mg/m^2. Systemic adverse effects were mild at doses <175 mg/m^2, but there was clear evidence of systemic absorption because white count suppression was noted and plasma levels of taxol were present in concentrations adequate to induce biological effects in vitro. Responses were noted, and pharmacology suggested a concentration advantage of nearly 3 logs. Intraperitoneal taxol levels were maintained for several days, suggesting very slow clearance. A trial is currently underway to evaluate lower doses of taxol given weekly.

With clear activity of taxol as a salvage therapy and with demonstration that taxol and cisplatin can be safely combined, it was logical that this new doublet (taxol/cisplatin) be compared to the current "standard doublet" (cytoxan/cisplatin). A multi-institutional trial was opened by the GOG in 1990 comparing these two doublets (taxol at 135 mg/m², cytoxan at 750 mg/m², and cisplatin at 75 mg/m²). The study is nearing its accrual goal, but because of the rapid rate of patient entry, no data are available regarding comparative efficacy at this time. It is possible to state, however, that there has not been any untoward or unexpected toxicity from the experimental arm as this regimen has been transferred to community hospitals participating in the trial.

Several other taxol doublets will be evaluated in phase I/II trials in the next year in preparation for the incorporation of taxol into combination treatment regimens in ovarian cancer. This incorporation will be supported firmly if the current national phase III trial shows that a taxol and cisplatin combination is better than the current "best" combination of cytoxan and cisplatin. Currently planned studies include taxol combined with ifosfamide, hexamethylmelamine, carboplatin, etoposide, and topotecan. It is unlikely that these studies will evaluate the role of drug sequencing or explore the pharmacology of the combinations. How these data will be utilized is unclear, but any acceptable combination from the toxicologic point of view will probably need to be prospectively tested against standard therapy because it is unlikely that any doublet will be so superior to current therapy that it can be accepted as the new standard without such testing.

Because of supply problems associated with taxol, other taxanes have had early clinical testing. The only one for which any data exist, however, is taxotere. Taxotere is a taxane similar to taxol. An isolate from the needles (a renewable resource) of the Western European yew, *Taxus baccata*, is 10-deacetyl baccatin III, which is synthetically converted into taxotere. This compound, like taxol, drives the tubulin/microtubule equilibrium toward microtubules (35,36). It is broadly active in the murine prescreen (37), and very early results from human trials in Europe and North America suggest it has some antitumor activity. Further phase I and II data are awaited.

Hexamethylmelamine (Hexalen)

One could include hexamethylmelamine (HMM) as part of the standard therapy of ovarian cancer, but its role in that regard remains unclear 25 years after its initial use in that tumor. HMM, a substituted melamine derived from cyanuric chloride, has demonstrated antineoplastic activity in untreated and alkylating agent-refractory ovarian cancer in numerous single agent and combination chemotherapy trials since 1964 (38) but has recently been marketed only as a salvage agent for epithelial ovarian cancer because of its unclear role as part of initial therapy. The principal dose-limiting toxicities are gastrointestinal, and a reversible peripheral neuropathy occurs with prolonged administration; this neuropathy is possibly more severe in patients treated with prior neurotoxic therapy. HMM's mechanism of action has not been firmly elucidated, but experimental evidence suggests that antineoplastic activity is mediated through the formation of carbinolamine intermediates during initial demethylation reactions, leading to the production of reactive species that covalently bind to macromolecules such as DNA (39).

HMM's exact role in the management of ovarian cancer has not been determined definitively by earlier studies and remains controversial. The shortcomings of these trials have been reviewed previously by Foster et al. (38). Some hints are emerging from the long-term follow-up of patients in early trials to suggest that HMM's potential has not been fully recognized, especially in patients with minimal residual disease.

The response data from two randomized phase II studies conducted at M. D. Anderson in the mid 1970s were combined, revealing overall response rates and CR rates of 40% and 19%, respectively (40,41). These results did not differ statistically from overall response and CR rates obtained with melphalan (35% and 15%, respectively), regarded at the time of the study as the standard therapy for advanced ovarian cancer. Additionally, a few patients (4/54) appreciated long-term (>120 months) survival, and each of these patients had minimal residual disease at the initiation of therapy.

Recently, the results of three large trials were reported, demonstrating impressive long-term survival in patients treated with combinations containing both cisplatin and HMM, especially in patients with minimal residual disease. These trials include two nonrandomized studies. The first, conducted at Vanderbilt, used HCAP (HMM 150 mg/m² PO days 1–8, cyclophosphamide 350 mg/m² IV days 1 and 8, doxorubicin 20 mg/m² IV days 1 and 8, and cisplatin 60 mg/m² IV day 1); a second study from Mount Sinai used CHAP II (cyclophosphamide 500 mg/m² IV day 3, HMM 100 mg/m² PO days 4–15, doxorubicin 50 mg/m² IV day 3, and cisplatin 50 mg/m² IV day 1) (42–45). HCAP produced objective responses in 53 of 55 patients (96%), and 19 patients (35%) had negative second-look laparotomies. In addition, ten patients (nine with minimal residual tumors) were reported to have been alive and disease-free at least 7 years after therapy. An updated report of the survival of patients receiving HCAP showed an overall median survival of 47 months, with a median survival of 101 months for patients with minimal residual disease. Similarly, CHAP-II yielded an overall response rate of 77%, a pCR rate of 18%, and a progression-free median survival of 43 months. The Vanderbilt researchers also compared their HCAP results with results obtained with CAP (cyclophosphamide 350 mg/m² IV days 1 and 8, doxorubicin 20 mg/m² IV days 1 and 8, and cisplatin 60 mg/m² IV day 1) in a similar but not prospectively randomized patient population. They observed a significant advantage of HCAP in terms of response, disease-free survival, and overall survival. This difference was particularly evident in patients with residual masses ≤3 cm (median survival for HCAP was 101 months and for CAP was 21 months). Care must be taken, however, in interpretation of these results, because both studies were small (sample size for HCAP was 55 patients and for CAP, 22 patients), and known prognostic factors were not balanced (more bulky disease in HCAP and more advanced stage and grade in CAP).

A reexamination of the long-term survival experience from a randomized controlled Mayo Clinic–North Central Cancer Treatment Group study showed distinct differences in the survival of patients with minimal residual disease favoring HCAP (HMM 150 mg/m^2 PO days 2–8, cyclophosphamide 400 mg/m^2 IV day 1, doxorubicin 30 mg/m^2 IV day 1, and cisplatin 60 mg/m^2 IV day 1) over CP (cyclophosphamide 1,000 mg/m^2 IV and cisplatin 60 mg/m^2 IV) (46). The two treatments were similar with respect to patient characteristics, survival, time to progression, and nadir white blood cell counts. Nevertheless, subset analyses demonstrated that good-risk patients exhibited significantly better progression-free survival and overall survival with HCAP (5 year survival: 46% for HCAP, 23% for CP), whereas CP appeared superior in poor-risk patients (47). This outcome was found in spite of patients on HCAP receiving greater dose reductions and treatment delays because of myelosuppression and despite more selective reductions in cisplatin in the HCAP arm owing to greater neurotoxic effects. Taken as a composite, these studies suggest strongly some synergistic reaction between HMM and cisplatin, cyclophosphamide, doxorubicin, or a combination of the three in ovarian cancer patients with small amounts of residual disease following primary surgery. Unfortunately, the data do not unequivocally show that hexamethylmelamine should be added to platinum-based primary chemotherapy.

Some cite a randomized study from Italy as evidence against HMM having significant activity in ovarian carcinoma. The long-term results of that prospective, randomized study in which HMM 150 mg/m^2 PO days 1–14, doxorubicin, and cyclophosphamide (HAC) were compared to cisplatin 50 mg/m^2 and similar doses of doxorubicin and cyclophosphamide (PAC) were recently reviewed (48). Although PAC produced more favorable results than HAC in terms of overall survival (25.5 months versus 23.1 months), survival in patients with minimal residual tumors (108 months versus 69 months), survival in patients with large-volume residual tumors (21.7 months versus 20 months), survival in patients who achieved a pCR (138+ months versus 126 months), and pCR rate (35% versus 28%), none of these differences were statistically significant. Unlike the previous studies, this study additionally failed to address whether HMM contributed to outcomes produced by cisplatin-based combinations. Another study, however, did prospectively evaluate the role played by HMM in combination chemotherapy. That study by Neijt et al. (49) compared CHAP-5 (cisplatin 20 mg/m^2 IV days 1–5, hexamethylmelamine 150 mg/m^2 PO days 15–28, doxorubicin 35 mg/m^2 IV day 1, and cyclophosphamide 100 mg/m^2 PO days 15–28) with CP (cyclophosphamide 750 mg/m^2 IV day 1 and cisplatin 75 mg/m^2 IV day 1). Median follow-up of 191 eligible patients is 7.7 years, and no advantage of the HMM-based regimen on any endpoint can be demonstrated. This is true for patients with both low- and high-volume disease.

Thus, the results on the efficacy of addition of HMM to primary platinum-based therapy are conflicting. Only a randomized clinical trial will answer the question of its value. Until that is performed, one must concur with the FDA in its withholding approval for HMM-based primary therapy, because there is potential for additive or synergistic toxicity and no definitive evidence of improved efficacy.

There have also been three encouraging reports of HMM as salvage chemotherapy after failure of cisplatin-based combination regimens (50–52), and it is as salvage therapy that HMM has been approved by FDA. Response rates in these studies were approximately 20%, and overall survival was significantly longer for responders than nonresponders. Gastrointestinal and peripheral neurotoxic effects were present but manageable. These salvage responses, however, are poorly documented because many patients had nonmeasurable disease at the start of therapy, and second-look assessment was not required for assignment of response. Additionally, many of the responders had not received any chemotherapy for long periods before HMM was initiated. Only the report by Moore et al. (52) states that no patient who progressed during prior cisplatin-based therapy responded to salvage HMM. If this is true, then one must question the value of HMM salvage therapy because most patients for whom such therapy would be entertained will be cisplatin-refractory. Nevertheless, the relatively favorable toxicity of HMM make it a reasonable alternative to more toxic drugs in the salvage therapy of ovarian cancer.

If HMM is to have a major role in the treatment of advanced ovarian cancer, available data suggest that it will likely be as first-line chemotherapy in good-risk patients with low-volume disease. Further studies are necessary before such a recommendation can be made. Additionally, future studies may explore the feasibility of HMM in combination with second-generation platinum analogues such as carboplatin, which may result in considerably less neurotoxicity than cisplatin-HMM combinations.

Finally, potentially significant interpatient differences in HMM's oral bioavailability and differences in tumor activation of HMM have led to the development of an intravenous formulation of HMM (53) as well as a trimethylol derivative that is suitable for intravenous administration and would not be expected to require metabolic activation for antineoplastic activity. This analogue has already demonstrated cytotoxic activity against various tumor cell lines in vitro as well as in human lung and ovarian xenografts (54).

NEW AGENTS WITH ANTICIPATED ACTIVITY IN OVARIAN CANCER

Topotecan

Topotecan, or hycamptamine, is a semisynthetic and water-soluble analogue of sodium camptothecin, a novel compound that forms a covalent complex with topoisomerase I and which subsequently leads to DNA cleavage. Topoisomerase also appears to be important in both transcription and replication of DNA (55). Perhaps most intriguing is the finding of high levels of topoisomerase in tumor tissues with low-growth fractions as well as those with high-growth fractions. Because topoisomerase-active drugs appear to be active in direct proportion to levels of the target enzyme (the opposite of most agents, which target enzyme systems such as the antimetabolites), topotecan is hoped to be just as effective on slowly dividing tumors as their more active counterparts (56).

Topotecan was less potent than the parent, camptothecin, against the L1210 model, but because higher doses of drug could be tolerated it improved by about 50% the increased life span (ILS) in L1210-bearing mice over that obtained with the parent (57). Validating these preclinical results, toxicologic studies of topotecan, the dose-limiting nonhematologic adverse effects that had precluded extensive testing of the parent (hemorrhagic cystitis) were not observed; the apparent dose-limiting toxicity of topotecan appeared to be myelosuppression, especially neutropenia.

Phase I studies of topotecan were initiated in 1989 at several institutions. In the study performed at Johns Hopkins (58), a schedule of daily × 5 administration every 21 days was employed with dose-limiting toxicity being noncumulative neutropenia. The maximal tolerated dose was 1.5 mg/m^2. Attempts at further dose escalation are underway with concomitant use of G-CSF. Other toxicities associated with topotecan include a hemolytic-like anemia (occasionally rapid and significant), alopecia, nausea, vomiting, diarrhea, and skin rash. During this phase I study, a partial response was noted in a patient with cisplatin-refractory ovarian carcinoma that had been maintained for over 18 months. The patient continues to receive topotecan without evidence of cumulative toxicity (25 courses, to date). This major response in cisplatin-refractory disease is unusual and has generated a phase II study in ovarian carcinoma. No results are yet available from that trial.

Tetraplatin

Tetraplatin is an organoplatinum IV analogue with preclinical data suggesting activity superior to that of cisplatin and carboplatin in human tumors (59) as well as lack of cross-resistance in ovarian cell lines made resistant to cisplatin (60). Some investigators, however, have seen moderate degrees of cross-resistance in similar cell lines and suggest that this partial cross-resistance is due to enhanced DNA repair mechanisms (61). Nevertheless, these same investigators are currently performing a phase I trial of this compound, and a phase II investigation in patients with cisplatin-refractory ovarian cancer will start soon thereafter.

Thigpen has discussed the relative values of the two currently available platinum coordination complexes in widespread clinical use in ovarian cancer (cisplatin and carboplatin). All current clinical data suggest near total cross-resistance between these two analogues, although some preclinical data with carboplatin had suggested otherwise. Obviously, then, a clinical trial in cisplatin-resistant (or carboplatin-resistant) disease should be required in phase I/II testing of tetraplafin.

APPROACHES TO OVERCOMING INTRINSIC AND ACQUIRED DRUG RESISTANCE

Because the classes of agents that are effective in the treatment of ovarian cancer remain small and because drug resistance continues to be a critical problem for the majority of patients, many researchers have been exploring novel approaches (A) to increase the dose intensity (mg/m^2/week) of active agents by blocking current dose-limiting toxicity or (B) to abrogate intrinsic or acquired drug resistance to improve the therapeutic index of available drugs. Table 1 summarizes these approaches and the predicted increase in dose intensity that each approach allows over standard platinum-based chemotherapy.

Increase in Dose Intensity

Retrospective data by Levin and Hryniuk (14) suggest that outcome in advanced ovarian cancer is directly correlated with intensity of therapy (mg/m^2/week) and that the relationship is strongest with cisplatin. Even the relationship with platinum, however, has rather poor correlation ($r^2 = 0.5$). A prospective

TABLE 1. *Effect on dose intensity of various maneuvers to abrogate dose-limiting toxicity*

Maneuver	Escalation factor	Organ protection
Carboplatin + cytokines	2	Marrow
Bone marrow transplantation	5–10	Marrow
Cisplatin + thiosulfate	2–3	Renal
Cisplatin + ethiofos (WR-2721)	1.5–2	Marrow, renal
Cisplatin + ORG.2766	1.5–2	Peripheral nervous
Organoplatinum + diethyldithiocarbamate	2	Renal, marrow, GI
Cisplatin + carboplatin	2–2.5	Marrow, renal

GOG trial (62) of the dose-intensity concept was carried out in patients with suboptimally debulked stage III and stage IV tumors. Total doses of cisplatin and cyclophosphamide were held constant, but one group received twice the intensity of the other (cisplatin 50 mg/m^2 IV and cytoxan 500 mg/m^2 IV Q3 weeks × 8 or cisplatin 100 mg/m^2 IV and cytoxan 1,000 mg/m^2 IV Q3 weeks × 4). In that study of 460 patients, still in the follow-up phase with >30% of the patients censored, the outcome measures (response rate, disease-free survival, and survival) were equal in both arms despite the actual achievement of twice the dose intensity in the experimental arm—0.47 (standard) and 0.93 (intense) received dose compared to the Greco standard. Some may argue that the intensity in both arms was too low and that no effect was seen for that reason. If there is in fact a linear dose-response relationship as suggested by Levin, however, one would expect to see some outcome effect over this clinically relevant dose range wherein the higher dose arm was associated with significantly greater toxicity. If, on the other hand, the relationship is nonlinear, then progressively larger increments in intensity (and its attendant toxicity) may be required for smaller and smaller gains. The data of Levin can be recalculated by separating average dose intensities ≤0.8 and >0.8, demonstrating that the slope of the relationship between dose intensity and outcome is significantly lower at the more intense doses. If, conversely, a certain minimum concentration of drug must be reached (exponential relationship) before any effect is noted, then approaches requiring significantly more than double dose intensity are likely to be necessary before improved clinical outcome is observed.

In a somewhat smaller study of 190 patients, however, Kaye (63) found the opposite result. In that study patients were randomized between cisplatin doses of 50 mg/m^2 and 100 mg/m^2, with a fixed cytoxan dose of 750 mg/m^2. All patients received six cycles at three weekly intervals so that both total dose and dose intensity varied. The trial was stopped before reaching its accrual goal because of a significant ($p = 0.0008$) survival advantage with the high-dose arm (73% 18-month survival for high dose versus 48% for low dose). Why a dissimilar outcome is seen in studies with similar though not equivalent designs will require further maturation of both studies and a more detailed examination of possible differences in the two patient populations regarding known prognostic factors. Of note, average postoperative disease volume in the study by Kaye was smaller than that in the GOG study, which may influence outcome. Subset analysis of outcome by disease volume may answer this question if mature data from both studies continue to reveal discordant results.

A final study by the Milan group (64) had a somewhat different design but seems to argue as well against a clinically relevant dose-response relationship. In that study 254 patients (stage and volume not stated) were randomized between standard therapy (cytoxan 750 mg/m^2 and cisplatin 75 mg/m^2 IV Q 3 weeks × 6) and intense therapy (cisplatin 50 mg/m^2 IV QW × 9). The weekly cisplatin is approximately 2.5 times more intense than standard therapy. With short follow-up there is no apparent difference in end results between the standard (pCR = 42%, RR = 77%) and intense (pCR = 34%, RR = 81%) arms of the study. The results are too early to assess differences in survival or disease-free survival.

Another approach designed to increase platinum dose intensity has been to combine cisplatin and carboplatin. The rationale for using platinum combinations is reasonable because both agents are active in ovarian cancer and neither share principal dose-limiting adverse effects. Two published studies utilizing schedules in which treatment with carboplatin preceded cisplatin suggest that nearly full doses of each platinum analogue can be combined with acceptable toxicity (65,66). This allows for an increment in dose intensity of 1.5 to 2 over that achieved with standard therapy. The sequence of platinum administration—carboplatin followed by cisplatin—potentially decreases the probability of cisplatin-induced renal dysfunction that may lead to higher plasma levels of carboplatin and greater myelosuppression (67). A phase II trial performed in Denmark (65) used carboplatin at a dose of 300 mg/m^2 on day 1 followed by 50 mg/m^2 of cisplatin on days 2 and 3 in 42 untreated ovarian cancer patients (80% with bulky residual disease). This study produced a pathologic response rate of 62% (pCR + pPR) and a pCR rate of 22%. The major dose-limiting toxicity was thrombocytopenia, although dose reductions were carried out in 22% and 7% of patients for nephrotoxicity and neurotoxicity, respectively. The Belgian Study Group (66) performed a phase I/II trial in 30 untreated patients with bulky residual ovarian cancer. These investigators recommended a starting dose of 300 mg/m^2 of carboplatin on day 1 and 100 mg/m^2 of cisplatin on day 2 with a vigorous 48-hour hydration scheme. The pCR rate, 22%, was equal to that of the Danish study. Toxicities were moderate but manageable, including dose-limiting myelosuppression (45% of patients delayed) as well as gastrointestinal (97%), ototoxic (39%), neurotoxic (21%), and nephrotoxic (12.5%) side effects. Although these studies demonstrated that cisplatin and carboplatin could be safely combined, the increase in organoplatinum dose intensity was only 1.8 to 2.0 times greater than that with conventional cisplatin-based regimens. Additionally, the results of these phase II trials were not obviously better than results achieved in similar groups of patients treated with either cisplatin alone or cisplatin-based combinations. Randomized studies that evaluate platinum dose intensity as the only variable are required to firmly address whether regimens with increased organoplatinum intensity lead to improved end results; however, the recent GOG experience (62) and Italian study (64) previously noted suggest that more intensity than is currently achievable by this mechanism will be necessary to see an effect.

Finally, the dose of carboplatin can be increased with the use of cytokines to abrogate marrow toxicity. Reed et al. described a phase I/II trial of high-dose carboplatin (800 mg/m^2 IV every 35 days) with escalating doses of recombinant granulocyte-macrophage colony-stimulating factor (rGM-CSF) in patients with refractory ovarian cancer (68). The response rate of 35% (2 CRs and 6 PRs) was similar to the rate (27%) achieved in a previous study of high-dose carboplatin without rGM-CSF (69). Patients who were treated at relevant rGM-CSF doses had significantly less febrile neutropenia than patients who did not receive rGM-CSF with carboplatin. Although hematopoietic growth factors such as rGM-CSF and G-CSF will not permit the escalation of doses of carboplatin and other alkylating agents to doses that could be achieved with autologous bone marrow transplant, the next generation of hematopoietic growth factors (e.g., interleukins 1, 3, and 6) may permit the use of more dose-intensive regimens. However, they are still unlikely to allow escalation to levels necessary to overcome resistance.

High-Dose Chemotherapy with Autologous Bone Marrow Transplantation

High-dose chemotherapy with autologous bone marrow transplantation (ABMT) is uniquely applicable to the management of ovarian carcinoma for many reasons. First, dose-response relationships have been demonstrated for platinum compounds as well as classic alkylating agents (14,70,71). Second, nonhematologic toxicities with such agents as carboplatin, melphalan, thiotepa, ifosfamide, and etoposide do not supervene until escalation to doses three- to fivefold higher than can be used in conventional therapy. Third, ovarian cancer rarely metastasizes to bone and bone marrow, making use of unpurged marrow feasible. Finally, ovarian cancer patients are commonly diagnosed in "low tumor burden states" or may be rendered so by cytoreductive surgery and/or standard doses of chemotherapy. If principals that apply to leukemias and lymphomas regarding the optimal use of high-dose chemotherapy with ABMT can be extrapolated to ovarian carcinoma, a significant proportion of patients should be rendered prognostically favorable with respect to high-dose chemotherapy and ABMT at some time in their disease course.

Unfortunately, few adequate studies of high-dose chemotherapy with ABMT in patients with ovarian cancer have been performed. These studies are summarized in Table 2. Early trials focused on the dose intensification of melphalan, cyclophosphamide, thiotepa, etoposide, and even chlorambucil (72–76), whereas more recent studies are intensifying doses of carboplatin, ifosfamide, and/or etoposide (77). To date, the data are largely uninterpretable owing to the pilot nature of the studies, small numbers of patients, brief follow-up durations, vast differences in cytoreductive regimens and pre-ABMT tumor burdens, and frequent use of patients with drug-resistant rather than drug-sensitive disease. As is the case with the leukemias and lymphomas, these studies suggest that high-dose chemotherapy with ABMT will be most effective at producing a high objective response rate and improved long-term survival in patients with minimal residual disease states and in tumors that are still relatively sensitive to cytotoxic therapy. Patients with minimal residual disease after second-look surgery have a highly variable long-term survival with either salvage therapy or no therapy (78) and will require long-term follow-up before any definitive conclusions can be made regarding efficacy. Use of adequate control arms in future studies will be necessary to determine the role of high-dose chemotherapy with ABMT. Currently, the major focus of high-dose chemotherapy ABMT trials involves the determination of optimal conditioning regimens that are principally carboplatin-based. These studies suggest that carboplatin can be safely escalated to approximately 1,500–2,000 mg/m^2 without undue nonhematologic toxicity. Ongoing phase I and II investigations include ABMT following high-dose chemotherapy in patients with refractory tumors. Preparative regimens include carboplatin/etoposide (Case West-

TABLE 2. *Phase I/II trials with high-dose chemotherapy and autologous bone marrow transplantation in advanced ovarian cancer*

Preparative regimen	Patient population	Published results
CTX 7 g/m² IV × 3 days VP-16 0.9–1.0 g/m² × 3 days MES 4 g/m² × 4 days ABMT day 7 (72)	11 patients with residual cancer after first-line therapy	5 pCRs/1 cCR in 8 pts (<2 cm) Median PFI: 15 mo
ALK 140–240 mg/m² IV ABMT day 2 (73)	35 patients: 60% low volume after initial Rx; only 5 progressed on initial Rx; most patients were nonmeasurable	75% response in measuring patients; 9 of 21 patients pCR or PR after initial Rx are NED at 9–32 mo
ALK 140 mg/m² IV ABMT day 2 (74)	14 patients: 60% low-volume disease after initial Rx	9 of 14 are NED at 32–60 mo
CBDCA 2,100 mg/m² IV VP-16 600 mg/m² IV ALK 125 mg/m² IV ABMT or ASCT (75)	5 patients: all low-volume disease after initial Rx	4 evaluated patients are NED at 3–29 mo
CBDCA 375–2400 mg/m² IV continuous infusion ABMT day 8 (77)	11 patients: treatment at relapse; 9 had prior sensitivity to cisplatin	5 PRs and 1 CR including 1 of 2 patients resistant to cisplatin
CTX 1,875 mg/m² IV × 3 days TSPA 300 mg/m² IV × 1 day CDDP 30 mg/m² IP × 5 days ABMT (76)	412 drug-resistant patients; most failed 3 regimens	3 Rx-related deaths; very short remission duration (3.5–7 mo)

CBDCA, carboplatin; VP-16, etoposide; ALK, melphalan; ABMT, autologous bone marrow transplant; MES, 2-mercaptoethane sulfonate (mesna); TSPA, thiotepa; PFI, progression-free interval; NED, no evidence of disease.

ern), carboplatin/ifosfamide plus mesna (Indiana University and GOG), carboplatin/etoposide/ifosfamide (ICE) plus mesna (NCI, Loyola, Dana Farber), thiotepa (University of Missouri), thiotepa/cytoxan/cisplatin (Duke) and etoposide/melphalan (Case Western and ECOG).

At this time ABMT must be considered a research procedure. Because of the toxicity associated with its use, patient selection should be judicious and generally limited to patients who fill the following criteria: age ≤55, small-volume disease (≤3 cm), good performance status (0 or 1), and drug-sensitive relapse. If any clear benefit can be shown in this group, then ABMT may have application as primary therapy in high-risk patients following initial cytoreduction.

Approaches to Reducing the Dose-Limiting Toxicities of Therapy

Several approaches to ameliorate the dose-limiting toxicities of platinum compounds and classical alkylating agents have been undertaken recently. It is hoped that these measures will not be associated with reduced antitumor efficacy and that further dose escalation may be possible to take advantage of the dose-response relationship with platinum compounds and less clearly with classic alkylating agents in ovarian cancer (14). As discussed previously, carboplatin can be safely escalated twofold when administered with cytokines and by fourfold to fivefold with autologous stem cell support.

New approaches to reducing cisplatin's principal and dose-limiting adverse effects—nephrotoxicity and peripheral neurotoxicity—are also being pursued. The most common approach designed to reduce nephrotoxicity without abrogating cytotoxic activity is use of sodium thiosulfate. Sodium thiosulfate neutralizes or prevents formation of the nephrotoxic aquated species of cisplatin in the renal tubule, thus abrogating renal dysfunction. Although cisplatin doses of 200 mg/m² can be administered with sodium thiosulfate without significant renal toxicity, neurotoxicity is not ameliorated by this approach and continues to be a major problem. This approach has been used exclusively with intraperitoneal cisplatin administration to date, and data from such trials suggest that regional platinum therapy can lead to further response in some 30% of patients with low-volume disease that has not shown absolute resistance to standard doses of platinum (79). Although an evaluation of intravenous cisplatin with intravenous sodium thiosulfate has not been performed, data suggest that not all the systemic antitumor activity of cisplatin administered in such a fashion is blocked by the concomitant administration of sodium thiosulfate (80). Protection from cisplatin-induced nephrotoxicity, however, is significant, and some studies suggest hypomagnesemia is abrogated as well.

Evidence from animal models indicates that another "neutralizing" agent, diethyldithiocarbamate (DDTC), can protect the kidney, gastrointestinal tract, and bone marrow from toxicities that are induced by both cisplatin and carboplatin. In the only clinical trial of this agent, however, DDTC used in conjunction with carboplatin produced substantial autonomic side effects consisting of diaphoresis, hypertension, anxiety, flushing, and conjunctival injection. There was also significant hematologic toxicity, which accounted for three treatment-related deaths. In addition, only a modest response rate of 19% occurred after concurrent treatment with 800 mg/m^2 carboplatin in previously treated patients (81).

Ethiofos (WR-2721), another modulator of cisplatin toxicity, was initially developed as a radioprotector. This organic thiophosphate may be useful in protecting normal tissues (except the CNS) from the toxic effects of alkylating agents and cisplatin by virtue of its selective uptake into normal tissue (82) and poorer uptake into tumor tissues. Preclinical studies demonstrated that ethiofos can protect hematopoietic tissues from alkylating agents or renal tubules from cisplatin injury by a factor of 1.5 to 2.0 (83) without decreasing antitumor efficacy. To date, ethiofos has been administered to patients to modulate the toxicities of cisplatin, cyclophosphamide, and nitrogen mustard. Short (15-minute) infusions of ethiofos in doses of 740–910 mg/m^2 have been associated with mild nausea and vomiting, sneezing, vasodilation, and rare allergic reactions and hypotension. A randomized clinical trial demonstrated that ethiofos can protect against cyclophosphamide-induced neutropenia, but the study did not address how much additional cyclophosphamide could be safely administered with concurrent ethiofos (84). Thus far, the data that indicate that ethiofos protects against renal toxicity are poor and inferential; however, transient elevations in creatinine were seen in only 5% of patients treated with cisplatin doses of 120–150 mg/m^2 in conjunction with ethiofos (85). The neuroprotective effect of ethiofos has not yet been adequately confirmed. Although it has been claimed that the agent offers protection from cisplatin-induced neuropathy based on the results of one study (86), the variety of treatment schemes, disease states, types of prior therapy, and lack of long-term and in-depth neurologic evaluations in this study makes this claim unconvincing. Preclinical studies have failed to show substantial uptake of ethiofos into the nervous system. Nevertheless, preliminary data from a randomized trial in ovarian cancer clearly suggest a protective effect on several organ systems (87). Seventy-two stage III/IV ovarian patients were randomly allocated to cyclophosphamide and cisplatin, 1,000 mg/m^2 and 100 mg/m^2, respectively, with or without ethiofos (940 mg/m^2). With very short follow-up, there were fewer episodes of febrile neutropenia (13% versus 24%), clinical peripheral neuropathy (10% versus 29%), loss of deep tendon reflexes (21% versus 42%), and ototoxicity (56% versus 80%) in the patients treated with ethiofos. Pathologic complete responses have occurred in 6 of 16 (38%) patients who received ethiofos and 4 of 17 (24%) patients who did not receive ethiofos (not statistically significant). At this juncture, additional trials and longer follow-up of ongoing studies are necessary to determine the magnitude of protection afforded by ethiofos and the extent to which ethiofos permits the dose escalation of active antineoplastic agents.

A final compound that may reduce the toxicities of cisplatin and/or allow escalation of cisplatin dose is the neuropeptide ORG.2766, a hexapeptide similar to α-MSH that has been shown in animal models to enhance the regrowth of neurons damaged by crush injury. This compound has been prospectively studied in a double-blind, placebo-controlled trial (88). In that study, women with ovarian cancer were treated with cisplatin and cyclophosphamide at doses of 75 mg/m^2 and 750 mg/m^2, respectively, and randomized to no neuropeptide, low-dose neuropeptide (0.25 mg), or high-dose treatment (1.0 mg). ORG.2766 was injected subcutaneously on two consecutive days at the start of each cycle. A neurologic exam, including a sensitive test of vibratory sense using a vibrameter that could be continuously varied, was performed before study and after every two cycles. The results in a small patient population suggested that ORG.2766 could abrogate the loss of vibratory discrimination that occurred after 4 to 6 cycles of cisplatin-based therapy. This modulatory effect appeared to be related to the dose of ORG.2766. There was also a decrease in neurotoxic signs and symptoms in patients treated with neuropeptide. The neuropeptide was not associated with toxicity, and no abrogation of tumor response was apparent in patients who were treated with the compound. However, randomized trials of standard dose cisplatin as used in this study with more dose-intensive schedules will be required to determine if ORG.2766 will be effective in allowing further dose intensification of cisplatin. Additionally, because higher doses of ORG.2766 appear to offer greater protection, evaluations of higher doses of the compound and/or more chronic dosing schedules seem appropriate.

Approaches to Reduce Intrinsic Resistance to Chemotherapy

Drug resistance appears to be a major factor in the inability to achieve and sustain complete responses. Although 75–80% of patients with ovarian carcinoma will initially respond to organoplatinum-based therapy, pCRs occur in only 30–35%, and 30–50% of these complete responders will eventually develop recurrent disease.

Initial attempts to overcome clinical drug resistance focused on adriamycin resistance, which is associated with the multidrug resistance phenotype (MDR). Ozols and co-workers found that adriamycin efflux from ovarian cancer cells could be blocked *in vitro* with high doses of verapamil, an inhibitor of the drug efflux pump (89). There was also a paucity of data to suggest that the MDR phenotype played any major role in drug resistance in ovarian neoplasms, although low levels of MDR expression could be detected in clinical tumor specimens (90). Finally, significant toxicity and little efficacy were observed in a clinical trial of high-dose verapamil and adriamycin in refractory ovarian cancer patients (91).

Buthionine Sulfoximine

Attention has recently turned to the significance of intracellular thiols, particularly glutathione (GSH) and glutathione-S-transferase (GST), in the development of resistance to both cisplatin and more classical alkylating agents. Another factor that may be operational in resistance to cisplatin is enhanced DNA repair mechanisms (92). Intracellular GSH can be depleted with buthionine sulfoximine (BSO), which inhibits the specific enzyme, Γ-glutamyl cysteine synthetase, involved in thiol production. The intracellular depletion of GSH by BSO leads to enhanced cytotoxicity in ovarian cell lines treated with melphalan (93) or cisplatin (94), although some investigators have been unable to confirm the relationship between GSH depletion and potentiation of cisplatin-induced cytotoxicity (95).

A phase I trial of BSO with melphalan is underway to determine if glutathione levels can be depleted sufficiently and if toxicity of the drug combination is acceptable (96). Comparative trials of organoplatinum compounds and classical alkylating agents with and without BSO are being planned to define the utility of BSO.

A final compound that has been shown to deplete intracellular thiols is ethacrynic acid (Edecrin), which competitively inhibits one or more of the GST isoenzymes. A phase I trial using ethacrynic acid (25–75 mg/m^2 PO every 6 hours × 3 doses) with thiotepa (30–40 mg/m^2 IV following the second dose of ethacrynic acid) has identified starting doses for subsequent phase II studies of 50 mg/m^2 and 40 mg/m^2 of ethacrynic acid and thiotepa, respectively (97). Dose-limiting toxicity of this combination is neutropenia, and the only side effect from ethacrynic acid is diuresis. Doses of ethacrynic acid used in this study induced >50% decrements in GST levels in circulating leukocytes in 42% of patients. Phase II studies will be initiated soon.

SUMMARY

The current therapy of advanced epithelial ovarian cancer is woefully inadequate. High response rates with platinum-based therapy are too often brief, and only 10% to 20% of patients with stage III and <3% of patients with stage IV disease will be alive 5 years after the diagnosis. Can the next decade push the therapeutic envelope to improve long-term results the same way short-term results were enhanced in the 1980s?

At least one new drug, taxol, holds that promise, reminiscent of cisplatin 15 years ago in terms of its ability to induce response in drug-resistant disease. One can only hope, as this new agent is incorporated into initial therapies, that not only response rates but also response durations will improve. The 1990s will most certainly answer this important question.

Recognition that intrinsic and/or acquired drug resistance is the major obstacle to successful tumor eradication in a tumor that is relatively drug sensitive is actually a new concept. Attempts to overcome this resistance by various mechanisms to increase dose intensity or to block resistance mechanisms are just beginning. Mechanisms that are currently clinically feasible are probably not of sufficient magnitude to overcome resistance, which is usually several-fold. Nevertheless, clinical trials in this area should continue along with further study of the genetic mechanisms that control this resistance. The 1990s and beyond are expected to be the era of gene therapy, so further basic understanding of these mechanisms will most likely lead to novel ways to circumvent this major cause for failure of current therapies.

REFERENCES

1. Perez RP, Godwin AK, Hamilton TC, et al. Ovarian cancer biology. *Semin Oncol* 1991;18:186–204.
2. Zalupski M, Baker LH. Ifosfamide. *J Natl Cancer Inst* 1988;80:556–566.
3. Bruhl P, Gunther U, Hoefer-Janker H, et al. Results obtained with fractionated ifosfamide massive-dose treatment in generalized malignant tumors. *Int J Clin Pharmacol* 1976;14:29–39.
4. Schnitker J, Brock N, Burkert H, et al. Evaluation of a cooperative clinical study of the cytotoxic agent ifosfamide. *Arzneimittelforschung* 1976;26:1783–1793.
5. Taki I, Kato T, Sekiba K, et al. Ifosfamide chemotherapy of gynecologic malignancies. *Jpn J Cancer Chemother* 1981;8:387–394.
6. Sutton GP, Blessing JA, Homesley HD, et al. Phase II trial of ifosfamide and mesna in advanced ovarian carcinoma: a Gynecologic Oncology Group trial. *J Clin Oncol* 1989;7:1672–1676.
7. Hakes T, Markman M, Reichman B, et al. Ifosfamide therapy of ovarian cancer previously treated with cisplatin and cytoxan. *Proc Am Soc Clin Oncol* 1991;10:A603.
8. Yazigi R, Wild R, Madrid J, et al. Ifosfamide treatment of advanced ovarian cancer. *Obstet Gynecol* 1984;63:163–166.
9. Perren TJ, Tan S, Fryatt I, et al. Carboplatin vs sequential ifosfamide carboplatin for patients with FIGO stage III epithelial ovarian carcinoma. *Br J Cancer* 1990;62:518.
10. Teufel G, Pfleiderer A. Ifosfamide in comparison with cyclophosphamide in advanced ovarian carcinomas. *Geburtshilfe Frauenheilkd* 1976;36:274–277.
11. Falkson G, Falkson HC. Further experience with ifosfamide. *Cancer Treat Rep* 1976;60:955–957.
12. Neijt JP. Salvage chemotherapy in advanced epithelial ovarian carcinoma. *Chemotherapia* 1983;2:815–819.

13. Lund B, Hansen M, Hansen OP, et al. Combined high-dose carboplatin and cisplatin, and ifosfamide in previously untreated ovarian cancer patients with residual disease. *J Clin Oncol* 1990; 8:1226–1230.
14. Levin L, Hryniuk WM. Dose intensity analysis of chemotherapy regimens in ovarian carcinoma. *J Clin Oncol* 1987;5:756–767.
15. Rowinsky EK, Cazenave LA, Donehower RC. Taxol: a novel investigational antimicrotubule agent. *J Natl Cancer Inst* 1990; 82:1247–1259.
16. Wani MC, Taylor HL, Wall ME, et al. Plant antitumor agents VI: the isolation and structure of taxol, a novel antileukemic and antitumor agent from *taxus brevifolia*. *Am Chem Soc* 1971;93: 2325–2327.
17. Manfredi JJ, Horwitz SB. Taxol: an antimitotic agent with a new mechanism of action. *Pharmacol Ther* 1984;25:83–125.
18. Schiff PB, Fant J, Horwitz SB. Promotion of microtubule assembly *in vitro* by taxol. *Nature* 1979;22:665–667.
19. Weiss RB, Donehower RC, Wiernik PK, et al. Hypersensitivity reactions from taxol. *J Clin Oncol* 1990;8:1263–1268.
20. Brown T, Havlin K, Weiss G, et al. A phase I trial of taxol given by a 6-hour intravenous infusion. *J Clin Oncol* 1991;9: 1261–1267.
21. Donehower RC, Rowinsky EK, Grochow LB, et al. Phase I trial of taxol in patients with advanced malignancies. *Cancer Treat Rep* 1989;71:1171–1177.
22. Kris MG, O'Connell JP, Gralla RJ, et al. Phase I trial of taxol given as a 3-hour continuous infusion every 21 days. *Cancer Treat Rep* 1986;70:605–607.
23. Wiernik PH, Schwartz EL, Straumann JJ, et al. Phase I clinical and pharmacokinetic study of taxol. *Cancer Res* 1987;47: 2486–2493.
24. Lipton RB, Apfel SC, Dutcher JP, et al. Taxol produces a predominately sensory neuropathy. *Neurology* 1988;39:368–373.
25. Einzig AI, Wiernik P, Sasloff J, et al. Phase II study of taxol in patients with advanced ovarian cancer. *Proc Am Assoc Cancer Res* 1990;31:1114.
26. McGuire WP, Rowinsky EK, Rosenshein NB, et al. Taxol: a unique antineoplastic agent with significant activity in advanced ovarian epithelial neoplasms. *Ann Intern Med* 1989;111: 273–279.
27. Thigpen JT, Blessing JA, Ball H, et al. Phase II trial of taxol as second-line therapy for ovarian carcinoma: a Gynecologic Oncology Group study. *Proc Am Soc Clin Oncol* 1990;9:604.
28. Rowinsky EK, Burke PJ, Karp JE, et al. Phase I study of taxol in refractory adult leukemia. *Cancer Res* 1989;49:4640–4647.
29. Sarosy G, Kohn E, Link C, et al. Taxol dose intensification in patients with recurrent ovarian cancer. *Proc Am Soc Clin Oncol* 1992;11:226.
30. Wiltshaw E, Subramarian S, Alexopoulos C, et al. Cancer of the ovary: a summary of experience with cis-dichlorodiammineplatinum (II) at the Royal Marsden Hospital. *Cancer Treat Rep* 1979; 63:1545–1548.
31. Rowinsky EK, Gilbert M, McGuire WP, et al. Sequences of taxol and cisplatin: a phase I/pharmacologic study. *J Clin Oncol* 1991;9:1692–1703.
32. Citardi MJ, Rowinsky EK, Schaefer KL, et al. Sequence-dependent cytotoxicity between cisplatin and the antimicrotubule agents taxol and vincristine. *Proc Am Assoc Cancer Res* 1990; 31:2431.
33. Rowinsky EK. *Personal communication*.
34. Markman M, Rowinsky E, Hakes T, et al. Phase I study of taxol by the intraperitoneal route: a GOG trial. *Proc Am Soc Clin Oncol* 1991;10:A601.
35. Barasoain I, de Ines C, Diaz F, et al. Interaction of tubulin and cellular microtubules with taxotere (RP56976), a new semisynthetic analog of taxol. *Proc Am Assoc Cancer Res* 1991;32: A1952.
36. Ringel I, Horwitz SB. Studies with RP 56976 (taxotere): a semi-synthetic analogue of taxol. *J Natl Cancer Inst* 1991;83:288–291.
37. Bissery MC, Renard A, Montay G, et al. Taxotere: antitumor activity and pharmacokinetics in mice. *Proc Am Assoc Cancer Res* 1991;32:A2386.
38. Foster BJ, Clagett-Carr K, Marsoni S, et al. Role of hexamethylmelamine in the treatment of ovarian cancer: where is the needle in the haystack? [Letter]. *Cancer Treat Rep* 1986;70:1003–1004.
39. Ames MM, Sanders ME, Tiede WS. Role of N-methylolpentamethylmelamine in the metabolic activation of hexamethylmelamine. *Cancer Res* 1983;43:500–504.
40. Wharton JT, Rutledge F, Smith JP, et al. Hexamethylmelamine: an evaluation of its role in the treatment of ovarian cancer. *Am J Obst Gynecol* 1979;13:833–844.
41. Wharton JT. Hexamethylmelamine activity as a single agent in previously untreated advanced ovarian cancer. *Cancer Treat Rev* 1991;18:15–21.
42. Hainsworth JD, Grosh WW, Barnett LS, et al. Advanced ovarian cancer: long-term results of treatment with intensive cisplatin-based chemotherapy of brief duration. *Ann Intern Med* 1988;108:165–170.
43. Greco FA, Johnson DH, Hainsworth JD, et al. A comparison of hexamethylmelamine (altretamine), cyclophosphamide, doxorubicin, and cisplatin (H-CAP) vs. cyclophosphamide, doxorubicin, and cisplatin (CAP) in advanced ovarian cancer. *Cancer Treat Rev* 1991;18:47–56.
44. Bruckner HW, Cohen CJ, Feuer E, et al. Modulation and intensification of a cyclophosphamide, hexamethylmelamine, doxorubicin, and cisplatin ovarian cancer regimen. *Obstet Gynecol* 1989;3:349–356.
45. Bruckner HW, Cohen C, Mandell J, et al. Hexamethymelamine for the treatment of ovarian cancer. The Mount Sinai experience. *Cancer Treat Rev* 1991;18:57–66.
46. Edmonson JH, McCormack GW, Fleming TR, et al. Comparison of cyclophosphamide plus cisplatin versus hexamethylmelamine, cyclophosphamide, doxorubicin, and cisplatin in combination as initial chemotherapy for stage III and IV ovarian carcinomas. *Cancer Treat Rep* 1985;69:1243–1248.
47. Edmonson JH, McCormack GW, Wieand HS. *Late emerging survival differences in a comparative study of HCAP vs. CP in stage III–IV ovarian carcinoma*. Sixth International Conference on the Adjuvant Therapy of Cancer. Tucson, 1990.
48. Sessa C, Colombo N. Randomized comparison of hexamethylmelamine, adriamycin, cyclophosphamide (HAC) versus cisplatin, adriamycin, cyclophosphamide in advanced ovarian cancer: long-term results. *Cancer Treat Rev* 1991;18:37–46.
49. Neijt JP, ten Bokkel Huinink WW, van den Burg MEL, et al. Long-term survival in ovarian cancer: mature data from the Netherlands study group for ovarian cancer. *Eur J Cancer* 1991; 27:1367–1372.
50. Rosen GF, Lurain JR, Newton M. Hexamethylmelamine in ovarian cancer after failure of cisplatin-based multiple agent chemotherapy. *Gynecol Oncol* 1987;27:173–179.
51. Manetta A, MacNeill C, Lyter JA, et al. Analysis of prognostic factors and survival in patients with ovarian cancer treated with second-line hexamethylmelamine (altretamine). *Cancer Treat Rev* 1991;18:23–29.
52. Moore DH, Fowler WC, Jones CP, et al. Hexamethylmelamine chemotherapy for persistent or recurrent epithelial ovarian cancer. *Am J Obstet Gynecol* 1991;165:573–576.
53. Ames MM, Richardson RL, Kovach JS, et al. Phase I and clinical evaluation of a parenteral hexamethylmelamine formulation. *Cancer Res* 1990;50:206–210.
54. Bowen E, Nanta MM, Schluper HM, et al. Superior efficacy of trimelamol to hexamethylmelamine in human ovarian cancer xenografts. *Cancer Chemother Pharmacol* 1986;18:124–128.
55. D'Arpa O, Liu LF. Topoisomerase-targeting antitumor drugs. *Biochim Biophys Acta* 1985;989:163–177.
56. Hsiang YH, Wu HY, Liu LF. Proliferation-dependent regulation of DNA topoisomerase II in cultured human cells. *Cancer Res* 1988;48:3230–3235.
57. Underberg WJM, Goosen RMJ, Smith BR, et al. Equilibrium kinetics of the new experimental anti-tumor compound SK&F 104864-A in aqueous solution. *J Pharm Biomed Anal* 1990;8: 681–683.
58. Rowinsky E, Grochow L, Hendricks C, et al. Phase I and pharmacologic study of topotecan: a novel topoisomerase I inhibitor. *Proc Am Soc Clin Oncol* 1991;10:A240.
59. Alberts DS, Garcia D, Roe D, et al. Lack of tetraplatin cross-resistance with cisplatin against epithelial ovarian cancers ob-

tained from more than 70 patients with advanced disease. *Proc Am Assoc Cancer Res* 1991;32:2434.
60. Perez RP, O'Dwyer PJ, Handel LM, et al. Comparative cytotoxicity of CI-973, cisplatin, carboplatin and tetraplatin in human ovarian carcinoma cell lines. *Int J Cancer* 1991;48:265–269.
61. Parker RJ, Vionnet JA, Bostick-Burton F, et al. Tetraplatin sensitivity/resistance in human ovarian cancer cells made resistant to cisplatin. *Proc Am Assoc Cancer Res* 1991;32:2105.
62. McGuire WP, Hoskin WJ, Brady MS, et al. A phase II trial of dose intense versus standard dose cisplatin and cytoxan in advanced ovarian cancer. *Proc Int Gynecol Cancer Soc* 1991;3:35.
63. Kaye SB. High dose cisplatin (100 mg/m^2) is more effective than low dose (50 mg/m^2) in combination with cycylophosphamide (750 mg/m^2) for the treatment of advanced ovarian cancer. *Proc Int Gynecol Cancer Soc* 1991;3:170.
64. Pecorelli S, Marsoni S, Belloni C, et al. Controlled clinical trial of two different dose-intensity induction regimens in advanced ovarian cancer patients. *Proc Int Gynecol Cancer Soc* 1991;3:215.
65. Lund B, Hansen M, Hansen OP, et al. High-dose platinum consisting of combined carboplatin and cisplatin in previously untreated ovarian cancer patients with residual disease. *J Clin Oncol* 1989;7:1469–1473.
66. Piccart MJ, Nogaret JM, Marcelis L, et al. Cisplatin combined with carboplatin: a new way of intensification of platinum dose in the treatment of advanced ovarian cancer. *J Natl Cancer Inst* 1990;82:703–707.
67. Calvert AH, Newell DR, Gumbrell LA, et al. Carboplatin dosage: prospective evaluation of a simple formula based on renal function. *J Clin Oncol* 1989;7:1748–1756.
68. Reed E, Janik J, Bookman M, et al. High-dose chemotherapy and rGM-CSF in refractory ovarian cancer. *Proc Am Soc Clin Oncol* 1990;9:157.
69. Ozols RF, Ostchega Y, Curt G, et al. High-dose carboplatin in refractory ovarian cancer patients. *J Clin Oncol* 1987;5:197–201.
70. Ozols RF, Ostchega Y, Myers CE, et al. Cisplatin in hypertonic saline in refractory ovarian cancer. *J Clin Oncol* 1987;5:1246–1250.
71. Frei E, Cucchi CA, Rosowsky A, et al. Alkylating agent resistance: *in vivo* studies with human cell lines. *Proc Natl Acad Sci USA* 1985;82:2158–2162.
72. Mulder POM, Willemese PHB, Aalders JG, et al. High-dose chemotherapy with autologous bone marrow transplantation in patients with refractory ovarian cancer. *Br J Cancer* 1989;25:645–649.
73. Viens P, Maraninchi D, Legros M, et al. High dose melphalan and autologous marrow rescue in advanced epithelial carcinomas: a retrospective analysis of 35 patients treated in France. *Bone Marrow Transplant* 1990;5:227–233.
74. Dauplat J, Legros M, Condat P, et al. High-dose melphalan and autologous bone marrow support for treatment of ovarian carcinoma with positive second-look operation. *Gynecol Oncol* 1989;34:294–298.
75. Barnett MJ, Swenerton KD, Hoskins PJ, et al. Intensive therapy with carboplatin, etoposide, and melphalan (CEM) and autologous stem cell transplantation (SCT) for epithelial ovarian carcinoma (EOC). *Proc Am Soc Clin Oncol* 1990;9:168.
76. Shpall EJ, Clarke-Pearson D, Soper JT, et al. High-dose alkylating agent chemotherapy with autologous bone marrow support in patients with stage III/IV epithelial ovarian cancer. *Gynecol Oncol* 1990;38:386–391.
77. Shea TC, Flaherty M, Elias A, et al. A phase I clinical and pharmacokinetic study of carboplatin and autologous bone marrow support. *J Clin Oncol* 1989;7:651–661.
78. Copeland LJ, Gershenson DM, Wharton JT, et al. Microscopic disease at second-look laparotomy in advanced ovarian cancer. *Cancer* 1985;55:472–478.
79. Markman M. Intraperitoneal chemotherapy. *Semin Oncol* 1991;18:248–254.
80. Goel R, Cleary SM, Horton C, et al. Effect of sodium thiosulfate on the pharmacokinetics and toxicity of cisplatin. *J Natl Cancer Inst* 1989;81:1552–1560.
81. Rothenberg ML, Ostchega Y, Steinberg SM, et al. High-dose carboplatin with diethyldithiocarbamate chemoprotection in treatment of women with relapsed ovarian cancer. *J Natl Cancer Inst* 1988;80:1488–1492.
82. Calabro-Jones PM, Aquilera JA, Ward JF, et al. Uptake of WR-2721 derivatives by cells in culture: identification of the transported form of the drug. *Cancer Res* 1988;48:3634–3640.
83. Yuhas JM, Spellman JM, Jordan SM, et al. Treatment of tumors with the combination of WR-2721 and cis-dichlorodiammine platinum or cyclophosphamide. *Br J Cancer* 1980;42:574–585.
84. Glover D, Glick JH, Weiler C, et al. WR-2721 protect against the hematologic toxicity of cyclophosphamide: a controlled phase II trial. *J Clin Oncol* 1986;4:584–588.
85. Glover D, Glick JH, Weiler C, et al. WR-2721 and high-dose cisplatin: an active combination in the treatment of metastatic melanoma. *J Clin Oncol* 1987;5:574–578.
86. Mollman J, Glover DJ, Hogan M, et al. Cisplatin neuropathy: risk factors, prognosis, and protection by WR-2721. *Cancer* 1988;61:2192–2195.
87. Kemp GM, Glover DJ, Schein PS. The role of WR-2721 in the reduction of combined cisplatin and cyclophosphamide toxicity. *Proc Am Soc Clin Oncol* 1990;9:67.
88. Gerritsen van der Hoop R, Vecht CJ, van der Burg MEL, et al. Prevention of cisplatin neurotoxicity with an ACTH (4-9) analogue in patients with ovarian cancer. *N Engl J Med* 1990;322:88–94.
89. Rogan AM, Hamilton TC, Young RC, et al. Reversal of adriamycin resistance by verapamil in human ovarian cancer. *Science* 1984;224:994–996.
90. Bourhis J, Goldstein LJ, Riou G, et al. Expression of a human multidrug resistance gene in ovarian carcinomas. *Cancer Res* 1989;49:5062–5065.
91. Ozols RF, Cunnion RE, Klecker RW, et al. Verapamil and adriamycin in the treatment of drug-resistant ovarian cancer patients. *J Clin Oncol* 1987;7:641–647.
92. Masuda H, Ozols RF, Lai GM, et al. Increased DNA repair as a mechanism of acquired resistance to cis-diamminedichloroplatinum (II) in human ovarian cell lines. *Cancer Res* 1988;48:5713–5716.
93. Ozols RF, Louie KG, Plowman J, et al. Enhanced melphalan cytotoxicity in human ovarian cancer in vitro and in tumor-bearing nude mice by buthionine sulfoximine depletion of glutathione. *Biochem Pharmacol* 1987;36:147–153.
94. Lai GM, Ozols RF, Young RC, et al. Effect of glutathione on DNA repair in cisplatin-resistant human ovarian cancer cell lines. *J Natl Cancer Inst* 1989;81:535–539.
95. Andrews PA, Murphy MP, Howell SB. Differential potentiation of alkylating agent cytotoxicity in human ovarian carcinoma cells by glutathione depletion. *Cancer Res* 1985;45:6250–6253.
96. Hamilton T, O'Dwyer P, Young R, et al. Phase I trial of buthionine sulfoximine (BSO) plus melphalan (L-PAM) in patients with advanced ovarian cancer. *Proc Am Soc Clin Oncol* 1990;9:73.
97. Schilder RJ, Nash S, Tew KD, et al. Phase I trial of thiotepa (TT) in combination with glutathione transferase (GST) inhibitor ethacrynic acid (EA). *Proc Am Assoc Cancer Res* 1990;31:177.

CHAPTER 22

Immunotherapy of Ovarian Cancer

Otoniel Martínez-Maza and Jonathan S. Berek

The immune system plays an essential role in host defense and in the maintenance of organismal integrity: Individuals with primary or acquired forms of immune deficiency are rapidly overwhelmed by viral or microbial infection, including infections by opportunistic infectious agents that do not normally cause clinical disease in healthy individuals. Also, the immune system can respond to host cells that have undergone transformation to become neoplastic cells. Many effective antitumor immune mechanisms exist, and these have been described in various study systems. However, the physiologic role of immune responses in controlling neoplastic growth, specifically as described in the concept of immune surveillance (1), is unclear (2). Although immune deficient patients have a higher frequency of clinically apparent tumors, the tumors that develop in these patients tend to be lymphoproliferative tumors, such as lymphoma, or unusual forms of cancer, such as Kaposi's sarcoma in the acquired immune deficiency syndrome (3). Therefore, the inherent role of the immune system in preventing cancer may be restricted to certain tumors.

Although the natural role of the immune system in the control of cancer is unclear, there is no doubt that the immune system can interact with tumor cells in various ways and that these responses, whether natural or induced, can in some cases lead to tumor regression. As more is learned about the regulation of immune responses, new opportunities are developed for the generation of novel immunotherapeutic approaches. Also, immunodiagnostic procedures, using antitumor marker antibodies, show great promise as diagnostic and/or prognostic tools.

In this chapter we present a brief introduction to the human immune system, a summary of immune effector mechanisms involved in antitumor responses, and a summary of experimental immunotherapeutic approaches to ovarian cancer.

IMMUNOLOGIC MECHANISMS INVOLVED IN THE ANTITUMOR RESPONSES

The human immune system has the potential to respond to tumor cells in various ways. Some of these immune responses occur in an innate, or antigen nonspecific, manner, but other immune responses are adaptive, or antigen-specific. Adaptive responses are specific for a given antigen and result in the establishment of memory, allowing a more rapid and vigorous response to that same antigen in future encounters (4,5). Various innate and adaptive immune mechanisms are involved in responses to tumors, including cytotoxicity directed to tumor cells mediated by cytotoxic T cells, natural killer (NK) cells, macrophages, or antibody-dependent cellular cytotoxicity (ADCC) (2,6).

Adaptive immune responses are made up of humoral and cellular responses. Humoral responses refer to the production of antibodies, which are antigen-reactive, soluble, bifunctional molecules composed of specific antigen-binding sites that react with foreign antigens. They are associated with a constant region that directs the biological activities of the antibody, such as the binding of antibody molecules to cells, including phagocytic cells, or the activation of complement. Cellular immune responses are antigen-specific immune responses mediated directly by activated immune cells, rather than by the production of antibodies. The distinction between humoral and cellular responses origi-

---

O. Martínez-Maza: Department of Obstetrics and Gynecology and Department of Microbiology and Immunology, Jonsson Comprehensive Cancer Center, UCLA School of Medicine, Los Angeles, California 90024-1740
J. S. Berek: Department of Obstetrics and Gynecology, Jonsson Comprehensive Cancer Center, UCLA School of Medicine, Los Angeles, California 90024-1740

nates from the experimental observation that humoral immune function can be transferred by serum, whereas cellular immune function requires the transfer of cells. In nature, responses to antigens usually involve both humoral and cellular responses.

Several types of cells, including cells from both the myeloid and lymphoid lineages, make up the immune system. Specific humoral and/or cellular immune responses to foreign antigens involve the coordinated action of populations of lymphocytes, operating in concert with each other and with phagocytic cells (macrophages). These cellular interactions include both direct cognate interactions, involving cell-cell contact, and cellular interactions involving the secretion of, and response to, cytokines or lymphokines. Lymphoid cells are found in lymphoid tissues, such as lymph nodes or spleen, or in the peripheral circulation. The cells that make up the immune system originate from stem cells in the bone marrow.

B Cells, Humoral Immunity, and Monoclonal Antibodies

The cells that synthesize and secrete antibodies are B lymphocytes (4,5). Mature, antigen-responsive B cells develop from pre-B cells (committed B cell progenitors) and differentiate to become plasma cells, which are cells that produce large quantities of antibodies. Pre-B cells originate from bone marrow stem cells in adults, following the rearrangement of immunoglobulin genes from their germ-cell configuration to that seen in B cells. Mature B cells express cell surface immunoglobulin molecules, which these cells use as their receptors for antigen. On interaction with antigen, mature B cells respond to become antibody-producing cells, in the presence of appropriate stimulatory signals and appropriate cell-cell interactions. Although the generation of antibodies directed to tumor cells does not appear to play a central role in antitumor immune responses, the production of monoclonal antibodies to tumor cell antigens has shown great potential for immunotherapy and tumor detection.

Kohler and Milstein developed monoclonal antibody technology more than 10 years ago (7). In recent years there has been considerable interest in the use of monoclonal antibodies for tumor detection, monitoring, and therapy. Monoclonal antibodies reactive with tumor-associated antigens may provide new therapeutic agents for ovarian cancer. Immunotoxin-conjugated monoclonal antibodies directed to human ovarian adenocarcinoma antigens can induce tumor cell killing and can prolong survival in mice implanted with a human ovarian cancer cell line (8).

However, many obstacles limit the clinical utility of monoclonal antibodies: tumor cell antigenic heterogeneity, modulation of tumor-associated antigens, and cross-reactivity of normal host and tumor-associated antigens. In fact, no unique tumor-specific antigens have been identified. All tumor antigens identified to date are tumor-related antigens, which have been expressed to some extent on nonmalignant tissues. However, normal tissues may display a lower level of antigen expression than tumor tissue, which can express high levels of these cell surface tumor antigens. Also, because most monoclonal antibodies are murine, the host's immune system can recognize and respond to these foreign mouse proteins. However, the use of genetically engineered monoclonal antibodies composed of human constant regions with specific antigen-reactive murine variable regions should result in reduced antigenicity to the host and might help eliminate many of the problems associated with the administration of murine monoclonal antibodies.

T Lymphocytes and Cellular Immunity

T lymphocytes play a central role in the generation of immune responses by acting as helper cells in both humoral and cellular immune responses and by acting as effector cells in cellular responses (4,5). T cell precursors originate in bone marrow and migrate to the thymus, where they mature into functional T cells. During this thymic maturation, T cells learn to recognize antigen in the context of the major histocompatibility type of the individual. Also, it appears that T cells with the capability of responding to self are removed during development.

T cells can be distinguished from other types of lymphocytes by their cell surface phenotype (the pattern of expression of various molecules on the cell surface) and by differences in their biological functions (4,5). All mature T cells express certain cell surface molecules. These include the CD3 molecular complex and the T cell antigen receptor (Ti), which is found in close association with the CD3 complex. The expression of these cell surface molecules can be quantified using monoclonal antibodies specific for these molecules. The availability of monoclonal antibody reagents specific for such markers has led to great progress in understanding the organization of the immune system in recent years. Certainly, such monoclonal antibodies are of great value in understanding the clinical immunology of immune deficiency disorders and in following the effects of experimental treatment, with biological response modifiers or cytokines, on the human immune system.

T cells recognize antigen via the cell surface T cell antigen receptor. In terms of its structure and molecular organization, this molecule is similar to antibody molecules, which are the B cell receptor for antigen. The T cell receptor gene undergoes gene arrangements during T cell development similar to those seen in B cells. However, there are important differences between the antigen receptors on B cells and T cells. For instance, the T cell receptor is not secreted, and its structure is different from that of antibody molecules in some ways. Also, the way in which the B cell and T cell receptors interact with antigens is quite different.

There are two major subsets of mature T cells, which are phenotypically and functionally distinct: T helper/inducer cells, which express the CD4 cell surface marker, and T suppressor/cytotoxic cells, which express the CD8 marker (4,5). The expression of these markers is acquired during the passage of T cells through the thymus. CD4 T cells can provide help to B cells, resulting in the production of antibodies by B cells. Also, CD4 T cells can act as helper cells for other T cells. CD8 T cells include cells that are cytotoxic (cells that can kill target cells bearing appropriate antigens). The CD8 T cell subset also contains suppressor T cells. Suppressor T cells can inhibit the biological functions of B cells or other T cells.

Although the primary biological role of cytotoxic T cells appears to be lysis of virus-infected autologous cells, cytotoxic immune T cells can directly mediate the lysis of tumor cells. Presumably, cytotoxic T cells first recognize antigens on tumor cells via their antigen-specific T cell receptor; a series of events then occurs that ultimately results in the lysis of the target cell.

Monocytes and Macrophages

Monocyte/macrophages, which are myeloid cells, play important roles in both innate and adaptive immune responses. In fact, macrophages can play a key role in the generation of immune receptors. T cells do not respond to foreign antigens unless these antigens are processed and presented by antigen-presenting cells. Macrophages (and B cells) can serve as antigen-presenting cells (4,5). After being processed, antigen is presented to T cells in an appropriate form on the surface of macrophages. Helper/inducer (CD4) T cells, bearing a T cell receptor of appropriate antigen and self-specificity, are activated by this antigen-presenting cell to provide help (various factors—lymphokines—that induce the activation of other lymphocytes).

In addition to their role as antigen-presenting cells, macrophages can play an important role in innate responses by ingesting and killing microorganisms. Also, activated macrophages, in addition to their many other functional capabilities, can act as cytotoxic, antitumor killer cells.

Natural Killer (NK) Cells

A third major population of lymphocytes includes NK cells (4,5). NK cells do not consistently bear cell surface markers characteristic of T or B cells, although they can share certain cell surface molecules with other types of lymphocytes. NK cells characteristically have a large granular lymphocyte morphology (9).

NK cells are effector cells in an innate type of immune response: the nonspecific killing of tumor cells and/or virus-infected cells. NK activity therefore represents an innate form of immunity that does not require an adaptive, memory response for optimal biological function. However, NK antitumor activity can be augmented by exposure to several agents, especially cytokines such as interleukin-2 (IL-2).

Although NK cells can express certain cell surface receptors, particularly a receptor for the Fc portion of antibodies and other NK-associated markers, it appears that cells with NK function are phenotypically heterogeneous, at least when compared to T or B cells. The cells that can carry out ADCC, or antibody-targeted cytotoxicity, appear to be NK-like cells. ADCC by NK-like cells has been shown to result in the lysis of tumor cell targets in vitro. The mechanisms of tumor cell killing in ADCC are not clearly understood, although close cellular contact between the ADCC effector cell and the target cell appears to be required.

Biological Response Modifiers

Most immunotherapeutic agents used in the treatment of cancer have been nonspecific agents, which when introduced into the human system elicit a generalized inflammatory reaction and immune response, probably mediated by the secretion of a spectrum of cytokines by many different types of cells. These agents have diverse and broad biological effects and often are referred to as immunomodulators or biologic response modifiers (BRM).

The response of a given patient to treatment with BRM depends on the patient's ability to react to treatment with a generalized immune response. In fact, it is possible that some elements of the immune response elicited by immunotherapeutic agents or BRM may be counterproductive, possibly causing immune suppression, inducing the production of cytokines that enhance tumor growth, and/or inducing an unfavorable or inappropriate immune response.

BCG (bacillus Calmette-Guérin) has been widely used in many tumor systems. BCG has been administered either systemically, by intralesional injection, or escarification (10). Occasionally BCG has been mixed with whole irradiated tumor cells and injected into the patient as a vaccine. In a large series (11), intracutaneous injection of melanoma lesions with BCG resulted in some tumor regression in patients with cutaneous recurrence. However, visceral or parenchymal metastatic disease has been resistant to this therapy. Although there have been some preliminary observations obtained examining the use of BCG as an adjuvant in children with acute lymphocytic leukemia and with stage II melanoma, randomized studies have not revealed significant responses.

Cytokines, Lymphokines, and Immune Mediators

Many events in the generation of immune responses and during the effector phase of immune responses appear to require or to be enhanced by cytokines, which are soluble mediator molecules (4). Cytokines are pleiotropic molecules: They have multiple biological functions, depending on the target cell type or the maturational status of the target cell. Also, cytokines are heterogeneous. Some cytokines appear to be related, in the sense that they share structural features, and appear to have evolved from a common ancestral precursor, but most cytokines share little structural or amino acid homology. Cytokines—also called monokines (cytokines from monocytes), lymphokines (cytokines from lymphocytes), interleukins (cytokines that exert their actions among leukocytes), or interferons (cytokines that have antiviral effects)—are produced by a wide variety of cells types and seem to play important roles in many biological responses outside of the immune response, such as hematopoiesis. Also, they may be involved in the pathophysiology of a wide range of diseases, and they show great potential as therapeutic agents in immunotherapy to cancer.

Although cytokines are a heterogeneous group of proteins, they share some characteristics. For instance, most cytokines are low-intermediate molecular weight (10–60 kDa), glycosylated secreted proteins. Also, cytokines are involved in immunity and inflammation, are produced transiently and locally (they do not generally act in an endocrine manner), are extremely potent on a molar basis, and interact with high-affinity cellular receptors that are specific for each cytokine. The cell surface binding of cytokines by specific receptors results in signal transduction, followed by changes in gene expression, and ultimately by changes in cellular proliferation and/or altered cell behavior. Also, the biological actions of cytokines overlap, and exposure of responsive cells to multiple cytokines can result in synergistic or antagonistic biological effects.

Interleukin-1 (IL-1) has a wide range of biological activities, including direct effects on several cells involved in immune responses (12). Also, IL-1 is involved in fever and inflammatory responses and may be involved in the pathogenesis of several diseases, such as rheumatoid arthritis. There are two defined forms of IL-1: IL-1α and IL-1β, which have similar biological activities. IL-1 can be released as a soluble form or can be found as a cell-associated molecule on the cell surface of macrophages. The primary sources of IL-1 production are macrophages, the phagocytic cells of the liver and spleen, some B cells, epithelial cells, certain brain cells, and the cells lining the synovial spaces. IL-1 has a broad range of target cells and biological activities, as do most lymphokines.

IL-2 is a lymphokine that was originally called T cell growth factor (TCGF), which indicates one of the major biological activities of this molecule. Failure of T cells to produce IL-2 results in the absence of a T cell immune response and a diminution of the antibody response. Natural human IL-2 is a 15 kDa glycoprotein and is produced primarily by activated T cells. In order for IL-2 to exert its proliferation-inducing effects, it has to interact with a specific receptor for IL-2 on the surface of the target cell. The high affinity receptor for IL-2 consists of two polypeptides, the α (75 kDa) and β (55 kDa) chains. After activation, T cells express greatly increased numbers of this high-affinity receptor for IL-2.

A principal role of IL-1 in immune responses is in the initiation of early events in immune responses. IL-1 induces antigen-responsive T cells to express the gene for IL-2; these T cells will then express the IL-2 receptor and will respond to IL-2 with increased proliferation. Therefore, stimulation of resting T cells with antigen presented in the context of self (i.e., antigen associated with an MHC molecule on the surface of an antigen-presenting cell) and with IL-1 induces the synthesis and secretion of IL-2. During this activation process, responding T cells undergo a change or alteration in their cell surface receptors, including the expression of cell surface receptors for IL-2. Continuing exposure to IL-2 then leads to the proliferation of T cells bearing the IL-2 receptor, thereby acting as an activation and response-amplification stage in the generation of immune responses. Activated T cells respond to and produce IL-2. Therefore, IL-2 can act in an autocrine manner, meaning that the cells producing the lymphokine then respond to it, or in a paracrine fashion, meaning that the IL-2 produced by a T cell is taken up and responded to by neighboring cells.

IL-1 has other direct effects on cells of the immune system. For instance, IL-1 can act as a B cell activation-inducing factor. Also, IL-1 can induce the production of other lymphokines that are involved in immune responses, such as IL-6. Since its original description as a T cell growth hormone, IL-2 has been shown to have a variety of other immune activities, including the promotion of B cell activation and maturation, and monocyte and NK cell activation. Also, IL-2 can lead directly or indirectly to the stimulation of the production of interferon and other cytokines.

IL-3 is a factor involved in the early differentiation of hematopoietic cells (13) and may find a role in immunotherapy in inducing hematopoietic differentiation in people undergoing aggressive chemotherapy or bone marrow transplantation.

Various cytokines are involved in the process of B cell activation and development from resting B cells to immunoglobulin-secreting plasma cells (4). T helper cells, as well as macrophages, induce and expand B cell responses by producing B cell activating factors, which include the lymphokines that are now called interleukin 4 (IL-4), interleukin 5 (IL-5), and interleukin 6 (IL-6), as well as IL-1 and IL-2. On exposure to antigen, mature B cells become receptive to these B cell stimulating factors, and in their presence proliferate and differentiate to become antibody-secreting cells. Although IL-4, IL-5, and IL-6 were originally described as B cell stimulatory factors, after further study it became clear that these cytokines are not involved exclusively in the process of B cell activation and differentiation. For instance, IL-4 can induce T cell differentiation. Also, these "B cell stimulating factors" have been seen to have a wider range of biological activities than originally envisioned, with biological effects extending outside of the immune system. For example, IL-6 can act as a potent inducer of the production of acute phase proteins by hepatocytes in addition to acting as a differentiation-inducing factor for B lymphocytes. IL-6, a 20–25 kDa factor that can induce B cell differentiation to immunoglobulin-secreting cells, is a particularly pleiotropic cytokine. The wide range of biological activities mediated by IL-6 includes the induction of the production of acute phase reactants by hepatocytes, the induction of thymocyte proliferation and differentiation to cytotoxic T cells, and activity as a colony-stimulating factor (CSF) for hematopoietic progenitor cells (14). IL-6 is produced primarily by activated monocyte/macrophages, although T or B cells can produce this lymphokine. As with IL-1, IL-6 can play an important role in autoimmune disease, including glomerulonephritis and rheumatoid arthritis. Interestingly, several types of tumor cells produce IL-6, and IL-6 has been proposed to act as an autocrine growth factor for different types of neoplasms (15). In spite of this, IL-6 may prove to be an effective antitumor agent by virtue of its ability to enhance antitumor immune responsiveness (16).

Other cytokines that have effects on the immune system include tumor necrosis factor (TNF-α) and interferons. TNF-α can enhance cellular cytotoxicity and is directly cytotoxic for sensitive tumor cells. Also, TNF-α can activate macrophages, resulting in the secretion of other cytokines such as IL-6. TNF-α can act synergistically with various cytokines, particularly with IL-1, with which it shares some biological properties. It is produced by activated macrophages. TNF-α also induces cachexia, plays a role in inflammation, is a pyrogen, and is an important mediator in endotoxin shock.

There are three types of interferon (IFN): IFN-α, IFN-β, and IFN-γ. In addition to interfering with viral production, these factors have a variety of effects on the immune system and direct antitumor effects (17). For example, IFN-γ, a T cell–produced lymphokine with direct effects on immune function, is a potent inducer of the expression of MHC class II molecules on monocyte/macrophages. Because of this activity, it has been implicated as an important factor in enhancing the activity of antigen-presenting cells. Therefore, IFN-γ could act as a positive feedback signal for T cell activation. IFN-γ also has effects on B cell activation and differentiation.

As research on the biological activities of cytokines has progressed, these factors have appeared to be more pleiotropic and to have a bewildering array of biological activities, including activities outside of the immune system (4,14). Some of these factors have potent antitumor and/or immune-enhancing effects, and several have been used in experimental treatment of cancer and immune deficiency.

Effects of Cytokines on Tumor Cells

Various cytokines appear to have antitumor effects in vitro and in vivo. Interferons have recently received much attention because of their ability to act as immunomodulators. These cytokines are natural cellular products that have been shown to be elicited by a variety of stimuli, particularly viral infections. Interferons are potent inducers of NK cell function in vitro and in vivo, and this has been associated with antitumor activity in animal models (18). The precise role of interferons in antitumor responses, in relation to other components of immune responses, has not been completely elucidated. The mechanisms by which these molecules exert antitumor effects could include both direct antitumor activities and induction of antitumor immune responses. Clinical trials of interferons have been undertaken in gynecologic malignancies.

Also, treatment of immune cells with cytokines could enhance their ability to respond to tumor cells. This treatment has been utilized in experimental adoptive immunotherapy by exposing patient immune cells to cytokines such as IL-2 in vitro to generate lymphokine-activated killer (LAK) cells; LAK cells are then reinfused along with additional IL-2.

Administration of cytokines also can enhance antitumor responses. Recent results in animal systems indicate that antitumor effects induced by cytokine treatment can involve the upregulation of host antitumor immune activity. For example, treatment of tumor-bearing mice with IL-6 has been seen to result in a notable decrease in metastasis, resulting from increased cytotoxic T cell function (16). Also, cytokines can exert direct antitumor effects. TNF can induce cell death in sensitive tumor cells.

However, in many instances it has been difficult to discern whether the antitumor effects of cytokines are the direct result of a cytokine-mediated antitumor effect or an indirect effect induced in some fashion by cytokine exposure, such as activation of immune effector cells or the induction of the secretion of other cytokines. Clearly, some cytokines, such as TNF, can have potent direct antitumor cytotoxic effects. Other cytokines, including some interferons, may inhibit tumor growth by cytostatic effects. Alternatively, cytokines could interact with tumor cells to make them more immunogenic to responding immune cells, resulting in an enhanced antitumor response.

Cytokines also can have growth-enhancing effects for tumor cells. Various cytokines have been seen to act as autocrine and/or paracrine growth factors for human tumor cells, including tumor cells of non-lymphoid origin. For instance, IL-6 has been seen to be produced by ovarian cancer cells (19) as well as various other types of tumor cells (15). IL-6 has been demonstrated to act as an autocrine growth factor for human myeloma (20), Kaposi's sarcoma (21), and renal carcinoma (22). Ovarian cancer cells also produce another cytokine, CSF-1 (23). The role of these cytokines as possible autocrine growth factors for ovarian cancer is currently under investigation.

The effects of cytokines in cancer patients may be modulated by soluble receptors or blocking factors. For instance, blocking factors for TNF and for lymphotoxin (LT) were found in ascites from patients with ovarian cancer (24). Such factors could inhibit the cytolytic effects of TNF or LT and should be taken into account in the design of clinical trials employing intraperitoneal administration of these cytokines.

The net effect of a given cytokine on tumor cell growth will reflect the sum of the biological effects of that cytokine, including induction of antitumor immune responses, direct antitumor cell cytotoxicity or cytostasis, enhancement of tumor cell antigenicity, and stimulation of tumor cell growth. Cytokines potentially have great value in inducing antitumor responses. However, because of the multiple biological effects of cytokines, a thorough understanding of these biological effects will be needed for the successful development of potentially useful experimental therapeutic approaches.

Adoptive Immunotherapy

Recently, the ex vivo enhancement of antitumor immune cell responses, including the generation of lymphokine-activated killer (LAK) cells or the activation of tumor-infiltrating lymphocytes (TIL), have provided new immune system-based approaches for antitumor responses. In particular, adoptive immunotherapy with IL-2 has been studied extensively and has been seen to produce tumor regression in a variety of animal and human tumors, such as melanoma and renal cell carcinoma, in conjunction with the adoptive transfer of autologous LAK cells (25,26).

Exposure of peripheral blood monoclonal cells (PBMC) to cytokines in vitro (particularly IL-2) leads to the generation of cytotoxic effect cells (LAK cells) (26). These cells are effective cytotoxic cells for a variety of tumor cells, including tumor cells resistant to NK cell–mediated or T cell–mediated lysis. The treatment of patients with such ex vivo–activated, autologous cells, along with the concomitant administration of IL-2, forms the basis of adoptive immunotherapy, a form of experimental antitumor immunotherapy that has been the subject of great interest.

Experimental treatment of human subjects with autologous, ex vivo–generated LAK cells and IL-2 has yielded tumor regression in some cases (25–28). This sort of treatment has resulted in some complete responses (27), with a combined response rate of 27% in 146 cancer patients treated in two separate studies (28–30). However, the overall response rate to LAK treatment is low, and this type of adoptive immunotherapy results in high morbidity (30). Also, the cost of LAK treatment is high, and this type of treatment is impractical in most medical settings.

Much current experimental work aims at developing more efficient and practical applications of adoptive immunotherapy. One approach involves the ex vivo generation of immune effector cells from tumor-infiltrating lymphocytes (TIL)—lymphocytes that are isolated from tumors and activated and expanded in vitro by exposure to IL-2—which are then administered concurrently with IL-2 (31,32). However, this approach is hampered by the need to expand a limited number of TIL in vitro, to generate enough effector cells for treatment. Also, much attention has been directed toward the development of new methods for the generation of LAK or TIL cells, including methods that utilize cytokines other than IL-2 for the stimulation of these cells.

Another promising approach that has been explored in recent animal studies involves the targeting of activated T lymphocytes with a bifunctional monoclonal antibody that binds to both the CD3/T cell receptor complex (on the activated effector T cell) and a tumor-associated antigen (on the target tumor cell) (33). This approach has the potential advantage of allowing a large fraction of the activated lymphocytes to target their effects directly on tumor cells, thereby reducing the need to amplify a large number of effector cells from TIL. Also, this approach has the potential to reduce some of the side effects associated with LAK treatment, which is a more nonspecific form of adoptive immunotherapy. Adoptive immunotherapy is a very active area of study and eventually may lead to effective forms of antitumor therapy.

IMMUNOTHERAPY IN OVARIAN CANCER

In recent years, increased clinical experience has been gained in immunotherapy for ovarian cancer, with various experimental immunotherapeutic approaches examined in ovarian cancer. Patients with small-volume, residual peritoneal disease remain an attractive target for immunotherapy, particularly regional peritoneal immunotherapy (34). Also, the rapid progress in molecular biology, biotechnology (monoclonal antibody production and conjugation), immunology, adoptive immunotherapy, and cytokine biology has resulted in the availability of many reagents for clinical evaluation in ovarian cancer.

Assessment of Immune Status in Patients With Gynecologic Cancers

The relative immune status of patients with gynecologic cancers has been examined in many studies. This has taken the form of the quantification of mitogen-induced in vitro proliferation of mononuclear cells, the use of skin tests to assess in vivo responses to microbial antigens or contact allergens, the enumeration of lymphocyte subsets, and the measurement of immunoglobulin levels (6,35).

The results of these studies have been difficult to assess, however, because of the complex and relatively insensitive nature of the tests used and the lack of appropriate controls. Also, the relative pretreatment immune status of patients may not be relevant to their subsequent response to immune-enhancing antitumor therapies. Future study of immune function and immune mechanisms in gynecologic cancers may benefit from new technologies and from more stringent experimental design and analysis, leading to insights relevant to treatment.

Monoclonal Antibodies and Immunotherapy

Monoclonal antibodies have the potential to kill tumor cells by complement activation and tumor cell lysis, direct antiproliferative effects, activity enhancement of nonspecific phagocytic cells that recognize the murine immunoglobulin on the surface of the tumor cell, or ADCC. However, most monoclonal antibodies (murine) are not directly cytotoxic and fail to activate human immune effector systems.

Studies evaluating the efficacy of monoclonal antibody–directed radiotherapy in gynecologic malignancies are limited. Radionuclide-conjugated monoclonal antibodies have been used as experimental treatment in patients with advanced ovarian cancer, given IP (36–38). This approach has the potential to reduce exposure of the monoclonal antibody to normal body tissue that might express antigens reactive with the monoclonal antibody. Prospective studies using new monoclonal antibody and different energy sources (particularly rhenium) are ongoing.

Another approach has been to link monoclonal antibodies to toxins, such as ricin A or *Pseudomonas* exotoxin (39), or detoxified *Salmonella* endotoxin, in combination with another biologic toxin (40). The efficacy of the clinical use of monoclonal antibodies and immunotoxins in humans requires further evaluation. The most successful studies using toxin-conjugated monoclonal antibodies in ovarian cancer have used an anti-transferrin receptor (a cell surface molecule expressed mainly by rapidly growing cells) antibody linked to *Pseudomonas* exotoxin (anti-TFR-PE) (41).

OC-125, a monoclonal antibody reactive with a molecule produced by human epithelial ovarian carcinoma cells, is widely used to monitor the blood CA-125 antigen level in women with ovarian cancer (42). Monoclonal antibodies have also been used in gynecologic oncology patients for radioimmunodetection. Monoclonal antibodies that recognize tumor-associated antigens on epithelial ovarian cancer cells, labeled with radioactive tracers, have been employed to detect primary and recurrent lesions (37,38,43,44).

Recent work has indicated that the HER-2/neu oncogene may play an important role in the pathogenesis of ovarian cancer: Elevated levels of HER-2/neu proto-oncogene expression were seen in about one-third of ovarian cancers (45). This alteration in HER-2/neu expression was seen to be associated with disease behavior. Also, the expression of HER-2/neu in ovarian cancer cells has been seen to be correlated with resistance to killing (46).

Because HER-2/neu is overexpressed in some cancer cells, it has been suggested that the HER-2/neu antigen, a transmembrane protein tyrosine kinase that is homologous to the human epidermal growth factor receptor, might be used as the target for immunotherapy (47). Very recently, a monoclonal antibody directed to HER-2/neu has shown promise as a potential immunotherapeutic agent (48). This monoclonal was seen to enhance human tumor cell susceptibility to TNF and to cisplatin in a nude mouse model system, suggesting that this anti-HER-2/neu monoclonal antibody could modulate the effects of HER-2/neu in vivo. Therefore, anti-HER-2/neu monoclonal antibody reagents may be valuable in the immunotherapy of HER-2/neu-expressing tumors, including ovarian cancer.

Immunotherapy with Biological Response Modifiers

There has been great interest in examining the potential role of immunotherapy in ovarian cancer. Because long-term survival in patients with ovarian epithelial malignancies is poor and most patients present with metastatic disease, there is a great need to develop useful biologic therapies. Furthermore, patients with advanced disease are significantly immunocompromised (49), suggesting a role for immune-enhancing therapies.

Most studies in metastatic ovarian cancer have utilized nonspecific immunotherapies. Such trials have involved inoculation with BRM, including inactivated bacterium, such as *Corynebacterium parvum* (a heat-killed, gram-negative anaerobic bacillus), bacillus Calmette-Guérin (BCG), which is a live, attenuated strain of *Mycobacterium bovis,* or Freund's complete adjuvant. Modifications of these agents can be produced by extracting fractions of these organisms using biochemical techniques. For instance, fractionation, typically by acid or phenol-extraction, can lead to the isolation of active components (glycolipids or carbohydrates) that might more selectively elicit desirable immunological responses while sparing less desirable immune reactions or side effects (50). For example, a methanol-extracted residue of BCG, MER, retains significant immunomodulatory activity while potentially avoiding some of the problems associated with viable BCG.

Exposure to *C. parvum* results in a variety of immune responses (51), including an acute inflammatory response, predominantly the induction and infiltration of neutrophils, and macrophage attraction, activation, and cytotoxicity. NK cytotoxicity is enhanced, and T lymphocyte activation also results from exposure (52). In animal systems, *C. parvum* has been shown to be active (53), with tumor rejection being temporally associated with a cellular immune response. Studies of a murine teratocarcinoma model examining biochemically fractionated *C. parvum* showed that tumor rejection in animals treated with intraperitoneal (IP) injection of the residue of pyridine-extracted *C. parvum,* a fraction that contains the bacterial cell walls (54), is comparable to the rejection observed after IP administration of whole, unmodified *C. parvum*. The sequential administration of these *C. parvum* fractions in combination with bacterial endotoxins resulted in an even greater antitumor effect (40). Interestingly, bacterial endotoxin is a potent inducer of the production of various cytokines that could mediate antitumor responses, particularly IL-1, IL-6, and TNF-α (14).

C. parvum and BCG have been used in the largest single retrospective series to date. Phase I studies of *C. parvum* have demonstrated that toxicity generally includes systemic chills, fever, malaise, nausea, and vomiting in most patients (55–59). Serious toxicity, including hypotension, prolonged elevated temperatures, and chest pain, is not common. In early studies in patients with ovarian cancer, subcutaneously administered *C. parvum* was combined with escalating doses of cyclophosphamide, doxorubicin, and 5-fluorouracil (CAF) administered monthly (59). Pretreatment immune parameters were normal in patients who responded to therapy, compared with decreased immune parameters in those who did not. However, immune function, as determined in these studies, was not augmented by therapy. A randomized trial of CAF chemo-immunotherapy with or without intravenously administered *C. parvum* showed no difference in response rates, disease progression-free intervals, or survival (60).

Creasman et al. reported a series of patients retrospectively treated with either melphalan or melphalan plus *C. parvum* (61). The study evaluated 108 patients with untreated stage III ovarian epithelial malignancies. The melphalan plus *C. parvum* combination group had 53% total response rate, compared to 29% in the group treated with melphalan alone. However, a prospective randomized study attempting to confirm these findings showed no significant differences between melphalan 7 mg/m^2 day × 5 days PO given every 4 weeks and the same regimen plus *C. parvum* given IV on day 7 after chemotherapy (62).

In a randomized prospective study by Alberts et al., 66 patients with stage III and IV epithelial ovarian carcinomas were treated with either a combination of cyclophosphamide and doxorubicin or these two agents plus concomitant intravenous BCG (55). Doxorubicin was given at 40 mg/m^2 on day 1, cyclophosphamide at 200 mg/m^2 on days 3 through 6, and BCG was given on day 8 and day 15. This cycle was repeated every 4 weeks. Of the 32 patients who were treated with a combination of chemotherapy and immunotherapy, the total response rate was 56%, with two of 32 evaluable patients having a complete response. The median duration of response was 45 weeks, and the median survival, 93 weeks. Of the 34 patients treated with doxorubicin and cyclophosphamide alone, only 11 patients (32%) had a partial response. The median duration of response in this group was 26 weeks, and the median survival was 59 weeks. Thus, the immunotherapy combined with chemotherapy did not improve the survival of patients with ovarian carcinoma. However, it is important to note that in most experimental animal systems where immunotherapy and chemotherapy are combined, tumor rejection is augmented most often when the administration of the immunostimulant precedes the administration of cytotoxic agents by a sufficient interval to permit some positive immunomodulation (63). We are awaiting the results of a prospective randomized GOG study that compares doxorubicin, cyclophosphamide, and cisplatin with or without BCG administered by escarification in patients with suboptimal stage III disease.

Only anecdotal evidence exists for responses using tumor vaccines in ovarian cancer. Graham and Graham treated 232 patients with gynecologic malignancies, 48 of whom had ovarian cancer, with Freund's complete adjuvant (64). Freund's complete adjuvant was mixed either with DNA-protein extract of the tumor or viable tumor cells. Systemic reactions to these agents were low in most patients who had tumor progression. However, this vaccine did not control tumor growth. BCG combined with an allogenic tumor cell vaccine was given to ten patients with stage III or IV ovarian cancer. Administration of alkylating agents along with the BCG and vaccine of 10^7 irradiated allogenic tumor cells resulted in prolonged survival, compared retrospectively to historical controls (65). Although these reports suggested some improvement in survival, they were all uncontrolled, retrospective studies involving a very small number of patients. Patients also have been treated with irradiated tumor cells injected intralymphatically, a technique referred to as active specific intralymphatic immunotherapy (ASILI) (66). A complete response, with the patient free of clinical evidence of disease at 13 months, was reported in seven patients with epithelial ovarian carcinoma treated with ASILI. Unfortunately, most patients with ovarian cancer have bulky, persistent tumors located in the peritoneal cavity and do not respond to this type of therapy.

Human leukocyte interferon has been seen to have antiproliferative effects on ovarian cancer cells in vitro (67). Purified or recombinant INF-α or INF-β has been administered systemically to ovarian cancer patients, most of whom had persistent or recurrent metastatic epithelial cancers, in five studies (68–70). The combined response rate of these phase I clinical trials was only 10%.

IL-2 has been used for experimental immunotherapy of ovarian cancer: Recombinant human IL-2 was administered intravenously to 23 patients with progressive melanoma, renal, colon, or ovarian cancer, by various regimens (71). IL-2 treatment was seen to induce lymphocytosis as well as significant increases in the number of cells expressing the IL-2 receptor, detectable circulating LAK cells, and augmented NK cytotoxicity.

Intraperitoneal Immunotherapy

Regional immunotherapy presents an appealing concept for the treatment of patients whose tumors are confined and have not yet metastasized beyond a definable body cavity. Malignancies that are isolated to the peritoneal cavity, such as residual ovarian cancer, have been treated in many clinical trials with IP drugs, most frequently with cytotoxic chemotherapy such as cisplatin alone or in combination with other agents (72,73). This approach is based on the premise that the residual tumor cells can be exposed to a higher concentration of the drug if brought into direct contact with the drug by IP administration and on the belief that this might provoke a response in malignancies that otherwise would be resistant. This approach has been promising as a salvage treatment for minimal residual ovarian cancer with complete responses of 20–30% when small disease persists after systemically administered, induction chemotherapy with a cisplatin combination (72,73).

The IP use of BRM or immunotherapy has been used for similar reasons, but also because it has been postulated that one might obtain the activation of regional effector mechanisms in the peritoneal cavity (35,56,74–77). Thus, regional immunotherapy could provide a means by which a biological therapy might be rendered effective, even when it has been found to be ineffective when administered intravenously. This might be particularly true for treatment with cytokines, or for adoptive immunotherapies, because activated immune effector cells may require direct contact with the malignant target cells in order to kill them (34,35, 56,74–76,78–82). In patients with minimal residual epithelial ovarian carcinoma after treatment with combination cytotoxic chemotherapy, Bast et al. (56) and Berek et al. (75) reported a total of 21 patients treated with IP immunotherapy. Of the 19 evaluable patients, there were 6 responders, including 2 complete responses. All of the responding patients had macroscopic disease of <5 mm maximum tumor diameter at the initiation of therapy. ADCC is significantly augmented during the course of therapy (56), as is NK cytotoxicity (74,83). The increase of cytotoxic effectors in the peritoneal cavity correlates well with the response to the agent *C. parvum* administered every 2 weeks in escalating doses starting at 0.25 mg/m^2 and rising to 4 mg/m^2.

The IP administration of *C. parvum* has been noted by Mantovani et al. to be useful for the palliation of ascites in women with advanced ovarian cancer (58). In eight patients, IP administration of 7 to 14 mg of *C. parvum* on days 0, 7, and 28 resulted in complete disappearance of ascites in three patients and a marked reduction of the effusion in two others. The palliative effect was noted to be sustained for 6–13 months. Hernandez et al. reported the treatment of nine patients with advanced ovarian epithelial malignancies with IP administration of sterile, pyrogen-free, rabbit-derived human ovarian antitumor serum (HOATS) (84). Although the study had short follow-up, the clinical response rate was 80%, with a 1-year survival of 87%. A trial of passive serotherapy utilizing the rabbit heteroantiserum is being studied prospectively (85). Patients are being treated with IP ^{32}P, total abdominal irradiation, and melphalan, with or without 150 to 200 ml of serum. After a 2-year follow-up in 13 patients, there is no difference in survival between the two groups.

Ohkawa and co-workers studied the use of IP administration of semisynthesized acid polysaccharides, BCG and OK432 (Picibanil, which is a *streptococcal* preparation) (86). These agents were administered IP for 4 days in a row, with weekly IP injections of doxorubicin, 5-fluorouracil, Endoxan, bleomycin, and mitomycin C. Although it was an uncontrolled study, the 60 evaluable patients treated between 1970 and 1977 had a 5-year survival of 40%. These results further suggest that locoregional immunotherapy combined with chemotherapy may play a role in the control of ovarian cancer confined to the peritoneal cavity.

However, treatment with *C. parvum,* as expected, induced a rather profound local reaction, and its toxicity precluded more widespread testing. *C. parvum* produced an appreciable amount of peritoneal fibrosis, presumably because it induces cells that promote the deposition of collagen. However, the attraction of these cells and the release of vasoactive molecules also might be responsible for the rejection of tumor cells via nonspecific killing, (i.e., the malignant cells are overwhelmed by the intense and massive outpouring of chemoattracted white cells and their products into the body cavity). In fact, the mechanism of tumor cell killing in these circumstances is unknown, although regional effector mechanisms such as ADCC are augmented after the administration of IP *C. parvum* (76).

The use of recombinant DNA technology has made it possible to obtain large quantities of defined cytokines. Several of these agents have been examined in phase I and II clinical trials, including recombinant alpha interferon (rIFN-α), recombinant gamma interferon (rIFN-γ), TNF, and IL-2.

Intraperitoneal Therapy with IFN-α

Treatment with rIFN-α is well tolerated locally but has significant systemic side effects. Interferon is a cytokine capable of the generation of cytotoxicity when autologous peripheral blood lymphocytes are incubated with human ovarian carcinoma cells (35,77). With IP rIFN-α, NK cytotoxicity is augmented, and this phenomenon is associated with tumor rejection (74–76). However, stimulation of NK is not invariably associated with clinical response. In vitro data suggest that the dominant mechanism responsible for killing tumor cells in the peritoneal cavity involves the direct effects of IFN on the cancer cells, similar to the cytotoxic chemotherapeutic agents (74). Exposure of tumor cells to rIFN-α may make them more vulnerable to the subsequent effects of cytotoxic drugs, such as cisplatin.

In phase II trials, systemically administered IFN-α has produced responses in up to 18% of patients with advanced ovarian cancer (69,82). Recombinant alpha-interferon, administered IP, also has demonstrated activity in patients with very small volume disease—that is, minimal residual disease (MRD) (microscopic disease or tumor nodules <5 mm) that is persistent ovarian cancer after first-line chemotherapy (82,87). The toxicity of IP IFN-α as a single agent also has been defined in these studies (82): Administration of the drug (25–50 million units three times a week) was not tolerated because of persistent general malaise, fever, and gastrointestinal toxicity. However, in patients treated with the same dose once a week, the treatment was tolerated for 8 to 16 consecutive weeks. Significant neurotoxicity and renal toxicity were notably absent. Although most of the side effects of single agent IFN-α appear to be complementary with cisplatin, the general malaise and gastrointestinal toxicity produced by each one could potentially be additive when the agents are combined. Willemse et al. (87) reported similar results in another trial of IP IFN-α in 20 patients with ovarian cancer, and of 17 who had a reassessment laparotomy, 5 (29%) had complete responses (CRs) and 4 (24%) had partial responses (PRs). Responses in both studies were confined to patients whose disease was minimal residual. The toxicity encountered in this trial was similar to that seen in the phase I GOG trial (82). Thus, overall, 28 surgically evaluated patients have been treated on these two trials, and 14 (50%) responded, with 9 (32%) complete responses. All of the responding patients had microscopic or small (<5 mm) residual disease. The combined surgically defined CR rate in patients with MRD was thus 50% (9 of 18 patients). These results suggest that the use of high-dose IP rIFN-α given frequently can produce the regional control of very small-volume disease confined to the peritoneal cavity. However, survival data are not available on these patients, so it is not clear if this approach can produce prolonged disease progression-free intervals.

Ample evidence suggests synergy between various interferons and standard cytotoxic agents (88–95). Interferon has been shown in vitro to act synergistically with cisplatin to kill ovarian cancer cells (90,94). In several reports, the synergy is seen only when the cells are exposed to the inteferon prior to the cytotoxic agent (88–90,92), presumably because the cytokine stimulates the proliferation of the cells, making them potentially more susceptible to the cytotoxic effects of the drug. In vivo studies have shown interferon to potentiate the cytotoxicity of cyclophosphamide and cisplatin in non–small lung cancer xenografts (94). Preclinical results suggest that enhancement of the cytotoxic effect can be achieved when the cancer cells are exposed to the antiproliferative effects of interferon prior to the administration of the cytotoxic agent (90–92,95). The results reported by Bezwoda and colleagues (96) confirm these prior observations in that the in vitro synergy observed between cisplatin and interferon, and the antitumor effect of interferon, is most likely related to the direct inhibitory effect of the molecule on tumor growth and not to its effects on modulating immune responses.

Because of the significant in vitro synergy between cisplatin and other agents, a search for clinically tolerable and effective combinations has been undertaken. Nardi et al. (97) reported 14 evaluable patients who were treated with weekly doses that alternated with 50 million units of IP rIFN-α and 90 mg/m² of cisplatin. In this trial, the surgically documented CR was 50% (7 of 14 patients), and all of these responses were confined to patients who started their treatment with MRD. The toxicity was similar to that seen in the phase I–II trials of alpha interferon alone, although the authors reported somewhat less general malaise and gastrointestinal toxicity. Therefore, the combination of IP cisplatin and interferon appeared to be tolerated in these patients and resulted in an appreciable response rate. The survival time of those patients who had a complete response was generally longer than those patients who were nonresponsive. However, since response rates are similar to those reported in other series of single-agent IP cisplatin, it was unclear whether the addition of the interferon to the cisplatin had any additive affect on the response rate. Another clinical phase I study (98), conducted at two institutions, demonstrated that combined IP therapy with cisplatin and rIFN-α can be administered safely to patients with residual ovarian carcinoma after systemic chemotherapy. The maximum tolerated doses (MTD) of the combination of rIFNα and cisplatin, as determined by the phase I trial, are 25×10^6 IU rIFNα and 60 mg/m² cisplatin. The therapy was best tolerated given as 1 cycle every 3 weeks, and of the eight patients who were treated with this precise dose, the median number of treatment cycles was 6 courses. The complete responses were noted in two patients after 5 and 6 treatment cycles, respectively; partial responses were seen in patients treated with 4 and 8 cycles, respectively.

When the two-institution trial schedule that combined IP rIFN-α and cisplatin was applied to the cooperative group setting, the Gynecologic Oncology Group (GOG), however, a very low response rate—only one (7%) partial response—was seen (99). This poor outcome can be compared with the other phase I–II trials of cisplatin-based or rIFN-α IP therapy in patients with persistent small-volume residual ovarian cancer (where response rates of 20–40% have been noted) (72,73,82). The difference probably can be accounted for by the fact that, in this series, most (15 of 18) evaluable patients had extensive carcinomatosis that was cisplatin-resistant. The maximum tumors were also larger.

In a phase I clinical trial presented by Bezwoda and colleagues (96), in which 35 patients with advanced ovarian cancer and ascites confined to the peritoneal cavity were treated with IP therapy with rIFN-α (some in combination with cisplatin), 7 responses in 19 (36%) patients were seen in this phase I trial of IP rIFN-α. This observation is intriguing and suggests that this mode of immunotherapy is appropriate in some patients with solid tumors, especially those whose tumors are localized to the peritoneal cavity (e.g., primary carcinomas of the ovary). In the phase II portion of the study, 16 patients were treated randomly with cisplatin with or without interferon. The combination of interferon and cisplatin produced a somewhat higher response rate than with interferon alone: five of the seven patients (77%) treated with the combination responded, while two of nine (22%) treated only with cisplatin responded. Furthermore, the responses correlated with the in vitro data in which the two agents produced synergy in the antitumor effect. The authors have concluded that the direct antitumor effect of cisplatin can be augmented by the concomitant exposure of the cancer cells to IFN-α.

Intraperitoneal Therapy with TNF

Various preclinical studies have shown significant antineoplastic activity for tumor necrosis factor (TNF) against various malignant cell lines (100–102). However, in phase I trials of the agent delivered systemically, there has been limited clinical activity, with considerable systemic toxicity being observed in these studies, especially fevers, rigors, and hypotension (103–106).

As with the application of all cytokines, the IP administration of TNF was hoped to produce an increased antitumor response and lower systemic side effects. In a phase I trial reported from the Memorial Sloan-Kettering Cancer Center, investigators showed that recombinant human TNF could be administered safely when given by the IP route and that this resulted in a marked pharmacokinetic advantage for IP exposure compared with that of the systemic compartment (107). After the administration of a 50 μg/m² IP dose of TNF, peak levels within the peritoneal cavity ranged between 15,000 to 59,000 pg/ml, compared with unmeasurable amounts in the systemic compartment (<50 pg/ml). In addition, levels between 14,000 and 33,000 pg/ml persisted within the compartment for up to 6 hours after a single dose of IP-administered TNF. Although the TNF was not measurable in the plasma, patients experienced mild emesis, temperature elevations, and chills, even with IP doses as low as 10 µg/m². Only one patient developed a hypotensive episode (BP 80/50), but treatment-related abdominal pain was common. No clinical responses were observed in this phase 1 trial (99).

In a study from the University of Heidelberg, IP recombinant human TNF was used to control malignant ascites formation and was shown to have a potential role in its management (107). Thirty-two patients with symptomatic malignant ascites were treated with a weekly infusion of TNF (80 µg/m²) in 1 l of fluid: 20 patients had ovarian cancer, and the other 12 had several nonovarian malignancies. Patients received an average of 2.6 infusions of recombinant TNF. Seventeen of the 31 evaluable patients (55%) experienced a complete resolution of ascites as determined by clinical and ultrasound examination at 30 days after the start of therapy, and 14 patients exhibited a partial control of malignant ascites reaccumulation. Interestingly, only one patient had relapsed during the follow-up of approximately 8 months. As observed in the Sloan-Kettering trial, the major side effects were fever, chills, abdominal pain, and emesis (107). On the basis of this report, further studies are indicated of IP TNF as an agent to control malignant ascites. It is possible that this treatment can be an important option for patients with malignant ascites when alternative systemic therapies have been ineffective.

The potential of this cytokine to augment the antitumor effect of a cytotoxic chemotherapeutic agent, cisplatin, offers a potential strategy for immunotherapy. There is evidence that even very low doses of TNF can significantly augment the antitumor properties of drugs such as cisplatin, doxorubicin, and cyclophosphamide (100). If this is the case, then the use of prolonged exposure, low-dose cytokine therapy administered in conjunction with cytotoxic chemotherapy could offer an advantage and minimize the toxicity of cytokine biotherapy. The IP route offers a means by which continuous exposure can be made practical.

Intraperitoneal Therapy with Gamma-Interferon

Recombinant IFN-γ has been shown to be active against malignant cell lines in vitro, including lines derived from patients with ovarian cancer (108–111). In a phase I trial of IP recombinant human IFN-γ conducted in patients with refractory ovarian cancer at the Memorial Sloan-Kettering Cancer Center, the agent was shown to be well tolerated when given weekly and to be associated with a 150-fold to 200-fold pharmacokinetic advantage for peritoneal cavity exposure compared with that of the systemic compartment (111). The major toxicity was fatigue and flu-like symptoms, and there was limited local toxicity at the highest dose level tested (8 million IU/m²). However, no clinical responses were observed.

In a cooperative trial performed in Europe, 40 patients with residual ovarian cancer after initial cisplatin-based chemotherapy were treated with IP recombinant human IFN-γ at a dose of 20 million IU/m² twice weekly for a maximum of 4 months (112). Of the 30 patients who were evaluable for response, 9 (30%) achieved a surgically-defined (laparoscopy or laparotomy) complete response. Ten of 23 patients (43%) whose largest residual tumor mass measured <2 cm responded to this treatment. Toxicity of the therapeutic regimen included fever (90%), leukopenia (45%), elevated transaminases (37%), abdominal discomfort (37%), and fatigue (10%). The response rate was similar to that observed with rIFN-α, as previously discussed. The difference between the high response rate noted in this trial and the failure of the Sloan-Kettering study to show activity for recombinant IFN-γ in a similar patient population may have been due to the much higher dose intensity employed in the European study (20 million units twice a week versus ≤8 million units weekly). Further studies will be needed to establish the potential of IP IFN-γ for therapy in ovarian cancer patients.

Intraperitoneal Adoptive Immunotherapy and Therapy with IL-2

Systemically administered IL-2 administration, with and without LAK cells or TIL, has been the subject of intense investigation in various forms of human cancer (27–32). In vivo studies that evaluate the response of ovarian tumor cells implanted in nude mice (113) or the effect of LAK cells in a murine model (114) have shown that treatment with LAK cells plus IL-2 can lead to a significant prolongation in survival. The IP administration of IL-2 has been the subject of several studies (81,115). A major justification for IP IL-2 is the finding in vitro that IL-2 activity against malignant tumors is enhanced with increasing drug concentrations (71,116).

In a phase I trial reported from the National Cancer Institute, IL-2 (25,000 U/kg every 8 hours) was administered IP route with LAK cells after systemic priming with IL-2 (79,80). A 100-fold increase in exposure of the peritoneal cavity to IL-2, compared with that of the systemic compartment, was observed (79). LAK activity was detectable in the peritoneal cavity during the entire period of treatment. Partial CRs were observed in several patients with both ovarian and colon cancers (80). However, toxicity was considerable and included fever, chills, emesis, hypotension, abdominal pain, fluid retention, bone marrow suppression, and liver function abnormalities. Infection was common. Several patients developed extensive peritoneal cavity fibrosis, probably resulting from the release by IL-2–activated cells of various growth factors and cytokines capable of inducing collagen synthesis by fibroblasts. These side effects might be reduced, either by modification of LAK plus IL-2 regimens, or by the development of more targeted and less nonspecific forms of adoptive immunotherapy (30).

The IP administration of IL-2 to patients, without LAK cells, has been tested (81,115). A major pharmacokinetic advantage for intracavity treatment was observed, with less local and systemic toxicity, compared with the NCI trial using LAK cells with IL-2. Researchers at the University of Pittsburgh performed a phase I–II study in refractory ovarian cancer and used two schedules of low-dose IP IL-2 (116). In a preliminary report, 13 patients were evaluable for response, and 2 patients had a complete response. Systemic toxicities were mild and included fever, fatigue, myalgias, diarrhea, emesis, and abdominal pain. These findings of antineoplastic activity and an acceptable toxicity suggest that IP IL-2 alone should be further investigated.

Aoki and co-workers reported a study that used TIL for immunotherapy in ovarian cancer (117). In seven patients with advanced or recurrent epithelial ovarian cancer treated with the adoptive transfer of TIL after a single dose of cyclophosphamide, one CR and four PRs were seen. Ten additional patients were treated with a cisplatin-containing chemotherapeutic regimen as well as TIL, and seven CRs and two PRs were seen. Four of the seven patients who had a complete response had no recurrence after 15 months of follow-up. Because TIL therapy was given without IL-2, it appears that TIL-based immunotherapy of ovarian cancer may achieve CR without IL-2 administration. Thus, this use of TIL may be more promising for adoptive immunotherapy than LAK-based immunotherapy.

CONCLUSIONS

Various immune mechanisms can play important roles in effective antitumor responses, including direct cytotoxicity directed against tumor cells as well as other mechanisms such as action of cytotoxic or immune-enhancing lymphokines. Immunotherapy for ovarian cancer has been limited in scope and responses. Preliminary studies indicate that immune enhancement leading to tumor rejection can most likely occur when the various biological response modifiers are brought into direct contact with tumors, when the tumor burden is minimal, such as in an adjuvant setting, and/or when combined with cytotoxic chemotherapy.

Recent advances in biotechnology have provided large amounts of relatively pure biologics that can be used for clinical trials. Thus, newly described cytokines and monoclonal antibodies will be available in sufficient quantities to permit appropriate clinical trials of these agents. However, much additional laboratory research will be needed to develop a complete understanding of the biological activities of these substances. Also, adoptive immunotherapy has created new opportunities for immunotherapy in ovarian cancer. Clearly, we are entering a period of extensive development and testing of these agents, both alone and in combination with adoptive immunotherapy, in the experimental therapy of ovarian cancer.

ACKNOWLEDGMENTS

This work was supported in part by grants from the NIH (CA01588), the California Institute for Cancer Research (CICR), the Ramona Moskovitz Memorial Cancer Research Fund, the June Hill Ovarian Cancer Research Fund, and the Brindell and Milton Gottlieb Gynecologic Oncology Laboratory.

REFERENCES

1. Burnet FM. The concept of immunological surveillance. *Prog Exp Tumor Res* 1970;13:1–27.
2. Benjamini E, Rennick DM, Sell S. Tumor immunology. In: Stites DP, Stobo JD, Fudenberg HH, Wells JV, eds. *Basic and clinical immunology*. Los Altos: Lange, 1984;223–241.
3. Martínez-Maza O. HIV-induced immune dysfunction and AIDS-associated neoplasms. In: Mitchell MS, ed. *The biomodulation of cancer*. Elsford, NY: Pergamon Press [in press].
4. Abbas AK, Lictman AH, Pober JS. *Cellullar and molecular immunology*. Philadelphia: WB Saunders Company, 1991.
5. Roitt I, Brostoff J, Male D. *Immunology*, 2nd ed. London: Gower Medical Publishing, 1989.
6. Boyer CM, Knapp RC, Bast RC. Immunology and immunotherapy. In: Berek JS, Hacker NF, eds. *Practical gynecologic oncology*. Baltimore: Williams & Wilkins, 1989;73–108.
7. Kohler G, Milstein C. Continuous cultures of fused cells secreting antibody of predefined specificity. *Nature* 1978;256:495–497.
8. Ettenson D, Sheldon K, Marks A, Houston LL, Baumal R. Comparison of growth inhibition of a human ovarian adenocarcinoma cell line by free monoclonal antibodies and their corresponding antibody-recombinant ricin A chain immunotoxins. *Anticancer Res* 1988;8:833–838.
9. Ortaldo JR, Herberman RB. Heterogeneity of natural killer cells. *Annu Rev Immunol* 1984;2:359.
10. Bast RC, Zbar B, Borsos T, Rapp RJ. BCG and cancer. *N Engl J Med* 1974;290:1413–1458.
11. Borstein RS, Mastrangelo MJ, Sulit H. Immunotherapy of melanoma with intralesional BCG. *Natl Cancer Inst Monogr* 1973;39:213–220.
12. Di Giovine FS, Duff GW. Interleukin 1: the first interleukin. *Immunol Today* 1990;11:13–20.
13. Shrader JW. The panspecific hemopoitin of activated T lymphocytes (interleukin-3). *Annu Rev Immunol* 1986;4:205.

14. Hirano T, Akira S, Taga T, Kishimoto T. Biological and clinical aspects of interleukin 6. *Immunol Today* 1990;11:443–449.
15. Martínez-Maza O, Berek JS. Interleukin 6 and cancer therapy. *In Vivo* [in press].
16. Mulé JJ, McIntosh JK, Jablons DM, Rosenberg SA. Antitumor activity of recombinant interleukin 6 in mice. *J Exp Med* 1990;171:629–636.
17. Golub SH. Immunological and therapeutic effects of interferon treatment of cancer patients. *Clin Immunol Allergy* 1984;4:377.
18. Stewart WE. *The interferon system.* New York: Springer-Verlag, 1979.
19. Watson JM, Sensintaffar JL, Berek JS, Martínez-Maza O. Epithelial ovarian cancer cells constitutively produce interleukin-6 (IL6). *Cancer Res* 1990;50:6959–6965.
20. Kawano M, Hirano T, Matsuda T, et al. Autocrine generation and requrienent of BSF-2/IL-6 for human multiple myelomas. *Nature* 1988;322:83–85.
21. Miles SA, Rezai AR, Salazar-Gonzalez JF, et al. AIDS Kaposi's sarcoma-derived cells produce and respond to interleukin-6. *Proc Natl Acad Sci USA* 1990;87:4068–4072.
22. Miki S, Iwano M, Miki Y, et al. Interleukin-6 (IL-6) functions as an in vitro autocrine growth factor in renal cell carcinomas. *FEBS Lett* 1989;250:607–610.
23. Ramakrishnan S, Xu FJ, Brandt SJ, Niedel JE, Bast RC Jr, Brown EL. Constitutive production of macrophage colony-stimulating factor by human ovarian and breast cancer cell lines. *J Clin Invest* 1989;83:921–926.
24. Cappuccini F, Yamamoto RS, DiSaia PJ, et al. Identification of tumor necrosis factor and lymphotoxin blocking factor(s) in the ascites of patients with advanced and recurrent ovarian cancer. *Lymphokine Cytokine Res* 1991;10:225–229.
25. Rosenberg SA. Immunotherapy of cancer by systemic administration of lymphoid cells plus interleukin-2. *J Biol Response Mod* 1984;3:501–511.
26. Rosenberg SA, Lotze MT. Cancer immunotherapy using interleukin-2 and interleukin-2 activated lymphocytes. *Annu Rev Immunol* 1986;4:681–709.
27. Rosenberg SA, Lotze MT, Muul LM, et al. Observations on the systemic administration of autologous lymphokine-activated killer cells and recombinant interleukin-2 to patients with metastatic cancer. *N Engl J Med* 1985;313:1485–1492.
28. Rosenberg SA, Lotze MT, Muul LM, et al. A progress report on the treatment of 157 patients with advanced cancer using lymphokine-activated killer cells and interleukin-2 or high-dose interleukin-2 alone. *N Engl J Med* 1987;316:889–897.
29. West WH, Tauer KW, Yannelli JR, et al. Constant-infusion recombinant interleukin-2 in adoptive immunotherapy of advanced cancer. *N Engl J Med* 1987;316:898–905.
30. Berek JS. Intraperitoneal adoptive immunotherapy for peritoneal cancer. *J Clin Oncol* 1990;8:1610–1612.
31. Topalian SL, Solomon D, Avis FP, et al. Immunotherapy of patients with advanced cancer using tumor infiltrating lymphocytes and recombinant interleukin 2: a pilot study. *J Clin Oncol* 1988;6:839–853.
32. Lotzova E. Role of human circulating and tumor-infiltrating lymphocytes in cancer defense and treatment. *Nat Immun Cell Growth Regul* 1990;9:253–264.
33. Garrido MA, Valdayo MJ, Winkler DR, et al. Targeting human T-lymphocytes with bispecific antibodies to react against human ovarian carcinoma cells growing in nu/nu mice. *Cancer Res* 1990;50:4227–4232.
34. Bookman MA, Bast RC Jr. The immunobiology and immunotherapy of ovarian cancer. *Semin Oncol* 1991;18:270–291.
35. Zighelboim J, Nio Y, Berek JS, Bonavida B. Immunologic control of ovarian cancer. *Nat Immun Cell Growth Regul* 1988;7:216–225.
36. Hammersmith Oncology Group and Imperial Cancer Research Fund. Antibody-guided irradiation of malignant lesions: three cases illustrating a new method of treatment. *Lancet* 1984;1:1441–1443.
37. Epenetos AA, Shepherd J, Britton KE, et al. [123]I radioiodinated antibody imaging of occult ovarian cancer. *Cancer* 1985;55:984–987.
38. Epenetos AA, Hooker L, Krausz T, Snook D, Bodmer WF, Taylor-Papadimitrion J. Antibody-guided irradiational malignant ascites in ovarian cancer: a new therapeutic method possessing specificity against cancer cells. *Obstet Gynecol* 1986;68(3):715–745.
39. Fitzgerald DJ, Willingham MC, Pastan I, et al. Antitumor effects of an immunotoxin made with *Pseudomonas* exotoxin in a nude mouse model of human ovarian cancer. *Proc Natl Acad Sci USA* 1986;83:6627–6632.
40. Berek JS, Lichtenstein AK, Knox RM, et al. Synergistic effects of combination sequential immunotherapies in a murine ovarian cancer model. *Cancer Res* 1985;45:4215–4218.
41. Pirker R, Fitzgerald DJP, Hamilton TC, Ozols RF, Willingham MC, Pasman J. Anti-transferrin receptor antibody linked to pseudomonas exotoxins as a model immunotoxin in human ovarian carcinoma cell lines. *Cancer Res* 1985;45:751–757.
42. Bast RC, Klug T, St. John E, et al. Monitoring growth of human ovarian carcinoma with a radioimmunoassay for antigen(s) defined by a murine monoclonal antibody (OC125). *N Engl J Med* 1983;309:883–887.
43. Granowska M, Britton KE, Shepherd JH, et al. A prospective study of ^{123}I-labeled monoclonal antibody imaging in ovarian cancer. *J Clin Oncol* 1986;4:730–736.
44. Symonds EM, Perkins AC, et al. Clinical implications for immunoscintigraphy in patients with ovarian malignancy: a preliminary study using monoclonal antibody 791T/36. *Br J Obstet Gynaecol* 1985;92:270–276.
45. Slamon DJ, Godolphin W, Jones LA, et al. Studies of the HER-2/neu proto-oncogene in human breast and ovarian cancer. *Science* 1989;244:707–712.
46. Lichtenstein A, Berenson J, Gera JF, Waldburger K, Martínez-Maza O, Berek JS. Resistance of human ovarian cancer cells to tumor necrosis factor and lymphokine-activated killer cells: correlation with expression of HER2/neu oncogenes. *Cancer Res* 1990;50:7364–7370.
47. Fendly BM, Kotts C, Vetterlein D, et al. The extracellular domain of HER2/neu is a potential immunogen for active specific immunotherapy of breast cancer. *J Biol Response Mod* 1990;9:449–455.
48. Shepard HM, Lewis GD, Sarup JC, et al. Monoclonal antibody therapy of human cancer: taking the HER2 protooncogene to the clinic. *J Clin Immunol* 1991;11:117–127.
49. Khoo SK, MacKay EV. Immunologic reactivity of female patients with genital cancer: status in preinvasive, locally invasive and disseminated disease. *Am J Obstet Gynecol* 1974;119:1018–1025.
50. Muruhata RI, Cantrell J, Lichtenstein AK, Zighelboim J. Disassociation of biological activities of *Corynebacterium parvum* by chemical fractionation. *Int J Immunopharmacol* 1980;2:47–53.
51. Halpern B. *Corynebacterium parvum. Applications in experimental and clinical oncology.* New York: Plenum, 1975.
52. Herberman RB. *Natural cell-mediated immunity against tumors.* New York: Academic Press, 1980.
53. Scott MT. *Corynebacterium parvum* as an immunotherapeutic anti-cancer agent. *Semin Oncol* 1984;1:367–378.
54. Berek JS, Cantrell JL, Lichtenstein AK, et al. Immunotherapy with biochemically dissociated fractions of proprionebacterium acnes in a murine ovarian cancer model. *Cancer Res* 1984;44:1871–1875.
55. Alberts DS, Salmon ES, Moon TE. Chemoimmunotherapy for advanced ovarian cancer with Adriamycin-cyclophosphamide ± BCG: early report of a Southwest Oncology Group study. *Recent Results Cancer Res* 1978;68:160–165.
56. Bast RC, Berek JS, Obrist R, et al. Intraperitoneal immunotherapy of human ovarian carcinoma with *Corynebacterium parvum*. *Cancer Res* 1983;43:1395–1401.
57. Gall SA, DiSaia PJ, Schmidt H, Mittlestaedt L, Newman P, Creasman W. Toxicity manifestation following intravenous *Corynebacterium parvum* administration to patients with ovarian and cervical carcinoma. *Am J Obstet Gynecol* 1978;132:555–560.
58. Mantovani A, Sessa C, Peri G, et al. Intraperitoneal administration of *Corynebacterium parvum* by chemical fractionation. *Int J Immunopharmacol* 1981;2:437–446.

59. Rao B, Wanebo HJ, Ochoa M, Lewis JL, Oettgen HF. Intravenous *C. parvum*: an adujvant to chemotherapy for resistant advanced ovarian carcinoma. *Cancer* 1977;39:514–526.
60. Wanebo HJ, Ochoa M. Randomized chemoimmunotherapy trial of CAF and intravenous *C. parvum* for resistant ovarian cancer-preliminary results. *Proc Am Assoc Cancer Res* 1977;18:225.
61. Creasman WT, Gall SA, Blessing JA, et al. Chemoimmunotherapy in the management of primary stage III ovarian cancer: a Gynecologic Oncology Group study. *Cancer Treat Rep* 1979;68:319–323.
62. Gynecologic Oncology Group (GOG) Statistical Report (1983).
63. Hanna MG, Key ME. Immunotherapy of metastases enhances subsequent chemotherapy. *Science* 1982;217:367–369.
64. Graham JB, Graham RM. The effect of vaccine on cancer patients. *Surg Gynecol Obstet* 1962;114:1.
65. Hudson CN, Levin L, McHaudy JE, et al. Active specific immunotherapy for ovarian cancer. *Lancet* 1976;2:877–879.
66. Julliard GJF, Boyer PJ, Yamashiro CH. A phase I study of active specific intralymphatic immunotherapy (ASILI). *Cancer* 1978;41:2215–2225.
67. Epstein LB, Shen JT, Abele JS, Reese CC. Sensitivity of human ovarian carcinoma cells to IFN and other antitumor agents as assessed by an in vitro semi-solid agar technique. *Ann NY Acad Sci* 1980;350:228–235.
68. Abdulhay G, DiSaia PJ, Blessing JA, Creasman WT. Human lymphoblastoid interferon in the treatment of advanced epithelial ovarian malignancies: a Gynecologic Oncology Group study. *Am J Obstet Gynecol* 1985;152:418–423.
69. Einhorn N, Cantrell K, Einhorn S, Strander H. Human leukocyte interferon for advanced ovarian carcinoma. *Am J Clin Oncol* 1985;5:167–172.
70. Niloff TM, Knapp RC, Jones G, et al. Recombinant leukocyte alpha interferon in advanced ovarian carcinoma. *Cancer Treat Rep* 1985;69:895–896.
71. Thompson JA, Lee DJ, Lindgren CG, et al. Influence of dose and duration of infusion of interleukin-2 on toxicity and immunomodulation. *J Clin Oncol* 1988;6:669–678.
72. Markman M, Howell SB. Intraperitoneal chemotherapy for ovarian cancer. In: Alberts DS, Surwit EA, eds. *Ovarian cancer*. Boston: Martinus Nijhoff, 1985;179–212.
73. Howell SB, Kirmani S, Lucas WE, et al. A phase II trial of intraperitoneal cisplatin and etoposide for primary treatment of ovarian epithelial cancer. *J Clin Oncol* 1990;8:137–145.
74. Berek JS, Bast RC, Hacker NF, et al. Lymphocyte cytotoxicity in the peritoneal cavity and blood of patients with ovarian cancer. *Obstet Gynecol* 1984;64:708–714.
75. Berek JS, Knapp RC, Hacker NF, et al. Intraperitoneal immunotherapy of epithelial ovarian carcinoma with *Corynebacterium parvum*. *Am J Obstet Gynecol* 1985;152:1003–1010.
76. Lichtenstein AK, Spina C, Berek JS, et al. Intraperitoneal administration of human recombinant alpha-interferon in patients with ovarian cancer: effects on lymphocytes, phenotype, and cytotoxicity. *Cancer Res* 1988;48:5853–5859.
77. Boyer P, Berek JS, Zighelboim J. Lymphocyte activation by recombinant interleukin-2 in ovarian cancer patients. *Obstet Gynecol* 1989;73:793–797.
78. Berek JS, Martínez-Maza O, Montz F. Immunology, immunotherapy and monoclonal antibodies. In: Coppleson M, Tattersall M, Morrow CP, eds. *Gynecologic oncology*. London: Churchill Livingstone 1992;119–134.
79. Urba W, Clark JW, Steiss RG, et al. Intraperitoneal lymphokine-activated killer cell/interleukin-2 therapy in patients with intra-abdominal cancer: immunologic considerations. *J Natl Cancer Inst* 1989;81(8):602–611.
80. Steiss RG, Urba WJ, Vander Molen LA, et al. Intraperitoneal lymphokine-activated killer cell and interleukin-2 therapy for malignancies limited to the peritoneal cavity. *J Clin Oncol* 1990;8:1618–1629.
81. Chapman PB, Kolitz JE, Hakes T, et al. A phase I trial of intraperitoneal recombinant interleukin-2 in patients with ovarian cancer. *Invest New Drugs* 1988;6:179–188.
82. Berek JS, Hacker NF, Lichtenstein AK, et al. Intraperitoneal recombinant alpha-interferon for salvage immunotherapy in stage III epithelial ovarian cancer: a Gynecologic Oncology Group study. *Cancer Res* 1985;45:4447–4453.
83. Lichtenstein A, Berek JS, Bast RC, et al. Activation of peritoneal lymphocyte cytotoxicity in patients with ovarian cancer by intraperitoneal treatment with *Corynebacterium parvum*. *J Biol Response Mod* 1984;3:1–8.
84. Hernandez E, Rosenshein NB, et al. IP immunotherapy and chemotherapy in advanced epithelial ovarian cancer. *Cancer Treat Rep* 1980;66:1981–1987.
85. Order SE, Rosenshein N, et al. The integration of new therapies and radiation in management of ovarian cancer. *Cancer* 1981;48:590–596.
86. Ohkawa K, Ohkawa R. Locoregional immunotherapy and chemotherapy in advanced ovarian cancer cytotoxicity. *Asian Oceania Fed Obstet Gynecol* 1981;Oct:352.
87. Willemse PHB, de Vries EGE, Mulder NH, Aalders JG, Bouma J, Sleijfer DTH. Intraperitoneal human recombinant interferon alpha-2b in minimal residual ovarian cancer. *Eur J Clin Oncol* 1990;26:353–358.
88. Balkwill FR, Moodie EM. Positive interactions between human interferon and cyclophosphamide or Adriamycin in a human tumor system. *Cancer Res* 1984;44:904–908.
89. Welander C, Gaines J, Homesley H, Rudnick S. In vitro synergistic effects of recombinant human interferon alpha 2(rIFN-α2) and doxorubicin on human tumor cell lines. *Proc Am Soc Clin Oncol* 1983;2:42.
90. Inoue M, Tan YH. Enhancement of actinomycin-D and cis-diamminedichloroplatinum (II) induced killing of human fibriblasts by human beta interferon. *Cancer Res* 1983;43:5484–5488.
91. Aapro MS, Salmon SE, Alberts DC. Schedule dependent synergism of vinblastine and cloned leukocyte interferon A. *Stem Cells* 1981;1:303–304.
92. Le J, Yip YK, Vilcek J. Cytologic activity of interferon gamma and its synergism with 5-FU. *Int J Cancer* 1984;34:495–500.
93. Harabayshi N, Nishiyama M, Yamaguchi M. Assessment of the combined effects of mitomycin C with alpha interferon by the clonogenic assay technique. *Gan To Kagaku Ryoho* 1982;12:1056–1062.
94. Carmichael J, Fergusson RJ, Wolf CR, Balkwill FR, Smyth JF. Augmentation of cytotoxicity of chemotherapy by human alpha interferons in human non-small cell lung cancer zenografts. *Cancer Res* 1986;46:4916–4920.
95. Aopro MS, Alberts DS, Salmon SE. Interaction of human leukocyte interferon with vinca alkaloids and other chemotherapeutic agents against human tumors in clonogenic assay. *Cancer Chemother Pharmacol* 1983;10:161–166.
96. Bezwoda WR, Golombick T, Dansey R, Keeping J. Treatment of malignant ascites due to recurrent/refractory ovarian cancer: the use of interferon-alpha or interferon-alpha plus chemotherapy. In vivo and in vitro observations. *Eur J Cancer* 1991;27:1423–1429.
97. Nardi M, Cognetti F, Pollera CF, et al. Intraperitoneal recombinant alpha-2-interferon alternating with cisplatin as salvage therapy for minimal residual disease ovarian cancer: a phase II study. *J Clin Oncol* 1990;8:1036–1041.
98. Berek JS, Welander C, Schink JC, Grossberg H, Montz FJ, Zighelboim J. A phase I–II trial of intraperitoneal cisplatin and alpha-interferon in patients with residual epithelial ovarian cancer. *Gynecol Oncol* 1991;40:237–243.
99. Markman M, Berek JS, Blessing JA, Mcquire WP, Bell J, Homesley HD. Characteristics of patients with small-volume residual ovarian cancer resistant to platinum-based intraperitoneal chemotherapy: lessons learned from a phase II Gynecologic Oncology Group trial of intraperitoneal cisplatin and alpha interferon. *Gynecol Oncol* 1991 1992;45:3–8.
100. Bonavida B, Tsuchitani T, Zighelboim J, Berek JS. Synergy is documented in vitro with low-dose tumor necrosis factor, cisplatin, and doxorubicin in ovarian tumor cells. *Gynecol Oncol* 1990;38:333–339.
101. Oettgen HF, Old LJ. Tumor necrosis factor. In: DeVita VT, Hellman S, Rosenberg SA, eds. *Important advances in oncology*. Philadelphia: Lippincott, 1987;105–130.
102. Old LJ. Tumor necrosis factor. *Science* 1985;230:630–632.

103. Chapman PB, et al. Clinical pharmacology of recombinant human tumor necrosis factor in patients with advanced cancer. *J Clin Oncol* 1987;5:1942–1951.
104. Creagan ET, Kovach JS, Moertel CG, Frytaks S, Kvols LK. A phase 1 clinical trial of recombinant human tumor necrosis factor. *Cancer* 1988;62:2467–2471.
105. Feinberg B, Kurzrock R, Talpaz M, Blick M, Saks S, Gutterman JU. A phase 1 trial of intravenously administered recombinant tumor necrosis factor-alpha in cancer patients. *J Clin Oncol* 1988;6:1328–1334.
106. Spriggs DR, Sherman MK, Michie H, et al. Recombinant human tumor necrosis factor administered as a 24-hr intravenous infusion. A phase 1 and pharmacologic study. *J Natl Cancer Inst* 1988;80:1039–1044.
107. Karymann M, Schmid M, Raeth U, et al. Therapy of ascites with tumor necrosis factor in ovarian cancer. *Geburt* and *Fravenheil* 1990;50:678–682.
108. Belardelli F, et al. Antitumor effects of interferon in mice injected with interferon-sensitive and interferon resistant Freund leukemia cells. *Int J Cancer* 1982;30:813–820.
109. Rubin BY, et al. Differential efficacies of human type I and type II interferons as antiviral and antiproliferative agents. *Proc Natl Acad Sci USA* 1980;77:5928–5932.
110. Crane JL, et al. Inhibition of murine osteogenic sarcomas by treatment with type I and type II interferons. *J Natl Cancer Inst* 1978;61:871–874.
111. D'Acquisto R, Markman M, Hakes T, Rubin S, Hoskins W, Lewis JL. A phase I trial of intraperitoneal recombinant gamma-interferon in advanced ovarian carcinoma. *J Clin Oncol* 1988;6:689–695.
112. Pujade-Lauraine E, et al. Intraperitoneal human recombinant interferon gamma in patients with residual ovarian carcinoma at second look laparotomy. *Proc Am Soc Clin Oncol* 1990;9:156 (abst).
113. Oomori K, Kikuchi Y, Miyauchi M, et al. Effects of lymphokine-activated killer cells and interleukin-2 on the ascites formation and the survival time of nude mice bearing human ovarian cancer cells. *J Cancer Res Clin Oncol* 1989;115:217–220.
114. Ottow RT, Steller EP, Sugarbaker PH, Wesley RA, Rosenberg SA. Immunotherapy of intraperitoneal cancer with interleukin 2 and lymphokine-activated killer cells reduces tumor load and prolongs survival in murine models. *Cell Immunol* 1987;104:366–376.
115. Lembersky B, et al. Phase I–II study of intraperitoneal low dose interleukin-2 in refractory stage III ovarian cancer. *Proc Am Soc Clin Oncol* 1989;8:163 (abst).
116. Mule JJ, et al. The anti-tumor efficacy of lymphokineactivated killer cells and recombinant interleukin 2 in vivo. *J Immunol* 1985;135:646–652.
117. Aoki Y, Takakuwa K, Kodama S, et al. Use of adoptive transfer of tumor-infiltrating lymphocytes alone or in combination with cisplatin-containing chemotherapy in patients with epithelial ovarian cancer. *Cancer Res* 1991;51:1934–1939.

CHAPTER 23

Intraperitoneal Chemotherapy

Maurie Markman

BASIC PRINCIPLES OF INTRAPERITONEAL ANTINEOPLASTIC DRUG DELIVERY

The administration of antineoplastic agents directly into the peritoneal cavity was first examined in the 1950s, with the introduction of alkylating agents and antimetabolites as therapy for malignant disease (1). This strategy was based on the idea that drugs administered into the region of the body containing the cancer might be more effective therapy than systemic drug delivery.

Unfortunately, the earliest clinical trials involving intraperitoneal therapy of ovarian cancer suffered from several serious difficulties. First, the drugs available during this time period had limited activity against ovarian cancer. Second, there was little if any appreciation of the importance of drug penetration in these studies, and patients with bulky intraabdominal disease rarely, if ever, achieved objective responses to this regional therapeutic strategy (1).

Thus, it is not surprising that limited evidence of efficacy was demonstrated in these early trials. The therapeutic strategy of direct intraperitoneal antineoplastic drug delivery in the management of ovarian cancer was effectively abandoned for more than a decade. However, in a now classic 1978 paper, Dedrick and colleagues at the National Cancer Institute (NCI) presented a pharmacokinetic model based on existing physiologic and pharmacologic data that strongly suggested that it might be possible to significantly increase the exposure of the peritoneal cavity to certain cytotoxic agents if the drugs were delivered directly into the body cavity (2).

The NCI group noted that previous investigative work had demonstrated that drug uptake from the peritoneal cavity is principally, although not exclusively, through the portal circulation (3,4). Thus, cytotoxic agents known to be rapidly and extensively metabolized in the liver during their first passage through the organ would be expected to demonstrate the greatest pharmacokinetic advantage following regional delivery. Drugs such as 5-fluorouracil and doxorubicin would fall into this category (5,6). The NCI group noted that, in attempting to maximize differences between peritoneal cavity and systemic exposure to cytotoxic agents following regional delivery, it was important to choose agents with slow clearance from the body compartment and rapid clearance from the systemic circulation.

Additional characteristics of drugs considered to be optimal for intraperitoneal delivery in the management of ovarian cancer are outlined in Table 1.

In the selection of agents for phase I clinical trials of intraperitoneal delivery in ovarian cancer, an important criterion is preclinical information suggesting that the activity of the drug against ovarian cancer is *concentration-dependent*. Simply stated, the only advantage of the intraperitoneal delivery of cytotoxic drugs over systemic administration is the opportunity to expose tumor to higher concentrations of the drug for longer periods of time. Thus, experimental evidence which suggests that higher concentrations of a particular drug could produce greater tumor cell kill would indicate drugs of greatest interest for intraperitoneal administration (7). In contrast, failure of preclinical investigation to reveal significant concentration-dependent cytotoxicity would suggest that the intraperitoneal route would have limited or no theoretical benefit over systemic delivery.

An extension of this argument supporting the importance of dose response is experimental data suggesting that tumor cell resistance to a number of cytotoxic agents may be relative rather than absolute. For example, in several preclinical experimental systems, it has been shown that resistance of ovarian cancer tumor

---

M. Markman: The Cleveland Clinic Cancer Center and the Department of Hematology/Medical Oncology, The Cleveland Clinic Foundation, Cleveland, Ohio 44195

TABLE 1. *Characteristics of the "optimal" chemotherapeutic agent to consider for intraperitoneal therapy of ovarian cancer*

1. Slow clearance from the peritoneal cavity and rapid clearance from the systemic circulation.
2. Rapid and extensive metabolism during first pass through the liver.
3. Not toxic to the peritoneal lining.
4. Drug does *not* require activation in the liver to become a cytotoxic agent.
5. Active against ovarian cancer following systemic delivery.
6. Experimental evidence for a dose response for the cytotoxic activity of the agent against ovarian cancer tumor cells.

TABLE 2. *Major concerns for intraperitoneal therapy of ovarian cancer*

1. Adequacy of drug distribution following intraperitoneal delivery.
2. Potential for decreased delivery of drug to tumor by *capillary flow* following intraperitoneal delivery.
3. Limited penetration of cytotoxic agents directly into normal or tumor tissue.

cells to cisplatin at concentrations of the agent achievable within the systemic compartment following intravenous administration can be overcome if twofold to fivefold higher concentrations of the cytotoxic agent are utilized (8,9).

Unfortunately, these concentrations are not achievable in plasma following systemic delivery owing to the known serious toxicities associated with higher dose cisplatin administration. However, concentrations reaching or exceeding those demonstrated to be required in experimental systems to overcome cisplatin resistance may be achievable within the peritoneal cavity following regional drug delivery.

An additional strategy that can be employed when administering drugs directly into the peritoneal cavity is simultaneous systemic delivery of neutralizing agents for intraperitoneally administered cytotoxic drugs. In theory, this approach may allow the intraperitoneal delivery of higher concentrations of cytotoxic drugs because some or all of the antineoplastic agent entering the systemic compartment may be neutralized into nontoxic metabolites prior to producing serious systemic side effects.

Several antagonist-agonist pairs have been investigated in both phase I and phase II clinical trials, including methotrexate with folinic acid (leucovorin) (10,11) and cisplatin with sodium thiosulfate (12). An important concern with this therapeutic strategy is the fact that the antagonist may inactivate the cytotoxic properties of the antineoplastic drug.

Through more than a decade of clinical investigation of intraperitoneal therapy in the management of ovarian cancer, several issues have emerged as the major points defining the limitations of this therapeutic strategy (Table 2).

First, in contrast to systemic drug delivery, in which the cytotoxic agent is assumed to reach tumor throughout the body by the mechanism of *capillary flow,* such an assumption cannot be made when patients are treated by the intraperitoneal route. After intraperitoneal therapy, drug uptake from the peritoneal cavity into tumor occurs by the mechanism of *free-surface diffusion,* and it is critical that the drug-containing treatment volume come in *direct* contact with tumor tissue. This goal is far more difficult to accomplish than might be anticipated after only a superficial examination of the problem.

Patients with ovarian cancer who are considered for an intraperitoneal treatment program will likely have undergone one or more exploratory laparotomies. This surgery may have resulted in the formation of significant intraabdominal adhesion. In addition, both the tumor itself and the intraperitoneal treatment can elicit an inflammatory response, with resultant adhesion formation. Even with drugs noted to cause little or no abdominal discomfort after intraperitoneal delivery, there may be subclinical cavity irritation leading to adhesions. The greater the extent of adhesion formation, the more concern there must be that the drug-containing intraperitoneal treatment volume will not be adequately distributed throughout the peritoneal cavity.

Fortunately, clinical experience gained to date suggests that the majority of patients considered for an intraperitoneal treatment program will be able to achieve adequate distribution of the drug-containing fluid following regional drug delivery. However, individual patients who may be considered ideal candidates for an intraperitoneal treatment approach (e.g., having small-volume residual disease following an initial excellent response to cisplatin-based therapy) may be ineligible for this therapeutic strategy because of excessive adhesion formation.

Although the adequacy of distribution can be assessed by an intraperitoneal distribution study prior to the initiation of the regional treatment program, we have found that patients who are able to tolerate the administration of a 2-l treatment volume with minimal discomfort generally have satisfactory distribution studies. In contrast, patients who develop pain with treatment or who have excessively slow fluid inflow into the peritoneal catheter will generally have inadequate distribution studies and will require repositioning or replacement of the catheter or discontinuation of treatment.

A second concern with intraperitoneal therapy of

ovarian cancer has been the potential for decreased delivery of drug to the cancer by capillary flow following regional drug delivery. Even if the high local drug concentrations in direct contact with tumor can be translated into a greater local cell kill, the overall effectiveness of the therapeutic program may be diminished if intraperitoneally administered drugs fail to reach the tumor through the vascular compartment. For agents that are *not* limited by local toxic effects, it should be possible to escalate the intraperitoneal dose to the point at which systemic toxicity is dose limiting. Thus, at this maximally tolerated dose, the amount of drug reaching the tumor by capillary flow through the vascular compartment should equal that achieved if the drug(s) had been delivered systemically.

In contrast, for agents which are limited by their local toxic effects, systemic exposure will be *less than* that achieved when the drugs are delivered intravenously. Although high local drug concentrations may significantly affect the overall results of treatment, there will be decreased delivery to tumor by the mechanism of capillary flow. Several methods are available to overcome this theoretical limitation of regional therapy. First, drugs can be delivered intravenously as well as by the intraperitoneal route. Second, additional drugs that do achieve significant systemic exposure following regional delivery can be employed, along with the intraperitoneal drug which has limited crossover into the plasma.

Although the issues of drug distribution and systemic exposure are important, the major factor defining the clinical situations in which intraperitoneal therapy is a rational therapeutic option is the known *limited penetration* of antineoplastic agents directly into tumor or normal tissues. Several experimental models, employing a number of cytotoxic agents, have confirmed the fact that the ability of drugs to penetrate into tissue is limited to from several cell layers to 1 to 2 mm (1,13–15).

Perhaps the most interesting series of experiments examining this important question has been presented by investigators at the Netherlands Cancer Institute (15). In a rat model, this group examined the concentration of cisplatin within the peritoneal cavity lining and compared intraperitoneal to systemic delivery. This experimental system was important because it not only evaluated the exposure of the peritoneal cavity to cisplatin following intraperitoneal administration but also examined the benefits of regional delivery compared to intravenous administration of the same drug.

In this experimental model, the Dutch investigators demonstrated cisplatin within the tissue of the peritoneal lining to depths in excess of 2 mm, but the *advantage* for direct peritoneal cavity administration was limited to a depth of 0.1 to 1 mm. As noted previously, certain agents, including cisplatin, enter the systemic compartment in significant concentrations following intraperitoneal delivery. Thus, it is not surprising that cisplatin will be found deep within the tissue of the peritoneal lining following intraperitoneal delivery because the agent reaches this area through capillary flow. However, near the surface of the peritoneal lining, cytotoxic drug concentrations are increased significantly following regional delivery.

TOXICITY OF INTRAPERITONEAL ANTINEOPLASTIC DRUG DELIVERY

The side effects associated with regional antineoplastic drug delivery can be divided into two general categories: systemic and local. As previously noted, for agents that are not limited by their local toxic effects, concentration can be escalated to the point at which systemic toxicities become dose limiting.

For cisplatin, an agent associated with minimal local toxicity, the dose-limiting side effects are emesis, neurotoxicity, and nephrotoxicity. These toxic effects are particularly relevant when intraperitoneal cisplatin is considered for administration in the salvage setting, in which the patient may have preexisting side effects from prior systemic cisplatin delivery.

Of greater concern are the unique local toxic effects associated with regional drug delivery. Drugs can cause local irritation leading to pain, adhesion formation, and even bowel obstruction. Even in the absence of severe abdominal pain, subclinical peritoneal cavity irritation can lead to adhesion formation, which may interfere with the adequacy of drug distribution in subsequent treatment courses.

Although the local toxicity associated with the intraperitoneal administration of certain antineoplastic agents (i.e., doxorubicin, mitomycin) can be predicted based on known vesicant properties, even nonvesicant medications may be associated with significant local toxicity at extremely high concentrations following regional delivery. All single drugs that are delivered intraperitoneally for the first time, as well as new combination regimens, must be administered with caution until it has been determined that an acceptable toxicity profile is associated with this unique route of drug delivery.

An additional concern with intraperitoneal administration is the establishment of a convenient and safe method of drug delivery. A peritoneal catheter can be placed percutaneously with each treatment course (16), but most investigators choose to deliver intraperitoneal therapy via a surgically implanted, semipermanent, indwelling catheter device (17). This method decreases the risk of bowel perforation with percutaneous catheter placement and minimizes the time required to administer each treatment course.

An additional refinement to the technology of intraperitoneal drug delivery has been the use of subcutaneous delivery systems attached to intraperitoneal catheters (18,19). These devices allow the catheter system to be completely protected from the external environment, except when treatment is administered. The risk of introducing infection is reduced with the subcutaneous "ports," and patient acceptance of these devices is improved.

CLINICAL EXPERIENCE WITH INTRAPERITONEAL CHEMOTHERAPY AS SALVAGE TREATMENT FOR OVARIAN CANCER

Numerous chemotherapeutic agents with known activity in ovarian cancer have been examined for safety, pharmacokinetic advantage, and efficacy following intraperitoneal delivery (Table 3) (5,6,10–12,20–28).

Cisplatin

Not surprisingly, the greatest experience with the intraperitoneal therapy of ovarian cancer has been with cisplatin. This drug is associated with limited adhesion formation and minimal or no abdominal pain following regional delivery. Several phase I pharmacokinetic studies have demonstrated that the peritoneal cavity is exposed to 10 to 20 times more drug than the systemic compartment following regional delivery of cisplatin (12,20,21). As noted previously, this increase in local exposure should not compromise delivery of cisplatin to the cancer by capillary flow, if treatment is delivered at or near the maximally tolerated intraperitoneal dose.

Several phase II trials of single agent intraperitoneal cisplatin or combination cisplatin-based salvage therapy of ovarian cancer have confirmed that approximately 25–30% of patients with small-volume disease (largest tumor mass ≤0.5–1 cm in diameter) can achieve a surgically documented complete response (CR) following intraperitoneal delivery (1). In a recent analysis of several cisplatin-based salvage intraperitoneal programs for patients with ovarian cancer conducted at the Memorial Sloan-Kettering Cancer Center, we have attempted to more critically define the patient population most likely to respond to a second-line, cisplatin-based intraperitoneal program (29). Overall, 16 of 50 patients (32%) whose largest tumor mass measured ≤1 cm demonstrated a surgically documented complete response to cisplatin-based therapy. However, when the responses were analyzed based on the patient's *prior* response to systemic therapy, this factor strongly influenced the potential for response to the salvage intraperitoneal cisplatin-based treatment program. Of 36 patients with small-volume disease who had previously demonstrated a response to systemic cisplatin, 15 (42%) achieved a surgically defined complete response, compared to only 1 of 14 patients (7%) who also had small-volume disease at the initiation of intraperitoneal therapy but had failed to demonstrate an objective response to the initial systemic treatment program.

This data strongly supports the argument that the ability of the high concentrations of cisplatin attainable within the peritoneal cavity following regional delivery to overcome clinically defined drug resistance is *relative* rather than *absolute*. The clinical relevance of these data is the conclusion that patients who have failed to respond to front-line platinum-based therapy with at least a partial response (PR) should not be treated with an intraperitoneal cisplatin-based treatment program, even if only small-volume disease remains at the initiation of the intraperitoneal treatment program. Such patients may still be considered for a salvage intraperitoneal treatment approach, but further therapy should not be platinum-based.

Carboplatin

The experience with intraperitoneal carboplatin as salvage therapy for ovarian cancer is less extensive than that of cisplatin, but several phase II clinical trials have demonstrated that approximately 25% of patients with small-volume residual disease following platinum-based systemic therapy who are treated with single agent intraperitoneal carboplatin can achieve a surgically defined CR (30,31). On the basis of the currently available literature, there is no reason to suspect that intraperitoneal carboplatin will be more active in small-volume platinum-resistant disease than cisplatin. Thus, salvage intraperitoneal carboplatin-based therapy should be employed only in patients who have demonstrated a prior sensitivity to platinum-based treatment administered systemically.

Two additional points should be made concerning the use of carboplatin by the intraperitoneal route. In

TABLE 3. *Pharmacokinetic advantage associated with intraperitoneal administration of selected cytotoxic agents*

Agent	Peak peritoneal cavity/plasma concentration ratio	Reference
Cisplatin	20	12,20,21
Carboplatin	18	22,23
Doxorubicin	474	6,24
Mitoxantrone	620	25,26
Mitomycin	71	27
5-fluorouracil	298	5
Methotrexate	92	10,11
Taxol	1,000	28

the salvage setting, carboplatin has been demonstrated to produce considerable bone marrow suppression, particularly in patients previously treated with systemic carboplatin. This may limit the amount of carboplatin that can be delivered by the intraperitoneal route, because the majority of the agent will ultimately enter the systemic compartment following regional delivery (22,23). Second, a recently reported experimental model has suggested that the concentration of platinum within tissue following intraperitoneal carboplatin administration is less than that achieved with cisplatin, presumably due to a lower degree of tissue penetration by carboplatin (32).

These two observations suggest that, in an initial treatment program for patients with ovarian cancer that includes the intraperitoneal route of drug delivery, the preferred sequence of platinum delivery would be systemic carboplatin-based treatment followed by intraperitoneal cisplatin-based therapy. Ultimately, however, this hypothesis will have to be tested in randomized controlled clinical trials to determine if such a treatment strategy is superior to standard systemic delivery alone.

Doxorubicin

Doxorubicin was initially explored for intraperitoneal delivery based on its known activity in ovarian cancer and on data demonstrating that, in a murine ovarian tumor model, intraperitoneal doxorubicin administration could "cure" the disease while systemic administration at the maximally administered dose was ineffective (33). Unfortunately, as predicted by clinical observations that doxorubicin is a vesicant and by preclinical data indicating that intraperitoneal administration of this drug produces sclerosis (34), regional doxorubicin delivery was associated with an unacceptable toxicity profile (abdominal pain) (6,24,35).

A recent report has suggested that the local toxicity of intraperitoneal doxorubicin delivery may be reduced while maintaining a high regional drug concentration by administering the agent in *liposomes* (36). In this small series, objective antitumor responses were reported. Further exploration of intraperitoneal doxorubicin in liposomes appears to be warranted.

Mitoxantrone

In most clinical situations, mitoxantrone appears to be similar to doxorubicin in terms of efficacy and toxicity (37). However, clinical observations and experimental data have demonstrated that mitoxantrone is *not* a vesicant (37,38). In addition, in the human tumor cloning assay, mitoxantrone was shown to be markedly cytotoxic to human ovarian cancer cells at concentrations potentially achievable with intraperitoneal delivery but not with standard systemic dosing regimens (7).

In several phase I clinical trials, the toxicity and pharmacokinetic advantage of intraperitoneal mitoxantrone delivery has been defined (25,26). In these studies exposure of the peritoneal cavity has been shown to exceed that of the systemic compartment by approximately 3 logs. However, the dose-limiting toxicity of intraperitoneally administered mitoxantrone has been found to be abdominal pain, and at the maximally tolerated dose, little active drug is found in the systemic circulation.

Several phase II trials have demonstrated activity for intraperitoneal mitoxantrone in patients with advanced ovarian cancer, including disease documented to be clinically resistant to cisplatin (39,40). As with salvage intraperitoneal therapy employing cisplatin or carboplatin, responses are almost exclusively limited to patients with small-volume residual disease when the second-line intraperitoneal mitoxantrone program is initiated.

The blue color of mitoxantrone persists within the peritoneal cavity for more than 2 to 3 months following the completion of regional therapy (39,40). This material may actually be active drug on the surface of the peritoneal lining. In a recent evaluation, native mitoxantrone was found in significant concentrations in this blue-staining material on the surface of the peritoneal lining in tissue obtained at the time of a response laparotomy following intraperitoneal mitoxantrone treatment (*unpublished data*).

Because any mitoxantrone present on the surface of the peritoneal lining is likely to be highly protein bound, it is uncertain if drug attached to protein will be cytotoxic. However, in the human clonogenic assay, mitoxantrone in the presence of 50% fetal bovine serum has been shown to be as cytotoxic to tumor cells as when the agent is mixed with 5% fetal bovine serum, which suggests that protein binding does not significantly interfere with the cytotoxic potential of mitoxantrone that persists within the peritoneal cavity following regional delivery (*unpublished data*).

It is uncertain how this potential "depot effect" following intraperitoneal mitoxantrone delivery may influence the effectiveness of this treatment regimen. However, in one experimental model, animals receiving intraperitoneal mitoxantrone were protected from the lethal effects of subsequent intraperitoneal tumor inoculation for up to 30 days following chemotherapy administration (41). In contrast, in the absence of intraperitoneal mitoxantrone delivery, a single tumor inoculation produced death.

Taxol

Taxol has been demonstrated to produce objective antitumor responses in approximately 20–30% of patients with platinum-refractory ovarian cancer (42,43). Thus, it is an important drug to examine for its potential role in intraperitoneal delivery. Experimental models have suggested that the activity of taxol against several human cancers depends on the *concentration and duration of exposure*. These features can potentially be optimized following intraperitoneal drug delivery (44).

In a recently completed phase 1 trial of single agent intraperitoneal taxol administered on a monthly schedule, the pharmacokinetics and toxicity of intraperitoneal delivery were defined (28). The maximally tolerated single intraperitoneal dose was approximately 125 mg/m^2, with local abdominal pain as the dose-limiting side effect. Peak and area-under-the-concentration-versus-time curve (AUC) ratios between peritoneal cavity and systemic circulation exposure to taxol were found to exceed 3 logs. In addition, the half-life in the peritoneal cavity of a single dose of intraperitoneal taxol exceeded 72 hours.

Both the concentration (peak and AUC) and duration of exposure of the peritoneal cavity to taxol, compared to the systemic compartment, were markedly enhanced following regional delivery. Of note, although the concentration of taxol within the peritoneal cavity was far greater than that in the systemic compartment, taxol concentrations achieved within the systemic circulation were found to be in the range in which both biologic and cytotoxic effects have been observed in in vitro and in vivo experimental systems.

Other Agents

Additional agents have been examined in phase I and phase II intraperitoneal clinical trials in individuals with ovarian cancer (Table 3). Unfortunately, although a pharmacokinetic advantage has been demonstrated for a number of drugs when delivered directly into the peritoneal cavity, little information is available regarding the efficacy of these agents. This is principally due to the fact that the most appropriate patients for an intraperitoneal regimen are those with small-volume residual disease. However, this is also the most difficult group of patients in whom to evaluate antitumor responses because of the major limitations in currently available noninvasive imaging technology.

Decreases in ascites formation and CA-125 serum levels, as well as improvements in a number of cancer-related symptoms, have been noted following treatment with a number of antineoplastic agents administered by the intraperitoneal route in early clinical trials. For some of these agents, further clinical exploration following regional delivery is indicated.

It is important to note that a decrease in ascites formation, perhaps the most readily apparent favorable response in a patient with advanced ovarian cancer receiving intraperitoneal therapy, may be due to a nonspecific sclerosing effect (secondary to peritoneal irritation) rather than to a direct cytotoxic effect of the agent (1). Thus, caution is advised in concluding that any antineoplastic agent is active following intraperitoneal delivery in the absence of surgically documented tumor regression or disappearance of microscopic residual disease.

IMPACT OF SALVAGE INTRAPERITONEAL THERAPY ON SURVIVAL

Several reports have examined the impact of salvage intraperitoneal therapy on the survival of patients with advanced ovarian cancer. Investigators at the University of California, San Diego, examining the survival of a group of patients treated on a series of phase I cisplatin/cytarabine-based intraperitoneal studies, noted an actuarial median survival of >4 years for a subgroup of patients with small-volume disease (largest tumor mass <2 cm in maximum diameter) when the salvage intraperitoneal therapy was initiated (45). For patients whose largest mass was >2 cm, the median survival was <1 year.

At the Memorial Sloan-Kettering Cancer Center we recently examined the survival of patients with small-volume residual (microscopic disease or macroscopic tumor ≤0.5 cm in diameter) ovarian cancer treated on one of three salvage intraperitoneal chemotherapy programs (cisplatin/etoposide {46}, cisplatin/cytarabine {47}, mitoxantrone {39}). The median duration of follow-up of the 58 patients included in this analysis was 43+ months (range 33+ to 58+ months). Of the 19 patients in the three trials who achieve a surgically documented CR, 12 (63%) have recurred, with all but 2 patients demonstrating evidence of recurrent disease in the abdominal cavity or pelvis.

In an attempt to avoid selection bias in evaluating survival of patients responding or failing to respond to the intraperitoneal treatment programs, any patient who lived for <6 months from the initiation of intraperitoneal therapy was excluded from the examination of survival. The median survival for the 18 patients with macroscopic (≤0.5 cm) residual disease who *responded* (completely or partially) to the intraperitoneal therapy was 40 months, compared to 19 for the 14 patients who failed to respond to the treatment regimen ($p = 0.009$).

The median survival of the ten patients with microscopic disease who achieved a surgically documented complete response to the intraperitoneal program has not been reached but will exceed 4 years, compared to 25 months for the 13 patients who failed to respond to this therapy ($p = 0.004$). The survival data for the group of patients with microscopic disease is particularly relevant because even those patients who failed to respond experienced a reasonable survival (>2 years), with the first death not occurring until 13 months following the initiation of the treatment program. Thus, the issue of selection bias in favor of the responding patients should be less relevant in this group of individuals. However, despite the relatively favorable survival of the nonresponding patients, the responding patients experienced a significantly superior survival.

Unfortunately, in the absence of a randomized controlled clinical trial, the ultimate impact of salvage intraperitoneal therapy on survival in patients with advanced ovarian cancer cannot be completely defined.

INTRAPERITONEAL THERAPY AS INITIAL CHEMOTHERAPY OF ADVANCED OVARIAN CANCER

Over the past 5 years, several groups have begun to explore intraperitoneal therapy as an integral component of the initial treatment strategy for individuals with advanced ovarian cancer. A major limitation of this therapeutic strategy is the fact that relatively few patients with advanced ovarian cancer begin an initial chemotherapy program with truly small-volume residual disease (microscopic, maximum diameter of residual tumor ≤0.5 cm). Thus, the optimal patient population for testing the concept of front-line intraperitoneal chemotherapy is limited in size.

The Southwest Oncology Group (SWOG) and the Gynecologic Oncology Group (GOG) are nearing completion of a randomized controlled clinical trial comparing a standard intravenous chemotherapy program (cisplatin and cyclophosphamide) with a regimen that employs the same drugs and dosages, but with the cisplatin delivered intraperitoneally. Preliminary results of this important trial, the first randomized test comparing intraperitoneal therapy to standard intravenous drug delivery, should be available within the next year.

Investigators at the University of California, San Diego, have recently reported their experience with initial chemotherapy of ovarian cancer employing intraperitoneal cisplatin (200 mg/m^2) with sodium thiosulfate nephroprotection and intraperitoneal etoposide (300 mg/m^2) (48). Although the overall response rate and survival in this preliminary report were quite good, it is unknown if the results of this trial are superior to what might have been accomplished with a standard cisplatin-based systemic chemotherapy program.

For the past few years, the Memorial Sloan-Kettering Cancer Center group has been exploring a program that calls for the administration of two cycles of high-dose cisplatin-based chemotherapy following initial surgery and tumor debulking (49). These two courses are followed by a second surgery designed to debulk patients to zero-volume residual disease. Finally, patients are then treated with four courses of organoplatinum-based intraperitoneal therapy. The goal of this approach is to add "chemical debulking" to aggressive surgery in an effort to minimize the amount of residual tumor present prior to the initiation of the intraperitoneal treatment program. Again, although the overall surgically defined complete response rate observed with this program is higher than our own institutional experience, the impact of this intensive treatment strategy cannot be clearly defined in the absence of a randomized controlled clinical trial.

TABLE 4. *Clinical situations in which intraperitoneal therapy may be considered in the management plan for patients with ovarian cancer*

1. Small-volume residual disease (microscopic disease or largest remaining tumor mass ≤0.5–1 cm) following initial systemic therapy.
   Patients who are demonstrated to be platinum-refractory should *not* be treated with an organoplatinum-based intraperitoneal program.
2. Initial treatment of patients with high-grade, stage I–II cancers.
3. Consolidation treatment for individuals with high-grade, stage III–IV cancers who achieve a surgically defined complete response (relapse rate approaches 50–60%).
4. Initial therapy of advanced ovarian cancer with all or some of the agents delivered by the intraperitoneal route.
5. Initial treatment of advanced disease following a limited number of courses (≤3) of systemic therapy designed to "chemically debulk" the tumor prior to intraperitoneal therapy.

CONCLUSION

Over the past decade, much has been learned about the potential clinical utility of intraperitoneal therapy and the important limitations of the approach (Table 4). Future efforts should be directed to finding and examining new agents with characteristics that allow for a superior therapeutic result following regional delivery as compared to systemic drug administration.

REFERENCES

1. Markman M. Intraperitoneal anti-neoplastic agents for tumors principally confined to the peritoneal cavity. *Cancer Treat Rev* 1986;13:219–242.
2. Dedrick RL, Myers CE, Bungay PM, DeVita VT Jr. Pharmacokinetic rationale for peritoneal drug administration in the treatment of ovarian cancer. *Cancer Treat Rep* 1978;62:1–9.
3. Lukas G, Brindle S, Greengard P. The route of absorption of intraperitoneally administered compounds. *J Pharmacol Exp Ther* 1971;178:562–566.

4. Kraft AR, Tompkins RK, Jesseph JE. Peritoneal electrolyte absorption: analysis of portal, systemic venous and lymphatic transport. *Surgery* 1968;64:148–153.
5. Speyer JL, Collins JM, Dedrick RL, et al. Phase I pharmacological studies of 5-fluorouracil administered intraperitoneally. *Cancer Res* 1980;40:567–572.
6. Ozols RF, Young RC, Speyer JL, et al. Phase 1 and pharmacological studies of adriamycin administered intraperitoneally to patients with ovarian cancer. *Cancer Res* 1982;42:4265–4269.
7. Alberts DS, Young L, Mason N, Salmon SE. In vitro evaluation of anticancer drugs against ovarian cancer at concentrations achievable by intraperitoneal administration. *Semin Oncol* 1985;12(3; suppl.4):38–42.
8. Andrews PA, Velury S, Mann SC, Howell SB. Cis-diamminedichloroplatinum(II) accumulation in sensitive and resistant human ovarian carcinoma cells. *Cancer Res* 1988;48:68–73.
9. Ozols RF, Corden BJ, Jacob J, Wesley MN, Ostchega Y, Young RC. High-dose cisplatin in hypertonic saline. *Ann Intern Med* 1984;100:19–24.
10. Howell SB, Chu BCF, Wung WE, Metha BM, Mendelsohn J. Long-duration intracavitary infusion of methotrexate with systemic leucovorin protection in patients with malignant effusion. *J Clin Invest* 1981;67:1161–1170.
11. Jones RB, Collins JM, Myers CE, et al. High-volume intraperitoneal chemotherapy with methotrexate in patients with cancer. *Cancer Res* 1981;41:55–59.
12. Howell SB, Pfeifle CE, Wung WE, et al. Intraperitoneal cisplatin with systemic thiosulfate protection. *Ann Intern Med* 1982;97:845–851.
13. Ozols RF, Locker GY, Doroshow JH, Grotzinger KR, Myers CE, Young RC. Pharmacokinetics of adriamycin and tissue penetration in murine ovarian cancer. *Cancer Res* 1979;39:3209–3214.
14. West GW, Weichselbau R, Little JB. Limited penetration of methotrexate into human osteosarcoma spheroids as a proposed model for solid tumor resistance to adjuvant chemotherapy. *Cancer Res* 1980;40:3665–3668.
15. Los G, Mutsaers PHA, van der Vijgh WJF, Baldew GS, deGraaf PW, McVie JG. Direct diffusion of cis-diamminedichloroplatinum(II) in intraperitoneal rat tumors after intraperitoneal chemotherapy: a comparison with systemic chemotherapy. *Cancer Res* 1989;49:3380–3384.
16. Runowicz CD, Dottino PR, Shafir MA, Mark MA, Cohen CJ. Catheter complications associated with intraperitoneal chemotherapy. *Gynecol Oncol* 1986;24:41–50.
17. Piccart MJ, Speyer JL, Markman M, et al. Intraperitoneal chemotherapy: technical experience at five institutions. *Semin Oncol* 1985;12(3; suppl.4):90–96.
18. Pfeifle CE, Howell SB, Markman M, Lucas WE. Totally implantable system for peritoneal access. *J Clin Oncol* 1984;2:1277–1280.
19. Rubin SC, Hoskins WJ, Markman M, Hakes T, Lewis JL Jr. Long term access to the peritoneal cavity in ovarian cancer patients. *Gynecol Oncol* 1988;33:46–48.
20. Casper ES, Kelsen DP, Alcock NW, Lewis JL. Ip cisplatin in patients with malignant ascites: pharmacokinetic evaluation and comparison with the iv route. *Cancer Treat Rep* 1983;67:325–328.
21. Lopez JA, Krikorian JG, Reich SD, Smyth RD, Lee FH, Issell BF. Clinical pharmacology of intraperitoneal cisplatin. *Gynecol Oncol* 1985;20:1–9.
22. Elferink F, van der Vijgh WJ, Klein I, ten Bokkel Huinink WW, Dubbelman R, McVie JG. Pharmacokinetics of carboplatin after intraperitoneal administration. *Cancer Chemother Pharmacol* 1988;21:57–60.
23. Deregorio MW, Lum BL, Holleran WM, Wilbur BJ, Sikic BI. Preliminary observations of intraperitoneal carboplatin pharmacokinetics during a phase I study of the Northern California Oncology Group. *Cancer Chemother Pharmacol* 1986;18:235–238.
24. Demicheli R, Bonciarelli G, Jirillo A, et al. Pharamcologic data and technical feasibility of intraperitoneal doxorubicin administration. *Tumori* 1985;71:63–68.
25. Alberts DS. Phase I clinical and pharmacokinetic study of mitoxantrone given to patients by intraperitoneal administration. *Cancer Res* 1988;48:5874–5877.
26. Blochl-Daum B, Eichler HG, Rainer H, et al. Escalating dose regimen of intraperitoneal mitoxantrone: phase I study—clinical and pharmacokinetic evaluation. *Eur J Cancer Clin Oncol* 1988;24:1133–1138.
27. Gyves J. Pharmacology of intraperitoneal infusion 5-fluorouracil and mitomycin-c. *Semin Oncol* 1985;12(3; suppl.4):29–32.
28. Markman M, Rowinsky E, Hakes T, et al. Phase 1 study of taxol administered by the intraperitoneal route. *Proc Am Soc Clin Oncol* 1991;10:185 (abst).
29. Markman M, Reichman B, Hakes T, et al. Responses to second-line cisplatin-based intraperitoneal therapy in ovarian cancer: influence of a prior response to intravenous cisplatin. *J Clin Oncol* 1991;9:1801–1805.
30. Speyer JL, Beller U, Colombo N, et al. Intraperitoneal carboplatin: favorable results in women with minimal residual ovarian cancer after cisplatin therapy. *J Clin Oncol* 1990;8:1335–1341.
31. Pfeiffer P, Bennedaek O, Bertelsen K. Intraperitoneal carboplatin in the treatment of minimal residual ovarian cancer. *Gynecol Oncol* 1990;36:306–311.
32. Los G, Verdegaal EME, Mutsaers PHA, McVie JG. Penetration of carboplatin and cisplatin into rat peritoneal tumor nodules after intraperitoneal chemotherapy. *Cancer Chemother Pharmacol* 1991;28:159–165.
33. Ozols RF, Grotzinger KR, Fisher RI, Myers CE, Young RC. Kinetic characterization and response to chemotherapy in a transplantable murine ovarian cancer. *Cancer Res* 1979;39:3202–3208.
34. Litterst CL, Collins JM, Lowe MC, Arnold ST, Powell DM, Guarino AM. Local and systemic toxicity resulting from large-volume Ip administration of doxorubicin in the rat. *Cancer Treat Rep* 1982;66:157–161.
35. Roboz J, Jacobs AJ, Holland JF, Deppe G, Cohen CJ. Intraperitoneal infusion of doxorubicin in the treatment of gynecologic carcinoma. *Med Pediatr Oncol* 1981;9:245–250.
36. Delgado G, Potkul RK, Treat JA, et al. A phase I/II study of intraperitoneally administered doxorubicin entrapped in cardiolipin liposomes in patients with ovarian cancer. *Am J Obstet Gynecol* 1985;160:812–819.
37. Shenkenberg TD, Von Hoff DD. Mitoxantrone: a new anticancer drug with significant activity. *Ann Intern Med* 1986;105:67–81.
38. Dorr RT, Alberts DS, Soble M. Lack of experimental vesicant activity for the anticancer agents cisplatin, melphalan, and mitoxantrone. *Cancer Chemother Pharmacol* 1986;16:91–94.
39. Markman M, George M, Hakes T, et al. Phase 2 trial of intraperitoneal mitoxantrone in the management of refractory ovarian carcinoma. *J Clin Oncol* 1990;8:146–150.
40. Markman M, Hakes T, Reichman B, et al. Phase 2 trial of weekly or biweekly intraperitoneal mitoxantrone in epithelial ovarian cancer. *J Clin Oncol* 1991;9:978–982.
41. Murdock KC, Wallace RE, White RJ, Durr FE. Discovery and preclinial development of Novantrone. In: Coltman CA, ed. *The current status of novantrone.* New York: Park Row, 1985;3–13.
42. McGuire WP, Rowinsky EK, Rosenshein NB, et al. Taxol: a unique antineoplastic agent with significant activity in advanced ovarian epithelial neoplasms. *Ann Intern Med* 1989;111:273–279.
43. Thigpen T, Blessing J, Ball H, Hummel S, Barret R. Phase II trial of taxol as second-line therapy of ovarian carcinoma: a Gynecologic Oncology Group study. *Proc Am Soc Clin Oncol* 1990;9:156 (abst).
44. Rowinsky EK, Donehower RC, Jones RJ, et al. Microtubule changes and cytotoxicity in leukemic cell lines treated with taxol. *Cancer Res* 1988;48:4093–4100.
45. Howell SB, Zimm S, Markman M, et al. Long term survival of advanced refractory ovarian carcinoma patients with small-volume disease treated with intraperitoneal chemotherapy. *J Clin Oncol* 1987;5:1607–1612.
46. Reichman B, Markman M, Hakes T, et al. Intraperitoneal cis-

platin and etoposide in the treatment of refractory/recurrent ovarian carcinoma. *J Clin Oncol* 1989;7:1327–1332.
47. Markman M, Hakes T, Reichman B, et al. Intraperitoneal cisplatin and cytarabine in the treatment of refractory or recurrent ovarian carcinoma. *J Clin Oncol* 1991;9:204–210.
48. Howell SB, Kirmani S, Lucas WE, et al. A phase II trial of intraperitoneal cisplatin and etoposide for primary treatment of ovarian epithelial cancer. *J Clin Oncol* 1990;8:137–145.
49. Hakes T, Markman M, Reichman T, et al. High intensity intravenous cyclophosphamide/cisplatin and intraperitoneal cisplatin for advanced ovarian cancer. *Proc Am Soc Clin Oncol* 1989;8:152 (abst).

CHAPTER 24

High-Dose Chemotherapy with Autologous Bone Marrow Support for the Treatment of Epithelial Ovarian Cancer

Elizabeth J. Shpall, Salomon M. Stemmer, Scott I. Bearman, Robert C. Bast, Jr., William P. Peters, Maureen Ross, and Roy B. Jones

Substantial improvements have been made in the treatment of advanced epithelial ovarian cancer in recent years. The majority of patients can achieve a minimal disease state following surgery and cisplatin-based chemotherapy. The unfortunate paradox of therapy with minimal residual disease, however, is the fact that further surgery and standard chemotherapy fail to eradicate tumor for the great majority of these patients. Thus, the single most common treatment experience for ovarian cancer patients is major tumor shrinkage, superior to that seen for most solid cancers, followed by relapse and death. This contrast of high response rates with major reductions in tumor burden and low numbers of durable complete remissions stimulated the development of high-dose marrow-supported chemotherapy regimens for advanced ovarian cancer.

This chapter elaborates on the rationale for using high-dose chemotherapy with autologous bone marrow support (ABMS) in the treatment of ovarian cancer and summarizes the relevant clinical data from Bone Marrow Transplant Centers in the United States and Europe.

Studies of high-dose chemotherapy with ABMS for ovarian cancer derive from considerations of tumor biology, extensive animal investigations, and previous clinical trials using this approach in other malignancies.

RATIONALE FOR DOSE INTENSIFICATION

Dose Intensification: General Principles

Studies in animal and human malignancies have quantitatively demonstrated that drug resistance appears to be relative to the dose employed and that absolute resistance is unusual. In experimental systems, a doubling of the administered dose will lead to a tenfold increase in tumor kill in most resistant animal tumors. With alkylating agents, which are the primary class of drugs used to treat ovarian cancer, this effect will continue over several log increases in drug dose. Furthermore, the slope of the killing curve among various ovarian cancer cell subpopulations remains constant and linear once the threshold had been reached. In vitro cell culture studies have demonstrated that cytotoxicity to resistant subpopulations appears to be relative and that it is possible to overcome this effect by dose escalation (1).

Clinical studies have confirmed a steep dose response for the treatment of a variety of malignancies (2–4), which implies that dose escalation of up to twofold may have a profound impact on therapeutic efficacy. The higher the dose administered, the greater the tumor killing and hopefully the greater chance of cure (5,6). The malignancies that exhibit high complete re-

---

E. J. Shpall, S. M. Stemmer, S. I. Bearman, R. B. Jones: The University of Colorado Bone Marrow Transplant Program, University of Colorado Health Science Center, Denver, Colorado 80262
R. C. Bast, Jr., W. P. Peters, M. Ross: The Duke University Bone Marrow Transplant Program, Durham, North Carolina 27710

TABLE 1. *Malignancies with high CR rates following high-dose chemotherapy and ABMS*

Acute leukemia
Non-Hodgkin's lymphoma
Hodgkin's disease
Neuroblastoma
Breast cancer

sponse rates following high-dose chemotherapy and ABMS are summarized in Table 1.

Dose Intensification: Ovarian Cancer

Levin and Hryniuk reviewed the importance of dose intensity in 33 different primary chemotherapy trials using cisplatin-based regimens for ovarian cancer. Both clinical response and survival rates correlated positively with the dose intensity of chemotherapy delivered (7). Several studies, summarized in Table 2, have demonstrated antitumor activity with 100–200 mg/m² of cisplatin in patients with ovarian cancer that was refractory to lower doses of the drug. In 1973, Hreshchyshyn reported an increased response rate in ovarian cancer as a result of increasing the dose of chemotherapy administered above the conventional range (8). Barker and Wiltshaw administered 100 mg/m² cisplatin to ovarian cancer patients who had progressive disease on lower doses of cisplatin, and they achieved a 21% response rate in that group (9). Using 120 mg/m² of cisplatin, Bruckner et al. demonstrated a 20% response rate in ovarian cancer patients who were refractory to standard doses of cisplatin (10). Ozols and colleagues demonstrated a 32% response rate with 200 mg/m² cisplatin in patients who were refractory to standard doses (11).

RATIONALE FOR THE USE OF ALKYLATING AGENTS

The alkylating agents are the most commonly used chemotherapeutic drugs in the treatment of ovarian

TABLE 2. *High-dose cisplatin in patients with advanced ovarian cancer refractory to lower doses*

Investigator	Cisplatin dose (mg/m²)	Response rate (%)	Ref.
Barker and Wiltshaw	100	21	9
Bruckner et al.	120	20	10
Ozols et al.	200	32	11

TABLE 3. *Alkylating agent activity in ovarian cancer*

Drug	Number of patients	Response rate (%)
Thiotepa	144	65
Cyclophosphamide	126	49
Cisplatin	34	27
Melphalan	494	47
Chlorambucil	280	50

cancer. Table 3 summarizes the significant antitumor activity of the alkylating agents against this disease. They have several properties that make them attractive for use in high-dose combinations (12).

Therapeutic Synergy

Preclinical Data

Heterogeneity in drug sensitivity is common and has been exhibited for a number of solid tumors in animals (13). Similar heterogeneity in sensitivity to chemotherapy has been demonstrated in vitro for a variety of human tumors, including ovarian cancer. The demonstration of heterogeneity in response to chemotherapy has greatly influenced those who practice modern oncology to administer combination rather than single agent chemotherapy. Multiple chemotherapeutic agents are combined to optimize the chances that one or more properties needed by drugs to show "therapeutic synergism" will be present in the combination. These properties are the following:

1. The drugs used in combination are less than additive in toxicity to normal cells.
2. The drugs have different biochemical mechanisms of cytotoxic activity for the sensitive tumor cells.
3. The tumor cells resistant to one or more drugs in the combination will be sensitive to other chemotherapeutic agents in the regimen.

If tumors contain subpopulations of cells that are relatively resistant to therapy at presentation, then combining non–cross-resistant drugs offers the best chance of a successful therapeutic outcome, particularly if the agents are subadditive in their toxicity to normal host cells.

Lidor and colleagues used isobolographic analysis to evaluate the ability of several combinations of alkylating agents to kill ovarian cancer cells (14). When the dose response curves for tumor cell killing are linear, isoboles fall on a diagonal line. When they are not linear, an envelope of additivity can be drawn. Synergistic isoboles fall beneath this curve. As shown in Figs. 1 and 2, respectively, therapeutic synergy was documented for cisplatin plus 4-hydroperoxycyclophospha-

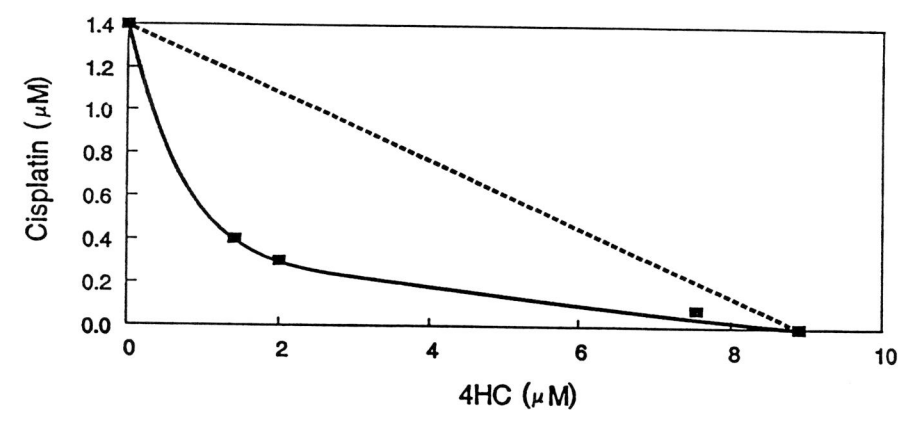

FIG. 1. Isobologram analysis of cisplatin plus 4-hydroperoxycyclophosphamide (4-HC): 2 log reduction in clonogenic growth of the OVCA 432 ovarian cancer cell line.

mide (4-HC), a cyclophosphamide derivative, and cisplatin plus thiotepa against the OVCA 432 ovarian cancer cell line. The synergy was exhibited at all concentrations of the drugs under evaluation. These data stimulated the design of the Duke University Bone Marrow Transplant protocol for ovarian cancer.

Non–Cross-Resistance

Alkylating agents are highly reactive compounds; they were previously considered to be relatively nonspecific and to possess similar mechanisms of action in inhibiting requisite biological functions in both normal and neoplastic cells. However, it has become clear that there are marked differences between alkylating agents, both in biological mechanism of action and in selective toxicity for tumor cells. In the early 1970s, certain investigators believed that tumor cells resistant to one alkylating agent would be resistant to all other alkylating agents. Extensive laboratory data have subsequently demonstrated that this is not the case for a variety of alkylating agent combinations (15). Schabel et al. demonstrated that cyclophosphamide, melphalan, and cisplatin are not cross-resistant to each other and appear to have subadditive toxicity in combination (16).

There are further intriguing aspects to using combinations of alkylating agents. The dose-response curve for many alkylating agents is steep and does not appear to be saturable at doses employed clinically (17). This makes them particularly attractive for use in programs attempting to escalate delivered drug dose.

Nonoverlapping Nonhematopoietic Toxicities

The dose-limiting toxicity of most alkylating agents other than cisplatin is myelosuppression. If myelosuppression is ameliorated with a bone marrow transplant, a three- to sevenfold increase above conventional doses can often be reached before serious nonhematologic toxicity develops. Single alkylating agents administered in high dose produce nonmyelosuppressive tox-

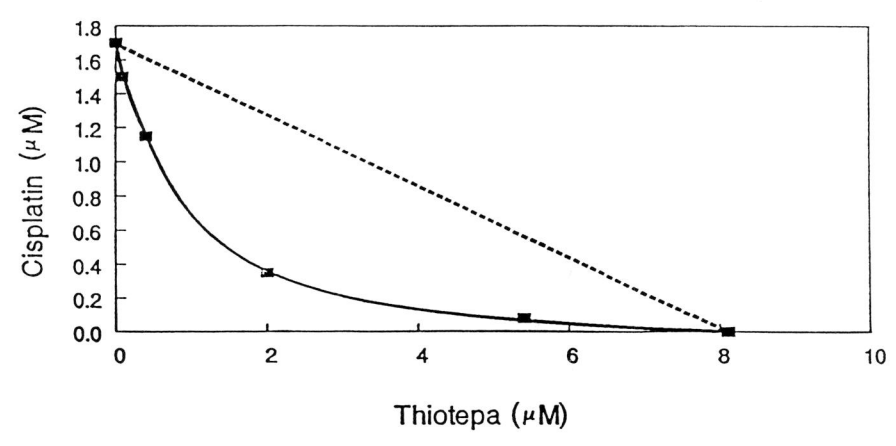

FIG. 2. Isobologram analysis of cisplatin plus thiotepa: 2 log reduction in clonogenic growth of the OVCA 432 ovarian cancer cell line.

TABLE 4. Toxicity of alkylating agents

Standard dose	Drug	High dose
Myelosuppression	Cyclophosphamide	Cardiac
Myelosuppression	Melphalan	GI
Myelosuppression	Thiotepa	Hepatic CNS
Myelosuppression Renal	Cisplatin	Renal
Myelosuppression	BCNU	Pulmonary Hepatic

GI, gastrointestinal; CNS, central nervous system; BCNU, carmustine.

icity, which often differs among the various agents. Table 4 lists representative alkylating agents and their dose-limiting nonhematopoietic toxicities. Hence, it is possible to select agents that possess nonoverlapping toxicities for use in combination.

CLINICAL STUDIES OF CONVENTIONAL CHEMOTHERAPY FOR POOR-PROGNOSIS OVARIAN CANCER

Table 5 describes the last 17 published phase II trials reported by the Gynecologic Oncology Group (GOG) for advanced ovarian cancer. These trials included women with recurrent or persistent disease following a maximum of one prior chemotherapy regimen. Patients who received more than one prior regimen were ineligible for treatment. Eleven trials evaluated drugs that showed no activity in ovarian cancer (response rate <10%). Five trials produced response rates of 11–17%. Sutton et al. reported the best GOG phase II evaluation in ovarian cancer to date, which was a 20% response rate for the ifosfamide/mesna regimen (18). The most promising anticancer agent to be evaluated in ovarian cancer recently is the diterpene plant product taxol, which promotes the assembly and stabilization of microtubules, thereby preventing cell division. McGuire reported a 30% response rate for this drug in patients with residual disease following cisplatin-based therapy (19). The response rate was decreased to 24% in cisplatin-refractory patients. The complete remission rates in all of these trials was less than 10%.

These relatively dismal results with the most promising agents available, in addition to the preclinical data suggesting improved therapeutic effect with high-dose combination alkylating agent therapy, stimulated the development of the marrow-supported trials for poor-prognosis advanced ovarian cancer patients.

CLINICAL STUDIES OF HIGH-DOSE CHEMOTHERAPY WITH ABMS FOR HIGH-RISK OVARIAN CANCER

Technical Aspects of Administering Marrow-Supported Therapy

Prior to high-dose chemotherapy administration, the patient undergoes a bone marrow harvest. A multilumen indwelling intravenous catheter is often inserted during the procedure. The bone marrow is aspirated from the posterior iliac crests of the patients under general or epidural anesthesia. Approximately 1 l of marrow (<5% of the patient's total marrow stores) is removed, concentrated, and cryopreserved in liquid nitrogen. The marrow can be used up to several years following cryopreservation. High-dose chemotherapy is generally administered over 2 to 5 days. The therapy is often administered in a specialized unit where procedures such as reverse isolation and laminar flow or High Efficiency Particulate Air (HEPA) filtration for severely myelosuppressed patients are implemented. A 2- to 5-day interval following high-dose chemotherapy administration (depending upon the regimen) is generally required for drugs to be eliminated from the systemic circulation. After this interval the marrow is rapidly thawed in a 37°C waterbath and reinfused through the patient's intravenous catheter. At the time of reinfusion, the patient's endogenous marrow is usually maximally suppressed from the intensive chemotherapy, with granulocyte counts of <50 cells/µl. The infused marrow will usually reconstitute, or "engraft," within approximately 3 to 4 weeks. The engraftment rates are faster when recombinant hematopoietic growth factors are also given to the patient.

Leukopheresed peripheral blood progenitor cells (PBPCs), which are collected after the patient receives several days of a recombinant hematopoietic growth factor such as granulocyte colony-stimulating factor (G-CSF) or granulocyte-macrophage colony-stimulating factor (GM-CSF), are being used with increasing frequency to support intensive chemotherapy. When administered in combination with autologous marrow, the patients receive additional blood product, which is enriched for hematopoietic progenitors (20). With marrow plus PBPCs, engraftment rates appear to be faster than in patients who receive marrow alone or marrow plus growth factor. At the University of Colorado, ovarian cancer patients receive ABMS plus G-

TABLE 5. Treatment studies in advanced ovarian cancer Phase II GOG Trials

	Response rate
11 trials	<10%
5 trials	11–17%
Ifosfamide/mesna	20%
Taxol[a]	30%

[a] Not a GOG study.

TABLE 6. Schema for Duke University protocol using high-dose intraperitoneal cisplatin with intravenous cyclophosphamide and thiotepa followed by ABMS for poor-prognosis advanced ovarian cancer

	Day from marrow infusion								
	−7	−6	−5	−4	−3	−2	−1	0	+1
CPA 1875 mg/M2/d		□	□	□					
cDDP 30 mg/M2d IP*		×	×	×					
Thiotepa 300 mg/M2	●								
Remove Tenchoff catheter				△					
Bone marrow infusion									△

cDDP will be escalated in cohorts of 3 patients.

* cohort #	dose (mg/M2/d)
2	40
3	50
4	60

CSF–primed PBPCs, followed by additional daily G-CSF until the marrow reconstitutes. The median time to engraftment, defined as a granulocyte count >500 cells/μl, is 9 days. This is an improvement over the median engraftment rate of 23 days in historically controlled ovarian cancer patients who received the same chemotherapy regimen and autologous bone marrow alone. Several investigators have used growth factor–primed PBPCs alone to support the patients following intensive therapy, with successful marrow reconstitution in most cases (21).

Duke University, Durham, North Carolina

The combination of cyclophosphamide (5,600 mg/m^2), cisplatin (165 mg/m^2), and escalating doses of thiotepa (150–450 mg/m^2) were initially studied intravenously in a phase I trial with ABMS for refractory solid tumors (22). In that trial with ABMS the thiotepa was escalated to the maximally tolerated dose (MTD) of (300 mg/m^2), and activity in ovarian cancer was demonstrated. The data of Lidor et al., which demonstrated synergistic killing of ovarian cancer with the alkylating agent combinations previously described (14), then stimulated the design of a phase I–II trial for advanced ovarian cancer patients who had residual peritoneal tumor following cisplatin-based chemotherapy. Table 6 shows the protocol schema in which cyclophosphamide (5,600 mg/m^2) and thiotepa (300 mg/m^2) were initially administered intravenously in the doses determined from the previous trial. The cisplatin was administered initially as an intraperitoneal bolus infusion (90 mg/m^2) and escalated by 30 mg/m^2/cohort. The rationale for using intraperitoneal cisplatin was based on the pharmacokinetic advantage of cisplatin administration in the peritoneal cavity demonstrated with this route of administration, with no major compromise in systemic levels of the drug (23). Clinical trials have suggested that intraperitoneal administration offers antitumor activity superior to that achieved with intravenous cisplatin administration in certain subsets of ovarian cancer patients (24–26).

Shpall et al. reported preliminary data from the Duke study (27). The demographic data are summarized in Table 7. This heavily pretreated group of patients had previously received a median of three prior chemotherapy regimens. All patients had bulky disease, with the majority having the largest tumor masses >3 cm at study entry. Seventy-five percent of the patients had pathologically documented partial responses (PRs) (>75% tumor reduction) of median 6-month duration (range 3–9 months). The toxicity of the treatment regimen, which was initially substantial, is summarized on Table 8. A patient from the first cohort received an

TABLE 7. Duke University BMTP High-dose IV/IP chemotherapy with ABMS for ovarian cancer: Patient demographics[a]

Stage at diagnosis: III/IV
Number of patients: 4 (stage III), 9 (stage IV)
Dominant metastases
Peritoneum/pelvis: 7/2
Lung or pleura/liver: 8/2
Age: mean = 45, range = 30–59
Months from initial diagnosis: mean = 21, range = 3–60
Number of prior regimens: mean = 3, range = 1–4

[a] n = 13.

TABLE 8. Duke University BMTP High-dose IV/IP chemotherapy with ABMS for ovarian cancer: Major toxicity[a]

Total dose of cisplatin (mg/m^2)	Number of patients	Toxic deaths
90	3	1[b]
120	3	0
150 (bolus)	3	2[c]
150 (continuous infusion)	7	0

[a] n = 13.
[b] infected platelets.
[c] renal failure/sepsis.

infected platelet transfusion that produced fatal septic shock within 2 hours. That complication was unique in the Duke Marrow Transplant experience comprising more than 400 patients. Another two patients from the third cohort, however, died from chemotherapy-related renal toxicity. These deaths prompted a change in the method of cisplatin administration from bolus intraperitoneal infusion daily for three days to continuous intraperitoneal infusion daily for three days (same total dose of 150 mg/m^2). This modification was made because of data suggesting that higher intravenous peak levels of cisplatin are more nephrotoxic than lower peak levels (28). Since the modification, an additional seven patients have been treated on the protocol with no evidence of renal insufficiency or other significant toxicity (29). The cisplatin has been escalated to the MTD of 165 mg/m^2, and the thiotepa to 600 mg/m^2. The response rate in the 16 patients treated thus far remains >60%, and accrual continues with further increases in thiotepa planned, to the MTD.

Serum CA-125 levels were evaluated daily from initiation of high-dose chemotherapy until discharge from the Transplant Unit (30). Three distinct patterns of CA-125 behavior were demonstrated.

1. One group of patients began chemotherapy with elevated baseline CA-125 levels (128–453 u/ml), as shown in Fig. 3. During the first week of chemotherapy, acute tenfold rises in the CA-125 levels (1,000–2,500 u/ml) were noted, which rapidly decreased to normal (two patients) or were continuing to decrease at the time of toxic death (two patients).
2. Patients began chemotherapy with elevated baseline CA-125 levels (109–2,581), which decreased rapidly either to normal (two patients) or remained elevated (two patients), as shown in Fig. 4.
3. Patients had normal (three patients) or slightly elevated (one patient) baseline CA-125 levels, which increased fivefold with chemotherapy but returned back to normal at the time of discharge from the Transplant Unit, as shown in Fig. 5.

Table 9 reveals that the only 2 patients of the initial 12 who left the Transplant Unit with elevated CA-125 levels experienced no antitumor effect.

University of Colorado, Denver, Colorado

The University of Colorado Bone Marrow Transplant Program (BMTP) initiated a phase I–II trial using

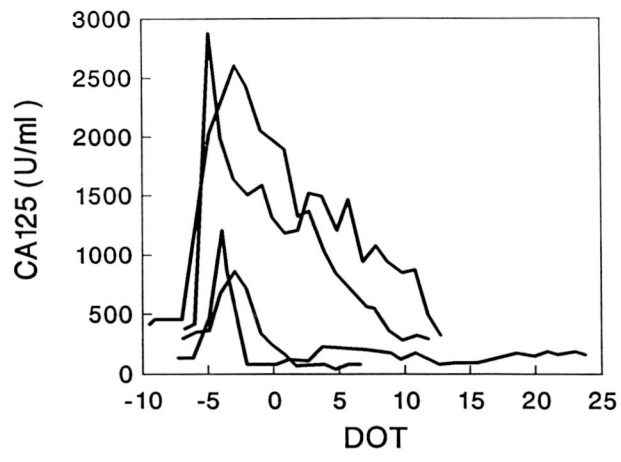

FIG. 3. Moderately elevated baseline Ca-125 levels that rose tenfold during the first week of therapy then rapidly decreased to normal (two patients) or were continuing to decrease at the time of death (two patients). Reprinted with permission from ref. 27.

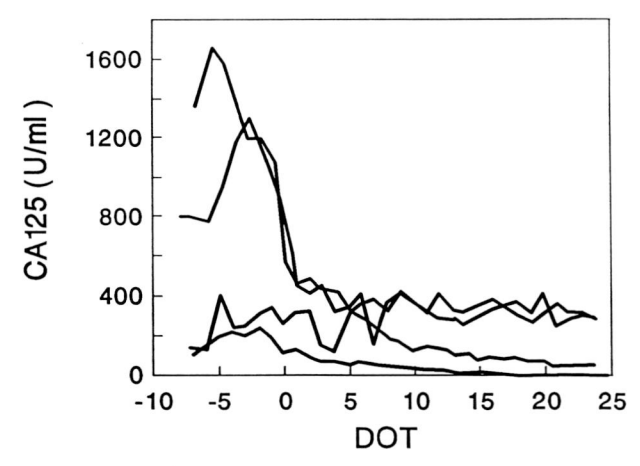

FIG. 4. High baseline CA-125 levels that decreased rapidly to normal (2 patients), or remained elevated (2 patients). Reprinted with permission from ref. 27.

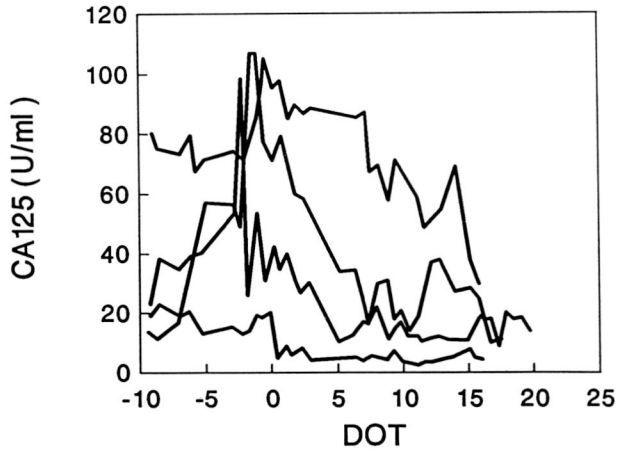

FIG. 5. Normal (three patients) or slightly elevated (one patient) baseline Ca-125 levels that increased acutely fivefold with chemotherapy and then returned to normal within 4 weeks of treatment. Reprinted with permission from ref. 27.

TABLE 9. Duke University High-dose chemotherapy with ABMT for refractory ovarian cancer: Serum CA-125 level post-BMT[a]

Last inpatient serum CA-125	Number	PR[b]	NR[c]	NE[d]	TD[e]
≤35 u/ml	7	6	0	1	0
≥35 u/ml	5	0	2	0	3[f]

[a] Reprinted with permission from ref. 27.
[b] PR, partial response.
[c] NR, no response.
[d] NE, not evaluable.
[e] TD, toxic death.
[f] CA-125 levels were decreasing at the time of death.

TABLE 10. High-dose cyclophosphonide cisplatin/thiotepa with ABMT for ovarian cancer

Patient	Size of tumor before BMT	Response	Duration (mo)
1	<1 cm	NED	14+
2	<1 cm	NED	6
3	<1 cm	CR	5+
4	<1 cm	NED	3+
5	<1 cm	NED	3+
6	<1 cm	NED	2+
7	<1 cm	NED	1+
8	>1 cm	NED	10+
9	>1 cm	PR	4

NED, no evidence of disease; PR, partial response.

the regimen developed at Duke University consisting of cisplatin, cyclophosphamide (5,600 mg/m^2), and escalating doses of thiotepa (300–600 mg/m^2) (31). Because of the technical difficulties of combining intraperitoneal therapy with bone marrow transplant, we elected to administer the cisplatin intravenously, as shown in Fig. 6. The dose of cisplatin, which is identical to the current intraperitoneal dose in the Duke regimen, is 55 mg/m^2/day, given as a continuous 72-hour infusion (165 mg/m^2 total dose). The study attempts to accrue patients who have persistent or progressive tumor following one prior cisplatin-based regimen and who have lesser disease volume at study entry (largest tumor <1 cm) than the patients treated previously. Table 10 summarizes the preliminary clinical results. Nine patients have been treated thus far, seven with the largest tumor <1 cm at study entry. The follow-up is short, but to date six of these seven patients (85%), and one of two with larger tumor volume, remain progression-free, although the longest patient is only 14 (range 1+ to 14+) months from transplant.

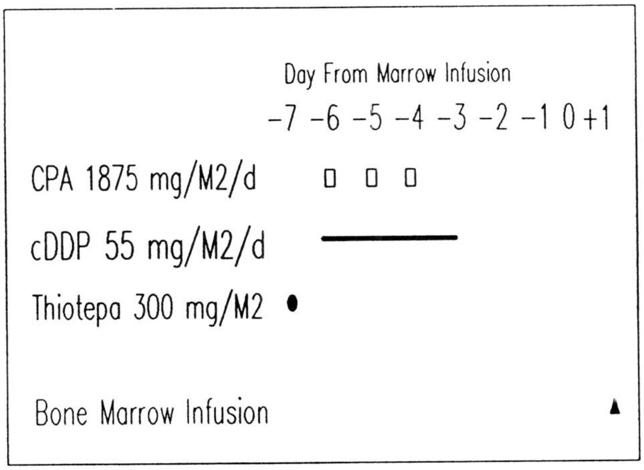

University of Gronigen, The Netherlands

This group initially reported results using ABMS in two refractory ovarian cancer patients who had persistent microscopic disease following cisplatin-based induction chemotherapy. The patients received high-dose cyclophosphamide, VP-16, and ABMS (32). At the time of the publication, the patients remained progression-free for 10 months following transplant. Mulder et al. from the same group subsequently described 11 refractory ovarian cancer patients (8 with the largest tumor <2 cm) who also received high-dose cyclophosphamide (7,000 mg/m^2), VP-16 (1,000–1,500 mg/m^2), and ABMS (33). They reported six complete remissions. Five of the eight low tumor volume patients experienced pathologically documented complete responses (CRs) (75%). The median duration of response was 15 months, with two patients who remained in CR at 43+ and 75+ months posttransplant. Only one of the patients with disease >2 cm responded.

The same investigators are evaluating other intensive chemotherapy regimens for patients with refractory tumors including ovarian cancer (34). Three of five refractory ovarian cancer patients (60%) responded to high-dose cyclophosphamide (7,000 mg/m^2) and mitoxantrone (30–75 mg/m^2) followed by ABMS. However, prohibitive hemorrhagic cystitis, despite the use of the protective agent mesna, precluded further evaluation of that regimen. More recently high-dose melphalan (180 mg/m^2) in combination with mitoxantrone (60 mg/m^2) produced CRs in two ovarian cancer patients who remained progression-free at 5+ and 9+ months, respectively, following therapy. Further evaluation of that regimen is in progress.

FIG. 6. Schema for University of Colorado protocol using high-dose intravenous cisplatin, cyclophosphamide, and thiotepa with ABMS for poor-prognosis advanced ovarian cancer. The thiotepa has been escalated to 600 mg/m^2 with no toxicity; accrual and thiotepa escalation continue.

Centre Jean Perrin, Clermont-Ferrand, France

Dauplat et al. administered high-dose melphalan (140 mg/m^2) and ABMS to 14 ovarian cancer patients with residual tumor following cisplatin-based induction therapy (35). Prior to study entry five patients had microscopic disease, and 9 of the 14 patients had macroscopic tumor that was surgically debulked before study entry. No significant toxicity was noted with the regimen. Five patients (37.5%) remained progression-free at a median of 43+ (range 30+ 60+) months following therapy. The status of the progression free survivors at second-look surgery was not documented in their report.

Dauplat et al. subsequently administered high-dose melphalan and ABMS to seven ovarian cancer patients who had no tumor at second-look surgery following cisplatin-based induction therapy but were thought to have tumors with prognostic features suggesting a high-risk of relapse. The therapy was well tolerated by all patients, but longer follow-up is necessary.

Centre Anticancer, Marseilles, France

Viens et al. reported promising results from 35 advanced stage ovarian cancer patients who received high-dose melphalan (140–200 mg/m^2) and ABMS following one cisplatin-based chemotherapy regimen and a second-look pathologic evaluation (36). The chemotherapy was extremely well-tolerated, with no fatal toxicity noted. The patients were stratified into three groups according to the amount of residual disease at second-look surgery. The first group included 16 patients with the largest residual tumor >2 cm. Seventy-five percent of the patients with measurable disease at study entry responded to the high-dose regimen. Five of the 16 (31%) remain progression-free at 8+ to 35+ months following transplant. The second group included ten patients with residual tumor <2 cm. Three of the ten, or 30%, remain progression-free 13+ to 23+ months posttransplant. The third group included nine patients with no residual cancer at second-look surgery (pathologic complete responders). Six of the nine, or 66%, remain progression-free at 10+ to 32+ months following intensive therapy.

Loyola University, Chicago, Illinois

McKenzie et al. reported results from six refractory ovarian cancer patients who received high-dose cyclophosphamide (120 mg/kg), mitoxantrone (30–75 mg/m^2) and carboplatin (1,500 mg/m^2) with ABMS (37). Mucositis was the limiting toxicity of mitoxantrone escalation, at 75 mg/m^2. Five of the six, or 82%, of the patients responded, four of them completely. An additional 11 ovarian cancer patients have been treated with the same regimen. The response rate remains high at 87% with 60% clinical complete responses (cCRs). All patients had bulky tumors (1–3 cm) prior to study entry. Forty percent remain progression-free at 2+ to 20+ months (38). Two patients experienced fatal treatment-related toxicity.

University of California, San Diego, California

Shea et al. treated eight advanced ovarian cancer patients with high-dose intraperitoneal carboplatin (1,600 mg/m^2), VP-16 (800 mg/m^2), intravenous thiotepa (300–400 mg/m^2), and mitoxantrone (24–30 mg/m^2), followed by autologous peripheral blood stem cell support (39). One patient received the therapy as consolidation for responding but bulky stage IV disease. The other patients had received a minimum of two prior cisplatin-based regimens and had progressive tumor at study entry. Six of the seven evaluable patients (84%) responded, four of them completely. The median duration of response was 6 months. The patient who received treatment as consolidation remains progression-free at 4+ months following therapy. No fatalities or serious nonhematologic toxicity were noted.

Tokai University, Kanagawa, Japan

Shinozuka et al. administered two cycles of high-dose cyclophosphamide (1,600–2,400 mg/m^2), adriamycin (80–100 mg/m^2), and cisplatin (100–150 mg/m^2) with ABMS to 42 patients with ovarian cancer following primary surgery that left all patients with <1 cm tumor masses (40). Seventy percent of the 23 patients with microscopic disease survived at 4 years. Fourteen percent of the other 19 patients with persistent macroscopic disease at study entry survived at 4 years. The disease-free survival rates were not discussed in their report.

Other Studies

Table 11 presents a summary of the clinical trials described in the preceding sections. Many other investigators have reported high response rates and in some studies have noted encouraging response durations for patients with refractory ovarian cancer. Table 12 summarizes these findings (41–47).

DISCUSSION

Although the numbers of patients in each of these marrow-supported studies are small, the therapeutic results are similar and quite consistent. When the data

TABLE 11. *Poor-prognosis ovarian cancer: summary of high-dose chemotherapy and ABMT studies*

Author (ref.)	Total number of patients	Number of prior regimens	Disease status prior to BMT	BMT regimen	Clinical responses (%)	Path responses (%)	Median response duration (mo)
Shpall (27)	12	3	mac	Cyt, Thio, IP Cis	PR[a] 6/8 (75)	PR 6/8 (75)	6
Univ. Colo (31)	9	2	mac	Cyt, Thio, Cis	CR 1/2 (50)	ND	4 (10+)
					NED 6/7 (85)	ND	6 (2+−14+) 85%
Mulder (34)	5	1	ND	Cyt, Mx/Mel, Mx	ND	PR 1/5 (20)	9+
						CR 2/5 (40)	6
Mulder (33)	11	1	mic 8, mac 3	Cyt, VP-16	CR 6/11 (55)	CR 5/11 (46)	15 (43+, 75+)
Dauplat (35)	14	1	mic 5, mac 9[a]	Mel	ND	ND	43 (30−60+) 35%
Viens (36)	35	1	mic 9, mac 26	Mel	ND	ND	ND (8+−54+) 45%
McKenzie (37)	17	3	mac	Cyt, Car, Mx	CR 11/17 (60)	ND	ND (2+−20+) 40%
					PR 4/17 (27)		
Shea (39)	8	3	mic 1, mac 7	IP Car, VP-16 +IV Thio, Mx	CR 4/7 (57)	ND	6
					PR 2/7 (29)		
Shinozuka (40)	42	0	mic 23, mac 19	Cyt, Adr, Cis (double BMT)	Alive 19/42 (45%)	ND	48+

[a] PR, partial response; CR, complete response; ND, no data; mic, microscopic; mac, macroscopic; NED, no evidence of disease; IP, intraperitoneal; IV, intravenous; Cyt, cyclophosphamide; Thio, thiotepa; Mel, Melphalan; Car, Carboplatin; Mx, Mitoxantron; Adr, Adriamicin; Cis, Cisplatin.
[b] Debulked prior to BMT.
[c] Disease status unknown.

are compiled, over 200 women with advanced stage ovarian cancer have received high-dose chemotherapy regimens with ABMS for their disease. A major feature of most studies is the strikingly high response rate achieved with intensive therapy.

The response rates of 70% to 82% achieved in several studies (27,33,35,36,38) (Table 13) with intensive marrow-supported therapy, usually in heavily pretreated ovarian cancer patients, are significantly higher than the standard phase II studies summarized in Table 5. In the majority of GOG trials, fewer than 10% of patients who had minimal prior chemotherapy (only one prior regimen) responded. The higher response rates for intensive, marrow-supported therapy suggest promise for this technique. However, the median duration of response in the majority of these trials is less than 9 months, suggesting that although large-volume tumor reduction occurred in these patients, substantial residual tumor remained.

If a 75% response rate can be obtained in patients with ovarian cancer refractory to standard therapy, then applying the same treatment earlier in the disease course when the tumors will be less resistant may produce more durable antitumor effects. This principle has been validated in the treatment of acute leukemia (48), Hodgkin's disease (49), non-Hodgkin's lymphoma (50), and more recently breast cancer (51). Studies of adjuvant, marrow-supported chemotherapy in patients with high-risk stage II breast cancer (≥10 axillary nodes containing tumor) have documented a 72% progression-free survival rate at three years (52). This result is superior to the 20% progression-free interval obtained at a similar time point in breast cancer patients transplanted with advanced, stage IV disease (53). Both results are superior to those achieved with standard therapy in the same setting. In addition to maximizing the response, toxicity is usually minimized when patients are treated earlier in their disease course, and with a minimal tumor burden.

It appears from the studies of Mulder, Dauplat, and

TABLE 12. *Poor-prognosis advanced ovarian cancer: summary of high-dose chemotherapy with ABMT studies*

Author (ref.)	Total number of patients	Number of prior regimens	Disease status prior to BMT	BMT regimen	Clinical responses (%)	Pathologic responses (%)	Response duration (mo)
Pierelli (42)	4	1	mac	Cis, VP-16, Car	ND[a]	ND	ND
Fields (43)	3	ND	mic 1, mac 2	Ifo, VP-16, Car	CR 2/3 (60)	ND	ND
Pico (47)	2	ND	mac	Cyt, Car, VP-16	CR 2/2 (100)	ND	ND
Nores (46)	1	1	mac[b]	Cyt, TBI	CR 1/1 (100)	ND	19+
Postmus (44)	2	1	mac	VP-16, Cyt	CR 2/2 (100)	CR 1/2 (50%)	12+, 16+
Vriesendorp (45)	2	2	mic	Cyt, VP-16	ND	CR 1/2 (50%)	10+, 10+
Panici (41)	13	1	ND	Cis, Car VP-16	ND	CR 6/11 (55%) PR 3/11 (27%)	ND

[a] ND, no data; mic, microscopic; mac, macroscopic; TBI, total body irradiation; CR, complete response; PR, partial response; Cis, cisplatin; Cyt, cyclophosphamide; Car, carboplatin; Ifo, Ifosfamide.
[b] Debulked prior to BMT.

TABLE 13. *Treatment studies in advanced ovarian cancer: High-dose chemotherapy with ABMS*

	Response rate	Ref.
Shpall	75%	27
Mulder	75%	33
Viens	75%	35
McKenzie	87%	36
Shea	84%	38

Viens and the preliminary data from the University of Colorado that the best results with poor-prognosis ovarian cancer patients will also be achieved when they are treated early and with minimal tumor burden. The long-term disease-free survival with standard salvage chemotherapy for advanced ovarian cancer is commonly reported to be less than 10% (54). Eighty percent of patients transplanted with less than 1 cm of tumor at the University of Colorado remain progression-free at 1+ to 14+ months posttransplant. Obviously, longer follow-up is needed to assess the ultimate impact of the regimen on disease-free survival. Mulder et al. reported a 55% response rate and a 20% long-term survival rate in a small number of ovarian cancer patients who were destined to fail standard salvage therapy (33). Their data demonstrate that meaningful progression-free survival can be achieved if refractory ovarian cancer patients are treated with intensive therapy at a time of minimal tumor burden. Dauplat et al. reported a 37% 2-year disease-free survival rate for ovarian cancer patients who received high-dose melphalan and ABMS for microscopic or macroscopic residual tumor following second-look surgery (35). Unfortunately, their report did not describe the status at study entry (microscopic versus macroscopic) of the 2-year disease-free survivors. The report of Viens et al. confirmed a high response rate or progression-free interval for patients with macroscopic and microscopic disease, respectively, prior to high-dose therapy (36). It is noteworthy that 50% of patients with >2 cm of disease in their study remained progression-free at a median of 24 months following melphalan administration. This result differs from the majority of studies discussed in this chapter. For patients with similar bulky disease, high response rates of short duration are common, with very few patients surviving disease-free at 2 years.

The most intriguing data reported by Dauplat et al. (35) and Viens et al. (36) involve the administration of high-dose therapy to patients with no tumor at second-look surgery. These patients had ovarian tumors with prognostic features suggesting a high risk of relapse. These features, described by Miller et al., included very large tumor burdens at initial diagnosis, large residual disease following initial surgery, and tumors of high histologic grade (55). Although the follow-up is short, 66% of patients reported by Viens et al. remained progression-free at 10+ to 32+ months following intensive therapy.

FUTURE DIRECTIONS

Follow-up of patients who are receiving intensive therapy for small volume (<1 cm) disease will be forthcoming in the next several years. More than one-half of ovarian cancer patients with negative second-look surgeries relapse and die of progressive disease. Definition of a poor-prognostic cohort, as Miller et al. described (55), might allow ethical application of ABM-supported therapy at a time of microscopic residual tumor when maximal antitumor effect is likely. Such trials could randomly assign patients to intensive therapy with ABMS, intraperitoneal therapy showing promise (26), or observation. CA-125 levels may be helpful in the future for defining patients with nonmeasurable tumor who may benefit from marrow-supported therapy. It appears from the Duke data previously cited that CA-125 levels may also be helpful in the early assessment of response to intensive therapy.

The toxicity of high-dose therapy should be low to justify its use in the early, minimal disease setting. The fatality rate of 8% in stage II ≥10 node positive breast cancer patients, who have a 70% to 80% chance of relapse following standard adjuvant therapy, may serve as a benchmark to define an acceptable relationship between relapse risk and fatal toxicity. However, the current >80% fatality rate for patients with poor-prognosis advanced ovarian cancer justifies significant risk in well-informed patients willing to participate in scientifically well-designed trials of high-dose therapy.

With experience and with improved supportive care such as recombinant hematopoietic growth factor administration and careful patient selection, the fatal toxicity rates are decreasing in the majority of major transplant centers. This should allow increasing numbers of patients with poor-prognosis, minimal tumor burden ovarian cancer to be treated in the future.

REFERENCES

1. Griswold DP, Trader MW, Freii E, Peters WP, Wolpert MK, Laster WR. Response of drug-sensitive and resistant L1210 leukemias to high-dose chemotherapy. *Cancer Res* 1987;47:2323–2327.
2. Peters WP. The rationale for high-dose chemotherapy with autologous bone marrow support in treating breast cancer. In: Dicke K, Spitzer G, Zander A, eds. *The first international symposium on ABMT*. The University of Texas M.D. Anderson Hospital and Tumor Institute, 1985;189–195.
3. Johnson LF, Thomas ED, Clark BS. A comparison of marrow transplantation with chemotherapy for children with acute lymphoblastic leukemia in second or subsequent remission. *New Engl J Med* 1981;305:846–852.

4. Appelbaum F, Dhalberg S, Thomas ED. Bone marrow transplantation or chemotherapy after remission induction for adults with acute nonlymphocytic leukemia. *Ann Intern Med* 1984;101: 581–588.
5. Shabel F. Animal models as predictive systems. In: *Cancer chemotherapy—fundamental concepts and recent advances*. Chicago: Yearbook Medical Publishers, 1975;323–355.
6. Steel G. Growth and survival of tumor cells. In: *Growth kinetics of tumors*. Oxford: Clarendon Press, 1977;244–267.
7. Levin L, Hryniuk WM. Dose intensity analysis of chemotherapy regimens in ovarian carcinoma. *J Clin Oncol* 1987;5:756–767.
8. Hreshchyshyn M. Single agent therapy in ovarian cancer: factors influencing response. *Gynecol Oncol* 1973;1:220.
9. Barker GH, Wiltshaw E. Use of high-dose cisplatin following failure on previous chemotherapy for advanced carcinoma of the ovary. *Br J Obstet Gynecol* 1981;88:1192–1199.
10. Bruckner H, Wallach R, Cohen CJ, et al. High-dose cisplatin for the treatment of ovarian cancer. *Gynecol Oncol* 1984;12:64–67.
11. Ozols R, Ostchega Y, Meyers C, Young RC. High-dose cisplatin in hypertonic saline in refractory ovarian cancer. *J Clin Oncol* 1985;3:1246–1250.
12. Ozols R, Young R. Ovarian cancer. *Curr Probl Cancer* 1987 Mar/Apr: 61–122.
13. Tsuruo T, Fidler IF. Differences in drug sensitivity among tumor cells from parental tumors, selected variants, and spontaneous metastases. *Cancer Res* 1981;41:3058–3064.
14. Lidor Y, Shpall EJ, Peters WP, Bast RC Jr. Synergistic cytotoxicity of different alkylating agents for epithelial ovarian cancer. *Int J Cancer* 1991;49:1–7.
15. Skipper HE, Schabel F. Quantitative and cytokinetic studies in experimental tumor systems. In: Holland J, Frei E, eds. *Cancer medicine*. Philadelphia: Lea and Febiger, 1982;663–685.
16. Schabel FM, Skipper HE, Trader MW, Laster WR, Griswold DP, Corbett TH. Establishment of cross resistant profiles for new agents. *Cancer Treat Rep* 1983;67:905–922.
17. Dykes D, Trader M, Griswold D, Peters W, Frei E, Laster W. Increased cytotoxic effect of high dose alkylating agent therapy in mice bearing drug sensitive resistant autologous leukemia. *Am Assoc Cancer Res* 1985;26:832.
18. Sutton GP, Blessing JA, Homesley HD, Berman ML, Malfetano J. Phase II trial of ifosamide and mesna in advanced ovarian carcinoma: a Gynecologic Oncology Group study. *J Clin Oncol* 1989;7:1672–1676.
19. McGuire WP, Rowinsky EK, Rosenshein NB, et al. Taxol: a unique antineoplastic agent with significant activity in advanced ovarian epithelial neoplasms. *Ann Intern Med* 1989;111: 273–279.
20. Peterson J, Kirkpatrick G, Ross M, Vredenbeurgh J, Peters WP, Kurtzberg J. Growth factor primed peripheral blood progenitor cells (PBPCs) are enriched for hematopoietic progenitor cells. *Proc Am Soc Clin Oncol* 1991;10:78.
21. Kessinger A, Armitage J, Landmark J, Smith D, Weisenburger D. Autologous peripheral hematopoietic stem cell transplantation restores hematopoietic function following myeloablative therapy. *Blood* 1988;71:723–727.
22. Shpall EJ, Peters WP, Jones RB, et al. A phase I trial of cyclophosphamide, cisplatin, and thiotepa with autologous bone marrow support in the treatment of resistant solid tumors. *Proc Am Soc Clin Oncol* 1986;6:139.
23. Howell S, Pfeile CE, Wung E, et al. Intraperitoneal cisplatin with systemic thiosulfate protection. *Ann Intern Med* 1982;97: 845–851.
24. McVie J, ten Bokkel H, Aarsten E, Simonetti G, Dubbelman R, Franklin H. Intraperitoneal chemotherapy in minimal residual ovarian cancer with cisplatin and intravenous sodium thiosulfate protection. *Proc Am Soc Clin Oncol* 1985;485:125.
25. Cohen C. Ovarian Cancer: New approaches with curative intent. In: Bruckner H, Cohen C, eds. *Pharma Libri*. Monographs in Medicine/Oncology, New York. 1984; pp. 37–50.
26. Markman M, Howell S, Lucas WE, Pfeifle CE, Green M. Combination intraperitoneal chemotherapy with cisplatin, cytarabine, and doxorubicin for refractory ovarian carcinoma and other malignancies principally confined to the peritoneal cavity. *J Clin Oncol* 1984;2:1321–1326.
27. Shpall EJ, Clarke-Pearson D, Soper J, et al. High dose alkylating agent therapy with autologous marrow support in patients with stage III/IV epithelial ovarian cancer. *Gynecol Oncol* 1990;38: 386–391.
28. Campbell AB, Kalman SM, Jacobs C. Plasma platinum levels: relationship to cisplatin dose and nephrotoxicity. *Cancer Treat Rep* 1983;67:169–172.
29. Peters W, Ross M. Duke University Bone Marrow Transplant Program. *Personal communication*.
30. Bast RC, Klug JL, St. John E, et al. A radioimmunoassay using a monoclonal antibody to monitor the cause of epithelial ovarian cancer. *N Engl J Med* 1983;309:383–387.
31. Shpall E. Preliminary results from the University of Colorado Bone Marrow Transplant Program, 1992 (*unpublished data*).
32. Vriesendorp R, Aalders JG, Sleijfer D, et al. Effective high-dose chemotherapy with autologous marrow infusion in resistant ovarian cancer. *Gynecol Oncol* 1984;17:271–276.
33. Mulder PO, Willemse B, Aalders JG, et al. High-dose chemotherapy with autologous bone marrow transplantation in patients with refractory ovarian cancer. *Eur J Cancer Clin Oncol* 1989; 25:645–649.
34. Mulder PO, Sleijfer D, Willemse P, De Vries E, Uges D, Nulder NH. High-dose cyclophosphamide or melphalan with escalating doses of mitoxantrone and autologous bone marrow transplantation for refractory solid tumors. *Cancer Res* 1989;49:4654–4658.
35. Dauplat J, Legros M, Condat P, Ferriere JP, Ben Ahmed S, Plagne R. High-dose melphalan and autologous bone marrow support for treatment of ovarian carcinoma with positive second look operation. *Gynecol Oncol* 1989;34:294–298.
36. Viens P, Maraninchi D, Legros M, et al. High dose melphalan and autologous marrow rescue in advanced epithelial ovarian carcinomas: a retrospective analysis of 35 patients treated in France. *Bone Marrow Transplant* 1990;5:227–233.
37. McKenzie RS, Alberts DA, Bishop MR, et al. Phase I trial of cyclophosphamide, mitoxantrone and carboplatin and autologous bone marrow transplantation in female malignancies: pharmacologic levels of mitoxantrone and high response rates in refractory ovarian cancer. *Proc Am Soc Clin Oncol* 1991;10:186.
38. Stiff P. Loyola University Bone Marrow Transplant Program. *Personal communication*.
39. Shea TC, Storniolo AM, Mason JR, Newton B, Mullen M, Hunger K. High-dose intravenous and intraperitoneal combination chemotherapy with autologous stem cell rescue for patients with advanced ovarian cancer. *Proc Am Soc Clin Oncol* [*submitted*].
40. Shinozuka T, Murakami M, Miyamoto T, et al. High-dose chemotherapy with autologous bone marrow transplantation in ovarian cancer. *Proc Am Soc Clin Oncol* 1991;10:193.
41. Panici PB, Scambia G, Baiocchi S, et al. High-dose chemotherapy and autologous peripheral blood stem cell support in advanced ovarian cancer. *Proc Am Soc Clin Oncol* 1991;10:195.
42. Pierelli L, Menichella G, Foddai ML, et al. High dose chemotherapy with cisplatin, VP16 and carboplatin with stem cell support in patients with advanced ovarian cancer. *Haematologica* 1991;76:63–65.
43. Fields KK, Zorsky PE, Saleh RA, et al. A Phase I-II study of high-dose ifosamide, carboplatin and etoposide (ICE) with autologous bone marrow rescue (ABMR): preliminary results. *Proc Am Soc Clin Oncol* 1991;10:70.
44. Postmus PE, DeVries EGE, DeVries-Hospers HG, et al. Cyclophosphamide and VP 16-213 with autologous bone marrow transplantation. A dose escalation study. *Eur J Cancer Clin Oncol* 1984;20:777–782.
45. Vriesendorp R, Aalders JG, Sleijfer DT, et al. Effective high-dose chemotherapy with autologous bone marrow infusion in resistant ovarian cancer. *Gynecol Oncol* 1984;17:271–276.
46. Nores JM, Dalayeun JF, Otmezguine Y, Folgoas C, Nenna AD. High-dose chemotherapy, total abdomen irradiation and autologous bone marrow infusion in ovarian cancer: an observation. *Gynecol Obstet Invest* 1989;27:55–56.
47. Pico JL, Zambon E, Sunderlan M, et al. Phase I clinical and pharmacokinetics study of high-dose carboplatin, in combination with etoposide and cyclophosphamide followed by autolo-

gous bone marrow transplantation. *Proc Am Soc Clin Oncol* 1990;9:80.
48. Cahn JY, Herve P, Flesch M, et al. Autologous bone marrow transplantation for acute leukemia in complete remission: a pilot study of 33 cases. *Br J Haematol* 1986;63:457–470.
49. Jagannath S, Dicke K, Armitage JO, et al. High-dose cyclophosphamide, carmustine, and etoposide and autologous bone marrow transplantation for relapsed Hodgkin's disease. *Ann Intern Med* 1986;104:163–168.
50. Philip T, Armitage JO, Spitzer G, et al. High-dose therapy and autologous bone marrow transplantation after failure of conventional chemotherapy in adults with intermediate-grade or high-grade non-Hodgkin's lymphoma. *N Engl J Med* 1987;316:1493–1498.
51. Peters WP, Shpall EJ, Jones RB, et al. High-dose combination alkylating agents with bone marrow support as initial treatment for metastatic breast cancer. *J Clin Oncol* 1988;6:1368–1375.
52. Peters WP, Davis R, Shpall EJ, et al. Adjuvant chemotherapy involving high-dose combination cyclophosphamide, BCNU, and cisplatin with bone-marrow support for stage II/II breast cancer involving ten or more lymph nodes (CALGB 8782): a preliminary report. *Proc Am Soc Clin Oncol* 1990;31:22.
53. Jones RB, Shpall EJ, Shogan J, et al. The Duke AFM program: intensive induction chemotherapy for metastatic breast cancer. *Cancer* 1990;66:431–436.
54. Ozols R, Young R. Chemotherapy of ovarian cancer. *Semin Oncol* 1984;11:251–263.
55. Miller DS, Balloon SC, Terry N, Seifer D, Soriero O. A critical assessment of second-look laparatomy in epithelial ovarian cancer. *Cancer* 1986;57:530–535.

CHAPTER 25

Hormone Therapy in Ovarian Cancer

Peter E. Schwartz and Joseph T. Chambers

Endocrine therapy for the management of epithelial ovarian cancers predated the identification of the presence of estrogen, progestin, and androgen receptors in epithelial ovarian cancer specimens. Nevertheless, hormone therapy for this malignancy has not been effective, perhaps due in part to the failure to use it routinely as part of primary therapy. For those few series where patients with epithelial cancer of the ovary were treated primarily with endocrine therapy, well-differentiated endometrioid carcinomas were most likely to be associated with substantial objective response rates. Efforts to combine tamoxifen with primary cytotoxic chemotherapy has failed to demonstrate beneficial effects. The overall failure of current standard treatment to cure advanced epithelial ovarian cancer supports the need to identify alternative therapy such as innovative hormonal manipulation to try to manage this devastating disease.

Hormonal therapy for the management of epithelial ovarian cancer has overwhelmingly been employed for treating refractory disease that has failed conventional surgery, cytotoxic chemotherapy, and radiation therapy. The presence of steroid receptor proteins in epithelial cancers of the ovaries has been well established and suggests therapeutic implications for endocrine therapy (1–47). This report will review the current methods for determining the presence of steroid receptor hormones in epithelial ovarian cancers and the role of endocrine therapy in the management of this disease.

DETERMINATION OF STEROID RECEPTOR PROTEINS

The evaluation of steroid receptor proteins in tissue traditionally has been done using biochemical ligand binding assays. Recently immunohistochemical techniques have been applied to determine their presence in tissue. The biochemical method usually measures the unoccupied receptor in a cytoplasmic fraction. Briefly, after the specimen is homogenized and centrifuged to produce a soluble fraction, the proteins in this cytoplasmic fraction and/or the DNA in the particulate fraction are quantified. The total bound steroid ligand levels are then obtained by incubating an aliquot of the cytosol with the appropriate radiolabeled steroid in order to reach binding equilibrium. Nonspecific bound steroid levels are obtained by simultaneously incubating with an excess of nonradiolabeled competitor. Because of the large concentration of the competitor, the radiolabeled steroid is displaced from the receptor binding sites that are present in a limited number, but not from the high capacity, nonspecific binding sites. Next, in an important step, the separation of the free radioligand from the receptor-bound radioligand is performed using various methods, e.g., sucrose density gradient sedimentation, selective adsorption of unbound steroid on dextran-coated charcoal, adsorption of the steroid-receptor complex, or gel filtration. The receptor binding capacity is calculated by subtracting the level of cytosol nonspecific bound steroid ligand from the total cytosol bound radioligand. The radioactivity associated with specific binding and the specific activity of the radiolabeled steroid are used to determine the steroid receptor levels. The receptor levels are expressed in femtomoles (10^{-15} moles) of radiolabeled steroid bound per milligram of cytosol protein or per milligram of DNA (48). Because of the different methods used in separating the bound and free proteins, the levels of receptor protein reported may vary.

There are limitations in the biochemical method. First, it is not possible to identify the source of the steroid receptor proteins since the specimen may contain both neoplastic and non-neoplastic tissues. Normal ovarian tissue contains receptor proteins coming

---

P. E. Schwartz and J. T. Chambers: Department of Obstetrics and Gynecology, Division of Gynecologic Oncology, Yale University School of Medicine, New Haven, Connecticut 06510

from a variety of cell types, e.g., epithelial cells, stromal cells, and germ cells (49). Also, it is not uncommon for a tumor to exhibit heterogeneity of dedifferentiation. Hence, the biochemical determination on a fragment may depend on the degree of dedifferentiation in the sample, which may not reflect the tumor as a whole. Second, this method measures principally cytoplasmic and unoccupied receptors, while the biological responses are mediated by nuclear receptors. It appears that simultaneous determination of both cytoplasmic and nuclear steroid receptor proteins could provide better information about the integrity of the hormone receptor system and the metabolic events activated by these hormones (50,51). Finally, the biochemical assay uses costly equipment and technician time, requires relatively large amounts of tissue (100 mg or more), and requires storage space for keeping tissue frozen until the assay is performed.

On the other hand, the availability of monoclonal antibodies to human estrogen and progestin receptor proteins and their applicability as immunohistochemical reagents in fresh frozen and formalin-fixed, paraffin-embedded sections has not only provided an opportunity to ascertain the exact localization of the receptors in the cell but has also offered an alternative and potentially more accurate way to perform steroid receptor determinations. Stained tissue is scored in a semi-quantitative method on the basis of a visual estimate of the percentage of tumor cells with positive nuclear staining and an estimate of the intensity of the nuclear staining. Numerous scoring systems have been proposed to weigh these parameters (45–47,52,53). Even though interobserver variability with these semi-quantitative systems has been reported as minimal (52), the use of an automated scale to visually assess immunostains has been recommended (54,55). The use of computerized image analysis may make such quantifications more objective but increases the cost and may make this technique less available in small laboratories. There are several advantages to the immunohistochemical method. It is more specific in measuring the receptor status of the individual tumor cells. Furthermore, the ability to use formalin-fixed, paraffin-embedded tissue enables determination of the receptor status on older specimens. Tissue composition is less a problem since the pathologist verifies both the source of the staining and the histological nature and composition of the specimen.

Comparisons of these biochemical and immunohistochemical methods have been reported for breast cancer, endometrial cancer, and in a few recent investigations for ovarian cancer. Parl and Posey (56) carefully outlined the possible explanation for discrepancies between these techniques in an extensive review article (56). When the biochemical analysis is positive but the immunohistochemical is negative, the fixative may have altered the antigenic site of the protein receptor and thus, immunohistochemically, the stain is negative (57). A delay in handling of the specimen may lead to a partial proteolysis of the tissue, consequently interfering with the immunohistochemical assay (58). The monoclonal antibodies may not be sensitive enough to recognize the molecular heterogeneity of the receptor (56). It may be that the nonmalignant component of the tissue contains the receptor that is correctly identified by the immunohistochemical stain. On the other hand, the biochemical analysis may be negative but the immunohistochemical analysis positive. If the biochemical assay is measuring an unoccupied receptor, circulating endogenous estrogen may be bound to the receptor, causing the biochemical analysis to be negative, but the immunohistochemical staining will react with the complex and thus be read as positive (59). Alternatively, the tissue may come from a hypocellular tumor that on biochemical analysis gives a low value; however, using the immunohistochemical techniques the specimen is positive (56). Through processing there may be an alteration in the hormonal binding site but a preservation of the immunoreactive epitope for the receptor. Others report there may be a false interpretation of the immunohistochemical analysis because of endogenous peroxidase of leucocytes or monophages present in the specimen (56).

Finally, an important factor to consider is the fact that the cutoff levels chosen for positivity by each method are arbitrary. This will influence the concordance rate between the two methods. Using the biochemically determined values for ovarian cancer, the positive range for estrogen receptor has been defined as from >1 fmol/mg to >35fmol/mg of protein, and the positive range for the progestin receptor as from >1 to >50 fmol/mg of protein (60–62). A similar situation can occur with the immunohistochemical method; the estimated percentage and the intensity of cells may vary with the observer and give different values for this semi-quantitative measure.

In the future, the application of the immunohistochemical method to the determination of steroid receptor status may better explain some of the conflicting clinical pathologic relationships which have been observed in the literature using biochemical determinations.

In the following review, unless otherwise stated, a biochemical method was used to determine the receptor status of the tumor under discussion.

Receptor Status and Clinic-Pathologic Features

Estrogen receptors were initially assayed in breast and then in endometrial cancers. Subsequently, progestin receptors were identified in these cancerous tissues (45,46). Hormonal manipulation of breast cancer may be predicted by the presence of each of these hormone receptors. The progestin receptor protein content of a cell reflects the successful interaction of estrogen with its own receptor (65,66). Quantification of the tumor progestin receptor content has proven to be a sensitive indicator for successful hormonal manipulation of breast cancer and for endometrial cancer (67–75).

In 1978, our laboratory was able to establish the presence of estrogen receptor in 16 of 30 specimens of previously untreated ovarian cancer patients (10). We subsequently identified progestin receptors, as well, in these tumors. However, the receptor content of primary tumors and their metastases were often heterogeneous in this initial series (10).

In an effort to identify whether estrogen receptor and progestin receptor content reflected histologic parameters, an analysis of 113 primary epithelial ovarian cancers was undertaken at Yale University (25). The histologic parameters studied included histologic grade, necrosis, fibrosis, lymphocyte infiltration, mitosis, and the presence of tumor giant cells, psammoma bodies, and stroma. Estrogen receptor content was statistically increased only in poorly differentiated cancers with abundant mitoses (25). Progestin receptor content was statistically associated with an increasing amount of lymphocyte infiltration. Overwhelmingly, it appeared that the estrogen and progestin receptor content of epithelial cancer cells was independent of the histologic parameters examined.

Subsequent studies at Yale University correlated the estrogen and progestin receptor content of epithelial ovarian cancers with patient survival (25). Patients with the International Federation of Gynecologists and Obstetricians (FIGO) stage I and II malignancies had improved survival if the progestin receptor levels were elevated, but the findings were not statistically significant, perhaps due to the low number of patients (twenty-two) in this series. Surprisingly, women with advanced disease (stage III and IV) and greater than 2 cm residual tumor associated with low progestin receptor content (less than 7 fmol/mg cp) did significantly better than those with tumors that contained elevated levels (more than 7 fmol/mg cp) of progestin receptor. Others have found varying correlations between estrogen receptor content and survival, as well as progestin receptor content and survival. For example, no difference in survival was demonstrated by Andrel et al. (31) when tumor samples were assayed for estrogen and progestin receptors. However, Sevelda et al. (41) were able to correlate survival with stage III disease and less than 2 cm residual tumor with progestin receptor content. Univariant analysis suggested an improved survival in another series associated with elevated progestin receptors but this could not be confirmed by multivariant analysis (38). Bizzi et al. (32) found a significant correlation between estrogen receptor content and survival, but was unable to establish more than marginal significance for progestin receptor content and survival. In yet another series, elevated levels of both receptors were associated with better survival (12), while others found no correlation between receptor status and survival (17,24,31).

Ploidy studies have failed to correlate estrogen receptor content with aneuploid or diploid tumors, but progestin receptor protein appears to be most highly expressed by diploid tumors (76,77). This may explain in part why progestin receptor status correlated with survival in some of the above series.

Several recent reports have explored the correlation between immunohistochemically determined steroid receptor protein and the biochemically determined assay in ovarian cancer. In a report by Nardelli et al. (45) of 29 malignant ovarian tumors (including 23 epithelial neoplasms), 72.5% of the cases stained positive for the estrogen receptor protein using immunohistochemical techniques, compared with only 58.8% positive using a biochemical method. Masood (46) evaluated the estrogen receptor status in 45 epithelial ovarian cancers with both methods and found a 91% concordance between the methods, with a 71% positivity for the estrogen receptor protein using immunohistochemical techniques. Kommoss et al. (47) evaluated both the estrogen and progestin receptor proteins in 79 epithelial ovarian cancers and found a 35% positivity for the estrogen receptor protein by immunohistochemistry and 65% by biochemical methods. For the progestin receptor protein, a 31% positivity was found for the estrogen receptor by immunohistochemistry and 66% positivity by biochemical methods.

Two recent abstracts (78,79) using immunohistochemical techniques for identifying estrogen receptor proteins in ovarian cancer have attempted to predict survival based on the positivity of the assay. In the first report (78), it is suggested that patients with nonserous epithelial tumors found to be immunohistochemically positive for estrogen receptor protein had a better prognosis than those with tumors lacking estrogen receptor proteins. In a subsequent report, the same authors used a more sophisticated approach by correcting the biochemically determined estrogen receptor content using immunohistochemical techniques for the percentage of tumor cells present in the specimen. This report showed that a cutoff level could be determined for ovarian serous tumors at which a significant prediction for better survival could be asserted. The authors employed the combined determinations from both techniques to give clinical information about the outcome of the patients with epithelial ovarian cancer depending upon the estrogen receptor proteins in the cancer.

Androgen Receptors

Androgen receptors have been established to be present in six different series to date (80). They have been correlated with the shift in the ratio of androgen to estrogen in postmenopause and with the regulation of androgen receptors by androgen (81). Data suggests that aromatase activity is inversely correlated with androgen receptor positivity (81).

Corticosteroid Receptors

There is only one reported series that has analyzed epithelial ovarian cancer specimens for corticosteroid receptor protein. Twelve of thirteen normal ovaries, two of four benign ovarian tumors, and eight of nine primary ovarian cancers had elevated levels of corticosteroid receptors (3). The therapeutic implications for this observation have yet to be evaluated.

Gonadotropin Receptors

Binding sites for gonadotropic hormones and luteinizing-hormone-releasing hormone (LHRH) have been demonstrated in ovarian tumors (82–84). One investigator has been able to inhibit ovarian cancer cell proliferation in vitro using leuprolide acetate (Lupron), a gonadotropin-releasing hormone agonist (85).

Hormonal Therapy

Progestin Therapy

Progestin therapy has been used for more than thirty years, yet has failed to demonstrate a significant response rate in the management of refractory epithelial ovarian cancers (Table 1). This is almost certainly due to withholding progestins until the patient develops disease that is refractory to standard therapy. Objective response rates vary from 0% to 17% with agents such as 17-alpha-hydroxyprogesterone caproate (Delalutin) (86–88), medroxyprogesterone acetate (Provera) (7,89–95), and megestrol acetate (Megace) (see Table 1) (96,97). Varying responses have been reported when high-dose megestrol acetate has been employed (96). However, most investigators, including ourselves, have failed to establish a role for high-dose Megace in the routine management of refractory epithelial ovarian cancer (97,98).

Progestin therapy as first-line therapy has been reported in three series (Table 2). The most significant series was that of Rendina et al. (95) who studied forty-eight women with endometrioid ovarian cancers, thirty of whom had advanced (stage III or IV) disease. Significantly, twenty-six of the thirty patients had well-differentiated cancers. Three complete and fourteen partial responses were seen in women treated with primary progestin therapy. All patients responding to progestin therapy had cancer that contained elevated levels of estrogen and progestin receptors. Bergqvist observed objective responses to Provera in three patients with mucinous carcinomas (7). Timothy (99) treated fifteen patients with intramuscular gestonorone caproate (Depostat). Seven patients with stage III and IV disease had a median progression-free interval of 12 months (range 9–48 months), two of whom had complete responses lasting 9 and 18 months (99).

The results of primary progestin therapy are difficult to interpret as none of these studies were prospective

TABLE 1. Progestin therapy in refractory ovarian cancer

Study	Year	Progestin[a]	Route of administration	No. of pts.	Response N	%
Jolles	1962	Delalutin	IM	10	1	10
Varga and Henrikson	1964	Delalutin	IM	6	1	17
Ward	1972	Delalutin	IM	23	3	13
Kaufman	1966	Provera	PO	11	1	9
Malkasian et al.	1977	Provera	PO	19	1	5
Mangioni et al.	1981	Provera	PO	30	0	0
Aabo et al.	1982	Provera	PO	27	1	4
Slayton, Paygano, and Creech	1981	Provera	IM	19	0	0
Mangioni et al.	1981	Provera	IM	33	5	15
Trope et al.	1982	Provera	IM	25	1	4
Geisler	1985	Megace	PO	31	10	32
Ahlgren et al.	1985	Megace	PO	26	1	4
Malkasian et al.	1985	NSC 123018	PO	9	2	22

From Jolles, ref. 86; Varga and Henrikson, ref. 87; Ward, ref. 88; Kaufman, ref. 89; Malkasian et al., ref. 90; Mangioni et al., ref. 91; Aabo et al., ref. 92; Slayton, Paygano, and Creech, ref. 93; Trope et al., ref. 94; Giesler, ref. 96; Ahlgren et al., ref. 97.
[a] Delalutin, 17-alpha-hydroxyprogesterone caproate; Provera, medroxyprogesterone acetate; Megace, megestrol acetate; NSC 123018, 6-alpha-dimethylprogesterone; IM, intramuscular; PO, per os (by mouth); N, number of patients responding; %, percent of patients responding.

TABLE 2. *Progestin therapy in previously untreated ovarian cancer*

Study	Year	Progestin[a]	Route of administration	Response		
				No. of pts.	N	%
Bergqvist et al.	1981	Provera	IM	4	3	75
Rendina et al.	1982	Provera	IM	31[b]	17	55
Timothy	1982	Depostat	IM	7[c]	3	43

From Bergqvist et al., ref. 7; Rendina et al., ref. 95; Timothy, ref. 99.
[a] Provera, medroxyprogesterone acetate; Depostat, gestonorone caproate.
[b] Each patient had an endometrioid ovarian carcinoma.
[c] Stage III/IV.
IM, intramuscular; N, number of patients responding; %, percent of patients responding.

randomized studies and patient selection criteria are not clear. The study done by Rendina et al. (95) was unique in that so many patients had well-differentiated endometrioid carcinomas.

Estrogen Therapy

Diethylstilbestrol therapy has been used in one series of patients with refractory cancer (100). Two of nine patients in this series apparently had objective responses lasting more than one year. An additional five patients were lost to follow-up. Small numbers and lack of objective response criteria make it a difficult study to evaluate.

Estrogen and Progestin Therapy

A combination of ethinyl estradiol and medroxyprogesterone acetate has been reported in the management of recurrent ovarian cancer, with nine of sixty-five patients experiencing an objective response (101,102). Reduction in ethinyl estradiol dose was necessary because of severe nausea associated with the treatment regimen.

Tamoxifen Therapy

Tamoxifen citrate (Nolvadex), an estrogen agonist-antagonist, was initially investigated in the management of patients with refractory ovarian cancer at Yale University based on our studies that demonstrated the presence of estrogen receptor protein in epithelial ovarian cancers (103). In a preliminary trial of thirteen patients with refractory disease, four had stabilization of rapidly advancing disease that lasted eleven to thirty weeks, and one had a partial remission (103). Other investigators have followed this program and established similar response rates (Table 3) (104–110). Generally, stabilization of disease has been observed for periods of three to eleven months. A Gynecologic Oncology Group study revealed an 17% objective response rate (ten complete, eight partial responses) in a group of 105 women with refractory ovarian cancers

TABLE 3. Tamoxifen therapy in recurrent ovarian cancer

Study	Year	Daily dosage	No. of pts.	Response			
				CR	PR	S	%
Schwartz et al.	1982	20+ mg	13	0	1	4	7.7
Pagel et al.	1983	NS	29	1	7	12	27.6
Hamerlynck et al.	1985	40 mg	18	0	1	2	5.6
Shirley et al.	1985	20 mg to 40 mg	23	0	0	19	0
Slevin et al.	1986	40 mg	22	0	0	1	0
Weiner et al.	1987	20 mg	37	1	2	6	8.1
Osborne et al.	1988	100 mg/m^2 × 1, 40 mg	53	0	1	5	1.9
Hatch et al.	1991	40 mg	105	10	8	40	17.1
Summary			300	12	20	89	10.7

From Schwartz et al., ref. 103; Pagel et al., ref. 105; Hamerlynck et al., ref. 108; Shirley et al., ref. 107; Slevin et al., ref. 104; Weiner et al., ref. 110; Osborne et al., ref. 109; Hatch et al., ref. 111.
NS, not specified; CR, complete response; PR, partial response; S, stable disease; %, percentage CR and PR to total number of patients treated.

treated with 20 mg tamoxifen twice a day (111). No correlation has been observed between those few patients with objective responses and the histologic grade of the malignancy.

Tamoxifen and Progestin Therapy

Two studies have now combined cyclic tamoxifen with progestin therapy (112,113). No objective responses to therapy have been identified to date, although stabilization of disease for four to sixteen months has been reported (113).

Tamoxifen Combined with Cytotoxic Chemotherapy

One hundred patients with stage III or IV epithelial ovarian cancers were initially treated with either doxorubicin hydrochloride (Adriamycin) and cisplatin (N = 51) or tamoxifen, Adriamycin, and cisplatin (N = 49) in a prospective randomized trial to determine whether the addition of tamoxifen to standard cytotoxic chemotherapy could prolong progression-free or overall survival (114). Unfortunately, no survival advantage accrued to those patients who received the tamoxifen, and no correlation could be made regarding steroid hormone receptor content and response to the tamoxifen, Adriamycin, and cisplatin treatment. Others have tried this strategy as well without identifying a survival advantage for the patient treated with tamoxifen and cytotoxic chemotherapy (31).

Progestins Combined with Cytotoxic Chemotherapy

Twenty-eight of thirty-three patients received melphalan and medroxyprogesterone acetate in the management of ovarian cancers in one series (7). Reportedly, twenty-eight patients responded to treatment, but the treatment details were incomplete (7). A subsequent report failed to demonstrate objective responses in five women with advanced ovarian cancer who received the combination of medroxyprogesterone acetate and cytotoxic chemotherapy (115).

Androgen Therapy

Two studies looking at androgen therapy for management of refractory ovarian cancer have failed to demonstrate objective responses (116,117).

Antiandrogen Therapy

Antiandrogen therapy is currently being evaluated by the EORTC Gynecologic Cancer Cooperative Group. This study is based on the observation that antiandrogens have an antiproliferative effect in ovarian cancer cell lines that are androgen receptor positive. Clinical trial results are not yet available (118).

LHRH Agonist

Scant data is available supporting the role of LHRH agonists in the management of epithelial ovarian cancer (Table 4) (119–124). There is a suggestion however, that women with histologically well-differentiated epithelial ovarian cancers may be most likely to respond to these agents (122). Overall duration of response of LHRH agonists in these series varies from 6 to 24 months, perhaps reflecting the natural history of well-differentiated tumors that grow slowly.

Corticosteroid Therapy

Only one series of eight patients with refractory ovarian cancer has been reported to specifically receive corticosteroid therapy for the management of their disease (116). No objective responses were observed.

TABLE 4. Gonadotropin-releasing hormone analogues in refractory ovarian cancer

Study	Year	Analogue	No. of pts.	Response CR	PR	S	%
Parmar et al.	1988	D-Trp-6 LHRH	39	0	6	5	15.4
Kavanagh et al.	1989	Leuprolide acetate[a]	23	0	4	2	17.4
Bruckner et al.	1989	Leuprolide acetate[a]	5	1	2	2	60.0
Summary			67	1	12	9	19.4

From Parmar et al., ref. 121; Kavanagh et al., ref. 122; Bruckner et al., ref. 124.
CR, complete response; PR, partial response; S, stable disease; %, percentage CR and PR to total number of patients treated; LHRH, luteinizing-hormone-releasing hormone.
[a] Dosage, 1 mg subcutaneously q.d. (daily).

CONCLUSION

The development of immunohistochemical techniques and their application to determining the steroid receptor status of ovarian cancer may identify a subpopulation of patients in whom the cancer is truly influenced by hormones and for whom the addition of endocrine therapy in their treatment may effect the outcome. However, the currently available clinical response data for hormonal therapy has been generated almost invariably in women with refractory ovarian cancers unlikely to respond to virtually any form of treatment. The few prospective randomized trials would suggest that progestin therapy may be effective for women with well-differentiated ovarian endometrioid carcinomas. Assessment of innovative hormonal therapy as part of the initial management of epithelial ovarian cancer must continue.

REFERENCES

1. Schwartz PE, Eisenfeld A. Steroid receptor proteins in epithelial ovarian cancer. Proceedings of the Ninth Annual Meeting of the Felix Rutledge Society. Washington, DC: June 21–24, 1978.
2. Holt JA, Caputo TA, Kelly KM, Greenwald P, Chorost S. Estrogen and progestin binding in cytosols of ovarian adenocarcinomas. *Obstet Gynecol* 1979;53:50.
3. Galli MC, DeGiovanni C, Nicolette G, Grilli S, Nanni P, Prodi G, Gola G, Rochetta R, Orcanda C. The occurrence of multiple steroid hormone receptors in disease-free and neoplastic human ovary. *Cancer* 1981;47:1297.
4. Creasman WT, Sasso RA, Weed JC, McCarty KS Jr. Ovarian carcinoma: histologic and clinical correlation of cytoplasmic estrogen and progesterone binding. *Gynecol Oncol* 1981;12:319.
5. Holt JA, Lyttle R, Lorincz MA, Stern SD, Press MF, Herbst AL. Estrogen receptor and peroxidase activity in epithelial ovarian carcinomas. *J Natl Cancer Inst* 1981;67:307.
6. Janne O, Kauppila A, Syrjala P, Vihko R. Comparison of cytosol estrogen and progestin receptor status in malignant and benign tumors and tumor-like lesions of the human ovary. *Int J Cancer* 1980;25:175.
7. Bergqvist A, Kullander S, Thorell J. A study of estrogen and progesterone cytosol receptor concentration in benign and malignant ovarian tumors treated with medroxyprogesterone acetate. *Acta Obstet Gynecol Scand* 1981;101[Suppl]:75.
8. Hamilton TC, Davies P, Griffith SK. Androgen and oestrogen binding in cytosols of human ovarian tumors. *J Endocrinol* 1981;90:421.
9. Hahnel R, Kelsall GRH, Martin JD, Masters AM, McCarthy AJ, Twaddle E. Estrogen and progesterone receptors in tumors of the human ovary. *Gynecol Oncol* 1982;13:145.
10. Schwartz PE, Livolsi VA, Hildreth N, MacLusky NJ, Naftolin FN, Eisenfeld AJ. Estrogen receptors in ovarian epithelial carcinoma. *Obstet Gynecol* 1982;59:229.
11. Quinn MA, Pearce P, Rome R, Funder JW, Fortune D, Pepperell RJ. Cytoplasmic steroid receptor in ovarian tumors. *Br J Obstet Gynaecol* 1982;89:754.
12. Kauppila A, Vierikko P, Kivien S, Stenback F, Vihko R. Clinical significance of estrogen and progestin receptors in ovarian cancer. *Obstet Gynecol* 1983;61:320.
13. Ford LC, Berek JS, Lagasse LD, Hackler NF, Heins Y, Malkasian F, Leuchter RS, DeLange RJ. Estrogen and progesterone receptors in ovarian neoplasms. *Gynecol Oncol* 1983;15:299.
14. Leibach S, Miller N, Slayton RE, Braham J, Miller A, Wilbanks G, Dunne C. Hormone receptors in ovarian carcinoma. *Proc Am Assoc Cancer Res* 1983;24:176.
15. Pollow K, Schmidt-Matthiesen A, Hoffman G, Schweikhart G, Krienberg R, Manz B, Grill HJ. ^{3}H-Estradiol and ^{3}H-R5020 binding in cytosols of normal and neoplastic human ovarian tissue. *Int J Cancer* 1983;31:603.
16. Spona J, Gitsch E, Salzer H, Karrer K. Estrogen- and gestagen-receptors in ovarian carcinoma. *Gynecol Oncol Invest* 1983;16:189.
17. Teuful G, Geyer H, DeGregorio G, Fuchs A, Kleine W, Pfleiderer A. Oestrogen and Progesteronereziptoren in malignan Ovarialtumoren. *Geburtshilfe Frauenheilkd* 1983;43:732.
18. Vierikko P, Kauppila A, Vihko R. Cytosol and nuclear estrogen and progestin receptors and 17 beta-hydroxysteroid dehydrogenase of the human ovary. *Int J Cancer* 1983;32:413.
19. Willcocks D, Toppila M, Hudson CN, Tyler WP, Baird PJ, Eastman CJ. Estrogen and progesterone receptors in human ovarian tumors. *Gynecol Oncol* 1983;16:246.
20. Wurz H, Wassner E, Citoler P, Schulz KD, Kaiser R. Multiple cytoplasmic steroid hormone receptors in benign and malignant ovarian tumors and in disease-free ovaries. *Tumor Diagn Ther* 1983;4:15.
21. Geyer H, Teuful G, DeGregorio G, Pfleiderer A. Steroidhormone-Rezeptoren beim Ovarialkarzinom und ihre klinische Bedeutung. *Onkologie* 1984;7[Suppl 2]:44.
22. Grosroos M, Kangras L, Maenpaa J, Vanharanta R, Paul R. Steroid receptor and response of ovarian cancer to hormone in vitro. *Br J Obstet Gynaecol* 1984;91:472.
23. Lantta M. Estradiol and progesterone receptors in normal ovaries and ovarian tumors. *Acta Obstet Gynecol Scand* 1984;63:497.
24. Richman CM, Holt JA, Lorincz MA, Herbst AL. Persistence and distribution of estrogen receptor in advanced epithelial ovarian carcinoma after chemotherapy. *Obstet Gynecol* 1985;65:257.
25. Schwartz PE, Merino MJ, LiVolsi VA, Lawrence R, MacLusky N, Eisenfeld A. Histopathologic correlations of estrogen and progestin receptor protein in epithelial ovarian carcinomas. *Obstet Gynecol* 1985;66:428.
26. Inverson O-E, Skarrland E, Utaaker E. Steroid receptor content in human ovarian tumors: survival of patients with ovarian carcinoma related to steroid receptor content. *Gynecol Oncol* 1986;23:65.
27. Sutton GP, Senior MB, Strauss JF, Mikuta JJ. Estrogen and progesterone receptors in epithelial ovarian malignancies. *Gynecol Oncol* 1986;23:176.
28. Toppila M, Tyler JPP, Fay R, Baird PJ, Craindon AJ, Eastman CJ, Hudson CN. Steroid receptors in human ovarian malignancy: a review of four years tissue collection. *Br J Obstet Gynaecol* 1986;93:986.
29. Kuhnel R, de Graaff J, Rao BR, Stolk JG. Androgen receptor predominance in human ovarian carcinoma. *J Steroid Biochem* 1987;26:393.
30. Kuhnel R, Delemarre JFM, Rao BR, Stolk JG. Correlation of multiple steroid receptors with histological type and grade in human ovarian cancer. *Int J Gynecol Pathol* 1987;6:248.
31. Andrel P, Fuith LC, Daxenbickler G, Marth C, Dapunt O. Correlation between steroid hormone receptors, histological and clinical parameters in ovarian carcinoma. *Gynecol Obstet Invest* 1988;25:135.
32. Bizzi A, Codegoni AM, Landoni F, Marelli G, Mansoni S, Spina AM, Torri W, Mangioni C. Steroid receptors in epithelial ovarian carcinoma: relation to clinical parameters and survival. *Cancer Res* 1988;48:6222.
33. Jakobsen A, Hansen V, Poulsen HS. DNA profile and steroid receptor content in ovarian cancer. *Eur J Gynaecol Oncol* 1988;9:461.
34. Nestok BR, Massod S, Lammert N. Correlation of hormone receptors with histologic differentiation in ovarian carcinoma. *J Fla Med Assoc* 1988;75:731.
35. Massod S. The potential value of imprint cytology in cytochemical localization of steroid hormone receptors in ovarian cancer. *Diagn Cytopathol* 1988;4:42.
36. Friedlander ML, Quinn MA, Fortune D, Foor MS, Toppila M,

Hudson CN, Russell P. The relationship of steroid receptor expression to nuclear DNA distribution and clinicopathological characteristics in epithelial ovarian tumors. *Gynecol Oncol* 1989;32:184.
37. Slotman BJ, Kuhnel R, Rao BR, Dijkhuizen GH, de Graaff J, Stolk JG. Importance of steroid receptors and aromatase activity in the prognosis of ovarian cancer: high tumor progesterone receptor levels correlate with longer survival. *Gynecol Oncol* 1989;33:76.
38. Harding M, Cowan S, Hole D, Cassidy L, Kitchener H, Davis J, Leake R. Estrogen and progesterone receptors in ovarian cancer. *Cancer* 1990;65:486.
39. Rao BR, Slotman BJ, Geldof AA, Dinjens WNM. Correlation between steroid receptors, tumor histology and adenosine deaminase complexing protein immunoreactivity in ovarian cancer. *Int J Gynecol Pathol* 1990;9:47.
40. Glavind K, Grove A. Estrogen and progesterone receptors in epithelial ovarian tumors. *Acta Pathol Scand* 1990;98:916.
41. Sevelda P, Denison U, Schemper M, Spona J, Vaura N, Salzer H. Oestrogen and progesterone receptor content as a prognostic factor in advanced epithelial ovarian carcinoma. *Brit J Obstet Gynaecol* 1990;97:706.
42. Slotman BJ, Nauta JJP, Rao BR. Survival of patients with ovarian cancer: apart from stage and grade, tumor progesterone receptor content is a prognostic indicator. *Cancer* 1990;66:740.
43. Rose PG, Peale FR, Longcope C, Hunter RE. Prognostic significance of estrogen and progesterone receptors in epithelial ovarian cancer. *Obstet Gynecol* 1990;76:258.
44. Harding M, Cowan S, Hole D, Cassidy L, Kitchener H, Davis J, Leake R. Estrogen and progesterone receptors in ovarian cancer. *Cancer* 1990;65:486.
45. Nardelli GB, Lamaina V, DaiPozzo M, Onnis GL. Determination of ER in ovarian cancer using monoclonal antibody technology. *Clin Exp Obstet Gynecol* 1987;3:185.
46. Masood S. Use of monoclonal antibodies in immunocytochemical localization of estrogen receptors in ovarian cancer. *Cancer Detect Prev* 1988;12:283.
47. Kommoss F, Pfisterer J, Geyer H, Thome M, Sauerberi W, Pfleiderer A. Estrogen and progesterone receptors in ovarian neoplasms: discrepant results of immunohistochemical and biochemical methods. *Int J Gynecol Cancer* 1991;1:147.
48. Milewich L. Steroid hormone receptors in gynecologic and mammary neoplasms. In: Buchsbaum HJ, Sciarra JJ, eds. *Gynecology and Obstetrics*. Hegerstown: Harper and Row, Inc. 1987;3–4.
49. Press MG, Holt JA, Herbst AL, Greene GL. Immunocytochemical identification of estrogen receptor in ovarian carcinomas: localization with monoclonal estrophilin antibodies compared with biochemical assays. *Lab Invest* 1985;53:349.
50. Welshons WV, Lieberman ME, Gorski J. Nuclear localization of unoccupied oestrogen receptors. *Nature* 1984;307:745.
51. Nardone FDC, Benedetto MT, Rossiello F, et al. Hormone receptor status in human endometrial adenocarcinoma. *Cancer* 1989;64:3572.
52. McCarty KS Jr, Miller LS, Cox EB, et al. Estrogen receptor analyses: correlation of biochemical and immunohistochemical methods using monoclonal antireceptor antibodies. *Arch Pathol Lab Med* 1985;109:716.
53. Carcangiu ML, Chambers JT, Voynick IM, et al. Immunohistochemical evaluation of estrogen and progesterone receptor content in 183 patients with endometrial carcinoma. I: Clinical and histologic correlations. *Am J Clin Pathol* 1990;94:247.
54. Bacus S, Flowers JL, Press MF, et al. The evaluation of estrogen receptor in primary breast carcinoma by computer-assisted image analysis. *Am J Clin Pathol* 1988;90:233.
55. Charpin C, Martin PM, DeVictor B, et al. Multiparametrics study (SAMBA 200) of estrogen receptor immunocytochemical assay in 400 human breast carcinomas: analysis of estrogen receptor distribution heterogeneity in tissues and correlations with dextran coated charcoal assays and morphological data. *Cancer Res* 1988;48:1578.
56. Parl F, Posey Y. Discrepancies of the biochemical and immunohistochemical estrogen receptor assays in breast cancer. *Hum Pathol* 1988;19:960.
57. Press M, Greene G. An immunocytochemical method for demonstrating estrogen receptor in human uterus using monoclonal antibodies to human estrophilin. *Lab Invest* 1984;50:480.
58. Pousette A, Gustafsson S, Thornblad A, et al. Quantification of estrogen receptor in seventy-five specimens of breast cancer: comparison between an immunoassay (Abbott ER-EIA monoclonal) and a [-^{3}H] estradiol binding assay based on isoelectric focusing in polyacrylamide gel. *Cancer Res* 1986;46:4308s.
59. Sarrif AM, Durant JR. Evidence that estrogen-receptor-negative, progesterone-receptor-positive breast and ovarian carcinomas contain estrogen receptor. *Cancer* 1981;48:1215.
60. Toppila M, Tyler JPP, Fay R, et al. Steroid receptors in human ovarian malignancy: a review of four years tissue collection. *Br J Obstet Gynaecol* 1986;93:986.
61. Richman CM, Holt JA, Lorincz MA, Herbst AL. Persistence and distribution of estrogen receptor in advanced epithelial ovarian carcinoma after chemotherapy. *Obstet Gynecol* 1985;65:257.
62. Sutton GP, Senior MB, Strauss JF, Mikuta JJ. Estrogen and progesterone receptors in epithelial ovarian malignancies. *Gynecol Oncol* 1986;23:176.
63. Jensen EV, Smith S, DeSombre ER. Hormone dependency in breast cancer. *J Steroid Biochem* 1976;7:911.
64. Knight WA, Livington RB, Gregory EJ, McGuire WL. Estrogen receptors as an independent prognostic factor for early recurrence in breast cancer. *Cancer Res* 1977;37:4669.
65. Horwitz KB, McGuire WL, Pearson OH, Segaloff A. Predicting response to endocrine therapy in human breast cancer: a hypothesis. *Science* 1975;189:726.
66. Fisher B, Redmond C, Brown A, et al. Influence of tumor estrogen and progesterone receptor levels on the response to tamoxifen and chemotherapy in primary breast cancer. *J Clin Oncol* 1983;1:227.
67. Kelley R, Baker WH. Progestational agents in the treatment of carcinoma of the endometrium. *N Engl J Med* 1961;264:216.
68. Ehrlich CE, Young PEM, Clearly RE. Cytoplasmic progesterone and estradiol in normal, hyperplastic and carcinomatosis endometria: therapeutic implications. *Am J Obstet Gynecol* 1981;141:539.
69. Martin PM, Rolland PH, Gammerre M, Serment H, Toga M. Estradiol and progesterone receptors in normal neoplastic endometrium: correlations between receptors, histopathological examination and clinical responses under progestin therapy. *Int J Cancer* 1979;23:321.
70. Bernard TJ, Friberg LG, Koenders AJM, Kullander S. Do estrogen and progesterone receptors (E_2R and PR) in metastasizing endometrial cancers predict the response to gestagen therapy? *Acta Obstet Gynecol Scand* 1980;59:155.
71. McGuire WL, Clark GM. The prognostic role of progesterone receptors in human breast cancer. *Semin Oncol* 1983;10[Suppl 4]:2.
72. Saez S, Chouvet C, Mayer M, Cheix F. Estradiol and progesterone receptor as prognostic factors in human primary breast tumors. Proceedings of AACR and ASCO: San Diego, May 28–31, 1980, p. 139.
73. Pichon MF, Paullud C, Brunet M, Milgrom E. Relationship of presence of progesterone receptors to prognosis in early breast cancer. *Cancer Res* 1980;40:3357.
74. Hubay CA, Pearson OH, Marshall JS, Stellato TA, Rhodes RS, DeBanne AM, Rosenblatt J, Mansour EG, Hermann RE, Jones JC, Flynn WJ, Eckert C, McGuire WL. Adjuvant therapy of stage II breast cancer: 48-month follow-up of a prospective randomized clinical trial. *Breast Cancer Res Treat* 1981;1:72.
75. Ehrich CE, Young PCM, Cleary RE. Progesterone receptor (PR) as a marker of progestin responsive human endometrial cancer. In: Witliff JL, Dapunt O, eds. *Steroid Receptors and Hormone-Dependent Neoplasia*. New York: Masson Publishing USA Inc.; 1980:95–100.
76. Slotman BJ, Baak JPA, Rao BR. Correlation between nuclear DNA and steroid receptor status in ovarian cancer. *Eur J Obstet Gynecol Reprod Biol* 1990;38:221.
77. Friedlander ML, Quinn MA, Fortune D, Foo MS, Toppila M, Hudson CN, Russel P. The relationship of steroid receptor expression to nuclear DNA distribution and clinicopathological

characteristics in epithelial ovarian tumors. *Gynecol Oncol* 1989;32:184.
78. Kieback DG, McCamant SK, Atkinson EN, Hajek RA, Edwards CL, Gallagher HS, Press, Jones LA. The impact of the histologic composition of tumor specimen on the prognostic significance of estrogen receptor assays in human ovarian cancer. *Meeting of Society of Gynecologic Investigation.* San Antonio, Texas: March 20–23, 1991;304.
79. Kieback DG, Press MF, McCamant SK, Atkinson EN, Edwards CL, Gallagher HS, Jones LA. Composition adjusted receptor level (CARL) for the estrogen receptor: a linear predictor of survival in serous ovarian carcinoma. *Meeting of the Endocrine Society.* Washington, D.C.: June 19–22, 1991, 428.
80. Friberg LG, Kullander S, Persijn JP, Korsten CB. On receptors for estrogen (E_2) and androgens (DHT) in human endometrial carcinoma and ovarian tumors. *Acta Obstet Gynecol Scand* 1978;57:261–264.
81. Kuhnel R, Delemarre JFM, Rao BR, Stolk JG. Correlation of aromatase activity and steroid receptors in human ovarian carcinoma. *Anticancer Res* 1989;6:889.
82. Kammerman S, Demopoulos RI, Raphael C, Ross J. Gonadotropin hormone binding to human ovarian tumors. *Hum Pathol* 1981;12:886.
83. Rajaniemi H, Kauppila A, Ronnberg L, Selander K, Pystynen P. LH (hCG) receptor in benign and malignant tumors of the human ovary. *Acta Obstet Gynecol Scan [Suppl]:* 1981;101:83.
84. Emons G, Pahwa GS, Brack C, Sturm R, Oberheuser F, Knuppen R. Gonadotropin releasing hormone binding sites in human epithelial ovarian carcinomata. *Eur J Cancer Clin Oncol* 1989;25:215.
85. Thompson MA, Adelson MD, Kaufman LM. Lupron retards proliferation of ovarian epithelial tumor cells cultured in serum-free medium. *J Clin Endocrinol Metab* 1991;72:1036.
86. Jolles B. Progesterone in the treatment of advanced malignant tumors of breast, ovary and uterus. *Br J Cancer* 1962;16:209–221.
87. Varga A, Henriksen E. Effect of 17-alpha-hydroxyprogesterone 17-n-caproate on various pelvic malignancies. *Obstet Gynecol* 1964;23:51.
88. Ward HW. Progestogen therapy for ovarian carcinoma. *J Obstet Gynaecol Br Commonw* 1972;79:555.
89. Kaufman RJ. Management of advanced ovarian carcinoma. *Med Clin North Am* 1966;50:845.
90. Malkasian GD, Decker DG, Jorgensen EO, Edmonson JH. Medroxyprogesterone acetate for the treatment of metastatic and recurrent ovarian carcinoma. *Cancer Treat Rep* 1977;61:913.
91. Mangioni C, Franceschi S, LaVecchia C, D'Incalci M. High-dose medroxyprogesterone acetate (MPA) in advanced epithelial ovarian cancer resistant to first- or second-line chemotherapy. *Gynecol Oncol* 1981;12:314.
92. Aabo K, Pedersen AG, Hald I, Dombernowski P. High-dose medroxyprogesterone acetate (MPA) in advanced chemotherapy-resistant ovarian carcinoma: a phase II study. *Cancer Treat Rep* 1982;66:407.
93. Slayton RE, Pagnano M, Creech RH. Progestin therapy for advanced ovarian cancer: a phase II Eastern Cooperative Group trial. *Cancer Treat Rep* 1981;65:895.
94. Trope C, Johnson JE, Sigurdsson K, Simonson E. High-dose medroxyprogesterone acetate for the treatment of advanced ovarian carcinoma. *Cancer Treat Rep* 1982;66:1441.
95. Rendina GM, Donadio C, Giovannini M. Steroid receptors and progestinic therapy in ovarian endometrioid carcinoma. *Eur J Gynaecol Oncol* 1982;3:241–246.
96. Geisler HE. The use of high-dose megestrol acetate in the treatment of ovarian adenocarcinoma. *Semin Oncol* 1985;12:20.
97. Ahlgren JD, Thomas D, Ellison N, Huberman M, Harvey J, Freeman A, Wilcosky T, Gillings D, Zaloudek C, Browder H, Noble S. Phase II evaluation of high-dose megestrol acetate in advanced refractory ovarian cancer (abst). *Proceedings of the Am Soc of Clin Oncol* 1985;4:124.
98. Schwartz PE, Eisenfeld AJ, MaclUsky NJ, Lazo JS, Hochberg RB, Naftolin FN. Hormonal therapy for epithelial ovarian cancer. In: Rutledge FN, Freeman RS, Gershenson DM, eds. *Gynecologic Cancer: diagnosis and treatment strategies, 1987.* Austin: University of Texas Press; 91.
99. Timothy I. Progestogen therapy for ovarian carcinoma. *Br J Obstet Gynaecol* 1982;89:561.
100. Long RTL, Evans AM. Diethylstilbestrol as a chemotherapeutic agent for ovarian carcinoma. *Mo Med* 1963;60:1125.
101. Jolles CJ, Freedman RS, Jones LA. Estrogen and progestogen therapy in advanced cancer: preliminary report. *Gynecol Oncol* 1983;16:352.
102. Freedman RS, Saul PB, Edwards CL, Jolles CJ, Gershenson DM, Jones LA, Atkinson N, Dana WJ. Ethinyl estradiol and medroxyprogesterone acetate in patients with epithelial ovarian carcinoma: a phase II study. *Cancer Treat Rep* 1986;70:369.
103. Schwartz PE, Keating G, MacLusky N, Naftolin FN, Eisenfeld A. Tamoxifen therapy for advanced ovarian cancer. *Eur J Cancer Oncol* 1982;59:583.
104. Slevin ML, Harvey VJ, Osborne RJ, Shepard JH, Williams CJ, Mead GM. A phase II study of tamoxifen in ovarian cancer. *Eur J Cancer Clin Oncol* 1986;22:309.
105. Pagel J, Rose C, Thorpe S, Hald I. Treatment of advanced ovarian carcinoma with tamoxifen: a phase II trial (abst). *Proceedings of the Second European Conference on Clinical Oncology.* Amsterdam: 5,1983.
106. Myers AM, Moore GE, Major FJ. Advanced ovarian carcinoma: response to antiestrogen therapy. *Cancer* 1981;48:2368.
107. Shirley ER, Kavanagh JJ, Gershenson DM, Freedman RS, Copeland LJ, Jones LA. Tamoxifen therapy of epithelial ovarian cancer. *Obstet Gynecol* 1985;66:575.
108. Hamerlynck JVTH, Vermorken JB, van der Burg MEL, ten Bokkel Huinink WW, Neijt JP, Carino F, Mangioni C, Rotmensz N, Veenhof CHN. Tamoxifen therapy in advanced ovarian cancer: a phase II study (abst). *Proc Am Soc Clin Oncol* 1985;4:115.
109. Osborne RJ, Malik S, Slevin ML, Harvey VJ, Spona J, Salzer H, Williams CJ. Tamoxifen in refractory ovarian cancer: the use of a loading dose schedule. *Br J Cancer* 1988;57:115.
110. Weiner SA, Alberts DS, Surwit EA, Davis J, Grosso D. Tamoxifen therapy in recurrent epithelial ovarian cancer. *Gynecol Oncol* 1987;27:208.
111. Hatch KD, Beecham JB, Blessing JA, Creasman WT. Responsiveness of patients with advanced ovarian carcinoma to tamoxifen: a gynecologic oncology group study of second-line therapy in 105 patients. *Cancer* 1991;68:269.
112. Jakobsen AJ, Bertelsen K, Sell A. Cyclic hormone treatment in ovarian cancer: a phase II trial. *Eur J Cancer Clin Oncol* 1987;23:915.
113. Belinson JL, McClure M, Badger G. Randomized trial of megestrol acetate vs. megestrol acetate/tamoxifen for the management of progressive or recurrent ovarian cancer. *Gynecol Oncol* 1987;28:151.
114. Schwartz PE, Chambers JT, Kohorn EI, Chambers SK, Wertzman H, Voynick IM, MacLusky N, Naftolin FN. Tamoxifen in combination with cytotoxic chemotherapy in advanced epithelial cancer. *Cancer* 1989;63:1074.
115. Kahanpaa KV, Karkkainen J, Nieminen U. Multi-agent chemotherapy with and without medroxyprogesterone acetate in the treatment of advanced ovarian cancer. *Excerpta Medica International Congress Series* 1982;611:477.
116. Kaufman RJ. Management of ovarian carcinoma. *Med Clin North Am* 1966;50:845.
117. Kavanagh JJ, Wharton JT, Roberts WS. Androgen therapy in the treatment of refractory epithelial ovarian cancer. *Cancer Treat Rep* 1987;71:537.
118. Rao BR, Slotman BJ. Endocrine factors in common epithelial ovarian cancer. *Endocrine Rev* 1991;12:14.
119. Parmer H, Micoll J, Stockdale A, Cassoni A, Phillips RH, Lightman SL, Schally AV. Advanced ovarian carcinoma: response to the agonist D-Trp-6-LHRH. *Cancer Treat Rep* 1985;69:1341.
120. Kullander S. LHRH agonist treatment in ovarian cancer. In: *Abstracts International Symposium on hormonal manipulation of cancer: peptides, growth factors and new (anti)steroidal agents.* Rotterdam, The Netherlands, 1986.
121. Parmar H, Rustin G, Lightman SL, Phillips RH, Hanham IW,

Schally AV. Response to D-Trp-6-luteinizing hormone releasing hormone (Decapeptyl) microcapsules in advanced ovarian cancer. *Br Med J* 1988;296:1229.
122. Kavanagh JJ, Roberts W, Twonsend P, Hewitt S. Leuprolide acetate in the treatment of refractory or persistent epithelial ovarian cancer. *J Clin Oncol* 1989;7:115.
123. Jager W, Wildt L, Lang N. Some observations on the effect of a GnRH analog in ovarian cancer. *Eur J Obstet Gynecol Reprod Biol* 1989;32:137.
124. Bruckner HW, Motwani BT. Treatment of advanced refractory ovarian carcinoma with a gonadotropin-releasing hormone analogue. *Am J Obstet Gynecol* 1989;161:1216.

CHAPTER 26

Complications of Chemotherapy

Maurie Markman

The use of cytotoxic chemotherapy in the management of ovarian cancer has resulted in a significant prolongation of survival for the majority of women with the malignancy and, for a smaller subset, the potential for cure. Unfortunately, all antineoplastic agents have side effects. These can range from the production of minimal, short-term interference with the patient's quality of life to severe, self-limited side effects, chronic, treatment-related morbidity, or even death. In this chapter the toxicities of chemotherapy for ovarian cancer will be discussed, along with methods to minimize both the short-term and long-term side effects associated with the use of the agents.

HEMATOLOGIC TOXICITY OF ANTINEOPLASTIC AGENTS

It is well known that one of the major toxicities of antineoplastic agents is their potential for production of bone marrow suppression. This should come as no surprise as bone marrow cells are among the most rapidly dividing in the human body; as such, they would be very susceptible to effects of cytotoxic chemotherapeutic agents.

Some degree of myelosuppression is observed following the administration of most chemotherapeutic drugs. The maximal white blood cell and platelet nadir period generally occurs between 7 and 14 days after drug administration, with complete recovery in the peripheral blood counts by 21 to 28 days following treatment.

There are a number of important exceptions to these general rules. In a patient who has been heavily pretreated with chemotherapy, there may be a considerable delay in marrow recovery. This delay can be measured in weeks and may necessitate considerable modification in second-line treatment strategies. Slow marrow recovery is generally due to cumulative toxicity on the earlier precursor cells present in the marrow.

Patients initially treated with a carboplatin-based regimen appear to be most susceptible to difficulties with bone marrow suppression when treated with second-line salvage chemotherapy programs. This is particularly true when carboplatin is also employed in the second-line treatment strategy. Carboplatin appears to exert a unique influence on marrow precursor cells compared to other drugs standardly used in ovarian cancer; patients treated with this drug in the salvage setting must be watched carefully for the possibility of excessive marrow suppression, particularly for pronounced and prolonged thrombocytopenia.

There are several chemotherapeutic agents which produce a delayed effect on the bone marrow, even when employed in front-line chemotherapy programs. These include the nitrosoureas, mitomycin C and L-phenylalanine mustard. While not commonly used at present in the treatment of ovarian cancer, the delayed bone marrow suppressive effects of these agents should be noted. The nadir may not be observed for three to four weeks following treatment, with complete recovery frequently not demonstrated until five to six weeks after the delivery of therapy.

Several chemotherapeutic agents are characterized by their production of minimal bone marrow cytotoxic effects at the standard dosing schedule. Though cisplatin can produce considerable bone marrow suppression, particularly when used at very high doses and in patients with limited bone marrow reserve, its administration will generally result in only limited bone marrow suppressive effects. This feature of the agent is one of the major reasons it has been so popular in combination chemotherapy regimens when administered with other agents which are far more myelosuppressive. In addition, relative lack of bone marrow suppres-

M. Markman: The Cleveland Clinic Cancer Center and the Department of Hematology/Medical Oncology, The Cleveland Clinic Foundation, Cleveland, Ohio 44195

sion is the only toxicity of cisplatin (ES) severer than that resulting from carboplatin.

MANAGEMENT OF HEMATOLOGIC COMPLICATIONS OF CHEMOTHERAPY

In general, the development of moderate, chemotherapy-associated bone marrow suppression is not a concern. In fact, many investigators recommend that a certain level of marrow suppression be aimed for to avoid the potential of undertreating the malignancy. However, severe bone marrow suppression (granulocyte count less than 1,000/mm^3) can be life-threatening.

If a patient develops fever in the presence of severe granulocytopenia (so-called nadir fever), broad spectrum antibiotics must be administered as soon as possible to prevent a fatal septic event. Most patients tolerate a short period of very low peripheral granulocyte counts remarkably well, even in the presence of fever. Thus, it is generally not necessary to administer prophylactic antibiotics for severe granulocytopenia, but rather only when fever accompanies the marrow suppression. Exceptions to this general rule include patients taking corticosteroids or other agents which may prevent a febrile reaction (e.g., aspirin, acetaminophen), and individuals who are already on antibiotics which may mask the presence of a more serious infectious process.

There is almost never a need to consider white blood cell transfusions in patients with ovarian cancer receiving cytotoxic chemotherapy. Even the most severe degrees of marrow suppression are generally of short duration, and the administration of appropriate broad spectrum antibiotics will allow a patient to get through the period of serious risk until her own granulocytes are able to recover and control any infection.

However, two new agents have been introduced into clinical practice which may significantly alter our approach to dealing with the granulocytopenia associated with chemotherapeutic agents. Both the granulocyte colony-stimulating factor (G-CSF) and the granulocyte-macrophage colony-stimulating factor (GM-CSF) have been shown to be capable of *shortening* the period of nadir following chemotherapy administration, although neither agent can actually prevent the nadir period (1–2).

Thus, it may be possible to significantly increase the intensity of chemotherapy programs for ovarian cancer without producing an unacceptable degree of granulocytopenia. Numerous clinical trials employing these bone marrow colony-stimulating factors are currently in progress. However, it remains to be determined whether the standard use of these new agents can result in an overall improvement in outcome of therapy for patients with ovarian cancer.

For the *individual* patient whose bone marrow will not tolerate the administration of what would be considered a standard chemotherapy dosing program, the administration of the colony-stimulating factors may be the only method available to safely deliver an appropriate dose intensity of chemotherapy for the disease. In general, outside the study setting, chemotherapy should initially be administered without a bone marrow colony-stimulating factor. If excessive marrow toxicity is observed, subsequent treatment courses may be administered with the bone marrow colony-stimulating factor. It must always be remembered that an alternative, and less expensive, approach would be the delivery of a lower dose of the chemotherapeutic drugs without the bone marrow colony-stimulating factor.

Thrombocytopenia is a potentially more serious toxicity than neutropenia. In most patients, fairly severe degrees of thrombocytopenia can be tolerated reasonably well. In general, platelet transfusions are not administered prophylactically (without evidence of bleeding) unless the platelet count is less than 10,000–20,000/mm^3. In patients who have recently undergone a surgical procedure or where there is greater than normal concern for bleeding (e.g., a patient with a large necrotic tumor mass), platelets may be administered prophylactically when the platelet count is less than 50,000/mm^3.

The major difficulty dealing with severe thrombocytopenia is that prediction cannot be made concerning exactly when bleeding will occur and, most importantly, where. Thus, while a large ecchymosis on the skin may not pose much of a hazard to the patient, a bleed into the lung or brain can be fatal. In addition, patients may become refractory to platelet transfusions, particularly individuals who have received numerous blood transfusions in the past, allowing alloimmunization to foreign blood products. Therefore, the use of platelets cannot be guaranteed to successfully get all patients through a period of severe chemotherapy-induced thrombocytopenia.

Unfortunately, neither of the two commercially available bone marrow colony-stimulating factors exert a significant impact on platelet recovery. In fact, the use of higher dose chemotherapy regimens with bone marrow colony-stimulating factor support of the granulocytes will almost certainly lead to the production of thrombocytopenia of greater severity in the treated population. Several of the colony-stimulating factors which have recently entered early phase clinical trials (e.g., interleukin-6) offer greater hope that the severity of thrombocytopenia may be reduced or its duration lessened through stimulation of marrow production of platelet formation.

Recent reports have suggested an alternative method of stimulating platelet recovery after intensive chemotherapy programs. Investigators have noted that the peripheral blood obtained from patients recovering from the bone marrow suppressive effects of cytotoxic chemotherapy contains factors or precursor cells which, when infused back into the patient with a subsequent chemotherapy course, leads to significantly *less* thrombocytopenia or more rapid platelet recovery than would have been anticipated if the infused "factor/cells" had not been employed (3). This platelet stimulatory effect associated with the peripheral blood of patients with recovering blood counts has not been well characterized at present. It also appears that the administration of either G-CSF or GM-CSF during the time of marrow recovery will increase the yield of the platelet stimulatory effect.

For the present, this treatment approach must be considered experimental. In addition, it is expensive and requires the patient to undergo multiple leukaphoreses to obtain the necessary material to reinfuse. However, the demonstrated presence of this platelet stimulatory activity gives hope that other less cumbersome approaches will be developed to prevent severe chemotherapy-induced thrombocytopenia.

Although generally not life-threatening, anemia can be a serious problem associated with both the underlying malignancy and the use of cytotoxic chemotherapy. It is not unusual for patients receiving cisplatin or carboplatin-based therapy for ovarian cancer to experience hemoglobin levels in the range of 7–9 g/dl range. While blood transfusions are generally avoided if possible, patients will frequently require transfusions, particularly if they are scheduled to undergo an elective or emergency laparotomy.

Preliminary evidence suggests that recombinant human erythropoietin may be helpful in both preventing and treating chemotherapy-induced anemia (4,5). There remain limited data in the literature regarding the use of this commercially available drug in patients with malignancy and treatment-related anemia, but it appears clear that patients may benefit from the use of the preparation.

Unfortunately, recombinant human erythropoietin is expensive, particularly if employed throughout the entire course of chemotherapy in a patient with ovarian cancer. It might be most appropriate to consider the use of this drug, outside a study setting, in patients who exhibit particularly severe anemia (e.g., hemoglobin levels less than 7–8 g/dl), where frequent transfusions are necessary, or where a patient's symptoms (e.g., fatigue) appear to be related to the degree of anemia.

A rare hematologic complication of chemotherapy is the development of the hemolytic uremic syndrome, which can be caused by mitomycin (6). In this process patients develop severe anemia caused by hemolysis, thrombocytopenia, and progressive renal insufficiency. Unfortunately, the process is frequently not reversible and there are no measures known which can reliably improve the clinical syndrome.

MUCOSITIS

Like the bone marrow, the epithelial lining of the gastrointestinal tract is highly susceptible to the effects of many cancer chemotherapeutic agents because the mucosal cells have a rapid turnover rate. When mucosal toxicity develops, it can be quite minor, leading to a small number of irritating mouth sores. It can also be severe, potentially leading to the patient's death, due principally to the development of secondary infection.

Mucosal damage can develop anywhere in the gastrointestinal tract, although most often patients will initially develop stomatitis. Loss of the integrity of the mucosal lining is particularly dangerous when the patient is also leukopenic, as these two factors significantly increase the risk of a serious infectious event.

Among chemotherapeutic agents administered to patients with ovarian cancer, doxorubicin is the drug most commonly associated with the development of mucositis. Taxol can also cause significant mucositis.

Management of this complication of chemotherapy is generally supportive. Topical anesthesia (viscous lidocaine) and saline mouthwashes can provide important symptomatic relief. It is also important for the patient receiving cancer chemotherapeutic agents to maintain good oral hygiene, to minimize the risk of serious infection if mucositis should develop.

CHEMOTHERAPY-INDUCED EMESIS

Although not a life-threatening toxic effect of chemotherapy, chemotherapy-induced emesis can have a significant negative impact on the quality of life of individuals receiving cytotoxic therapy. The organoplatinum agents (cisplatin, carboplatin), the most important drugs in the management of ovarian cancer, are among the most emetogenic of the commercially available antineoplastic agents (7).

Experience with the management of this toxicity of cisplatin and carboplatin has led to the important observation that the goal of therapy should be *prevention* of emesis rather than treatment of nausea and vomiting once it has occurred. The major justification for this therapeutic strategy is the development of *anticipatory emesis* in patients who have experienced significant nausea and vomiting with a previous treatment cycle.

Anticipatory emesis can be a serious clinical problem. In patients receiving cisplatin-based systemic therapy, its incidence approaches 100%. While the symptoms of anticipatory emesis will vary, in its most severe form patients may experience significant emesis upon entering the hospital or physician's office prior to the placement of an intravenous line to administer therapy. In some patients the disability associated with this process can lead to their withdrawal from active treatment, despite evidence of an objective response to therapy.

Treatment of anticipatory emesis can be extremely difficult. Lorazepam can reduce anxiety associated with treatment, which may allow a patient to continue with therapy. In individuals with the most severe symptoms of anticipatory emesis, behavioral modification techniques have been employed with some success.

It has recently been recognized that the nausea and vomiting associated with certain chemotherapeutic agents, including cisplatin, is characterized by two distinct patterns: acute and delayed emesis (7). Acute emesis develops during the first 24 hours following chemotherapy administration. Delayed emesis develops more than 24 hours after drug delivery and can persist for several days. Drugs which are utilized to control acute emesis appear to have limited activity in preventing the delayed emetogenic process, leading to the hypothesis that different mechanisms are responsible for the two physiologic processes.

Until recently, metoclopramide had been the standard antiemetic agent employed to prevent cisplatin-induced emesis. The drug was shown in several clinical trails to be effective in either reducing the severity of acute emesis or completely preventing it in 50–70% of patients receiving cisplatin. Unfortunately, metoclopramide can be associated with considerable toxicity, including extrapyridimal side effects, restlessness, anxiety, and diarrhea. Metoclopramide can be administered in several treatment schedules, but one popular regimen calls for the drug to be delivered at a dose of 3 mg/kg every two hours for two doses, starting just prior to cisplatin administration. This regimen allows for the delivery of cisplatin in the outpatient setting.

The recent availability of a new class of agents, the serotonin S-3 receptor antagonists, has significantly improved the therapeutic ratio associated with the use of antiemetic therapy in patients receiving highly emetogenic chemotherapy. It has been hypothesized that serotonin S-3 receptor antagonists block both peripheral and central nervous system signals associated with the emetic process. Of particular importance, this class of agents has no dopaminergic-blocking properties, thus reducing the potential for toxicity.

Several randomized, controlled, double-blind clinical trials have compared ondansetron, the first commercially available serotonin S-3 receptor antagonist, to metoclopramide (8). These studies have confirmed both a *decrease* in the severity of emesis (nausea and vomiting) with ondansetron (compared to metoclopramide) and a striking *reduction* in the incidence of antiemetic-associated side effects, including extrapyrimidal reactions, restlessness, and anxiety.

A recently reported randomized double-blind trial has further suggested that the use of dexamethasone along with ondansetron significantly improves the results of antiemetic therapy in patients receiving cisplatin-based therapy (9). Thus, at the present time, a combination regimen of ondansetron plus dexamethasone would appear to be the most effective antiemetic regimen available for patients receiving highly emetogenic chemotherapy.

Unfortunately, in the only reported clinical trial specifically examining the value of ondansetron in the control/treatment of cisplatin-induced delayed emesis, the agent was shown to be relatively ineffective (8). An oral regimen of metoclopramide plus dexamethasone had previously been demonstrated to produce at least moderate benefit in a subset of patients receiving cisplatin and might be considered a reasonable prophylactic regimen when sending patients home following cisplatin therapy. This regimen calls for metoclopramide to be administered at a dose of 30 mg four times a day for a total of four days following cisplatin administration, with dexamethasone given at 8 mg/day for two days, and 4 mg/day for an additional two days.

In the initial clinical trials of carboplatin, it had been suggested that the drug caused significantly less emesis than cisplatin. While it is probably appropriate to state that overall carboplatin causes less emesis, particularly the development of severe delayed emesis, the newer cytotoxic chemotherapeutic agent can produce considerable discomfort secondary to intense nausea and vomiting (9). Thus, it is important that *all* patients being treated with carboplatin receive the *same* intensive prophylactic antiemetic regimen employed with cisplatin. At the present time this will most probably include the use of ondansetron and dexamethasone.

Although there has been only limited investigation of ondansetron when used in conjunction with carboplatin, it is likely the new antiemetic agent will be at least as effective with carboplatin as it has been shown to be with cisplatin. This is due to the fact that although carboplatin can cause severe acute emesis, delayed emesis is, in general, not as serious a problem with carboplatin as it is with cisplatin. One small study has demonstrated that a significant number of a group of patients experiencing severe emesis secondary to carboplatin were able to receive additional courses of the cytotoxic drug when ondansetron was added to the therapeutic program (10).

Other agents used in the treatment of ovarian cancer can also result in significant emesis, including doxorubicin, ifosfamide and hexamethylmelamine. Hexamethylmelamine-induced emesis is a particular problem, as the agent is administered orally. Agents such as mitomycin, etoposide, tamoxifen, and progestional agents which have been used as salvage therapy in patients with ovarian cancer are generally associated with minimal or no emesis.

NEPHROTOXICITY

Nephrotoxicity is a potentially serious side effect of a number of chemotherapeutic agents, including cisplatin (11). Until recently, the potential renal toxicity of cisplatin was considered to be the dose-limiting side effect of this important antineoplastic drug. Cisplatin-induced nephrotoxicity is dose-related, and its incidence and severity increase with higher total cumulative doses. Rarely, irreversible cisplatin-induced renal insufficiency can develop following a single treatment with the drug, delivered at a standard dose.

The major change in the management of cisplatin administration which has allowed for the safe delivery of this agent has been the recognition that *vigorous hydration* prior to, during, and following cisplatin instillation will markedly reduce the nephrotoxic potential of the agent. Urine output should be closely monitored and maintained at a minimum rate of 100 ml/hr for at least four hours before to four hours after cisplatin delivery. In experimental systems, the use of normal saline has been demonstrated to be superior to either a dextrose and water solution or a hypotonic saline solution in preventing cisplatin-induced renal injury.

The major pathologic finding associated with cisplatin-induced renal insult is tubular damage. A number of tubular abnormalities have been noted, including degeneration of the basement membrane of the tubules, hyaline droplets in the proximal tubules, and tubular necrosis. Glomerular and vascular injury is not observed.

Patients developing cisplatin-induced renal dysfunction may experience a number of abnormalities, including increases in the blood urea nitrogen (BUN) and serum creatinine levels and decreases in serum magnesium, phosphorus, and calcium. Hypomagnesemia, hypophosphatemia, and hypocalcemia are caused by tubular defects which lead to renal wasting.

Hypomagnesemia is particularly common following cisplatin administration, with several series suggesting almost 100% of individuals receiving at least 2–3 cycles of therapy will experience laboratory evidence of hypomagnesemia (11,12). Fortunately, few patients develop clinical symptoms directly attributable to the decreased serum magnesium level. However, it remains uncertain whether some of the nonspecific symptoms commonly ascribed to cisplatin administration (e.g., fatigue, weakness) may at least in part result from the hypomagnesemic state.

Treatment of hypomagnesemia is far from satisfactory. While the serum magnesium level will rise following intravenous infusions of magnesium, they will generally fall rapidly after the infusions are stopped. It is difficult to replace magnesium orally, and quantities of magnesium in the gastrointestinal tract sufficient to result in a significant rise in serum magnesium levels will usually result in diarrhea. It should also be noted that a recent report has suggested hypomagnesemia can persist more than 1–2 years following the last dose of cisplatin, and retreatment with this agent can result in a further fall in the serum magnesium level (12).

Patients treated with cisplatin who experience evidence of renal damage (increase in serum creatinine, decrease in creatinine clearance) will generally have the dose reduced with future courses in an effort to prevent further damage. This is not an unreasonable strategy in the absence of firm evidence that the dose of cisplatin delivered impacts significantly on ultimate patient survival in ovarian cancer.

It is important to note that, as with hypomagnesemia, persistent abnormalities of renal function, as measured by the serum creatinine or creatinine clearance, can be observed in a subgroup of patients with ovarian cancer more than 1–2 years following the last dose of the agent (13). Fortunately, late renal failure developing after acute cisplatin-induced renal injury does not appear to be a major clinical problem.

Very high dose cisplatin regimens (200 mg/m^2 over 5 days) have been administered to patients with ovarian cancer with limited evidence of renal dysfunction when extensive hydration and hypertonic saline infusions are employed. As will be discussed in the next section of this chapter, this therapeutic strategy is limited by the severity of cisplatin-induced neurotoxicity.

While carboplatin can cause renal injury, it is much less likely to do so than cisplatin. Thus, one of the major advantages associated with the use of carboplatin is the fact that extensive hydration is not required, and outpatient drug administration is easier to facilitate. However, it must be remembered that carboplatin-induced bone marrow toxicity is greatly influenced by the renal function. Ovarian cancer patients receiving salvage carboplatin who have previously been treated with cisplatin and have developed evidence of renal dysfunction must have their carboplatin dose adjusted appropriately to avoid unacceptable myelosuppression, particularly thrombocytopenia.

Ifosfamide can also be associated with renal dysfunction, although a more significant concern with the use of this agent is the development of hemorrhagic cystitis (14). The incidence of ifosfamide-induced renal injury is less than that of cisplatin, but it also appears to involve the renal tubules. Patients with pre-existing renal dysfunction, which may develop following cisplatin administration, may have a higher risk for the development of ifosfamide-induced renal toxicity. Due to the renal toxic potential of both cisplatin and ifosfamide, there has been some concern regarding the use of the two important cytotoxic agents in combination. However, it appears that if adequate precautions are taken which include the administration of appropriate levels of both pretreatment and posttreatment hydration, the drugs can be administered together with acceptable toxicity.

BLADDER TOXICITY

As noted above, ifosfamide can be associated with significant bladder toxicity because the drug concentrates at high levels in the bladder (14). This toxicity can also be observed with cyclophosphamide, but usually only when the drug is administered at very high dose levels. Prevention of ifosfamide-induced bladder toxicity, which is usually manifested initially by microscopic hematuria but can progress to hemorrhagic cystitis, is the therapeutic strategy of choice rather than treatment of an established toxic event.

In patients receiving ifosfamide, adequate pretreatment and post-treatment hydration must be provided. In addition, all patients must be treated with mesna, which has been shown to successfully prevent ifosfamide-induced bladder toxicity in most patients. Two general approaches to the use of mesna in patients receiving ifosfamide have been employed in clinical practice. In one program, mesna is administered at the time of ifosfamide delivery, with the dose repeated four and eight hours later. In the second regimen, the mesna is administered as a continuous infusion along with the ifosfamide. Both methods have been shown to successfully reduce the risk of bladder toxicity.

Patients receiving ifosfamide must have daily urinalyses performed to reveal the presence of hematuria before it develops into a serious clinical problem. In general, if treatment is stopped when significant microscopic hematuria is demonstrated, more serious consequences can be avoided. However, once hemorrhagic cystitis develops, treatment can be difficult. Such patients should be treated with vigorous hydration to eliminate the toxic compound from the bladder as quickly as possible. Hydration will also remove blood clots. If the hemorrhagic cystitis is severe, local sclerosing agents may be employed to prevent even more serious consequences.

NEUROTOXICITY

Following the demonstration that the renal toxic effects of cisplatin could be avoided or minimized by providing adequate hydration, it became possible to administer higher single and cumulative dose levels of the cytotoxic agent. Unfortunately, it soon became apparent that the total cumulative dose level which could be delivered was limited by the development of neurotoxicity, principally a peripheral sensory neuropathy (15).

Generally, patients developing this toxic effect of cisplatin will initially note numbness and tingling of the hands and feet. This can progress up the arms and legs and become very painful. Patients developing a severe neuropathy may require narcotic analgesia, may be unable to write or to button their clothes, and may even become confined to a wheelchair secondary to severe peripheral sensory dysfunction.

Unfortunately, even if cisplatin is discontinued when only mild or moderately serious symptoms are noted, the severity may worsen over future weeks or months. However, it would be very unusual for a patient who has experienced only mild numbness and tingling when cisplatin is stopped to progress to the point that symptoms become this severe.

Another interesting and important feature of cisplatin-induced peripheral neuropathy is the fact that symptomatic recovery can occur over a period of months to several years. Thus, it is possible for the physician to be at least moderately reassuring to the individual who develops this toxic effect of therapy that with time the symptoms will significantly improve, even if they do not disappear entirely. How much of the subjective improvement is due to actual repair of damaged nervous tissue as opposed to an individual patient's ability to learn to live with the dysfunction remains an unanswered question.

Carboplatin is associated with a far lower incidence of peripheral neurotoxicity than is cisplatin. However, the safety of carboplatin in patients with pre-existing cisplatin-induced neuropathy is not well defined. Patients with a cisplatin-induced neuropathy may have their symptoms wax and wane over a period of months. Thus, it is often difficult to know whether the symptoms of numbness and pain which increase following the use of carboplatin in an individual previously treated with cisplatin are secondary to the current or previous treatment regimen.

Ifosfamide can cause a reversible encephalopathy in approximately 10–15% of treated patients (14). This is usually manifested by mild confusion, but severe disorientation can be observed. Poor performance status and renal function, as well as low serum albumin levels and the use of narcotic analgesia have all been correlated with ifosfamide central nervous system toxicity. When this side effect of therapy is observed, treatment with ifosfamide should be discontinued. Symptoms usually resolve within 24–48 hours, though longer recovery time may be required.

SECONDARY MALIGNANCIES

A particular concern with the use of chemotherapeutic agents is the development of secondary malignancies, particularly acute, nonlymphocytic leukemia (16,17). In fact, it was the chronic use of alkylating agents in responding patients with advanced ovarian cancer that first brought to medical attention the significant risk of the development of secondary leukemia following the use of cytotoxic chemotherapy. However, the risk of this extremely serious complication of chemotherapy appears to be minimized by delivering treatment over a limited period of time (five to ten months), rather than the use of low doses of the drugs for two or more years.

Isolated reports suggest that cisplatin can also be associated with the development of secondary acute leukemia (18,20). Etoposide, an agent used with cisplatin in patients with germ cell tumors, also appears to have a significant association with acute nonlymphocytic leukemia (20).

CARDIOTOXICITY

While cardiac complications of chemotherapeutic agents are uncommon, they can lead to serious consequences. Doxorubicin is the antineoplastic agent most frequently associated with cardiac dysfunction. The cardiac toxic effects of doxorubicin can be present in two forms: acute and chronic.

Serious acute doxorubicin-induced cardiotoxicity is far less common than chronic toxicity and is characterized by reversible arrhythmias, usually premature atrial and ventricular contractions. Patients may also demonstrate nonspecific ST- and T-wave changes on the electrocardiogram. These abnormalities may occur immediately after doxorubicin delivery or during the infusion. There is no relationship between total cumulative dose of doxorubicin and the development of acute cardiac changes. In addition, the appearance of acute cardiac toxicity does *not* predict for the more serious doxorubicin-induced chronic cardiomyopathy.

In sharp contrast, the incidence of chronic cardiac toxicity caused by doxorubicin is dramatically influenced by the cumulative dose of the agent administered (21). At a total cumulative doxorubicin dose of 550 mg/m^2 or less, the overall incidence of cardiomyopathy is approximately 1%. However, at total dose levels greater than 550 mg/m^2, the incidence of cardiomyopathy has been reported to approach 30%. Additional risk factors for the development of doxorubicin-induced cardiomyopathy include: age over 70 years, prior mediastinal radiation, pre-existing cardiac disease, and concurrent treatment with cyclophosphamide, particularly if this agent is administered at high dose levels.

The severity of doxorubicin-induced cardiomyopathy will vary significantly from one individual to another. In some, it will only be documented at the time of formal cardiac function testing (generally, tests examining left ventricular ejection fraction), while in others, symptoms of severe intractable heart failure may develop. Thus, patients with any evidence of asymptomatic compromise in left ventricular function should have further therapy with this agent discontinued. In general, unless a patient has other risk factors (see above) for the development of doxorubicin-induced cardiomyopathy, it is not necessary to formally evaluate cardiac function when administering doxorubicin if it is anticipated that a maximum of 400–450 mg/m^2 of the drug will be delivered.

Other agents known to be associated with the development of cardiac dysfunction include high-dose cyclophosphamide (as used in bone marrow transplant programs) and taxol (22). Cyclophosphamide can produce a hemorrhagic myocardial necrosis. Taxol can be associated with the development of severe bradycardia, with heart rates of 40–50 being observed in patients treated in the early clinical trials. It has been recommended that patients with underlying cardiac conduction abnormalities should not be treated with taxol.

PULMONARY TOXICITY

A number of chemotherapeutic agents are known to produce pulmonary toxic effects. Bleomycin, commonly used in patients with germ cell tumors, and mitomycin, used in patients with epithelial ovarian cancer in the salvage setting, are two of the agents most commonly associated with this complication of therapy.

The drugs can cause a diffuse interstitial pneumonitis characterized by dyspnea, a dry cough and bibasilar rales. The chest radiograph generally demonstrates bibasilar infiltrates. Treatment of this condition is generally supportive. If chemotherapy-induced pulmonary toxicity is suspected, the offending agent should be discontinued immediately. Corticosteroids may provide symptomatic benefit, although a precise role for this class of agents in this condition has not been clearly defined.

HYPERSENSITIVITY REACTIONS

A number of chemotherapeutic agents, including the organoplatinum drugs and doxorubicin, have been associated with the development of hypersensitivity reactions. In general, these events are very uncommon and prophylaxis to prevent their development is not indicated.

However, a high incidence of hypersensitivity reactions have been noted with the use of taxol (22). It remains unclear if these events are a direct effect of the taxol itself or its vehicle, cremaphor. As taxol is poorly soluble in water, it is necessary for the drug to be administered in the cremaphor base. Of note, the incidence and severity of taxol-associated hypersensitivity reactions appears to have been dramatically reduced through the standard use of a pretreatment regimen of dexamethasone (20 mg, 14 and 7 hours prior to taxol), benadryl, and either cimetidine or ranitidine. This regimen is administered before each dose of taxol.

CYTOTOXIC DRUG EXTRAVASATION

One of the more serious (but essentially completely preventable) side effects of cytotoxic chemotherapy delivery is extravasation of *vesicant* medications into the subcutaneous tissue following intravenous administration. Several antineoplastic agents with clinical utility in ovarian cancer can produce this toxic effect, including doxorubicin and mitomycin. Extravasation injury can lead to full thickness loss of tissue, including severe damage to muscles, tendons, and peripheral nerves.

Great care must be exercised when administering vesicant medications. Assuring a blood return from an intravenous line which is freely flowing is the best method to ensure the drug delivery is into only the vascular compartment rather than into the subcutaneous tissue. In addition, from the perspective of safety, *bolus* injections are preferred to long-term infusions as the method of delivering vesicant medications. Semipermanent, surgically-implanted venous access devices should be *strongly* encouraged for use in patients receiving vesicants where there is any question of the safety of drug delivery through the individual's peripheral veins.

For an established vesicant extravasation there is no optimal management strategy. Attempts must be made to minimize tissue damage. This includes the immediate discontinuation of the infusion. Some investigators have recommended the use of ice packs over the involved area to decrease the spread of drug into the surrounding tissue. Other researchers have suggested tissue infiltration of hydrocortisone to reduce local inflammation. Surgical debridement may also be required.

ALOPECIA

Hair loss is one of the most common side effects of cancer chemotherapy and among the most distressing to women with ovarian cancer receiving these medications. Alopecia is caused by an effect of the cytotoxic drugs on the rapidly dividing tissue of the hair follicle. Inhibition of growth leads to a decrease in the diameter of the shaft of hair, significantly weakening the strand and causing breakage with minimal pressure. Scalp hair is the most susceptible to this effect as it is the most rapidly growing body hair. Hair loss generally begins 1–2 weeks following the initial chemotherapy administration and will usually worsen with each cycle of therapy.

A number of cancer chemotherapeutic agents can cause significant hair loss, including doxorubicin and cyclophosphamide, two drugs commonly used in the treatment of ovarian cancer. Taxol is also associated with rather profound hair loss which can involve all body hair, not just scalp hair.

Several measures have been attempted to reduce the severity of chemotherapy-induced hair loss, including scalp hypothermia and the application of a tight tourniquet around the scalp during drug delivery. Although such strategies have been reported to be of some clinical utility, they are rarely successful in patients with ovarian cancer receiving standard programs which employ moderately high doses of cyclophosphamide or doxorubicin. In addition, there is a reasonable theoretical argument *against* the decrease of cytotoxic drug delivery to any region of the body where there may be circulating tumor cells present. A more reasonable approach to the management of chemotherapy-induced alopecia is to encourage the patient to obtain an acceptable hair prosthesis to use during this course of chemotherapy.

REFERENCES

1. Gabrilove JL, Jakubowski A, Scher H, et al. Effect of granulocyte colony-stimulating factor on neutropenia and associated morbidity due to chemotherapy for transitional-cell carcinoma of the urothelium. *N Engl J Med* 1988;218:1414–1422.
2. Antman KS, Griffin JD, Elias A, et al. Effect of recombinant human granulocyte-macrophage colony-stimulating factor on chemotherapy-induced myelosuppression. *N Engl J Med* 1988; 319:593–598.
3. Wasserheit C, Crown J, Hakes T, et al. High dose cyclophosphamide plus leukapheresis followed by intensive peripheral blood progenitor cell-rescued carboplatin chemotherapy in ovarian cancer. *Proc Am Assoc Cancer Res* 1991;33:243.
4. Oster W, Herrmann F, Gamm H, et al. Erythropoietin for the treatment of anemia of malignancy associated with neoplastic bone marrow infiltration. *J Clin Oncol* 1990;8:956–962.
5. Miller CB, Platanias LC, Mills SR, et al. Phase I–II trial of erythropoietin in the treatment of cisplatin-associated anemia. *J Natl Cancer Inst* 1992;84:98–103.
6. Hamner RW, Verani R, Weinman EJ. Mitomycin-associated renal failure: case report and review. *Arch Intern Med* 1983;143: 803–807.
7. Kris MG, Gralla RJ, Clark RA, et al. Incidence, course, and severity of delayed nausea and vomiting following the administration of high-dose cisplatin. *J Clin Oncol* 1985;3:1379–1384.
8. DeMulder PHM, Seynaeve C, Vermorken JB, et al. Ondansetron compared with high-dose metoclopramide in prophylaxis of acute and delayed cisplatin-induced nausea and vomiting: a multicenter, randomized, double-blind, crossover study. *Ann Intern Med* 1990;113:834–840.
9. Roila F, Tonato M, Cognetti F, et al. Prevention of cisplatin-induced emesis: a double-blind multicenter randomized crossover study comparing ondansetron and ondansetron plus dexamethasone. *J Clin Oncol* 1991;9:675–678.

10. Harvey VJ, Evans BD, Mitchell PLR, et al. Reduction of carboplatin-induced emesis by ondansetron. *Br J Cancer* 1991;63:942–944.
11. Blachley JD, Hill JB. Renal and electrolyte disturbances associated with cisplatin. *Ann Intern Med* 1981;95:628–632.
12. Markman M, Rothman R, Reichman B, et al. Persistent hypomagnesemia following cisplatin chemotherapy in patients with ovarian cancer. *J Cancer Res Clin Oncol* 1991;117:89–90.
13. Markman M, Rothman R, Hakes T, et al. Late effects of cisplatin-based chemotherapy on renal function in patients with ovarian carcinoma. *Gynecol Oncol* 1991;41:217–219.
14. Brade WP, Herdrich K, Varini M. Ifosfamide: pharmacology, safety and therapeutic potential. *Cancer Treat Rev* 1985;12:1–47.
15. Mollman JE. Cisplatin neurotoxicity. *N Engl J Med* 1990;322:126–127.
16. Green MH, Boice JD, Greer BE, et al. Acute nonlymphocytic leukemia after therapy with alkylating agents for ovarian cancer: a study of five randomized clinical trials. *N Engl J Med* 1982;307:1416–1421.
17. Kaldor JM, Day NE, Petterson F, et al. Leukemia following chemotherapy for ovarian cancer. *N Engl J Med* 1990;322:1–6.
18. Bassett WB, Weiss RB. Acute leukemia following cisplatin for bladder cancer. *J Clin Oncol* 1986;4:614.
19. Reed E, Evans MK. Acute leukemia following cisplatin-based chemotherapy in a patient with ovarian cancer. *J Natl Cancer Inst* 1990;82:431–432.
20. Pedersen-Bjergaard J, Daugaard G, Hansen SW, et al. Increased risk of myelodysplasia and leukaemia after etoposide, cisplatin, and bleomycin for germ-cell tumours. *Lancet* 1991;338:359–363.
21. Von Hoff DD, Layard MW, Basa P, et al. Risk factors for doxorubicin-induced congestive heart failure. *Ann Intern Med* 1979;91:710–717.
22. Rowinsky EK, Cazenave LA, Donehower RC. Taxol: a novel investigational antimicrotubule agent. *J Natl Cancer Inst* 1990;82:1247–1259.

CHAPTER 27

Management of Early Stage Ovarian Cancer

Robert C. Young

Approximately one-third of the 21,000 new epithelial ovarian cancers reported annually in the United States present with apparently localized disease [International Federation of Gynecology and Obstetrics (FIGO) stages I and II] (1). While the prognosis of these 7,000 women is much better than their counterparts with advanced disease, the five-year survivals reported for patients with early stage disease has been quite variable. Published five-year survival rates for stage I patients range from 50% to 95% and from 30% to 80% for patients with stage II disease (2–3). These widely variable results are undoubtedly related to the admixtures of patients with differing prognostic factors included in these studies. Complicating this is the fact that true early ovarian cancer is uncommon and published studies have tended to be small and nonrandomized. They have employed variable and often ill-defined selection criteria and have employed a variety of adjuvant therapies or none at all. All of these problems have made it difficult to determine which patients, if any, require postoperative adjuvant therapy and which form of adjuvant therapy is most effective.

A major advance in the management of early ovarian cancer has been the identification of prognostic factors which predict those patients at high risk for relapse. Multiple studies have demonstrated the need for thorough surgical staging to define the extent of disease and for prospective comparisons of treatments in groups of patients balanced for known prognostic factors. Unfortunately, most of the published studies are still nonrandomized and most contain patients with variable risks of recurrence.

Notwithstanding these obstacles, a body of evidence is emerging which allows us to distinguish with reasonable accuracy those good prognosis patients with early disease who do not require adjuvant therapy from the poor prognostic group which clearly could benefit from effective adjuvant therapy if it could be identified.

CLINICAL EVALUATION AND STAGING

A standardized approach to evaluation and staging has developed which now defines appropriate staging for the individual patient while allowing comparisons between groups of women who have been similarly staged. Women with a pelvic mass should have an expedited but complete workup prior to surgical staging. All perimenopausal or postmenopausal women with either pelvic or abdominal symptoms should have a careful physical and pelvic examination, with particular attention to the adnexa. Many women are subjected to prolonged and expensive diagnostic x-ray studies when a careful pelvic examination would have identified a pelvic mass at the first office visit.

An adnexal mass in a premenarchal or postmenopausal woman generally must be evaluated with an exploratory laparotomy. Functional ovarian cysts rarely occur in these age groups, and these masses are commonly neoplastic. Barber and colleagues (4) have pointed out that a normal ovary in the postmenopausal patient should be 2.0 × 1.0 × 0.5 cm or less, and therefore would not ordinarily be easily palpable. As a general rule, palpation of an ovary in a postmenopausal woman is unusual and should be further evaluated using a pelvic or vaginal probe ultrasound. If a complex mass is identified on ultrasound, this is usually an indication for surgery. Occasionally one finds a simple cyst of less than 4 cm. These can be observed by serial ultrasound examination and operation should be performed only if growth occurs.

Ovarian enlargement in a premenopausal woman is usually benign. Most enlargements result from either functional follicular or corpus luteum cysts. Most will regress over several menstrual cycles. Patients should

---

R. C. Young: Fox Chase Cancer Center, Philadelphia, Pennsylvania 19111

be followed carefully with repeat pelvic examination and pelvic or vaginal probe ultrasound.

Papanicolaou smears are uncommonly positive in patients with ovarian cancer, and when they are, they usually indicate advanced disease. However, a patient with adenocarcinoma cells on a Pap smear and a negative evaluation of the vulva, vagina, cervix, and endometrium should be carefully evaluated further for carcinoma of the ovary, fallopian tube, or other intraabdominal malignancy. Routine screening with culdocentesis and peritoneal lavage has been done, but the yield is low and patient acceptance is poor (5).

Ultrasound is a safe, noninvasive procedure which is useful in evaluating intrapelvic disease. Solid elements and prominent papillary projections suggest a malignant process. Ultrasound is also useful in distinguishing ascites from a large ovarian cyst. It can also be used to guide direct percutaneous needle aspirations of suspected metastasis and aspiration biopsies of aortic nodes (6,7). However, abdominal ultrasound is time-consuming, requires that the patient remain for a prolonged period with a full bladder, and is not particularly sensitive.

Vaginal probe ultrasound has become increasingly useful in evaluating pelvic abnormalities. It is more accurate than an abdominal ultrasound and does not require a full bladder. It is also faster and more comfortable for the patient. Studies at the University of Kentucky on 1,000 asymptomatic women (40 years of age or older) found abnormal transvaginal sonograms in 3% (8,9). Twenty-four women had a laparotomy and 70% had tumors, although only one was malignant. Doppler color flow imaging may improve the accuracy of sonography but little more than anecdotal data exists at present (10). It is not clear that transvaginal ultrasound with or without Doppler imaging will have an important role in screening for early ovarian cancer. The major problem is the high frequency of false-positive findings which, if evaluated surgically, would result in an excessive number of unnecessary laparotomies.

Lymphangiography may be helpful in initial staging and is positive in about 30% of patients (11,12). In patients with a positive lymphangiogram, 32% have disease in pelvic nodes only, and 46% have both pelvic and para-aortic disease (13). Lymphangiography by an experienced radiologist is accurate when the lymph nodes are enlarged or replaced by tumor, but cannot identify microscopic disease. In one study, positive preoperative lymphangiograms were histologically confirmed in 100% of patients. In sixty-three patients with negative preoperative lymphangiograms, 87% were confirmed negative and the others had microscopic nodal involvement at surgery. The overall accuracy of the study was 92% (11).

Computed axial tomography (CT) can sometimes add useful information to the findings of ultrasound and lymphangiography. CT can delineate liver and pulmonary nodules, large abdominal and pelvic masses, and retroperitoneal nodal involvement. However, CT is expensive and cannot reliably detect masses less than 2 cm in diameter. CT is sometimes useful when bowel gas makes the ultrasonogram difficult to interpret (14). The typical presurgical evaluation performed in patients with suspected early ovarian carcinoma is listed in Table 1.

Accurate surgical staging is required in order to correctly identify true stage I and II patients. Knowledge of the natural history of early disease spread has provided information about sites at highest risk for occult metastasis and has defined the surgical evaluation most likely to detect this occult disease.

Epithelial cancers arise from the ovarian surface epithelium. Eventually, the tumor penetrates the ovarian capsule and malignant cells are exfoliated into the peritoneal cavity and into the posterior gutter. Normal respiration produces negative intraabdominal pressure, which causes malignant cells to flow up the posterior gutters, over the domes of the diaphragms, and through the diaphragmatic lymphatics. All of these sites are at high risk for early disease spread.

Direct spread from the malignant mass on the surface of the ovary to the omentum can occur as one of the initial steps in early spread of disease. The omentum is therefore an important additional site to evaluate for occult metastasis.

The lymphatic drainage of the ovaries evolved from their embryonic origin as midline structures, and primary drainage is to the lymph nodes in the region of the renal hilus. Secondary drainage is to the iliac nodes, with tertiary drainage to the inguinal nodes. Any of these three sites can be involved with early spread. Approximately 10% of patients with apparent early disease are found to have positive aortic nodes at staging laparotomy (4).

TABLE 1. *Presurgical evaluation of patients with suspected early stage ovarian carcinoma*

Required	Required if symptoms or signs indicate
Careful history and physical examination including pelvic and rectal examination	Cystoscopy Proctoscopy Barium enema Upper GI series
Complete blood count, routine blood chemistries, and CA-125	
Chest X-ray	
CT, MRI, or ultrasound	
Intravenous urogram	

CT, computed tomography; MRI, magnetic resonance imaging.

TABLE 2. *Proper surgical staging for early stage ovarian carcinoma*

Vertical incision adequate to evaluate entire abdomen
Complete abdominal exploration
Multiple washings for cytology
Intact tumor removal
Total abdominal hysterectomy and bilateral oophorectomy
Partial infracolic omentectomy
Pelvic, iliac, and para-aortic lymph node sampling
Peritoneal and diaphragmatic sampling

Careful evaluation of all of these sites at risk is necessary for the proper surgical staging of patients with early disease (Table 2). Surgery should be performed through a vertical incision of adequate length to evaluate the entire peritoneal cavity. The surface of the ovary should be carefully inspected to determine the integrity of the capsule. Any ascitic fluid should be collected and, if none is present, washings should be collected and examined cytologically. Routine biopsies of all known sites of high risk should be performed including para-aortic, iliac, and pelvic lymph nodes and peritoneal surfaces. The diaphragms should be carefully inspected and biopsied if any suspicious lesions are present. Finally, a total abdominal hysterectomy (TAH), bilateral salpingo-oophorectomy (BSO) and partial infracolic omentectomy completes the staging procedure. The FIGO stages of early ovarian carcinoma are summarized in Table 3.

If accurate surgical staging is performed in the first place, there is little need for additional postsurgical staging. Unfortunately, appropriate comprehensive surgical staging is frequently not completed at initial operation (15–17). In one typical study of patients referred with supposedly early disease, only 25% of patients had an incision that allowed full exploration of the abdominal cavity. At restaging, about one-third were upstaged and three-fourths of these had stage III disease (17) (Table 4). Similar results have been reported by others. In a study of 291 women with ovarian cancer (15), only 54% had complete surgical evaluation. Accurate surgical staging was most often done by gynecologic oncologists (97%) but they performed the initial surgery in only 12% of patients. The clear implication of these data is that frequently patients with stage I and II disease are inadequately staged. This not only results in the selection of inappropriate or inadequate therapy, but when such patients are included in clinical trials, as often occurred in early studies, the results can be inaccurate or even erroneous.

If the upper abdomen was not properly evaluated at the initial operation, postoperative reevaluation by either laparotomy or laparoscopy may be necessary before initial treatment is begun. Several laparoscopy studies have documented upper abdominal spread in 30% to 40% of patients with apparently early (FIGO stage I and II) disease (18–20). Other investigators found diaphragmatic metastases in 11% and aortic lymph node metastases in 13% of patients otherwise felt to have stage I disease (20). The use of laparoscopy can be helpful both to enhance initially incomplete staging and as a means to monitor therapeutic response (18,19). In the National Cancer Institute (NCI) studies, laparoscopy documented undetected disease in 42% of

TABLE 3. *FIGO grouping for early stage ovarian carcinoma*

Stage I		Stage II	
Growth limited to the ovaries		Growth involving one or both ovaries with pelvic extension	
Ia	Growth limited to one ovary; no ascites. No tumor on the external surface; capsule intact.	IIa	Growth involving one or both ovaries with pelvic extension
Ib	Growth limited to both ovaries; no ascites. No tumor on the external surfaces; capsule intact.	IIb	Extension and/or metastasis to the uterus and/or tubes.
Ic*	Tumor either stage Ia or Ib but with tumors on the surface of one or both ovaries, or with capsule ruptured, or with ascites present containing malignant cells, or with positive peritoneal washings.	IIc*	Tumor either stage IIa or IIb but with tumor on the surface of one or both ovaries, or with capsule(s) ruptured, or with ascites present containing malignant cells, or with positive peritoneal washings.

* To evaluate the impact on prognosis of the different criteria for advancing cases to Ic or IIc, it would be of value to know if rupture of the capsule was (1) spontaneous or (2) caused by the surgery, and if the source of the malignant cells detected was (1) peritoneal washings or (2) ascites.
FIGO, International Federation of Gynecology and Obstetrics.

TABLE 4. *Comprehensive restaging in patients with apparent stage I and II disease*

Apparent stage	No. of patients	Percent upstaged
Ia	37	16
Ib	10	30
Ic	2	0
IIa	4	100
IIb	38	39
IIc	9	33
TOTAL	100	31

Modified from Young et al., ref. 17.

patients (21). Laparoscopy also provided the only evidence of disease in 38% of patients. Twenty to thirty percent of patients referred with apparent stage I and II disease were documented to have stage III disease based on diphragmatic metastases detected at laparoscopy. Laparoscopy is feasible and relatively safe, even after prior laparotomies. In only 6% of patients did technical problems preclude complete evaluation. Of 159 procedures performed in the NCI studies, there were few serious complications. Only 2.5% of the patients required medical therapy to manage a complication. There were no deaths or viscus perforations, and no patient required surgical exploration because of a complication of laparoscopy. Other institutions have had similar experiences with laparoscopy in ovarian cancer patients. Another report of 112 laparoscopies (22) documented that the entire peritoneal cavity was visualized in 71%, and visualization was totally inadequate in only 14%. There were no serious complications in this study as well.

TABLE 5. *Prognostic groups in early ovarian cancer*

Group	Prognostic factors
Good Prognosis	Intact capsule
	No tumor excrescences
	No malignant ascites
	Negative peritoneal cytology
	Stage Ia and Ib disease
	Grade 1 and 2 disease
Poor Prognosis	Ruptured capsule
	Tumor excrescences
	Positive peritoneal cytology
	Malignant ascites
	Stage Ic–II disease
	Grade 3 disease
	Clear cell histology
	Tumor residuum

PROGNOSTIC FACTORS

Stage is not the only prognostic factor of importance in early stage disease. In addition to stage, the most important prognostic variables are tumor residuum, grade, histologic subtype, and the age of the patient at diagnosis (23–25). One multivariate analysis of 430 ovarian carcinoma patients indicated that residual disease and tumor grade were most important ($p < 0.001$), followed by stage ($p = 0.002$), age ($p = 0.004$) and histologic type ($p = 0.058$) (24). Residual tumor is significantly more important in predicting therapeutic outcome than FIGO stage. The histologic type of malignant epithelial ovarian cancer has limited significance independent of clinical stage, extent of residual disease, and histologic grade. Although several studies suggest clear cell carcinomas to have a worse prognosis (26), others do not (27) and the matter remains unsettled. The better survival rates for mucinous and endometrioid carcinomas can be explained because these tumors are frequently better differentiated. Poorly differentiated mucinous tumors have a very poor prognosis, and poorly differentiated endometrioid carcinomas are often misdiagnosed as undifferentiated adenocarcinomas.

In contrast to histologic type, histologic grade is an important independent prognostic factor for response to treatment and survival (28–31). Studies from the Mayo Clinic, using a modified Broder's grading classification in stage II serous cystadenocarcinoma, documented an 80% survival for patients with grade 1 tumors, 47% survival for grade 2, and 10% survival for grade 3 and 4 tumors (29). Studies from M.D. Anderson Hospital (30) using the pattern grading system show that for stages I and II serous carcinoma of the ovary, patients with grade 1 tumors had a 78% seven-year survival compared to a 35% seven-year survival for grade 2 and a 0% seven-year survival for grade 3.

Dembo and Bush (32) have proposed a more complex interaction between grade and histologic type. For patients with serous tumors, grade was highly significant. In contrast, grade was not significant for patients with mucinous, endometrioid, or clear cell tumors. When the two variables of grade and histologic type were combined, significant survival differences were seen between patients with "favorable" pathologies (serous, well-differentiated; and mucinous, endometroid, and clear cell types of all grades). The five-year survival in patients with "favorable" pathology was 59% compared to a five-year survival of 19% in patients with "unfavorable" pathology (serous, moderately and poorly differentiated; and the unclassified type).

Histologic grading of ovarian tumors has not been accepted enthusiastically by pathologists, primarily because no standardized, easily reproducible, and objective classification exists. Nevertheless, although different classifications have been used, most studies document the prognostic impact of grade on survival. Grading of epithelial ovarian tumors should be a part of every carefully designed clinical study.

Using these prognostic variables, it is possible to divide early ovarian cancer patients into those with good prognosis features which probably do not require adjuvant therapy and those with poor prognosis features who should receive additional therapy (Table 5).

SCREENING FOR EARLY DISEASE

The majority of patients with localized ovarian cancer (stages I and II) are curable with surgery and for certain groups of patients, relatively simple adjuvant therapy. Clearly, a dramatic change in overall survival in ovarian cancer could be achieved if more patients were discovered when the disease was still localized. This has led to an intensive effort to identify screening programs capable of detecting early disease in asymptomatic women. Unfortunately, most of these screening programs have not been evaluated prospectively in large groups of women, and as yet none are known to be reliable in consistently detecting early disease. Many patients with early disease are first identified when a routine pelvic examination discloses a pelvic mass, but there is no data on the frequency with which routine pelvic examinations are successful in consistently identifying early disease. Just as frequently, routine physical examination discloses advanced disease, and it is not clear that the routine use of pelvic examination alters either mortality or morbidity.

The use of the tumor marker CA-125 common to most nonmucinous epithelial ovarian tumors has been of considerable interest as a possible screening tool. The OC-125 antibody recognizes multiple antigen determinants on a high-molecular-weight glycoprotein. These antigens are found on coelomic epithelium during development as well as on fetal tissues, müllerian duct remnants, amnion and amniotic fluid. The antigen is not found in normal ovarian tissues but it is found in nonmucinous epithelial ovarian carcinomas. Over 80% of ovarian cancer patients react positively, as do 25% of patients with nongynecologic malignancies, 5% of patients with benign disease, and 1% of apparently healthy women.

Several studies have tried to use CA-125 to screen for early disease. One study (33) looked at over 900 asymptomatic women. CA-125 ranged from 0 to 574 u/ml. Thirty-six women (3.9%) had CA-125 levels greater than 35 u/ml, and seven (0.8%) had levels greater than 65 u/ml. Five of these seven women had neoplasms but only one was malignant (colon carcinoma), and none had ovarian cancer. False-positive tests have been reported in peritonitis, pancreatitis, renal failure, alcoholic hepatitis, endometriosis, and even in normal pregnancy (34). Because of the low incidence of ovarian cancer and its occasional elevation in nonmalignant disease, a single CA-125 assay is not a useful routine screening test.

Other studies have attempted to use serial CA-125 screening to detect early disease. Einhorn and colleagues (35) studied one hundred women with palpable adnexal masses with prelaparotomy CA-125. The CA-125 levels were greater than 35 u/ml in 61% of women with some form of ovarian cancer, and greater than 65 u/ml in 80% of those positive.

Two other screening studies using CA-125 have been published, one from England and one from Sweden. Jacobs and associates (36) evaluated over one thousand asymptomatic women. CA-125 had a specificity of 97%. The Swedish study (35) screened 5,500 apparently healthy women and found CA-125 levels greater than 30 u/ml in 175 (3.2%). Laparotomies were eventually performed on twelve women and six were found to have ovarian cancer, although only two of the six had stage I disease. To date, only 50% of patients with clinically detectable ovarian cancer will have an elevated CA-125 (37), and this makes it unlikely that it will be found to be consistently elevated in patients with FIGO stage I and II disease.

Ultrasound has also been evaluated as a potential screening tool for early ovarian carcinoma. Transabdominal ultrasound is easy, painless, and is essentially without complications. However, it is not specific enough to be a good screening test for ovarian cancer. Bourne and colleagues (38) studied over five thousand asymptomatic women. Only five patients with ovarian cancer were identified from over 15,000 scans, and four of these five already had advanced disease. They estimated the odds of an abnormal abdominal sonogram being due to ovarian cancer at 67 to 1.

Transvaginal ultrasound has been proposed as a potentially more accurate screening procedure. It is faster than the transabdominal procedure, does not require a full bladder, and is more comfortable for the patient. In studies of one thousand asymptomatic patients, 3.1% had abnormal sonograms and twenty-four patients underwent laparotomy. Eight cystadenomas, two cystic teratomas, six endometriomas, and one adenocarcinoma were found.

The addition of the color flow doppler imaging may improve the screening accuracy and reduce the high frequency of false-positives now seen with ultrasound. As yet, however, there are no prospective studies of the technique published. This procedure identifies neovascularization, which is characteristic of neoplasms. Combining both ultrasound and doppler appears to increase the specificity and accuracy. In the English studies which utilized both, an increase in the specificity to 99.6% was documented (36).

In spite of the interest and the media publicity, these screening procedures either alone or in combination have not yet been shown to be effective or cost-effective procedures for routine screening of asymptomatic women with no family history of risk. Further studies will have to be completed before any routine screening can be recommended.

EARLY STAGE PATIENTS NOT REQUIRING ADJUVANT TREATMENT

The extent of surgical intervention in stage I ovarian cancer is influenced by the histologic grade of the tumor and the reproductive desires of the patient. While most women require comprehensive surgical staging as described in the previous section, unique circumstances allow certain patients to be managed more conservatively. Scully (39,40) retrospectively analyzed three studies in which disease was confined to one ovary and reported a 75% survival with oophorectomy alone. No improvement in survival was seen in those women managed with aggressive surgery. An earlier study by Munnell (41) also reported a 75% survival in similar groups of women. Webb and colleagues (42) found a 90% survival in stage I patients without capsular rupture but 57% survival when rupture or penetration of the capsule was noted. These studies suggest that there are small groups of women who present with uniquely limited disease who can be safely managed with limited surgery alone.

Several recent randomized trials have sought to define which patients with early disease can be treated with conventional surgery alone. Dembo (43) randomized fifty-four patients with stage Ia disease to receive either observation or pelvic radiation and included patients with all histologic grades. There were no relapses in either arm in the twenty-four patients with well-differentiated tumors. Studies from the Gynecologic Oncology Group (GOG) (26,46) in patients with Ia–b disease with well- or moderately well-differentiated tumors reported only one relapse in fifty-six patients. In the later GOG study (26), patients in this good prognosis group were randomized to receive either oral melphalan (forty-three patients) or no further therapy (thirty-eight patients). With a median followup in excess of six years, there are only six deaths (7%). The deaths were equally distributed in the two arms and not all were tumor-related. The five-year disease-free survival (91% vs. 98%) and the overall survival (94% vs. 98%) are similar for the two groups.

These studies indicate that women with disease confined to one ovary, with a grade 1 or 2 tumor, and a negative comprehensive surgical exploration, do not require further therapy if the patient desires children.

In patients who have unilateral oophorectomy, the opposite ovary should be biopsied. However, in patients with grade 3 tumors or for those who do not want further children, TAH and BSO should be performed. Based upon the data from these studies, stage I patients who have moderately or well-differentiated (grade 1 and 2) tumors, negative peritoneal cytology, no densely adherent tumors, and no tumor rupture or spill, can be managed without postoperative therapy.

Patients with stage II disease or with stage I disease and incomplete surgical staging or poor prognostic findings require complete surgical staging, as outlined earlier, and are candidates for adjuvant therapy. During complete surgical staging of these patients, particular care must be taken to identify potential spread to the upper abdomen or retroperitoneal space.

Stage I and II Borderline Tumors

Tumors of low malignant potential (borderline tumors) are a unique histologic group displaying cytologic evidence of malignancy but no stromal invasion (45). They have a different, and generally significantly better, natural history and there is presently little evidence that any adjuvant therapy is required if appropriate surgical evaluation has been carried out. Long-term survivals of stage I and II patients with borderline tumors are generally reported to be 90–100% and since many of these women are in childbearing years, conservative surgery is particularly relevant.

In one study of stage I women with borderline tumors, the survival after unilateral oophorectomy was similar to survival with TAH and BSO (95% vs. 94%), even though the recurrence rate was higher after limited surgery (15%) than after aggressive resection (5%) (46).

Evidence suggests that patients with stage II borderline tumors should be managed with TAH and BSO and careful staging of the abdominal cavity. However, there is no evidence that their survival can be improved with adjuvant therapy. Several nonrandomized trials have used adjuvant chemotherapy, radiation, or radioisotopes to treat patients with borderline stage I disease, but there is little evidence of its benefit. In a retrospective analysis of eighty patients treated with various adjuvants, only three relapsed and died of their disease. In 450 patients with stage I borderline tumors who received no treatment, there were only two deaths (0.4%). A randomized trial has been carried out in stage I borderline tumors with patients randomized to observation, pelvic irradiation, or intermittent oral melphalan (47). In the fifty-five patients randomized, only one patient had a recurrence, confirming that adjuvant therapy in this group of patients is not required.

One other randomized trial provides additional data. In the adjuvant randomized GOG trial (26) mentioned previously, all patients were supposed to have invasive epithelial tumors. However, central pathology review concluded that fifty-one patients had tumors of borderline malignancy. Only two of these fifty-one patients, thirty-six of whom received adjuvant treatment, died (4%) and neither died directly of ovarian cancer. These trials, taken as a whole, provide strong evidence that patients with stage I borderline tumors should not receive adjuvant therapy.

There is very little data on the use of any form of adjuvant therapy for patients with stage II borderline tumors; as yet, there is no evidence that adjuvant therapy prolongs survival or is required (48).

NONRANDOMIZED TRIALS IN STAGE I AND II OVARIAN CANCER

Many published nonrandomized or retrospective trials attempt to document the worth or lack of worth of adjuvant therapy of various types for patients with early disease (49–55). Virtually all of these publications have reported good results, whether they gave additional therapy or not; it is difficult to use these trials to make therapeutic decisions. Nonrandomized trials in early ovarian cancer are not likely to be definitive because the events (recurrence and death) are so uncommon. As a result, very small, subtle selection processes (either planned or unplanned) markedly affect results.

For example, the clinical trials group of the National Cancer Institute of Canada followed sixty-eight women (stages Ia–c) without adjuvant therapy and reported excellent results (three-year disease-free survival of 94%) (49). In contrast, a study from the Mayo Clinic (50) looked at fifty-five stage I patients, virtually all (93%) treated with adjuvant therapy and also reported excellent results (85% five-year survival for stage Ic, grades 3 and 4; and 95% for all other stage I patients). One can account for these seemingly different conclusions on the basis of the small size of the trials and selection factors, both recognized and unrecognized. The Mayo Clinic trial (50) is a retrospectively constructed collection of fifty-five patients who had second-look laparotomy after initial stage I classification. Only 49% had their original staging at Mayo. In the NCI Canada trial (49), ten institutions entered patients and the authors point out that "the low incidence of poorly differentiated tumors and the small number of excrescences suggest that not all institutions were registering all patients (presumably because of reluctance to withhold treatment) making this not only a small but somewhat selected patient population." These well-analyzed and well-presented trials illustrate clearly the problems involved in interpreting nonrandomized trials in early ovarian cancer.

Gallion et al. (51) treated fifty stage I patients with oral melphalan. All histologic grades except borderline tumors were included and comprehensive surgical staging was used. The five-year actuarial survival was 94% although twenty of fifty (40%) of the patients had grade 1 tumors and had an excellent prognosis without treatment. In this study, twenty-eight patients received only six to eleven cycles of melphalan, and there was no difference in relapse rate compared to those receiving a full twelve cycles. The optimal duration of adjuvant therapy in appropriate patients has not been determined in any trial.

Chiara et al. (55) have used combination chemotherapy with cisplatin and cyclophosphamide in FIGO stage I and II patients in a nonrandomized trial. Eighty-seven patients at "high risk" of recurrence were treated with six cycles of therapy. Although only stages I grade 3, Ic, and IIa–c, were included, 31% of patients had grade 1 tumors. The seven-year relapse-free survival and overall survival were 61% and 76%, respectively. A significant difference in outcome was noted by grade but not by stage. Although the authors conclude that the therapy is tolerable and effective, the outcomes are not clearly different from studies where single agent chemotherapy, isotopes, whole abdominal irradiation, or observation alone were used. With some known short-term toxicity and the risk of late leukemia (not observed in their trial), this approach needs evaluation in a large randomized trial.

ADJUVANT RADIATION THERAPY IN EARLY OVARIAN CANCER

Radiation therapy was the first adjuvant therapy used to treat patients with localized disease. In the 1960s, the published five-year survivals for patients with stage I and II disease after surgery alone were 70% and 21%, respectively (56–58). Although undoubtedly these early studies included patients with unappreciated stage III disease, they suggested a need for effective adjuvant therapy.

A series of studies from the Princess Margaret Hospital (PMH) has provided much of the background information which defines the preferred techniques for adjuvant therapy using irradiation. In an early randomized stage I patient trial (59), pelvic irradiation was compared to observation alone. This study showed that irradiation reduced pelvic recurrences but made no impact on survival. In a subsequent trial from PMH, 190 patients with stages Ib, II, and asymptomatic stage III disease were randomized to receive either pelvic irradiation, pelvic irradiation plus oral chlorambucil for two years, or pelvic irradiation with whole abdominal irradiation (WAR) (60). There were no differences in survival for patients who did not have complete surgical resection of disease, but for those who did, WAR produced a 78% five-year survival compared to 51% for patients with pelvic irradiation with or without chlorambucil. The better survival with WAR appeared to be related to the reduction in upper abdominal relapses. Unfortunately, several problems make interpretation of this trial difficult. Comprehensive surgical staging was not performed. Therefore, the true distribution of stage and extent of residual disease in the three arms cannot be determined. Second, chlorambucil in modest doses is inadequate chemotherapy by modern standards and is unlikely to control disease in areas not irradiated.

Two studies have compared the moving strip technique with the open field technique to determine the optimum technique for whole abdominal irradiation. In studies from the PMH (61) and from Fazekas and Maier (62), the acute toxicity was similar from the two procedures, but late bowel injury requiring surgery was more common with the moving strip technique. In both studies, the five-year survivals for the two techniques were equivalent, and in the PMH study the techniques were still comparable when the patients were matched for stage, histology, grade, and tumor residuum. Other studies have compared whole abdominal irradiation with subtotal abdominopelvic irradiation. In one hundred six women with disease staged I–IIIa and minimal (less than 2 cm) residual disease, Fuller and colleagues (63) in a nonrandomized trial achieved a 71% ten-year survival with WAR compared to 40% for patients treated with subtotal abdominopelvic irradiation. The difference in survival was more dramatic when the patient populations were adjusted for imbalances in stage, grade, and residual disease. Patients with ascites fared worse with subtotal irradiation than with WAR. Bowel injury requiring surgical intervention occurred in 8.1% of patients treated with subtotal irradiation compared to 7.1% for patients treated with WAR. The addition of intraperitoneal P^{32} increased the bowel complication rate 33% over irradiation alone. Unfortunately, even with WAR, the predominant site of failure was in the abdomen and pelvis in sixty-one of sixty-two (98%) of those who relapsed and died. Other retrospective reviews (64,65) of various radiation approaches have produced similar results, although differences in patient populations, extent of surgery, and radiation techniques make these nonrandomized studies difficult to compare. On the basis of the randomized comparisons and other data, the open field technique has become the standard in most centers because of the shorter treatment course, technical simplicity, and reduced long-term toxicity.

Gastrointestinal toxicity is the most common complaint after WAR, and about three-fourths of patients develop nausea, abdominal cramping, and diarrhea. Hematologic toxicity is common but rarely dose-limiting, although thrombocytopenia can be a significant problem in about 10% of all patients (66).

The acute side effects of WAR usually resolve within several weeks after completing therapy. Chronic toxicity occurs in a minority of patients. Because the lower lung fields are included in the radiation ports, 15–20% of patients develop basalar fibrosis, which is usually asymptomatic. Radiation of the liver produces abnormalities of liver function tests in about half of the patients but jaundice is rare (66). The most serious complication is bowel injury with fibrosis and obstruction which sometimes requires surgical intervention. Several large studies totaling over one thousand patients have estimated the frequency of this injury to be slightly over 5% (range 1.4% to 14%) (66–69). Fatal bowel injury occurred in only four patients (less than 0.5%). The frequency of bowel injury is related to the total dose administered, the extent of previous surgery, the dose per fraction, and the concomitant use of radioisotopes (70,71) and appears to be increased when extensive lymph node sampling has been performed.

ADJUVANT RADIOISOTOPES IN EARLY DISEASE

Early studies commonly employed intraperitoneal installation of radioactive colloidal Au^{198} or P^{32} to irradiate the peritoneal cavity (72,73). In recent years, most investigators have used P^{32} because of higher beta particle energy, tissue penetration, longer half-life, and the absence of gamma irradiation which provides a better safety index (74).

One of the early randomized trials (75) done at the Norwegian Radium Hospital compared pelvic irradiation alone (5000 cGy) with pelvic irradiation (3000 cGy) and intraperitoneal Au^{198}. Although this trial demonstrated that there were fewer cancer deaths in the arm receiving Au^{198}, the therapeutic advantage was outweighed by a higher number of deaths from complications. Radioactive gold is no longer available for therapy in the United States. With radioisotope therapy in general, the radiation dose distribution to the peritoneal surface is quite variable and the dose to lymph nodes and the retroperitoneum is generally negligible (74). The colloidal particles increase isotope uptake by the mesothelial peritoneal cells and lymph nodes and reduce radioisotope elution. P^{32} in the form of chromic phosphate has a half-life of 14.2 days and emits only high energy beta particles (1.7 MeV). The range of tissue penetration of these particles is 3–5 mm and the irradiation may sterilize microscopic peritoneal implants but is inadequate to treat macroscopic disease of any size because of this limited penetration. Adequate distribution of the isotope within the peritoneal cavity is sometimes compromised by adhesions or loculation (76). The patency of the peritoneal cavity can be evaluated by injecting dilute hypaque or by instilling 99 technetium into the peritoneal cavity. Follow-up scans can then be done to assess the adequacy of isotope distribution.

Intraperitoneal isotopes can be associated with small bowel obstruction and bowel stenosis. One analysis of 104 patients treated with intraperitoneal isotopes reported that 11% required surgery for adhesions or fibrosis of the small intestine (77). In patients treated with radioactive colloidal gold, only one patient in forty-five (2.2%) developed small bowel complications, compared to twelve of fifty (24%) patients treated with both radioisotopes and pelvic irradiation. Most studies have shown that bowel complications are significantly increased when isotopes are used with external beam irradiation (78). Overall, P^{32} produces fewer bowel complications than radiogold, but complications are more frequent in patients with uneven distribution of the radioisotope in the peritoneal cavity.

A multivariate retrospective analysis of stage I and II tumors at the Norwegian Radium Hospital demonstrated a slightly higher relapse rate in patients treated with radioisotopes compared to pelvic irradiation or no treatment, but the differences were not significant (79). Piver et al. treated twenty-five stage I patients with intraperitoneal P^{32} (80). Pretreatment surgery included a TAH and BSO with or without omentectomy. The estimated ten-year disease-free and overall survival rates were 84% and 75%, respectively. Those patients with stages Ia and Ic, nonruptured cysts, and grade 1 or 2 tumors had an excellent prognosis. In contrast, poor survival was achieved in patients with Ib disease, ruptured cysts, and grade 3 tumors. Similar results for grade 3 tumors treated with intraperitoneal P^{32} were achieved by Powell and colleagues compared to patients with grade 1 tumors (33% vs. 88%) (81). It is not clear from these studies whether intraperitoneal isotopes improve survival compared to untreated controls in patients with ruptured cysts, grade 3 histology, or other poor prognostic features.

RADIATION THERAPY VERSUS SINGLE AGENT CHEMOTHERAPY IN EARLY DISEASE

Several studies have compared radiotherapy to single agent chemotherapy. The first randomized trial was conducted by the GOG in the late 1970s (82). This study randomized patients to receive either pelvic irradiation, oral melphalan chemotherapy, or observation. There was no significant difference in survival among the three groups. However, the recurrence rate was higher after pelvic irradiation (30%) and observation (17%) compared with melphalan (6%). Unfortunately, this study is marred by the lack of uniform staging or stratification by known prognostic variables, and almost half of the enrolled patients were eventually inevitable. Reevaluation of the trial with a different statistical analysis suggested that melphalan was no better than observation (83).

A study from the M.D. Anderson Hospital randomized patients with stages I, II, and minimal residual stage III disease to receive either whole abdominal irradiation or oral melphalan (84). The two- and five-year survivals for the two groups of patients were 87% and 72% for radiation and 90% and 78% for melphalan. At ten-year follow-up there are still no differences between the two groups (85). The M.D. Anderson group concluded that chemotherapy is as effective as irradiation, has fewer serious side effects, and is less expensive. This trial has also been seriously criticized because the radiation therapy techniques used did not fully include the domes of the diaphragms and shielded the liver, and because patients with borderline tumors were not excluded. In addition, the patients were not stratified for stage and extent of residual disease, and twice as many stage I patients were treated with chemotherapy as were treated with radiation.

Two small trials evaluated WAR or pelvic irradiation followed by one year of oral melphalan in stage II patients (86). Neither of these treatments improved survival over historical results with surgery alone.

A Danish study randomized early ovarian cancer patients to either WAR or pelvic irradiation and cyclophosphamide (87). With about sixty patients in each arm of the trial, there was no difference in four-year relapse-free or overall survival. Furthermore, there was no difference in the frequency of abdominal recurrences between the two approaches, although pelvic relapse with upper abdominal or distant recurrence was more common in the pelvic irradiation–cyclophosphamide-treated group. Diarrhea and leukopenia occurred with equal frequency in the two arms but nausea, vomiting, and thrombocytopenia were more common with WAR. The dose-limiting toxicity of the irradiation-chemotherapy regimen was hemorrhagic cystitis which occurred in 17% of patients. No secondary leukemias occurred in either arm but eight patients (6%) developed bowel injury which required surgery (five patients on WAR and three on pelvic irradiation-cyclophosphamide). Although the radiation approach was modeled after the approach of the Princess Margaret group, the Danish investigators were not able to demonstrate the superiority of WAR over pelvic irradiation and chemotherapy, although a different alkylating agent was used. Table 6 summarizes some of the studies comparing adjuvant radiation with chemotherapy.

Davy and colleagues (88) randomized 301 patients with stage I and II disease to either thio-TEPA or observation, with both arms subsequently receiving either intraperitoneal P^{32} or pelvic irradiation (4000 cGy) if adhesions prevented installation of P^{32}. The relapse frequencies in the two arms were the same (25%), suggesting that neither adjuvant regimen was particularly effective.

An English study (89) employed WAR using the Princess Margaret technique but was unable to reach the degree of control reported by the Canadian group. In patients with stage I (grade 2 or above), stage II, and minimal residual stage III patients they were able to achieve a five-year relapse-free survival of 49% and an overall survival of 57%. There was no correlation between survival and FIGO stage, but survival did cor-

TABLE 6. Radiation therapy versus chemotherapy in early disease

Study design	No. of patients	Stage	Results
Pelvic RT vs.	43	I–III	Better five-year survival for WAR
WAR vs.	76		
Pelvic & chlorambucil	76		
WAR vs.	60	I–II	Same four-year survival
Pelvic RT and cyclophosphamide	60		
WAR vs.	74	I–III	Same five-year and ten-year survival
Melphalan	75		
WAR vs.	85	I–III	[a] No survival difference
Melphalan vs.	86		
IP P^{32}	86		

From Dembo et al., ref. 60; Sell et al., ref. 87; Smith et al., ref. 84; Klaassen et al., ref. 91.
[a] 62% vs. 61% vs. 66%.
RT, radiation therapy; WAR, whole abdomen irradiation; IP, intraperitoneal.

relate with grade. Bowel toxicity occurred in 7% of patients (higher than in the Princess Margaret studies).

As data have accumulated on the results of radiation therapy in early ovarian cancer, it has become possible to define the group of patients that is potentially appropriate for such treatment. Selection of therapy depends upon stage, volume and site of residual disease, and histology (66). In order to be candidates for radiation therapy, patients should have no macroscopic disease in the upper abdomen; they should not have any residual disease greater than 2 cm in cross-sectional diameter. In addition, the Princess Margaret Group has emphasized that WAR is only indicated for primary treatment of patients with stage I to III disease, minimal residual disease (less than 2 cm), and no high-grade tumors. If any two or more of these bad prognostic factors are present, the ten-year disease-free survival is less than 20% (66,90). If these criteria are applied to ovarian cancer patients, less than one-third will even be potential candidates for WAR as a curative modality. When patients are selected appropriately for this therapy and the therapy is administered by radiation therapists skilled in the technique, then 50% to 60% of these patients survive ten years or more free of disease (83,90).

The Ovarian Cancer Study Group and the Gynecologic Oncology Group published two prospective randomized trials in which standardized and comprehensive surgical staging was performed to ensure that all patients were truly stage I and II (26) (Table 7). Patients with early disease were divided into good (stage Ia, Ib; and well- or moderately well-differentiated histologic grade) and poor (stages Iaii, Ibii, Ic, II; and poorly differentiated histologic grade) prognostic groups. In the first trial, eighty-one patients were randomized to either melphalan (forty-eight patients) or observation (forty-four patients). The two groups were well matched for histologic type, grade, and stage. The five-year survival (91% vs. 98%) and the overall survival (94% vs. 98%) were not statistically different. Since the survival in both arms was excellent and one arm was observation only, this trial defines a group of patients with early disease who do not require adjuvant therapy after comprehensive surgical staging. This trial sought to include only patients with true invasive disease, but central pathology review concluded that 33% of these patients had borderline tumors. As mentioned earlier, none of these patients died of ovarian cancer, whether treated with adjuvant chemotherapy or not. The five-year survival in this trial was unchanged if the borderline tumor patients in the two arms of the trial are excluded.

The second part of this randomized prospective trial included patients with poorer prognostic features. One hundred forty-one patients were randomized after comprehensive surgical staging to receive either melphalan (sixty-eight patients) or P^{32} (seventy-three patients). These two groups were also well balanced for histologic type, histologic grade, stage, extent of residual disease, and age. The five-year disease-free survival was 80% in both arms of the trial, and the overall survival was 81% with melphalan and 78% with P^{32} (p = 0.48). In this trial, 17% of patients were reclassified as having tumors of borderline malignancy, and they were equally balanced in the two arms. The five-year survival for the two arms was 76% rather than 80% if

TABLE 7. OCSG/GOG Trials of good and poor prognosis early ovarian carcinoma

	Good risk trial		Poor risk trial	
	Observation	Melphalan	IP P^{32}	Melphalan
Patient numbers	38	43	73	68
Recurrences	4	1	16	18
Deaths	4	2	16	15
Disease-free survival	91%	98%	80%	80%
Overall survival	94%	98%	78%	81%

IP, intraperitoneal; OCSG, Ovarian Cancer Study Group; GOG, Gynecologic Oncology Group.

those patients are excluded, and the conclusions from the trial are unchanged. These trials also confirmed the risk of upper abdominal recurrence. The majority (71%) of the recurrences were either abdominal (39%) or distant (32%). In these trials, the presence of clear cell histology was associated with a poor prognosis. Forty percent of all the relapses contained clear cell elements, although only 17% of patients had clear cell features in their tumor. These two trials established that comprehensive surgical staging in patients with early ovarian cancer defines a group of patients who do not require adjuvant therapy and allows the selection of suitable adjuvant therapy for those patients who do require additional treatment.

The National Cancer Institute of Canada clinical trials group performed a three-arm randomized study which focussed primarily on patients with poor prognosis early disease (91). Two hundred and fifty-seven patients with stage I, IIa "high risk" (rupture of cyst, extracystic excrescences, positive peritoneal cytology, or grade 3 histology), stage IIb or III disease (minimal disease involving the bowel or pelvic side wall) were randomized to receive either WAR, melphalan, or intraperitoneal P^{32}. However, all patients received pelvic irradiation (2250 cGy in those treated with WAR and 4500 cGy for those receiving either melphalan or P^{32}). Median duration of follow-up was eight years. There were no significant differences between the overall survivals in the three arms (62%, 61%, 66%) although there was a marginally significant difference in disease-free survival, with the melphalan-treated group superior to those treated by WAR. A multivariate analysis indicated that stage, grade, and histologic subtype were important predictors of survival. The arm which included pelvic irradiation and intraperitoneal P^{32} was closed early because of unacceptably high incidence of bowel toxicity (29% vs. 10% and 11% for the other two arms). This trial confirms the experience of others that pelvic irradiation cannot be combined with intraperitoneal P^{32} without a significant increase in bowel toxicity. Four patients in the arm receiving melphalan developed a myelodysplastic syndrome or acute leukemia which confirms the experience of many studies reporting an excess of leukemia in patients with ovarian cancer treated with long-term alkylating agents (92–94).

Unfortunately, this study was compromised by the report that one-third of the patients had significant field violations in the pelvis and the abdomen. Nevertheless, the survival of those patients treated with WAR who had no field violations was not superior to those treated with pelvic irradiation and melphalan or P^{32}.

ADJUVANT THERAPY WITH CISPLATIN

Because cisplatin is felt to be the most active single agent for ovarian cancer (95), there has been increasing interest in its use as an adjuvant therapy for early disease. Several trials by the Italian Interegional Cooperative Group for Gynecologic Oncology have focussed on patients with stage I disease and looked at various prognostic groups (96). Their first study included stage Ia and Ib patients with grade 1 disease who received no treatment and had a three-year disease-free survival rate of over 94%. The second study randomized patients with stage Ia and Ib disease and grade 2–3 tumors to receive either cisplatin (50 mg/M^2 every 28 days for 6 cycles) or observation alone. At three years, there was no significant difference in disease-free survival (85%) between the cisplatin-treated patients and those with no treatment in this group of patients. The third group of patients (those with stage Ic disease) were randomized to either intravenous cisplatin or P^{32}. Patients treated with cisplatin in this study had a better disease-free survival (78% vs. 62%) than those with P^{32}, but the difference did not reach statistical significance, partly due to small numbers and partly because 20% of those patients randomized to P^{32} received cisplatin instead because of peritoneal adhesions which prevented intraperitoneal therapy.

These trials have now been updated with five-year follow-up (97). For the ninety-two patients with stage Ia, Ib grade 1 tumors followed off-treatment, the five-year disease-free survival is 90% [four patients relapsed (three extrapelvic) and three have died]. The data from the second trial are unchanged (85% five-year survival for either cisplatin or observation) and for the trial in patients with stage Ic, cisplatin is more effective than intraperitoneal P^{32} (disease-free survival 82% vs. 70%, p = 0.006).

Several nonrandomized trials using cisplatin as an adjuvant have now been reported. Piver et al. (98,99) have used cisplatin as an adjuvant in stage I and II disease. Patients received weekly cisplatin for four weeks followed by cyclophosphamide, doxorubicin hydrochloride (Adriamycin), and cisplatin (CAP) monthly for five cycles. The disease-free and overall survival for stage I patients was 93% and 97%, respectively. Unfortunately, only half of the patients had been completely surgically staged, and twenty of the thirty stage I patients had grade 1–2 disease and may not have required adjuvant chemotherapy at all. Piver's results in stage II disease were less encouraging where this adjuvant approach produced a 45% five-year progression-free survival. These results are similar to results from trials using WAR or pelvic irradiation and melphalan (86) where the five-year survivals were 40% and 50%, respectively.

A nonrandomized trial from the Netherlands used CAP in patients with stage Ic and II disease and reported a five-year relapse-free survival of 60% (100,101). Of note, no late leukemias were reported with cisplatin in contrast to the data with alkylating agents.

A large trial was recently reported from the Norwegian Radium Hospital in which 347 patients with early disease were randomized to either intraperitoneal P^{32} or six courses of cisplatin at 50 mg/M² (102). Patients with stages I–III were included but none had residual disease. All invasive histologies and mucinous borderline tumors were included. Surgical staging included TAH and BSO but peritoneal washings, para-aortic lymphadenectomy or scrapings of the diaphragms were not routinely performed. One hundred sixty-nine patients were randomized to P^{32} but twenty-eight had adhesions which prevented the isotope administration and they were treated with WAR. The dose of P^{32} ranged from 7–10 mCi, depending upon body weight. One hundred seventy-one patients were randomized to cisplatin. Median follow-up now exceeds five years. Sixteen percent of patients treated with P^{32} have died compared to 18% of those receiving cisplatin. Estimated five-year disease-free survival (81% for P^{32} vs. 75% for cisplatin) and overall survivals (83% for P^{32} vs. 81% for cisplatin) show no significant differences in either group. Estimated five-year disease-free survival for all stage I patients were 86% for patients treated with P^{32} and 83% for those receiving cisplatin. If borderline tumors are excluded, the survivals for stage I are 82% versus 79% (p = 0.79). Stage II patients fared less well with five-year survivals of 55% for those on P^{32} and 68% for patients receiving cisplatin. Both regimens were relatively well tolerated but patients with P^{32} had more bowel toxicity (9% vs. 2%). There were no late second malignancies reported in either arm. Multivariate analysis demonstrated that degree of differentiation and FIGO stage were both significant (p = <.001). Disease-free survival was not influenced by ascites, capsular rupture, tumor excrescences, or location of the primary tumor. Although there was a difference in actuarial survival between clear cell tumors and serous, mucinous, and endometroid tumors (p = 0.02), this was not confirmed in the multivariate analysis. In patients with stage I disease, degree of differentiation was the only significant prognostic variable among FIGO substage, histologic type, age, ascites, capsular rupture, dense adhesions, and tumor excrescences. These authors conclude that cisplatin should become the standard for adjuvant therapy for early disease because of its equivalent effect and reduced incidence of late bowel complications compared with intraperitoneal P^{32}.

The GOG, the North Central Cancer Treatment Group, and the Southwest Oncology Group have an ongoing randomized prospective trial in patients with poor prognosis (stage I grade 3, Ic, and II with no macroscopic residua) early disease comparing intraperitoneal P^{32} with three monthly courses of cyclophosphamide (1,000 mg/M²) and cisplatin (100 mg/M²). Over one hundred twenty patients have been randomized but no interim results are available at the present time. This trial should provide important information about the relative worth of P^{32} versus a cisplatin-containing combination.

INTRAPERITONEAL CHEMOTHERAPY IN EARLY DISEASE

Intraperitoneal chemotherapy is now being studied as an adjuvant therapy for early ovarian cancer. Such an approach has good pharmacokinetic rationale because of the high drug concentrations achievable and the slow peritoneal clearance (103,104). The approach is most likely to be effective in small volume disease due to the limited penetration of most chemotherapeutic agents. A derivative of cisplatin, carboplatin has been shown to be equally effective but has less overall renal toxicity, ototoxicity, and neurotoxicity (105). Intraperitoneal carboplatin has little local toxicity and has a pharmacologic advantage compared to intravenous administration since the peak peritoneal/systemic concentration ratio is around 18. One trial of intraperitoneal carboplatin has been reported in patients with early ovarian cancer (106). The dose-limiting toxicity was thrombocytopenia and leukopenia. The maximum tolerated dose is 500 mg/M² every 28 days. No response data were reported but the approach is now being evaluated in a phase II trial.

CONCLUSIONS

Careful and comprehensive surgery provides the cornerstone of proper management of early ovarian cancer. Much of the confusion in the literature results from groups of patients with "apparent" early disease who have been inadequately staged or from nonrandomized retrospective analyses of small admixed groups of patients not balanced for known prognostic factors. It is now clear that patients with stage Ia or Ib disease and borderline, well-differentiated or moderately differentiated (grade 1 and 2) tumors do not require adjuvant therapy of any kind and have a five-year survival in excess of 90%. In contrast, patients with poor prognostic features such as stage Ic and II disease, poorly differentiated histology, massive ascites, clear cell histology or dense adhesions are at significant (20% or more) risk for subsequent relapse and death from ovarian cancer. These patients would benefit from effective adjuvant therapy. Currently, several therapies appear to be useful, including whole abdominal irradiation, intraperitoneal P^{32}, short-term alkylating agent therapy or platinum-based combination chemotherapy. As yet, all of them appear to be equally effective, but several earlier therapies such as radioactive gold, pelvic irradiation or intraperitoneal P^{32} with pelvic irradiation should be abandoned because of poorer results or excessive toxicity. The results of the ongoing GOG trial comparing intraperitoneal P^{32} to the cyclophosphamide-cisplatin combination should clarify the relative roles of these two approaches. Although there has been substantial reluctance to include a untreated control arm (because of the 20% mortality), it has still not been demonstrated that any of these therapies significantly improve survival in early disease.

REFERENCES

1. Boring CC. Cancer statistics 1992. *CA Cancer J Clin* 1992;42: 19.
2. Young RC, Knapp RC, Fuks Z, et al. Cancer of the ovary. In: DeVita VT Jr, Hellman S, Rosenberg S, eds. *Cancer: Principles and Practice of Oncology*. 3rd ed. New York: JB Lippincott; 1989;1162–1196.
3. Richardson GS, Scully RE, Nikuri N, Nelson JH Jr. Common epithelial cancer of the ovary. *N Engl J Med* 1985;312:415–424.
4. Barber HRK, Graber EA. The PMPO syndrome. *Obstet Gynecol* 1971;38:921.
5. Bolandgray A, Mehellati KA, Ardekany MS. Early detection of ovarian malignancy by culdocentesis. *J Reprod Med* 1971;9: 32.
6. Samuels BI. Usefulness of ultrasound in patients with ovarian cancer. *Semin Oncol* 1975;2:229–233.
7. Berkowitz RS, Leavitt TJ, Knapp RC. Ultrasound directed percutaneous aspiration biopsy of periaortic lymph nodes in cervical carcinoma recurrence. *Am J Obstet Gynecol* 1978;131: 906–908.
8. Higgins RV, van Nagell JR, Donaldson ES, et al. Transvaginal sonography as a screening method for ovarian cancer. *Gynecol Oncol* 1989;34:402.
9. Van Nagell JR, Higgins RV, Donaldson ES, et al. Transvaginal sonography as a screening method for ovarian cancer. A report of the first 1000 cases screened. *Cancer* 1990;65:573.
10. Bourne T, Campbell S, Steer C, et al. Transvaginal colour flow imaging: a possible new screening technique for ovarian cancer. *Br Med J* 1989;299:1367.
11. Musumeci R, DePalo G, Kenda R, Tesoro-Tess JD, et al. Retroperitoneal metastases from ovarian carcinoma: reassessment of 365 patients studied with lymphography. *Am J Radiol* 1980; 134:449–452.
12. Parker BR, Castellino RA, Fuks ZY, Bagshawe MA. The role of lymphography in patients with ovarian cancer. *Cancer* 1974; 34:100–105.
13. Fuks Z. Patterns of spread of ovarian carcinoma: relation to therapeutic strategies. *Adv Biosci* 1980;26:39–51.
14. Schaner EG, Head GL, Kalman MA, et al. Whole body computed tomography in the diagnosis of abdominal and thoracic malignancy: review of 600 cases. *Cancer Treat Rep* 1977;61: 1537–1560.
15. McGowan L, Lesher LP, Norris HJ, et al. Misstaging of ovarian cancer. *Obstet Gynecol* 1985;65:568.
16. Piver MS, Barlow JJ, Lele SB. Incidence of subclinical metastasis in stage I and II ovarian carcinoma. *Obstet Gynecol* 1976; 52:100.
17. Young RC, Decker DG, Wharton JJ, et al. Staging laparotomy in early ovarian cancer. *JAMA* 1983;250:3072.
18. Bagley CM, Young RC, Schein PS, Chabner BA, DeVita VT. Ovarian carcinoma metastatic to diaphragm: frequently undiagnosed at laparotomy. *Am J Obstet Gynecol* 1973;116:397–400.
19. Rosenoff SH, DeVita VT, Hubbard S, Young RC. Peritoneoscopy in the staging and follow-up of ovarian cancer. *Semin Oncol* 1975;2:223–228.
20. Knapp R, Friedman E. Aortic lymph node metastases in early ovarian cancer. *Am J Obstet Gynecol* 1974;110:1013
21. Ozols RF, Fisher RI, Anderson T, Makuch R, Young RC. Peritoneoscopy in the management of ovarian cancer. *Am J Obstet Gynecol* 1981;140:611–619.
22. Berek JS, Griffiths CT, Leventhal JM. Laparoscopy for second-look evaluation in ovarian cancer. *Obstet Gynecol* 1981; 58:192–198.
23. Bjorkholm E, Pettersson F, Einhorn N, et al. Long term follow-up and prognostic factors in ovarian carcinoma: the Radiumhemmet series 1953–1973. *Acta Rad Oncol* 1982;21: 413–419.
24. Dembo AJ, Bush RS. Choice of postoperative therapy based on prognostic factors. *Int J Radiat Oncol Biol Phys* 1982;8: 893–897.
25. Martinez A, Schray MF, Hoes AE, Bagshaw MA. Postoperative radiation therapy for epithelial ovarian cancer: the curative role based on a 24-year experience. *J Clin Oncol* 1985;3: 901–922.
26. Young RC, Walton LA, Ellenberg SS, Homesley HD, Wilbanks GD, Decker DG, Miller A, Park R, Major F Jr. Adjuvant therapy in stage I and stage II epithelial ovarian cancer: results of two prospective randomized trials. *N Engl J Med* 1990;322: 1021–1027.
27. Jenison EL, Montag AG, Griffiths CT, et al. Clear cell adenocarcinoma of the ovary: a clinical analysis and comparison with serous carcinoma. *Gynecol Oncol* 1989;32–65.
28. Munnell EW, Taylor HC. Ovarian carcinoma: a review of 200 primary and 51 secondary cases. *Am J Obstet Gynecol* 1949;58:943.
29. Decker DG, Mussey E, Williams TJ. Grading of gynecologic malignancy: epithelial ovarian cancer. In: *Proceedings of the 7th National Cancer Congress Philadelphia*. JB Lippincott; 1972:223–231.
30. Day TG, Gallagher HS, Rutledge F. Epithelial carcinoma of the ovary: prognostic importance of histologic grade. *Monogr Natl Cancer Inst* 1975;42:15–18.
31. Ozols RF, Garvin WJ, Costa J, et al. Advanced ovarian cancer: correlation of histologic grade with response to therapy and survival. *Cancer* 1980;45:572–581.
32. Dembo AJ, Bush RS. Choice of postoperative therapy based on prognostic factors. *Int J Radiat Oncol Biol Phys* 1982;8: 893–897.
33. Zurawski VR, Broderick SF, Pickens P, et al. Serum CA-125 levels in a group of nonhospitalized women: relevance for the early detection of ovarian cancer. *Obstet Gynecol* 1987;69:606.
34. Olt GJ, Berchuck A, Bast RC. Gynecologic tumor markers. *Semin Surg Oncol* 1990;6:305.
35. Einhorn N, Sjovall K, Knapp R, et al. Prospective evaluation of the specificity of serum CA-125 levels for detection of ovarian cancer in a normal population. *Obstet Gynecol* [in press].
36. Jacobs I, Bridges J, Reynolds C, et al. Multimodal approach to screening for ovarian cancer. *Lancet* 1988;2:268–271.
37. VanNagell JR, DePriest PD. Early diagnosis of ovarian cancer. In: Markman M, Hoskins WJ, eds. *Cancer of the Ovary*. New York: Raven Press; [in press]
38. Campbell S, Bhan V, Royston P, et al. Transabdominal ultrasound screening for early ovarian cancer. *Br Med J* 1989;299: 1363.
39. Scully RE. Recent progress in ovarian cancer. *Hum Pathol* 1970;1:73–98.
40. Scully RE. Ovarian tumors. *Am J Pathol* 1977;87:686–720.
41. Munnell EW. Is conservative therapy ever justified in stage I (Ia) cancer of the ovary? *Am J Obstet Gynecol* 1969;103: 641–650.
42. Webb MJ, Decker DG, Massey, et al. Factors influencing survival in stage I ovarian cancer. *Am J Obstet Gynecol* 1973;166: 222.
43. Dembo AJ, Bush RS, Beale FA. Ovarian carcinoma: improved survival following abdominopelvic irradiation in patients with a completed pelvic operation. *Am J Obstet Gynecol* 1979;134: 793–800.
44. Hreshchyshyn MM, Park RC, Blessing JA, et al. The role of adjuvant therapy in stage I ovarian cancer. *Am J Obstet Gynecol* 1980;138:139–145.

45. Bell DA, Rutgers JL, Scully RE. Ovarian epithelial tumors of borderline malignancy. *Prog Rep Urinary Tract Pathol* 1989;1:1.
46. Ozols RF, Rubin SC, Dembo AJ, Robboy S. Epithelial ovarian cancer. In: Hoskins WJ, Perez CA, Young RC, eds. *Principles and Practice of Gynecologic Oncology*. Philadelphia: JB Lippincott; 1992;731–781,
47. Creasman WT, Park R, Norris H, et al. Stage I borderline ovarian tumors. *Obstet Gynecol* 1982;59:93.
48. Chambers JT. Borderline ovarian tumors: a review of treatment. *Yale J Biol Med* 1989;62:351.
49. Monga M, Carmichael JA, Shelley WE, et al. Surgery without adjuvant chemotherapy for early epithelial ovarian carcinoma after comprehensive surgical staging. *Gynecol Oncol* 1991;43(3):195–197.
50. Lentz SS, Cha SS, Wieand HS, Podratz KC. Stage I ovarian epithelial carcinoma: survival analysis following definitive treatment. *Gynecol Oncol* 1991;43(3):198–202.
51. Gallion HH, van Nagell JR, Donaldson ES, et al. Adjuvant oral alkylating chemotherapy in patients with stage I epithelial ovarian cancer. *Cancer* 1989;63:1070.
52. Piver MS, Malfetano J, Baker TR, et al. Adjuvant cisplatin-based chemotherapy for stage I ovarian adenocarcinoma: a preliminary report. *Gynecol Oncol* 1989;35:69.
53. Dottino PR, Plaxe SC, Cohen CJ. A phase II trial of adjuvant cisplatin and doxorubicin in stage I epithelial ovarian cancer. *Gynecol Oncol* 1991;43(3):203–205.
54. Wils J, van Gevns H. Chemotherapy consisting of cisplatin, doxorubicin and cyclophosphamide as an adjunct to surgery in Stage Ic-II epithelial ovarian carcinoma. *Am J Clin Oncol* 1989;12:251–254.
55. Chiara S, Mammoliti S, Oliva C, et al. Adjuvant cisplatin-based chemotherapy for stage I and II ovarian cancer: a 7-year experience. *Eur J Cancer* 1991;27(10):1211–1215.
56. Fuks Z. The role of radiation therapy in the management of ovarian carcinoma. *Ir J Med Sci* 1977;13:815.
57. Bagley CM Jr, Young RC, Canellos GP, DeVita VT. Treatment of ovarian carcinoma: possibilities for progress. *N Engl J Med* 1972;287:856–862.
58. Tobias JS, Griffiths CT. Management of ovarian carcinoma: current concepts and future prospects. *N Engl J Med* 1976;294:818–823, 877–882.
59. Bush RS, Allt WEC, Beale FA, et al. Treatment of epithelial carcinoma of the ovary: operation, irradiation and chemotherapy. *Am J Obstet Gynecol* 1977;127:692.
60. Dembo AJ, Bush RS, Beale FA, et al. Ovarian carcinoma: improved survival following abdominopelvic irradiation in patients with completed pelvic operation. *Am J Obstet Gynaec* 1979;134:793.
61. Dembo AJ. Radiotherapeutic management of ovarian cancer. *Semin Oncol* 1984;11:238.
62. Fazekas T, Maier JG. Irradiation of ovarian carcinomas: a prospective comparison of the open-field and moving strip techniques. *Am J Roentgenol Rad Ther Nucl Med* 1974;120:118.
63. Fuller DB, Sause WT, Plenk HP, et al. Analysis of postoperative radiation therapy in Stage I through III epithelial ovarian carcinoma. *J Clin Oncol* 1987;5:897.
64. Hart S, Ben-Baruch G, Herczeg E, et al. Abdominopelvic radiation for stage I-II ovarian cancer. *Eur J Gynaecol Oncol* 1989;106:416.
65. Weiser EB, Burke TW, Heller PBV, et al. Determinants of survival of patients with epithelial ovarian carcinoma following whole abdomen irradiation (WAR). *Gynecol Oncol* 1988;30:2012.
66. Dembo AJ. Abdominopelvic radiotherapy in ovarian cancer: a 10-year experience. *Cancer* 1985;55:2285.
67. Weiser EB, Burke TW, Heller PB, et al. Determinants of survival of patients with epithelial ovarian carcinoma following whole abdominal irradiation (WAR). *Gynecol Oncol* 1988;30:201.
68. Goldberg N, Peschel RE. Postoperative abdominopelvic radiation therapy for ovarian cancer. *Int J Radiat Oncol Biol Phys* 1988;14:425.
69. Dubois JB, Joyeux H, Solassol CL, et al. Les tumeurs epitheliales de l'ovaire. Resultats therapeutiques a propos de 165 stades II et III. *J Gynecol Obstet Biol Reprod* 1985;14:627.
70. Perez CA, Korba A, Zivnuska F, et al. ^{60}Co moving strip technique in the management of carcinoma of the ovary: analysis of tumor control and morbidity. *Int J Radiat Oncol Biol Phys* 1978;4:379.
71. Schray MF, Martinez A, Howes AE. Toxicity of open field whole abdominal irradiation as primary post-operative treatment in gynecologic malignancy. *Int J Radiat Oncol Biol Phys* 1989;16:397.
72. Aure JC, Hoeg K, Kolstad P. Radioactive colloidal gold in the treatment of ovarian carcinoma. *Acta Radiol* 1971;10:399–407.
73. Potter ME, Partridge EE, Shingleton HM, et al. Intraperitoneal chromic phosphate in ovarian cancer: risks and benefits. *Gynecol Oncol* 1989;32:314–318.
74. Rosenshein NB. Radioisotopes in the treatment of ovarian cancer. *Clin Obstet Gyn* 1983;10:279.
75. Kolstad P, Davy M, Hoeg K. Individualized treatment of ovarian cancer. *Am J Obstet Gynecol* 1977;128:617–625.
76. Spencer TR, Marks RD, Fenn JO, et al. Intraperitoneal P-32 after negative second-look laparotomy in ovarian carcinoma. *Cancer* 1989;63:2434.
77. Pezner RD, Stevens KRJ, et al. limited epithelial carcinoma of the ovary treated with curative intent by intraperitoneal installation of radiocolloids. *Cancer* 1978;42:2563–2671.
78. Klassen D, Starreveld A, Shelly W, et al. External beam pelvic radiotherapy plus intraperitoneal radioactive chromic phosphate in early stage ovarian cancer: a toxic combination: a National Cancer Institute of Canada Clinical Trials Group Report. *Int J Radiat Oncol Biol Phys* 1985;11:1801–1804.
79. Dembo AJ, Davy S, Stenwig AE, Berle EJ, Bush RS, Kjorstad K. Prognostic factors in patients with stage I epithelial ovarian cancer. *Obstet Gynecol* 1990;75:263–273.
80. Piver MS, Lele SB, Bakshi S, et al. Five and ten year estimated survival and disease-free rates after intraperitoneal chromic phosphate; stage I ovarian adenocarcinoma. *Am J Clin Oncol* 1988;11:515.
81. Powell JL, Burrell MO, Kirchner AB, et al. Intraperitoneal radioactive chromic phosphate P32 in the treatment of ovarian cancer. *Southern Med J* 1987;80:1513.
82. Hreshchyshyn MM, Park RC, Blessing JA, et al. The role of adjuvant therapy in stage I ovarian cancer. *Am J Obstet Gynecol* 1980;138:139.
83. Dembo AJ, Bush RS, De Boer G. Therapy in stage I ovarian cancer. *Am J Obstet Gynecol* 1981;14:231.
84. Smith JP, Rutledge FN, Delclos L. Postoperative treatment of early cancer of the ovary: a random trial between postoperative irradiation and chemotherapy. *Monogr Natl Cancer Inst* 1975;42:149.
85. Delclos L. International symposium on combined modalities approach on gynecologic cancer. Mexico City, Mexico, 1985:61.
86. Piver MS, Lele SB, Patsner B, et al. Stage II invasive adenocarcinoma of the ovary: results of treatment by whole abdominal radiation plus pelvis boost versus pelvic radiation plus oral melphalan chemotherapy. *Gynecol Oncol* 1986;23:168.
87. Sell A, Bertelsen K, Andersen JE. Randomized study of whole-abdomen irradiation versus pelvic irradiation plus cyclophosphamide in treatment of early ovarian cancer. *Gynecol Oncol* 1990;37:367.
88. Davy M, Stenwig AE, Kjorstad KE, et al. Early stage ovarian cancer. *Acta Obstet Gyn Scand* 1985;64:531.
89. MacBeth FR, MacDonald H, Williams CJ. Total abdominal and pelvic radiotherapy in the management of early stage ovarian carcinoma. *Int J Radiat Oncol Biol Phys* 1988;15:353.
90. Dembo AJ. Radiotherapeutic management of ovarian cancer. *Semin Oncol* 1984;11:238.
91. Klaassen D, Shelley W, Starreveld A, et al. Early stage ovarian cancer: a randomized clinical trial comparing whole abdominal radiotherapy, melphalan, and intraperitoneal chromic phosphate: a National Cancer Institute of Canada Clinical Group Report. *J Clin Oncol* 1988;6:1154.
92. Reimer RR, Hoover R, Fraumeni JF, Young RC. Acute leuke-

mia after alkylating agent therapy in ovarian cancer. *N Engl J Med* 1977;297:117.
93. Greene MH, Boice JD Jr, Greer Be, Blessing JA, Dembo AJ. Acute non-lymphocytic leukemia after therapy with alkylating agents for ovarian cancer: a study of five randomized clinical trials. *N Engl J Med* 1982;307:1416–1421.
94. Pedersen-Bjergaard J, Nissen NI, Sorensen HM, et al. Acute non-lymphocytic leukemia in patients with ovarian carcinoma following long-term treatment with Treosulfan (=dihydroxybusulfan). *Cancer* 1980;45:19–29.
95. Ozols RF, Young RC. Chemotherapy of ovarian cancer. *Semin Oncol* 1984;11:251.
96. Bolis G, Marsoni S, Chiari N, et al. Cooperative randomized clinical trial for stage I ovarian carcinoma (OC). In: Conte PF, Ragni N, Rosso R, Vermorken JB, eds. *Multimodal treatment of ovarian cancer*. New York: Raven Press; 1989. p. 87.
97. Bolis G, Torri V, Babilonti L, Colombo N, et al. Multicenter controlled trial in patients with stage I epithelial ovarian cancer. Gruppo Interregionale Cooperative Oncologia Ginecologica, Via Eritrea 62, Milan, Italy (abst) Int. Soc. Gynecol. Cancer Meeting, Cairns, Australia, 1991.
98. Piver MS, Malfetano J, Baker TR, et al. Adjuvant cisplatin-based chemotherapy for stage I ovarian adenocarcinoma: a preliminary report. *Gynecol Oncol* 1989;35:69.
99. Piver MS, Malfetano J, Hempling RE, et al. Cisplatin-based chemotherapy for stage II ovarian adenocarcinoma: a preliminary report. *Gynecol Oncol* 1990;39:249.
100. DePree W, Wils J. Chemotherapy consisting of cisplatin, doxorubicin and cyclophosphamide as an adjunct to surgery in stage Ic-II epithelial ovarian carcinoma. *Anticancer Res* 1989;9:1873.
101. Wils J, van Geuns H. Chemotherapy consisting of cisplatin, doxorubicin and cyclophosphamide as an adjunct to surgery in stage Ic-II epithelial ovarian carcinoma. *Am J Clin Oncol* 1989;12:251.
102. Vergote IB, Vergote-De Vos LN, Abeler VM, et al. Randomized trial comparing cisplatin with radioactive phosphorus or whole-abdomen irradiation as adjuvant treatment of ovarian cancer. *Cancer* 1992;69:741–749.
103. Dedrick RL. Theoretical and experimental bases of intraperitoneal chemotherapy. *Semin Oncol* 1985;12:1–6.
104. Ozols RF. Intraperitoneal chemotherapy in the management of ovarian cancer. *Semin Oncol* 1985;12:75–80.
105. Ozols RF, Young RC. Chemotherapy of ovarian cancer. *Semin Oncol* 1991;18:222.
106. Malmstrom H, Larsson D, Simonsen E. Phase I study of intraperitoneal carboplatin as adjuvant therapy in early ovarian cancer. *Gynecol Oncol* 1990;39:289.

CHAPTER 28

Management of Germ Cell Tumors of the Ovary

Stephen D. Williams and David M. Gershenson

The last two decades have seen great improvements in the diagnosis and management of patients with ovarian germ cell tumors. Most obvious are the improvements in chemotherapy. However, it must be realized that the care of these patients requires the contributions of several specialties and is an excellent example of multidisciplinary collaboration. As will be seen, a substantial majority of these patients will survive and suffer little long-term morbidity of treatment. The staging of these tumors is identical to that used for epithelial ovarian cancer and will not be discussed in this chapter. Likewise, the pathologic classification is discussed elsewhere.

CLINICAL FEATURES

Malignant germ cell tumors of the ovary occur principally in girls and young women. In the UT M.D. Anderson Cancer Center (UTMDACC) series, the age of the patients ranged from 6 to 46 years. These tumors are known to be associated with pregnancy in a small percentage of cases. For example, approximately 15–20% of all dysgerminomas are diagnosed during pregnancy or in the immediate postpartum period.

Signs and symptoms in these patients are rather consistent and frequently rapidly progressive. About 85% of patients will have abdominal pain associated with a palpable pelvic-abdominal mass. Approximately 10% of patients will present with acute abdominal pain, usually caused by rupture, hemorrhage, or torsion of the tumors. This finding may be somewhat more common in patients with endodermal sinus tumor or mixed germ cell tumors and is frequently misdiagnosed as acute appendicitis. Less common signs and symptoms include abdominal distension (35%), fever (10%), and vaginal bleeding (10%). A few patients will exhibit isosexual precocity, presumably due to human chorionic gonadotropin production by the tumor.

Many germ cell tumors possess the unique property of producing biologic markers which can be detected in the serum. The development of specific and sensitive radioimmunoassay techniques for measuring human chorionic gonadotropin (HCG) and alpha fetoprotein (AFP) has led to dramatic improvement in the monitoring of patients with these tumors.

Measurement of these serum markers aids in the diagnosis and, more importantly, may be used in monitoring response to treatment and in the detection of subclinical disease recurrence. Endodermal sinus tumor and choriocarcinoma are the prototypes of AFP and HCG production, respectively. Embryonal carcinoma is capable of producing both HCG and AFP, more commonly the former. Mixed tumors and immature teratoma may produce either, both, or none. Dysgerminoma is commonly considered to be void of any hormonal production, although a small percentage of these tumors do produce low levels of HCG from the multinucleated syncytiotrophoblastic giant cells. An elevation of AFP in a patient who otherwise appears to have pure dysgerminoma connotes the presence of other elements, and that patient should be considered to have a tumor other than dysgerminoma and treated accordingly.

A third serologic marker that has recently received increasing attention is the glycolytic enzyme lactic dehydrogenase (LDH). Certain LDH isoenzymes have been reported to be elevated in patients with testicular cancer as well as in ovarian dysgerminomas. Further

---

S. D. Williams: Indiana University School of Medicine, Indianapolis, Indiana 46202
D. M. Gershenson: Department of Gynecology, The University of Texas M.D. Anderson Cancer Center, Houston, Texas 77030

study of these substances in ovarian germ tumors is warranted. Other serum tumor markers that may be elevated in patients with malignant ovarian germ cell tumors include CA-125 and neuron-specific enolase. Altaras et al. (1) noted elevations of serum CA-125 in five patients with germ cell tumors (three mixed germ cell tumors, one dysgerminoma, and one immature teratoma). Kuzmits et al. (2) observed elevations of serum neuron-specific enolase in eight of eleven (73%) patients with metastatic seminoma. This tumor marker is also likely elevated in a high percentage of patients with ovarian dysgerminoma.

OPERATIVE FINDINGS

Malignant germ cell tumors of the ovary tend to be quite large. In the UTMDACC series, they ranged in size from 7–40 cm with a median of 16 cm. Bilateral tumor involvement, especially true stage IB disease, is exceedingly rare except in the case of dysgerminoma. In dysgerminoma, as many as 10–15% of patients will have bilateral involvement. With the nondysgerminomatous tumors, bilateral involvement almost always signifies advanced disease with metastatic spread to the contralateral ovary or a mixed germ cell tumor with a dysgerminoma component. Contralateral occult ovarian disease may also be seen with dysgerminoma but is rare in tumors other than dysgerminoma except in the case of mixed tumors containing this element.

Ascites is be noted in approximately 20% of cases. Tumor rupture, either preoperatively or intraoperatively, also occurs in approximately 20% of cases. Torsion of the ovarian pedicle is seen infrequently. Benign cystic teratoma is associated with 5–10% of malignant germ cell tumors. It may occur in the ipsilateral ovary, the contralateral ovary, or bilaterally. Likewise, a preexisting gonadoblastoma may be noted in some patients. These patients will generally have dysgenetic gonads with a Y chromosome present.

Malignant germ cell tumors generally spread by peritoneal surface spread or lymphatic dissemination. Although the relative frequency of these two principal mechanisms is difficult to discern, it is generally accepted that these neoplasms more commonly metastasize to lymph nodes than epithelial ovarian cancer. The frequency of poor staging makes the true incidence of lymph node involvement unclear. Hematogenous metastases to liver or lung also occurs. The likelihood of this is much less than in testicular germ cell tumors but probably more than in epithelial tumors. The stage distribution is also very different from that of epithelial ovarian cancer. In most large series, approximately 60–70% of tumors will be stage I. The next most common stage is III, accounting for 25–30% of tumors. Stages II and IV are relatively uncommon.

EXTENT OF PRIMARY SURGERY

The initial treatment approach for a patient suspected of having a malignant ovarian germ cell tumor is surgery, which confirms the diagnosis and initiates therapy. After an adequate vertical midline incision, a thorough determination of disease extent should be made by inspection and palpation. If the disease seems to be confined to one or both ovaries, it is imperative that proper staging biopsies be performed (see below).

The type of primary operative procedure depends upon the surgical findings. As noted previously, bilateral ovarian involvement with tumor is rare except in pure dysgerminoma. Bilateral involvement may also be found in cases of advanced disease (stages II–IV), in which there is metastasis from one ovary to the opposite and in cases of mixed germ cell tumors with a dysgerminoma component. Therefore, unilateral salpingo-oophorectomy with preservation of the contralateral ovary and the uterus can be performed in most patients, thus preserving the potential for fertility. If the contralateral ovary appears grossly normal on careful inspection, it should be left undisturbed. However, biopsy may be considered in the case of pure dysgerminoma, because occult tumor involvement does occur in a small percentage of patients. Unnecessary biopsy, however, may theoretically result in future infertility due to peritoneal adhesions or ovarian failure. If the contralateral ovary appears abnormally enlarged, a biopsy or ovarian cystectomy should be performed. If frozen section analysis reveals malignant disease or a dysgenetic gonad, then bilateral salpingo-oophorectomy is indicated. If a benign cystic teratoma is found (which occurs in approximately 5–10% of cases), then only ovarian cystectomy with preservation of normal ovarian tissue is recommended.

The development of in vitro fertilization technology should also have an impact on intraoperative management. Convention has dictated that if a bilateral salpingo-oophorectomy is necessary, a hysterectomy should also be performed. However, with current technology involving donor oocyte and hormonal support, a woman without ovaries may still sustain a normal intrauterine pregnancy. Similarly, if the uterus and one ovary are resected because of tumor involvement, current techniques provide the opportunity for retrieval of oocytes from the patient's remaining ovary, in vitro fertilization with sperm from her male partner, and implantation of the embryo into a surrogate's uterus. Therefore, traditional guidelines concerning fertility no longer necessarily apply in the surgical treatment of young patients with these tumors.

SURGICAL STAGING

Surgical staging information is important to determine the extent of disease, to provide prognostic information, and to guide postoperative management. A meticulous approach is important for every patient but is of particularly critical importance in those patients with apparent early disease in order to detect the presence of occult or microscopic metastatic disease. Proper staging procedures are analogous to those used in epithelial ovarian cancer and should consist of the following:

1. A vertical midline incision is usually necessary for adequate exposure, for appropriate staging biopsies, or for resection of large pelvic tumors or metastatic disease in the upper abdomen.
2. Ascites, if present, should be evacuated and submitted for cytologic analysis. If no peritoneal fluid is noted, cytologic washings of the pelvis and bilateral paracolic gutters should be performed.
3. The entire peritoneal cavity and its structures should be carefully inspected and palpated in a methodical manner. If any suspicious areas are noted, they should be submitted for biopsy or excised.
4. The primary ovarian tumor and pelvis should next be examined. Both ovaries should carefully be assessed for size, presence of visible tumor involvement, capsular rupture, external excrescences, or adherence to surrounding structures.
5. If disease seems to be confined to the ovary or localized to the pelvis, then random staging biopsies of structures at risk should be performed. Included should be the omentum (with generous biopsies from multiple areas) and the peritoneal surfaces of the following sites: bilateral paracolic gutters, cul-de-sac, lateral pelvic walls, vesicouterine reflection, and subdiaphragmatic areas. Any adhesions should also be generously sampled.
6. The para-aortic and bilateral pelvic lymph-node-bearing areas should be carefully palpated. Any suspicious nodes should be excised or sampled. If no suspicious areas are detected, these areas should be sampled, but there is no evidence that a complete pelvic or retroperitoneal node dissection is beneficial.
7. If obvious gross metastatic disease is present, it should be excised if feasible or at least biopsied. The concept of cytoreductive surgery and evidence to support it will be discussed subsequently.

Unfortunately, many patients with these tumors are inadequately initially staged. Upon referral of such a patient to a university or tertiary center, the oncologist is faced with the dilemma of inadequate staging information. In such cases, postoperative studies, including markers and computed tomography of the abdomen, may provide additional data. It is probably inadvisable to consider re-exploration of these patients with chemosensitive tumors for the purpose of obtaining more precise staging information. As the majority will be treated with chemotherapy, it is important to initiate this without delay.

CYTOREDUCTIVE SURGERY

If metastatic disease is encountered at initial surgery, it is recommended that, as in epithelial ovarian cancer, as much tumor as is technically feasible and safe be resected. It must be remembered, however, that it is difficult to prove the worth of "debulking" surgery and the seeming benefit of it may be related to tumor biology and not the surgery. Slayton et al. (3), in a study of the Gynecologic Oncology Group (GOG), found that fifteen of fifty-four (28%) patients with completely resected disease at primary surgery failed chemotherapy with a combination of vincristine, dactinomycin, and cyclophosphamide (VAC). Of twenty-two (68%) patients with incompletely resected disease treated with the same regimen, fifteen (68%) failed. Furthermore, a higher percentage of patients with bulky residual disease (82%) failed chemotherapy compared to those with small volume residual disease (55%). In a subsequent GOG study in which patients received the combination of cisplatin, vinblastine, and bleomycin (PVB), patients with tumors other than dysgerminoma who had clinically nonmeasurable disease had a greater likelihood of remaining progression-free than those with measurable disease (65% vs. 34%). In addition, patients who had been surgically debulked to optimal disease had an outcome intermediate between patients with suboptimal disease and those with optimal disease without debulking (4).

Even with epithelial tumors, the relative influences of tumor biology and surgical skill and aggressiveness remain uncertain. Germ cell tumors are much more chemosensitive than are epithelial tumors. Therefore, the advisability of aggressive resections of metastatic disease, especially bulky retroperitoneal nodes, is questionable. Certainly, the mainstay of treatment is prompt chemotherapy. The surgeon must exercise thoughtful and mature intraoperative judgment when encountering such situations, carefully weighing the risks and benefits of each cytoreductive maneuver. There is no substitute for surgical experience and a clear understanding of the biologic behavior of these neoplasms in their surgical management. Even in the face of extensive metastatic disease, it is not uncommon for the surgeon to be able to preserve a normal contralateral ovary.

CHEMOTHERAPY OF ADVANCED DISEASE

One of the great triumphs of cancer treatment in the decades of the 70s and 80s has been the development of effective chemotherapy for testicular germ cell tumors and its subsequent application to similar tumors of ovarian origin (5–6). The overwhelming majority of patients with these tumors will survive their disease with the judicious use of surgery and cisplatin-based combination chemotherapy. The lessons learned from prospective, frequently randomized trials in testis cancer have been applied to ovarian germ cell tumors. There are many similarities and a few important differences.

Patients with established unresected metastatic ovarian germ cell tumors other than dysgerminoma all should receive combination chemotherapy. In the past, these patients were usually treated with VAC or VAC-type regimens. Indeed, such treatment would induce complete remission, even in patients with advanced disease. However, the number of such patients who were long survivors was under 50%. In a GOG trial, only seven of twenty-two patients were long survivors (3). In a more recent GOG trial using the combination of cisplatin, vinblastine, and bleomycin (PVB), forty-seven of eighty-nine (53%) patients with advanced and recurrent ovarian germ cell tumors were continuously disease-free with a median follow-up of 52 months (4). The latest treatment failure occurred at 28 months. Eight other patients had durable remissions with second-line therapy. Thus, four-year survival was about 70%. In this trial, 29% had had prior radiation or chemotherapy. These factors appeared to adversely effect outcome, as did amount of residual disease. Of note, however, fully 27% (eight of thirty) who had no previous treatment and nonmeasurable (and presumably small volume) tumor failed. As discussed previously, patients who were debulked to optimal disease fared better than those who were not. Cell type and marker elevation were not associated with outcome.

In testis cancer, a more recent trial has documented that the substitution of etoposide for vinblastine in this regimen gives at least equivalent and actually superior results in patients with high tumor volume (7). Further, the use of etoposide has reduced neurologic toxicity, abdominal cramps, and constipation. The latter two adverse effects are particularly important in these patients as many will have had recent surgery. It also would appear that bleomycin is an important component of the regimen (8) and that carboplatin should not be substituted for cisplatin (9). Thus, most investigators feel that the combination of cisplatin, etoposide and bleomycin (BEP; Table 1) is the preferred regimen.

TABLE 1. *The BEP regimen: three to four courses given at 21-day intervals*

Cisplatin 20 mg/m² days 1–5
* Etoposide (VP-16) 100 mg/m² days 1–5
Bleomycin 30 units i.v. weekly

* Etoposide dose reduced 20% for patients with prior radiotherapy or episode of granulocytopenic fever

TABLE 2. *Chemotherapy of advanced disease*

Institution	Regimen	Prognosis free of total	Prognosis free percent of total
GOG	PVB	47 of 89	53
Stanford	PVB	4 of 4	100
Cross Cancer Institute	PVB	8 of 10	80
M.D. Anderson Cancer Center	PVB	7 of 11	64
M.D. Anderson Cancer Center	BEP	5 of 6	83

From Williams et al., ref. 4; Carlson et al., ref. 35; Taylor et al., ref. 36; Gershenson et al., refs. 37, 22.
GOG, Gynecologic Oncology Group; PVB, cisplatin-vinblastine-bleomycin combination; BEP, cisplatin-etoposide-bleomycin combination.

The results of representative series of patients treated with cisplatin-based treatment is shown in Table 2.

Acute adverse effects of chemotherapy can be substantial and the management of these patients should be done by experienced physicians. About 25% will have febrile neutropenic episodes during chemotherapy and require hospitalization and broad-spectrum antibiotics. Cisplatin can be associated with nephrotoxicity, which can almost always be avoided by ensuring adequate hydration and avoidance of aminoglycoside antibiotics. Bleomycin can cause pulmonary fibrosis. Pulmonary function testing is frequently used in the follow-up of these patients. However, the value of carbon monoxide diffusion capacity to predict early lung disease has recently been challenged (10). Possibly the most useful follow-up technique is careful physical examination of the chest. Findings of early bleomycin pulmonary fibrosis are a lag in or diminished expansion of one hemi-thorax or fine basilar rates that do not clear with cough. These findings can be very subtle but, if present, mandate immediate discontinuation of bleomycin.

In general, these patients should receive four courses of treatment given in full dose and on schedule. There is presumptive evidence in testicular germ cell tumors that treatment delays are associated with a worse outcome. Thus, chemotherapy courses should be given regardless of hematologic parameters on the scheduled day of treatment. Etoposide dose is reduced 20% for previous febrile neutropenic episodes or radiotherapy and bleomycin discontinued as noted above. Modern antiemetic therapy has substantially lessened chemotherapy-induced emesis. By following these guidelines and supportive care as indicated, virtually all patients can be treated on schedule in full or nearly full dose. Chemotherapy-related mortality in earlier times in patients with advanced disease occurred in 4–5% but more recent GOG experience is that this should occur in less than 1%. Late effects are discussed subsequently.

Current clinical trials in testicular germ cell tumors separate patients with small tumor volume and a resultant excellent prognosis from those with bulky tumor or liver or brain involvement. Patients in the former group will almost always be chemotherapy complete responders and long survivors whereas only about 50–60% of patients with bulky tumor will survive. Trials in good prognosis patients investigate shorter or less toxic chemotherapy; trials in advanced disease patients are evaluating more intensive chemotherapy in an effort to improve the likelihood of cure. However, as noted above, in patients with incompletely resected ovarian germ cell tumors other than dysgerminoma, to date there has not yet been a group defined that has a sufficiently high cure rate to warrant less intensive therapy. Whether this is an inherent biologic difference or merely underestimation of tumor volume because of intraperitoneal spread is not clear.

ADJUVANT CHEMOTHERAPY

The increased level of understanding of systemic therapy for advanced and recurrent tumor has had profound implications for the management of patients with completely resected tumor. Unfortunately, even when tumor is completely resected, the likelihood for recurrence in most situations is substantial.

Most well-staged patients with grade 1, stage I immature teratoma will survive progression-free, but the failure rate of less well-differentiated immature teratoma is appreciable. As many as 75% with grade 3, stage I patients will recur after initial surgery, as will a similar number of patients with resected endodermal sinus tumor, embyronal carcinoma, or mixed germ cell tumors. Thus, all patients except those with grade 1 stage I immature teratoma should receive adjuvant chemotherapy. Traditionally, VAC or VAC-like regimens were used. In an early GOG trial employing VAC as a postoperative surgical adjuvant, fifteen of fifty-four (28%) patients experienced disease recurrence (3). In more recent GOG experience that required precise surgical staging, twenty-four of one hundred patients treated with six months of VAC recurred (11).

Because of successes of cisplatin-based chemotherapy in testicular cancer and in advanced stage ovarian germ cell tumors, similar regimens have been given to patients after surgery with complete resection of an ovarian germ cell tumor. Multiple anecdotal reports have suggested that virtually all patients will remain progression-free after such treatment. In an ongoing prospective trial of the GOG, fifty of fifty-two stage I,

TABLE 3. Adjuvant chemotherapy

Institution	Regimen	Progressions free total	Percent of total
GOG	BEP	50 of 52	96
Standford	PVB	5 of 5	100
Cross Cancer Institute	PVB	4 of 4	100
MD Anderson Cancer Center	PVB	4 of 4	100
MD Anderson Cancer Center	BEP	20 of 20	100

From Williams et al., ref. 11; Carlson et al., ref. 35; Taylor et al., ref. 36; Gershenson et al., refs. 37, 22.
GOG, Gynecologic Oncology Group; PVB, cisplatin-vinblastine-bleomycin combination; BEP, cisplatin-etoposide-bleomycin combination.

stage II, and stage III patients with completely resected tumor are disease-free after three courses of BEP (11). The only two failures had grade 1 immature teratoma at second-look laparotomy and both have had no further progression. One was treated with VAC and the other received no additional treatment. Thus, all fifty-two patients are currently clinically free of disease. These and the results of others are summarized in Table 3.

These results provide convincing evidence that BEP is superior to VAC as a surgical adjuvant. With modern supportive care, acute toxicity is manageable and in the GOG study there have been no treatment-related deaths or severe short-term toxicity. As opposed to the situation in resected stage II testis cancer, in which chemotherapy can be deferred until the time of relapse in patients destined to do so, the relapse rate of ovarian patients is higher and the ability to salvage them at recurrence lower. Thus, all such patients should receive adjuvant chemotherapy given as soon as possible after their initial surgical treatment. It should be emphasized that some of these patients will recur very rapidly and every effort should be made to initiate treatment rapidly, preferably within 7–10 days of surgery. Because of these time constraints, serial marker studies are less useful; chemotherapy is frequently initiated before markers have had time to normalize.

TREATMENT OF PERSISTENT OR RECURRENT TUMOR

The management of patients with persistent or recurrent active tumor after initial chemotherapy is a complex topic. It is important to distinguish between patients truly cisplatin-resistant (i.e., no response or progression within six weeks of chemotherapy) and cisplatin-sensitive (progression later than six weeks off treatment). In the latter group, it is appropriate to administer further cisplatin-based treatment, usually cisplatin, vinblastine, and ifosfamide (12). This approach, however, makes little sense in cisplatin-resistant patients and high-dose chemotherapy with autologous bone marrow rescue should be considered in these patients (13).

SECOND-LOOK LAPAROTOMY

Since 1960, second-look laparotomy has been incorporated into the routine management of patients with epithelial ovarian cancer to assess disease status after chemotherapy. It was only natural that such an approach would be extrapolated to the management of patients with ovarian germ cell tumors who have no clinical evidence of disease after chemotherapy. In a review of the experience with second-look laparatomy at UTMDACC, findings were negative in fifty-two of fifty-three patients (14). One patient with no tumor subsequently relapsed and died. Thirteen patients had mature teratoma—the so-called chemotherapeutic retroconversion—at second-look laparotomy; treatment was discontinued in all patients and none have developed recurrence.

In testis cancer, as many as 25–40% of patients will have a clinically or radiographically apparent residual mass after chemotherapy. This finding is much less common in ovarian germ cell tumors than in testicular cancer. At completion of chemotherapy, men with nonseminomatous tumors or seminoma may have persistent mature teratoma or fibrosis. Although a number of patients with pure ovarian immature teratomas or mixed germ cell tumors have persistent mature teratoma at the completion of chemotherapy, as documented by second-look laparotomy, the majority have multiple small peritoneal implants rather than a true mass. The latter phenomenon, however, has been observed. Likewise, some patients with dysgerminoma will have a persistent mass which is likely, in the vast majority, to be fibrosis.

For patients with persistent masses after completion of chemotherapy, options for diagnosis and management include surgical intervention, fine needle aspiration, or surveillance with serial imaging studies. In view of the above discussion, it is recommended that the latter two options be considered initially. It currently seems appropriate to limit the use of second-look laparotomy in this patient population as much as possible. Patients with early stage disease almost always have negative findings and should not have this procedure. Likewise, as will be discussed subsequently, patients with dysgerminoma will routinely have negative findings. It is conceivable that enough patients with advanced disease, particularly those with initially negative serum tumor markers, will benefit in a meaningful way and warrant this procedure. Further study is needed in this area. Nevertheless, as better therapies are developed and refined, second-look laparotomy will inevitably become obsolete except in unusual situations.

DYSGERMINOMA

Dysgerminoma is the female equivalent of seminoma. This disease differs from its nondysgerminomatous counterpart in several respects. First, it is probably more likely to be localized to the ovary at the time of diagnosis. Bilateral involvement is more common, as is spread to retroperitoneal lymph nodes. Most notable, however, is its sensitivity to radiotherapy.

The literature of dysgerminoma is difficult to interpret because much of it was developed in a time when careful surgical staging was not done. It was thought that about 75% of patients would have stage I disease. With careful surgical staging, this number is certainly less, but it has been estimated that about two-thirds of such patients will have disease confined to one ovary at diagnosis. These women were traditionally treated with postoperative radiotherapy. However, as pelvic radiotherapy is associated with a high incidence of sterility, some patients have been observed after surgery and have not received radiation. It has been stated that those women with primary tumors less than ten centimeters and with no evidence of contralateral ovarian involvement could be observed; those patients with a primary tumor greater than ten centimeters should receive adjuvant radiotherapy (15). However, the distinction based upon size has been called into question (16). Currently, the majority of investigators feel that size should not be used to decide between the options of observation or postoperative radiotherapy and that observation is a reasonable option regardless of the size of the primary tumor. It is particularly attractive in those patients who wish to retain potential for childbearing. Careful follow-up is required as 15–25% will recur, but because of the sensitivity of this tumor to chemotherapy or radiotherapy, virtually all patients should be successfully salvaged by chemotherapy given at the time of recurrence, assuming follow-up has been careful and the recurrence is diagnosed at a time when the tumor volume is relatively small.

In the past, many stage I patients and all patients of higher stage have been treated with radiotherapy. The specifics of the radiation are beyond the scope of this discussion. In general, doses required are relatively modest. In patients with disease confined to one ovary, radiation is typically given to the ipsilateral hemipelvis and para-aortic nodes. For IB tumors, the whole pelvis is treated. In patients with para-aortic involvement, in addition to the treatment of this area, many have advocated prophylactic mediastinal radiation. Patients with intraperitoneal tumor have received whole abdomen radiation with or without mediastinal treatment.

The role of prophylactic treatment of the mediastinum should be discussed further, particularly considering the recent improvements in chemotherapy to be discussed subsequently. In testicular seminoma, dogma taught that similar therapy should be given. This thinking, however, was challenged and most investigators now feel mediastinal radiation is not necessary (17). It is difficult to know whether this line of reasoning applies to dysgerminoma. However, it seems now to be a moot point as it is clear that most, if not all, of these patients are best treated primarily with chemotherapy.

Results of radiation therapy are reasonably good. DePalo and associates (18) report that all thirteen stage I patients (twelve stage IA and one stage IB) are alive and free of disease with a median follow-up of 77 months. The five-year relapse-free survival of the twelve stage III patients was 61.4%, and the overall survival was 89.5%. Median follow-up was 67 months. Only one death is reported in this group. A recent series from Sweden reported the results of therapy of a heterogeneous group of sixty patients of all stages of dysgerminoma. Fifty-five percent had stage IA disease, but 22% had stage III, and 3% stage IV tumors. Nearly all received external radiation. Only eleven died of tumor; five-year disease-free and overall survivals (excluding intercurrent illness) were approximately 70% and 83%, respectively (19).

Recent data have shown that dysgerminoma is quite sensitive to cisplatin-based chemotherapy. The analogous disease in male patients is seminoma. Patients with advanced seminoma have a substantial complete remission and cure rate (20). Prognostic factors in testicular seminoma include extent of disease and amount of previous radiation therapy. Those patients who have had radiation therapy to both retroperitoneum and the mediastinum fare substantially worse than those with limited or no previous radiotherapy. It is unknown, however, whether this is because of reduced chemotherapy tolerance or inherent biologic differences.

The GOG has recently reviewed its experience with dysgerminoma patients entered on its ovarian germ cell protocols. All had advanced incompletely resected tumor. Treatment was PVB in the first protocol (4). The second and ongoing study is induction chemotherapy with BEP, followed by consolidation with VAC. To date, twenty dysgerminoma patients are evaluable on these two protocols (21). All had stage III or IV disease and most had greater than 2 cm residual tumor. Eleven of twelve patients with measurable disease responded completely. Fourteen patients underwent second-look laparotomy and all were negative. Overall, nineteen are disease-free with follow-up of 9–66 months (26 month median). These results, as well as those from other studies (22), suggest that high-stage or recurrent dysgerminoma patients should receive BEP, just as do their nondysgerminomatous counterparts.

As in other germ cell tumors, these results have implications for management of patients with resected early stage dysgerminoma. As noted earlier, three courses of BEP will essentially always prevent relapse in patients with completely resected tumors other than dysgerminoma. There is limited experience with "adjuvant" chemotherapy of dysgerminoma, but the information that is available is equally favorable (22). Further, metastatic dysgerminoma is more sensitive to chemotherapy than tumors other than dysgerminoma. All things considered, it seems likely that the appropriate adjuvant therapy for resected dysgerminoma of stages IB to III is chemotherapy with three courses of BEP. It is difficult to know what the natural history of tumors of these stages are if adjuvant therapy is not given, but it seems likely that the vast majority will recur. In patients with IA tumors, the risk of recurrence is 15–20%, and compliant patients can be followed without adjuvant treatment. On occasion, it may be deemed appropriate to administer adjuvant treatment to such a patient because of patient wishes or concerns about compliance. In this situation, chemotherapy seems the best choice, considering the limited impact of it on fertility (see below).

The role of tumor markers (HCG and AFP) should be discussed further. These tumor markers are useful methods to follow the clinical course in patients with tumors other than dysgerminoma. It is likely that, as in seminoma, an AFP elevation connotes the presence of elements other than dysgerminoma and treatment should be given accordingly. However, as in seminoma, an elevated HCG is seen occasionally in pure dysgerminoma and should not alter therapy.

LATE EFFECTS

As the prognosis of patients with malignant ovarian germ cell tumors has dramatically improved with the evolution of modern combination chemotherapy, attention has increasingly been focussed on late effects of therapy. Although there is a considerable body of literature on late effects in testicular cancer patients, there is little available information concerning their female counterparts. However, many analogies can be drawn.

One potentially important cause of late morbidity is surgery. Young patients with malignant ovarian germ cell tumors undergo at least one and, not uncommonly, multiple procedures. Although there is not available information on the long-term effects of surgery, future infertility related to pelvic surgery with consequent peritoneal and tubal adhesions is well-described. Therefore, it seems prudent for the surgeon to practice meticulous surgical technique and to avoid unnecessary operative maneuvers, including unnecessary biopsy of the contralateral ovary (23). Another cause of infertility in this patient population is unnecessary bilateral salpingo-oophorectomy and hysterectomy. This phenomenon will hopefully diminish in frequency as information concerning the natural history of ovarian germ cell tumors and the effectiveness of chemotherapy is more widely appreciated.

As with any group of patients with a history of pelvic surgery, patients with ovarian germ cell tumors may subsequently develop functional cysts in their remaining ovary. Muram et al. (24) reported their experience with twenty-seven patients with ovarian germ cell tumors who underwent unilateral salpingo-oophorectomy and were followed for 12–215 months after completion of therapy. Of the eighteen patients who maintained ovarian function, thirteen (72%) developed a functional ovarian cyst during the follow-up period.

Most of the available literature on the late effects of radiotherapy on long-term survivors of childhood or adolescent cancer involves patients with Hodgkin's disease or nonHodgkin's lymphoma. It is now well-appreciated that premature ovarian failure may be avoided in some young females undergoing abdominal radiotherapy by the use of oophoropexy or shielding techniques. There is, however, less information about the late effects of radiotherapy in patients with dysgerminoma. In one series from UTMDACC, the late effects of radiation were studied in forty-three patients (25). Somewhat surprisingly, none developed small intestinal obstruction 3.3 to 34.6 years later (median follow-up is 12.4 years). Furthermore, there were no other significant bowel or bladder problems noted. No patients have conceived since receiving radiotherapy, although three have spontaneously resumed menses. The number of patients attempting pregnancy is unknown. The current strong trend away from radiation and toward chemotherapy as a postoperative adjuvant will likely allow many more patients to retain fertility.

One of the earliest recognized effects of chemotherapy was the risk of secondary malignancies, usually acute leukemia. Several studies have clearly documented the development of nonlymphocytic leukemia in patients who received alkylating agent chemotherapy for ovarian cancer (26). There are several reports of the development of acute leukemia in testicular cancer patients who received PVB (27). However, treatment-related leukemia has been rarely seen in patients who have received neither classic alkylating agents nor radiotherapy (28). In the UTMDACC series, one female patient has thus far developed acute nonlymphocytic leukemia (14). She had stage Ic immature teratoma and received 12 cycles of VAC. She then did well for 26 months, at which time she was diagnosed as having acute leukemia.

A recently published study has described the occurrence of leukemia in testis tumor patients treated with etoposide in combination with bleomycin and cisplatin (29). The evidence would indicate that etoposide is the responsible agent, considering its mechanism of action and other studies. Interestingly, this finding was not seen in patients receiving less than 2000 mg/m^2 total cumulative dose of etoposide. By current standards, few patients would receive more than this dose except in those who are heavily treated and require high-dose chemotherapy with autologous bone marrow rescue. Thus, while etoposide probably is a leukemogenic drug, there seems no reason not to use it in these patients. Further, it does not appear that leukemia is associated with modern therapy of ovarian germ cell tumors, with this one exception.

There also continues to be considerable focus on the long-term effects of chemotherapy on gonadal function. Studies of patients with a variety of cancers suggest that, although ovarian dysfunction or failure is a risk of chemotherapy, the majority of survivors can anticipate normal menstrual and reproductive function (30–32). Factors such as older age at initiation of therapy, greater cumulative drug dose, and longer duration of therapy have an adverse effect on future gonadal function. Successful pregnancies after treatment with chemotherapy have been well documented in other types of malignancies. There are also anecdotal reports in patients with ovarian germ cell tumors (4).

In a recent review of the UTMDACC series, twenty-seven (68%) of forty patients who had retained a normal contralateral ovary and uterus after successful treatment with combination chemotherapy for ovarian germ cell tumors maintained regular menses consistently after completion of chemotherapy, and thirty-three (83%) were having regular menses at the time of follow-up (33). Many of these patients had been treated with VAC and a relatively small number had received cisplatin-based treatment. Of sixteen patients who had attempted to become pregnant, twelve did so. One patient had an elective first-trimester abortion, and the other eleven patients over time bore twenty-two healthy infants.

Although no reports of other late effects of chemotherapy on patients with ovarian germ cell tumors are available, there are several articles on this topic involving patients with testicular cancer. Anecdotal care reports have described various late toxicities, including stroke, myocardial infarction, peripheral vascular disease, Raynaud's phenomenon, hypertension, and chronic renal failure. However, in a retrospective review of the Indiana University experience in a large number of patients with relatively long follow-up, the only common toxicities were peripheral neuropathy and Raynaud's phenomenon, both of which tended to be relatively mild (28). Furthermore, the late follow-up experience of the Testicular Cancer Intergroup Study has been recently reviewed (34). In this study, patients with completely resected stage II disease were randomized to two courses of adjuvant PVB or observation. At the time of recurrence, the latter patients were treated with four courses of PVB. Thus, this prospective random study has groups of patients that received no, two, or four courses of chemotherapy. The chemotherapy patients had a more frequent incidence of paresthesias, but there were no differences in the frequency of cardiovascular events.

SUMMARY

Virtually all patients with early stage, completely resected tumors other than dysgerminoma will survive after careful surgical staging and cisplatin-based adjuvant chemotherapy. In addition, over 50% to perhaps as high as 80% of patients with advanced disease will also survive their disease. There are, however, areas of improvement and the role of ifosfamide, consolidation noncrossresistant chemotherapy, and the use of high-dose chemotherapy with autologous marrow rescue are being investigated. The late consequences of chemotherapy are modest and efforts should be made to preserve reproductive organs in patients who are desirous of subsequent pregnancy, as many patients so treated will resume menses and childbearing potential. All of these patients are potential candidates for clinical trials.

The majority of dysgerminoma patients have stage I disease at diagnosis. These patients usually can be treated with unilateral salpingo-oophorectomy and if fertility is an issue, they can be observed carefully with regular pelvic exams, abdominal computerized tomography, and tumor markers, including LDH. Relapsing patients are treated with chemotherapy. In patients with more advanced but resected disease, risk of recurrence is significant enough to warrant adjuvant treatment, which for most patients should be chemotherapy because of its universal effectiveness and limited impact on fertility. In patients with incompletely resected tumor or for patients who recur after previous radiation, chemotherapy similar to that given for tumors other than dysgerminoma is also appropriate.

Surgery continues to have a pivotal role in the management of all patients with ovarian germ cell tumors. Initial careful surgical staging is important for selection of appropriate subsequent therapy. The role of cytoreductive surgery is under study but the evidence supports the judicious use of this. However, an operation done strictly for debulking when the diagnosis is established does not seem warranted. The role of second-look surgery is also under study. It clearly is not indicated in patients with early stage nondysgerminoma or in all patients with dysgerminoma. The impact of this procedure in patients with high stage nondysgerminoma who are clinically disease-free is under study but may allow the early administration of "salvage" chemotherapy.

REFERENCES

1. Altaras MM, Goldberg GL, Levin W, Darge L, Block B, Smith JA. The value of cancer antigen-125 as a tumor marker in malignant germ cell tumors of the ovary. *Gynecol Oncol* 1986;25:150.
2. Kuzmits R, Schernthaner G, Krisch K. Serum neuron-specific enolase: a marker for response to therapy in seminoma. *Cancer* 1987;60:1017.
3. Slayton RE, Park RC, Silverberg SG, Shingleton H, Creasman WT, Blessing JA. Vincristine, dactinomycin, and cyclophosphamide in the treatment of malignant germ cell tumors of the ovary: a Gynecologic Oncology Group study (a final report). *Cancer* 1985;56:243–248.
4. Williams SD, Blessing JA, Moore DH, Homesley HD, Adcock L. Cisplatin, vinblastine, and bleomycin in advanced and recurrent ovarian germ-cell tumors. *Ann Intern Med* 1989;111:22–27.
5. Bosl GJ, Gluckman R, Geller NL, Golbey RB, Whitmore WF, Herr H, Sogani P, Morse M, Martini N, Bains M, McCormack P. VAB-6: an effective chemotherapy regimen for patients with germ-cell tumors. *J Clin Oncol* 1986;4(10):1493–1499.
6. Loehrer PJ, Williams SD, Einhorn LH. Testicular Cancer: the quest continues. *J Natl Cancer Inst* 1989;80:1373–1382.
7. Williams SD, Birch R, Einhorn LH, Irwin L, Greco FA, Loehrer PJ. Disseminated germ cell tumors: chemotherapy with cisplatin plus bleomycin plus either vinblastine or etoposide. *N Engl J Med* 1987;316:1435–1440.
8. Loehrer PJ, Elson P, Johnson DH, Williams SD, Trump DL, Einhorn LH. A randomized trial of cisplatin plus etoposide with or without bleomycin in favorable prognosis disseminated germ cell tumors: an ECOG study. *Proc Am Soc Clin Oncol* 1991;10:169.
9. Bajorin DF, Sarosdy MF, Bosl GJ, Weisen S, Heller G. A randomized trial of etoposide + carboplatin vs. etoposide + cisplatin in patients with metastatic germ cell tumors. *Proc Am Soc Clin Oncol* 1991;10:168.
10. McKeage MJ, Evans BD, Atkinson C. Carbon monoxide diffusing capacity is a poor predictor of clinically significant bleomycin lung. *J Clin Oncol* 1990;8:779–783.
11. Williams SD, Blessing J, Slayton R, Homesley H, Photopolus G. Ovarian germ cell tumors: adjuvant trials of the Gynecologic Oncology Group. *Proc Am Soc Clin Oncol* 1989;8:150.
12. Loehrer PJ, Lauer R, Roth BJ, Williams SD, Kalasinski L, Einhorn LH. Salvage therapy with VP-16 or vinblastine plus ifosfamide plus cisplatin in recurrent germ cell cancer. *J Clin Oncol* 1988;109:540–546.
13. Nichols CR, Tricot G, Williams SD, Von Besien K, Loehrer PJ, Roth BJ, Akard L, Hoffman R, Goulet R, Wolff SN, Giannone L, Greer J, Einhorn LH, Jansen J. Dose-intensive chemotherapy in refractory germ cell cancer: a phase I/II trial of high-dose carboplatin and etoposide with autologous bone marrow transplantation. *Ann Int Med* 1989;7:932–999.
14. Gershenson DM, Copeland LJ, Del Junco G. Second-look laparotomy in the management of malignant germ cell tumors of the ovary. *Obstet Gynecol* 1986;67:789.
15. Krepart G, Smith JP, Rutledge F, Delclos L. The treatment for dysgerminoma of the ovary. *Cancer* 1978;41:986–990.
16. Thomas GM, Dembo AJ, Hacker NF, DePetrillo AD. Current

therapy for dysgerminoma of the ovary. *Obstet Gynecol* 1987; 70:268–275.
17. Thomas GM, Rider WD, Dembo AJ, et al. Seminoma of the testis: results of treatment and patterns of failure after radiation therapy. *Int J Radiot Oncol Biol Phys* 1982;8:165–174.
18. DePalo G, Lattuada A, Kenda R, Musumeci RMZ, Pilotti S, Bellani FF, Re, FD, Banfi A. Germ cell tumors of the ovary: the experience of the National Cancer Institute of Milan. I. Dysgerminoma. *Int J Radiat Oncol Biol Phys* 1987;13:853–860.
19. Bjorkholm E, Lundell M, Gyftodimos A, Silfversward C. Dysgerminoma: the Radiumhemmet series 1927–1984. *Cancer* 1990; 65:38–44.
20. Loehrer PJ, Birch R, Williams SD, Greco FA, Einhorn LH. Chemotherapy of metastatic seminoma: the Southeastern Cancer Study Group experience. *J Clin Oncol* 1987;5:1212–1220.
21. Williams SD, Blessing JA, Hatch KD, Homesley HD. Chemotherapy of advanced dysgerminoma: trials of the Gynecologic Oncology Group. *J Clin Oncol* 1991;1950–1955.
22. Gershenson DM, Morris M, Cangir A, Kavanagh JJ, Stringer CA, Edwards CL, Silva EG, Wharton JT. Treatment of malignant germ cell tumors of the ovary with bleomycin, etoposide, and cisplatin. *J Clin Oncol* 1990;8:715–720.
23. Trimobs-Kemper T, Trimbos B, Van Hall E. Etiological factors in tubal infertility. *Fertil Steril* 1982;37:384.
24. Muram D, Gale C, Thompson E. Functional ovarian cyusts in patients cured of ovarian neoplasms. *Obstet Gynecol* 1990;75: 680.
25. Mitchell MF, Gershenson DM, Soeters RP, Eifel PJ, Delclos L, Wharton JT. The long-term effects of radiotherapy on patients with ovarian dysgerminoma. *Cancer* 1991;67:1084–1090.
26. Reimer RR, Hoover R, Fraumeni JF, Young RC. Acute leukemia after alkylating-agent therapy of ovarian cancer. *N Engl J Med* 1977;297.
27. Van Imhoff GW, Sleijfer D, Breuning MH, Anders G, Mulder NH, Halie MR. Acute nonlymphocytic leukemia 5 years after treatment with cisplatin, vinblastine, and bleomycin for disseminated testicular cancer. *Cancer* 1986;57:984.
28. Roth B, Greist A, Kubilis PS, Williams SD, Einhorn LH. Cisplatin-based combination chemotherapy for disseminated germ cell tumors: long-term follow-up. *J Clin Oncol* 1988;6: 1239–1247.
29. Pedersen-Bjergaard J, Hansen SW, Larsen SO, Daugaard G, Philip P, Rorth M. Increased risk of myelodysplasia and leukaemia after etoposide, cisplatin, and bleomycin for germ-cell tumours. *Lancet* 1991;338:359–363.
30. Siris E, Leventhal BG, Vaitukaitis JL. Effects of childhood leukemia and chemotherapy on puberty and reproductive function in girls. *N Engl J Med* 1976;294:1143.
31. Horning SJ, Hoppe RT, Kaplan HS, Rosenberg SA. Female reproductive potential after treatment for Hodgkin's disease. *N Engl J Med* 1981;304:1377.
32. Byrne J, Mulvihill JJ, Myers MH, Connelly RR, Naughton MD, Krauss MR. Effects of treatment on fertility in long-term survivors of childhood or adolescent cancer. *N Engl J Med* 1987;317: 1315.
33. Gershenson DM. Menstrual and reproductive function after treatment with combination chemotherapy for malignant ovarian germ cell tumors. *J Clin Oncol* 1988;6:270–275.
34. Nichols C, Roth B, Williams S, Muggia F, Gill I, Stablein D, Weiss R, Einhorn L. Cardiovascular complications of chemotherapy for testicular cancer. *Proc Am Soc Clin Oncol* 1990;9: 132.
35. Carlson RW, Sikic BI, Turbow MM, Ballon SC. Combination cisplatin, vinblastine, and bleomycin chemotherapy (PVB) for malignant germ-cell tumors of the ovary. *J Clin Oncol* 1983;1: 645–651.
36. Taylor MD, Depetrillo AD, Turner AR. Vinblastine, bleomycin, and cisplatin in malignant germ cell tumors of the ovary. *Cancer* 1985;56:1341–1349.
37. Gershenson DM, Kavanaugh JJ, Copeland LJ, Junco GD, Cangir A, Saul PB, Stringer A, Edwards CL, Wharton TJ. Treatment of malignant nondysgerminomatous germ cell tumors of the ovary with vinblastine, bleomycin, and cisplatin. *Cancer* 1986;57:1731–1737.

CHAPTER 29

Sex Cord-Stromal Tumors of the Ovary

Walter B. Jones

Sex cord-stromal tumors and sex cord-mesenchymal tumors are terms used to describe a complex group of ovarian neoplasms that are derived from coelomic and mesonephric epithelium. This same general group of neoplasms is also referred to as mesenchymomas and gonadal stromal tumors by investigators who are of the view that these tumors are derived from the mesenchyme or specialized stroma of the genital ridge. The term *sex cord-stromal tumors*, at any rate, has been adopted by the World Health Organization (WHO) (1-2) and, according to Young and Scully (3), has the advantage of acknowledging the presence of derivatives of either or both the sex cords and the stroma. These derivatives include neoplasms containing granulosa cells, theca cells, collagen-producing stromal cells, Sertoli cells, Leydig cells, and/or cells resembling their embryonic precursors, singly or in varying combinations. The generic term *sex cord-stromal tumors* will be used in this chapter to describe ovarian tumors containing these cell types.

Sex cord-stromal tumors are reported to account for 3% to 9% of all ovarian neoplasms (3-6). Tumors of stromal origin such as thecoma, stromal luteoma, and Leydig cell tumors typically follow a benign course while sex cord tumors of granulosa or Sertoli cell types are generally of a low order of malignancy, tending to late recurrence, and only rarely to distant metastasis (7). Sex cord-stromal tumors, while uncommon before menarche, account for approximately 6% of malignant tumors in childhood (8). As a group, sex cord-stromal tumors receive a disproportionate amount of attention from pathologists relative to their incidence, because they are often difficult to diagnose. Therapeutic decisions depend in large measure on the histopathologic interpretation of these tumors; thus, an experienced pathologist is required to establish the correct diagnosis.

For purposes of organization, the classification of sex cord-stromal tumors will be given first (Table 1). The classification is that of the WHO, modified by Young and Scully to include several tumors recognized since the WHO classification was adopted (3). Following this, each of the tumors according to this classification will be discussed. The histogenesis, where known, the clinical presentation, and the gross and cytopathologic features leading to the diagnosis will be presented. In the last two decades, ultrastructural and immunohistochemical studies have played a significant role in establishing the origin of the cell type and in clarifying certain functional correlations of these tumors. Finally, current management and prognosis of sex cord-stromal tumors will be presented. The recent introduction of platinum-based chemotherapy regimens for certain advanced and recurrent sex-cord stromal tumors has resulted in improved survival rates.

GRANULOSA CELL TUMORS

The origin of granulosa cell tumors is not universally agreed upon. Whether they arise in the ovarian stroma or are derived from the germinal epithelium is still disputed (9). That the granulosa cells differentiate from the primitive sex cords of the indifferent gonad is generally accepted, but the origin of these cords remains uncertain (10). Granulosa cell tumors account for up to 10% of all ovarian malignancies (11), with the incidence of malignancy estimated to be as low as 7% and as high as 53% of cases (12). However, all granulosa cell tumors are considered by some authorities to be actually or potentially malignant. Granulosa cell tumors, the most common type of functioning ovarian neoplasm, are almost always estrogenic when endocrine manifestations are present (13). In most cases, both granulosa and theca cells are present (14). The tumors,

---

W. B. Jones: Gynecology Service, Department of Surgery, Memorial Sloan-Kettering Cancer Center, New York, New York 10021

TABLE 1. *Classification of sex cord-stromal tumors*

Granulosa-stromal tumor
  Granulosa cell tumor
    Adult type
    Juvenile type

Tumors in the thecoma-fibroma group
  Thecoma
    Typical
    Luteinized
  Fibroma-fibrosarcoma
    Fibroma
    Cellular fibroma
    Fibrosarcoma
  Stromal tumor with minor sex cord elements
  Sclerosing stromal tumor
  Unclassified

Sertoli-stromal cell tumors
  Sertoli cell tumor
  Leydig cell tumor
  Sertoli-Leydig cell tumors
    Well-differentiated
    Of intermediate differentiation
    Poorly differentiated
    With heterologous elements

Gynandroblastoma

Sex cord tumor with annular tubules

Unclassified

although encountered in all age groups, principally occur in women between 30 and 70 years old, with a peak incidence between 45 and 55 years (10). The age-specific incidence rates increase almost linearly after age 35 (15). According to Roth and Czernobilsky (13), the incidence rates increase in a fashion similar to that of epithelial tumors. As indicated previously, these tumors are uncommon before puberty (5% to 7%), but when they occur, isosexual precocity develops in most cases (13,16).

Granulosa Cell Tumor (Adult Type)

Clinical Features

Adult granulosa cell tumors account for approximately 1–2% of all ovarian tumors and 95% of all granulosa cell tumors (3). Approximately 3% of granulosa cell tumors are asymptomatic chance findings (12). In the reproductive age group, granulosa cell tumors may cause a variety of symptoms related to estrogen effects. These generally include menometrorrhagia and oligomenorrhea. However, a significant number of women develop prolonged amenorrhea, which may be their only complaint. Postmenopausal patients frequently complain of postmenopausal bleeding. This was the initial symptom in 48% of patients in a review reported by Westholm (11). Rarely, breast tenderness and enlarging abdomen may be the chief complaint (17). Reactivated libido may also occur. Nonspecific tumor symptoms such as abdominal pain, backache, abdominal swelling, dysuria, and dyspareunia have been reported in 30% to 40% of patients. Five percent of patients present with an acute onset of abdominal pain due to either hemorrhage into the tumor or to rupture of a cystic tumor resulting in hematoperitoneum (10). Uterine abnormalities are common in women with granulosa cell tumors, usually manifested as myohypertrophy and leiomyomata. Endometrial hyperplasia has been noted in up to 56% of patients, and coexistent endometrial adenocarcinoma may be present in 6% to almost 30% of patients (10). Virilizing granulosa cell tumors are rare. They may cause oligomenorrhea, underdeveloped breasts, clitoromegaly, deepening of the voice, and hirsuitism. In reported cases, elevated preoperative plasma testosterone levels either regressed or returned to normal after removal of the tumor, symptoms of masculinization did not progress, and ovulation resumed (18–20).

Diagnosis

Granulosa cell tumors are usually unilateral. Bilateral tumors occur in 5% to 8% of cases and are thought by some investigators to be the result of metastasis from the primary tumor because of the poor prognosis associated with bilateral tumors. The tumors vary in size from a few millimeters to huge masses which fill the pelvis. The mean diameter of tumors studied by Fox and Langley (10) was approximately 13 cm. The gross appearance of granulosa cell tumors is quite variable. Young and Scully describe the gross appearance of these tumors as solid and gray, tan, or yellow, or predominantly cystic with loculi containing hemorrhagic fluid. Large areas of hemorrhage may also be present in the solid specimens. Rarely, the tumor appears as a unilocular or multilocular thin-walled cyst, which may simulate a serous or mucinous cystadenoma (3). Granulosa cell tumors are frequently encapsulated with a smooth or lobulated outer surface. The solid tumors may be hard, rubbery, or soft, and their cut surface can be white, brown, pink, yellow, or grey. Foci of hemorrhage or necrosis are common (10).

Microscopic features of granulosa cell tumors are also variable and tend to occur in combinations of patterns. The most differentiated forms of granulosa cell tumors may show a *microfollicular pattern* containing the characteristic Call-Exner bodies (Fig. 1). These consist of granulosa cells in a radial arrangement around a small cystic cavity containing a central rounded mass of eosinophilic material and often a few nuclear fragments. They are thought to represent small

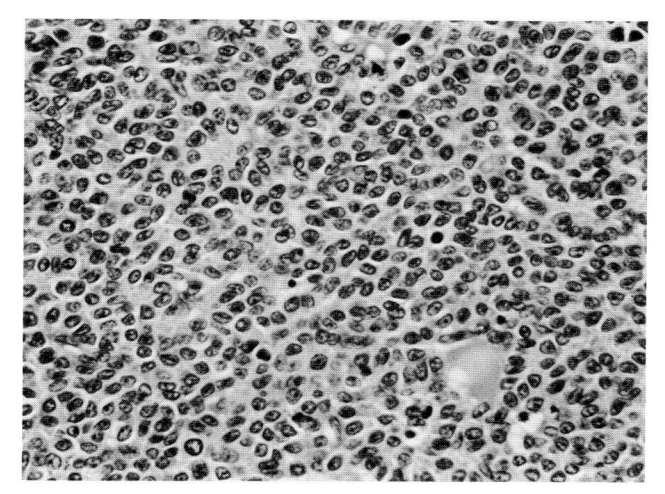

FIG. 1. Adult granulosa cell tumor showing nuclear grooving and Call-Exner bodies.

areas of cystic liquefaction and constitute the most distinctive feature of granulosa cell tumors (14). The other common patterns are the *macrofollicular pattern*, characterized by the presence of large, relatively uniform follicles which resemble follicle cysts. The tumor cells in the *insular* and *trabecular patterns* form islands and broad bands of granulosa cells separated by a fibromatous or thecomatous stroma. The *moire silk pattern* (watered silk) consists of a zigzag arrangement of thin winding cords. In the *diffuse luteinized pattern* (sarcomatoid), the cells grow in sheets. Occasionally, solid *tubular* structures and, rarely, tubules with lumina are present (3). A *cylindromatous* form of granulosa cell tumor consisting of a trabecular pattern in which the connective tissue stroma has undergone a hyaline or mucoid change has also been described (10).

The diagnosis of granulosa cell tumor depends upon recognition of the characteristic appearance of cell nuclei. They are described by various pathologists as pale, angular, round, oval, or slightly spindle-shaped, and as being haphazardly oriented with respect to one another; nuclear grooves are common and significant pleomorphism is lacking in most cases (13). Nuclei are also described as large, round, ovoid, or spindle-shaped with longitudinal grooving, and often contain a single nucleolus (10).

Several tumors may be confused with or misinterpreted as granulosa cell tumors. The most common of these include insular carcinoid, undifferentiated and poorly differentiated adenocarcinoma, metastatic endometrial stroma sarcoma, small cell carcinoma, fibroma, and thecoma. Clinical and histopathological features of specific tumors that are taken into account in the differential diagnosis have been outlined by previous authors (3,10). It is worth emphasizing again that definitive therapy should be based on frozen section diagnosis rendered by an experienced pathologist, or delayed pending study of paraffin-embedded material if necessary.

Immunohistochemical studies of intermediate filament expression by granulosa cell tumors have not consistently provided information of diagnostic value. As an example, the presence of cytokeratins and vimentin in granulosa cell tumors as well as in some ovarian carcinomas limits their value in the differential diagnosis of these two tumor groups (21). Similarly, thecomas and fibromas have been shown to express vimentin. On the other hand, desmin reactivity was not detected in a study of granulosa cell tumors but was commonly present in fibromas and thecomas (22). In a group of tumors primarily diagnosed as poorly differentiated malignant granulosa cell tumors, immunohistochemical studies for vimentin were negative but intensely positive with the anti-epithelial membrane antigen, thus allowing these tumors to be subsequently diagnosed as undifferentiated ovarian carcinomas (23).

It has been reported that granulosa cell tumors in general have a slightly higher mean nuclear contour, which is a measure of the nuclear indentation or grooving, and a lower mean nuclear area than do adenocarcinomas. These findings suggest that objective morphometric nuclear criteria may be useful in the diagnosis of granulosa cell tumors (24). Immunohistochemical localization of estradiol in granulosa cells may also be useful in the differential diagnosis. Similarly, the presence of polygonal cells with abundant smooth endoplasmic reticulum found at the ultrastructural level has provided further evidence establishing the granulosa cell as the cell type responsible for the production of estrogens (25,26).

Treatment

The standard treatment of granulosa cell tumors is total hysterectomy and bilateral salpingo-oophorectomy. Since the tumor is bilateral in less than 10% of cases, as indicated previously, patients in whom the preservation of fertility is a consideration can be treated by unilateral oophorectomy or salpingo-oophorectomy. It is essential to ascertain, however, whether the tumor is well-encapsulated and confined to the one ovary. This is accomplished by performing a thorough intraabdominal examination, biopsy of the contralateral ovary, selective biopsies of pelvic and para-aortic lymph nodes, biopsy of the omentum, and cytologic evaluation of peritoneal washings.

The value of adjunctive radiotherapy in the management of resected granulosa cell tumors has not been proven in randomized clinical trials. However, postoperative irradiation after hysterectomy bilateral adenectomy given to twelve patients in one study resulted in all of the patients surviving without evidence of tumor in follow-up that averaged ten years (27). In a similar study of fifty-four patients, the majority of whom were stage I, forty-eight of fifty patients treated primarily by surgery also received adjuvant external radiotherapy (11). No clear evidence was demonstrated that adjuvant radiotherapy improved the outcome compared to that reported in studies of early stage tumors treated by surgery alone. In another study of twenty-seven patients with granulosa cell tumors, five of the twenty-seven patients who had polymorphic tumors with a high mitotic count died. Simultaneous radiotherapy and chemotherapy has therefore been suggested in such cases (28).

A variety of chemotherapeutic agents administered alone or in combination regimens have been shown to be effective against granulosa cell tumors. Single-agent alkylating chemotherapy has been known to be effective against granulosa cell tumors for more than a decade. As an example, L-phenylalanine mustard (melphalan) administered to a patient with an unresectable granulosa tumor that recurred 18 years after initial diagnosis produced a prolonged complete remission (29). The same agent given to another patient with an unresectable tumor seven years after initial surgical therapy also resulted in complete tumor regression confirmed by laparoscopy (30). More recent studies have included cisplatin-based regimens (31,32). The combination consisting of cisplatin, vinblastine, and bleomycin (PVB) administered to eleven previously untreated patients with recurrent and/or metastatic disease achieved six pathologically complete responders at a median follow-up of fourteen months from the start of treatment. Hematologic and nonhematologic toxicity in this study were severe, with two drug-related deaths reported (33). This same combination of drugs administered to seven patients with advanced and/or recurrent tumors produced three complete responses (one pathologically documented) and one partial response, for an overall response rate of 66%. As in the previous study, drug toxicity was significant, with one death due to sepsis in agranulocytosis and peripheral neurotoxicity documented in three patients. The drug dosages and schedule in the latter study consisted of cisplatin, 20 mg/m^2 on days 1–5; vinblastine, 6 mg/m^2 on days 1 and 2; and bleomycin, 18 mg/m^2 on days 2, 9, and 16 (34). No patients in these two studies had received prior radiotherapy or chemotherapy.

A phase II study performed to assess the activity of PVB in patients with advanced or recurrent granulosa cell tumors further supports the efficacy of this drug combination in the treatment of granulosa cell tumors. The drug dosages and schedule in this study consisted of cisplatin, 20 mg/m^2 on days 1–5; vinblastine, 0.15 mg/kg or 0.10 mg/kg in previously irradiated patients on days 1 and 2; bleomycin, 30 mg (24-hour infusion) on day 2 and 15 mg intravenously or intramuscularly on day 15. This schedule was given every 28 days for 5 cycles. Twelve of thirteen evaluable patients (92%) responded to PVB for a duration of 4 to 27+ months in cases of complete response (CR = 7), and 4+ to 19+ months for partial responders (PR = 5). The results indicate that PVB may produce long remissions, with six out of thirteen fully evaluable patients disease-free at a follow-up of eight to twenty-seven months. Again, hematologic and nonhematologic complications were considered to be severe (35).

The current Gynecologic Oncology Group study utilizing bleomycin, etoposide, and cisplatin (BEP) as first-line therapy of malignant tumors of the ovarian stroma is expected to provide important new data when completed. In this study, etoposide replaces vinblastine based on its reduced toxicity without compromise of anticipated efficacy. Eligible patients include those with histologically confirmed primary stage II, III, and IV, with incompletely resected disease, recurrent or persistent tumors. The dosages and schedule of drugs consist of bleomycin, 20 units/m^2 on days 1, 8, 15, etc. (weekly for 9 weeks; total dose not 270 units or more); etoposide, 75 mg/m^2 intravenously on days 1–5, every three weeks for four courses; cisplatin, 20 mg/m^2 intravenously on days 1–5, every 3 weeks for four courses. For complete responders, reassessment laparotomy is recommended. The optimal chemotherapeutic regimen for treating advanced and recurrent granulosa cell tumors remains to be established. We are hopeful that prospective randomized clinical trials in the future will identify new drugs and new drug combinations that are less toxic and at the same time result in improved survival rates.

It is of interest that serum estradiol levels have been observed to fall during treatment of patients with advanced granulosa cell tumors, suggesting its value as a tumor marker (31). Follicle regulatory protein (FRP), a growth factor involved in intraovarian regulation of folliculogenesis, may potentially be a more sensitive tumor marker. Levels of FRP were elevated in the serum of 79% of patients compared to normal controls (36). Serial levels of FRP, which were measured in nineteen patients with granulosa cell tumors, paralleled the clinical course, including predicting disease status at second look laparotomy (37). Inhibin is a peptide hormone normally produced by ovarian granulosa cells. Serum concentrations of the hormone measured in six patients with granulosa cell tumors were abnormally elevated at five and twenty months in two patients before the clinical manifestations of recurrence became evident, suggesting that measurements of inhibin may also function as a marker for primary disease and for recurrent disease (38).

Survival and Prognosis

Crude survival rates over a short period of time are known to be of little value in assessing the malignant potential of granulosa cell tumors. The ten-year survival rate of patients with stage I tumors averages 90%, compared to 30% to 40% in advanced stages. Reports indicate however, that a decrement in survival occurs in all stages over time. Indeed, as noted previously, recurrent disease many years after primary therapy is not uncommon (39). Overall five-year survival rates range between 80% and 90% (28,40–43). Ten-year survival rates average 70% (28,40), while twenty-year survival rates indicate that 50% of patients died of their disease (44,45). Several adverse prognostic factors have been reported, but little concensus exists with respect to the ability to predict the outcome for a particular patient based on any one factor or combination of factors. From a clinical perspective, rupture of the tumor appears to have an adverse effect on outcome. This is demonstrated by an 86% 25-year relative survival reported in a group of patients with intact stage I tumors compared to 60% survival in patients with ruptured tumors of the same stage (3). In other studies, however, rupture had no relationship to survival (44).

Tumor size has been found by several investigators to be consistently related to prognosis. Tumors 5 cm or less in diameter have an excellent prognosis when compared to those of greater dimensions. Moreover, survival rates appear to decrease as size of the tumor increases (45,46). The available data however, fail to demonstrate a relationship between tumor size and prognosis independent of the stage of disease.

Investigators have evaluated tumor cellular patterns and differentiation in an effort to determine whether a particular tumor is likely to be associated with a poor prognosis. For example, survival of patients with well-differentiated tumors with follicular or cylindromatous patterns has been shown to be significantly higher at ten years than in patients with sarcomatoid tumors (82% versus 29%) (47,48). Conversely, some authors have not found any particular pattern associated with an unusually poor prognosis. Fox and Langley (10) reported that tumors with a diffuse pattern behave no differently than those showing an insular or follicular arrangement of cells (10). In general, most authorities agree that there is little correlation between the clinical course and the histologic pattern of the tumor. Several reports indicate however, that tumor grade may be an independent prognostic variable. Patients with well-differentiated tumors appear to enjoy a survival advantage over patients with high-grade tumors, with five-year survival rates 10% to 20% higher for patients with grade one tumors, compared to patients with less well-differentiated tumors (46,49).

Flow cytometric DNA analyses in some studies indicate that survival of patients with euploid tumors is more favorable than that of patients with aneuploid tumors (50). Other studies, however, fail to show any correlation between the risk of recurrence and ploidy. At present, it appears that the clinical course of granulosa cell tumors cannot be reliably predicted by DNA flow cytometry analysis (51,52). Similarly, survival of patients with two or fewer mitotic figures per ten high-power fields has been shown to be associated with a 70% ten-year survival, compared to a 37% ten-year survival when three or more mitotic figures were present. Yet most authorities agree that while numerous mitotic figures may portend a relatively poor prognosis, it is not possible to predict the behavior of a granulosa cell tumor. As Fox and Langley point out, the most apparently benign tumor should be considered as having a malignant potential (10). It seems likely, therefore, that the only reliable criterion of a poor outcome is the presence of extraovarian spread at the time of diagnosis.

It is worth noting that granulosa cell tumors diagnosed during pregnancy or puerperium do not appear to worsen the prognosis (53). Androgenic granulosa cell tumors of the adult type are also highly curable by surgery in early stage disease. They are not unlike estrogenic tumors, however, in their capacity to recur months after treatment and ultimately cause the patient's death (54).

In patients with recurrent disease, resection of tumor masses followed by radiotherapy and/or chemotherapy, depending on the extent of residual disease, is the usual treatment, but the prognosis for patients with recurrent granulosa cell tumors is poor, irrespective of treatment. This is clearly demonstrated in a recent study of twenty-eight patients in which six of seven patients who developed recurrence died of disease. Significantly, five of the seven patients were older than 40 years, which agrees with previous reports indicating that patients of higher ages are at high risk for recurrent disease (55).

Granulosa Cell Tumor (Juvenile Type)

Clinical Features

Juvenile granulosa cell tumors account for approximately 5% of all granulosa cell tumors. While various clinical and histopathologic features of these tumors differ from adult granulosa cell tumors, it is because of their common occurrence in young females that they have been termed *juvenile granulosa cell tumors* (Table 2). Although the literature contains many reports on juvenile granulosa cell tumors, the clinicopathological analysis of 125 cases reported by Young, Dickersin, and Scully (56) remains the principal source

TABLE 2. *Comparison of juvenile and adult granulosa cell tumors*

Juvenile type	Adult type
Almost always before age 30	All ages but mostly postmenopausal
Rarely malignant	Indolent course if malignant
Usually estrogenic	Usually estrogenic
Follicles large, irregular, often contain mucin	Follicles usually small, round (Call-Exner bodies)
Thecomatous component common	Fibrothecomatous component common
Cytoplasm usually abundant	Cytoplasm usually scanty
Nuclei, dark, ungrooved, and often pleomorphic	Nuclei pale and often grooved
Mitoses usually numerous	Mitoses variable

Modified from Young and Scully, ref. 3.

of knowledge about these tumors. The overwhelming majority of juvenile granulosa cell tumors occur before age 30, and of those that occur in premenarchal girls, approximately 80% are associated with isosexual precocity (57–59). In this review of the relevant literature, the youngest patient with a granulosa cell tumor was an eleven-week-old infant who developed bilateral tumors, although in this case sexual precocity did not occur (60). When present, the syndrome is designated pseudoprecocity because ovulation does not occur and progesterone is not produced. This is in contrast to precocity that may result from premature release of pituitary gonadotropins. The typical findings include breast development, appearance of pubic and axillary hair, enlargement of the labia, and irregular uterine bleeding. Accelerated somatic and skeletal development also occur. The syndrome of precocious pseudopuberty caused by a juvenile granulosa cell tumor has also been reported in association with Ollier's disease (enchondromatosis) (61,62) and with Maffucci's syndrome (enchondromatosis and hemangiomatosis) (56). Rare androgenic juvenile granulosa cell tumors may cause virilization (63). In the reproductive age group, abdominal pain, menometrorrhagia, amenorrhea, and, rarely, postmenopausal bleeding are presenting symptoms.

Diagnosis

Juvenile granulosa cell tumors are rarely bilateral (2%) and, due to an average size of more than 10 cm, they are nearly always palpable on pelvic examination (56). The vast majority of patients are found to have stage I disease, but 10% of the tumors are noted to have ruptured at operation. The gross appearance of the tumors is variable, but they are commonly described as solid and cystic. The cysts may contain hemorrhagic fluid, and the solid component is typically yellow-tan or gray (3).

Microscopically, juvenile granulosa cell tumors usually contain granulosa cells arranged in nodules, which may be solid or contain follicular spaces. The cytological features are characterized by the presence of round nuclei, abundant cytoplasm, pleomorphism, and mitotic activity (Fig. 2). Both the granulosa cells and the theca cells are frequently luteinized with abundant eosinophilic cytoplasm commonly observed. Notably absent in most juvenile granulosa cell tumors is nuclear grooving. While the mitotic activity is usually greater than that seen in adult granulosa cell tumors and suggests a more malignant tumor, the juvenile-type tumor has an excellent prognosis. A comparison of some microscopic and clinical features of adult granulosa cell and juvenile granulosa cell tumors is shown in Table 2.

The differential diagnosis of juvenile granulosa cell tumor includes several tumors that may also occur in young females, such as embryonal carcinoma, choriocarcinoma, and endodermal sinus tumor. Other tumors that may be misdiagnosed as juvenile granulosa cell tumor include small cell carcinoma, thecoma, Sertoli cell tumor, and clear cell carcinoma. Histopathologic criteria used to differentiate these tumors have been comprehensively described elsewhere (56). Immunohistochemical studies of intermediate filament expression by juvenile granulosa cell tumors show prominent positivity for vimentin and cytokeratin, which is similar to the findings in the adult type of tumor (64). These

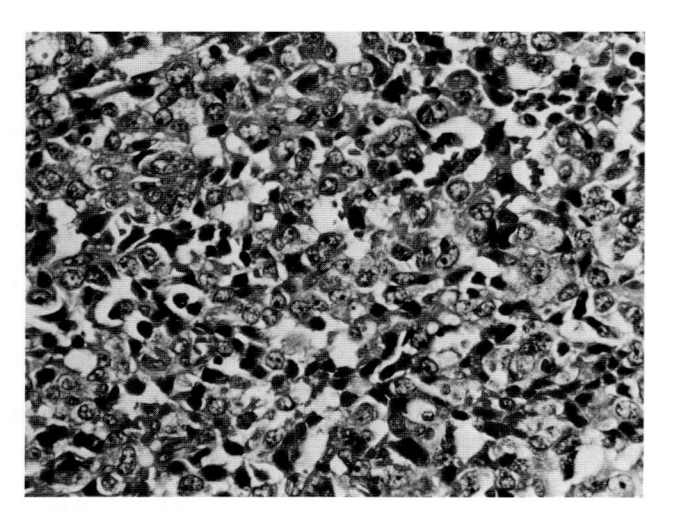

FIG. 2. Juvenile granulosa cell tumor. High-power view showing round nuclei, abundant cytoplasm, pleomorphism, and mitotic activity.

studies also demonstrate that the steroid hormones produced by juvenile granulosa cell tumors are localized mainly in the stromal cells, but also in the follicular cells. Ultrastructural studies identify three types of tumor cells, polygonal, spindle, and transitional cells. Well-developed smooth endoplasmic reticulum, mitochondria with tubulovesicular cristae, and lipid droplets in the cytoplasm, typically found in steroid synthesis, have been described as conspicuous in juvenile type tumors (65).

Treatment

The recommended treatment for patients with juvenile granulosa cell tumor confined to the ovary is unilateral oophorectomy or salpingo-oophorectomy. This recommendation is based on the fact that these tumors are rarely bilateral and in the age group in which they typically occur, the preservation of reproductive potential is often a consideration. It is worth reiterating that certain criteria for conservative therapy should be met. First, the diagnosis must be rendered by an experienced pathologist; and second, a thorough intraabdominal exploration as described for adult granulosa cell tumors must disclose no tumor beyond the involved ovary. More advanced tumors require total hysterectomy with bilateral salpingo-oophorectomy.

The best treatment for advanced and recurrent juvenile granulosa cell tumors has yet to be determined. Chemotherapy is essentially that recommended for adult granulosa cell tumors and stromal tumors in general. A recent prospective phase II study of stromal tumors was carried out to determine the efficacy of a combination regimen consisting of cisplatin, doxorubicin, and cyclophosphamide (CAP). The drug dosages and schedule consisted of cisplatin, 40–50 mg/m^2 intravenously; doxorubicin, 40–50 mg/m^2 intravenously; and cyclophosphamide, 400–500 mg/m^2 intravenously; all given on day one, every 28 days. Of the eight patients entered in the study, two had stage II disease, one had stage III, and five had recurrent disease. The overall response rate was 63%. Toxicity was minimal, and four patients were disease-free at 13+ to 48+ months. The authors concluded that the combination of cisplatin, doxorubicin, and cyclophosphamide had modest activity in the treatment of metastatic stromal tumors (66). When considering chemotherapy for juvenile granulosa cell tumors, this regimen and the regimens previously outlined for the treatment of adult granulosa cell tumors (consisting of PVB and BEP) all seem worthy of further study. The CAP regimen, it should be noted, appears to be the least toxic regimen.

Inhibin, previously described as a useful marker of adult granulosa cell tumors, may also function as a marker for the juvenile-type tumor. Extremely high preoperative levels have been observed to return to normal after resection of the tumor (67).

There is no data evaluating the value of FRP as a tumor marker in juvenile granulosa cell tumors. However, in a study of immunohistochemical staining of juvenile granulosa cell tumors with anti-FRP antisera, expression of FRP was demonstrated throughout the tumor. In addition, treatment of these tumors injected into nude mice slowed the rate of tumor growth, suggesting the need for further study of FRP in patients with this tumor (68).

Survival and Prognosis

The cure rate of juvenile granulosa cell tumors by surgery averages 95% (56,69,70). Unlike adult granulosa cell tumors, which tend to follow an indolent course with late recurrences, malignant juvenile granulosa cell tumors typically recur within two to three years after surgery and frequently follow a rapidly fatal course (56,71–73). As with adult granulosa cell tumors, rupture of juvenile granulosa cell tumors at the time of operation also does not appear to have an adverse effect on prognosis (3,69).

Flow cytometric studies of DNA content of juvenile granulosa cell tumors also have not been shown to correlate with outcome. In one study in which flow cytometry revealed that 46% of the tumors had abnormal DNA content and increased average growth fraction, all of the patients remained free of disease in follow-up, leading the authors to conclude that despite such findings these tumors may yet behave benignly (74). This observation is consistent with that of Young and Scully (3), who found that both mitotic rate and the degree of nuclear atypicality correlated with the prognosis when tumors of all stages were considered, but no such correlation could be demonstrated when only stage I tumors were evaluated. For most patients, the stage of the disease at the time of diagnosis is the best indicator of prognosis.

TUMORS IN THE THECOMA-FIBROMA GROUP

Tumors in this group are usually benign, typically occur in older women, may be hormonally active, and generally have distinctive histopathological features that facilitate their recognition. They are of interest because of their relative frequency, possible effect on the uterus, and the charge to the pathologist of identifying the occasional malignant variant.

Thecoma

Clinical Features

Thecomas are estimated to account for approximately 1% of all ovarian tumors and are about one-third as common as granulosa cell tumors (10). They are rarely bilateral (2–3%) and almost never malignant. The average age of patients with a thecoma is 53 years and more than half of those women are postmenopausal. Thecomas are extremely rare in childhood, and are in fact uncommon before the age of 30 years. Estrogenic effects of these tumors are manifested in menopausal or postmenopausal patients as menstrual aberrations, which is frequently the initial complaint. However, the presenting sign or symptoms in 86% of patients in a reported series of twenty-two patients with pure thecomas was an abdominal/pelvic mass (75). Thecomas are associated with a high incidence of myohypertrophy and leiomyomata, with the reported incidence of coexistent endometrial hyperplasia and endometrial carcinoma as high as 78% and 21%, respectively (3,10). It is worth noting that the incidence of endometrial neoplasia appears to be higher in patients with a thecoma than it is in those with a granulosa cell tumor (14).

Thecomas vary in size from minute seedlings to large masses. They average 10 cm diameter and are described as smooth or lobulated, and well-demarcated but not encapsulated. On cut section they characteristically display a yellow mass. However, they may be white, brown, grey, or dull orange-yellow (3,10). Microscopic examination reveals masses of cells, most of which are ill-defined and oval or rounded. The cytoplasm is pale and vacuolated, containing moderate to abundant amounts of lipid. The nuclei exhibit little or no atypia and mitoses are absent or infrequent (3). *Luteinized thecoma* is a term applied to tumors that are predominantly fibromatous or thecomatous but also contain collections of steroid-type cells resembling luteinized theca and stromal cells. In a report of fifty cases, they were considered to be distinctive, due to the relatively high frequency of masculinization and their occurrence in a significant percentage of women under the age of 30 years (76). These tumors are similar to typical thecomas in that they are almost always unilateral and both follow a clinically benign course (77).

Immunohistochemical studies of thecomas have demonstrated localization of estradiol in a small number of tumor cells, which suggests that thecoma cells are capable of steroid synthesis. Such observations support the assertion that hyperestrogenism in patients with thecomas may be the result of estradiol secretion by these tumors. There appears to be a continuous spectrum of ultrastructural findings where the cells are those of a typical highly-collagenised fibroma and that of a typical thecoma (10). According to Gaffney and associates (78), two principle cell types are present: type I immature mesenchymal cells that differ from typical steroid-secreting cells in that only a minority had conspicuous smooth endoplasmic reticulum although mitochondria often had tubular cristae; and type II cells which are distinguished by abundant intermediate microfilaments and round mitochondria with incomplete cristae and empty centers.

Diagnosis

The differential diagnosis of thecoma and fibroma is the usual consideration when thecoma is suspected. According to Fox and Langley (10), the diagnosis of thecoma rests principally upon the presence of large pale cells that usually contain abundant lipid. It is worth noting from a clinical diagnostic perspective that true thecomas may produce signs of hyperestrogenism, while fibromas do not (79).

Treatment

The treatment of patients with thecomas is oophorectomy or salpingo-oophorectomy when preservation of fertility is desired. For menopausal and postmenopausal patients, hysterectomy and bilateral salpingo-oophorectomy is the usual treatment. It would seem prudent to evaluate the endometrium prior to operation in all cases, but especially where conservative management has been elected.

Survival and Prognosis

Thecomas have an excellent prognosis and are considered to be benign (80,81). While no fewer than 19 malignant thecomas have been reported (10), critical analysis of such cases indicates that most are diffuse granulosa cell tumors or fibrosarcomas (82).

Fibroma-Fibrosarcoma

Clinical Features

Fibromas are the most common of the sex cord-stromal tumors, accounting for 4% of all ovarian neoplasms. They occur in all ages but are more common in adults than children and range in size from microscopic to large masses. They are infrequently bilateral. Two uncommon syndromes are associated with ovarian fibromas and merit brief mention. Meigs' syndrome, which occurs in 1% of fibromas, is characterized by the presence of ascites and pleural effusion. Ascites alone is present in 10% to 15% of cases in which the fibroma is greater than 10 cm in size (83). Gorlin's syndrome is characterized by the occurrence of ovarian fibromas, usually bilateral, in association with a spectrum of hereditary abnormalities, the most notable of which is basal cell nevi appearing early in life. Recurrent ovarian fibromas associated with this syndrome have been reported (84).

Diagnosis

The benign fibroma must be differentiated from the cellular fibroma, fibrosarcoma, and a rare, low-grade endometrial stromal sarcoma. The typical benign fibroma is described as hard, flat, chalky-white, with a whorled appearance on cut section. There may be areas of edema and calcification. Microscopic findings include intersecting bundles of spindle cells producing collagen. Many tumors show varying degrees of intercellular edema and some cells may contain small quantities of lipid (3). *Cellular fibromas* contain one to three mitotic figures per ten high-power fields (HPF) with only slight nuclear atypia, and are considered to be of low malignant potential. Tumors with four or more mitotic figures per ten HPF, and significant nuclear atypica are almost always malignant and are designated *fibrosarcoma* (85).

Treatment

Benign fibromas can be treated by oophorectomy or salpingo-oophorectomy. Cellular fibromas in patients who have completed their families should be treated with total hysterectomy and bilateral salpingo-oophorectomy, especially if the tumor is adherent or has ruptured (85). A recent case report of a patient with a cellular fibroma who presented with ascites and an elevated CA-125 mimicking ovarian adenocarcinoma emphasizes the need for frozen section diagnosis prior to definitive therapy (86). Fibrosarcomas require total hysterectomy and bilateral salpingo-oophorectomy. The value of radiotherapy and combination chemotherapy has not been established for fibrosarcomas, but adjuvant therapy may have a role, considering the aggressive behavior of these tumors.

Survival and Prognosis

The prognosis for the vast majority of patients with tumors in the thecoma-fibroma category is excellent because malignant variants of these tumors are exceedingly rare. In a review of 38 ovarian sarcomas treated at Memorial Hospital between 1977 and 1990, no patient had a diagnosis of malignant thecoma or fibrosarcoma (R. Barakat et al., *submitted for publication*). Of the six ovarian fibrosarcomas reported by Prat and Scully (85), four were found to be adherent or had ruptured. One patient with distant metastases was lost to follow-up; the remaining five died of disease.

Stromal Tumor with Minor Sex Cord Elements

Young and Scully (87) were the first investigators to report on an unusual group of seven tumors with thecomatous or fibromatous features that contained small aggregates of epithelial cells of sex cord derivation, including indifferent or granulosa cells and tubules lined by Sertoli cells. The report, published in 1983, indicated that the behavior of these tumors appeared to be more like that of a fibroma or thecoma than that of a sex cord-stromal tumor.

Sclerosing Stromal Tumor

Clinical Features

Sclerosing stromal tumors are a unique group of neoplasms that originate from the ovarian stroma and differ from the typical thecoma and fibroma by the characteristic tendency of their cellular areas to undergo collagenous sclerosis (88). These are relatively rare tumors, as evidenced by a recent review of 168 sex cord-stromal tumors in which there were only four sclerosing stromal tumors (89). The tumors are typically unilateral and occur at an earlier age than thecoma and fibroma, with an average age at diagnosis of 27 years. In contrast to thecoma, sclerosing stromal tumors are not usually hormonally active; there were none in the ten cases originally described. Recent studies indicate, however, that these tumors can rarely secrete estradiol, progesterone, and testosterone. In one report of a patient with anovulation and infertility, removal of the tumor was followed by reversal of the abnormalities (90). Similar results were achieved by operation in a masculinized female with elevated free testosterone levels (91).

Diagnosis

The gross description of sclerosing stromal tumors includes the presence of a discrete, sharply demarcated mass that is white with yellow areas, edema, and cyst formation (3). Microscopic examination reveals a well-developed vascularity, prominent pseudolobulation with lobules composed of cellular areas separated by sclerotic or edematous cell-poor areas (92). It is of interest that the presence of partially or completely obstructed vessels has been suggested as a possible cause of the edema in the tumor (93). Two cell types are described: spindle cells producing collagen and round or oval cells containing lipid. Immunohistochemical demonstration of desmin and smooth muscle actin-positive spindle cells in sclerosing stromal tumors and their absence in thecofibromas is useful in differential diagnosis (94). Ultrastructural studies reveal a diverse cellular population composed of conspicuous lipid-laden cells, fibroblast-like and undifferentiated primitive mesenchymal cells. These findings are thought to confirm the stromal origin of these tumors (95).

Treatment

Total hysterectomy with bilateral salpingo-oophorectomy is the treatment recommended for most patients who have completed their families. Simple oophorectomy or salpingo-oophorectomy is adequate treatment for patients in the childbearing age group.

Survival and Prognosis

There were no reported deaths resulting from malignant sclerosing tumors found in this review of the literature.

Unclassified

This group of tumors is rare and appears to possess histologic and clinical features intermediate between thecomas and fibromas.

SERTOLI-STROMAL CELL TUMORS

Sertoli Cell Tumor

Clinical Features

The term *androblastoma* has been used to describe neoplasms composed of Sertoli cells, Leydig cells, or precursors of either, alone or in combination. Androblastomas may produce androgens, estrogens, or both; or they may be endocrinologically inert (14). Pure Sertoli cell tumors, sometimes described as well-differentiated androblastomas, are associated with symptoms caused by an estrogenic effect in over 70% of cases (10). These tumors account for 4% of Sertoli-stromal cell tumors and may present at any age. The most common symptoms related to the hyperestrogenism caused by the tumor are menstrual aberrations, including postmenopausal bleeding. Isosexual precocious puberty and increased libido have also been associated with Sertoli cell tumors. In approximately 20% of patients, virilization occurs, characterized by amenorrhea or oligomenorrhea, hirsutism, deepening of the voice, and clitoral hypertrophy. Rarely, hyperaldosteronism, shown by hypertension and hypokalemia, has been reported (96,97).

Diagnosis

Sertoli cell tumors are almost always unilateral and on gross examination appear as well-encapsulated, lobulated, solid, yellow, or brown masses. The tumors range in size from 2 to 18 cm in diameter, with the majority measuring less than 5 cm (10). Microscopic examination reveals that the tumors are composed entirely of Sertoli cells, with uniform hollow or solid tubules lined by a single layer of radially arranged cells with clear cytoplasm. Well-differentiated Sertoli cell tumors may contain abundant intracytoplasmic lipid, resulting in the designation "lipid-rich Sertoli cell tumor." Ultrastructural examinations have demonstrated the presence of Böttcher's filaments unequivocally identifying the Sertoli differentiation as the predominant cell in the neoplasm (98). In one study, the basal part of the cells were observed to rest on a nonfibrillary basement membrane layer, while the free border showed occasional cilia, considered to be a manifestation of focal metaplasia of the neoplastic Sertoli cell (99).

Differential diagnosis generally includes lipid cell tumors, which are usually masculinizing and Sertoli-Leydig cell tumors which contain Leydig cells as well as Sertoli cells.

Treatment

Conservative treatment is appropriate since these tumors appear to be totally benign. Simple oophorectomy is curative and those with hormonally active tumors are noted to have their symptoms ameliorated by excision of the neoplasm.

Survival and Prognosis

The prognosis is excellent, with only one known death due to this tumor. In this case, the tumor was described as focally poorly differentiated and reported to have metastasized, resulting in the death of a sexually precocious child (100).

Leydig Cell Tumor

Clinical Features

Leydig cell tumors are rare and are also considered to be a form of androblastoma. The majority of these tumors are androgenic (80%), while the remainder are estrogenic (10%), or nonfunctional. The tumors may occur at any age, but peak between the ages of 50 and 70. They are typically of small size and do not cause local symptoms; thus the clinical presentation is almost always due to endocrinological disturbance. In premenarchal girls, the presentation is that of virilization manifested by short stature, growth of pubic and axillary hair, and clitoral hypertrophy. Women in the reproductive years demonstrate defeminization, mild virilism, oligomenorrhea or amenorrhea, atrophy of the breast, loss of scalp hair, deepening of the voice, acne, and clitoral hypertrophy. In postmenopausal women, alopecia, hirsutism, and clitoromegaly are seen (10).

Virilized patients are characteristically found to have markedly elevated plasma testosterone levels (101–104). Recent radiographic studies demonstrate that the Leydig cells are the steroid-secreting cells in the tumors (105). Leydig cell tumors are sometimes difficult to diagnose but should be considered in any elderly female with signs of virilization. Patients may not have a detectable mass on pelvic examination or sonography because of the small size of these tumors. Recent studies indicate that nuclear scanning techniques such as 131I-19 iodocholesterol scintigraphy are capable of localizing functioning Leydig cell tumors which are too small to palpate or localize by other means (106). Careful intraoperative examination of even normal-appearing ovaries is therefore recommended in virilized patients, particularly when no adrenal disease is found (107).

Diagnosis

It should be noted that ovarian Leydig cell tumors have been divided by Roth and Sternberg (108) into two subgroups, the hilus cell tumor and the rare Leydig cell tumor. The two tumors differ only in their location and proposed cell of origin, and not in their clinical and pathological features. An ovarian stromal cell derivation has been proposed for the Leydig cell tumor and hilar cells for the hilus cell tumor (109).

The majority of Leydig cell tumors measure less than 5 cm in diameter and are almost always unilateral. In a patient with the rare finding of bilateral tumors, one tumor measured 7 mm and the other 6 mm (110). The tumors are described as well-circumscribed but not encapsulated, usually soft, fleshy, and reddish-brown to yellow in color.

Microscopically, the cells are arranged in sheets or cords with markedly eosinophilic cytoplasm (Fig. 3). The cytoplasm of some of the cells may contain abundant lipochrome pigment. The nuclei are described as large and centrally placed. Occasionally, the nuclei cluster and are separated by a nucleus-free eosinophilic zone which is highly suggestive of a hilus cell tumor in the absence of Reinke crystalloids (3). Light and electron microscopic investigations typically reveal polygonal cells containing intracytoplasmic Reinke crystalloids (111). It is of interest that these structures,

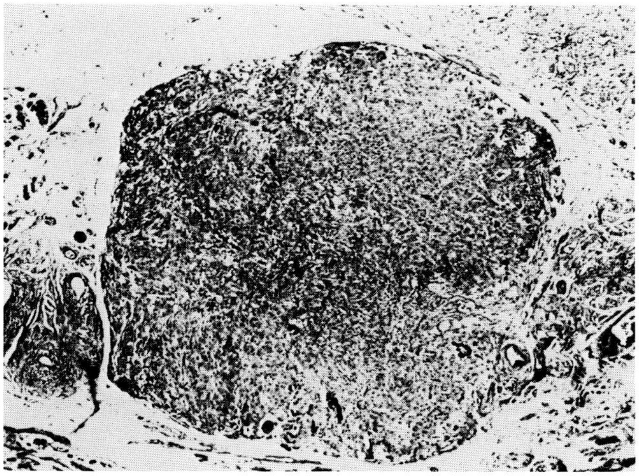

FIG. 3. Hilus cell tumor showing a circumscribed mass of cells with abundant eosinophilic cytoplasm. In this case, Reinke crystals were not observed.

described as slender, rodlike bodies with rounded, square, or tapering ends, have been shown on electron microscopy to be true crystals (10). Although the crystals are present in approximately 50% of cases and not essential for the diagnosis, their presence is usually pathognomonic.

Treatment

Leydig cell tumors are almost always benign, thus simple oophorectomy is curative. In the patient beyond the childbearing years, total hysterectomy and bilateral salpingo-oophorectomy is recommended, since 15% of patients have an associated cystic hyperplasia of the endometrium (10). Virilizing symptoms regress promptly after surgery, but in 50% of cases symptoms do not completely disappear (112).

Survival and Prognosis

Metastasizing Leydig cell tumors are exceedingly rare. Radiotherapy and estrogen therapy appear to have no effect on the tumors' growth. Chemotherapy consisting of doxorubicin and mitotane given to a patient with widespread Leydig cell tumor originating in the testes did not produce a response (113).

Sertoli-Leydig Cell Tumors

Clinical Features

Sertoli-Leydig cell tumors are extremely rare (less than 0.5% of all ovarian tumors), but are of considerable interest because of their varied clinical presentations and unique histopathologic features. These tumors, previously also termed *androblastomas* or *arrhenoblastomas* because of their androgenic properties, are known to be masculinizing in only about 50% of cases and many are nonfunctioning, while some are estrogenic. The masculinized patients present with hirsutism or virilization, and typically give a history of oligoamenorrhea followed by amenorrhea. This is followed by atrophy of the breasts, loss of body fat, acne, hirsutism, and later, deepening of the voice, cliteromegaly, and recession of the hairline (109). It is noteworthy that 40% of the cases are discovered during investigation of androgen excess (114). The laboratory findings in the virilized patients characteristically demonstrate elevated plasma levels of testosterone and androstenedione, and normal 17-ketosteroid levels. Testosterone typically predominates over androstenedione in Sertoli-Leydig cell tumors and has been shown to be of value in differential diagnosis (114,115). It is of interest that in patients with increased androgen production there appears to be little correlation between endocrine function, cellular composition or degree of differentiation of these tumors (116).

Diagnosis

Factors related to the diagnosis and behavior of Sertoli-Leydig cell tumors have been detailed in a comprehensive clinicopathological analysis of two hundred seven cases by Young and Scully (114). Because the tumors are discovered in a significant number of young women (60%) (10) and in certain cases are malignant, an accurate diagnosis and knowledge of the prognosis becomes of great therapeutic importance.

Several recent reports indicate that some Sertoli-Leydig cell tumors are capable of secreting alpha fetoprotein (AFP) and thus may be misdiagnosed as a germ cell tumor (117–118). High serum levels of AFP have been seen in association with tumors of intermediate differentiation (119) as well as in those that are poorly differentiated (120). While the mechanism by which these tumors produce AFP is not clearly established, immunohistochemical studies indicate that the Leydig cell is the probable source (121). Immunohistochemical evaluation of tumors with heterologous mesenchymal elements, however, have also localized AFP in hepatocytes (122). One patient found to have AFP within liver cells experienced a rapidly fatal course despite radiation therapy and chemotherapy (123).

The tumors have been divided into four categories by the WHO: well-differentiated, intermediate differentiation, poorly differentiated, and those with heterologous elements (1). Clinicopathologic features of the four groups will be discussed separately, as they differ with respect to the frequency of occurrence, average age at diagnosis, histopathology, and incidence of malignancy.

Well-Differentiated Sertoli-Leydig Cell Tumors

These are the least common of the tumors in the Sertoli-Leydig cell group (11%) (114) and their average age of occurrence of 40 years is 10 years older than the overall average. Defeminization and virilization is encountered in two-thirds of the patients (10). Previously termed *tubular adenoma of Pick*, they are the smallest tumors in the group, with an average size of approximately 5 cm. The tumors are rarely bilateral and on gross inspection appear to be encapsulated. On cut section they are described as firm, yellow, yellow-white, or yellow-grey, and typically lobulated (10).

Microscopic findings of the well-differentiated tumors are characterized by a predominantly tubular differentiation with little nuclear atypia or mitotic activity. The tubules are lined or filled with benign-appearing Sertoli cells separated by variable numbers of Leydig cells. Reinke crystals are identified in the Leydig cells in approximately 20% of cases (3). Electron microscopic study of well-differentiated tumors reveals cylindrically shaped cells with round to oval nuclei with a thin basement membrane. The cytoplasm is described as fibrillary, showing rough and smooth endoplasmic reticulum, lipid droplets and secretory granules. At the luminal borders, the cells are often irregular and display apocrine-like activity (124). Differential diagnosis includes well-differentiated endometrioid carcinoma with luteinized stroma (125) and granulosa cell tumors.

Intermediately Differentiated Sertoli-Leydig Cell Tumors

Tumors in this group are defined by their degree of differentiation and by the great admixture of patterns, including the presence of endodermal heterologous elements (20%) and foci with retiform components (15%) (114). They are the most common of the Sertoli-Leydig cell tumors, accounting for 54% of the group. The patients are typically younger than those with well-differentiated tumors (average age 25 years), and approximately one-third of the tumors are associated with androgen excess. The gross description of intermediately differentiated tumors is that of a solid mass in one-third of the cases, while 50% are solid and cystic. They vary in size from very small to 35 cm, with an average size of approximately 10 cm. On cut section they are described as yellow or yellow-tan (114).

Microscopic examination reveals immature Sertoli cells with small, round or angular nuclei arranged typically in ill-defined masses, often creating a lobulated appearance. They are further described by Young and Scully (3) as containing solid and hollow tubules, nests, thin cords resembling the sex cords of the embryonic testis, and broad columns are often present. The stroma typically contains clusters of well-differentiated Leydig cells.

Formations simulating the rete of the testis (retiform pattern) are present in approximately 10% of Sertoli-Leydig cell tumors and are almost always limited to those of intermediate or poor differentiation. These patterns consist of an irregular anastomosing network of spaces lined with cuboidal cells, often with papillary formations, and sometimes with tubules compressed to form slitlike spaces (126). It should be noted that the retiform pattern appears to be specific for Sertoli-Leydig tumors and is of prognostic significance.

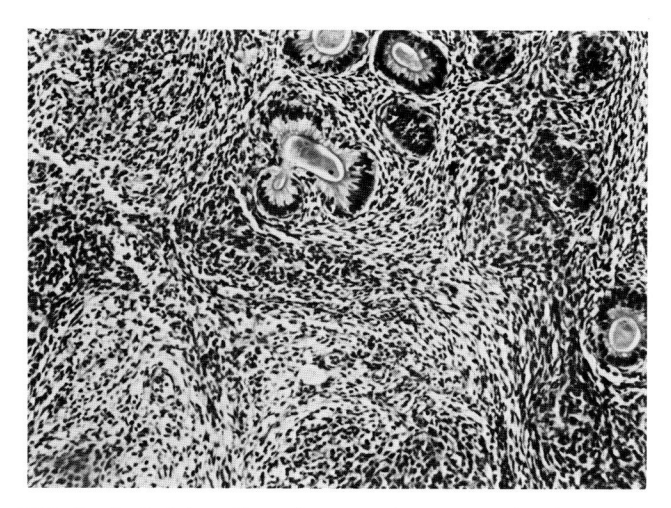

FIG. 4. Sertoli-Leydig cell tumor demonstrating heterologous elements. In this case, gastrointestinal epithelium.

Poorly Differentiated Sertoli-Leydig Cell Tumors

The poorly differentiated tumors typically consist of sheets of closely packed, spindle-shaped cells in which occasional irregular cord-like structures or imperfectly formed tubules may be seen. Small groups of Leydig cells may also be seen. These tumors appear highly malignant cytologically because of their diffuse or sarcomatoid features. Mesenchymal heterologous elements, when encountered in Sertoli-Leydig cell tumors, are most often in tumors in which the homologous component is poorly differentiated.

Sertoli-Leydig Cell Tumors with Heterologous Elements

Approximately 20% of Sertoli-Leydig cell tumors contain heterologous elements. In the intermediately differentiated tumors, the heterologous component, as indicated above, is usually of the endodermal variety such as mucinous epithelium of gastrointestinal type (Fig. 4). Microscopic carcinoid tumors are also encountered. In approximately 5% of Sertoli-Leydig cell tumors, mesenchymal heterologous elements are present, and they are almost always associated with poorly differentiated tumors. The findings in these tumors include foci of immature skeletal muscle, and cartilage arising on a sarcomatous background, or areas of embryonal rhabdomyosarcoma, or both (Figs. 5–6) (3).

Treatment

The treatment of Sertoli-Leydig cell tumors depends on several factors primarily related to prognosis. In the older patients, hysterectomy with bilateral salpingo-oophorectomy is the treatment of choice. In the young patient who desires preservation of fertility, unilateral salpingo-oophorectomy is appropriate, provided the tumor is in stage Ia1, is not ruptured, and is well-differentiated. Patients with intermediately differentiated tumors in stage Ia1 that are intact and do not demonstrate a significant retiform pattern may also be managed conservatively. Poorly differentiated tumors require hysterectomy with bilateral salpingo-oophorectomy and consideration for adjuvant therapy. Evidence of androgen excess regresses after removal of the tumor and menses return in amenorrheic patients. The management of patients whose tumors contain heterologous elements should be based on the degree of differentiation of the homologous component. Some clinical and

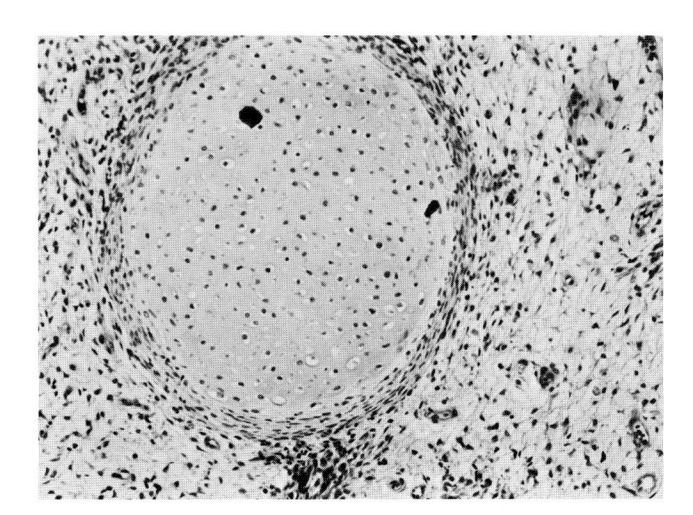

FIG. 5. Sertoli-Leydig cell tumor showing a focus of cartilage.

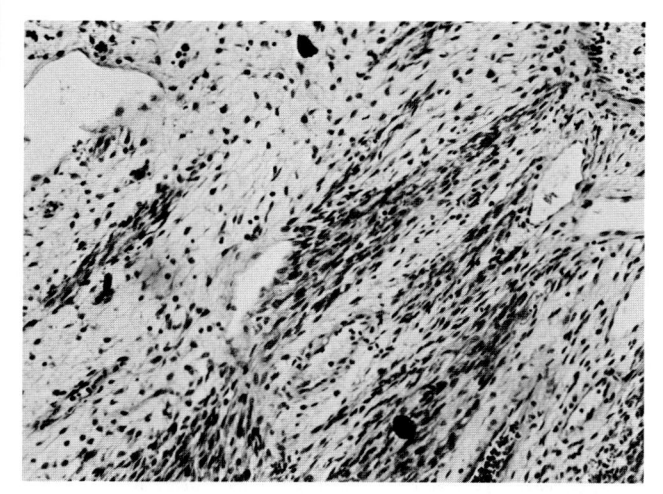

FIG. 6. Poorly differentiated Sertoli-Leydig cell tumor with spindled cells.

pathologic characteristics of Sertoli-Leydig cell tumors are shown in Table 3.

Survival and Prognosis

The prognosis for patients with Sertoli-Leydig cell tumors is clearly related to the stage of disease and the degree of differentiation of the tumor. For patients with well-differentiated tumors, the prognosis is excellent. In the report by Young and Scully (114) on 207 cases, all of the well-differentiated tumors were diagnosed in stage Ia1, and none were malignant (114).

For patients with intermediately differentiated tumors, the prognosis is quite favorable, with the majority diagnosed in stage Ia1 (83%). More advanced stages are encountered, however, and overall, 11% are malignant. Rupture of the tumor also adversely affects the outcome in intermediately differentiated tumors; 30% that are clinically ruptured are malignant, in contrast to 7% of those that are intact. The presence of the retiform pattern has an adverse prognostic effect on these tumors, as evidenced by a malignancy rate of 25% in patients who have a significant retiform component, compared to 10% of those with no retiform component. Approximately 10% of tumors in this category contain heterologous mesenchymal elements which also adversely affect prognosis.

More than half of the poorly differentiated tumors are clinically malignant, and rupture of the tumor is associated with malignant behavior in the vast majority of cases. Among a group of ten patients with tumors containing heterologous mesenchymal elements, seven died of their disease; in 90% of them, the homologous component of the tumor was poorly differentiated (109). When the heterologous element is rhabdomyosarcoma, the prognosis is as poor as that of rhabdomyosarcoma in general (127).

Unlike granulosa cell tumors, in which late recurrences are common, recurrent Sertoli-Leydig cell tumors typically are diagnosed within three years after surgery and the course thereafter is often rapidly fatal (128–129). Pathologic factors that correspond with the development of recurrence can be summarized as follows: poor tumor differentiation, presence of mesenchymal heterologous elements, significant retiform pattern, and rupture of the tumor (130).

The optimal chemotherapy for advanced or recurrent Sertoli-Leydig cell tumors remains to be established. In the mid 1970s, Schwartz and Smith (131) recommended chemotherapy for ovarian stromal tumors utilizing a combination chemotherapy regimen consisting of vincristine (1.5 mg/m^2 intravenously) weekly for 10 to 12 consecutive weeks, actinomycin D (0.5 mg intravenously), and cyclophosphamide (5–7 mg/kg intravenously) (VAC) for five consecutive days every 4 weeks. In their report, two patients with Sertoli-Leydig cell tumors were long-term survivors with VAC administered monthly for 18 and 24 months, with the addition of pelvic radiation therapy in one of the patients. In a 1980s report, a patient with stage III disease treated with bleomycin, vincristine, cyclophosphamide, doxorubicin, and cisplatin (BV-CAP) was found to be free of disease at second-look laparotomy. She subsequently received additional vincristine, cyclophosphamide, and cisplatin and remained free of disease 22 months following treatment (132).

There is, in fact, relatively little knowledge about chemotherapy or radiotherapy in the management of advanced or recurrent Sertoli-Leydig cell tumors. Anecdotal experience indicates that while initial re-

TABLE 3. *Clinical and pathological features of Sertoli-Leydig cell tumors*

Histopathology	Average age (years)	Percent androgenic	Percent stage Ia1	Size (cm)	Percent malignant
Well Differentiated	34	40	100	5.3	0
Intermediately Differentiated	25	35	83	12.5	11
Poorly Differentiated	25	38	52	17.5	59
Heterologous Elements	23	28	80	15–18	19

Modified from Young, Scully, ref. 114.

sponses to chemotherapy occur, relapses are common and complete remissions are rare. The VAC regimen appears to be a common initial treatment strategy, but survival is usually poor (126,133). In one patient with stage III disease who received VAC plus pelvic irradiation, a second-look operation did not disclose residual disease and the patient was free of disease more than three years after treatment (130). Two patients with stage III disease reported by Talerman and associates (134) showed an initial response to vinblastine, cisplatin, etoposide, bleomycin, and vincristine, but in both cases the patients' tumors became refractory and they died. In another report of a patient whose tumor demonstrated a predominant retiform pattern and mesenchymal heterologous elements, a pelvic recurrence was noted three months after receiving two courses of vincristine, bleomycin, and cisplatin. She was then treated with whole abdominal radiotherapy as well as cyclophosphamide, actinomycin D, and doxorubicin but died nine months postoperatively (123).

In summary, there is no good evidence that current chemotherapy is effective in eradicating recurrent or metastatic Sertoli-Leydig cell tumors. Similarly, radiotherapy has not been proven to be of value in an adjuvant setting or for advanced or locally recurrent disease. Although randomized trials are not feasible because of the rarity of these tumors, it is hoped that prospective multi-institutional trials, such as that employing BEP chemotherapy or new drugs and drug combinations for malignant ovarian stromal tumors, will provide new approaches to management of these unusual tumors.

GYNANDROBLASTOMA

The diagnosis of gynandroblastoma is based entirely on morphologic criteria that require the presence of both granulosa-theca and Sertoli-Leydig cell types (10). The diagnosis further requires that the minor component account for at least 10% of a tumor in the sex-cord stromal category (3). The tumors may cause virilization, estrogen excess, or exhibit no endocrinological disturbance. Gynandroblastomas are typically small in size (1.4–6 cm) (10), but a tumor weighing 37 pounds was removed from a virilized 18-year-old patient (135). They are unilateral and on gross inspection are described as solid, brown, yellow, or white. Microscopic examination reveals typical mature granulosa cells intermingling or alternating with hollow tubules lined by mature Sertoli cells. Leydig cells are also seen (10), and in some cases Reinke crystals have been identified in the Leydig cell component (136). Electron microscopy shows Call-Exner bodies of the hyaline type, composed of multiple layers of basal lamina resembling Call-Exner bodies of the normal graffian follicle (137).

Gynandroblastomas are considered to be benign, and thus may be treated conservatively in young patients. There are, however, too few cases to be certain of their malignant potential.

SEX CORD TUMOR WITH ANNULAR TUBULES

In 1970, Scully (138) reported on a rare but morphologically distinct group of ten ovarian sex cord tumors characterized by the presence of simple and complex annular tubules, a tendency to calcification, and an unusually high association with the Peutz-Jeghers syndrome (gastrointestinal polyposis, oral and cutaneous melanin pigmentation). Over the last two decades, numerous reports on sex cord tumors with annular tubules, including Young and colleagues on seventy-four cases (139), have further documented the association between these tumors and the Peutz-Jeghers syndrome.

The characteristics of sex cord tumors with annular tubules in patients with and without Peutz-Jeghers syndrome will be reviewed separately since the tumors differ in their clinical and pathological features, depending on the presence or absence of the syndrome.

Sex Cord Tumor with Annular Tubules with Peutz-Jeghers Syndrome

The overwhelming majority of patients with the Peutz-Jeghers syndrome who have had their ovaries examined microscopically are found to have sex cord tumors with annular tubules. In almost all cases, the tumors have been incidental findings in ovaries removed for other reasons. The age of the patients varies (mean, 27 years) and those that exhibit endocrine activity (50%) appear to be usually estrogenic, manifested by menstrual irregularity or postmenopausal bleeding (3). In approximately two-thirds of the cases, the tumor is bilateral (109). They are typically small in size (3 cm or less) and are seen on gross inspection of the ovaries in about one-fourth of the patients. They are described as single or multiple nodules appearing yellow on their sectioned surfaces (139).

On microscopic examination, the tumors are characterized by sharply circumscribed, rounded epithelial nests composed of ring-shaped tubules encircling hyalinized basement-membranelike material. Simple annular tubules encircling a central hyaline mass and complex communicating tubules encircling several hyaline masses are both seen (Fig. 7). In approximately one-half of the cases, foci of calcification occupy the site of the hyaline masses (139). An ultrastructural study of a tumor from a patient with the syndrome revealed numerous solid cords of cells surrounded by fibrillary layers of basal lamina, as well as central hya-

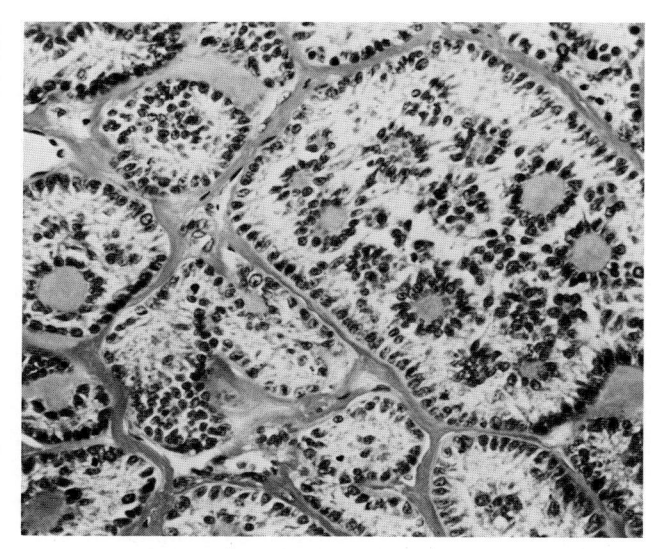

FIG. 7. Sex cord tumor with annular tubules. Shown here are sharply circumscribed, rounded epithelial islands composed of ring-shaped tubules. Hyaline masses are encircled by simple and complex tubules. (Courtesy of Robert E. Scully, M.D.)

line bodies. In that case, Böttcher filaments were not seen. Immunohistochemistry of the same tumor showed staining for estradiol and testosterone similar to that of Sertoli and granulosa cell tumors (140).

In a review of cases of sex cord tumors with annular tubules by Young and associates (139), four of twenty-seven patients with the Peutz-Jeghers syndrome had adenoma malignum of the cervix, and two of them died of it. Since that report, additional cases of adenocarcinoma of the cervix in these patients have been encountered (141), and some have been associated with other pelvic tumors such as granulosa cell tumors, mucinous and serous ovarian tumors (142–144).

It has been suggested that the Peutz-Jeghers gene may also be associated with an increased risk of malignant lesions in other organ systems (145). In the case of breast cancer, this view is supported by the finding of sex cord tumor with annular tubules, Peutz-Jeghers syndrome, and bilateral breast cancer in both a patient and her paternal grandmother (146).

The relevant literature indicates that sex cord tumors with annular tubules associated with the Peutz-Jeghers syndrome do not behave in a malignant fashion and thus may be treated conservatively (109). It is imperative, however, that a coexistent endocervical tumor is not present and that the patient remain under surveillance after treatment.

Sex Cord Tumor With Annular Tubules Without Peutz-Jeghers Syndrome

In patients without the Peutz-Jeghers syndrome, the tumors are almost always unilateral and usually form palpable masses (3). The mean age of these patients (34 years) is somewhat older than those with the syndrome and the average size of the tumors is greater and may reach 18 cm in diameter (139,147). The gross appearance of the tumors is round to oval, generally solid, with various degrees of cystic degeneration (148). The microscopic pattern is similar to the Peutz-Jeghers lesion but may show focal differentiation toward typical granulosa cell tumor, typical Sertoli cell tumor, or both. Ultrastructural features show a striking similarity between the predominant cell type and the granulosa cell, as well as the presence of fibrillary material of the type seen in Call-Exner bodies (149). Such findings, along with the absence of Böttcher filaments have led some authors to the conclusion that sex cord tumors with annular tubules should be considered to be a variant of the granulosa cell tumor (150,151). It is of interest that 40% of the patients have manifestations of estrogen secretion (3) and preoperative and postoperative endocrine profiles have been shown to resemble a granulosa cell tumor (152). In contrast, ultrastructural studies showing cells joined by specialized junctions along their lateral and adjacent borders and the presence of Böttcher filaments are thought to support the hypothesis of the Sertoli nature of these neoplasms (148,153).

Unilateral salpingo-oophorectomy is appropriate therapy in the young patient who does not have the Peutz-Jeghers syndrome, because of the rarity of bilateral ovarian involvement. In contrast to patients with the syndrome in whom malignancy of the ovarian tumor almost never occurs, the tumor in 20% of those without the syndrome is clinically malignant (139). Total hysterectomy with bilateral salpingo-oophorectomy is the recommended treatment for older patients.

Well-defined prognostic criteria are not available; however, the tumor size is considered by some authors to be an important prognostic indicator, as are atypia, stromal invasion, and the mitotic index (154,155). In an unusual case in which synchronous invasive adenocarcinoma of the cervix, mucinous tumor of the ovary, and concurrent bilateral sex cord tumors with annular tubules were found, the patient did not exhibit stigmata of the Peutz-Jeghers syndrome. She was treated with bilateral salpingo-oophorectomy and omentectomy for symptomatic relief and referred for radiotherapy, but the outcome was not stated (156).

Sex cord tumors with annular tubules are capable of widespread dissemination, as evidenced by the incidental finding of metastatic tumor in a patient's umbilicus. This patient was treated with total hysterectomy, bilateral salpingo-oophorectomy, pelvic lymph node biopsies, and omentectomy. Histologic examination revealed foci of tumor limited to the omentum and peritoneal washings without evidence of a primary ovarian tumor. Second-look laparotomy following six courses of chemotherapy consisting of cyclophosphamide, actinomycin D, and vincristine, revealed multiple microscopic intraperitoneal deposits. She was subsequently treated with whole abdominal radiotherapy and was reported to have been rendered clinically free of disease (157).

In another case, needle biopsy of a left-sided neck mass in a 38-year-old woman revealed a metastatic sex cord tumor with annular tubules. Müllerian-inhibiting substance, a glycoprotein hormone produced by fetal Sertoli cells, causes regression of the müllerian ducts in males during sexual differentiation. In its absence, the müllerian ducts give rise to the fallopian tubes, uterus, and upper third of the vagina. In the patient reported above, serum concentrations of müllerian-inhibiting substance correlated with the degree of tumor burden throughout her course. After two courses of cyclophosphamide, doxorubicin, and cisplatin, which produced no response, multiple major surgical procedures were performed. At 16 months after her last operation there was no evidence of recurrence, and the level of müllerian-inhibiting substance was undetectable (158). It is noteworthy that the production of müllerian-inhibiting substance is specific to cells of sex cord origin. Measurement of the hormone, therefore, is not considered to be of value in the management of epithelial or germ cell tumors of the ovary.

In summary, the use, and therefore the value, of chemotherapy and radiotherapy in patients with malignant sex cord tumors with annular tubules is based solely on anecdotal experience. We are hopeful that effective therapy will become available in the future. At present, surgical resection remains the treatment of choice.

UNCLASSIFIED

Tumors in this category are histologically diverse and await further study for clarification of their biology.

SUMMARY

Sex cord-stromal tumors of the ovary are a fascinating group of neoplasms that may occur in any age group, may be endocrinologically active and, in some cases, frankly malignant. Prior to making a decision concerning surgical management and possible preservation of reproductive capacity in a patient with a unilateral, clinically localized sex cord-stromal tumor of the ovary, it is mandatory to obtain a frozen section diagnosis by an experienced pathologist. In young patients with unilateral tumors and no clinical or histopathological evidence of malignancy, conservative salpingo-oophorectomy is recommended. Stromal tumors otherwise should be treated with total hysterectomy and bilateral salpingo-oophorectomy whenever possible. If the tumor is potentially malignant and may metastasize, the surgeon must inspect the diaphragm, remove the omentum for histological evaluation, take biopsies of any suspicious para-aortic lymph nodes, and obtain washings for cytological evaluation from the pelvis and paracolic gutters.

Recurrent stromal tumors are generally treated with surgical resection whenever possible. The usual practice is to resect as much tumor as possible and treat the patients with residual disease limited to the pelvis with postoperative radiotherapy. The approach to the chemotherapeutic management of patients with bulky, unresectable tumors, or for patients with metastatic disease, should be individualized based on the histopathology of the tumor.

REFERENCES

1. Serov SF, Scully RE, Sobin LH. International histological classification of tumours, no. 9; Histological Typing of Ovarian Tumours. *Bull World Health Organ*, Geneva, 1973.
2. Scully RE. World Health Organization Classification and Nomenclature of Ovarian Cancer. *Monogr Natl Cancer Inst* 1975; 42:5–7.
3. Young RH, Scully RE. Sex cord-stromal, steroid cell, and other ovarian tumors with endocrine, paraendocrine, and paraneoplastic manifestations. Kurman RJ, ed., *Blaustine's pathology of the female genital tract*, 3rd Ed, New York: Springer-Verlag, 1987;607–58.
4. Slayton RE. Management of germ cell and stromal tumors of the ovary. *Semin Oncol* 1984;11:299–313.
5. Scully RE. The pathology of incipient neoplasia: The ovary. In: Henson DE, Albores-Saavedra J, eds. *The pathology of incipient neoplasia*. Phildelphia: WB Saunders Company, 1986; 279–293.
6. Gee DC, Russell P. The pathological assessment of ovarian neoplasms. IV: the sex cord-stromal tumours. *Pathology* 1981; 13:235–255.
7. Sternberg WH, Dhurandhar HN. Functional ovarian tumors of stromal and sex cord origin. *Hum Pathol* 1977;8:565–582.
8. Makni MK, Mzabi-Regaya S, Kattech A, Chadli A. Anatomopathological aspects of malignant ovarian tumors in children. Apropos of 16 cases. *Arch Inst Pasteur Tunis* 1988;65:87–98.
9. Murphy ED, Blawer WG. Biology of ovarian neoplasm. *UICC Technical Report Series*. report no. 4. 1980; Geneva: 50.
10. Fox H, Langley FA. Tumours of the ovary. Chicago: Year Book Medical Publishers, Inc., 1976.
11. Westholm B. Granulosa cell tumors of the ovary. A retrospective analysis (Meeting Abstract). ECCO-4. *Fourth European Conference on Clinical Oncology and Cancer Nursing*. Federation of European Cancer Societies, Madrid: 1987;229.
12. Diddle AW, O'Connor KA. Feminizing ovarian tumors and pregnancy. *Am J Obstet Gynecol* 1951;62:1071–1078.
13. Roth LM, Czernobilsky B. Tumors and tumorlike conditions of the ovary. New York, Edinburgh, London, Melbourne: Churchill Livingstone; 1985.
14. Teilum G. Special tumors of ovary and testis and related extragonadal lesions. Philadelphia and Toronto: JP Lippincott; 1976.
15. Bjorkholme E, Silfversward C. Granulosa- and theca-cell tumors. Incidence and occurrence of second primary tumors. *Acta Radiol* 1980;19(3):161–167.
16. Lack EE, Perez-Atayde AR, Murthy AS, Goldstein DP. Granulosa theca cell tumors in premenarchal girls: a clinical and pathologic study of ten cases. *Cancer* 1981;48(8):1846–1854.

17. McCormack TP, Riddick DH. Hormonal function of a granulosa cell tumor. *Obstet Gynecol* 1976;48[suppl 1]:18s–21s.
18. Wilansky DL, Scott BH, Lachance RC. Masculinizing granulosa cell tumor. *Can Med Assoc J* 1976;115(6):545–546.
19. Jarabek J, Talerman A. Virilization due to a metastasizing granulosa cell tumor. *Int J Gynecol Pathol* 1983;2(3):316–324.
20. Taylor HC, Velasco ME, Flores SG, Berg G, Brown TR. Amenorrhea and failure to virilize in a patient with a testosterone secreting granulosa cell tumor. *Clin Endocrinol (Oxf)* 1982;17(6):557–567.
21. Benjamin E, Law S, Bobrow LG. Intermediate filaments cytokeratin and vimentin in ovarian sex cord-stromal tumours with correlative studies in adult and fetal ovaries. *J Pathol* 1987;152:253–263.
22. Lastarria D, Sachdev RK, Babury RA, Yu HM, Nuovo GJ. Immunohistochemical analysis for desmin in normal and neoplastic ovarian stromal tissue. *Arch Pathol Lab Med* 1990;114(5):502–505.
23. Chadha S, Cornelisse CJ, Schaberg A. Flow cytometric DNA ploidy analysis of ovarian granulosa cell tumors. *Gynecol Oncol* 1990;36(2):240–245.
24. Sassen RJ, Baak JD. Morphometry in the differential diagnosis of granulosa-cell tumors of the ovary. *Anal Quant Cytol Histol* 1986;8(3):245–249.
25. Gaffney EF, Majmudar B, Hertzler GL, Zane R, Furlong B, Breding E. Ovarian granulosa cell tumors—immunohistochemical localization of estradiol and ultrastructure, with functional correlations. *Obstet Gynecol* 1983;61(3):311–319.
26. Klempi PJ, Gronroos M. An ultrastructural and clinical study of theca and granulosa cell tumors. *Int J Gynecol Obstet* 1979;17(3):219–225.
27. Alberti W, Bamberg M, Schulz U. Granulosa cell tumor. The results of postoperative irradiation. *Deutsche Medizinische Wochenschrift* 1984;109(19):750–752.
28. Bartl W, Spernol R, Breitenecker G. The significance of clinical and morphological parameters for the prognosis of granulosa cell tumors of the ovaries. *Geburtshilfe Frauenheilkunde* 1984;44(5):295–299.
29. Lusch CJ, Mercurio TM, Runyeon WK. Delayed recurrence and chemotherapy of a granulosa cell tumor. *Obstet Gynecol* 1978;51:505–507.
30. Lomax CW, May HV Jr, Panko WB, Thornton WN Jr. Progesterone production by an ovarian granulosa cell carcinoma. *Obstet Gynecol* 1977;50(Suppl 1):39s–40s.
31. Kaye SB, Davies E. Cyclophosphamide, adriamycin, and cis-platinum for the treatment of advanced granulosa cell tumor, using serum estradiol as a tumor marker. *Gynecol Oncol* 1986;24(2):261–264.
32. Jacobs AJ, Deppe G, Cohen CJ. Combination chemotherapy of ovarian granulosa cell tumor with cis-platinum and doxorubicin. *Gynecol Oncol* 1982;14:294–297.
33. Colombo N, Sessa C, Landoni F, Sartori E, Pecorelli S, Mangioni C. Cisplatin, vinblastine, and bleomycin combination chemotherapy in metastatic granulosa cell tumor of the ovary. *Obstet Gynecol* 1986;67(2):265–268.
34. Zambetti M, Escobedo A, Pilotti S, DePalo G. Cis-platinum/vinblastine/bleomycin combination chemotherapy in advanced or recurrent granulosa cell tumors of the ovary. *Gynecol Oncol* 1990;36(3):317–320.
35. Pecorelli S, Wagener P, Bonazzi C, ten Bokkel Huinink W, Kobierska A, Ploch E, Veenhoff CH, Vermorken JB, Willemse A, Rotmensz N. Cisplatin (P), vinblastine (V), and bleomycin (B) combination chemotherapy in recurrent or advanced granulosa cell tumor of the ovary (GCTO) an EORTC Gynecol Cancer Coop Group Study. *Proc Am Soc Clin Oncol* 1988;7:A567.
36. Rodgers KE, Marks JF, Ellefson DD, Yanagihara DL, Tonetta SA, Vasilev SA, Morrow CP, Montz FJ, diZerega GS. Follicle regulatory protein: a novel marker for granulosa cell cancer patients. *Gynecol Oncol* 1990;37(3):381–387.
37. Montz FJ, Rodgers KE, diZerega GS, Berek JS. Follicle regulatory protein (FRP): a new tumor marker for granulosa cell tumors (GCT) of the ovary (Meeting Abstract). *Proc Am Soc Clin Oncol* 1989;8:A589.
38. Lappohn RE, Burger HG, Bouma J, Bangah M, Krans M, de Bruijn HW. Inhibin as a marker for granulosa-cell tumors (see comments). *N Engl J Med* 1989;321(12):790–793.
39. Li MK, van der Wait JD. Recurrent granulosa cell tumor of the ovary 22 years after primary excision. *J R Coll Surg Edin* 1984;29:192–194.
40. Ptackov B, Kucera F, Kopecny J. Granulosa cell tumor of the ovary; evaluation of therapeutic results. *Cesk Gynekol* 1989;54(4):263–267.
41. Bjorkholme E, Pettersson F. Granulosa-cell and theca-cell tumors. The clinical picture and long-term outcome for the Radiumhemmet series. *Acta Obstet Gynecol Scand* 1980;59(4):361–365.
42. Bjorkholm E. Granulosa cell tumors: A comparison of survival in patients and matched control. *Am J Obstet Gynecol* 1980;138(3):329–331.
43. Pankratz E, Boyes DA, White GW, Galliford BW, Fairey RN, Benedet JL. Granulosa cell tumors. A clinical review of 61 cases. *Obstet Gynecol* 1978;52(6):718–723.
44. Chang CY, Yeh WR, Chao KC, Ng HT. Granulosa cell tumor of the ovary. *Chin Med J* 1990;46(3):172–176.
45. Fox H, Agrawal K, Langley FA. A clinicopathologic study of 92 cases of granulosa cell tumor of the ovary with special reference to factors influencing prognosis. *Cancer* 1975;35:231–241.
46. Stenwig JT, Hazekamp JT, Beecham JB. Granulosa cell tumors of the ovary. A clinicopathological study of 118 cases with long term follow-up. *Gynecol Oncol* 1979;7:136–152.
47. Kottmeier HL. Carcinoma of the female genital tract. *The Abraham Flexner Lectures*, Ser. no. 11. Baltimore: Williams and Wilkins, 1953.
48. Santesson L, Kottmeier HL. General classification of ovarian tumors. In: Gentil F, Junqueira AC, *UICC Monograph Series*, Vol. II. Berlin, Heidelburg, New York: Springer-Verlag; 1968;1–8.
49. Bjorkholme E, Silfversward C. Prognostic factors in granulosa cell tumors. *Gynecol Oncol* 1981;11:261–274.
50. Klemi PF, Joensuu H, Salmi T. Prognostic value of flow cytometric DNA content analysis in granulosa cell tumor of the ovary. *Cancer* 1990;65(5):1189–1193.
51. Suh KS, Silverberg SG, Rhame JG, Wilkinson DS. Granulosa cell tumor of the ovary. Histopathologic and flow cytometric analysis with clinical correlation. *Arch Pathol Lab Med* 1990;114:496–501.
52. Hitchcock CL, Norris HJ, Khalifa MA, Wargotz ES. Flow cytometric analysis of granulosa tumors. *Cancer* 1989;64(10):2127–2132.
53. Young RH, Dudley AG, Scully RE. Granulosa cell, Sertoli-Leydig cell, and unclassified sex cord-stromal tumors associated with pregnancy: a clinicopathological analysis of thirty-six cases. *Gynecol Oncol* 1984;18(2):181–205.
54. Nakashima N, Young RH, Scully RE. Androgenic granulosa cell tumors of the ovary. A clinicopathologic analysis of 17 cases and review of the literature. *Arch Pathol Lab Med* 1984;108(10):786–791.
55. Petru E, Pickel H, Heydarfadai M, Tamussino K, Lahousen M, Schaider H. Experience with stromal tumors and germ-cell tumors of the ovary. *Int J Gynecol Cancer* 1991;1:9–14.
56. Young RH, Dickersin GR, Scully RE. Juvenile granulosal tumor of the ovary. A clinicopathological analysis of 125 cases. *Am J Surg Pathol* 1984;8:575–596.
57. Fernandez F, Jordan J, Carmona M, Oliver A, Gracia R, Gonzalez M, Peralta A. Precocious pseudopuberty secondary to granulosa cell tumor. *An Esp Pediatria* 1984;21:822–886.
58. McCann EC, Zerner J. Granulosa cell tumor of the ovary in a 7-year-old female with late (12-year) lung metastases. A case report and discussion. *J Maine Med Assoc* 1973;564:201–203.
59. Bonnevalle M, Mazinque F, Necken B, Vaast P, Lecomte-Houcke M, Debeugny P. Precocious pseudo-puberty in granulosa cell tumor in children less than 1 year old. 2 Cases. *Chir Pediatr* 1990;3:32–34.
60. Hollenbeck JI, Rodgers BM, Talbert JL, Donnelly WH. Bilateral granulosa cell tumors of the ovaries in infancy. *J Pediatr Surg* 1978;13:542–543.
61. Vaz RM, Turner C. Other disease (enchondromatosis) associ-

ated with ovarian juvenile granulosa cell tumor and precocious pseudopuberty. *J Pediatr* 1986;108:945–947.
62. Velasco-Oses A, Alonso-Alvaro A, Blanco-Pozo A, Nogales FF Jr. Ollier's disease associated with ovarian juvenile granulosa cell tumor. *Cancer* 1985;62:222–225.
63. Betta P, Bellingeri D. Androgenic juvenile granulosa cell tumor. Case report. *Eur J Gynaecol Oncol* 1985;6:71–74.
64. Biscotti CV, Hart WR. Juvenile granulosa cell tumor of the ovary. *Arch Path Lab Med* 1989;113:40–46.
65. Hisaoka M, Horie A, Kajiawara Y. Juvenile granulosa cell tumor in a three-year-old infant. An immunohistochemical and ultrastructural study. *Acta Pathol Jpn* 1990;40:616–621.
66. Gershenson DM, Copeland LJ, Kavanagh JJ, Stringer CA, Saul PB, Wharton JT. Treatment of metastatic stromal tumors of the ovary with cisplatin, doxorubicin, and cyclophosaphide. *Obstet Gynecol* 1987;60:765–769.
67. Niishida M, Jimi S, Haji M, Hayashi I, Kai T, Tasaka H. Juvenile granulosa cell tumor in association with a high serum inhibin level. *Gynecol Oncol* 1991;40:990–994.
68. Rodgers KE, Montz FJ, Scott L, Condon S, Fujimori K, DiZerega GS. Inhibition of ovarian cancer cell proliferation in vivo and incorporation of 3H-thymidine in vitro after follicle regulatory protein administration. *Obstet Gynecol* 1989;73:66–74.
69. Lack EE, Perez-Atayoe AR, Murthy AS, Gozstein DP, Grigler JF Jr, Vanter GI, Granulosa theca cell tumors in premenarchal girls: A clinical and pathologic study of ten cases. *Cancer* 1981; 48:1846–1854.
70. Zaloudek C, Norris HJ. Granulosa tumors of the ovary in children. A clinical and pathologic study of 32 cases. *Am J Surg Pathol* 1982;6:513–522.
71. Vassal G, Flamant F, Caillaud JM, Demeocq F, Nihoul-Fekete C, Lemerie J. Juvenile granulosa cell tumor of the ovary in children: A clinical study of 15 cases. *J Clin Oncol* 1988;6: 990–995.
72. Takeuchi H, Hamada H, Sodemoto Y, Ushigome S. Juvenile granulosa cell tumor associated with rapid distant metastases. *Acta Pathol Jpn* 1983;33:537–545.
73. Ricci P, Mazza D. A clinical pathological study of a granulosa cell tumor with a fatal course: Case report. *Eur J Gynecol Oncol* 1985;4:107–111.
74. Swanson SA, Norris HJ, Kelsten ML, Wheeler JE. DNA content of juvenile granulosa tumors determined by flow cytometry. *Int J Gynecol Pathol* 1990;9:101–109.
75. Stage AH, Grafton WD. Thecomas and granulosa cell tumors of the ovary—an analysis of 51 tumors. *Obstet Gynecol* 1977; 50:21–27.
76. Zhang J, Young RH, Arseneau J, Scully RE. Ovarian stromal tumors containing lutein or Leydig (luteinized thecomas and stromal Leydig cell tumors). A clinicopathological analysis of fifty cases. *Int J Gynecol Pathol* 1982;1:270–285.
77. Roth LM, Sternberg WH. Partly luteinized theca cell tumor of the ovary. *Cancer* 1983;51:1697–1707.
78. Gaffney EF, Majmudar B, Hewan-Lowe K. Ultrastructure and immunohistochemical localization of estradiol in three thecomas. *Hum Pathol* 1984;15:153–160.
79. Robert HG, Dutranoy Vu J, Dupre-Froment J. Thecal tumors of the ovary. 14 cases. *Nouvelle Presse Medicale* 1976;6: 1459–1462.
80. Bjorkholm E, Silfversward C. Theca cell tumors. Clinical features and prognosis. *Acta Radiol* 1980;19:241–244.
81. Spinelli A, Morf P, Genton C. Granulosa cell and theca cell tumors in 25 cases. *Geburtshilfe Frauenheilk* 1979;39:882–887.
82. Waxman M, Vuletin JC, Urcuyo R, Belling CG. Ovarian low grade stromal sarcoma with thecomatous features. A critical reappraisal of the so-called malignant thecoma. *Cancer* 1979; 44:2206–2217.
83. Samanth KK, Black WC. Benign ovarian stromal tumors associated with free peritoneal fluid. *Am J Obstet Gynecol* 1970; 107:538–545.
84. Raggio M, Kaplan AL, Harberg JF. Recurrent ovarian fibromas with basal cell nevus syndrome (Gorlin syndrome). *Obstet Gynecol* 1985;61:95–96.
85. Prat J, Scully RE. Cellular fibromas and fibrosarcomas of the ovary. A comparative clinicopathologic analysis of seventeen cases. *Cancer* 1981;47:2663–2670.
86. Walker JL, Manetta A, Mannel RS, Liao SY. Cellular fibroma masquerading as ovarian carcinoma. *Obstet Gynecol* 1990;76: 530–531.
87. Young RH, Scully RE. Ovarian stromal tumors with minor sex cord elements. A report of seven cases. *Int J Gynecol Pathol* 1983;2:227–234.
88. Chalvardjian A, Scully RE. Sclerosing stromal tumors of the ovary. *Cancer* 1973;31:664–670.
89. Gee DC, Russell P. The pathological assessment of ovarian neoplasms. IV: The sex cord-stromal tumours. *Pathology* 1981; 13:235–255.
90. Ho YB, Robertson DI, Clement PB, Mincey EK. Sclerosing stromal tumor of the ovary. *Obstet Gynecol* 1982;60:252–256.
91. Cashell AW, Cohen ML. Masculinizing sclerosing stromal tumor of the ovary during pregnancy. *Gynecol Oncol* 1991;43: 281–285.
92. Katsube Y, Iwaoki Y, Silverberg SG, Fujiwara A. Sclerosing stromal tumor of the ovary associated with endometrial adenocarcinoma: A case report. *Gynecol Oncol* 1988;29:392–398.
93. Shah KH, Steele HD. Sclerosing stromal tumor of the ovary. A case report and further observations. *Diag Gynecol Obstet* 1981;3:155–159.
94. Saitoh A, Tsutsumi Y, Osamura RY, Watanabe K. Stromal tumor of the ovary. Immunohistochemical and electron-microscopic demonstration of smooth-muscle differentiation. *Arch Pathol Lab Med* 1989;113:372–376.
95. Lam RM, Geittman P. Sclerosing tumor of the ovary. A light, electron microscopic, and enzyme histochemical study. *Int J Gynecol Pathol* 1988;7:280–290.
96. Erhlich EN, Dominguez OV, Samuels LT, Lynch D, Oberhelman H, Warner NE. Aldosteronism and precocious puberty due to an ovarian androblastoma (Sertoli cell tumor). *J Clin Endocrinol Metab* 1963;23:358–367.
97. Korzets A, Nouriel L, Steiner Z, Griffel B, Kraus L, Freund U, Klajman A. Resistant hypertension associated with a renin-producing ovarian Sertoli cell tumor. *Am J Clin Pathol* 1986; 85:242–247.
98. Tavassoli FA, Norris HJ. Sertoli tumors of the ovary. A clinicopathologic study of 28 cases with ultrastructural observations. *Cancer* 1980;46:2281–2297.
99. Ramzy I, Bos C. Sertoli cell tumors of the ovary: Light microscopic and ultrastructural study with histogenetic considerations. *Cancer* 1976;38:2447–2256.
100. Young RH, Scully RE. Ovarian Sertoli cell tumors. A report of ten cases. *Int J Gynecol Pathol* 1984;2:349–363.
101. Bonaventura LM, Judd H, Roth LM, Cleary RE. Androgen, estrogen, and progesterone by a lipid cell tumor of the ovary. *Am J Obstet Gynecol* 1978;131:403–409.
102. Janson PO, Hamberger L, Damber JE, Dennefors B, Knutson F. Steroid production in vitro of a hilus cell tumor of the human ovary. *Obstet Gynecol* 1980;55:662–665.
103. Nagamani M, Gonzalez-Vitale JC. Steroid secretion patterns of a hilus cell tumor of the ovary. *Obstet Gynecol* 1981;58: 521–527.
104. Mandel FP, Voet RL, Weiland AJ, Judd HL. Steroid secretion by masculinizing and "feminizing" Hilus cell tumors. *J Clin Endocrinol Metab* 1981;52:779–784.
105. Hiura M, Muta M, Nogawa T, Nagai N, Katoh K, Fujiwara A. Histogenesis, cytodifferentiation, and its subcellular steroidogenic sites in the virilizing ovarian Leydig cell tumor: light microscopic dry-mounting radioauthography for [3H] cholesterol and electron microscopic cytochemistry for 3 beta-hydroxysteroid dehydrogenase activity. *Gynecol Oncol* 1984;17:175–184.
106. Glaser B, Weill S, Lurie M, Kahana L, Abramovici H, Sheinfeld M. Leydig-cell tumor of the ovary: visualization using 131I-19-iodocholesterol scintigraphy. *Eur J Nucl Med* 1985;11: 13–16.
107. Raaf JH, Bajorunas DR, Smith DH, Woodruff J. Virilizing hilus (Leydig) cell tumor of the ovary: the challenge of an accurate preoperative diagnosis. *Surgery* 1983;94:951–954.
108. Roth LM, Sternberg WH. Ovarian stromal tumors containing

108. Leydig cells. II. Pure Leydig cell tumor, non-hilar type. *Cancer* 1973;32:952–960.
109. Young RH, Scully RE. Ovarian Sex-Cord Stromal and Steroid Cell Tumors. In: Roth LM, Czernobilsky B, eds. *Tumors and Tumor-like Conditions of the Ovary*. New York, Edinburgh, London, and Melbourne: Churchill Livingstone, 1985;43–73.
110. Baramki TA, Leddy AL, Woodruff JD. Bilateral hilus cell tumors of the ovary. *Obstet Gynecol* 1983;62:128–131.
111. Paradisi R, Venturoli S, Martinelli G, Serra L, Govoni E, Fabbri R, Flamigni C. In vivo endocrine studies and morphological features in a case of hilus cell tumor in mesovarium. *Gynecol Obstet Inv* 1982;14:184–194.
112. Paraskevas M, Scully RE. Hilus cell tumor of the ovary. A clinicopathological analysis of 12 Reinke crystal-positive and nine crystal-negative cases. *Int J Gynecol Pathol* 1989;8:299–310.
113. Bertram KA, Bratloff B, Hodges GF, Davidson H. Treatment of malignant Leydig cell tumor. *Cancer* 1991;68:2324–2329.
114. Young RH, Scully RE. Ovarian Sertoli-Leydig cell tumors. A clinicopathological analysis of 207 cases. *Am J Surg Pathol* 1985;9:543–569.
115. Wiebe RH, Morris CV. Testosterone/androstenedione ratio in the evaluation of women with ovarian androgen excess. *Obstet Gynecol* 1983;61:279–284.
116. Munemura M, Inoue S, Himeno R, Koyama N, Mizumoto J, Maeyama M, Iwamasa T. Endocrine studies on ovarian androblastomas (Sertoli-Leydig tumors). *J Endocrinol* 1984;7:615–622.
117. Mann WJ, Chumas J, Rosenwaks Z, Merrill JA, Davenport D. Elevated serum alpha-fetoprotein associated with Sertoli-Leydig cell tumors of the ovary. *Obstet Gynecol* 1986;67:141–144.
118. Sekiya S, Inaba N, Iwasawa H, Kobayashi O, Takamizawa H, Matsuzaki O, Nagao K. AFP-producing Sertoli-Leydig cell tumor of the ovary. *Arch Gynecol* 1985;236:187–196.
119. Larsen WG, Felmar EA, Wallace ME, Frieder R. Sertoli-Leydig cell tumor of the ovary: A rare cause of amenorrhea. *Obstet Gynecol* 1992;79:831–833.
120. Tetu B, Ordñez NG, Silva EG. Sertoli-Leydig cell tumor of the ovary with alpha-fetoprotein production. *Arch Pathol Lab Med* 1986;110:65–68.
121. Gagnon S, Tetu B, Silva EG, McCaughey TE. Frequency of alpha fetoprotein production by Sertoli-Leydig cell tumors of the ovary: An immunohistochemical study of 8 cases. *Mod Pathol* 1989;2:63–67.
122. Chadha S, Honnebier WJ, Schaberg A. Raised serum alpha-fetoprotein in Sertoli-Leydig cell tumor (androblastoma) of ovary: report of two cases. *Int J Gynecol Pathol* 1987;6:82–88.
123. Young RH, Perez-Atayde AR, Scully RE. Ovarian Sertoli-Leydig cell tumor with retiform and heterologous components. Report of a case with hepatocyte differentiation and elevated serum alpha-fetoprotein. *Am J Surg Pathol* 1984;8:709–718.
124. Kooijman CD, Strakes W. Sertoli-Leydig cell tumors of the ovary. A report of three cases with ultrastructural findings. *Eur J Obstet Gynecol Reprod Biol* 1982;13:93–104.
125. Dardi LE, Miller AW, Gould VE. Sertoli-Leydig cell tumor with endometroid differentiation. Case report and discussion of histogenesis. *Diagn Gynecol Obstet* 1984;4:227–234.
126. Roth LM, Slayton RE, Brady LW, Blessing JA, Johnson G. Retiform differentiation in ovarian Sertoli-Leydig cell tumors. A clinicopathologic study of six cases from a Gynecologic Oncology Group study. *Cancer* 1985;55:1093–1098.
127. Gúrard MJ, Ferenczy A, Arguelles MA. Ovarian Sertoli-Leydig cell tumor with rhabdomyosarcoma: an ultrastructural study. *Ultrastruct Pathol* 1982;3:347–358.
128. Nolan T, Gallup DG, Dufour DR. Recurrence of a gonadal stromal cell tumor (Sertoli-Leydig cell with heterologous elements) in a teenager. *Gynecol Oncol* 1983;15:111–119.
129. Dicker D, Dekel A, Feldberg D, Goldman JA, Kessler E. Bilateral Sertoli-Leydig cell tumor with heterologous elements: report of an unusual case and review of the literature. *Eur J Obstet Gynecol Reprod Biol* 1986;22:175–181.
130. Zaloudek C, Norris HJ. Sertoli-Leydig tumors of the ovary. A clinicopathologic study of 64 intermediate and poorly differentiated neoplasms. *Am J Surg Pathol* 1984;8:405–418.
131. Schwartz PE, Smith JP. Treatment of ovarian stromal tumors. *Am J Obstet Gynecol* 1976;125:402–411.
132. Pride GL, Pollock WJ, Norgard MJ. Metastatic Sertoli-Leydig cell tumor of the ovary during pregnancy treated by BV-CAP chemotherapy. *Am J Obstet Gynecol* 1982;143:231–233.
133. Reddick RL, Walton LA. Sertoli-Leydig cell tumor of the ovary with teratomatous differentiation: clinicopathologic considerations. *Cancer* 1982;50:1171–1176.
134. Talerman A. Ovarian Sertoli-Leydig cell tumor (androblastoma) with retiform pattern. A clinicopathologic study. *Cancer* 1987;60:3056–3064.
135. Cantor B, Pierson KK, Kalra PS. Hormone studies in a gynandroblastoma. *Fertil Steril* 1978;29:681–685.
136. Anderson MC, Rees DA. Gynandroblastoma of the ovary. *Br J Obstet Gynecol* 1975;82:68–73.
137. Chalvardjian A, Derzko C. Gynandroblastoma: its ultrastructure. *Cancer* 1982;50:710–721.
138. Scully RE. Sex cord tumor with annular tubules a distinctive ovarian tumor of the Peutz-Jeghers Syndrome. *Cancer* 1970;25:1107–1121.
139. Young RH, Welch WR, Dickersin GR, Scully RE. Ovarian sex cord tumor with annular tubules. Review of 74 cases including 27 with Peutz-Jeghers Syndrome and four with adenoma malignum of the cervix. *Cancer* 1982;50:1384–1402.
140. Benagiano G, Bigotti G, Buzzi M, D'Allesandro P, Napolitano C. Endocrine and morphological study of a case of ovarian sex-cord tumor with annular tubules in a woman with Peutz-Jeghers syndrome. *Int J Gynecol Obstet* 1988;26:441–452.
141. Costa J. Peutz-Jeghers syndrome: case presentation. *Obstet Gynecol* 1977;50:15–17.
142. Clement S, Efrusy ME, Dobbins WO, Palmer RN. Pelvic neoplasia in Peutz-Jeghers syndrome. *J Clin Gastroent* 1979;1:341–343.
143. Chen KT. Female genital tract tumors in Peutz-Jeghers Syndrome. *Hum Pathol* 1986;17:858–861.
144. Dolan J, Al-Timimi AH, Richards SM, Jeffs JB, Mason GC, Smith DB, Hasleton PS. Does ovarian sex cord tumour with annular tubules produce progesterone? *J Clin Pathol* 1986;39:29–35.
145. Rodu B, Martinez MG, Peutz-Jeghers syndrome and cancer. *Oral Surg, Oral Med, Oral Path* 1984;58:584–588.
146. Riley E, Swift MY. A family with Peutz-Jeghers syndrome and bilateral breast cancer. *Cancer* 1980;46:815–817.
147. Anderson MC, Govan AD, Langley FA, Woodcock AS, Tyagi SP. Ovarian sex cord tumours with annular tubules. *Histopathology* 1980;4:137–145.
148. Ahn GH, Chi JG, Lee SK. Ovarian sex cord tumor with annular tubules. *Cancer* 1986;57:1066–1073.
149. Hertel BF, Kempson RL. Ovarian sex cord tumors with annular tubules: an ultrastructural study. *Am J Surg Pathol* 1977;1:145–153.
150. Crissman JD, Hart WR. Ovarian sex cord tumors with annular tubules. An ultrastructural study of three cases. *Am J Clin Pathol* 1981;75:11–17.
151. Kalifat R, de Brux J. Ovarian sex cord tumor with annular tubules: an ultrastructural study. *Int J Gynecol Pathol* 1987;6:380–388.
152. Crain JL. Ovarian sex cord tumor with annular tubules: Steroid profile. *Obstet Gynecol* 1986;58:75S–79S.
153. Astengo-Osuna C. Ovarian sex-cord tumor with annular tubules. Case report with ultrastructural findings. *Cancer* 1984;54:1070–1075.
154. Metamala MF, Nogales FF, Lardelli P, Navarro N. Metastatic granulosa cell tumor with pattern of sex cord tumor with annular tubules. *Int J Gynecol Pathol* 1987;6:185–193.
155. Gloor E. Ovarian sex cord tumor with annular tubules. Clinicopathologic report of two benign and one malignant cases with long follow-ups. *Virchows Arch* [A] 1979;384:185–193.
156. Matseoane S, Moscovic E, Williams S, Huang JC. Case Re-

157. Baron BW, Schraut WH, Azizi F, Talerman A. Extragonadal sex cord tumor with annular tubules in an umbilical hernia sac: port: Mucinous neoplasm in the cervix associated with a mucinous neoplasm in the ovary and concurrent bilateral sex cord tumors with annular tubules: Immunohistochemical Study. *Gynecol Oncol* 1991;43:300–304.

a unique presentation with implications for histogenesis. *Gynecol Oncol* 1988;30:71–75.

158. Gustafson ML, Lee MM, Scully RE, Moncure AC, Hirakawa T, Goodman A, Muntz HG, Donahoe PK, MacLaughlin DT, Fuller AF. Müllerian inhibiting substance as a marker of ovarian sex-cord tumor. *N Engl J Med* 1992;326:466–471.

CHAPTER 30

Metastatic Tumors to the Ovary

Richard R. Barakat

A review of the histopathologic features of metastatic tumors to the ovary has been presented in a previous chapter. In this chapter we shall deal with the clinical aspects of these tumors that may aid the gynecologist in suspecting metastatic disease and thereby carry out the appropriate surgical procedure.

Although difficult to establish, the frequency of secondary ovarian neoplasms has been estimated at 5–10% (1–4). There are four possible mechanisms of spread to the ovary from other primary sites (5). These include direct extension from contiguous organs, hematogenous spread, lymphatic spread, and transperitoneal spread from other organs. The gross features of tumors that tend to metastasize to the ovary closely resemble those of primary ovarian neoplasms. Several features may raise the index of suspicion for metastatic disease. First, tumors that metastasize to the ovary are bilateral in up to 75% of cases. Secondly, the surface of the ovary may contain multiple nodules, while on cut section the parenchyma may be spared. Finally, if the distribution of disease at the time of laparotomy is atypical for ovarian cancer (i.e., distant metastases in the absence of peritoneal disease), a metastatic source should be suspected.

METASTASES FROM THE GENITAL TRACT

Fallopian Tube

Because of the close proximity of the tube and ovary, fallopian tube cancer involves the ovary in 33% of cases (6). These rare cancers comprise approximately 1% of all gynecologic malignancies. Histologically, tubal cancers are often serous or undifferentiated adenocarcinomas, making the distinction between a tubal and ovarian primary difficult. A conglomerate mass involving both tube and ovary is more likely to be classified as an ovarian primary than a much rarer tubal cancer. The term *tubo-ovarian carcinoma* has been suggested in these cases (7). Prognosis with metastatic tubal cancer depends on residual disease following cytoreductive surgery (8). These cancers appear to respond favorably to cisplatin-based chemotherapy, and are therefore managed clinically in a manner similar to epithelial ovarian cancer.

UTERUS

Endometrium

The endometrium has been shown to be the most frequent primary site of genital tract malignancies metastatic to the ovary (9). Scully (10) reported that 5–15% of hysterectomy specimens for endometrial cancer had ovarian involvement. Eifel et al. (11) suggested that tumors with endometrioid features at both sites had a good prognosis and were most likely independent, while if other histologies such as papillary, clear cell, or mixed cell type were present at both sites, the prognosis was poor and probably represented single primary tumors and metastases. Ulbright et al. (12) considered cancers to be metastatic from endometrium to ovary if the ovary had a multinodular pattern or if two or more of the following were present: (1) small ovaries (less than 5 cm), (2) bilateral ovarian involvement, (3) deep myometrial invasion, (4) vascular invasion, or (5) tubal lumen involvement. Tumors considered metastatic had a significantly higher incidence of disease outside of the uterus and ovary than those felt to be independent primaries. Both tumors considered to be metastatic and independent primaries had a high incidence of associated endometrial hyperplasias, support-

R. R. Barakat: Gynecology Service, Department of Surgery, Memorial Sloan-Kettering Cancer Center, New York, New York 10021

ing the belief that the endometrium was the primary site in both groups. Only one case in thirty-four was felt to represent metastasis from ovary to endometrium. This study differed with Eifel's in that the group of tumors considered to be independent contained a variety of nonendometrioid tumor types which did not confer a worse prognosis. Distinguishing the origin of simultaneously occurring carcinoma in the ovary and endometrium can be a difficult task. Recently the use of flow cytometric DNA-ploidy analysis has been advocated as being useful in determining the lineage of multiple malignancies of the female genital tract. The DNA index of the primary tumor tends to be maintained in the metastases, while independent tumors would likely differ in their DNA content. Smit et al. (13) evaluated DNA content from paraffin-embedded tissue of six patients with endometrial and ovarian cancer. Histologic review suggested an independent uterine primary in only one case; analysis of DNA content revealed two cases to have independent primaries, while the similar DNA content of the other cases suggested metastatic disease.

CERVIX

The incidence of ovarian metastasis from cervical carcinoma, although small, may be higher with adenocarcinomas than with squamous cell carcinomas. The two largest series (14–15) reported a 0.6% and 1.3% incidence, respectively, of ovarian metastases from cervical adenocarcinomas. Kaminski and Norris (16) noted a higher incidence of ovarian metastases with mucinous cervical adenocarcinomas than with other histologic types. Of thirty-nine patients with this histology, 10% had ovarian metastases. Eight percent of fifty-one patients with endometrioid cervical carcinomas had synchronous or subsequent primary endometrioid ovarian carcinomas, leading the authors to postulate diffuse Müllerian neoplasia as the causative mechanism of these multiple primary neoplasms. Brown et al. (17) reported their experience with ovarian metastases in stage I adenocarcinoma of the cervix and reviewed the literature on this subject. They noted a 1.8% incidence of ovarian metastases in four hundred patients with adenocarcinoma of the cervix. All of the patients with ovarian metastasis had at least one of the following characteristics: postmenopausal status, adnexal pathology, or positive pelvic lymph nodes.

Squamous cell carcinoma of the cervix metastatic to the ovary is indeed an even rarer entity. In a review of 524 squamous cell carcinomas of the cervix, Toki et al. (18) found only one patient with ovarian metastasis. Tabata et al. (19) noted no ovarian metastases in 278 patients with stage IB to stage III epidermoid carcinoma of the cervix, whereas six (12%) of forty-eight similarly staged patients with adenocarcinomas or adenosquamous carcinomas had ovarian metastases. Two cases of recurrent cervical squamous cell carcinoma in an ovary at 16 and at 23 months (20–21) following radical hysterectomy have been reported. The low incidence of ovarian metastasis from squamous cell carcinoma of the cervix does not justify prophylactic oophorectomy at the time of surgery in younger women. This also applies to cervical adenocarcinomas with the possible exception of mucinous tumors, which may have a higher incidence of ovarian metastases. Glassy cell carcinoma of the cervix is a poorly differentiated variety of adenosquamous cancer that accounts for approximately 1% of all cervical cancers (22). Two cases of glassy cell carcinoma of the cervix metastatic to the ovary have been reported in the literature to date (23–24), raising the issue of prophylactic oophorectomy in these patients. There are not enough cases, however, to conclusively answer this question.

VULVA AND VAGINA

It is exceedingly rare for vulvar or vaginal cancers to metastasize to the ovary unless they are associated with advanced disease and diffuse intraabdominal metastases. Robboy et al. (25) reported on four patients with recurrent clear cell adenocarcinoma of the vagina involving the ovaries. Two were detected at the time of recurrence laparotomy and two at autopsy. In all four cases there was extensive tumor dissemination throughout the pelvis.

EXTRAGENITAL TRACT

Virtually any malignancy arising outside the genital tract can metastasize to the ovary but, according to three recent large series, most commonly originate in the colon, breast, and the remainder of the gastrointestinal tract (9,12,26) (Table 1).

In one of the largest reports on genital tract metastases from extragenital sites, Mazur et al. (9) noted that in 149 cases, the primary tumor was diagnosed pre-

TABLE 1. *Site of origin of extragenital ovarian metastases*

Organ site	Number	Percent
Colon	64	37
Breast	61	36
Stomach	12	7
Appendix	3	2
Miscellaneous	20	12
Uncertain	11	6
Total	171	100

vious to or concurrent with the discovery of the metastasis in 86% of the cases, while 14% required a subsequent search for the primary neoplasm. The ovary was the most frequent site of metastases (76%), followed by the vagina (13%). In forty cases (35%), the metastatic extragenital tumors presented as a possible ovarian primary, and 58% of these originated in the gastrointestinal tract. The difficulty in suspecting metastatic ovarian disease was outlined by Yazigi and Sandstadt (26). In a review of twenty-nine patients with ovarian involvement from extragenital cancer, almost half of them presented with abdominal pain and increasing abdominal girth. In addition, 93% presented with a pelvic mass and 41% had ascites, making the gynecologist the most likely physician involved. Furthermore, preoperative tomographic imaging has not been found to be useful in differentiating primary from metastatic ovarian neoplasms. The CT appearance of thirty-four patients with ovarian metastases was shown to resemble a wide variety of ovarian neoplasms, particularly mucinous cystadenocarcinomas (27).

GASTROINTESTINAL CARCINOMA

Colon

Three to eight percent of women operated on with colorectal cancer will be found to have ovarian metastases at the time of surgery (28), while autopsy data reveal a 4–14% incidence (29–30). In compiled series (28,31), the rectosigmoid colon represents the most common primary tumor site in patients with ovarian metastases (Table 2). Additionally, the majority of patients with ovarian metastases from colorectal cancer presented with advanced disease. Only 3% were Dukes' A, while 69% were either Dukes' B or C.

The role of prophylactic oophorectomy in colorectal carcinoma has not been clearly established. Blamely et al. (32) feel that the incidence of ovarian metastases is too low to justify the procedure while Cutait et al. (33) recommended prophylactic oophorectomy in postmenopausal women to prevent later recurrences and the possibility of developing ovarian cancer. Rendleman and Gilchrist (34) advocated bilateral oophorectomy in patients with serosal extension of colonic cancer, when peritoneal disease was present, and in all palliative cases. Graffner et al. (28) reported on fifty-eight patients who underwent prophylactic oophorectomy at the time of surgery for colorectal cancer. Six patients (10.3%) had metastatic ovarian disease, four microscopic and two with gross disease. This, in addition to the risk of subsequent ovarian neoplasms, led the authors to recommend prophylactic oophorectomy at the time of surgery for colorectal carcinoma. Ballantyne et al. (35) retrospectively reviewed 571 patients who had undergone a curative resection for colon cancer at the Mayo Clinic. Of these women, seventy-five had undergone bilateral oophorectomy while 496 had not. There was no difference in survival or disease-free survival between the two groups. This confirmed the findings of Cutait et al. (33), who also noted no survival advantage for 201 patients undergoing prophylactic oophorectomy at the time of surgery for colon cancer versus 134 patients who did not.

Morrow and Enker (31) reviewed sixty-three patients with metachronous ovarian metastases from colorectal cancer treated at Memorial Sloan-Kettering Cancer Center. The mean duration to recurrence was 12 months, with a mean survival following surgery of 16.6 months. For those patients with disease localized to the ovary, the mean survival was 55 months versus 30 months if disease was confined to the pelvis. A group of seven patients with localized disease outside the pelvis who were surgically rendered free of disease had a mean survival of 32 months, while those with diffuse disease only survived a mean of 7.7 months. The most important determinant of survival was whether or not the patient could be surgically rendered free of gross disease. In 51% of the cases, the ovarian metastases were bilateral. The authors emphasized the role of bilateral oophorectomy at the time of palliative resection in advanced colorectal cancer, as 27% of the patients had previously undergone a palliative procedure without oophorectomy and now required a second procedure to remove large ovarian metastases. Although survival may not be improved, significant palliation occurs from removing such large masses.

Differentiating between primary ovarian tumors and gastrointestinal metastases can be difficult when conventional pathological criteria are used. In one series, approximately two-thirds of metastatic colon cancers were classified as ovarian primaries (1). Histologically, the ovarian metastases resemble primary intestinal carcinomas with gland formation and occasional mucin-containing goblet cells (5). Necrosis is a common and sometimes extensive finding. Ulbright et al. (1) noted that the consistent presence of intracellular mucin in the metastatic lesions creates a difficulty in distinguish-

TABLE 2. *Site of colonic primary in patients with ovarian metastases*

Primary tumor site	Percent
Rectum	23.0
Sigmoid colon	51.1
Ascending colon	10.8
Transverse colon	7.2
Cecum	1.4

ing these from primary mucinous adenocarcinoma of the ovary. The presence of a predominant mucus cell pattern along with a transition from benign to malignant epithelium, however, allows the diagnosis of an ovarian primary to be made. Lash and Hart (36) noted a 10:1 preponderance of a "pseudoendometrioid" pattern over mucinous carcinoma in colonic cancer metastatic to the ovary, reflecting the fact that the typical adenocarcinoma of the large bowel is basically a non-mucinous, gland-forming carcinoma. This makes misdiagnosis of colonic metastases to the ovary as a primary endometrioid adenocarcinoma much more likely. The authors felt that the key to the histologic diagnosis of colonic metastases to the ovary included the presence of prominent garland and cribriform structures with intraluminal necrosis, often accompanied by aggregates of rounded glands with segmental necrosis of their walls.

Carcinoembryonic antigen (CEA) serum levels may be evaluated in up to 70% of patients with ovarian cancer, depending on the histologic cell type (37). Immunohistochemistry, however, may be helpful in differentiating between primary ovarian tumors and intestinal metastases. Using monospecific anti-CEA antibodies, Fleuren et al. (38) noted that metastatic ovarian tumors originating from the digestive tract showed intense and diffuse staining comparable to the staining of CEA in primary colon cancer (38).

On the contrary, the glandular endometrioid ovarian tumors failed to stain for CEA, and the focal apical membranous staining of mucinous tumors differed markedly from the diffuse cytoplasmic staining of intestinal metastases. As newer, more specific monoclonal antibodies directed against CEA continue to be developed, differentiating between primary ovarian neoplasms and intestinal metastases will continue to improve. Pavelic et al. (39) recently reported on D-14 mAb, a monoclonal antibody directed against a specific epitope of CEA. Colonic carcinoma metastases to the ovary reacted strongly, while two of eighty-seven epithelial ovarian cancers had weak immunoreactivity.

KRUKENBERG TUMORS

In 1896, Krukenberg (40) described an interesting group of ovarian neoplasms which he termed *fibrosarcoma ovarii mucocellulare* (carcinomatides). Originally believed to be an unusual type of mucin-producing sarcoma of the ovary, the true metastatic nature of these tumors was pointed out several years later by Schlagenhaufer (41). They are now known to be signet-ring cell carcinomas within a cellular non-neoplastic stroma, usually metastatic from the gastrointestinal tract. The term *Krukenberg tumor,* however, has been loosely applied by some physicians to all metastatic tumors to the ovary.

TABLE 3. *Site of origin of Krukenberg tumor*

Organ site	Number	Percent
Stomach	120	77.4
Colon	12	7.7
Breast	7	4.5
Gallbladder	1	0.1
Unknown	15	9.7
Total	155	100

Krukenberg tumors account for approximately 3–5% of all ovarian tumors (42–43). The stomach is the most frequent site of origin for these tumors (Table 3) (42–45).

Histologically, the tumors are characterized by mucin-laden, signet-ring cells arranged individually or in small clusters within a cellular ovarian stroma which occasionally has a storiform pattern. Variations commonly seen include small glands, prominent tubular architecture, mucin-poor tumor cells in trabeculae and large masses, abundant collagen formation, marked stromal edema, and cell-free pools of mucin in the stroma (5).

In general, signet-ring cell carcinomas display a greater propensity to metastasize to the ovary (46). In an autopsy series of thirty-four women with advanced gastric carcinoma, ovarian metastases were noted in 40.9% of twenty-two patients with signet-ring cell type of carcinoma versus 16.7% of twelve patients with an intestinal type of carcinoma (47). Additionally, 60% of the uncommon signet-ring cell carcinomas of the colon reportedly metastasized to the ovary (48).

Clinically, the patients present in a manner similar to patients with primary ovarian carcinoma; symptoms include bloating, abdominal pain, and gastrointestinal discomfort, with physical examination usually revealing a pelvic mass (43–45). The diagnosis of the primary tumor site is often not determined preoperatively. In a report of twenty cases, Holtz and Hart (45) noted that the primary carcinoma was detected prior to the ovarian tumor in only 25% of cases, while 50% were diagnosed synchronously, and 25% at the time of autopsy. Both ovaries were usually involved in cases evaluated for bilaterality.

The existence of a primary Krukenberg tumor of the ovary has been debated in the pathology literature. Joshi (49) reviewed the literature with regard to this entity and accepted seventeen cases as being primary Krukenberg tumors. Briefly, the criteria used for this diagnosis required that:

1. The ovarian tumors were solid growths which retained the general shape of the ovary. They have

a firm capsule and no tendency to adhere to the surrounding structures.
2. On microscopic examination the tumor is composed of mucin containing cells embedded in cellular collagenous or myxomatous stroma. The cells have peripheral flattened nuclei (signet-ring cells).
3. If an autopsy is performed, an absence of a primary tumor in any organ except the ovary is noted.
4. If alive, the patient should survive more than five years after resection of the ovarian tumor.

These criteria are not infallible and it is known that small carcinomas of the stomach are often difficult to detect, even at autopsy. In addition, primary gastric and mammary carcinomas may remain undetectable for years. In general, however, patients with metastatic Krukenberg tumors survive an average of only 7.1 months from the time of diagnosis (44).

APPENDICEAL TUMORS

Adenocarcinoma of the appendix compromises only 0.2–0.5% of all gastrointestinal tumors (50–51) and consequently accounts for only a small percentage of metastatic tumors to the ovary. The reported incidence of ovarian metastases in patients with appendiceal primaries, however, ranges from 7–88% (52–54). Conte et al. (53) noted that ovarian metastases were present in seven out of eight patients with appendiceal primaries. In six of the cases, carcinomatosis was present. However, it was the presence of an ovarian mass that led to laparotomy in four of the cases. The authors recommended oophorectomy for palliation in patients with metastases and possibly as prophylaxis against future recurrences. Mucinous adenocarcinoma of the appendix can also metastasize as a signet-ring cell carcinoma of the Krukenberg type. De Graff et al. (55) reported a case where the primary site was initially missed because the appendix appeared grossly normal. The authors recommended performing an appendectomy if Krukenberg tumors of the ovary are diagnosed on frozen section and there is no obvious primary site.

Appendiceal adenocarcinoid is a rare tumor that has histologic features of both carcinoid and adenocarcinoma. Chen (54) reviewed the literature and reported such a case that was metastatic to the ovary. He noted a 32% incidence of ovarian metastasis in eighteen patients. In thirteen patients the metastases were present initially, while the remaining five developed 6 months to 8 years after the initial diagnosis. The high incidence of ovarian metastases led the author to advise bilateral oophorectomy as part of the initial surgical management in all patients with appendiceal adenocarcinoma.

CARCINOID

Carcinoids metastatic to the ovary are extremely rare tumors that usually originate in the small intestine (56). Histologically it is difficult to distinguish these tumors from the more common primary ovarian carcinoids which, following epidermoid carcinomas, are the most frequent neoplasms originating in benign cystic teratomas of the ovary (57). Although usually impossible to determine the teratomatous structure that gives rise to the primary ovarian carcinoid, it is generally assumed that they originate from neuroendocrine stem cells. Alternatively, cells programmed to produce neurohormonal peptides arise in the neural crest and migrate to the ovary, where they may eventually form carcinoid tumors (58). Robboy et al. (59) reported on thirty-five cases of carcinoid metastatic to the ovary, of which twenty-five were discovered at the time of laparotomy, while ten were discovered at autopsy. In 40% of the patients, symptoms of the carcinoid syndrome, including diarrhea, were present prior to surgery. None of these patients had preoperative 5-HIAA levels. The majority of patients were found to have extraovarian involvement at the time of surgery. However, a primary site could not be determined before or at surgery in twelve of the patients. Interestingly, six of the patients with carcinoid syndrome preoperatively became and remained asymptomatic postoperatively despite extensive disease residual in four. Surgery usually consisted of a bilateral salpingo-oophorectomy often accompanied by a hysterectomy and bowel resection as needed. The five-year actuarial survival in the patients with metastatic ovarian carcinoid was 25%.

The histologic features of metastatic carcinoids are similar to primary ovarian carcinoid except for the presence of teratomatous elements in the former. Young and Scully (5) further differentiate the two by the presence of bilateral multinodular ovaries in the case of metastatic disease in addition to the presence of extraovarian metastases. Postoperative 5-HIAA levels usually remain elevated in the case of ovarian metastases but return to normal following removal of a primary ovarian carcinoid.

BREAST CARCINOMA

Next to the gastrointestinal tract, the breast is the second most common site of origin for ovarian metastases (9,12,26). The two most common histologic subtypes of breast cancer are infiltrating ductal carcinoma and lobular carcinoma. Lobular breast cancer has been shown to metastasize more frequently to the ovary (36%) than ductal cancers (2.6%) (60). The majority of information regarding involvement of the ovaries with metastatic breast cancer is obtained from reports of patients undergoing therapeutic oophorectomy for palliation of advanced breast cancer (61–64), where microscopic metastases are noted in 23.9–30.7% of cases. Autopsy data reveal a 6.4–23.4% incidence of ovarian involvement by metastatic breast cancer (60,65–68). Gagnon and Tetu (69) recently reported on fifty-nine patients with ovarian metastases from breast cancer, of which twenty-two were autopsy cases, twenty-eight were incidental findings at therapeutic oophorectomy, and five patients were operated on for a pelvic mass. In 75% of surgical cases the diagnosis of breast cancer was made prior to the diagnosis of ovarian metastasis by a median of 11.5 months. In only one case was the diagnosis of breast disease made following the discovery of ovarian metastasis, while in 22% the diagnosis was made simultaneously. The majority of patients with ovarian metastases had advanced-stage breast disease and survived a median of 16 months following their metastatic diagnosis.

In 64% of the patients, the ovarian metastases were bilateral, which is consistent with other reports in the literature (62,64,67). Histologically, 75% of the cases had features suggestive of mammary cancer, with 57% having features of ductal carcinoma and 43% lobular. Twenty-five percent of the cases resembled primary ovarian tumors including stromal luteoma, hyperthecosis, dysgerminoma, carcinoid, and granulosa cell tumor. No tumors in this series resembled Krukenberg tumors, which is consistent with the low incidence of breast primaries noted in reports on Krukenberg tumors (42–45).

Differentiating between an ovarian primary and metastatic mammary cancer can be difficult, especially when the tumors are poorly differentiated. Monoclonal antibodies such as OC-125 are useful in the management of ovarian cancer but are not specific for ovarian origin on tissue sections (70). Immunohistochemistry may be helpful in differentiating between an ovarian primary and metastatic breast cancer. Alpha-lactalbumin (AL) is a milk protein synthesized by differentiated breast epithelium that has been widely used as an immunohistochemical marker for breast cancer. Although the presence of AL may suggest the diagnosis of adenocarcinoma of breast origin, 20% of epithelial ovarian neoplasms also react with AL antisera (71). Gross cystic disease fluid protein 15 (GCDFP-15) is a highly specific and sensitive breast cancer marker (72). Monteagudo et al. (73) demonstrated that ten of fourteen cases of breast cancer metastatic to the ovary displayed strong cytoplasmic immunostaining for GCDFP-15, while thirty-two primary ovarian tumors and seven tumors metastatic to the ovary from other sites were negative (73).

RARE TUMORS METASTATIC TO THE OVARY

Several other tumors have been reported to metastasize to the ovary on rare occasions. These are briefly presented out of interest rather than clinical relevance.

Genitourinary

Bladder (74), ureteral (75), and urethral (76) cancers have been reported to metastasize to the ovary. Renal cell carcinomas rarely spread to the ovary and would be extremely difficult to differentiate from ovarian clear cell carcinoma.

Lung

Carcinoma of the lung spreads to the ovary very uncommonly. Young and Scully (77) reported on seven such cases. The diagnosis of a pulmonary neoplasm preceded the diagnosis of ovarian metastases in only one case, while three were diagnosed synchronously and three were discovered 2 to 26 months following removal of the ovarian mass. The authors noted that the evidence for the pulmonary origin of the tumors was provided by the resemblance to known lung cancers (oat cell, large cell undifferentiated, carcinoid) and the relative rarity of similar histologic types in the ovary.

Malignant Melanoma

Metastasis to the ovary may occur in 18% of patients with disseminated melanoma, usually of cutaneous origin (78) although occult extragonadal sources of melanoma, including the choroid of the eye, choroid plexus, and adrenal glands have been reported (79). Cases of secondary melanoma appearing in an ovary 14 years after removal of the primary from the choroid have been reported (80). Melanoma metastatic to the ovary is far more common than primary ovarian melanoma, which usually originates in a benign cystic teratoma (81). Marcial-Rojas and Ramirez de Arellano (82) required that junctional changes in the squamous epithelium adjacent to a malignant melanoma arising in a dermoid cyst be present as evidence of the tumor's origin. Failure to identify this junctional change does not necessarily rule out an ovarian origin, as the tumor itself may destroy any evidence of junctional change.

Gallbladder and Pancreas

Although gallbladder carcinoma is very rare, one autopsy study revealed that 12% of thirty-four women had ovarian metastases (83). Pancreatic cancer has also been reported to metastasize to the ovary. Cubilla and Fitzgerald noted seven patients with ovarian metastases in a review of 380 patients with pancreatic duct cancer (84).

REFERENCES

1. Ulbright TM, Roth LM, Stehman FB. Secondary ovarian neoplasia. *Cancer* 1984;53:1164–1174.
2. Kepson RL, Hendrickson MR. The female reproductive system. In: Coulsen WF, ed. *Surgical Pathology*, vol. 1. Philadelphia: J.B. Lippincott Co; 1978;725–727.
3. Santesson L, Kottmeier HL. General classification of ovarian tumors. In: Gentil F, Junqueira AC, eds. *Ovarian Cancer*. UICC Monograph series, vol. 11. Berlin: Spinger-Verlag, 1968;1–8.
4. Fox H, Langley FA. *Tumors of the Ovary*. Chicago: Year Book Medical Publishers; 1976;293–305.
5. Young RH, Scully RE. Metastatic Tumors of the Ovary. In: Kurman RJ, ed. *Blaustein's Pathology of the Female Genital Tract*. New York: Springer-Verlag; 1987, 742–764.
6. Sedlis A. Primary carcinoma of the fallopian tube. *Obstet Gynecol* 1961;16:209–226.
7. Greene HJ, Grusetz MW, Mackles A. Subsequent second primary and metastatic cancer of the ovary. *Clin Obstet Gynecol*. 1969;12:972–979.
8. Barakat RR, Rubin SC, Saigo PS, et al. Cisplatin-based combination chemotherapy in carcinoma of the fallopian tube. *Gynecol Oncol* 1991;42:156–160.
9. Mazur MT, Swei HS, Gersell DJ. Metastases to the female genital tract. *Cancer* 1984;53:1978–1984.
10. Scully RE. Tumors of the ovary and maldeveloped gonads. In: *Atlas of Tumor Pathology, Second Series, Fascicle 16*. Washington DC: Armed Forces Institute of Pathology; 1979;323–352.
11. Eifel P, Hendrickson, M Ross J, Ballon S, Martinez E, Kempson R. Simultaneous presentation of carcinoma involving the ovary and the uterine corpus. *Cancer* 1982;50:163–170.
12. Ulbright TM, Roth TM. Metastatic and independent cancers of the endometrium and ovary. *Hum Pathol* 1985;16:28–34.
13. Smit VTHBM, Fleuren GJ, vanHouwelingen JC, Zegveld ST, Kuipers-Dijkshoorn NJ, Cornelisse CJ. Flow cytometric DNA-ploidy analysis of synchronously occurring multiple malignant tumors of the female genital tract. *Cancer* 1990;66:1843–1849.
14. Tamimi HK, Figge DC. Adenocarcinoma of the uterine cervix. *Gynecol Oncol* 1982;13:335–344.
15. Kjorsted KE, Bond B. Stage IB adenocarcinoma of the cervix: metastatic potential and patterns of dissemination. *Am J Obstet Gynecol* 1984;150:297–299.
16. Kaminski PF, Norris HJ. Coexistence of ovarian neoplasms and endocervical adenocarcinoma. *Obstet Gynecol* 1984;64:553–556.
17. Brown JV, Fu YS, Berek JS. Ovarian metastases are rare in stage I adenocarcinoma of the cervix. *Obstet Gynecol* 1990;76:623–626.
18. Toki N, Tsukamoto, Kaku T, et al. Microscopic ovarian metastasis of the uterine cervical cancer. *Gynecol Oncol* 1991;41:46–51.
19. Tabata M, Ichinoe K, Sakuragi N, Shina Y, Yamaguchi T, Mabuchi Y. Incidence of ovarian metastases in patients with cancer of the uterine cervix. *Gynecol Oncol* 1987;28:255–261.
20. Cassidy LJ, Kennedy JH. Ovarian metastasis from stage Ib squamous cell cancer of the cervix: case report. *Br J Obstet Gynaecol* 1986;93:1169–1170.
21. Johnston CM, Dottino PR, Heller DS, Cohen CJ. Recurrent cervical squamous cell carcinoma in an ovary following ovarian conservation and radical hysterectomy. *Gynecol Oncol* 1991;41:64–66.
22. Seltzer V, Sall S, Castadot MJ, Muradian-Davidian M, Sedlis A. Glassy cell cervical carcinoma. *Gynecol Oncol* 1979;8:141–151.
23. Nahhas WA, Abt AB, Mortel R. Stage IB glassy cell carcinoma of the cervix with ovarian metastases. *Gynecol Oncol* 1977;5:87–91.
24. Reisinger SA, Palazzo JP, Talerman A, Carlson J, Jahshan A. Stage Ib glassy cell carcinoma of the cervix diagnosed during pregnancy and recurring in a transposed ovary. *Gynecol Oncol* 1991;42:86–90.
25. Robboy SJ, Herbst AL, Scully RE. Clear-cell adenocarcinoma of the vagina and cervix in young females. *Cancer* 1974;34:606–614.
26. Yazigi R, Sandstadt J. Ovarian involvement in extragenital cancer. *Gynecol Oncol* 1989;34:84–87.
27. Megibow AJ, Hulnick DH, Bosniak MA, Balthazar EJ. Ovarian metastases: computed tomographic appearances. *Radiology* 1985;156:161–164.
28. Graffner HOL, Alm POA, Oscarson JEA. Prophylactic oophorectomy in colorectal carcinoma. *Am J Surg* 1983;146:233–235.
29. Buirge RE. Carcinoma of the large intestine: review of four hundred and sixteen autopsy records. *Arch Surg* 1941;42:807–818.
30. Abrams HL, Spiro R, Goldstein N. Metastases in carcinoma: analysis of 1000 autopsied cases. *Cancer* 1950;3:74–85.
31. Morrow M, Enker WE. Late ovarian metastases in carcinoma of the colon and rectum. *Arch Surg* 1984;119:1385–1388.
32. Blamely S, McDermott F, Pihl E, et al. Ovarian involvement in adenocarcinoma of the colon and rectum. *Surg Gynecol Obstet* 1981;153:42–44.
33. Cutait R, Lesser M, Enker WE. Prophylactic oophorectomy in surgery for large bowel cancer. *Dis Colon Rectum* 1983;26:6–11.
34. Rendleman DF, Gilchrist RK. Indications for oophorectomy in carcinoma of the gastrointestinal tract. *Surg Gynecol Obstet* 1959;109:364–366.
35. Ballantyne GH, Reigel MM, Wolff BG, Ilstrup M. Oophorectomy and colon cancer. *Ann Surg* 1985;202:209–214.
36. Lash RH, Hart WR. Intestinal adenocarcinomas metastatic to the ovaries. *Am J Surg Pathol* 1987;11(2):114–121.
37. Stall KE, Martin DW. Plasma carcinoembryonic antigen levels in ovarian cancer patients: a chart review and survey of published data. *J Reprod Med* 1981;26:73–79.
38. Fleuren GJ, Marius N. Carcinoembryonic antigen in primary and metastatic ovarian tumors. *Gynecol Oncol* 1988;30:407–415.
39. Pavelic ZP, Pavelic L, Pavelic K, Peacock JS. Utility of anti-carcinoembryonic antigen monoclonal antibodies for differentiating ovarian adenocarcinomas from gastrointestinal metastasis to the ovary. *Gynecol Oncol* 1991;40:112–117.
40. Krukenberg F. Ueber das Fibrosacoma mucocellulare (carcinomatodes). *Arch Gynaekol* 1896;50:287–321.
41. Shlagenhaufer F. Ueber das metastatische Ovarialcarcinom nach Krebs des Magens, Darmes und anderer Bauchorgane. *Monatsschr Gerbrtshulfe Gynaekol* 1902;15:485–528.
42. Soloway I, Latour JPA, Young MHV. Krukenberg tumors of the ovary. *Obstet Gynecol* 1956;8:636–638.
43. Woodruff JD, Novak ER. The Krukenberg tumor: study of 48 cases from the Ovarian Tumor Registry. *Obstet Gynecol* 1960;15:351–360.
44. Hale RW. Krukenberg tumors of the ovaries: A review of 81 records. *Obstet Gynecol* 1968;32:221–225.
45. Holtz F, Hart WR. Krukenberg tumors of the ovary: a clinicopathologic analysis of 27 cases. *Cancer* 1982;50:2438–2447.
46. Saphir O. Signet-ring cell carcinoma. *Mill Surg* 1951;109:360–369.
47. Duarte I, Llanos O. Patterns of metastases in intestinal and diffuse types of carcinoma of the stomach. *Hum Pathol* 1981;12:237–242.
48. Amorn Y, Kight WA Jr. Primar linitis plastica of the colon: report of two cases and review of the literature. *Cancer* 1978;41:2420–2425.
49. Joshi VV. Primary Krukenberg tumor of the ovary: review of literature and case report. *Cancer* 1968;22:1199–1207.
50. Mehzad M, Aflaki B, Afghari H. Adenocarcinoma of the appendix: report of an unusual case. *Dis Colon Rectum* 1978;21:205–206.
51. Gamble HA. Adenocarcinoma of the appendix: an unusual case and review. *Dis Colon Rectum* 1976;19:621–625.
52. Fichera AP, Petty WM, Park RC, Muir RW. Primary adenocarcinoma of the vermiform appendix in a gynecologic patient. *Am J Obstet Gynecol* 1976;124:663–664.

53. Conte CC, Petrelli NJ, Stulc J, Herrera S, Mittelman A. Adenocarcinoma of the appendix. *Surg Gynecol Obstet* 1988;166:451–453
54. Chen KTK. Appendiceal adenocarcinoid with ovarian metastasis. *Gynecol Oncol* 1990;38:286–288.
55. De Graff J, Puyenbroek JI, VanDer Harten JJ. Primary mucinous adenocarcinoma of the appendix with bilateral krukenberg tumors of the ovary and primary adenocarcinoma of the endometrium. *Gynecol Oncol* 1984;19:358–364.
56. Luisi A. Metastatic Ovarian Tumors. In: Gentil F, Junqueira C, eds. *Ovarian Cancer;* UICC monograph series #11. New York: Springer-Verlag, 1968;87–104.
57. Falkmer S, Frankendal B, Hassler O, Angstrom T. Carcinoid tumour in a benign cystic teratoma of the ovary. *Acta Pathol Scand [Suppl]* 1972;80:233:91–97.
58. Pearse AGE. The cytochemistry and ultrastructure of polypeptide hormone-producing cells of the APUD series and the embryologic, physiologic, and pathologic implications of the concept. *J Histochem Cytochem* 1969;17:303–313.
59. Robboy SJ, Sculy RF, Norris HJ. Carcinoid metastatic to the ovary. *Cancer* 1974;33:798–811.
60. Harris M, Howell A, Chrissohou M, Swindell RIC, Hudson M, Sellwood RA. A comparison of the metastatic pattern of infiltrating lobular carcinoma and infiltrating duct carcinoma of the breast. *Br J Cancer* 1984;50:23–30.
61. Lee YTN, Hori JM. Significance of ovarian metastasis in therapeutic oophorectomy for advanced breast cancer. *Cancer* 1971;27:1374–1378.
62. Puga FJ, Gibbs CP, Williams TJ. Castrating operations associated with metastatic lesions of the breast. *Obstet Gynecol* 1973;41:713–719.
63. Haagensen CD. *Diseases of the Breast,* 2nd ed. Philadelphia: WB Saunders; 1971;448.
64. Lumb G, Mackenzie DH. The incidence of metastasis in adrenal glands and ovaries removed for carcinoma of the breast. *Cancer* 1959;12:521–526.
65. Turksoy N. Ovarian metastasis of breast carcinoma: a surgical surprise. *Obstet Gynecol* 1960;15:573–578.
66. Viadana E, Bross IDJ, Pickren JW. An autopsy study of some routes of dissemination of cancer of the breast. *Br J Cancer* 1973;27:336–340.
67. Cifuentes N, Pickren JW. Metastases from carcinoma of mammary gland: an autopsy study. *J Surg Oncol* 1979;11:193–205.
68. Harris JR, Hellman S, Canellos GP, Fisher B. Cancer of the breast. In: DeVita VT Jr, Hellman S, Rosenberg SA, eds. *Cancer: Principles and Practices of Oncology,* 2nd ed. Philadelphia: JB Lippincott, 1985;1119–1177.
69. Gagnon Y, Tetu B. Ovarian metastases of breast carcinoma: a clinicopathologic study of 59 cases. *Cancer* 1989;64:892–898.
70. Bast RC, Knapp RC. Recent advances in the immunodiagnosis of epithelial ovarian carcinoma. In: Alberts DS, Surwit EA, eds. *Ovarian Cancer,* Boston: Nijhoff, 1985;23–25.
71. Doira MI Jr, Adamec T, Talerman A. Alpha-lactalbumin in "common" epithelial tumors of the ovary. *Am J Clin Pathol* 1987;87:752–756.
72. Wick MR, Lilleome TJ, Copland GT, et al. Gross cystic disease fluid protein-15 as a marker for breast cancer: immune histochemical analysis of 690 human neoplasms and comparison with alpha-lactalbumin. *Hum Pathol* 1989;20:281–287.
73. Monteaugudo C, Merino MJ, LaPorte HT, Neumann RD. Value of gross cystic disease fluid protein-15 in distinguishing metastatic breast carcinomas among poorly differentiated neoplasms involving the ovary. *Hum Pathol* 1991;22:368–372.
74. Kishi K, Hirota T, Matsumoto K, Kakizo ET, Murase T, Fujita J. Carcinoma of the bladder: a clinical and pathological analysis of 87 autopsy cases. *J Urol* 1981;125:36–39.
75. Batata MA, Whitmore WF, Hilaris BS, Tokita N, Grabstald H. Primary carcinoma of the ureter: a prognostic study. *Cancer* 1975;35:1616–1632.
76. Posso MA, Berg GA, Murphy AI, Totten RS. Mucinous adenocarcinoma of the urethra: report of a case associated with urethritis glandularis. *J Urol* 1961;85:944–948.
77. Young RH, Scully RE. Ovarian metastases from cancer of the lung: problems in interpretation: a report of seven cases. *Gynecol Oncol* 1985;21:337–350.
78. Das Gupta T, Brasfield R. Metastatic melanoma: a clinicopathological study. *Cancer* 1964;17:1323–1329.
79. Morrow CP, DiSaia PJ. Malignant melanoma of the female genitalia: a clinical analysis. *Obstet Gynecol Surv* 1976;31:233–271.
80. Dawson HGW. Melanotic sarcoma of the choroid and ovary. *Brit Med J* 1992;2:757.
81. Tham KT, Ma PH, Kung TM. Malignant melanoma in an ovarian cystic teratoma. *Hum Pathol* 1981;12:577–579.
82. Marcial-Rojas RA, Ramirez de Arellano GA. Malignant melanoma arising in a dermoid cyst of the ovary. *Cancer* 1956;9:523.
83. Brandt-Rauf PW, Pincus M, Adelson S. Cancer of the gallbladder. A review of forty-three cases. *Hum Pathol* 1982;13:48–53.
84. Cubilla Al, Fitzgerald PJ. Pancreas cancer: I. duct adenocarcinoma: a clinical-pathologic study of 380 patients. *Pathol Annu* 1978;1:241–289.

CHAPTER 31

Epithelial Ovarian Tumors of Low Malignant Potential

Edward L. Trimble and Cornelia Liu Trimble

Epithelial ovarian tumors of low malignant potential (LMP) have long perplexed gynecologic pathologists and oncologists. A majority of patients with these tumors have the same long-term survival as age-matched peers. Up to a quarter of them, however, may encounter late recurrences and death from progressive disease. A host of questions remain unanswered. Do serous tumors of LMP behave differently from mucinous tumors of LMP? Can reliable conclusions be made about the behavior of the rare subtypes of LMP tumors? What are the roles of hereditary and environmental factors in tumors of LMP? Is there a way to distinguish between the tumor which will recur and that which will not? What is the best surgical management for tumors of LMP? Can ovarian and reproductive function be safely preserved in a premenopausal patient? Does subsequent pregnancy affect the recurrence rate? Is adjuvant chemotherapy or radiotherapy effective in preventing recurrences or in prolonging survival? Is estrogen replacement safe in a woman with a history of a tumor of LMP?

It is difficult to answer many of these questions. Most institutional series report fewer than one hundred patients. Mucinous and serous tumors are frequently combined, both in epidemiologic surveys and in series reported from single institutions. Endometroid, Brenner, and mixed-type tumors are encountered in such small numbers so as to preclude meaningful statistical analysis; some studies include them, while others omit them entirely. Long-term follow-up is rarely available. We have delineated differences between mucinous and serous tumors of LMP as much as possible. We have also endeavored to place these tumors in perspective amid the broader range of epithelial ovarian neoplasia and peritoneal müllerian neoplasia.

EPIDEMIOLOGY

Incidence

Epithelian ovarian tumors of LMP have been reported in Caucasian, black African, Chinese, Japanese, and Indian populations (1–7). Among predominantly Caucasian populations, they are reported to comprise approximately 4–14% of all ovarian malignancies (1,8,9). In the absence of evidence to the contrary, it is possible that tumors of LMP comprise a similar proportion of epithelial ovarian malignancies in other populations. The highest incidence of invasive epithelial ovarian malignancies is found among affluent, predominantly Caucasian populations (10). By extension, these same populations may well have the highest incidence of tumors of low malignant potential. In their survey of ovarian tumors in western Washington State, Harlow et al. (11) found the incidence of tumors of LMP to be 26.2 per million women per year in the white population, and 16.5 per million women per year in the nonwhite population. In this part of the state of Washington, the nonwhite population was predominantly African-American and Asian. They also noted a temporal trend in incidence. Between 1975 and 1983, the incidence of serous and mucinous ovarian tumors of low malignant potential rose from 7.1 per million women per year to 39 per million women per year. This increase appears too large to be attributable solely to an increase in diagnosis.

E. L. Trimble: Clinical Investigation Branch, Cancer Therapy Evaluation Program, Division of Cancer Treatment, National Cancer Institute, Bethesda, Maryland 20892
C. L. Trimble: Department of Gynecologic Pathology, The Johns Hopkins Hospital, Baltimore, Maryland 21205

Age

Mean age at diagnosis in 5 combined series ranged from 39 to 45 years (6,12–15), in contrast to patients with invasive epithelial ovarian cancer, whose tumors were diagnosed at a mean age of 52 approximately 10 years later (16). Mean age of diagnosis of serous tumors of LMP falls close to 40 years (12,14,15,17–20), as does mean age for mucinous tumors of LMP (12,14,15,17,21). Series focussing on ovarian tumors in adolescence, pregnancy, and young adulthood have also noted a high proportion of tumors of LMP (22–25). Although these studies suggest that the highest incidence of tumors of LMP falls among women aged 35 to 50 years, Harlow et al. (11), in their epidemiologic study of ovarian malignancies in western Washington State, found otherwise. Among women aged 35 to 49 years, the incidence of tumors of LMP was 25.8 per million women per year. The highest incidence of tumors of LMP was in the group aged 65 to 79 years, 45.9 cases per million women per year. This study did not include a standardized review of all histologic diagnoses, however. Katsube et al. (14) carried out a histologic review of all primary ovarian tumors diagnosed in the Denver metropolitan area during two six-month periods in 1969 and 1979. During the entire 12 months studied, 18.8% of all malignant tumors were of LMP. Using their figures, one can calculate the incidence of tumors of LMP in the Denver area in 1969 to be 37.5 per million women per year. Of 18 tumors of LMP Katsube et al. discovered, 8 (44%) were diagnosed in women aged 20 to 39 years, and 8 (44%) in women aged 40 to 59 years. Thus, their findings support the hospital-based reports, which suggest a higher incidence of tumors of LMP among younger women.

Pregnancy and Lactation

Harlow et al. (26) found that, as with invasive ovarian malignancies, pregnancy had a protective effect against serous and mucinous tumors of LMP. The relative risk of women who had given birth to one to two children was 0.7 that of nulliparous women. No consistent trend was noted for increasing age at first birth. Breastfeeding for one or more months led to a 50% reduction in risk, controlling for age, parity, and use of oral contraceptives.

Exogenous Hormones

Harlow et al. (26) discovered that the use of oral contraceptives had a protective effect against tumors of LMP, as has been demonstrated with invasive ovarian malignancies. Women who had used oral contraceptives had a relative risk of 0.4 compared to those who had never used such hormones. No significance was found for the use of postmenopausal estrogens.

Menstrual History

Harlow et al. (26) found no significance for age at menarche or menopause as a risk factor to tumors of serous and mucinous tumors of LMP.

Family History

Schildkraut and Thompson (27), in a population-based case-control study, found that women with tumors of LMP did not report ovarian cancer in relatives, in contrast to women with invasive epithelial ovarian cancer.

Plasma Alpha-L-Fucosidase Activity

A deficiency of plasma alpha-L-fucosidase activity has been reported to be associated with an increased risk of epithelial ovarian cancer (28). Harlow et al. (29) compared plasma activity of alpha-L-fucosidase in 106 women with serous and mucinous tumors of LMP and in 134 controls. They found a slightly higher mean activity in cases, and concluded that plasma alpha-L-fucosidase had little to no bearing on the risk of ovarian tumors of LMP.

Environmental Factors

Harlow and Weiss (30) found no appreciably altered risk of serous and mucinous tumors of LMP associated with the perineal application of corn starch or baby powder. Women who used deodorizing power, as distinct from corn starch or baby powder, whether alone or in combination with talc-containing powder, had nearly three times the risk of women without perineal exposure to powder.

CLINICAL FEATURES

Symptoms

Serous and mucinous tumors of LMP share the same presenting symptoms as those of any ovarian enlargement, benign or malignant. In general, the most commonly reported symptoms are a feeling of abdominal enlargement or sensation of a mass, as well as abdominal discomfort or pain (17,31,32).

Diagnosis

Achiron et al. (33) found that carcinomas of LMP had a sonographic appearance similar to that of benign tumors. Buy et al. (34) compared ultrasonographic (US), computerized tomographic (CT), and pathologic findings in 130 women with 170 epithelial ovarian tumors. Of these, fourteen (8%) were of LMP. All the tumors of LMP were noted on CT and US. Using CT evaluation, a diagnosis of malignancy based on endocystic vegetation, wall thickening and irregularity, as well as on contrast material uptake, was made in nine (64%) of the fourteen cases of LMP. Transabdominal ultrasound noted positive findings of malignancy in five (36%) of the fourteen. They concluded that CT was more sensitive than US in detecting malignant tumors (both invasive and those of LMP) as well as in distinguishing benign serous ovarian tumors from malignant serous tumors. Neither CT nor US was reliable in predicting the malignancy of mucinous tumors.

Rice et al. (35) found that six of eight patients with advanced stage disease (all but one serous) had elevated CA-125 levels. Chambers et al. (36) found four of eighteen patients to have levels of CA-125 above 35 U/ml. No value was above 54 U/ml. Chien et al. (37) measured serum levels of CA-125 in sixteen patients. Five patients had elevated levels preoperatively, ranging from 35–114 U/ml. All levels fell to the normal range within 2 weeks of the initial debulking procedure. Although only Rice et al. report tumor subtype, it is likely that as with invasive carcinomas, tumor expression of CA-125 is found predominantly in serous lesions of LMP, rather than in mucinous tumors of LMP. Kudlacek et al. (38) screened ovarian tumor specimens for CA-125 tissue expression using immunohistochemistry. CA-125 was noted in 50% of benign serous tumors, in 75% of serous tumors of LMP, and in 84% of malignant serous tumors. No expression of CA-125 was noted in mucinous tumors, whether benign, malignant, or of LMP.

Survival

As mentioned above, long-term follow-up is rare. In addition, many studies lump serous and mucinous subtypes together. We summarize combined survival statistics for serous and mucinous tumors of LMP in Table 1 (1,6,9,11,12,17,24,31,36,39,40). A review of these figures suggests that deaths due to disease may occur even in patients with stage I disease. At 20 years, however, survival is above 90% for this group. Close to 70% of patients with stage III disease may face a 20-year survival. Survival statistics for serous tumors of LMP are outlined in Table 2 (1,4,11,12,31,41) and mucinous tumors of LMP in Table 3 (1,6,11,12,31).

TABLE 1. *Survival in patients with epithelial ovarian tumors of LMP*

Author and stage	5-year (%)	10-year (%)	15-year (%)	20-year (%)
Aure (1)				
stage Ia	98	95	95	95
stage Ib	95	90	90	88
Barnhill (12)				
all stages	95	87		
stages I–II	97			
stages III–IV	88			
Carter (24)				
all stages	100			
Chambers (36)				
all stages	83			
Dgani (39)				
all stages	100			
Harlow (11)				
all stages	93.1			
local	94.3			
regional and distant	93.5			
Kliman (17)				
all stages	95	85	85	85
stage I	100	93	93	
stage III	70	70	70	
Nakashima (6)				
all stages	75	65		
Nikrui (31)				
all stages	85	78	63	
Russell (9)				
stage I	95	78		
stage II	78			
stage III	66	52		
Sutton (40)				
stage III	96			

PATHOLOGY

The impetus for the initial segregation of this group of epithelial lesions of the ovary came with the clinical recognition of a subset of patients with ovarian tumors who fared relatively well. In 1929, Howard Taylor (42) was the first to note the different pathologic and biologic nature of these tumors. This distinction was recognized by the International Federation of Gynecology and Obstetrics (FIGO) in 1971, when tumors of LMP were included in the categorization of epithelial tumors of the ovary (43). The World Health Organization followed suit in 1973 (44). These tumors have been designated *low-grade noninvasive carcinoma, proliferating cystadenoma without stromal invasion, tumor of borderline malignancy, carcinoma of low-grade malignant potential, intermediate tumor, tumor of low ma-*

TABLE 2. *Survival in patients with serous tumors of LMP, all stages*

	Survival			
Author	5-year (%)	10-year (%)	15-year (%)	20-year (%)
Aure (1)	94	92	90	90
Barnhill (12)	97			
Harlow (11)	92			
Julian (41)	92			
Nikrui (31)	91	83	73	
Tang (4)	94	88	86	

lignant potential, and, most recently, *proliferating common epithelial tumor*, an appellation intended to imply a continuum of neoplastic potential. For the sake of consistency, in this chapter they will be called *tumors of low malignant potential* (LMP).

In the course of the years following Taylor's observations, it has become increasingly clear that a certain proportion of patients with lesions classified as LMP do poorly. The great majority, however, especially those diagnosed at an early stage with either serous and mucinous tumors, do well. Heretofore, histological classification has been grounded in the traditional dogma of a single primary lesion, with ensuing metastasis which is typically intraperitoneal. More recently, it has been proposed by some that peritoneal epithelial tumors arise from coelomic mesothelial cells retaining the potential for müllerian differentiation (45–51).

Müllerian metaplasia of various types has been documented in the peritoneal cavity. Could synchronous metaplasia explain peritoneal "implants"? Adenocarcinomas, stromal sarcomas, and even a few cases of müllerian mixed tumors arising in extraovarian sites (without ovarian involvement) have been documented. One can speculate that they may have arisen in foci of intraperitoneal endometriosis. The Arias-Stella reaction is also found throughout the peritoneum during pregnancy. It is plausible that such foci of müllerian metaplasia might undergo malignant transformation similar to that which occurs in the ovary.

The criteria currently used to make a diagnosis of LMP include the presence in an ovarian tumor with any two of the following histologic features:

1. epithelial budding
2. multilayering of epithelium
3. mitotic activity
4. nuclear atypia

By definition, an additional criterion is the absence of stromal invasion. Currently, histological diagnoses are made solely on the basis of the neoplastic process in the ovary, without consideration of the appearance of extraovarian "implants." If even a fraction of intraperitoneal disease is in fact due to multifocal, extraovarian primaries, then this system of classification may be inappropriate.

Reproducibility

Several studies assessing both intraobserver and interobserver reproducibility of diagnoses of the full spectrum of ovarian epithelial lesions—from benign to tumors of LMP to frank carcinomas—have yielded comparable results (52–56). Overall, intraobserver reproducibility ranges from 50% to 75%. Similarly, interobserver reproducibility was uneven, with agreement among three or more pathologists ranging from 40% to 97%. Although the largest variability was in the distinction between poorly differentiated serous and poorly differentiated not-otherwise-specified carcinomas, comparable variations were reported in the diagnosis of tumors of LMP from well-differentiated carcinomas.

SEROUS TUMORS OF LMP

Of all serous ovarian tumors, approximately 50–65% are benign. Tumors of LMP comprise between 7–15%, while the rest are carcinomas (1,8,9). Thus, about one-third of malignant serous ovarian tumors are of LMP.

Pathology

Gross

The mean greatest diameter of serous tumors of LMP in four series ranged between 6.7 cm and 12.2 cm (13,14,35,39). Bilaterally ranged from 33.5–74% (4,14,15,17,19,31,57,58). They are cystic, with mural

TABLE 3. *Survival in mucinous tumors of LMP, all stages*

	Survival			
Author	5-year (%)	10-year (%)	15-year (%)	20-year (%)
Aure (1)	98	95	90	82
Barnhill (12)	78			
Harlow (11)	95			
Nakashima (6)	69			
Nikrui (31)	80	73	57	

clusters of rounded papillations. These papillary structures are often more prominent than those in benign serous cystadenomas. Many have multiple loculations. The intracystic fluid is generally clear.

Microscopic

The cyst walls are lined by low cuboidal cells which resemble those normally found in fallopian tubes. Within a given tumor, the epithelium may undergo various types of metaplasia. Because of variations, at least one block of tissue for every 1 cm of maximum tumor diameter should be submitted. Histologic criteria for the diagnosis of serous tumors of LMP include stratification of the papillary epithelial lining, microscopic projections or "tufting" arising from the epithelium, nuclear atypia, and mitotic activity. A characteristic serous tumor of LMP is shown in Figs. 1–2. Throughout the peritoneum, one can also see a full spectrum of cytologic and architectural changes ranging from simple serous cysts (also called "endosalpingiosis") to serous carcinoma (19,20,59–61). This spectrum of changes can be seen both in association with ovarian serous tumors and in the complete absence of any ovarian lesions. Great care must be taken to distinguish "endosalpingiosis," which may be found even in lymph nodes, from true metastatic ovarian disease.

Invasion in implants is difficult to diagnose, particularly in structures which have lobulated contours, such as the omentum. In general, in noninvasive implants, the interface between the tumor and underlying tissue is smooth or pushing. In contrast, invasive implants are characterized by an irregular interface with a concomitant desmoplastic stromal reaction. As surface implants may engender desmoplastic stroma, the presence of underlying normal tissue is necessary to make a diagnosis of invasion. Studies to date do not concur on the prognostic significance of invasive implants (see below).

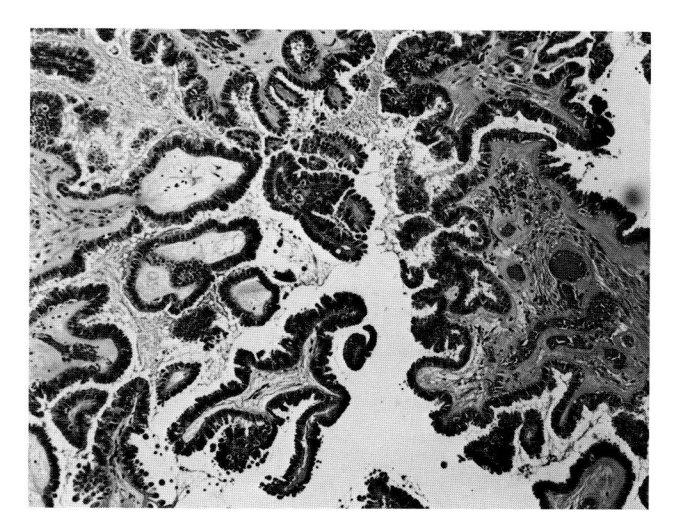

FIG. 2. Serous tumor of LMP, hematoxylin and eosin, 40 X.

MUCINOUS TUMORS OF LMP

Seventy to eighty percent of all mucinous tumors of the ovary are benign. About 10% are of LMP; the rest are adenocarcinomas (8,9,14). Tumors of LMP, therefore, may comprise more than half of all mucinous ovarian malignancies.

Pathology

Gross Findings

The mean greatest diameter in five series ranged between 17 cm and 20 cm (13,14,35,54,62). Bilaterality in mucinous tumors ranged from 0–12.8% (13–15,17). Grossly they resemble benign mucinous cystadenomas, being large cystic tumors with multiple loculations. The inner surfaces may show papillations and solid thickening.

Microscopic Findings

The cystic spaces are lined by tall, columnar, mucin-secreting cells which resemble those normally found in the endocervix or intestines. Unlike benign mucinous tumors, their epithelial linings are marked by stratification, cellular atypia, hyperchromatic nuclei, and en-

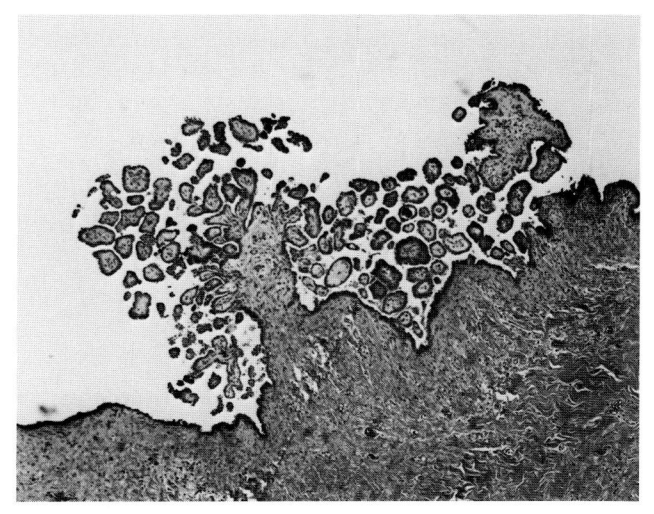

FIG. 1. Serous tumor of LMP, hematoxylin and eosin, 10 X.

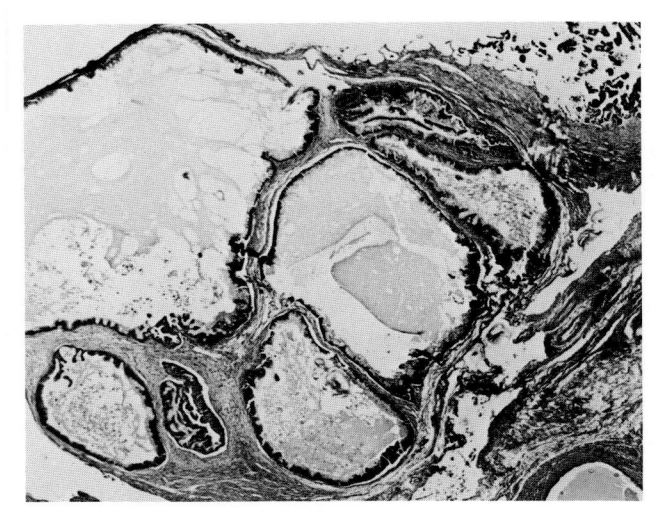

FIG. 3. Mucinous tumor of LMP, hematoxylin and eosin, 10 X.

larged nucleoli. Figs. 3–4 demonstrate a typical mucinous tumor of LMP. As with their serous counterparts, these changes can also be found throughout the peritoneum. Advanced-stage disease is less common with mucinous tumors of LMP, however, than with serous tumors of LMP.

Recent clinicopathologic studies of mucinous tumors have suggested a subclassification to tumors composed of endocervical-type epithelium (müllerian) and those which resemble intestinal-type epithelium (63). Histologically, "endocervical-type" mucinous tumors of LMP typically exhibit papillae and extensive epithelial tufting without fibrovascular cores. The epithelial cells themselves are tall, regular, and columnar. Areas which are less differentiated may appear to be lined with serous epithelium. Some tumors previously categorized as mixed type or "seromucinous" may in fact fall into this category (64). The peritoneal lesions associated with endocervical-type tumors of LMP are discrete nodules which appear to sit atop the underlying tissue. They may or may not provoke a desmoplastic response.

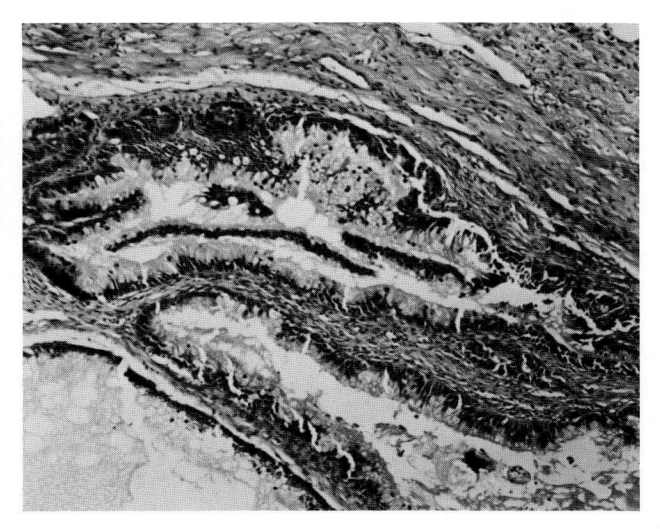

The presence of goblet cells, Paneth cells, or argyrophil cells suggests an intestinal-type mucinous tumor of LMP. The intraperitoneal disease associated with these tumors is typically in the form of dissecting mucinous pools with scant epithelial lining. The presence of pseudomyxoma peritonei should prompt examination of the appendix. Young et al. (65) recently reported twenty-two patients with mucinous ovarian tumors and pseudomyxoma peritonei. Twenty-one of the twenty-two had a synchronous appendiceal primary. Sixteen patients had unilateral tumors; twelve of the sixteen were right-sided, again suggesting the possibility of an appendiceal origin.

BRENNER, ENDOMETRIOID, AND CLEAR CELL TUMORS OF LMP

Brenner

Brenner tumors of LMP have generally been termed *proliferating Brenner tumors*. Although the histologic criteria for a Brenner tumor of LMP are fairly strict, it is frequently overdiagnosed. The differential diagnosis includes poorly differentiated adenocarcinoma and transitional cell carcinoma. To make the diagnosis of Brenner tumor of LMP, areas of benign or proliferating Brenner tumor must be identified within the lesion. Histologically, these tumors are cystic and are lined by broad, blunt papillae in a low-power configuration which is vaguely cerebriform. The epithelium is many cell layers thick, generally at least seven, and resembles that of noninvasive papillary urothelial cell carcinoma. The epithelial cells themselves are fairly regular, with a moderate amount of cytoplasm. Atypia may be present. As is the case with other tumors of LMP, no invasion is present. Only a few Brenner tumors of LMP have been reported (66,67). As far as we were able to ascertain, their behavior has been benign in all cases.

Endometrioid

Endometrioid tumors of LMP are relatively uncommon, and as such neither the histologic criteria nor the clinical behavior of these lesions is well-documented. There appear to be two distinct types. The more common subtype occurs in an adenofibromatous background and displays focal low-grade epithelial atypia (68,69). Invasion, by definition, is not present. These have been classified as benign proliferating neoplasms

FIG. 4. Mucinous tumor of LMP, hematoxylin and eosin, 40 X.

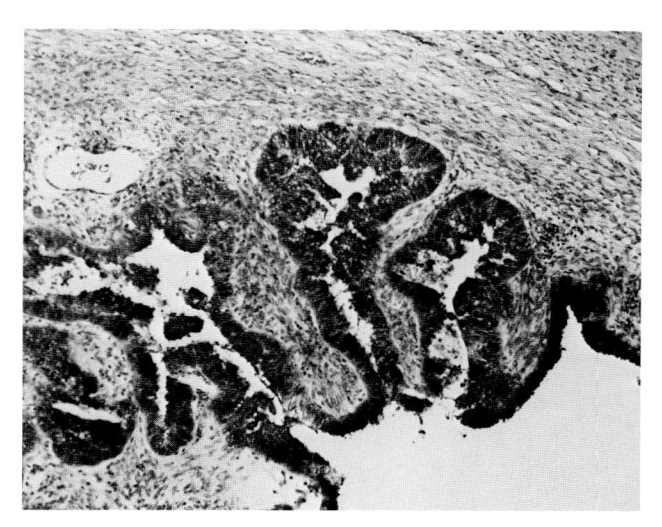

FIG. 5. Endometrioid tumor of LMP, adenofibromatous background, hematoxylin and eosin, 40 X.

by Roth and Czernobilsky (70,71). Fig. 5 shows an endometrioid tumor of LMP of this more common subtype. The second subtype, described by Colgan and Norris (72), lacks the adenofibromatous matrix, and consists of crowded, back-to-back glands with atypia and low mitotic activity. Both of these types tend to be cystic. No recurrences are reported in two small series (73,74).

Clear Cell

Clear cell adenofibromas are also rare and not well-characterized. They are predominantly fibrous tumors with tubular or glandular elements lined with a single layer of hobnail or clear cells. In tumors of LMP, the tubules show epithelial stratification, budding, and proliferation. There is no stromal invasion. Three deaths from tumor are reported among twenty-two patients with this diagnosis (75,76).

SPECIAL TECHNIQUES

Immunohistochemistry

The technique of immunohistochemistry has been in use longer than the others, and confers the advantage of being able to visualize the distribution of a given antigen within the lesion of interest. Many investigators have assessed the presence of CA-125, CEA, estrogen and progesterone receptors, CA-19-9, and various other markers in ovarian lesions (77–79). The presently available battery of markers seems to be of some use in distinguishing between types of epithelium (e.g., less-differentiated mucinous from serous) but does not appear to be of much prognostic value.

Morphometry

In 1981, Baak et al. (80) proposed the use of computer-assisted quantitative microscopic analysis to distinguish between benign tumors, those of LMP, and malignancies. After analyzing 42 mucinous tumors (22 malignant, 10 benign, and 10 of LMP), they found 5 features useful in this classification: the mean nuclear area, the mean nuclear perimeter, the mean of the short axis of the nucleus, the volume percentage of the epithelium, and the mitotic activity. Subsequently, they applied this analysis in blinded fashion to 20 ovarian tumors (19 of LMP and one invasive carcinoma) (81). Morphometry identified the adenocarcinoma and the two tumors of LMP which had led to patients' deaths as having a "poor" prognosis. A fourth patient who also was identified as having a poor prognosis had been treated with chemotherapy. She was alive and well at time of analysis. They concluded that morphometry might be used to identify those patients with tumors of LMP who might benefit from adjuvant treatment. They have reported one case of a patient managed in this way (82). The small number of patients in these studies makes it difficult to draw meaningful conclusions from them.

Flow Cytometry

For years, flow cytometric techniques have enhanced the diagnosis of hematogenous malignancies by automating the process of quantification and tabulation of various cytologic parameters. This process, however, required fresh tissue. In 1983, Hedley et al. (83) adapted this technique to solid, paraffin-embedded tissues, thus rendering archival tissues available for study. Since then, many investigators have examined the prognostic significance of DNA content and cell cycle in epithelial tumors of the ovary. Unfortunately, the heterogeneity in DNA content in different parts of a tumor, even within the same block, limits our ability to understand the implications of ploidy data.

Most studies report a greater frequency of DNA aneuploidy in stage III and IV disease versus stage I and II. Kaern et al. (84) reported greater frequency of aneuploidy of mucinous (47%) as opposed to serous tumors of LMP (15%). Patients with aneuploid tumors had shorter survival than did those with diploid tumors. However, in this series, patients with mucinous tumors presented with later stage disease than did patients with serous tumors. Although the staging distribution may offset some of the significance of ploidy, the difference in survival is worth noting.

Klemi et al. (85) attempted to correlate nuclear DNA content, defined as proportion of aneuploid to diploid tumor cells within a single tumor, with prognosis in patients with serous ovarian tumors. They found aneuploidy in 1% of benign lesions, 17% of tumors of LMP, and 66% of serous carcinomas. They were unable to find any evidence of aggressive behavior associated with aneuploidy in the tumors with LMP.

Erhardt et al. (86) analyzed DNA content in tissue from seventy-three patients with serous ovarian carcinomas and serous tumors of LMP. They found no abnormal DNA content in the tissue from the twenty-six patients with tumors of LMP. As no deaths or recurrences were noted in this group, they concluded that this analysis was not helpful in tumors of LMP.

Friedlander et al. (87,88) performed flow cytometric analysis on tissue from forty-four patients with tumors of LMP. Forty-two tumors were diploid; all were associated with a good prognosis. One of the two patients with an aneuploid tumor died within 7 months of diagnosis.

Magnetic Resonance

Malignant cells display a characteristic high-resolution protein magnetic resonance (MR) spectrum, largely due to a high plasma membrane content of triglyceride molecules (89). These neutral lipids have been compared with a recently characterized RNA-proteolipid complex found in the serum of patients with malignant disorders (90,91). Early studies attempting to identify those ovarian epithelial lesions with metastatic potential suggest that this complex may be the cause for the magnetic resonance signals that indicate the tumor's biological status. Mountford et al. (92) examined tissue from three benign ovarian tumors, six tumors of LMP, and ten invasive carcinomas. None of the benign lesions, five of the six tumors of LMP, and all ten of the invasive carcinomas yielded MR signals indicating metastatic potential.

Oncogene Expression

Expression of c-*myc*, an oncogene coding for a DNA-binding protein which plays a role in the regulation of cell growth, has been documented in both hematopoietic and solid neoplasms. Increased expression of c-*myc* has been found in advanced ovarian carcinomas (93,94). Sasano et al. (95) were unable to find expression of c-*myc* in three mucinous tumors and one endometrioid tumor of LMP. Using in situ hybridization, Kacinski et al. (96) were able to find expression of c-*myc* greater than the level of beta-actin, a housekeeping gene, in one of three tumors of LMP. Polacarz et al. (97) examined 60 mucinous tumors for cellular distribution of the c-*myc* oncogene product $p62^{c-myc}$. Using a monoclonal antibody, they were able to demonstrate three patterns of immunostaining: (1) nuclear staining alone; (2) staining of the nucleus and basal cytoplasm; and (3) staining of the entire cell. The benign mucinous cystadenomas showed nuclear staining alone. Sixteen of the seventeen tumors of LMP showed staining of the nucleus and basal cytoplasm. All twenty-two cases of invasive carcinomas showed staining of the cell nucleus and entire cytoplasm. Six of the tumors of LMP also had focal staining of the apical cytoplasm; these patients did not have a different clinical course from those without such staining.

Tumor Suppressor Genes

The retinoblastoma gene (Rb), found on chromosome 13q14, is perhaps the most well-characterized tumor suppressor gene to date. Mutations have been documented in mesenchymal and epithelial tumors in addition to cases of familial retinoblastoma. Sasano et al. (98) examined 16 ovarian tumors and found homozygous deletion of Rb in one tumor classified histologically as an endometrioid tumor of LMP. This neoplasm proved to be highly aggressive despite its benign histologic appearance.

Summary

There remains a small but constant proportion of tumors whose clinical behavior belies their histologic appearance. To date, no techniques have been identified to consistently isolate this group of tumors of LMP.

STAGING

Ovarian tumors of LMP are staged surgically in accordance with the same FIGO guidelines as invasive ovarian malignancies (99). A complete staging procedure should include examination of all pelvic and peritoneal surfaces, pelvic and para-aortic lymph node sampling, pelvic and intraabdominal washings for cytologic examination, biopsies of all suspicious lesions as well as random biopsies of the omentum, both paracolic gutters, the pelvic sidewalls, bladder peritoneum, and posterior cul-de-sac.

The distribution of stage at diagnosis in four hundred sixty-eight patients with serous tumors of LMP, compiled from ten studies, is shown in Table 4 (4,9,17,31,32,35–37,39,41). Sixty-five percent are diagnosed with stage I disease as opposed to 89% of those with mucinous tumors of LMP. Fully one-fifth had stage III disease; a total of four patients were noted to have stage IV disease. Table 5 demonstrates staging distribution of 236 patients with mucinous tumors of LMP reported in eight series (9,17,31,32,35–37,39).

TABLE 4. Stage at diagnosis in 468 patients with serous tumors of LMP

Stage	Percent of patients	Total percent of patients
I		65.0
Ia	41.7	
Ib	17.1	
Ic	6.2	
II		13.9
IIa	4.5	
IIb	7.5	
IIc	1.9	
III		20.3
IV		0.8

Eighty-nine percent of them were diagnosed with stage I disease. Only one case of a patient with stage IV disease was reported.

Leake et al. (100) recently reported on thirty-four patients with tumors of LMP. Seven, or 21%, had metastatic disease in the pelvic or paraaortic lymph nodes. Tazelaar et al. (101), in their series of sixty-one patients with stage I mucinous and serous tumors of LMP, found no microscopic tumors in grossly normal ovaries which were bivalved and biopsied. They concluded that, due to the risk of infertility, [reportedly 14% after ovarian wedge biopsy (102)], a grossly normal ovary should not be sampled in a young woman interested in retaining fertility. Tumor implants have been reported at abdominal trocar sites after laparoscopic biopsies (103). Careful inspection of abdominal laparoscopic scars is also advised. As mucinous ovarian tumors have been reported to present with synchronous appendiceal primaries (63), the appendix should be removed as part of staging. Ideally, staging and appropriate debulking should be done at the time of initial laparotomy. Should the initial laparotomy be made via a transverse incision, a second midline incision may be necessary to expose the upper abdomen for examination and biopsy.

Restaging Procedures

Many patients with tumors of LMP are young women in whom cancer is not suspected. The initial diagnostic procedure may well have been laparoscopy or ovarian cystectomy via a transverse incision. The difficulty of making a pathologic diagnosis of tumor of LMP has been discussed above. Many patients and their physicians learn of the diagnosis only after a diagnostic procedure inadequate for staging. Several investigators have examined the efficacy of restaging procedures in patients with tumors of LMP. Yazigi et al. (104) reported twenty-nine patients with presumed stage I or II disease who underwent restaging procedures. Seven of twenty-nine were upstaged to stage II on the basis of omental disease or pelvic and paraaortic lymph node metastasis. Hopkins and Morley (105) reported restaging fifteen patients. Seven were noted to have further disease; five were upstaged to either stage II or III. Snider et al. (106) upstaged five of twenty-seven patients with clinical stage I disease. None of twelve patients with mucinous tumors of LMP were upstaged, while four of thirteen patients with serous tumors were upstaged. They concluded that restaging procedures were not indicated in mucinous tumors of LMP. In the series reported by Leake et al. (100), 21% were upstaged on the basis of metastatic disease in retroperitoneal lymph nodes. We believe that the decision to restage must be individualized, taking into consideration the adequacy of the previous abdominal exploration, the tumor subtype, potential recommendations for adjuvant therapy, as well as the level of concern of both the patient and the physician.

TREATMENT

In general, the recommended therapy for patients with all-stage tumors of LMP is total abdominal hysterectomy (TAH), bilateral salpingo-oophorectomy (BSO), and tumor debulking. No randomized, prospective study has compared conservative therapy to TAH/BSO. Only one prospective, randomized study has compared TAH/BSO alone to TAH/BSO with adjuvant therapy. Creasman et al. (107) reported fifty-five patients with stage I disease, initially treated with TAH/BSO. Postoperatively, patients were randomized to no further therapy, pelvic irradiation (5,000 rads), or oral melphalan (0.2 mg/kg for 5 days every 4 weeks for 18 months). One recurrence was noted on the radiation arm. They concluded that TAH/BSO was adequate

TABLE 5. Stage at diagnosis in 236 patients with mucinous tumors of LMP

Stage	Percent of patients	Total percent of patients
I		89.4
Ia	80.1	
Ib	3.4	
Ic	5.9	
II		0.8
IIa	0.4	
IIb	0.0	
IIc	0.4	
III		9.3
IV		0.4

therapy for stage I disease. The Gynecologic Oncology Group is conducting an ongoing study in which patients without clinical evidence of disease after initial surgical therapy are followed prospectively. Melphalan chemotherapy is only begun for disease progression.

Conservative Therapy

Conservative therapy, as defined by that which preserves some ovarian tissue, has been reported in several series of younger patients. Tazelaar et al. (99) reported twenty patients with stage Ia serous and mucinous ovarian tumors of LMP who were treated conservatively, either with an ovarian cystectomy or unilateral salpingo-oophorectomy. After a mean follow-up of 89 months, three recurrences were noted, all in patients with serous tumors of LMP. The risk of recurrence for a patient with stage Ia serous or seromucinous tumor of LMP, treated conservatively, was not significantly different from patients with the same tumors treated with TAH/BSO. Rice et al. (35) reported on thirty-two patients with tumors of LMP (18 mucinous, 15 serous) managed conservatively. Ten with stage I disease had ovarian cystectomies alone. Follow-up was available in thirty patients, all of whom were alive and free of disease. Lim-Tan et al. (108) reported on the experiences of thirty-five patients initially treated with unilateral or bilateral ovarian cystectomy. Recurrent or persistent disease was noted in four patients (12%). Involvement of the resection margin or multiple cystectomies from one ovary were almost always associated with persistent or recurrent disease. In twenty-one patients, they could document preservation of ovarian tissue for a "relatively long period of observation" without clinical evidence of recurrence. Fort et al. (109) report one patient who developed papillary serous adenocarcinoma in a conserved ovary five years after diagnosis. Chambers et al. (36) reported two recurrences among twenty patients treated conservatively. Wienold et al. (110) demonstrated a 74.4% ten-year survival in women treated with TAH/BSO as opposed to a 51.9% ten-year survival in women treated with unilateral adnexectomy. These reports suggest that conservative therapy may be a viable option for young women interested in preserving fertility. The incidence of recurrent or persistent disease, at least 10%, mandates close follow-up of these patients. Patient and physician anxiety may also suggest a TAH/BSO once childbearing has been completed.

Postoperative Adjuvant Therapy

A variety of postoperative regimens for adjuvant therapy have been reported. Patients have been treated with single-agent alkylators and combination chemotherapy, sometimes platinum based. They have been treated with intraperitoneal radioactive phosphorus and external whole pelvic irradiation. No study has documented efficacy for postoperative treatment in prolonging survival.

As mentioned above, Creasman et al. (105) found no advantage to adjuvant external radiation therapy or chemotherapy in patients with stage I disease. Chambers et al. (36) found no statistical difference in survival between patients with serous and mucinous tumors of LMP treated with surgery alone and those receiving additional therapy. Gershenson and Silva (19) found no difference in survival rate in eighty-two patients with serous tumor of LMP according to the type of initial postoperative treatment. Bell et al. (20) found no impact on survival in patients with serous tumors of LMP from the presence or absence of postoperative therapy or its type. In making recommendations for postoperative therapy, therefore, oncologists must make clear to patients the lack of evidence supporting such efforts.

Second-look Procedures; Response to Adjuvant Treatment

Findings at second-look laparotomy following therapy in ten studies are shown in Table 6 (12,13,16,19,36,37,40,107,111,112). Treatment included a variety of regimens, including single-agent alkylators, noncisplatin combinations, cisplatin-containing combinations, and radiotherapy. These results suggest that these tumors are responsive to therapy. The Gynecologic Oncology Group is conducting a study to evaluate the effectiveness of melphalan chemotherapy in patients whose disease progresses after primary surgery.

Concurrent Pregnancy

A total of twenty-one patients were diagnosed with tumors of LMP during pregnancy; an additional three were diagnosed in the postpartum period. No recurrences or deaths from disease are recorded in this group of patients (13,17,24,36,61,62,106). There is no evidence to suggest, therefore, that concurrent pregnancy adversely affects prognosis in this disease.

Pregnancy After Initial Conservative Therapy

Twelve patients have conceived and delivered term infants after conservative therapy for tumors of LMP (13,36,98,106). Only one recurrence in this group has been reported (36). This patient, with stage I disease,

TABLE 6. *Findings at second-look laparotomy*

Author	Stage	Residual	Treatment	No. patients undergoing second look	No. patients with negative findings
Barnhill (12)				10	5
			melphalan	6	4
Bostwick (13)				18	15
Chambers (36)				10	8
			melphalan	7	5
Chien (37)				10	6
	II, III			9	5
			melphalan	6	3
			CAP	3	2
Fort (109)				25	21
	I			10	9
	II–IV			15	12
		gross		19	12
Gallup (111)				9	5
Gershenson (19)				32	13
		no gross		12	5
			single agent	5	3
			non-Pcomb	2	0
			Pcomb	5	2
		gross		20	8
			single agent	12	5
			non-Pcomb	4	1
			Pcomb	4	2
Hopkins (15)				18	15
	I–II			12	12
	III			8	5
			RT	4	4
			CAP	3	1
O'Quinn (112)			melphalan	11	0
Sutton (40)					
	III				
			CP/CAP	14	6

RT, radiotherapy; CAP, cyclophosphamide/doxorubicin/cisplatin; CP, cyclophosphamide/cisplatin; non-Pcomb, non-cisplatin-containing combination; Pcomb, cisplatin-containing combination.

seems to have been treated initially with laparoscopic ovarian cystectomy. She underwent a repeat laparoscopy with negative washings 3 months after initial diagnosis. She subsequently became pregnant. One year later, an exploratory laparotomy showed recurrent tumor of LMP. In this small sample there is no evidence that subsequent pregnancy increases the risk of recurrence above the baseline 10%.

Invasive Carcinoma After a Tumor of LMP

Only four cases of invasive epithelial ovarian carcinoma following treatment of a tumor of LMP have been documented (19,31,107). In addition, Chambers et al. (36) report one patient who was discovered to have a poorly differentiated adenocarcinoma along the transverse colon after initial therapy. They suspected that this might represent a new primary. The vast majority of patients with recurrent or persistent disease had recrudescent tumors which continued to meet histologic criteria for tumors of LMP.

Leukemia After Chemotherapy

Nine cases of acute myelogenous leukemia have been reported after chemotherapy (15,19,36,106). Patients who have received chemotherapy (particularly alkylating agents) for treatment of this disease should be monitored regularly for development of hematologic abnormalities.

Recurrent Disease

Hopkins and Morley (103) describe 22 exploratory laparotomies for suspected disease in thirteen patients. In 19 of 22, malignancy was encountered. They concluded that in patients with a history of ovarian tumors of LMP, symptoms or signs of recurrent disease should be investigated promptly.

Synchronous Primaries

Twelve patients are reported to have second primary cancers synchronous with ovarian tumors of LMP (17,36,62). Second primaries were as follows: endometrial adenocarcinoma, 7; colon carcinoma, 2; appendiceal carcinoma, 1; fallopian tube carcinoma, 1; squamous cell carcinoma of the cervix, 1.

Post-Treatment Estrogen Replacement

We were unable to find any study which reports retrospective or prospective experience in giving estrogen replacement therapy to women with a history of an ovarian tumor of LMP. In the absence of evidence to the contrary, these women should be given estrogen replacement when medically appropriate.

Risk of Recurrence

A variety of clinical and histopathologic factors have been examined to identify prognostic factors associated with the risk of recurrent disease. Table 7 outlines the associations found (13,15,17–20,57,58,99,102,113). What can we glean from these reports? First, unlike in invasive ovarian cancer, age at diagnosis of ovarian tumors of LMP does not seem to affect survival. Neither does size of the primary ovarian tumor. Patients with stage III disease do not do as well as those with stage I. Gross residual disease has been associated with a higher risk of persistent or recurrent disease, suggesting the importance of primary cytoreduction. Of a variety of histopathologic factors examined, only implant invasion, mitotic activity in implants, nuclear and cytologic atypia, and tumor grade have been associated with an increased risk of recurrence. Although Bell et al. (20) have suggested that adjuvant therapy be reserved for those with invasive implants, no prospective study has evaluated these recommendations. It is possible that further pathologic analysis of tissue from tumors of LMP, using some of the special techniques outlined above, may provide additional clues as to which tumors are at high risk of recurrence.

TABLE 7. *Risk of recurrence associated with histolopathologic factors*

Factor	Study documenting an association	Study finding no association
Patient age		Bostwick (13)
		Tazelaar (101)
		Bell (20)
Tumor size		Bostwick (13)
		Tazelaar (101)
		Lim-Tan (108)
Advanced stage	Bostwick (13)	Bell (20)
	Hopkins (15)	Gershenson
	Kliman (17)	(19)
Residual disease	Bostwick (13)	Gershenson
	Bell (20)	(19)
Implant invasion	McCaughey (60)	Gershenson
	Bell (20)	(19)
		Michael (59)
Capsular status		Hopkins (15)
Tumor spillage		Hopkins (15)
Cystadenofibroma		Hopkins (15)
Surface growth	Bostwick (13)	
Nuclear atypia	Hopkins (15)	Lim-Tan (108)
	Bell (20)	Tazelaar (101)
Cytologic atypia	Bell (20)	Bostwick (13)
Mitotic counts	Bell (20)	Bostwick (13)
		Tazelaar (101)
		Lim-Tan (108)
		Katzenstein (18)
Necrosis		Bostwick (13)
		Tazelaar (101)
		Lim-Tan (108)
		Katzenstein (18)
Psammoma bodies		Tazelaar (101)
		Hopkins (15)
		Katzenstein (18)
Cellular budding		Lim-Tan (108)
Grade	Hopkins (15)	
	Russell (9)	
	Sumithran (113)	
Number of nucleoli		Hopkins (15)
		Katzenstein (18)
Stratification		Hopkins (15)
		Katzenstein (18)
		Bostwick (13)
Cribriform pattern		Hopkins (15)
		Katzenstein (18)
Cellular acantholysis		Bostwick (13)
		Katzenstein (18)
Tufting/papillae		Katzenstein (18)
		Bostwick (13)
Stromal inflammation		Katzenstein (18)

CONCLUSION

Many questions remain unanswered. We do know that these tumors of LMP comprise about 10–15% of epithelial ovarian tumors. Among affluent, predominantly Caucasian populations, they seem to occur most commonly in women aged 35 to 50 years. Pregnancy, lactation, and oral contraceptives have a protective effect against them, as they do for other ovarian epithelial tumors. They do not have a hereditary component. Mucinous tumors present at an earlier stage than do serous tumors. Both subtypes may be accompanied by intraperitoneal müllerian neoplasia ranging from benign rests to invasive carcinoma. Twenty-year survival for patients with serous and mucinous tumors of LMP ranges between 90% with stage I disease to 70% for stage III disease. There is insufficient data on which to base survival statistics for Brenner, endometrioid, and clear cell tumors of LMP. Young women with stage I disease may be safely treated conservatively to preserve reproductive potential. Advanced stage disease should be treated with TAH/BSO. Both groups should have close follow-up, as late recurrences are not uncommon. Although these tumors seem to be sensitive to chemotherapy and radiation therapy, the adjuvant value of either has not been demonstrated. The safety of estrogen replacement has not been evaluated. We await further pathologic investigation, using a variety of special techniques, to tell us which tumors are truly of no malignant potential and which are at risk for recurrence.

REFERENCES

1. Aure JC, Hoeg K, Kolstad P. Clinical and histologic studies of ovarian carcinoma. *Obstet Gynecol* 1971;37:1–9.
2. England MJ, Sonnendecker EWW, Margolius KA. Epithelial ovarian tumours of low malignant potential. *S Afr Med J* 1986; 70:543–8.
3. Tiltman J, Sweerts M. Ovarian neoplasms in the Western Cape. *S Afr Med J* 1982;61:342–5.
4. Tang M, Lian L, Liu T. The characteristics of ovarian serous tumors of borderline malignancy. *Chin Med J* 1980;93:459–64.
5. Singh P, Arunchalam I, Singh P, Tan B-Y, Tock EPC, Ratnam SS. Ovarian cancer in oriental women from Singapore: disease pattern and survival. *Int Surg* 1990;75:115–22.
6. Nakashima N, Nagasaka T, Oiwa N. Ovarian tumors of borderline malignancy in Japan. *Gynecol Oncol* 1990;38:90–8.
7. Prabhakar BR, Maingi K. Ovarian tumours—prevalence in Punjab. *Indian J Pathol Microbiol* 1989;32:276–81.
8. Koonings PP, Campbell K, Mishell DR, Grimes DA. Relative frequency of primary ovarian neoplasms: a 10-year review. *Obstet Gynecol* 1989;74:921–6.
9. Russell P. The pathological assessment of ovarian neoplasms: I. Introduction to the common 'epithelial' tumors and analysis of benign 'epithelial' tumors. *Pathology* 1979;11:5–26.
10. Whelan SL, Parkin DM, Masuyer E, eds. *Patterns of Cancer in Five Continents*. Lyons: IARC; 1990.
11. Harlow BL, Weiss NS, Lofton S. Epidemiology of borderline ovarian tumors. *J Natl Cancer Inst* 1987;78:71–4.
12. Barnhill D, Heller P, Brozozowski P, Advani H, Gallup D, Park R. Epithelial ovarian carcinoma of low malignant potential. *Obstet Gynecol* 1985;65:53–9.
13. Bostwick DG, Tazelaar HD, Ballon SC, Hendrickson MR, Kempson RL. Ovarian epithelial tumors of borderline malignancy. *Cancer* 1986;58:2052–65.
14. Katsube Y, Berg JW, Silverberg SG. Epidemiologic pathology of ovarian tumors: a histopathologic review of primary ovarian neoplasms diagnosed in the Denver standard metropolitan statistical area, 1 July–31 December 1969 and 1 July–31 December 1979. *Int J Gynecol Pathol* 1982;1:3–16.
15. Hopkins MP, Kumar NB, Morley GW. An assessment of pathologic features and treatment modalities in ovarian tumors of low malignant potential. *Obstet Gynecol* 1987;70:923–9.
16. Berek JS, Hacker NF, eds. *Practical Gynecologic Oncology*. Baltimore: Williams & Wilkins, 1989.
17. Kliman L, Rome RM, Fortune DW. Low malignant potential tumors of the ovary: a study of 76 cases. *Obstet Gynecol* 1986; 68:338–44.
18. Katzenstein A-LA, Mazur MT, Morgan TE, Kao M-S. Proliferative serous tumors of the ovary. *Am J Surg Pathol* 1978;2: 339–55.
19. Gershenson DM, Silva EG. Serous ovarian tumors of low malignant potential with peritoneal implants. *Cancer* 1990;65: 578–85.
20. Bell DA, Weinstock MA, Scully RE. Peritoneal implants of ovarian serous borderline tumors. *Cancer* 1988;62:2212–22.
21. Hart WR, Norris HJ. Borderline and malignant mucinous tumors of the ovary. *Cancer* 1973;31:1031–45.
22. Dgani R, Shoham, Schwartz Z, Atar E, Zosmer A, Lancet M. Ovarian carcinoma during pregnancy: a study of 23 cases in Israel between the years 1960 and 1984. *Gynecol Oncol* 1989; 33:326–31.
23. Diamond MP, Baxter JW, Peerman CG, Burnett LS. Occurrence of ovarian malignancy in childhood: a community-wide evaluation. *Obstet Gynecol* 1988;71:858–60.
24. Carter J, Atkinson K, Coppleson M, et al. A comparative study of proliferating (borderline) and invasive epithelial ovarian tumors in young women. *Aust N Z J Obstet Gynaecol* 1989;29: 245–9.
25. Gallup DG, Cody WM, Metheny WP, Talledo OE. Epithelial tumors of the ovary in women less than 40 years old. *South Med J* 1988;81:10–4.
26. Harlow BL, Weiss NS, Roth GL, Chu J, Daling JR. Case-control study of borderline ovarian tumors: reproductive history and exposure to exogenous female hormones. *Cancer Res* 1988;48:5849–52.
27. Schildkraut JM, Thompson WD. Familial ovarian cancer: a population-based case-control study. *Am J Epidemiol* 1988; 128:456–66.
28. Barlow JJ, DiCioccio RA, Dillard PH, Blehenson LE, Matta KL. Frequency of an allele for low activity of alpha-L-fucosidase in sera: possible increae in epithelial ovarian cancer patients. *J Natl Cancer Inst* 1981;67:1005–9.
29. Harlow BL, Weiss NS, Holmes EH. Plasma alpha-L-fucosidase activity and the risk of borderline epithelial ovarian tumors. *Cancer Res* 1990;50:4702–3.
30. Harlow BL, Weiss NS. A case-control study of borderline ovarian tumors: the influence of perineal exposure to talc. *Am J Epidemiol* 1989;130:390–4.
31. Nikrui N. Survey of clinical behavior of patients with borderline epithelial tumors of the ovary. *Gynecol Oncol* 1981;12: 107–19.
32. Nation JG, Krepart GV. Ovarian carcinoma of low malignant potential: staging and treatment. *Am J Obstet Gynecol* 1986; 154:290–3.
33. Achiron R, Schejter E, Malinger G, Zakut H. Observations on the ultrasound diagnosis of ovarian neoplasms. *Arch Gynecol Obstet* 1987;241:183–90.
34. Buy JN, Ghossain MA, Sciot C, et al. Epithelial tumors of the ovary: CT findings and correlation with US. *Radiology* 1991; 178:811–8.
35. Rice LW, Berkowitz RS, Mark SD, Yavner DL, Lage JM. Epithelial ovarian tumors of borderline malignancy. *Gynecol Oncol* 1990;39:195–8.
36. Chambers JT, Merino MJ, Kohorn EI, Schwartz PE. Borderline ovarian tumors. *Am J Obstet Gynecol* 1988;159:1088–94.
37. Chien RTY, Rettenmaier AM, Micha JP, DiSaia PJ. Ovarian epithelial tumors of low malignant potential. *Surg Gynecol Obstet* 1989;169:143–6.
38. Kudlacek S, Schider K, Kolbl H, Neunteufel W, Nowotsny C. Use of CA 125 monoclonal antibody to monitor patients with ovarian cancer. *Gynecol Oncol* 1989;35:323–9.
39. Dgani R, Blickstein I, Shoham Z, et al. Clinical aspects of ovarian tumors of low malignant potential. *Eur J Obstet Gynecol* 1990;35:251–8.
40. Sutton GP, Bundy BN, Omura GA, Yordan YL, Beecham JB, Bonfiglio T. Stage III ovarian tumors of low malignant potential treated with cisplatin combination therapy (a Gynecologic Oncology Group study). *Gynecol Oncol* 1991;41:230–233.
41. Julian CG, Woodruff JD. The biologic behavior of low-grade papillary serous carcinoma of the ovary. *Obstet Gynecol* 1972; 40:860–7.
42. Taylor HC. Malignant and semimalignant tumors of the ovary. *Surg Gynecol Obstet* 1929;48:204–30.
43. International Federation of Gynecology and Obstetrics. Classi-

fication and staging of malignant tumors in the female pelvis. *Acta Obstet Gynecol Scand* 1971;50:1–7.
44. Serov SF, Scully RE, Sobin LH. International histological classification and staging of tumors. No. 9 Histologic Typing of Ovarian Tumors. Geneva: World Health Organization, 1973.
45. Woodruff JD, Julian CG. Multiple malignancy in the upper genital canal. *Am J Obstet Gynecol* 1969;103:810–22.
46. Parmley TH, Woodruff JD. The ovarian mesothelioma. *Am J Obstet Gynecol* 1974;120:234–41.
47. Genadry R, Parmley T, Woodruff JD. The origin and clinical behavior of the parovarian tumor. *Am J Obstet Gynecol* 1977;129:873–80.
48. Russell P. The pathological assessment of ovarian neoplasms. II: the proliferating 'epithelial' tumors. *Pathology* 1979;11:251–82.
49. Russell P. Borderline epithelial tumors of the ovary: a conceptual dilemma. *Clin Obstet Gynecol* 1984;11:259–77.
50. Russell P, Bannatyne PM, Solomon HJ, Stoddard LD, Tattersall MHN. Multifocal tumorigenesis in the upper female genital tract—implications for staging and management. *Int J Gynecol Pathol* 1985;4:192–210.
51. Bell D. Ovarian surface epithelial-stromal tumors. *Hum Pathol* 1991;22:750–62.
52. Hernandez E, Bhagavan BS, Parmley TH, Rosenshein NB. Interobserver variability in the interpretation of epithelial ovarian cancer. *Gynecol Oncol* 1984;17:117–23.
53. Baak JP, Langely FA, Talerman A, Delemarre JF. Interpathologist and intrapathologist disagreement in ovarian tumor grading and typing. *Anal Quant Cytol Histol* 1986;8:354–7.
54. Cramer SF, Roth LM, Ulbright TM, et al. Evaluation of the reproducibility of the World Health Organization classification of common ovarian cancer. *Arch Pathol Lab Med* 1987;111:818–29.
55. Stalsberg H, Abeler V, Blom GP, Bostad L, Sklarland E, Westgaard G. Observer variation in histologic classification of malignant and borderline ovarian tumors. *Hum Pathol* 1988;19:1030–5.
56. Taylor CW, Lee NC, Robboy SJ, et al. The diagnosis of ovarian cancer by pathologists: how often do diagnoses by contributing pathologists agree with a panel of gynecologic pathologists? *Am J Obstet Gynecol* 1991;164:65–70.
57. Julian CG, Woodruff JD. The biologic behavior of low-grade papillary serous carcinoma of the ovary. *Obstet Gynecol* 1972;40:860–7.
58. Tasker M, Langley FA. The outlook for women with borderline epithelial tumors of the ovary. *Br J Obstet Gynaecol* 1985;92:969–73.
59. Michael H, Roth LM. Invasive and noninvasive implants in ovarian serous tumors of low malignant potential. *Cancer* 1986;57:1240–7.
60. McCaughey WTE, Kirk ME, Lester W, Dardick I. Peritoneal epithelial lesions associated with proliferative serous tumors of ovary. *Histopathology* 1984;8:195–208.
61. Robey SS, Silva EG. Epithelial hyperplasia of the fallopian tube: its association with serous borderline tumors of the ovary. *Int J Gynecol Pathol* 1989;8:214–220.
62. Hart WR, Norris HJ. Borderline and malignant mucinous tumors of the ovary. *Cancer* 1973;31:1031–45.
63. Rutgers JL, Scully RE. Ovarian Müllerian mucinous papillary cystadenomas of borderline malignancy. *Cancer* 1988;61:340–8.
64. Rutgers JL, Scully RE. Ovarian mixed-epithelial papillary cystadenomas of borderline malignancy of Müllerian type. *Cancer* 1988;61:546–45.
65. Young GH, Gilks CB, Scully RE. Mucinous tumors of the appendix associated with mucinous tumors of the ovary and pseudomyxoma peritonei. *Am J Surg Pathol* 1991;15:415–29.
66. Roth LM, Czernobilsky B. Ovarian Brenner tumors. *Cancer* 1985;56:592–601.
67. Trebeck CE, Friedlander ML, Russell P, Baird PJ. Brenner tumours of the ovary: a study of the histology, immunohistochemistry and cellular DNA content in benign, borderline, and malignant ovarian tumours. *Pathology* 1987;19:241–6.
68. Kao GF, Norris HJ. Unusual cystadenofibromas: endometrioid, mucinous, and clear cell types. *Obstet Gynecol* 1979;54:729–36.
69. Kao GF, Norris HJ. Cystadenofibromas of the ovary with epithelial atypia. *Am J Surg Pathol* 1978;2:357–63.
70. Roth LM, Czernobilsky B, Langley FA. Ovarian endometrioid adenofibromatous and cystadenofibromatous tumors: benign, proliferating, and malignant. *Cancer* 1981;48:1838–45.
71. Czernobilsky B. Endometrioid neoplasia of the ovary: a reappraisal. *Int J Gynecol Pathol* 1982;1:203–5.
72. Colgan TJ, Norris HJ. Ovarian epithelial tumors of low malignant potential: a review. *Int J Gynecol Pathol* 1983;1:367–82.
73. Bell DA, Scully RE. Atypical and borderline endometrioid adenofibromas of the ovary. *Am J Surg Pathol* 1985;9:205–14.
74. Snyder RR, Norris HJ, Tavassoli F. Endometrioid proliferative and low malignant potential tumors of the ovary. *Am J Surg Pathol* 1988;12:661–71.
75. Bell DA, Scully RE. Benign and borderline clear cell adenofibromas of the ovary. *Cancer* 1985;56:2922–31.
76. Roth LM, Langley FA, Fox H, Wheeler JE, Czernobilsky B. Ovarian clear cell adenofibromatous tumors. *Cancer* 1984;53:1156–63.
77. Neunteufel W, Breitenecker G. Tissue expression in malignant lesions of ovary and Fallopian tube: a comparison with CA 19-9 and CEA. *Gynecol Oncol* 1989;32:297–302.
78. Neunteufel W, Gitsch G, Scheider K, Kolbl H, Breitenecker G. Ovarian tumors of low malignant potential (borderline tumors); immune morphology and current status. *Anticancer Res* 1989;9:993–8.
79. Einhorn N, Knapp RC, Bast RC, Zurawski VR. CA 125 assay used in conjunction with CA 15-3 and TAG-72 assays for discrimination between malignant and non-malignant disease of the ovary. *Acta Oncol* 1989;28:655–7.
80. Baak JPA, Agrafojo-Blanco A, Kurva PHJ, et al. Quantitation of borderline and malignant mucinous ovarian tumors. *Histopathology* 1981;5:353–60.
81. Baak JPA, Fox H, Langley FA, Buckley CH. The prognostic value of morphometry in ovarian epithelial tumors of borderline malignancy. *Int J Gynecol Pathol* 1985;4:186–91.
82. Baak JPA, Van der Ley G. Borderline or malignant ovarian tumour: a case report of decision making with morphometry. *J Clin Pathol* 1984;37:1110–3.
83. Hedley DW, Friedlander ML, Taylor IW, Rugg CA, Musgrove EA. Method for analysis of cellular DNA content of paraffin-embedded pathological material using flow cytometry. *J Histochem Cytochem* 1983;31:1333–5.
84. Kaern J, Trope C, Kjorstad KE, Abeler V, Pettersen EO. Cellular DNA content as a new prognostic tool in patients with borderline tumors of the ovary. *Gynecol Oncol* 1990;38:452–7.
85. Klemi PJ, Joensuu H, Kilholma P, Maenpaaa J. Clinical significance of abnormal nuclear DNA content in serous ovarian tumors. *Cancer* 1988;62:2005–10.
86. Erhardt K, Auer G, Bjorkholm E et al. Prognostic significance of nuclear DNA content in serous ovarian tumors. *Cancer Res* 1984;44:2198–2202.
87. Friedlander ML, Russell P, Taylor IW, Hedley DW, Tattersall MHN. Flow cytometric analysis of cellular DNA content as an adjunct to the diagnosis of ovarian tumours of borderline malignancy. *Pathology* 1984;16:301–6.
88. Friedlander ML, Hedley DW, Swanson C, Russell P. Prediction of long-term survival by flow cytometric analysis of the cellular DNA content in patients with advanced ovarian cancer. *J Clin Oncol* 1988;6:282–90.
89. Mountford CE, Grossman G, Reid G, Fox RM. Characterization of transformed cells and tumors by proton nuclear magnetic resonance spectroscopy. *Cancer Res* 1982;42:2270–6.
90. Wieczorek AJ, Rhymer C, Block LH. Isolation and characterization of an RNA-proteolipid complex associated with the malignant state in humans. *Proc Natl Acad Sci USA* 1985;82:3455–59.
91. Wright LC, Sullivan DR, Muller M, Dyne M, Tattersal MHN, Mountford CE. Elevated apolipoprotein (a) levels in cancer patients. *Int J Cancer* 1989;43:241–44.
92. Mountford CE, May GL, William PG, et al. Classification of

tumors by high-resolution magnetic resonance spectroscopy. *Lancet* 1986;i:651–3.
93. Zhou DJ, Gonzalez-Cadavid N, Ahuja H, et al. A unique pattern of proto-oncogene abnormalities in ovarian adenocarcinomas. *Cancer* 1988;62:1573–6.
94. Baker VV, Borst MP, Dixon D, Hatch KD, Singleton HM, Miller D. C-*myc* amplification in ovarian cancer. *Gynecol Oncol* 1990;38:340–2.
95. Sasano H, Garrett CT, Wilkinson DS, Silverberg S, Comerford J, Hyde J. Protooncogene amplification and tumor ploidy in human ovarian neoplasms. *Hum Pathol* 1990;21:382–91.
96. Kacinski BM, Carter D, Kohorn EI, et al. Oncogene expression *in vivo* by ovarian adenocarcinomas and mixed-mullerian tumors. *Yale J Biol Med* 1989;62:379–92.
97. Polacarz SV, Hey NA, Stephenson TJ, Hill AS. C-*myc* oncogene product P62 in ovarian mucinous neoplasms: immunohistochemical study correlated with malignancy. *J Clin Pathol* 1989;42:148–52.
98. Sasano H, Comerford J, Silverberg SG, Garret CT. An analysis of abnormalities of the retinoblastoma gene in human ovarian and endometrial carcinoma. *Cancer* 1990;66:2150–4.
99. International Federation of Gynecology and Obstetrics. Annual report and results of treatment in gynecologic cancer. *Int J Gynecol Obstet* 1989;28:189–90.
100. Leake JF, Rader JS, Woodruff JD, Rosenshein NB. Retroperitoneal lymphatic involvement with epithelial ovarian tumors of low malignant potential. *Gynecol Oncol* 1991;42:124–30.
101. Tazelaar HD, Bostwick DG, Ballon SC, Hendrickson MR, Kempson RL. Conservative treatment of borderline ovarian tumors. *Obstet Gynecol* 1985;66:417–22.
102. Weinstein D, Polishuk WZ. The role of wedge resection of the ovary as a cause for mechanical sterility. *Surg Gynecol Obstet* 1975;141:417–21.
103. Hsiu J-G, Given FT, Kemp GM. Tumor implantation after diagnostic laparoscopic biopsy of serous ovarian tumors of low malignant potential. *Obstet Gynecol* 1986;68S;90S–93S.
104. Yazigi R, Sandstad J, Munoz AK. Primary staging in ovarian tumors of low malignant potential. *Gynecol Oncol* 1988;31:402–8.
105. Hopkins MP, Morley GW. The second-look operation and surgical reexploration in ovarian tumors of low malignant potential. *Obstet Gynecol* 1989;74:375–8.
106. Snider DD, Stuart GCE, Nation JG, Roberston DI. Evaluation of surgical staging in stage I low malignant potential ovarian tumors. *Gynecol Oncol* 1991;40:129–32.
107. Creasman WT, Park R, Norris H, DiSaia PJ, Morrow CP, Hreshchysyn MM. Stage I borderline ovarian tumors. *Obstet Gynecol* 1982;59:93–6.
108. Lim-Tan SK, Cajigas HE, Scully RE. Ovarian cystectomy for serous borderline tumors: a follow-up study of 35 cases. *Obstet Gynecol* 1988;72:775–81.
109. Fort MG, Pierce VK, Saigo PE, Hoskins WJ, Lewis JL. Evidence of the efficacy of adjuvant therapy in epithelial ovarian tumors of low malignant potential. *Gynecol Oncol* 1989;32:269–72.
110. Wienold J, Sarembe B, Richter P. Therapie und verlauf bei 105 bordrline-tumoren des ovars. *Zenbl Gynakol* 1989;111:721–7.
111. Gallup DG, Talledo OE, Dudzinski MR, Brown KW. Another look at the second-assessment procedure for ovarian epithelial carcinoma. *Am J Obstet Gynecol* 1987;157:590–6.
112. Quinn AG, Hannigan EV. Epithelial ovarian neoplasms of low malignant potential. *Gynecol Oncol* 1985;21:177–85.
113. Sumithran E, Susil BJ, Looi L-M. The prognostic significance of grading in borderline mucinous tumors of the ovary. *Human Pathol* 1988;19:1915–8.

Subject Index

A

Adenosarcoma
  of cervix, 42
  as ovarian mesodermal mixed tumor, 28–29
Adnexal masses
  asymptomatic, 153
  CA-125 detection, 156,157
  clinical evaluation, 359
  CT imaging, 143,144
  Doppler evaluation of, 137–138
  IVP findings in, 157
  malignancy of, 136
  MRI detection, 148,149
  predictive factors, 136,157
  preoperative studies, 156–158
  radiographic evaluation, 157–158
  sonography of, 136,137,138
  TAS of, 137
Adriamycin, resistant cell line, 263,264
Age
  benign/malignant tumors and, 153,155
  cancer risk and, 109,153
  cancer screening guidelines for, 108
  epithelial tumors and, 80,81
  ovarian tumors and, 80–82,95,153–154, 155
  as prognostic factor, 118,121,122,123,170
Alpha fetoprotein (AFP)
  in clear cell carcinoma, 29
  in EST, 35
  in germ cell tumors, 375
  in SLT, 396
Alpha-L-fucosidase, as prognostic factor, 416
Androgens
  in Leydig cell tumors, 394,395
  ovarian production, 13
  in SLT, 396
Androstenedione
  FSH and, 13
  ovarian production, 13,15
Antibodies. *See also* Monoclonal antibodies
  bifunctional, 56
  in immunotherapy, 55–56
  to ovarian tumors, 47,54–55
  in radiolocalization of tumors, 54–55
Antibody-dependent cellular cytotoxicity (ADCC), response to neoplasms, 301,303
Aphidicolin
  AZT treatment and, 270
  cisplatin toxicity enhancement, 270
  clinical trials, 273
  DNA repair inhibition, 269–270,273
Appendiceal tumors, metastasis to ovary, 408,411
Appendix
  metastasis to, 160
  removal, 160
Ascites
  BRM treatment, 309–311
  CT imaging, 141–142,143,144,145,148, 224
  in fibromas, 393
  IP chemotherapy of, 322
  palliative surgery for, 224
  pathophysiology of, 224
  as prognostic factor, 118,136,153–154
  sonography of, 136,140
  sources of, 153–154
  treatment, 224,312
Autologous bone marrow support (ABMS) therapy
  in advanced ovarian cancer, 330–334
  clinical trials, 295–296
  dose-limiting drug toxicity and, 329
  drug resistance and, 295–296
  in high-dose chemotherapy, 295–296,327,330–334,351
  patient care in, 330–331
  technique for, 330–331
Autologous stem cells, use in dose-limiting drug toxicity, 296

B

Bacillus Calmette-Guèrin (BCG)
  as BRM agent, 303–304,308–309,310
  chemotherapy combination, 308–309
  semisynthesized, 310
  tumor treatment, 303–304,308–309,310
Biologic response modifiers (BRM)
  in ascites treatment, 309–310
  BCG as, 303–304,308–309,310
  as immunotherapeutic agents, 303–304, 308–309
  inactivated bacteria as, 308,309–310
Bleomycin
  adverse effects, 378
  cisplatin,vinblastine therapy, 378–379, 388
  germ cell tumor treatment, 378–379
  granulosa cell tumor treatment, 388
Blood group antigens
  ABO group, 51–52
  determinants of, 51,52
  Lewis group, 51,52
  in ovarian carcinoma, 51–53
  T/Tn group, 52
B lymphocytes, response to tumors, 302, 303
Borderline malignancies
  of advanced nature, 199,200
  conservative surgery in, 199
  prognosis in, 199
Breast carcinoma
  histologic subtypes of, 411–412
  metastasis to ovary, 408,411–412
  prophylactic mastectomy and, 109
  screening effectiveness, 107–108
Brenner tumors
  histopathology, 30,420
  incidence of, 30,420
  of LMP, 420
Buthionine sulfoximine
  clinical trials, 298
  drug resistance,overcoming of, 271–272, 298
  GSH intracellular levels and, 271–272, 298

C

Cancer antigen-125 (CA-125)
  adnexal mass and, 125
  assay for, 49
  biochemical characterization, 49
  in chemotherapy assessment, 119, 332–333
  efficacy of, 129,155–156,363
  germ cell tumors and, 376
  in high-dose chemotherapy + ABMS, 332–333,336
  LMP tumors and, 417
  metastatic ovarian tumors and, 410
  normal serum levels, 97
  OSE and, 49
  as ovarian tumor antigen, 48–49,50,97
  in ovarian tumor screening, 48–49,54, 97–98,110,129,155–156,177,363
  predictive value of, 155–156
  as second-look laparatomy alternative, 177
  sensitivity/specificity of, 97–98,129,177, 363
Carboplatin
  ABMS and, 295–296
  advantages of, 255
  in celomic carcinoma, 279,280–281
  cisplatin combination, 255,259
  cisplatin comparison, 281
  cytokine combination, 261
  DI studies of, 255–256
  ifosfamide and, 288
  IP administration, 320–321
  in multiagent treatments, 255,281–282
  myelosuppressive effect, 255,261,349
  in salvage therapy, 320–321
  toxicity reduction, 255,261–262,296–297, 351–352
Carcinoembryonic antigen (CEA), in ovarian carcinoma, 51,54
Carcinoids
  metastatic to ovary, 411
  teratomas and, 38,39
Carcinomas. *See also* specific types
  anaplastic, 26
  Brenner tumors as, 30
  classification, 21
  of cervix, 42
  differential diagnosis, 41–42
  embryonal, 36,37
  endometrial, 41–42
  immunohistochemistry of, 26
  leukemia and, 42
  lymphomas and, 42
  origin of, 21,40

433

Carcinomas (contd.)
　rare, 40
　undifferentiated, 30
Cell cycle
　alkylating agent effects on, 268–269
　arrest of, 268–269
　growth factors and, 61
　phases of, 164
　sequence of events in, 61
Celomic epithelial carcinoma, chemotherapy
　in advanced stages, 277–284
　carboplatin in, 279,281–283
　cisplatin in, 279,280–284
　combination therapy in, 280–284
　cyclophosphamide in, 279,280–282
　DI in, 278,282
　doxorubicin in, 279,280–282
　IP therapy in, 283–284
　in limited disease stage, 284–285
　melphalan in, 280,285
　patient assessment for, 277,278
　in recurrence, 277,284
　residual tumor volume and, 277,278
　single agent treatment, 277–280
　staging for, 277,278
　survival rates in, 278,279,281,282
　taxol in, 279
Central venous access
　advantages/limitations of, 205,206–207, 214–215
　autologous stem cell infusion, 214
　catheter maintenance, 210–211
　catheter placement technique, 206–208
　catheter selection for, 205–206
　complications of, 208–210
　implantable ports for, 206,207,210,214
　infection in, 209–210,214–215
　long-term, 205
　removal indications, 209
　subcutaneous port placement, 207–208
Cervix
　metastasis to ovary, 408
　squamous cell carcinoma, 408
Chemotherapeutic agents, in vitro evaluation
　clinical status of, 247–248
　dose response curves in, 245,246
　of drug combinations, 245–246,247
　of drug resistance, 245,246
　future directions of, 248
　for individual patients, 246–247
　in vitro/in vivo correlations, 244
　methodology for, 243–244
　of new drugs, 244
　therapeutic response and, 243,247
Chemotherapy. See also Drug resistance
　administration route, 205
　central venous access for, 205–211
　course of, 237–238
　cytoreduction and, 235–236
　dose-limiting toxicities and, 329–330
　dose response curves, 245,256–258
　drug resistance in, 165,245,258–259, 261–274,287
　experimental, 287–298
　high-dose, 295–296,327–336
　immunotherapy combination, 308–309
　IP delivery of, 211–214,261,283–284, 317–323
　long-term effects of, 382–383
　multiagent, 253–254,256,259,280–284, 322,378–379,388
　non-cross-resistant drugs in, 284

number of cycles of, 258
primary cytoreduction effects on, 165, 169,171,172
radiotherapy combination, 235–237
radiotherapy comparison, 367–369
in salvage therapy, 287–293,322–323
secondary cytoreduction and, 190,192, 194–195
in second-line therapy, 178
second-look laparotomy based, 176
single agent, 246,278–280
toxicity of, 329–330,382–383
Chemotherapy, complications of
　alopecia, 356
　bladder toxicity
　　prevention, 354
　　treatment, 354
　cardiotoxicity, 355
　emesis
　　acute, 352
　　anticipatory, 351–352
　　delayed, 352
　　management, 352
　extravasation as, 356
　hematologic
　　ABMS in, 351
　　delayed effects, 349
　　leukemia, 382,425
　　management, 350–351
　　myelosuppression and, 255,261,349
　　neutropenia and, 350
　　thrombocytopenia and, 350
　hypersensitivity reactions, 355–356
　mucositis as, 351
　neurotoxicity as, 354
　pulmonary, 355
　secondary malignancies as, 354–355
Chemotherapy, dose intensity (DI)
　average DI and, 251,252,253–254
　calculation of, 251,252
　carboplatin studies, 255–256
　circadian rhythm effects, 256
　cisplatin studies, 252–254,278,282
　clinical determination of, 252–254
　clinical response and, 253, 278
　cyclophosphamide studies, 252–254,256
　definition of, 251
　dose response curves, 256–258
　doxorubicin studies, 256
　drug combinations and, 252–254,256
　drug resistance and, 258–259,293–295
　in multiagent testing, 253–254,256,259
　projected/received DI and, 251–252
　relative DI and, 251–252,253–254,259
　scheduling effects on, 256
　survival times and, 254
　taxol studies, 256
　total dose effects, 256–257,259
Chemotherapy, high dose + ABMS
　in advanced cancer, 335–336
　alkylating agents in, 328–330
　CA-125 levels in, 332–333,336
　cisplatin in, 328–329,331–333,334
　cisplatin, cyclophosphamide combination in, 331,334
　clinical response in, 333–336
　clinical trials of, 330–336
　dose intensification principles in, 327–328
　dose-limiting toxicity and, 329–330,336
　drug resistance and, 328,329
　future directions of, 336
　in high-risk patients, 330–334
　melphalan use in, 333,334

mitoxantrone use in, 333,334
non-cross resistance and, 329
patient demographics in, 331
in poor prognosis patients, 330–335,336
rationale for, 327–328
in refractory patients, 333–334
response rate in, 328–336
techniques in, 330–331
therapeutic senergy in, 328–329
thiotepa use in, 328–329,331,333,334
toxicity in, 331–332,334,336
VP-16 use in, 333,334
Chlorambucil, radiation therapy and, 232, 365
Chromosomes
　for growth factors, 62
　fragmented, 105
Cisplatin
　bleomycin combination, 378–379,388
　carboplatin combination, 255,294
　carboplatin comparison, 281
　cell line sensitivity to, 262
　in celomic epithelial carcinoma, 279,280, 283
　cyclophosphamide combination, 252–254,256,331,365,369
　cytoxan and, 291
　DDTC use and, 296–297
　DI studies of, 252–254,256,293–295
　DNA lesion induction, 267–270
　dose response curves for, 245,282
　in dysgerminomas, 381
　in early stage carcinoma, 365,369–370
　efficacy of, 176
　in germ cell tumors, 378–379
　in granulosa cell tumors, 388
　GSH cell levels and, 265–266
　hexamethylmelamine and, 291–292
　in high dose + ABMS therapy, 328–329, 331–334
　IFN and, 310–311
　ifosfamide and, 288
　individual patient, in vitro testing of, 246–247
　IP administration of, 283,320,322,323,331
　in LMP tumors, 425
　in multiagent therapy, 235,252,256, 280–282,322
　nephrotoxicity reduction, 296
　nonresponders to, 197–198
　ORG.2766 use and, 297
　radiotherapy and, 235–237,369–370
　recurrence rate on, 120,190,192,194–196, 365,369
　resistance to, 237,238,262–271,293–295
　in salvage treatment, 322–323
　secondary cytoreduction and, 190,192, 194–198
　in secondary treatment, 178
　side-effects of, 349,351,353,354
　taxol use and, 290–291
　thiotepa use and, 328–329
　toxicity reduction, 296–297,351–352,353
　vinblastine combination, 378–379,388
Clear cell carcinoma
　differential diagnosis, 29–30
　histopathology of, 29,30,421
　incidence of, 21,29
　LMP type, 29,421
　of vagina, 21
Colorectal cancer screening, efficacy of, 108
Color-flow Doppler. See also Doppler
　in malignancy detection, 96,97

in ovarian tumor screening, 96,97,
128–129,130,141,363
TVS use and, 141
Computed tomography (CT)
advantages of, 141,156,360
ascites detection, 141–142,143–145,148
in benign/malignant differentiation,
141–142
cystic mass detection, 142
as laparotomy replacement, 146
lesion size for detection, 143
limitations of, 141,156,177,360
metastasis detection, 143–144,145,146,
147,148
MRI complementation, 150
negative findings interpretation, 146–147
of pseudomyxoma peritoneal, 143,144
recurrence detection, 146–147,177
as second-look laparotomy alternative,
177
sensitivity/specificity of, 141–142,146,
147
sonography effectiveness comparison,
138,141
of teratoma, 143
Contraceptives
composition/dosage, 84
duration of use, 83–84,106
nonoral, 85
oral, 83–85,106
ovarian cancer risk and, 83–85,106
for ovarian cancer preventiion, 106
Cyclophosphamide
in celomic epithelial carcinoma, 280–281
cisplatin combination, 252–254,256,
280–281,283,331–334
DI determination, 252–254,256,282
hexamethylmelamine use and, 291–292
in high-dose chemotherapy + ABMS,
332–334,354,355
IFN combination, 310–311
side-effects of, 354,355
as single agent, 256
Cystadenomas
CT detection, 141
differential diagnosis, 24
Cytokines
antitumor response, 305–306
in carboplatin therapy, 304,305
IL as, 304,305
lymphokines and, 304
TNF as, 305

D
Diethyldithiocarbamate (DDTC), platinum
drug toxicity reduction, 296–297
DNA analysis
of dysgerminomas, 34–35
flow cytometry in, 23,24,118–119,389,
421–422
in LMP tumors, 421–422
in metastasis origin determination, 408
in prognosis determination, 118–119,121,
123
of serous carcinoma, 23,24
for S-phase fraction, 119,121
DNA banking, clinical value of, 109
DNA repair
alkylating agents effect on, 267–270
cell cycle arrest and, 268
cisplatin effects on, 267–270
clinical trials of inhibitors of, 273
in drug resistance, 367–270

GSH enhancement of, 268,269
mechanisms for, 267–269
suppression of, 269–270
Doppler. *See also* Color-flow Doppler
in adnexal mass imaging, 137–138
in chemotherapy evaluation, 138
specificity/sensitivity of, 138
Dose intensity (DI). *See* Chemotherapy,
dose intensity (DI)
Doxorubicin
analogues of, 244
cardiotoxicity of, 355
in celomic carcinoma, 279,280
cisplatin combinations, 253–254
DI determination for, 253–254,256
hexamethylmelamine use and, 291–292
in vitro evaluation, 244
in liposomes, 321
IP administration of, 320,321
Drug resistance, acquired
to alkylating agents, 262–265,267–270,
328–329
biochemical mechanisms in, 262–271
cell lines for study of, 263
to cisplatin, 237,238,262,263–272
clinical reversal trials, 271–273
cytoreduction and, 165
DI and, 258–259,317–318
DNA repair and, 267–270,273
GSH and, 265–266,271–272
GST inhibition and, 272–273
GST isozymes and, 266–267
high-dose therapy and, 262
in vitro drug testing and, 245
in vivo models for, 263–264
mdr-1 gene expression and, 120,273
metallothioneins and, 266
non-cross resistance and, 329
to platinum compounds, 262–265,
267–270
relative, 261–262,317,320
signal transduction pathways and,
270–271
to sulfhydral compounds, 265–266
survival and, 165
Drug resistance, overcoming
ABMS in, 295–296
autologous stem cells in, 296
BSO and, 271–272,298
clinical trials of, 294–296
cytokines use in, 296
by DI increase, 262,293–295
dose-limiting toxicities and, 296–297
drug sequence and, 294
GSH use in, 265–266,271–272
GST and, 266–267,272–273,298
MDR and, 120,297–298
to platinum compounds, 293–295
Dysgerminomas. *See also* Germ cell
tumors
characterization of, 17,34–35,375,380
chemotherapy of, 380–381
cisplatin sensitivity of, 381
differential diagnosis, 34,375
DNA analysis of, 34–35
histopathology, 34
incidence, 17,34
management, 380–381
prognosis in, 35
radiation therapy of, 380,381
risk factors for, 82
secondary cytoreduction in, 200–201
serum markers for, 381
staging of, 380

E
Early stage ovarian cancer. *See* Ovarian
cancer, early stage
Embryonal carcinoma
characteristics of, 36,37
histopathology in, 36,37
Endodermal sinus tumor (EST) (yolk sac
tumor)
gross features of, 35
histopathology, 35–36
incidence of, 35
teratomas in, 35
Endometrioid carcinoma
adenocarcinoma and, 28
adenofibromas and, 26
differential diagnosis, 28
epidemiology of, 80,82
estrogen therapy of, 85–86
histopathology of, 26,27,28,421
incidence of, 21,27
of LMP, 26–27,420–421
sex cord stromal tumors and, 28
squamous cells in, 27–28
staging of, 116
subtypes of, 420–421
TVS screening for, 108
Epidemiology of ovarian cancer
age and, 80,81,82,95,416
alcohol use and, 87
breast cancer and, 88
chemical exposure and, 89
coffee consumption and, 87
diet and, 86–87
drug use and, 89
environmental factors, 16,416
family factors, 88–89,102–105,109–110,
416
fertility and, 79,80
genetic factors, 98–102
geographic factors, 79
histologic subtypes and, 80–82
incidence, 79–82,415
industrial exposure and, 89
infectious diseases and, 87–88
lactose intolerance and, 87
menstrual history and, 83,89,416
non-ovarian neoplasms and,88
oral contraceptives and, 83–85,90,416
postmenopausal estrogen therapy and,
85–86
race/religion and, 79
reproductive history, 83,89,416
risk factors, 82–88,109–110
smoking and, 87
sterilization and, 85,90,409,412
talc use and, 86,90,416
temporal trends in, 415
time trends in, 79–80
Epidermal growth factor (EGF)
growth regulation by, 66
malignant transformation and, 63,66–67
in ovary, 63
properties of, 62,63,66
receptor for, 62,63
TGF-α and, 63
Epithelial ovarian cancer. *See also*
Celomic epithelial carcinoma
ABMS use in, 327–336
age and, 80–81,153,154,155
antigenic markers for, 48–51
CA-125 serum elevations in, 155–156
drug resistance in, 261
early diagnosis, 127–130,359–362
EGF in, 63
epidemiology of, 15,16,80

Epithelial ovarian cancer (contd.)
  estrogenic influences, 16
  growth regulation in, 66–67
  histogenesis of, 15–16
  histopathology, 116
  hormone receptor determination in, 119
  hormone therapy in, 339–345
  immune response to, 47–54
  immunotherapy of, 55–56
  incidence of, 15,80–81
  inclusion cysts and, 16
  intraoperative management, 158–166
  IP access for, 211–215
  laparotomy in, 158–160
  localization of, 54–55
  lymph nodes in, 160–161
  monoclonal antibodies to, 50–55
  oncogenes and, 67–72
  oral contraceptive use and, 85
  peptide growth factor production in, 66
  pleural infusions in, 157
  preoperative evaluation, 156–158
  prognostic factors for, 73,115–116,119
  radiotherapy of, 229–238
  risk factors for, 82–88
  secondary cytoreduction efficacy in, 190,193
  secondary therapy effectiveness in, 178
  second-look laparotomy in, 176
  staging of, 153
  surgery in, 158–161
  survival rates in, 194–196,261,341,359
  taxol treatment, 289
  tumor antigens to, 48–54
  tumor-suppressor genes and, 73
  TVS in, 156,360
Epithelial ovarian cancer, of LMP
  adjunct therapy in, 424
  Brenner tumor as, 420
  chemotherapy in, 425
  clinical features of, 416–417
  conservative therapy of, 424,427
  diagnosis, 417,418
  endometroid tumors as, 26–27,420–421
  epidemiology of, 415–416
  flow cytometry of, 421
  immunohistochemistry of, 415–416
  incidence of, 415–416
  invasive carcinoma after, 425
  metastasis in, 423
  morphometry in, 421
  MRI in, 422
  mucinous, 24–25,416,417,418,419–420, 426–427
  oncogene expression in, 422
  pathology in, 417–420,426
  pregnancy and, 424,425
  prognosis in, 424,425,426
  recurrence in, 425–426
  restaging of, 423
  second-look laparotomy in, 424
  serous, 22–24,416,417,418–419,422, 426–427
  staging of, 422–423
  survival in, 415,417,418,426–427
  treatment, 423–426,427
  tumor suppressor genes in, 422
Epithelial surface antigens (ESA)
  monoclonal antibodies to, 53
  in ovarian carcinoma, 53
Estradiol
  follicular maturity and, 13
  granulosa cell production, 13,388
  ontogeny of secretion, 11,12,13
  in reproductive ovary, 13–15
  in thecomas, 392
  two-cell theory of follicular production, 13–14
Estrogen receptors, prognosis and, 119,123
Estrogen therapy, ovarian cancer risk and, 85–86
Ethiofos (WR-2721), cisplatin toxicity reduction by, 297
Experimental chemotherapeutic agents
  hexamethylmelamine as, 291–293
  ifosfamide as, 287–289
  in salvage treatments, 287–293
  taxol as, 289–291
  tetraplatin as, 293
  topotecan as, 293

F

Fallopian tube, metastasis to ovary, 407
Family cancer syndromes
  breast cancer pedigree in, 103,104
  cancer types in, 103
  characterization of, 102–103
  genetic basis for, 102
  linkage analysis of, 103–105
  ovarian cancer pedigree in, 103–104
  scoring susceptibility for, 103–105, 109–111
Fibroblast growth factors (FGFs)
  characterization of, 64
  functions of, 64,67
Fibroma-fibrosarcoma
  clinical features of, 392–393
  diagnosis, 393
  prognosis in, 393
  treatment, 393
Fibromas
  characterization of, 32
  histopathology in, 32
Flow cytometry
  of dysgerminomas, 35
  of granulosa cell tumors, 389
  of LMP tumors, 421–422
  in metastasis origin determinations, 114
  in prognosis determinations, 118–119, 121
  of serous carcinomas, 24
  S-phase fraction determination, 119,121
Follicle regulatory protein (FRP)
  as granulosa cell tumor marker, 388
  as juvenile granulosa cell tumor marker, 391
Follicle stimulating hormone (FSH)
  in fetal development, 11
  GnRH and, 10,11
  LH and, 12–13
  ontogeny of secretion, 11–13
  ovarian differentiation and, 5
  in reproductive ovary, 13–14,15
Folliculogenesis
  gene action effects on, 4
  gonadotropin effects on, 3
Frozen section diagnosis
  in initial tumor staging, 158–159,160
  of primary/metastatic cancer, 161

G

Gadolinium-DTPA (Gd-DTPA), as MR contrast agent, 148–149
Gastrointestinal tract carcinoma, metastasis to ovary, 408–411
Genetics of ovarian cancer, *see also* Family cancer syndromes
  associated genetic conditions, 105
  chromosome deletion and, 101–102
  chromosome translocation and, 101–102
  cytogenetic studies, 101–102
  family history in, 105
  in first-degree female relatives, 98
  fragmented Y chromosomes and, 105
  gene amplification and, 102
  gene identification in, 98,99
  linkage analysis in, 99,100–102
  loss of heterozygosity and, 98,100–102
  molecular basis for, 98,100,102
  oncogene identification and, 98,99
  retinoblastoma and, 98,100–101
  testing for, 105–106
  two-hit hypothesis, 98,100
  white blood cell studies, 102
Germ cell tumors. *See also* Dysgerminomas
  ascites in, 376
  CA-125 elevations in, 376
  clinical features, 375–376
  cytogenetics of, 16
  diagnosis, 3
  embryonal carcinoma as, 36,37
  epidemiology of 16,80,81
  gonadoblastomas as, 16–17,39
  incidence of, 16,34,35
  LDH serum levels in, 375–376
  malignant, 16,34–38,165
  metastasis of, 376
  mixed, 39
  operative findings in, 376
  serum markers for, 376
  teratomas as, 36–39,376,380
  testicular tumors and, 377–378,379
  types, 16
Germ cell tumors, management
  adjuvant chemotherapy in, 379,383
  in advanced disease, 377
  bleomycin,vinblastine treatment, 378–379
  chemosensitivity of, 277
  chemotherapy of, 166,377–379
  cisplatin multidrug therapy in, 378–379
  courses of therapy for, 378–379
  ifosfamide treatment, 287
  late effects of therapy, 381–382
  lymph nodes in, 377
  primary cytoreduction of, 165–166,377
  prognosis in, 377,378,379,381
  radiation treatment, 378, 382
  recurrence treatment, 379–380,383
  reproductive capacity conservation in, 165–166
  secondary cytoreduction of, 200–201
  second-look laparotomy in, 380,383
  surgical staging techniques in, 376–377, 382,383
Glutathione (GSH)
  BSO synthesis inhibition, 271–272,298
  cisplatin resistance and, 265–266
  DNA repair enhancement, 268,269
  drug resistance and, 265–266,271–272, 298
  melphalan resistance and, 265–266
  metabolic functions, 265
Glutathione S-transferase (GST) isozymes
  clinical trials of inhibitors of, 272–273
  drug resistance and, 266–267,272–273, 298
  inhibition of, 272–273
  metabolic functios of, 266
  in ovarian cancer, 266,272–273
Gonadal dysgenesis. *See also* Pure gonadal dysgenesis

hermaphroditism and, 8
intraabdominal testis as, 8–9
malignant tendencies in, 5,6,7
in sex chromosome aneuploidy, 5–6
in Turner's syndrome, 6
in X chromosome aneuploidy, 6–7
in XY phenotypic females, 8–9
in Y chromosome aneuploidy, 7–8
Gonadoblastomas
characterization of, 16–17,39
in gonadal dysgenesis, 5
gross features of, 39
histopathology, 39
karyotypes in, 17
Gonadotropin
in female life cycle, 12–13
folliculogenesis and, 3
GnRH and, 12
ontogeny of, 11–12
receptors, 342
reproduction and, 13–15
Gonadotropin-releasing hormone (GNRH)
in fetus, 11
LH and, 10
MBH synthesis of, 10
menstrual cycle and, 12–13
opioid neurons and, 12
receptors, 10
Gonads
abnormal development, 5–9
accessory structures, 2–3
differentiation of, 1–5
G proteins
adenylate cyclase activation, 70–71
in ovarian cancer
properties of, 70–71
ras family of, 68,71
Granulocyte colony-stimulating factor (G-CSF), bone marrow stimulation, 350,351
Granulosa cells
histology of, 31,32
in reproductive ovary, 13–14
Granulosa cell tumors
adjunctive radiotherapy in, 387–388
age and, 386
chemotherapy, 388
clinical features, 31,386–387
diagnosis, 386–387
differential diagnosis, 387
FRP serum levels in, 388
histopathology in, 31–32,386–387
incidence of, 31,385
malignancy of, 385
origin of, 385
prognosis in, 389
secondary cytoreduction in, 200
serum estradiol levels in, 388
surgery in, 387
Granulosa cell tumors, juvenile
adult form comparison, 389–390
clinical features of, 389–390
diagnosis, 390–391
FRP serum levels in, 391
histopathology in, 31–32,390–391
prognosis, 391
treatment, 391
Growth factors. See Peptide growth factors
Growth regulation. See also Tumor growth
ILs and, 66
nuclear transcription factors and, 71–72
oncogenes and, 67–72
ovarian cancer and, 70,73

peptide growth factors and, 66–67
tumor-suppressor genes and, 67,72–74
Gynandroblastoma
characterization of, 399
diagnosis, 399
SLT and, 33

H
Hermaphroditism, true, clinical presentation, 8
Her-2/neu oncogene
growth regulation, 68–70
as immunotherapy target, 307–308
monoclonal antibody to, 307–308
overexpression in cancer, 69–70,119–120
as prognostic factor, 70,119–120
Hexamethylmelamine (Hexalen)
adverse effects of, 280,291
in celomic carcinoma treatment, 280
cisplatin combination, 291–292
clinical trials of, 291–292
cyclophosphamide combination, 291–292
DI analysis for, 256
doxorubicin use and, 291–292
indications for use, 291
intervenous use, 293
as salvage agent, 291–293
Histopathology
classification system for, 116–117
of epithelial tumors, 116
as prognostic indicator, 116–117
Hormone therapy
androgens in, 344
chemotherapy and, 344
clinical trials of, 342–344
corticosteroids in, 344
in endometrial cancer, 342–343
in epithelial ovarian caner, 339–345
estrogen in, 343
estrogen-progestin combination in, 343
estrogen receptors and, 341
LHRH agonists in, 344
progestin in, 342–343
progestin receptors in, 341,342
steroid receptor determination in, 339–340,345
tomoxifen use in, 343–344
Human chorionic gonadotropin (HCG), as marker for germ cell tumors, 375

I
Ifosfamide (Ifex)
adverse effects of, 280,287–288,353,354
in celomic carcinoma, 280,284
cisplatin combination, 288
dose schedule for, 287
efficacy of, 288–289,330
in germ cell tumors, 287
as salvage agent, 287–289
Immune response, to tumors
ADCC in, 301,303
antibodies in, 47,301
autoimmunity and, 47
B cells in, 302
cellular immunity and, 302–303
cytokines and, 304–306
humoral immunity and, 302
IFN and, 305
Ils and, 304–305
lymphocytes in, 47,302–303
monocytes/macrophages in, 303
in ovarian cancer, 47–54
specificity of, 47
TILs in, 47

Immunotherapy of tumors
activated T lymphocytes in, 306–307
adoptive, 306–307
BCG use in, 303–304,308–309,310
BRM use in, 303–304,308–310
chemotherapy combination, 308–309
cytokines in, 305–306
in gynecologic cancers, 307
IFN use in, 305,309,310–311,312
IL-2 use in, 309,312–313
IL-6 use in, 306
inactivated bacterium use in, 308, 309–310
IP administered, 309–313
LAK cells in, 306,313
melphalan combination, 308
monoclonal antibodies in, 54–55,302, 307–308
in ovarian cancer, 54–55,307–313
TILs use in, 56,306,313
TNF use in, 311–312
tumor vaccines and, 309
Insulin-like growth factors (IGFs)
binding proteins,63–64
functions, 64
properties of, 63–64
Interferon (IFN)
adverse effects of, 310,312
antitumor effects, 305,310,312
cisplatin combination, 310–311
clinical trials of, 310–311,312
dose response curve for, 245
dose schedules, 310,312
immune response and, 305
immunotherapy use, 309,310–311,312
IP use, 310–311,312
NK cell induction, 305,310
Interleukins (ILs)
adverse effects, 312–313
biologic activities of, 304
clinical trials, 312–313
growth regulation and, 66,156
IL-1 and, 304
IL-2 and, 304–305
IL-6 and, 304,305,306
immune response and, 304–305
immunotherapy use, 309,312–313
in ovarian cancer, 156
International Federation of Gynocology and Obstetrics (FIGO)
ovarian cancer staging system, 116,153, 159,278
Intestinal fistula
clinical presentation, 223
diagnosis/management, 223–224
palitive surgery for, 223–224
Intestinal obstruction
clinical presentation
etiology of, 217
incidence of, 217
of large bowel, 219
nonoperative management, 219–220
pallitive surgery for, 217–223
patient selection for surgery, 221–222
PEG in, 222
radiology in, 218–219
sites of, 218–219
of small bowel, 218,219
surgical complications, 221
surgical morbidity in, 221
surgery, efficacy of, 220–221
TPN role in, 222–223
Intraperitoneal access
for chemotherapy, 211–214,319–320
external type, 212

Intraperitoneal access (*contd.*)
  function failure in, 212–213
  infection complications, 212,214
  intestinal complications in, 214
  methods for, 211–212
  semipermanent catheter use in, 211,212
  totally implantable, 211,212
Intraperitoneal (IP) chemotherapy
  access for, 211–214,319–320
  advantages of, 317–318,320
  in ascites treatment, 322
  carboplatin administration in, 320–321
  cisplatin administration in, 319,320,323
  clinical trials of, 320–321,322,323
  doxorubicin administration in, 320,321
  drug distribution/uptake in, 317,318
  in early stage cancer, 370
  indications for, 323
  major concerns in, 318–319
  mitoxantrone administration in, 320,321
  optimal drug characteristics for, 317,318,320
  pharmokinetic advantages of, 320
  as salvage treatment, 322–323
  systemic exposure in, 318–319
  taxol administration in, 321–322
Intraperitoneal colloidal radioisotopes
  efficacy of, 233–235
  indications for, 323–325
  isotopes for, 233
  ^{32}P use in, 233–234,235
  tumor stage and, 233,234
Intraperitoneal immunotherapy
  BRM use in, 309–310
  indications for, 309
  IFN use in, 310–312
  TNF use in, 311–312
Intravenous pyelography (IVP)
  in adnexal mass evaluation, 156
  CT augmentation by, 134
  efficacy of, 133–134

K

Krukenberg tumors
  clinical presentation, 410
  diagnosis, 410–411
  origin of, 410
  of ovary, 410–411

L

lactic dehydrogenase (LDH), as germ cell tumor marker, 375–376
Laparoscopy
  complications of, 177,362
  in early tumor staging, 361–362
  efficacy of, 361–362
  as second-look laparotomy alternative, 177
Laparotomy. *See also* Second-look laparotomy
  frozen section studies during, 158,159
  palliative, 217,218
  procedures for, 158–160
  staging during, 159
Leukemia
  as chemotherapy side effect, 382,425
  ovarian sarcoma and, 42
Leydig cell tumors
  clinical features, 394–395
  diagnosis, 395
  histopathology, 395
  prognosis in, 395
  treatment, 395

Liver function tests (LFTs), preoperative, 156–157
Low malignant potential (LMP) tumors.
    See also Epithelial LMP tumors
  clear cell, 29,421
  clinical course of, 198–199,415
  definition of, 21,415
  diagnostic criteria for, 23–24,418
  in endometrioid carcinoma, 26–27, 420–421
  epidemiology of, 415–416
  of epithelial origin, 198–199,415–427
  fertility-sparing surgery in, 161
  histopathology of, 198
  incidence of, 198
  in mucinous carcinoma, 24–25,416–417, 418–420
  secondary cytoreduction of, 198–199,200
  in serous carcinoma, 22–24,416,417–418
  survival rate for, 417–418
Luteinizing hormone (LH)
  in fetal development, 11
  FSH levels and, 13
  GnRH and, 10
  ontogeny of secretion of, 11–13
  ovarian function and, 10
  in puberty, 12,13
  in reproductive ovary, 13–14
  thecal cells and, 13
Lymphangiography, efficacy in tumor staging, 360
Lymph nodes
  in germ cell tumors, 377
  metastasis to, 160
  in ovarian cancer, 154,160–161
  resection of, 160,161
  sampling of, 160–161
  in tumor staging, 160,161
Lymphokine-activated killer (LAK) cells
  IL-2 effect on, 305,306
  in tumor treatment, 306,313
Lymphomas
  histopathology in, 42
  ovarian, 42

M

Macrophage colony-stimulating factor (M-CSF)
  ovarian production of, 65
  as tumor marker, 65
Magnetic resonance imaging (MRI)
  advantages/limitations of, 148,149
  in adnexal mass imaging, 148,149
  CT complementation, 150
  Gd-DTPA use in, 148–149
  of LMP tumors, 422
  of metastatic ovarian cancer, 150
  ovarian cancer detection, 148–150,156
Malignant transformation
  by EGF, 63
  oncogenes and, 67–72,74
  TGF- and, 63
Medial basal hypothalamus (MBH)
  GnRH release and, 10
  neuromodulation of, 10–11
Melphalan
  in celomic epithelial carcinoma, 280,285
  cytoreduction and, 190
  dose response curve for, 245
  in early stage cancer, 365,367,369
  in epithelial carcinomas, 190
  GSH cell levels and, 265
  in high-dose chemotherapy + ABMS, 333,334

  immunotherapy combination, 308
  in LMP tumors, 425
  progestins and, 344
  radiation treatment and, 231,368
  resistance to, 263,264,265
Menstrual cycle
  FSH and, 12–13
  GnRH and, 12–13
  LH and, 12–13
Mesodermal mixed tumor(MMT)
  adenosarcoma as, 28–29
  gross features, 28
  histopathology of, 28,29
  rhabdomyosarcoma as, 28,29
Metallothionein
  cisplatin and, 266
  heavy metal detoxification and, 266
Metastasis
  of appendiceal origin, 408,411
  of breast origin, 408,411–412
  of carcinoid origin, 411
  of cervical origin, 408
  of colon origin, 408,409–410
  environment for, 164
  of fallopian tube origin, 407
  of germ cell tumor origin, 376
  IL-6 effect on, 306
  incidence of, 407,408,409
  of Krukenberg tumors, 411
  of LMP tumors, 423
  of lung origin, 412
  of melanoma origin, 412
  origin determination, 408,409–410,412
  to ovary, 407–413
  of rare tumor origin, 412–413
  in sex cord tumor, 400–401
  second-look laparotomy detection of, 176
  tumor growth kinetics and, 164
  tumor stage and, 176
Mitoxantrone
  clinical trials of, 321,333,334
  drug persistance, 321
  efficacy of, 321
  in high dose chemotherapy + ABMS, 333,334
  IP administration, 320,321
Monoclonal antibodies
  to CA-125, 48,50
  clinical utility of, 302
  drug conjugates of, 55,56,302,307
  to ESA, 53
  to folate-binding protein, 53
  to HER-2/neu oncogenes, 307–308
  in immunotherapy, 55–58,302,307–308
  L6 as, 55
  to mucins, 49,50
  MX35 as, 53–54
  to ovarian carcinoma, 50–54
  for radiolocalization of tumors, 54–55
  to steroid receptors, 340
  toxicity of, 55
  to tumor antigens, 48,49,302
  uses for, 48,49
MUC-1 antibodies
  epitopes of, 50–51
  to ovarian carcinoma, 50–51
Mucinous carcinoma
  of appendix, 26
  characterization of, 25
  colorectal carcinoma and, 41
  differentail diagnosis, 26,41
  gross features of, 24–25
  histopathology of, 24–25,26,419–420
  incidence of, 21,24

of LMP, 24–25,416,417,418,419–420,426
pathology in, 419–420
pseudomyxoma peritonei and, 26
sonography of, 136
staging of, 24–25,116,426
survival rates for, 417,418,426–427
Mucins
antibodies to, 49–50
characterization of, 49
MUC-1 antibodies to, 50–51
as ovarian tumor antigens, 49–51
Müllerian-inhibiting substance (MIS)
function, 2
gene for, 2–3
in gonadal dysgenesis, 5
Multidrug resistance gene (MDR1)
drug resistance and, 120,297–298
as prognostic factor, 120

N

Natural killer(NK) lymphocytes
in ovarian cancer, 47,48
response to cancer, 301,303
Nuclear transcription factors
in cancer, 71–72,74
myc oncogenes and, 71,74
oncogenic activation, 71–72

O

Oncogenes
activation of, 74
amplification of, 102
cancer development and, 67,102
classification of, 68
function of, 67,422
G proteins and, 68,70–71
HER-2/neu and, 102
identification methods, 98,99
in LMP tumors, 422
nuclear, 68,71–72
ovarian cancer and, 67–72,74,102
proto-oncogenes and, 67
in retroviruses, 67,68
serine/threonine kinases and, 68
tyrosine kinases and, 67,68–70
Oocyte
embryology of, 4
germ cell tumors and, 16
reactivation of arrested, 16
Oog
differentiation, 3–4
oocytes and, 4
Oophorectomy
vs aggressive surgery, 364
bilateral, 376
in breast carcinoma, 412
in colorectal carcinoma, 409
in early cancer, 364,365,376
in germ cell tumors, 166,376,377
in LMP tumors, 423–424
prophylactic, 106–107,110–111,409,412
prognosis in, 364,365
in sex cord tumor, 400
unilateral, 364
Oral contraceptives (OCP). See
Contraceptives
ORG.2766, in cisplatin toxicity reduction, 297
Ovarian cancer. See also specific
neoplasms
advanced, 160–161
age and, 80–81,95,153,154,155
of borderline malignancy, 199

death rates in, 1
epidemiology of, 79–90
etiology of, 89–90,106
family history and, 88–89,102–105, 109–110
frozen section analysis in, 158–159,160
genetic basis for, 98–102
genetic conditions associated with, 105
genetic testing and, 105–106
GI tract metastasis in, 165
growth factors for, 61–67
histological classification of, 116–117
immune response to, 47–54
immunotherapy of, 15,80–82,95,127
lymph nodes in, 154,160–161,377
menopausal status and, 153
metastatic, 40,41–42,153
physical examination for, 153–156
preclinical phases of, 127
prevention, 106–107
prognostic factors in, 70,73,115–124
prophylactic surgery in, 106–107,110–11
recurrence rate of, 187
risk assessment, 82–88,95, 109–110
secondary cytoreduction in,187–201
statistical definitions in, 127–128
survival rates, 95,121,127,163,187, 191–192,196–194
Ovarian cancer, early stage
adjuvant therapy indications for, 363–365
adnexal mass in, 359
biopsies in, 364
carboplatin therapy in, 370
chemotherapy/radiotherapy in, 368
cisplatin therapy in, 369–370
CT use in, 360
IP chemotherapy in, 370
IP radiotherapy in, 366–367
laparoscopy in, 361–362
lymphangiography in, 360
melphalan therapy in, 365,368,369
presurgical evaluation, 360
prognosis/prognostic factors in, 359,362, 364,368
radiation therapy in 365–366,367–369
restaging of, 361–362
screening for, 362–363
stage I treatment, 363–364,365–370
stage II treatment, 364–370
staging of, 360,361–362,364,368
survival rates in, 359,362,364,365,366, 368
TVS evaluation in, 360,363
unilateral oophorectomy in, 364
Ovarian cancer screening
cancer registries and, 109
CA-125 serum levels and, 48–49,50, 97–98,110,127,155–156,177,363
color-flow Doppler use in, 96,128–129, 141,363
counseling and, 95–96
DNA banking and, 109
for early stage cancer, 362–363
MRI use in, 148–150
objectives in, 95,127,363
patient selection for, 130
predictive value of, 96,363
risk assessment and, 95,109–111
sonography in, 96–97,140–141
TAS in, 96
trial design for, 129–130
TVS in, 96,128–129,130,140–141,360,363
Ovarian cancer surgery. See also Primary
cytoreduction

fertility-sparing, 364–365
frozen section staging in, 158–159,160
historical aspects of, 163
laparotomy as, 158–160
lymph nodes in, 160,161
palliative, 217–226
procedures in, 158–160
secondary cytoreduction as, 187–201
second-look laparotomy as, 175–182
Ovarian organogenesis
abnormal, 5–9
accessory structure development in, 2–3
cortical dominance in, 3–4
differentiation in, 1–5
folliculogenesis in, 3–4
gonadal differentiation in, 1–2
male gonads and, 1–3
sexual differentiation and, 2–3
X and Y chromosomes and, 4–5
Ovarian surface epithelium (OSE)
antigenic markers to, 48,49
peritoneal lining and, 48
Ovaries
accessory, 10
anatomy of, 9–10
blood supply of, 9
ectopic, 10
embryology of, 1–5
lymphatic drainage of, 9,360
measurements of,128, 135,141,359
postmenopausal, 9
at puberty, 10
in reproduction, 13–15
in senescence, 15
supernumerary, 10
OVCAR cell lines
drug resistance studies in, 262–265
GSH metabolism in, 265

P

Palliative surgery
for ascites, 224
in bowel obstruction, 220–221
efficacy of, 220–221
incidence of, 217,218
indications for, 217,218–220
for intestinal fistula, 223–224
for intestinal obstruction, 217–223
laparotomy in, 217,218
operative techniques, 220
for pericardial effusions, 225
for pleural effusions, 224–225
in ureteral obstruction, 225–226
Peptide growth factors. See also specific
factors
autocrine, 61–62,66
chromosomes for, 62
EGF as, 63,66,67,102
FGFs as, 64
G-CSF as, 350
growth regulation by, 63–64
IGFs as, 63–64
juxtacrine, 62
listing of, 62
M-CSF as, 65
mechanism of action, 61–62
paracrine, 62,67
PDGF as, 64–65
receptors for, 62–63
TGF-β as, 65–66
Percutaneous endoscopic gastrostomy (PEG)
efficacy of, 222
in intestinal obstruction, 222

Percutaneous nephrostomy (PCN)
  efficacy of, 225–226
  in ureteral obstruction management, 225–226
Pericardial effusions, management of, 225
Peutz-Jeghers syndrome (PJS)
  characterization of, 105,400
  ovarian cancer association, 105
  in sex cord tumor, 399–401
Platelet-derived growth factor (PDGF)
  characterization of, 64
  functions, 64–65,66
  receptors for, 64,65
Pleural effusions
  chemotherapy for, 225
  incidence of, 224
  management of, 224–225
  palliative surgery for, 225
Ploidy
  determination of, 118
  as prognostic factor, 118,119,121–122
Postmenopausal palpable ovary (PMPO), malignancy incidence in, 9
Postmenopausal women
  adnexal cysts in, 136,137,138
  cancer risk in, 153,154
  ovary dimensions in, 135,141
  sonography of, 136
Primary cytoreduction. *See also* Secondary cytoreduction
  in advanced ovarian cancer, 166–170
  benefits of, 164–165,1680170,172, 187–188
  bladder in, 166–167
  bowel resection in, 167
  chemotherapy and, 169,171,172
  criticism of, 170–172
  of germ cell tumors, 165–166
  hysterectomy in, 166,167
  objectives in, 167–168,187
  peritoneal surface in, 167
  progression-free interval after, 169,170
  quality of life after, 171,172
  residual mass after, 168–169
  response rate after, 168
  retroperitoneal approach in, 166–167
  second-look reassessment of, 169–170,171
  in stage III cancer, 171
  survival and, 168,169,170,171
  techniques in, 165–168
  theoretical basis for, 163–165,187
  tumor- bearing omentum removal in, 166
  ureter in, 167
Proctosigmoidoscopy, in ovarian cancer, 158
Progesterone, luteinized cell production, 13
Progestin
  chemotherapy and, 344
  in epithelial carcinoma, 341–343,344
  hormone therapy, 342–343,344
  receptors, 341
  tamoxifen combination, 344
  therapy response, 342–343
Prognostic factors
  adherence as, 120,121
  age as, 118,121,122,123,170
  ascites presence as, 118,121,122,123
  CA-125 elevations as, 119,120,155–156
  cancer volume as, 115,116
  in celomic carcinoma, 277–278
  clonogenic cell growth as, 120
  DNA index as, 118–119,121,123
  endpoints for, 115
  grading of, 117,121
  in granulosa cell tumors, 389
  HER-2/neu overexpression as, 70, 119–120
  histology as, 116–117,121,122,123,170, 180,181,362,389,426
  initial tumor mass as, 117
  in LMP tumors, 426
  MDRI gene as, 120
  penetration as, 121
  performance status as, 118,121,122,123
  p53 gene expression as, 73
  ploidy as, 118,121–122,123,389
  post-treatment variables as, 120
  in primary cytoreduction, 168–170
  ranking of, 121–124
  response rate as, 168
  in second-look laparotomy, 179–182
  S-phase cells as, 119,122
  in stage I, 120–121,362
  in stage II, 122
  in stage III/IV, 122–124
  steroid hormone receptors as, 341
  tumor residium as, 115,116,117–118,122, 123,163,164,168,170,180,181,277, 362,389
  tumor stage and, 116,179–182,362
Proopiomelanocortin (POMC), in puberty, 12
Prophylactic oophorectomy
  counseling for, 110–111
  efficacy of, 106
  patient selection for, 107,110–111,409, 412
  premalignant lesion detection in, 106–107
  prophylactic mastectomy and, 109
Pseudomyxoma peritonei
  CT imaging of, 143,144
  incidence of, 26
  mucinous tumors and, 26
p53 tumor suppressor gene
  characterization of, 72–73
  malignancy and, 72–74
  mutations in, 73–74
  sequence analysis of, 73,74
Puberty
  extragonadal constraint and, 10
  GnRH in, 12
  LH secretion in, 11,12
  POMC in, 12

R

Radiolocalization of tumor, antibody use in, 54–55
Radiology. *See also* specific imaging techniques
  in adnexal mass evaluation, 157–158
  advantages/limitations of, 133–134,151
  barium studies in, 134,135,151
  in intestinal obstruction, 218–219
  IVP in, 133–134,157
  lymphangiography and, 134,136,151, 156–157
  in metastatic disease, 133–134
  plain film studies in, 133
Radiotherapy
  in celomic carcinoma, 285
  chemotherapy and, 367
  chemotherapy comparison, 367–369
  chemotherapy + cytoreduction and, 235–237
  chlorambucil and, 232,365
  of epithelial tumors, 229–238
  external beam therapy as, 231–232
  field shape in, 230
  fractionation schemees for, 230
  of germ cell tumors, 378,382
  of granulosa cell tumors, 387–388
  historical aspects of, 229
  IP colloids in, 233–235,366–367
  long-term toxic effects of, 231,366–367
  ^{32}P use in, 366,367,368,370
  prognosis in, 232–233,285
  radiation dose in, 229–230
  radiosensitizing agents in, 238
  recomendations for, 237–238
  relapse rate in, 231–232,367
  site of relapse in, 232
  in stage I, 233,234,285,365–369
  in stage II, 365–369
  in stage III, 235–237
  survival rates in, 229,230,231,365,366, 367
  techniques for,230–231,365–366
  tumor residuum and, 231–233
  tumor size and, 229,232,236,237
  tumor stage and, 229,230,231
  WAR in, 365–366,367–369
Receptors
  chromosomes for, 62
  for growth factors, 62–63
  in hormone therapy, 339–345
  monoclonal antibodies to, 340

S

Sarcomas
  chondrosarcoma as, 28,29
  fibrisarcoma as, 39
  granulocytic, 42
  histopathology of, 28,29
  immunohistochemistry of, 26
  incidence of, 39
  leukemia and, 42
  MMT type, 28–29
  of ovary, 39,42
Secondary cytoreduction
  benefits of, 188
  in borderline malignancies, 199
  chemotherapy and, 190,192,194–195
  complications of, 192–193
  concepts in, 187–188
  of epithelial tumors, 190,193,198–199
  of germ cell tumors, 200–201
  of granulosa cell tumors, 200
  as interval procedure
    chemotherapy and, 193,194–196
    definition of, 193
    success rate in, 193–196
    survival impact, 194–196
  of LMP tumors, 198–199
  of nonresponders, 197–198
  rationale for, 178,187–188
  in recurrent disease, 196–198,199,200
  residual disease following, 189–190,191
  in second-look laparotomy, 178,188–189, 190–192
  in salvage treatment, 196–197
  in stromal tumors, 199–200
  success rate in, 189
  survival, impact on, 189–192
  tumor size and, 189,190,191,192,198
Second-look laparotomy
  alternatives to, 176–177
  in chemotherapy evaluation, 176
  clinical correlates of, 178–179
  complications of, 180–181
  CT comparison, 177

cytological specimens in, 179
in germ cell tumors, 380
histologic grade of tumor and, 180,181
historical aspects of, 175
laparoscopy as alternative to, 177
metastasis detection, 176
morbidity in, 180–181
prognostic significance of findings in, 181–182
rationale for, 175–178,182,188–189
residual tumor and, 180,181
results in, 179–182
secondary cytoreduction during, 178, 188–189,190–191
serum tumor markers as alternative to, 177
in stage I cancer, 365
technique, 178–179
Serine/threonine kinases
mitogenic transduction and, 68
role of, 68–69
Serous ovarian carcinoma
cubodial cells of, 22,23
differential diagnosis, 23
DNA analysis of, 23,24
epidemiology, 80,82
frank, papillary, 24
histopathology of, 22,23,24,419
incidence, 21–22
invasive, 23
of LMP, 22–24,416,417–418,422,426–427
metastasis of, 23
prognostic features of, 23,24,422
sonography of, 136
staging of, 22–23,24,116
survival rates in, 417–418,426–427
Sertoli cell tumors (SCT)
characterization of, 32
clinical features, 394
estrogen secretion in, 32
prognosis in, 394
stromal cell, 394
treatment, 394
Sertoli-Leydig cell tumors (SLT)
AFP serum levels in, 396
characterization of, 33
chemotherapy ineffectiveness in, 398–399
classification, differentiation based, 396–397
clinical features, 395–396
diagnosis, 396
histopathology, 33,396–397,398
incidence of, 33,395–396
masculinization in, 396
treatment, 397–398,399
Sex cord-stromal tumors. *See also* Granulosa cell tumors
characterization of, 17,31–32,385,393
classification of, 385,386
diagnosis, 385,393–394
endometroid carcinoma and, 28
epidemiology of, 80,81
fibrosarcoma as, 32,393
FSH receptors in, 17
of granulosa cells, 31–32,393
histopathology of, 31–32,393
incidence of, 17,30–31,32,385
juvenile, 31,32
prognosis in, 394
sclerosing, 393
secondary cytoreduction of, 199–200
theca cells of 31,32
treatment, 394
unclassified type, 33–34

Sex cord tumor with annular tubules
characterization of, 34,399,401
histopathology of, 399–400
incidence of, 34
metastasis in, 400–401
PJS and, 399–400
PJS absence in, 400–401
treatment, 400–401
Small cell carcinoma
differential diagnosis, 40
histopathology in, 40
Sodium thiosulfate, in cisplatin toxicity reduction, 296
Sonography. *See also* Color-flow Doppler
of adenocarcinomas, 140
of ascites, 136,140
CT effectiveness comparison, 138,141
of hepatic metastasis, 138,140
malignancy diagnostic capability, 135–141
ovarian imaging by, 134–141,151
of ovarian leiomyosarcoma, 138
of pelvis, 134–135,137,139–140
of postmenopausal patients, 135,136
in recurrent disease detection, 138–139
screening use of, 96–97,140–141
as second-look laparotomy alternative, 177
specificity/sensitivity of, 136,137,138,139
transrectal, 139–140
in young females, 137
Squamous carcinoma
histopathology in, 37
teratoma and, 37
Staging. *See* Tumor staging
Steroid receptors
for androgens, 342
assay procedures, 339–340,345
for corticosteroids, 342
detection limits for, 340
determination of, in specimens, 339–342
in epithelial cancer, 339–345
for estrogen, 340–341
for gonadotropin, 342
hormone therapy and, 339–345
monoclonal antibodies to, 340
for progestin, 341
survival predictions and, 341
Sulfoximine (BSO)
carboplatin and, 272
clinical trials of, 271–272
DNA repair suppression, 269
GSH cell level reduction, 265,271–272
toxic effects of, 271

T
Tamoxifen
chemotherapy combination, 344
clinical trials of, 343–344
as estrogenagonist/antagonist, 343
progestin and, 344
in refractory ovarian cancer, 343–344
Taxol
adverse effects of, 280,289,355–356
in celomic carcinoma, 279–280
cisplatin and, 290–291
clinical trials of, 289–291,322
DI analysis for, 256
dose-response relations, 290
drug resistance and, 273
efficacy of, 321–322
in epithelial carcinoma, 289
IP administration of, 321–322
mechanism of action, 279,289

mdr-1 gene product and, 273
response rate, 289,330
as salvage agent, 289–291
as single agent, 290
Teratomas
carcinoids in, 38,39
classification of, 36–37
CT imaging of, 143
in EST, 35–36
in germ cell tumors, 36–39,376,380
gross features of, 37,38
histopathology of, 37–39
immature, 37–38
mature, 37
monodermal, 38–39
MRI of, 149
risk factors for, 82
squamous carcinoma and, 37
Testosterone, in senescent ovary, 15
Tetraplatin, preclinical testing of, 293
Thecal cells
androgen production and, 13
estrogen production and, 13,14
in granulosa cell tumors, 31,32
LH receptors of, 13
Thecoma
clinical features of, 391–392
immunohistochemistry of, 392
incidence of, 391–392
prognosis in, 392
treatment, 392
Thiotepa
drug resistance inhibition and, 272–273
cisplatin, cyclophosphamide and, 331
GST inhibition and, 272–273
in high dose chemotherapy + ABMS, 331,333,334
therapeutic synergy of, 328–329
T lymphocytes
cytotoxic, 303
immune response and, 302–303
in immunotherapy, 306–307
in ovarian cancer, 47,48
receptors, 302–303
response to malignancy, 302–303
Topotecan
clinical trials of, 293
DNA cleavage by, 293
Total parenteral nutrition (TPN)
efficacy of, 222–223
in intestinal obstruction, 222–223
PEG as alternative to, 223
Transabdominal sonography (TAS)
of adnexal mass, 137
efficacy of, 96
in ovarian screening, 96,135,137
sensitivity/specificity of, 96,135–137, 139–140
transrectal sonography comparison, 139–140
TVS imaging comparison, 135,137
Transforming growth factor-alpha (TGF-α)
EGF homology, 63
TGF-B and, 65
Transforming growth factor-B (TGF-B)
genes for, 65
growth regulation by, 66
ovarian production, 66
properties of, 65–66
Transvaginal sonography (TVS)
color-Doppler and, 141
efficacy of, 96,128,129,360,363
of endodermal sinus tumor, 139
of endometrial cancer, 108
in epithelial cancer screening, 108,156

Transvaginal sonography (TVS) (contd.)
  increasing sensitivity of, 128
  in ovarian screening, 96,128–129,135, 137,140–141
  ovarian volume and, 128
  patient selection for, 130
  sensitivity/specificity of, 96,108,128, 129–130,135–137
  TAS imaging comparison, 135,137
Tumor antigens
  for blood group, 51–53
  CA-125 as, 48–49,97–98
  CEA as, 51,54
  characteristics of, 50
  in diagnosis/monitoring, 54
  epitheleal surface, 53
  folate-binding, 53
  monoclonal antibodies to, 48,49–54
  mucins as, 49–51
  to OSE, 48
  to ovarian carcinomas, 48–54
Tumor growth
  curve for, 164
  immune response to, 301–306
  kinetics of, 163–165
  metastasis and, 164
  mutations and, 164,165
  renewal tissue growth and, 164
  time frame for, 164,165
Tumor-infiltrating lymphocytes (TILs)
  in ovarian cancer, 47
  therapeutic applications for, 56,306,313
Tumor necrosis factor (TNF)
  adverse effects of, 312
  in ascites treatment, 312
  chemotherapy and, 312
  IL-1 interaction, 305
  immune response and, 305
Tumor staging
  adequacy of, 361

of dysgerminomas, 380
in early cancer, 361–362
FIGO system for, 116,159,278,361,422
of germ cell tumors, 377
at initial diagnosis, 153,360,361
of LMP tumors, 422–423
lamphangiography in, 360
lymph nodes in, 60
of primary ovarian cancer, 159,278, 360–362
as prognostic factor, 116,121–124,187
restaging findings in, 159,361–362,423
in surgery, 158–159,376–377
technique/requirements for, 361
Tumor-suppressor genes
  function of, 67,72
  in LMP tumors, 422
  loss of function by, 72,73
  mutation of, 73,74
  p53 gene/gene product and, 72–73
Turner's syndrome, gonadal dysgenesis in, 6
Two-cell theory, of follicular estrogen production, 13–14
Tyrosine kinases
  activation of, 69
  cancer survival and, 70
  FGFs and, 64
  as growth factor receptors, 62,68,69
  HER-2/neu expression and, 69–70,74
  oncogenes, 67,68–70
  ovarian cancer and, 68–70

U

Ultrasound, 9–10,360. *See also* Sonography; Color-flow Doppler; malignancy detection
Ureteral obstruction
  diagnostic evaluation, 225
  PCN in, 225–226

Uterus
  endometrium of, 407–408
  metastasis to ovary, 407–408

V

Vinblastine
  cisplatin,bleomycin therapy, 378–379, 388
  germ cell tumor therapy, 378–379
  granulosa cell tumor therapy, 388

W

Whole abdominal irradiation (WAR)
  clinical trials of, 367–369,370
  in eary stage cancer, 365–366,367–368, 370

X

X chromosome
  aneuploidy, 6–7
  malignant tendencies and, 5,6
  ovarian development and, 5
  in Turner's syndrome, 6
XY pure gonadal dysgenesis (Swyers syndrome)
  developmental failure in, 5
  malignant tendencies in, 5

Y

Y chromosome
  absence in ovarian development, 4
  aneuploidy, 7–8
  gonadal dysgenesis and, 7–8
  testicular determination and, 2